Perspectives for Occupation-Based Practice

Foundation and Future of Occupational Therapy,
3rd Edition

Edited by Rita P. Fleming-Castaldy, PhD, OT/L, FAOTA

AOTA Centennial Vision
We envision that occupational therapy is a powerful, widely recognized, science-driven, and evidence-based profession with a globally connected and diverse workforce meeting society's occupational needs.

Mission Statement
The American Occupational Therapy Association advances the quality, availability, use, and support of occupational therapy through standard-setting, advocacy, education, and research on behalf of its members and the public.

AOTA Staff
Frederick P. Somers, *Executive Director*
Christopher M. Bluhm, *Chief Operating Officer*

Chris Davis, *Director, AOTA Press*
Caroline Polk, *Digital Manager*
Ashley Hofmann, *Development/Acquisitions Editor*
Barbara Dickson, *Production Editor*
Joe King-Shaw, *Business and Customer Service Administrator*

Rebecca Rutberg, *Director, Marketing*
Amanda Goldman, *Marketing Manager*
Jennifer Folden, *Marketing Specialist*

American Occupational Therapy Association, Inc.
4720 Montgomery Lane
Bethesda, MD 20814
Phone: 301-652-AOTA (2682)
TDD: 800-377-8555
Fax: 301-652-7711
www.aota.org
To order: 1-877-404-AOTA or store.aota.org

Disclaimers
This publication is designed to provide accurate and authoritative information in regard to the subject matter covered. It is sold or distributed with the understanding that the publisher is not engaged in rendering legal, accounting, or other professional service. If legal advice or other expert assistance is required, the services of a competent professional person should be sought.
—*From the Declaration of Principles jointly adopted by the American Bar Association and a Committee of Publishers and Associations*

It is the objective of the American Occupational Therapy Association to be a forum for free expression and interchange of ideas. The opinions expressed by the contributors to this work are their own and not necessarily those of the American Occupational Therapy Association.

ISBN: 978-1-56900-360-2

Library of Congress Control Number: 2014948125

Cover Design by Jennifer Folden, AOTA, Bethesda, MD
Composition by Rella Sessa, Maryland Composition, White Plains, MD
Printed by Automated Graphic Systems, Inc., White Plains, MD

I dedicate this work to my brother,
Kevin Michael Fleming (1954–1989).
Although Kevin could not win
his battle with Friedrich's ataxia,
his tenacious fight to live a self-directed
life remains my inspiration.

Contents

About the Editor...ix

List of Active Reflections, Exhibits, Figures, Tables, and Appendixes xi

Preface xv
    Rta P. Fleming-Castaldy, PhD, OT/L, FAOTA

Introduction... xix
    Rita P. Fleming-Castaldy, PhD, OT/L, FAOTA

Part I. Occupational Therapy's Heritage: Historical and Philosophical Foundations for
    Occupation-Based Practice.. 1

Chapter 1. Moral Treatment: Contexts Considered 7
    Suzanne M. Peloquin

Chapter 2. Occupational Therapy Revisited: A Paraphrastic Journey.. 17
    Robert K. Bing

Chapter 3. Occupational Therapy Service: Individual and Collective Understandings of the Founders 37
    Suzanne M. Peloquin

Chapter 4. The Philosophy of Occupation Therapy 63
    Adolf Meyer

Chapter 5. Pragmatism and Structuralism in Occupational Therapy: The Long Conversation............................ 69
    Barb Hooper and Wendy Wood

Chapter 6. Occupational Therapy and Rehabilitation: An Awkward Alliance 83
    Judith Friedland

Chapter 7. Occupational Therapy Can Be One of the Great Ideas of 20th-Century Medicine 93
    Mary Reilly

Appendix I.A. The Philosophical Base of Occupational Therapy 103

Appendix I.B. Setting the Stage—Address in Honor of Eleanor Clarke Slagle 105
    Adolf Meyer

Part II. Theoretical and Conceptual Frameworks to Guide Occupation-Based Practice 109

Chapter 8. Why the Profession of Occupational Therapy Will Flourish in the 21st Century 115
    David L. Nelson

Chapter 9. Uniting Practice and Theory in an Occupational Framework 131
    Anne G. Fisher

Chapter 10. Putting Occupation Into Practice: Occupation as Ends, Occupation as Means 147
    Julie McLaughlin Gray

Chapter 11. Occupation: Purposefulness and Meaningfulness as Therapeutic Mechanisms............................ 159
    Catherine A. Trombly

Chapter 12. Mindfulness and Flow in Occupational Engagement: Presence in Doing 175
Denise Reid

Chapter 13. Occupational Well-Being: Rethinking Occupational Therapy Outcomes 183
Susan E. Doble and Josiane Caron Santha

Chapter 14. Sacred Texts: A Sceptical Exploration of the Assumptions Underpinning Theories of Occupation .. 191
Karen Whalley Hammell

Chapter 15. A Monistic or a Pluralistic Approach to Professional Identity? 201
Anne Cronin Mosey

Appendix II.A. Position Paper: Broadening the Construct of Independence 207

Part III. Contextual Considerations for Engagement in Occupation and Participation **209**

Part III.A. Temporal Contexts ***225***
Chapter 16. What Happened to Time? The Relationship of Occupational Therapy to Time 227
Sue Pemberton and Diane Cox

Chapter 17. Flow and Occupation: A Review of the Literature 237
Heather Emerson

Chapter 18. Sleep, Occupation, and the Passage of Time 247
Andrew Green

Chapter 19. Exploring Balance as a Concept in Occupational Science 259
Penelope Westhorp

Chapter 20. Balancing the Boat: Enabling an Ocean of Possibilities 269
Annette Majnemer

Chapter 21. A Proposed Model of Lifestyle Balance 279
Kathleen M. Matuska and Charles H. Christiansen

Part III.B. Cultural Contexts ***295***
Chapter 22. Culture: A Factor Influencing the Outcomes of Occupational Therapy 297
Ruth Levine Schemm

Chapter 23. Culture Emergent in Occupation 305
Bette R. Bonder, Laura Martin, and Andrew W. Miracle

Chapter 24. The Kawa Model: The Power of Culturally Responsive Occupational Therapy 317
Michael K. Iwama, Nicole A. Thomson, and Rona M. Macdonald

Part III.C. Sociopolitical Contexts ***329***
Chapter 25. Building Inclusive Community: A Challenge for Occupational Therapy 331
Ann P. Grady

Chapter 26. Occupational Deprivation: Global Challenge in the New Millennium 345
Gail Whiteford

Chapter 27. Occupational Justice and Client-Centered Practice: A Dialogue in Progress 353
Elizabeth Townsend and Ann A. Wilcock

Chapter 28. Well-Being and Occupational Rights: An Imperative for Critical Occupational Therapy 367
Karen R. Whalley Hammell and Michael K. Iwama

Part III.D. Personal Contexts ***379***
Chapter 29. Eudaimonic Well-Being: Its Importance and Relevance to Occupational Therapy for Humanity 381
Claire Hayward and Jackie Taylor

Chapter 30. A Theory of the Human Need for Occupation 391
Ann Wilcock

Chapter 31. Health and the Human Spirit for Occupation 399
    Elizabeth J. Yerxa

Chapter 32. Resilience and Human Adaptability: Who Rises Above Adversity? 407
    Susan B. Fine

Chapter 33. Spirituality, Occupation and Occupational Therapy Revisited: Ongoing Consideration
    of the Issues for Occupational Therapists 421
    Lesley Wilson

Chapter 34. Defining Lives: Occupation as Identity: An Essay on Competence, Coherence,
    and the Creation of Meaning 425
    Charles H. Christiansen

Appendix III.A. Position Statement: Human Rights 441

Appendix III.B. Occupational Therapy's Commitment to Nondiscrimination and Inclusion 443

Appendix III.C. AOTA's Societal Statement on Livable Communities 445

Appendix III.D. Occupational Therapy's Perspective on the Use of Environments and Contexts
    to Support Health and Participation in Occupations 447

Part IV. The Conscious Use of Self: Joining With People to Enable Occupational Engagement ... 461

Chapter 35. Occupational Therapy's Challenge: The Caring Relationship 469
    Elizabeth B. Devereaux

Chapter 36. Client-Centered Practice: What Does It Mean and Does It Make a Difference? 477
    Mary Law, Sue Baptiste, and Jennifer Mills

Chapter 37. Client-Centered and Family-Centered Care: Refinement of the Concepts 485
    Panelpha (Penny) L. Kyler

Chapter 38. Understanding the Family Perspective: An Ethnographic Framework for Providing
    Occupational Therapy in the Home 497
    Laura N. Gitlin, Mary Corcoran, and Susan Leinmiller-Eckhardt

Chapter 39. Enhancing Occupational Performance Through an Understanding of Perceived Self-Efficacy 507
    Marie Gage and Helene Polatajko

Chapter 40. Constructions of Disability: A Call for Critical Reflexivity in Occupational Therapy 519
    Shanon K. Phelan

Part V. Tools of Practice That Enable Occupational Engagement 531

Chapter 41. Clinical Reasoning: The Ethics, Science, and Art 541
    Joan C. Rogers

Chapter 42. The Therapist With the Three-Track Mind 555
    Maureen Hayes Fleming

Chapter 43. The Narrative Nature of Clinical Reasoning 565
    Cheryl Mattingly

Chapter 44. A Framework of Strategies for Client-Centred Practice 575
    Gayle Restall, Jacquie Ripat, and Marlene Stern

Chapter 45. Linking Purpose to Procedure During Interactions With Patients 585
    Suzanne M. Peloquin

Chapter 46. The Origin and Evolution of Activity Analysis 593
    Cynthia Creighton

Chapter 47. Tools of Practice: Heritage or Baggage? 599
    Kathlyn L. Reed

Chapter 48. Ethical Decision-Making Challenges in Clinical Practice 609
  Beverly P. Horowitz

Appendix V.A. Physical Agent Modalities 617

Appendix V.B. Complementary and Alternative Medicine 621

Appendix V.C. Telehealth 627

Part VI. The Scholarship of Occupation-Based and Evidence-Based Practice **649**

Chapter 49. Our Mandate for the New Millennium: Evidence-Based Practice.. 661
  Margo B. Holm

Chapter 50. Heterarchy and Hierarchy: A Critical Appraisal of the "Levels of Evidence"
        as a Tool for Clinical Decision Making.. 675
  Linda Tickle-Degnen and Gary Bedell

Chapter 51. The Process of Evidence-Based Decision Making in Occupational Therapy............................. 681
  Christopher J. Lee and Linda T. Miller

Chapter 52. Informing Client-Centred Practice Through Qualitative Inquiry:
        Evaluating the Quality of Qualitative Research 689
  Karen Whalley Hammell

Chapter 53. Sharing the Agenda: Pondering the Politics and Practices of Occupational Therapy Research 703
  Karen R. W. Hammell, William C. Miller, Susan J. Forwell, Bert E. Forman, and Brad A. Jacobsen

Part VII. Envisioning the Future of Occupation-Based Practice **711**

Chapter 54. Old Values—New Directions: Competence, Adaptation, Integration....................................... 721
  Jerry A. Johnson

Chapter 55. Creating Excellence in Patient Care 733
  Kathleen Barker Schwartz

Chapter 56. Dreams, Dilemmas, and Decisions for Occupational Therapy Practice
        in a New Millennium: An American Perspective 739
  Elizabeth J. Yerxa

Chapter 57. Dreams, Dilemmas, and Decisions for Occupational Therapy Practice
        in a New Millennium: A Canadian Perspective 743
  Helene J. Polatajko

Chapter 58. Professional Responsibility in Times of Change 749
  Wilma L. West

Chapter 59. Reexamining Concepts of Occupation and Occupation-Based Models:
        Occupational Therapy and Community Development 757
  Leanne L. Leclair

Chapter 60. Change: Creating Our Own Reality.. 765
  Virginia G. Fearing

Chapter 61. Occupation by Design: Dimensions, Therapeutic Power, and Creative Process........................ 775
  Doris Pierce

Chapter 62. Embracing Our Ethos, Reclaiming Our Heart 789
  Suzanne M. Peloquin

Chapter 63. A Fork in the Road: An Occupational Hazard?.. 807
  Glen Gillen

Appendix A. *Occupational Therapy Practice Framework: Domain and Process, 3rd Edition* 821

Subject Index.. 869

Citation Index... 875

About the Editor

Rita P. Fleming-Castaldy, PhD, OT/L, FAOTA, has been an occupational therapist for more than 35 years. She began her career in acute psychiatry, expanding her practice into community mental health, case management, and transitional living programs. In each of her clinical positions, Dr. Fleming-Castaldy developed and maintained an active fieldwork program. Her love of teaching the next generation of occupational therapy practitioners motivated her to obtain post-professional master of arts and doctor of philosophy degrees in occupational therapy and assume the role of full-time academic educator. Currently, she is an associate professor of occupational therapy at the Panuska College of Professional Studies at the University of Scranton.

Dr. Fleming-Castaldy is a staunch advocate for the development of public policies and professional practices that enable full societal participation for persons with disabilities. In her written work and presentations, Dr. Fleming-Castaldy combines her personal experience as a family caregiver with her professional expertise to promote occupational therapy's role in ensuring that all persons with disabilities are able to pursue meaningful occupations within their environments of choice. She is strongly committed to promoting the development of historical literacy within the field and ensuring that the relevance of the profession's heritage to current and future occupational therapy practice is recognized.

Dr. Fleming-Castaldy has authored and edited 18 textbooks. She is the author or coauthor of more than 200 book chapters, peer-reviewed national and international journal articles, and peer-reviewed national and international occupational therapy and interdisciplinary conference presentations. Dr. Fleming-Castaldy is considered a leading expert on the national occupational therapy certification examination. Her research interests include examining the relationships among occupation, social participation, and quality of life for persons with significant disabilities who reside in the community.

Dr. Fleming-Castaldy is an active member in several professional and consumer associations. She serves on the editorial boards of the *American Journal of Occupational Therapy* and *Occupational Therapy in Mental Health*. In 2002, she received the honor of being named a Fellow to the American Occupational Therapy Association for innovation and leadership in education and advocacy. Many of Dr. Fleming-Castaldy's works are referenced under her former name of Fleming Cottrell.

Active Reflections, Exhibits, Figures, Tables, and Appendixes

Active Reflections

Active Reflection I.1. Occupational Therapy's Founding Principles and Philosophical Base 2
Active Reflection I.2. Major Influences on the Profession's Development 4
Active Reflection I.3. Occupational Therapy's Professional Identity 4
Active Reflection I.4. Lessons From the Past 5
Active Reflection II.1. Commonalities in Theoretical and Conceptual Frameworks 110
Active Reflection II.2. Relevance of Theory to the *Occupational Therapy Practice Framework* 111
Active Reflection II.3. Challenges to Traditional Theoretical Conceptualizations 112
Active Reflection II.4. Monism or Pluralism in Occupational Therapy Practice 113
Active Reflection III.1. Balance, Harmony, and Flow 211
Active Reflection III.2. Life: A Balancing Act 213
Active Reflection III.3. Cross-Cultural Awareness 214
Active Reflection III.4. Inclusive Communities and Occupational Justice 216
Active Reflection III.5. Willpower, Occupation, and Well-Being 218
Active Reflection III.6. Virtual and Personal Contexts: A Symbiotic or Parasitic Relationship? 219
Active Reflection III.7. Personal Perspectives on Spirituality and Resilience 221
Active Reflection III.8. The Contexts of Personal Identity and Subjective Well-Being 221
Active Reflection IV.1. Personal, Cultural, and Societal Influences on Caring 462
Active Reflection IV.2. Impact of Practice Realities on Client-Centered Practice 463
Active Reflection IV.3. Application of the Ethnographic Approach 463
Active Reflection IV.4. Comparative Analysis of Social and Medical Models 465
Active Reflection IV.5. Conscious Use of Self and the *Centennial Vision* 465
Active Reflection V.1. Clinical Reasoning 532
Active Reflection V.2. Client-Centered Strategic Framework 533
Active Reflection V.3. Linking Purpose to Procedure 533
Active Reflection V.4. Tools of Practice in Occupational Therapy 535
Active Reflection V.5. Clinical Application of Practice Tools 535
Active Reflection V.6. Ethical Decision Making 536
Active Reflection VI.1. Science and the Scholarship of Practice 649
Active Reflection VI.2. Hierarchy of Evidence for Occupation-Based Practice 652
Active Reflection VI.3. Patterns and Possibility 653
Active Reflection VI.4. The Contextualized Nature of Research 654
Active Reflection VI.5. The Quality of Quantitative Research 655
Active Reflection VI.6. Politics, Power, and Research 655
Active Reflection VII.1. Professional Association Membership 714
Active Reflection VII.2. Macro-Level Thinking for Community Development 715
Active Reflection VII.3. Reclaiming the Heart of Practice 717
Active Reflection VII.4. Taking the Right Fork 718

Exhibits

Exhibit I.1. Dunton's Principles of Occupational Therapy 1
Exhibit I.2. Basic Principles of Occupational Therapy 2
Exhibit III.1. McColl's Spirituality Research Questions.. 221
Exhibit V.1. Helen and the Disappearing Pegs 536
Exhibit VI.1. Principal Purposes of Statistics in Occupational Therapy.. 651
Exhibit VII.1. Occupational Therapy at Its Best 718

Figures

Figure 8.1. Occupation as the meaningful, purposeful occupational performance of a person
in the context of an occupational form. 116
Figure 8.2. Occupation depicted with the occupational dynamics of impact and adaptation. 117
Figure 8.3. A Conceptual Framework for Therapeutic Occupation (for therapeutic adaptation). 118
Figure 8.4. A Conceptual Framework for Therapeutic Occupation (for therapeutic compensation). 119
Figure 9.1. Schematic relationship between the Model of Human Occupation and sensory
integration theory... 132
Figure 9.2. Interrelationship between meaning and purpose when applied to occupation..................... 133
Figure 9.3. Four continua that can be used to evaluate the characteristics of any activity used
as occupational therapy intervention... 134
Figure 9.4. Schematic representation of the Occupational Therapy Intervention Process Model. 137
Figure 9.5. Schematic representation of occupational performance unfolding as a transaction
between the person and the environment as he or she enacts a task. 137
Figure 11.1. Conceptualization of occupational performance.. 161
Figure 11.2. Nesting of levels of occupation.. 162
Figure 11.3. Dynamical systems theory of motor control hypothesizes that goal-directed action
emerges from a synthesis of goal or purpose and contextual constraints.. 165
Figure 11.4. Velocity profiles for reaches to a 4-centimeter disk, after which the goal was to fit
the disk into a slot or to throw it into a basket.. 166
Figure 11.5. Phase planes (velocity × displacement) of two trials of two conditions (natural
and simulated) by one normal subject.. 167
Figure 11.6. Pictorial description of r^2. 169
Figure 12.1. Two-dimensional model of flow. 176
Figure 19.1. Proposed cycle for achieving occupational balance.. 265
Figure 21.1. Visual depiction of the model of lifestyle balance. 288
Figure 24.1. Schematic box and arrow rendition of the Kawa model.. 318
Figure 24.2. Diagrammatic representation of Western, rational, in which the self and environs
are regarded to be discrete, separate entities.. 319
Figure 24.3. Diagrammatic representation of an alternate worldview in which the self, deities,
and all parts of nature are inseparably inter-related 320
Figure 24.4. "Life is like a river"; the river used metaphorically to represent the life journey............... 321
Figure 24.5. Four basic components of the Kawa (River) model; listed first in Japanese,
followed by the English translation. 321
Figure 24.6. Specific problems have a tendency to combine with other aspects of the client's
context of daily living and compound the overall impediment to life flow.. 323
Figure 24.7. Each potential foci for intervention is multi-faceted, ideally requiring an
inter-disciplinary, combined approach, resulting in decreasing impeding factors and
ultimately increasing life flow. 325
Figure 25.1. Circle of Friends petroglyph. 332
Figure 25.2. Personal community building. 333
Figure 25.3. Celebrating diversity: Individual and society... 336

Figure 25.4. The person in life span. 337
Figure 25.5. Environment–person relationships. 338
Figure 25.6. Linking past experiences. 340
Figure 25.7. The link of past experience with personal community. 341
Figure 25.8. Linking current information. 341
Figure 25.9. The link of current situation with personal community. 342
Figure 25.10. Exploring future possibilities. 342
Figure 25.11. The link of hopes, dreams, and future expectations with personal community. 342
Figure 27.1. Client-centered activism for occupational justice. 362
Figure 30.1. Needs: Three-way role in health. 393
Figure 30.2. Occupation: Three major functions in species survival. 394
Figure 30.3. Capacities and needs are subjugated to external purpose. 397
Figure 31.1. Formula for satisfaction. 400
Figure 34.1. Hierarchy of identity concepts. 427
Figure 34.2. Reflexive self-consciousness—The dialogue between the *I* and the *me*. 429
Figure 34.3. Concepts that link sense of coherence to identity. 434
Figure 37.1. Client-centered care model. 485
Figure 37.2. Family-centered care model. 488
Figure 37.3. Relationship-centered care model. 491
Figure 37.4. *ICF* conceptual framework. 491
Figure 38.1. Ethnographic framework for service delivery. 500
Figure V.1. Insights on the therapeutic value of occupational therapy tools of practice from 1922 535
Figure 44.1. Client-centered Strategies Framework. 577
Figure 47.1. Relative influence of organismic and mechanistic models on occupational therapy practice. 604
Figure 49.1. Factors affecting the performance of evidence-based practice. 670
Figure 51.1. The evidence-based occupational therapy process. 684
Figure 57.1. World Health Organization disablement model. 743
Figure 57.2. Occupational competence model. 745
Figure 57.3. Ability and environment interaction. 746
Figure 57.4. Changes for occupational therapy in the coming millennium 747
Figure 61.1. Three bridges required to rapidly translate knowledge of occupation into powerful
    occupation-based practice. 776
Figure 61.2. The occupational design approach: Conceptual tools for building occupation-based practice. 778
Figure 63.1. Comparison of occupational therapy's normalcy and current evidence-based practice. 811
Figure 63.2. Timeline related to our involvement in motor control training and cognitive assessment. 812

Tables

Table 11.1. Mean Number of Repetitions as a Result of Preference and Purpose in Assigned Tasks 168
Table 11.2. Effects of Product-Oriented and Nonproduct-Oriented Activities 168
Table 11.3. Average Effects of Materials-Based Occupation, Imagery-Based Occupation, and
    Rote Exercise 169
Table 18.1. References to (Adult) Sleep Found in Indexes of Occupational Therapy Textbooks 248
Table 18.2. Some Definitions of *Occupation* and Relationship of Sleep 251
Table 21.1. Comparison of Need-Based Theories Related to the Model of Lifestyle Balance 283
Table 27.1. Two Foundations to Explore Occupational Justice 354
Table 27.2. Word Associations: *Occupation, Justice,* and *Occupational Justice* 355
Table 27.3. An Exploratory Theory of Occupational Justice 357
Table 27.4. Proposed Occupational Rights 358
Table 27.5. Working for Occupational Justice Through Client-Centered Practice 361
Table 38.1. Ethnographic Principles, Definitions, and Clinical Applications 498

Table 47.1. Factors in the Selection and Use of Media and Methods.. 600
Table 47.2. Types of Sanding Blocks 604
Table 47.3. Purposes or Objectives of Sanding Blocks.. 604
Table VI.1. Historical Perspectives on the Scholarship of Practice.. 650
Table VI.2. Scholarship in Occupational Therapy 651
Table 49.1. Hierarchy of Levels of Evidence for Evidence-Based Practice 662
Table 49.2. Hierarchy of Evidence Applied to Articles Published in the *Occupational Therapy*
     Journal of Research, 1995–1999.. 668
Table 51.1. Evidence Matrix: Varieties of Evidence Classified by Method and Perspective................ 684
Table 52.1. Framework of Guidelines for Evaluating Qualitative Research 691
Table 59.1. Definitions of *Occupation*.. 758
Table 59.2. Community Development Models 760
Table 63.1. Changing Descriptions of Occupational Therapy for Clients With Impaired
     Motor Control Across the Life Course.. 809

Appendixes

Appendix I.A. The Philosophical Base of Occupational Therapy 103
Appendix I.B. Setting the Stage—Address in Honor of Eleanor Clarke Slagle 105
Appendix II.A. Position Paper: Broadening the Construct of Independence 207
Appendix 38.A. Examples of Useful Questions 503
Appendix 45.A 591
Appendix V.A. Physical Agent Modalities 617
Appendix V.B. Complementary and Alternative Medicine.. 621
Appendix V.C. Telehealth 627
Appendix VI.A. Guide to Evaluating Research Evidence: Guiding Questions..................................... 660
Appendix VI.B. Resources to Appraise Evidence 660
Appendix 57.A. *Occupational Therapy Values Statement* 747
Appendix A. *Occupational Therapy Practice Framework: Domain and Process, 3rd Edition* 821

Preface

RITA P. FLEMING-CASTALDY, PHD, OT/L, FAOTA

Typical of many occupational therapy practitioners, my entry into our field was deeply rooted in personal life experience. My life was forever changed and greatly enriched by my brother Kevin and his lifelong struggle with a degenerative neuromuscular disorder (Fleming-Castaldy, 2010). Therefore, I begin this text by describing my subjective experience with the profession of occupational therapy. I share this story because it highlights the meaningfulness of occupation and is a major precipitant for this publication and my life work as an occupational therapist.

When I was a young child, my older brother Kevin was diagnosed with Friedreich's ataxia, a progressive neuromuscular disorder. Because we were only 2 years apart in age, his lifelong journey through the disease process became my journey. Initially, my childhood naiveté prompted me to decide to become a physician who would cure my brother and all others with devastating illnesses. However, with age comes realism, and as I grew older, I began to recognize that cures were infrequent, particularly for such rare diseases as my brother's. While I realized that extensive research might one day find a cure (or at least an effective treatment), my brother needed something done during his lifetime to help him manage his progressive illness. As an adolescent, I began to explore the profession of physical therapy. Throughout high school, I formalized my decision to become a physical therapist and entered New York University (NYU) as a "pre-PT" student. At this point, Kevin's disease had progressed significantly, and he could not participate in many activities. He was an avid reader and a music aficionado, but many hours were filled with boredom and depression.

After my first introductory PT class, I realized that physical therapy would not sufficiently meet my brother's needs because he had lost all gross motor abilities. Fortunately, in my ongoing search to find ways to improve the quality of Kevin's life, I discovered the field of occupational therapy. It was a perfect match. Occupational therapy's holistic approach, which maximized abilities, minimized disabilities, and provided adaptive strategies and compensation methods to enable the individual to live a productive, satisfying life, was just what Kevin and I had sought.[1] I quickly changed my major to occupational therapy and became a sponge, absorbing all of the information and skills we had been seeking for so many years (without even knowing what we had been looking for).

With the field of occupational therapy finally discovered, I promptly had Kevin's physician refer him to an internationally known hospital for rehabilitation. The initial care my brother received seemed highly competent. He was given a customized wheelchair and scads of adaptive equipment. As an occupational therapy student, I was impressed with these obviously skilled practitioners and their thoughtful interventions. However, it quickly became evident that Kevin's greatest needs were not being addressed by the rehabilitation team. Most striking was the total lack of interest in who Kevin was or what he wanted to achieve. As a 22-year-old living at home with no job or social network, Kevin clearly needed a complete occupational therapy evaluation. Unfortunately, his entire evaluation and treatment focused on his motor functioning, wheelchair mobility, and the self-care task of dressing. Increasing his strength and coordination were generally helpful to Kevin, but wheelchair mobility and dressing were difficult and extremely exhausting for him. Also, due to the nature of his illness, it was likely that these difficulties would increase as his disease progressed. Dressing in

---

[1] Kevin had the misfortune to be born before the development of early childhood intervention programs and the expansion of occupational therapy into community, home, and school-based settings. Therefore, his childhood contact with therapists consisted only of periodic sessions in medical clinics focused largely on measuring his deficits. Fortunately, today's children with disabilities and their families do not have to wait a lifetime to receive appropriate and essential services.

the morning took a frustrating 2 hours to complete and left him so fatigued that he could not even hold a book to read or put a record on his turntable. This was devastating to Kevin because he was extremely intelligent and craved the fine literature and music that still filled his life with meaning. To be so weary that one cannot enjoy life's pleasures is sad; to have this fatigue brought on by an ill-conceived intervention plan is tragic.

My brother's assertive nature fortunately remedied this unproductive situation. He quickly (and loudly!) refused to independently dress himself and threw out all of the adaptive equipment. This act of self-preservation was viewed by his occupational therapist and rehabilitation team as a clear indication that he was a "difficult, unmotivated" client, and he was promptly discharged from the occupational therapy program. He was "allowed" to continue in the wheelchair clinic, "as needed." Not once during the time he was involved with this treatment program did anyone fully assess his values, interests, or goals; they assessed only his muscle strength, range of motion, coordination, and sensory awareness. Nor did any therapist ever see Kevin's high intelligence, sharp wit, and brilliant smile (when earned).

Fortunately, I was continuing in my occupational therapy studies and developing a strong appreciation for the holistic and therapeutic use of occupation. After consulting with Kevin (and using him as a guinea pig for several of my school assignments), we decided that he would become a student at NYU during my senior year so that I would be available to assist him with his transition to independent living. His choice of a political science major was, as he stated, one of "pure selfish interest." It would have questionable use after graduation, but Kevin did not care, because the progressive nature of his illness precluded employment at the time (this was pre–Americans with Disabilities Act [ADA]). Kevin's primary goals for attending college were to be intellectually stimulated, develop a social network, and live independently. He accomplished all of these goals, with me serving as a novice occupational therapist and adapting his dormitory room and activities to meet his needs.

Kevin's success was truly a testament to his character, but I often found myself wondering what would have happened to him and his ability to attain his goals if his sister had not been an occupational therapist? Why was it so difficult for the occupational therapists working with him to see him as a whole person with interests, hopes, and dreams, not just a set of weak, unco-

ordinated muscles? Years went by and Kevin pursued a successful academic career, typing his papers from memory with one finger while proudly maintaining a B average. He obtained his bachelor's and master's degrees within 5 years, developed friendships, attended concerts, dined in restaurants, and traveled to England and a multitude of American states. A definite quality of life had replaced the boredom and depression of our "pre-OT" years.

The question about the lack of holism and the absence of occupation in actual occupational therapy clinical practice came back to haunt us many times. To preserve our sibling relationship, I tried not to act as Kevin's therapist, and periodically we obtained physician's referrals for occupational therapy to meet his needs as his disease progressed. During these forays into the rehabilitation world, I was always available as the family representative when a new therapist began working with Kevin. I never initially mentioned that I was an occupational therapist because I was serving as a family member, not as a professional colleague. Invariably, each occupational therapist would competently assess Kevin's physical status, prescribe built-up handled and weighted utensils, and begin a morning dressing program. Only one occupational therapist ever asked Kevin what he did for leisure, work, or meaningful occupation. This same occupational therapist was the only one to question if there were any psychosocial needs that were not being met for Kevin and our family. Unfortunately, this gifted therapist did not stay in her position for long due to a lack of administrative support for her holistic approaches.[2]

Kevin responded to all of these reductionistic occupational therapists by discontinuing treatment after only a few sessions because, as Kevin accurately noted, "it's pointless." This served to perpetuate his reputation as a difficult, unmotivated client. Invariably, I resumed my dual role of sister–OT, adapting activities and modifying Kevin's environment according to his interests and needs. Again, we asked ourselves in frustration, *What if*

---

[2] Years later, I met this therapist at a conference and learned that she had been a student in her third month of fieldwork when she asked Kevin and me these critical questions. After completing her fieldwork, she accepted a position at this facility hoping to effect changes that would enable client-centered practices. When her enthusiasm was crushed by the cynicism that surrounded her, she questioned if occupational therapy was the right profession for her. Fortunately, she decided to change jobs rather than leave the field and reported that she eventually found a setting that supported the practice of occupational therapy in the manner she had sought to provide to my brother and our family.

I were not an occupational therapist? How could our family help Kevin manage a devastating progressive illness and maintain quality of life? My occupational therapy professional literature was replete with holistic views about the therapeutic use of occupation and client-centered practices, but why we did not see this in in my brother's occupational therapy interventions?

Kevin passed away in 1989. Decades later, the lessons he taught me about life and the questions he raised about my profession continue to influence me and my teaching. In many respects, I cannot separate my personal self from my professional self because they were intertwined for so long. I often use my brother and our life experiences as examples to underscore fundamental occupational therapy principles to my students.

Kevin's life journey also taught me the critical need to be astute about the social, economic, and political issues that influence the reality of living with a disability in the United States. Therefore, the role of the occupational therapy practitioner as an advocate is also central to my teachings. Our parents' struggle to obtain basic medical care for Kevin because of our family's low socioeconomic status provided me with many early childhood memories that reflect societal inequities. My brother's battle to acquire an education that was equal to the education of students without disabilities enabled me, as a teenager, to appreciate the monumental significance of the Rehabilitation Act of 1973. In 1975, my brother and I celebrated the enactment of the Education for All Handicapped Children Act, which finally mandated free and appropriate education for all children, regardless of ability or disability. This act's passage was of special significance to our family because, as Staten Island residents, my parents were told that my brother should be institutionalized at the infamous Willowbrook State School (Riveria, 1972). Fortunately, my parents resisted the status quo, and as previously noted, my brother successfully attained a graduate degree from NYU. However, this path was fraught with obstacles, so we carefully followed all subsequent legislation related to disability rights.

Regrettably, my brother passed away 6 months before the passage of the ADA. Although Kevin did not witness this milestone in disability rights history, I toasted this landmark legislation in his honor with the hope that others with disabilities would not have to fight as hard as he did to fully participate in society. Regrettably, the reality that the ADA has not removed many of the social, economic, and political barriers to full community participation has to be acknowledged.

Nearly a quarter-century post-ADA, millions of Americans with disabilities remain unemployed, institutionalized, and segregated from society (National Council on Disability, 2010; U.S. Department of Labor, 2012). Because the final 2 years of my brother's life had to be spent in a skilled nursing facility due to a lack of funding for home-based care, I have focused my scholarship on examining and confronting barriers to full community participation (Cottrell, 2003, 2005, 2007; Fleming-Castaldy, 2009, 2011, 2014). This work has deepened my understanding of the relationships among personal choice, control, occupation, and quality of life and the role of occupational therapy in empowering people to live self-directed lives in environments *they* choose.

I have been heartened by our profession's reaffirmed commitment to the promotion of full community participation for *all* people as put forth in the *Occupational Therapy Practice Framework: Domain and Process* (American Occupational Therapy Association [AOTA], 2002) and its subsequent revisions (AOTA, 2008, 2014), the most recent of which is reprinted in this text's appendix. As an advocate, I applaud the *Framework's* inclusion of the political, economic, and social contexts that can support or hinder full societal participation and self-determined engagement in desired occupations. The *Framework's* focus on occupational justice and its adoption of the World Health Organization's (WHO) definition of disability to include participation restrictions resulting from attitudinal, physical, and social environmental factors are indicative of our profession's abandonment of past reductionistic practices dominated by the medical model (which had so negatively affected my brother's life).

The identification of a primary role of "occupational therapy practitioners to advocate for the well-being of all persons, groups and populations with a commitment to inclusion and non-discrimination" (AOTA, 2008, p. 630); the delineation of advocacy as a major type of occupational therapy intervention to empower clients and promote occupational justice; and the inclusion of participation, social well-being, quality of life, role competence, self-advocacy, and occupational justice as desired outcomes of occupational therapy are welcome changes from the singular focus on the remediation of deficits that dominated my brother's therapy sessions. I hope that by providing this accessible compilation of outstanding occupational therapy literature and promoting the use of critical reflexivity to those who read this volume, I can contribute to a renewed commitment to the use of occupation as a means of empowerment to enable people with disabilities (and their families) to attain and maintain a satisfying self-determined life. Based on my life experiences, this is the true purpose of authentic occupational therapy and the gift that my brother and I embraced many years ago. It is a legacy worth perpetuating.

References

American Occupational Therapy Association. (2002). Occupational therapy practice framework: Domain and process. *American Journal of Occupational Therapy, 56,* 609–639. http://dx.doi.org/10.5014/ajot.56.6.609

American Occupational Therapy Association. (2008). Occupational therapy practice framework: Domain and process (2nd ed.). *American Journal of Occupational Therapy, 62,* 625–683. http://dx.doi.org/10.5014/ajot.62.6.625

American Occupational Therapy Association. (2014). Occupational therapy practice framework: Domain and process (3rd ed.). *American Journal of Occupational Therapy, 68*(Suppl.), S1–S48. http://dx.doi.org/10.5014/ajot.2014.682006

Cottrell, R. P. (2003). The Olmstead decision: Fulfilling the promise of ADA? *OT Practice, 8*(5), 17–21.

Cottrell, R. P. (2005). The Olmstead decision: Landmark opportunity or platform for rhetoric? Our collective responsibility for full community participation. *American Journal of Occupational Therapy, 59,* 561–567. http://dx.doi.org/10.5014/ajot.59.5.561

Cottrell, R. P. (2007). The New Freedom Initiative: Transforming mental health care—Will OT be at the table? *Occupational Therapy in Mental Health, 23*(2), 1–24.

Fleming-Castaldy, R. (2009). *Disability. Personal care assistance, and quality of life: A study of the relationships between consumer-direction and life satisfaction of people with disabilities who use home-based personal care assistance.* Saarbrucken, Germany: VDM Verag Dr Muller.

Fleming-Castaldy, R. (2010). Honoring a life of loss, resilience, and meaning: Kevin. In A. Hofmann & M. Strzelecki (Eds.), *Living life to its fullest: Stories of occupational therapy* (pp. 24–35). Bethesda, MD: AOTA Press.

Fleming-Castaldy, R. P. (2011). Are satisfaction with and self-management of personal assistance services associated with the life satisfaction of persons with physical disabilities? *Disability and Rehabilitation, 33*(15–16), 1447–1459.

Fleming-Castaldy, R. (2014). Occupations, activities, and empowerment. In J. Hinojosa, & M. L. Blount (Eds.), *The texture of life: Purposeful activities in the context of occupation* (4th ed., pp. 393–416). Bethesda, MD: AOTA Press.

National Council on Disability. (2010). *The state of housing in America in the 21st century: A disability perspective.* Washington, DC: Author.

Riveria, G. (1972). *Willowbrook: A report on how it is and why it doesn't have to be that way.* New York: Random House.

U.S. Department of Labor, Office of Disability Employment Policy. (2012). *Current disability employment statistics.* Retrieved from http://www.dol.gov/odep/topics/DisabilityEmploymentStatistics.htm

Introduction

RITA P. FLEMING-CASTALDY, PhD, OT/L, FAOTA

Archives [of Occupational Therapy] *is also playing a large part in making occupational therapy better known generally from the fact that it is to be found in practically all medical libraries today. There are also numerous subscriptions from foreign countries. Quite recently our secretary treasurer received a most appreciative letter from the head of a large institution in Glasgow, Scotland, who said that he read each number from cover to cover.*

Kidner (1924, p. 429)

As I describe in this text's preface, growing up with my brother Kevin influenced my life in countless ways. One of the most rewarding is the love of reading that we shared. Throughout our childhood, we often sought to escape the crueler aspects of life by finding refuge in books (Fleming-Castaldy, 2010). While I remained an avid reader into adulthood, my passion for the literature of my chosen profession was not fully ignited until I became an educator. In striving to ensure that I was providing my students with the most relevant and meaningful resources, I would assemble article packets and reserve readings to supplement course textbooks. Each semester, I would review these compilations and complete extensive literature reviews to update them. My aim was to include the "latest and greatest" in the profession's current literature while retaining historical classics.

In 1996, I formalized my course compilation habit into the editorship of an anthology, *Perspectives on Purposeful Activity: Foundation and Future of Occupational Therapy* (Cottrell, 1996), which was published by the American Occupational Therapy Association (AOTA). My aim was to provide an "at your fingertips" library to occupational therapy educators and students and save them the time and effort needed to access these foundational readings. To place this work in context, it is important to note that this time period was before the advent of digital libraries. In 2005, the second edition of this text was published by AOTA Press (Cottrell, 2005). At that time, the text's name was changed to the current title, *Perspectives for Occupation-Based Practice: Foundation and Future of Occupational Therapy,* to reflect the changes that had occurred in our profession's language since the publication of the first edition.

Over the ensuing years, electronic access to the profession's literature has become an invaluable asset to students, educators, practitioners, and scholars. However, one unforeseen consequence of the digital age is that electronic searches on a given topic typically results in hundreds (and often thousands) of citations. Finding the gold among the dross can be an overwhelming, time-consuming, and frustrating process. This third edition seeks to continue the vision of the past two editions by providing a meaningful and *easily accessible* compilation of the occupational therapy literature related to occupation-based practice. To complete this publication, I conducted an extensive literature review to gather the best of the best in the profession's literature. These works reflect multiple perspectives from the inception of occupational therapy to its envisioned future. I selected original literary classics from the founding and ensuing years of the field that have had a global impact to thought-provoking recent works from national and international peer-reviewed journals to provide readers with a solid theoretical and philosophical foundation, as well as realistic and relevant guidelines for occupation-based practice throughout the occupational therapy process.

In recognition of the globalization of occupational therapy and the increased emphasis in our field to integrate and use "international resources in education, research, practice, and policy development (and to) utilize national and international resources in making assessment or intervention choices" (Accreditation Council for Occupational Therapy Education [ACOTE], 2012, p. 28), I have greatly expanded content from international occupational therapy journals. To meet AOTA's *Centennial Vision's* call for a "globally connected and diverse workforce meeting society's occupational needs" (2007, p. 613) and to address the latest ACOTE (2012) standards concerned with occupational injustice and service disparities, I have added substantial content on sociopolitical contexts that influence occupation-based practice. It is my hope that this enhanced global perspective will help readers appreciate the potential contribution occupational therapy practitioners can make to the attainment of social and occupational justice throughout the world. To provide readers with resources to help attain the AOTA vision for our field to be a "science-driven, and evidence based profession" (AOTA, 2007, p. 613) and to meet the strengthened professional educational standards for research (ACOTE, 2012), I have added a new section on the scholarship of occupation-based practice.

I begin each part of the text with an introductory chapter that highlights the relevance of the section's focus to the AOTA (2014) *Occupational Therapy Practice Framework: Domain and Process* (subsequently called the *Framework*) and the AOTA (2007) *Centennial Vision*. In these chapters, I strive to provide a philosophical, yet practical, link between occupational therapy's heritage, current practice realities, and future practice opportunities. This continuity of thought is expressed in the quotes from the profession's historical literature that I present at the start of each chapter and intersperse throughout my narratives. To help readers develop personal insights into key issues and challenge their perceptions about person-directed, occupation-based practice, I provide a diversity of reflective exercises. It is my hope that active participation in these reflections and thoughtful consideration of the questions posed will strengthen the readers' commitment to the core values and ethos of occupational therapy.

Readers should note that because all the chapters in this text are reprinted from other sources, they vary in style. Due to the need to comply with copyright laws, all of the chapters in this text were reprinted as originally published. While editorial efforts were made to ensure grammatical accuracy and gender-neutral language, readers will note some inconsistencies in several chapters. These chapters contain relevant content, but their formats do not always adhere to the AOTA Press's publication guidelines. Areas of concern include various styles of referencing and usage and non–gender-neutral language. In addition, because these writings have been culled from 100 years of occupational therapy professional literature, some concepts and terms will be understandably dated. These historical pieces were included because they were significant works during their respective time and they remain a vital part of our profession's literary history and ongoing development.

While I carefully selected articles for the text chapters that accurately reflect the philosophical foundations, contextual influences, practical application, and scholarship of occupation-based practice, there are realistic parameters to the text. Due to space constraints, many strong works were omitted. The resulting compilation is representative of the wealth of literature in our field, but it is not an exhaustive anthology. Because there are several excellent publications available that provide in-depth information on specific occupational therapy frames of reference, models of practice, evaluation methods, and intervention approaches, I have not included works on these professional topics. Readers are urged to use the reference lists at the end of each chapter to identify works that study these topics and other relevant issues further. The text also includes appendices to supplement the text's chapters and/or areas of focus and serve as an additional resource for readers.

Since the publication of this text's first edition in 1996, I have had the privilege to work with hundreds of students and many practitioners and educators who have used these foundational readings in their coursework and research. It has been most gratifying to observe the development of their strong appreciation for our profession's literature and its relevance to their current and future practice. In 1955, Stattel observed "We have been given a wonderful professional heritage of courage and wisdom and as we continue to extend our hand to benefit mankind, may we continue to believe and search for further knowledge" (1956, p. 194). I hope this text will foster an increased awareness and appreciation of the rich heritage Stattel spoke of, and that which is reflected in this text's chapters. I believe that those who critically reflect on these readings and participate in engaged discourse about their relevance will be able to positively meet professional challenges and develop a rich occupational therapy career dedicated to the provision of person-directed occupation-based practice.

References

Accreditation Council for Occupational Therapy Education. (2012). *ACOTE standards and interpretive guide*. Retrieved from http://www.aota.org/Educate/Accredit/Draft-Standards/50146.aspx?FT=.pdf

American Occupational Therapy Association. (2007). AOTA's *Centennial Vision* and executive summary. *American Journal of Occupational Therapy, 61*, 613–614. http://dx.doi.org/10.5014/ajot.2007.61.6.613

American Occupational Therapy Association. (2014). Occupational therapy practice framework: Domain and process (3rd ed.). *American Journal of Occupational Therapy, 68*(Suppl.), S1–S48. http://dx.doi.org/10.5014/ajot.2014.682006

Cottrell, R. (Ed.). (1996). *Perspectives on purposeful activities: Foundation and future of occupational therapy.* Bethesda, MD: American Occupational Therapy Association.

Cottrell, R. P. (Ed). (2005). *Perspectives for occupation-based practice: Foundation and future of occupational therapy* (2nd ed.). Bethesda, MD: AOTA Press.

Fleming-Castaldy, R. (2010). Honoring a life of loss, resilience, and meaning: Kevin. In A. Hofmann & M. Strzelecki (Eds.), *Living life to its fullest: Stories of occupational therapy* (pp. 24–35). Bethesda, MD: AOTA Press.

Kidner, T. B. (1924). President's address. *Archives of Occupational Therapy, 3,* 423–432.

Stattel, F. (1956). 1955 Eleanor Clarke Slagle Lecture: Equipment designed for occupational therapy. *American Journal of Occupational Therapy, 10,* 194–198.

Part I. Occupational Therapy's Heritage: Historical and Philosophical Foundations for Occupation-Based Practice

That occupation is as necessary to life as food and drink
That every human being should have both physical and mental occupation
That all should have occupations which they enjoy.

—"Credo for Occupational Therapists," Dunton (1919b, p. 10)

The founders of occupational therapy were comprised of professionals from the fields of architecture, education, medicine, nursing, psychiatry, and social work. They established occupational therapy as a singular profession because they believed in the inherent healing power of occupation (Law, 2002; Quiroga, 1995; Schwartz, 2009). This commitment is strongly illuminated in the above statement by William Dunton (1919b). The founders emphasized the therapeutic value of engagement in occupation throughout their writings and in their work, providing a rich heritage and a strong basis for occupation-based practice.

Over the years, this commitment to occupation has been challenged and weakened by reductionist practices based on allegiance to the medical model (Schwartz, 2009; Shannon, 1977; Whiteford, Townsend, & Hocking, 2000). Fortunately, many of the profession's leaders and best practitioners have recognized the invaluable contribution occupational therapy can make to health and wellness—*if* the profession rejected reductionism and retained its unique legacy of occupation (Fidler, 2000; Kielhofner, 2008; Law, 2002; Schwartz, 2009).

This commitment to occupation was re-affirmed when the American Occupational Therapy Association (AOTA) adopted the *Occupational Therapy Practice Framework: Domain and Process* in 2002 (AOTA, 2002). Over the ensuing decade, the *Framework* has become fully integrated into the profession's literature, official documents, and educational standards (Accreditation Council for Occupational Therapy Education [ACOTE], 2012; Gutman, Mortera, Hinojosa, & Kramer, 2007). Revised in 2008 and 2014,[1] the *Framework* asserts that "occupational therapy's distinct perspective and contribution to promoting the health and participation of people, groups, and populations [are] through *engage-*

ment in occupation" (AOTA, 2014, p. S2, italics added). The actualization of this affirmed link among occupation, life participation, and well-being holds the promise of ensuring that current and future occupational therapy practice will reflect the core tenets and values of the profession as first put forth in the early 1900s.

As Schwartz (2009) noted, there is a strong congruence between the profession's founding vision and the AOTA *Centennial Vision* (AOTA, 2007). These commonalities provide continuity to link our heritage to the present and afford philosophical consistency to guide our future. The similarities between many of occupational therapy's founding principles and the profession's current values become evident when one reviews the nine cardinal principles of occupational therapy that Dunton presented in 1918 to guide the developing profession (see Exhibit I.1) and the 15 principles of occupational therapy delineated by the National Society to Promote Occupational Therapy (NSPOT) in 1919 (Dunton, 1919a; see Exhibit I.2 and Active Reflec-

---

Exhibit I.1. Dunton's Principles of Occupational Therapy

1. The work should be carried on with cure as the main object.
2. The work must be interesting.
3. The patient should be carefully studied.
4. The one form of occupation should not be carried to the point of fatigue.
5. That it should have some useful end.
6. That it preferably should lead to an increase in the patient's knowledge.
7. That it should be carried on with others.
8. That all possible encouragement should be given the worker.
9. The work resulting in a poor or useless product is better than idleness.

Source. Dunton, W. R. (1919a). Appendix. In Reconstruction therapy (p. 229). Philadelphia: Saunders. *Original source:* Dunton, W. R. (1918). The principles of occupational therapy. *Public Health Nurse, 18,* 316–321. *As cited in:* Reed, K., & Peters, C., (2006). Occupational therapy values and beliefs, the formative years: 1904–1929. *OT Practice,* pp. 21–21.

---

[1]The complete *Occupational Therapy Practice Framework: Domain and Process* (AOTA, 2014) is provided in Appendix A at the end of this volume.

Exhibit I.2. Basic Principles of Occupational Therapy

To members of the National Society for the Promotion of Occupational Therapy: Your Committee on Principles has agreed upon the following as representing the basic principles of occupational therapy:

1. Occupational therapy is a method of treating the sick or injured by means of instruction and employment of productive occupation.
2. The objects sought are to arouse interest, courage, and confidence; to exercise mind and body in health activity; to overcome functional disability; and to re-establish capacity for industrial and social usefulness.
3. In applying occupational therapy, system and precision are as important as in other forms of treatment.
4. The treatment should be administered under constant medical advice and supervision and correlated with the other treatment of the patient.
5. The treatment should, in each case, be specifically directed to the individual's needs.
6. Though some patients do best alone, employment in groups is usually advisable because it provides exercise in social adaptation and the stimulating influence of example and comment.
7. The occupation selected should be within the range of the patient's estimated interests and capability.
8. As the patient's strength and capability increase, the type and extent of occupation should be regulated and graded accordingly.
9. The only reliable measure of the value of the treatment is the effect on the patient.
10. Inferior workmanship or employment in an occupation which would be trivial for the healthy may be attended with the greatest benefit to the sick or injured. Standards worthy of entirely normal persons must be maintained for proper mental stimulation.
11. The production of well-made, useful, and attractive articles, or the accomplishment of a useful task, requires healthy exercise of mind and body, gives the greatest satisfaction, and thus produces the most beneficial effects.
12. Novelty, variety, individuality, and utility of products enhance the value of an occupation as a treatment measure.
13. Quality, quantity and salability of the products may prove beneficial by satisfying and stimulating the patient but should never be permitted to obscure the main purpose.
14. Good craftsmanship and ability to instruct are essential qualifications in the occupational therapist; understanding, sincere interest in the patient and an optimistic, cheerful outlook and manner are equally essential.
15. Patients under treatment by means of occupational therapy should also engage in recreational or play activities. It is advisable that gymnastics and calisthenics, which may be given for habit training, should be regarded as work. Social dancing and all recreational and play activities should be under the definite head of recreations.

Source. Dunton, W. R. J. (1919a). N.S.P.O.T. *Maryland Psychiatric Quarterly, 13*(3), 68–73. *As cited in:* Reed, K., & Peters, C., (2006). Occupational therapy values and beliefs, the formative years: 1904–1929. *OT Practice*, pp. 21–25.

tion I.1). Appendix I.A at the end of this part elucidates these principles for contemporary practice as put forth in the AOTA's official statement on the *Philosophical Base of Occupational Therapy.*

In this section, occupational therapy's philosophical base, founding principles, and core beliefs are explored in depth in the first four chapters. These scholarly writings examine the lives, times, values, and philosophies that influenced the development of the profession. Subsequent chapters by esteemed scholars build on this historical base to highlight the danger of adopting conflicting ideologies and reductionistic approaches. These works provide solid philosophical and practical arguments, which support the therapeutic use of occupation. Many of these chapters are considered classics in the field. It is an honor to include them in this text.

Active Reflection I.1. Occupational Therapy's Founding Principles and Philosophical Base

Consider each principle put forth by Dunton in Exhibit I.1 and the NSPOT in Exhibit I.2, and reflect on your personal beliefs about the philosophical base of occupational therapy.

- Which of these founding principles do you believe have withstood the test of time?
- Which principles are consistent with the profession's current values?
- Are any principles dated or incongruent with the profession's contemporary beliefs and present global views of occupational well-being?
- If you were a client, which principles would you want an occupational therapy practitioner to use to guide his or her work with you?

The treatment, under medical direction, of physical and mental disorders by the application of occupation and recreation with the object of promoting recovery, of creating new habits and of prevention deterioration. Its object is twofold; the first, to keep occupied, during at least part of the long, tiresome period of invalidism, the minds of those who are temporarily swept aside from healthy living by the ravages of disease. Second, to adapt the method of treatment to the needs of the individual so that, by active occupation, maimed limbs and minds may be once more restored to health.

—deBrisay (1933, p. 120)

In Chapter 1, Peloquin explores a social movement that began in the 18th century and greatly influenced the founders of occupational therapy in the early 19th century. Her presentation describes the moral treatment movement, its characteristics, and the course of its practice, detailing the successful therapeutic use of occupation within the asylums. Peloquin analyzes the tremendous impact that historical contexts and societal trends can have on a profession's development. The societal changes, ideological conflicts, and lack of leadership, which ultimately led to the demise of this movement, are clearly traced. The resulting inequity in treatment, the decrease in quality of care, and the often total lack of care are carefully considered, leading Peloquin to call for occupational therapy practitioners to reaffirm a humanistic view of practice that is committed to the effective use of occupation.

The influence of moral treatment on the development of occupational therapy is further explored by Bing in Chapter 2. In his 1981 Eleanor Clarke Slagle Lecture, Bing postulates that occupational therapy is a retitled form of moral treatment. He supports this viewpoint with a comprehensive analysis of the beginnings of moral treatment in Europe, its expansion in the United States, its disappearance in the last quarter of the 19th century, and its re-emergence in the early 20th century as occupational therapy. The occupation-based principles and definitions of occupational therapy identified by the founders of the profession are reviewed. Bing elaborates on this holistic heritage of occupation in his presentation of the second generation of occupational therapy practitioners, as exemplified in the life and work of Beatrice Wade. This work is replete with personal vignettes and quotes from the founders of occupational therapy and Wade, offering a unique perspective on the rich history of occupational therapy. Bing ends his historical analysis with a thoughtful summation of his views on the lessons current occupational therapy practitioners can learn from the first and second generation of the profession's leaders.

In Chapter 3, Peloquin further contributes to the understanding of the profession's history by analyzing the writings of the founders of NSPOT. Peloquin's comprehensive literature review provides readers with an insightful inquiry into the contemporary historical events and the shared beliefs that influenced the founders of occupational therapy and resulted in the development of our multifaceted profession. She discusses the founders' understanding of service with respect to three primary agents: (1) the person, (2) the therapist, and (3) the occupation. The interrelationships among these agents are emphasized throughout the chapter. The personal narratives, life stories, and unique perspectives of the founders are explored and supported by numerous quotes from their original writings, enabling readers to share their vision for a profession rooted in care and function.

This personalization of the early years of occupational therapy is continued in Chapter 4, which presents Adolf Meyer's landmark speech to the attendees of the Fifth Annual Meeting of NSPOT in 1921. Although the profession was very young at that time, and many years have since passed, readers will be struck by the timelessness of much of Meyer's *Philosophy of Occupation Therapy*. His call for the individuation of activity based on the personal interests and the natural capacities of the individual and the provision of opportunities for meaningful occupation, rather than the use of predetermined treatment prescriptions, has remained relevant despite the passage of many decades. Meyer's presentation traces the development of the therapeutic use of occupation from the 1890s to his time and looks toward a future in which all individuals will be able to engage in gratifying activity to productively use their time.

> *And, after all, what is occupational therapy? It is merely a means of mental contact whereby the patient is gradually brought back to reality and all existent energy is held and increased, or non-existent energy is generated. An occupation—simple or complicated—is not therapeutic unless it holds all available power and reason and tends to increase it, to restore self-confidence by giving the feeling that accomplishment alone can give.*
> —Melrose (1927, p. 45)

Meyer's eloquence is further evident in an *Address in Honor of Eleanor Clarke Slagle*, which is included as Appendix I.B to this part of the text. Meyer delivered this testimonial at a banquet on the eve of Slagle's retirement in 1937. This event also featured a speech by First Lady Eleanor Roosevelt (Quiroga, 1995). Regrettably, Mrs. Roosevelt's complete testimony to Slagle is not available, but fortunately Meyer's remains accessible. Meyer's intimate knowledge of Mrs. Slagle's significant contributions to our profession, and to the clients she worked with, led to this stirring tribute to the woman who personified occupational therapy (see Active Reflection I.2).

In Chapter 5, Hooper and Wood continue the exploration of the development of occupational therapy as

Active Reflection I.2. Major Influences on the Profession's Development

Reflect on the historical trends, sociocultural issues, and sociopolitical forces that have influenced the evolution of the profession of occupational therapy.
- How have ideological conflicts influenced this development?
- How do these trends, issues, forces, and conflicts continue to influence current occupational therapy practice?

a profession. They provide a thought-provoking analysis of the influence that pragmatism and structuralism had on the field. Hooper and Wood present a clear historical and conceptual overview of these two discordant philosophies, highlighting their implications for occupational therapy practice. Readings in occupational therapy that reflect pragmatist and structuralist discourse are reviewed. Hooper and Wood examine the pragmatist and structuralist assumptions about humanity and knowledge, which resulted in divergent and conflicting views about the purpose and focus, tools and methods, and goals and outcomes of occupational therapy. They propose that following these two disparate discourses has contributed to an ongoing professional identity struggle for occupational therapy. Most importantly, they place this pragmatism–structuralism discourse into the broader contexts of society and culture. They conclude that practitioners must become literate in the field's shared language to critically examine our assumptions about knowledge and develop a consciousness about how what we know influences our practice. In addition, Hooper and Wood advocate for the development of cultural literacy to ensure that occupational therapy joins with an ethos that is congruent with our profession's varied practices, multiple theories, and numerous viewpoints so that occupational therapy practitioners' contribution to society is unequivocal and rich.

When we gain the interest of patients we also have their conscious attention; we preclude the preconscious stimuli which otherwise interfere with the progress we are making. Occupational therapy will be far more beneficial when we arouse the patient's interest in the form prescribed. This fact is recognized by every well trained therapist but continues to be ignored by some. Perhaps the question of convenience plays too dominant a role in the selection of occupations for the patient.

—Dunton (1951, p. 384)

Hooper and Wood's examination of the impact of occupational therapy's historical acquiescence to medical authority and the resultant persistent struggle to establish the profession's identity is further explored by Friedland in Chapter 6. In this work, Friedland provides a brief review of early philosophical influences on occupational therapy and reflects on the emerging profession's commitment to occupation and activity. Friedland's discussion about the origins and history of our profession and the development of physical medicine underscores the inevitability of the conflict in values that resulted between occupational therapy and rehabilitation. After World War II, the profession's assumption of the physical rehabilitation model led to the erosion of occupational therapy's core values, as evident in the abandonment of the use of occupation to achieve health and well-being. Friedland realistically discusses the contextual influences that contributed to the demise of occupation-based practices. She honestly discusses the complete lack of fit between authentic occupational therapy and the medical model and questions why we strive to fit into an environment that is intrinsically counter to our very being. She challenges practitioners to cease this abdication to the medical model and align ourselves with newer models of rehabilitation that emphasize social integration. Most significantly, Friedland concludes that the profession must reconnect to occupation-based practice if we are to establish a unique identity as contributors to health and well-being through the therapeutic use of occupation (see Active Reflection I.3).

The impact that practice specialization and the rehabilitation movement had on occupational therapy's growth and development is provocatively explored in

Active Reflection I.3. Occupational Therapy's Professional Identity

Consider the impact of occupational therapy's adoption of structuralistic views and the field's alignment with physical medicine and rehabilitation on the profession's developing identity.
- Do you think these alliances helped or hindered the development of occupational therapy's professional identity?
- Does the profession's historic adoption of structuralism and the medical model continue to affect the therapeutic use of occupation in current practice? Describe this influence.
- How can the concepts put forth in the *Centennial Vision* and *Framework* be used to develop a professional identity that promotes occupational therapy's unique contribution to society?

the final chapter of Part I, which contains Mary Reilly's oft-quoted 1962 Eleanor Clarke Slagle Lecture. In this seminal address in Chapter 7, Reilly critically asks, "Is occupational therapy a vital and unique service for medicine to support and for society to reward?" Reilly's discourse in answer to this question is typically recognized in the field as a literary classic and contains one of the most widely cited passages in our profession's literature. Reilly answers her query with a decisive "yes" in the form of her hypothesis: "That man, through the use of his hands as they are energized by mind and will, can influence the state of his own health."

Because more than 50 years have passed since Reilly presented her Slagle lecture, her postulate reflects a dated view of health that has been critiqued as not inclusive of the reality that well-being can be attained and sustained by people with grave disabilities (see Chapter 14). I personally believe Reilly would embrace this critique because she describes herself as a staunch critic and identifies public criticism in a profession as essential to its progress. Particularly relevant, given the growing competition from other professions (Gutman, 1998; Hinojosa, 2007), is Reilly's concern that occupational therapy will dissolve if the profession does not apply its unique body of knowledge to meet societal needs.

The intrinsic worth of occupation for adaptation, health, and wellness is emphasized by all of this part's authors, from the profession's founders to its leading scholars. The historical perspectives and philosophical tenets they present provide a wealth of thought-provoking writings on the foundations of occupation in our profession. Historian Daniel Boorstin advised that "Trying to plan for the future without a sense of the past is like trying to plant cut flowers."[2] It is my hope that critical reflection on the seminal literature presented in Part I facilitates readers' ability to develop a personal commitment to the therapeutic use of occupation that is congruent with the unique heritage of occupational therapy; cognizant of the missteps that the profession took when its core values and founding principles were abandoned, and consistent with the *Centennial Vision's* and *Framework's* support of society's need for full participation and occupational well-being for all (see Active Reflection I.4).

Active Reflection I.4. Lessons From the Past

Friedland and Rais (2005) have stated "We believe that by examining our roots, we can understand our present more readily, and approach our future more confidently" (p. 131).
- Which perspectives put forth in this section can help inform your understanding of the profession and guide your future practice?
- When you describe occupational therapy to others, does your personal explanation reflect these foundational perspectives?

References

Accreditation Council for Occupational Therapy Education. (2012). 2011 Accreditation Council for Occupational Therapy Education (ACOTE) standards. *American Journal of Occupational Therapy, 66,* S6–S74. http://dx.doi.org/10.5014/ajot.2012.66S6

American Occupational Therapy Association. (2002). Occupational therapy practice framework: Domain and process. *American Journal of Occupational Therapy, 56,* 609–639. http://dx.doi.org/10.5014/ajot.56.6.609.

American Occupational Therapy Association. (2007). *Centennial Vision* and executive summary. *American Journal of Occupational Therapy, 61,* 613–614. http://dx.doi.org/10.5014/ajot.61.6.613

American Occupational Therapy Association. (2008). Occupational therapy practice framework: Domain and process (2nd ed.). *American Journal of Occupational Therapy, 62,* 625–683. http://dx.doi.org/10.5014/ajot.62.6.625

American Occupational Therapy Association. (2014). Occupational therapy practice framework: Domain and process (3rd ed.). *American Journal of Occupational Therapy, 68*(Suppl.), S1–S48. http://dx.doi.org/10.5014/ajot.2014.682006

---

[2]This quote by Boorstin is on the first page of the syllabus for a graduate course I teach on leadership in occupational therapy. In this course, students complete extensive archival research and author comprehensive analyses of the profession's historical influences and their relationships to current and emerging trends in occupational therapy leadership. They critically analyze the application of the profession's core values, founding philosophy, past and current practice standards, and professional ethics to the current state of the profession. These reflective analyses provide the opportunity for students to link their emerging professional identities to the foundational principles and core concepts of occupational therapy as envisioned by the profession's leaders. Consistently, students report that the completion of this assignment is one of the most enlightening and rewarding experiences of their professional education. Although an admittedly challenging experience, student reflections on the outcomes of this capstone project strongly describe their commitment to the actualization of the profession's heritage in their future practice. Post-graduation, many students retain contact with me, and it is heartening to learn that this commitment has been fulfilled in their daily practice and pursuit of leadership opportunities within the field.

deBrisay, A. (1933). Preliminary scheme for the organization of occupational therapy at the Astley Ainslie Institute. In C. Paterson (2010), *Opportunities not prescriptions: The development of occupational therapy in Scotland 1900–1960*. Aberdeen, Scotland: Aberdeen History of Medicine.

Dunton, W. R. J. (1919a). N.S.P.O.T. *Maryland Psychiatric Quarterly, 13*(3), 68–73

Dunton, W. R. (1919b). *Reconstruction therapy*. Philadelphia: W. B. Saunders.

Dunton, W. R. (1951). The importance of interest in occupational therapy. *Occupational Therapy and Rehabilitation, 30*(6), 341–435.

Fidler, G. (2000). The Issue Is—Beyond the therapy model: Building our future. *American Journal of Occupational Therapy, 54*, 99–101. http://dx.doi.org/10.5014/ajot.54.1.99

Friedland, J., & Rais, H. (2005). Helen Primrose Le Vesconte: Occupational therapy clinician, educator and maker of history. *Canadian Journal of Occupational Therapy, 74*, 131–141. http://dx.doi.org/10.1177/000841740507200301

Gutman, S. (1998). The domain of function: Who's got it? Who's competing for it? *American Journal of Occupational Therapy, 52*, 684–689. http://dx.doi.org/10.5014/ajot.52.8.684

Gutman, S., Mortera, M., Hinojosa, J., & Kramer, P. (2007). The Issue Is—Revision of the *Occupational Therapy Practice Framework*. *American Journal of Occupational Therapy, 63*, 119–126. http://dx.doi.org/10.5014/ajot.61.1.119

Hinojosa, J. (2007). Becoming innovators in an era of hyperchange [2007 Eleanor Clarke Slagle Lecture]. *American Journal of Occupational Therapy, 61*, 629–637. http://dx.doi.org/10.5014/ajot.61.6.629

Kielhofner, G. (2008). *Model of Human Occupation* (4th ed.). Philadelphia: Lippincott Williams & Wilkins.

Law, M. (2002). Participation in the occupation of everyday life [Distinguished Scholar Lecture]. *American Journal of Occupational Therapy, 56*, 640–649. http://dx.doi.org/doi:10.5014/ajot.56.6.640

Melrose, A. H. (1927). Occupational therapy department: Report of Lanark District Asylum. In A. Wilcock (2002), *Occupation for health: A journey from prescription to self-health*. London: British Association and College of Occupational Therapists.

Quiroga, V. A. (1995). *Occupational therapy: The first 30 years—1900 to 1930*. Bethesda, MD: AOTA Press.

Reed, K., & Peters, C. (2006, April 17). Occupational therapy values and beliefs, the formative years: 1904–1929. *OT Practice*, pp. 21–25.

Schwartz, K. B. (2009). Reclaiming our heritage: Connecting the *Founding Vision* to the *Centennial Vision* [Eleanor Clarke Slagle Lecture]. *American Journal of Occupational Therapy, 63*, 681–690. http://dx.doi.org/10.5014/ajot.63.6.681

Shannon, P. (1977). The derailment of occupational therapy. *American Journal of Occupational Therapy, 31*, 229–234.

Whiteford, G., Townsend, E., & Hocking, C. (2000). Reflections on a renaissance of occupation. *Canadian Journal of Occupational Therapy, 67*, 61–70. http://dx.doi.org/10.1177/000841740006700109

CHAPTER 1

Moral Treatment: Contexts Considered

SUZANNE M. PELOQUIN

M oral treatment is intriguing in its emergence, its essence, and its decline. The fascination with moral treatment deepens when one encounters the 20th-century term *occupational therapy* used in historical commentaries about the 19th-century practice. Digby (1985), in discussing moral treatment, noted that "occupational therapy took a variety of forms" (p. 63). Bell (1980) and Grob (1973) both identified occupational therapy as a component of moral treatment. Although this identification is incorrect in the strict historical sense, it is perhaps apt in other ways.

Three views provide different representations of the nature of the relationship between moral treatment and occupational therapy. Bing (1981) (see Chapter 2), an occupational therapist, described the relationship as evolutionary: "Occupational therapy's roots are in the subsoil of the moral treatment developed in Europe during the Age of Enlightenment. . . . Moral treatment came to the U.S. as part of the Quaker's religious and intellectual luggage. . . . During the last quarter of the 19th century moral treatment disappeared. It re-emerged in the early decades of the 20th century as Occupational Therapy" (p. 499). In contrast, Bockoven (1971), a psychiatrist, insisted that "the history of moral treatment in America is not only synonymous with, but is the history of occupational therapy before it acquired its 20th century name of 'occupational therapy'" (p. 225). Engelhardt (1977), a philosopher familiar with Bockoven's work, suggested a similarity between moral treatment and occupational therapy in the attempt to "effect more successful adaptation to society through organizing certain activities for patients in special environments" (p. 668). These divergent views suggest that

a clearer understanding of the nature of moral treatment is relevant for occupational therapy professionals. Such an understanding seems particularly valuable in light of the continued desire within the profession to clarify its identity and its lineage.

A Definition of Moral Treatment

Dr. Thomas Kirkbride (1880/1973), a physician and the superintendent of the Pennsylvania Hospital for the Insane from 1841 to 1883, described moral treatment in terms of daily efforts to provide "system, active movements, and diversity of occupation" to the patients (referred to then as "inmates") (p. 275). Dr. Amariah Brigham (1847), a contemporary of Kirkbride, interpreted moral treatment as "the removal of the insane from home and former associations, with respect and kind treatment upon all circumstances, and in most cases manual labor, attendance on religious worship on Sunday, the establishment of regular habits of self control, [and] diversion of the mind from morbid trains of thought" (p. 1).

More than 150 years later, Dain and Carlson (1960) characterized the theory and practice of moral treatment as the psychological medicine that constituted milieu therapy in the 19th century. Tomes (1984) believed that moral treatment was based on the assumption that one could appeal to the patient's innate capacity to live an ordered and rational existence. To allay any concern that moral treatment meant the enforcement of moral standards, Bockoven (1963) argued that early psychiatrists used the word moral to mean psychological or emotional. He viewed moral treatment as "the first practical effort made to provide systematic and responsible care for an appreciable number of the mentally ill" (p. 12).

Other interpretations articulate various goals and principles underlying moral treatment. Several of these

This chapter was previously published in the *American Journal of Occupational Therapy, 43,* 537–544. Copyright © 1989, American Occupational Therapy Association. Reprinted with permission. http://dx.doi.org/10.5014/ajot.43.8.537

suggest that moral standards were, in fact, guiding principles. Grob (1973) described the goal of moral treatment as the "inculcation, through habit and understanding, of desirable moral traits and values" (p. 12). Rothman (1971) viewed the process of moral treatment as the arrangement of a disciplined routine that provided stability for a person suffering from environmentally generated ills. Bell (1980) considered moral treatment to be a distinct method of therapy that enabled the patient to understand right from wrong within a total therapeutic community. Through moral treatment, the physician manipulated both the environment and the patient to help the patient overcome past associations and to create an atmosphere in which natural restorative elements could assert themselves (Grob, 1983). The image of moral treatment emerging from these interpretations is one of a treatment of the mentally ill that occurred in virtually all institutions; it included humane treatment, a routine of work and recreation, an appeal to reason, and the development of desirable moral traits.

Moral Treatment Within Its Various Contexts

An understanding of certain 19th-century conditions is crucial to an appreciation of the significance of moral treatment's emergence. Two environments—the medical community and 19th-century society as a whole—did much to influence the characteristics of moral treatment and its emergence in institutions.

The medical community's perception of insanity greatly influenced the development of moral treatment. A shift in 19th-century thinking revolutionized medical thought: persons with mental disorders, then labeled "the insane," were capable of reason. Before this awareness, insane persons had been considered subhuman because they were believed to be devoid of reason (Deutsch, 1949). Torturous methods were used to treat insane persons. These methods were used not to inflict pain, but to frighten the irrational beast. Methods congruent with contemporary theory included chaining the patients, placing them in cold showers, and lowering them into water-filled wells. The physician's goal was to dominate patients to cure them (Carlson & Dain, 1960). Only when it was acknowledged in the early 19th century that insane persons retained intellectual and rational capacities could treatment methodologies change.

The new philosophy of insanity generated the first humane systems for treatment in Europe. Philippe Pinel, a physician in France, and William Tuke, a Quaker in England, established the specific regimen of moral treatment. Pinel first used the term *moral treatment (traitement morale)* in 1801, but it was not until 1817 that a hospital was founded in the United States expressly for the purpose of providing moral treatment. This hospital, built by Pennsylvania Quakers for members of their Society and patterned after Tuke's York Retreat in England, was named the Friend's Asylum. Within 7 years, three more privately endorsed mental asylums (called *corporate asylums*) were built: McLean Hospital in Massachusetts, Bloomingdale Hospital in New York, and the Hartford Retreat in Connecticut. All of these corporate asylums practiced moral treatment (Bockoven, 1963).

This humane system of moral treatment became identified with institutional care. Its character was shaped by the medical men of these early institutions. Scull (1981) called the first four asylums the "earlier generation of asylums" (p. 151). Many developments among this earlier generation significantly influenced later institutions. The first influence related to lines of authority for providing treatment. The Bloomingdale Hospital and the Friend's Asylum, which were patterned after the York Retreat in England, were initially managed by lay superintendents, a custom prevalent in Europe. These superintendents oversaw the provision of moral treatment, and resident physicians provided mild medical treatments for physical conditions. At the Hartford Retreat, a physician named Eli Todd was superintendent. Todd endorsed and supervised traditional therapeutics as well as an increasing use of opium and morphine to complement moral treatment. He campaigned for medical treatment at the other three asylums. As a result of his efforts, medical treatment came to figure more prominently at all of these institutions. Over time, an uneasy relationship developed between the medical leadership and the moral leadership. In 1850, the tension culminated in a codification: An asylum superintendent would be a well-qualified physician. This new role that combined moral and medical functions became the leadership model adopted by the second generation of asylums (Scull, 1981).

A second early asylum influence was the adoption of public relations measures in the community. Superintendents realized that the negative image of European "madhouses" was powerful. They made a point of using annual reports to communicate the advantages of asylum treatment. The widespread communication of these messages was continued by later superintendents.

A final measure through which early superintendents ensured their influence on second-generation asylums was their personal involvement in the establishment of the first state asylums: Worcester State Hospital and Utica Asylum. These two facilities, though designed more for public than for private use, were patterned after the early asylums. These second-generation asylums, in turn, became models for later state facilities. The consolidated physician–superintendent role, the public relations efforts, and the tutelage of second-generation superintendents solidified the manner in which moral treatment would be practiced. The setting would continue to be institutional, the overseers would be physicians, and the public would remain convinced of the utmost practicality of this arrangement.

Changing social patterns during the 19th century helped to place the practice of moral treatment in institutions. America was industrializing, and many people moved from farms to urban centers. The urban family clustered into smaller units and became less able to deal effectively with its ill members. Not surprisingly, the new view of insanity was linked to these changing social patterns of industrialization and urbanization. Dr. Isaac Ray (1861), superintendent of the Butler Hospital, noted that many of his patients displayed deranged moral faculties of the will and of the emotions, although their intellectual faculties remained apparently intact. Deranged moral faculties could be attributed to societal tensions and chaos in the community, which social observances and institutions of the time were unable to handle. The result, for some, was moral insanity (Rothman, 1971).

Given the environmental causes of insanity and the family unit's growing inability to keep a family member with insanity at home, upper- and middle-class members of the community saw the asylum as a new, less chaotic, and more effective environment that could first halt and then reverse the process of insanity. The acceptance of institutions was not a desperate measure. With physician–superintendents and asylum supporters advertising their effectiveness in curing insanity, families admitted the insane with a sense of optimism (Rothman, 1971). The community supported physicians in this new movement toward institutionalization of a class of the population heretofore treated at home. Poor persons, commonly housed in local jails and poorhouses, were minimally affected during the early years of moral treatment (Dain, 1964; Deutsch, 1949; Galt, 1846/1973).

American superintendents shaped the practice of moral treatment. In Europe, the prevalent belief was that moral treatment alone cured insanity; in the United States, some form of medical treatment accompanied moral treatment (Scull, 1981). Tomes (1984) claimed that American superintendents reworked Pinel's original concept of moral treatment to justify treatment by medical doctors. This reworking is evident in Brigham's (1844) writings. He believed that deranged moral and intellectual faculties were generally the result of a diseased brain, although he thought that emotions and great trials of affection could derange brain function and cause insanity. Treatment of insanity stayed within the province of medical practice because physicians continued to link insanity to a disease process. Additionally, moral treatment in the United States was considered most appropriate for recent cases of insanity; more chronic cases (often the long-standing cases among the poor) were considered less likely to be reversed. The chronicity of disease among the poor made them less suitable candidates for moral treatment. For the most part, the asylum community consisted mainly of upper-middle-class doctors treating upper- and middle-class patients.

The Asylum: Structuring a New Environment

American physicians became involved in the design of the new therapeutic environments. As asylum superintendents, they were responsible for individual patient care, management of daily operations, and supervision of asylum personnel. Largely from the upper middle class, they were said to prefer treating patients from their own social stratum (Bell, 1980). They enforced the admission policies specific to their asylums, although they sometimes made concessions to local authorities and accepted a few poor people. Admission policies varied widely. Many corporate institutions totally excluded the poor; others, such as the Quaker asylums, admitted them more freely.

The standards set by the private asylums also set the example for state institutions eager to attract curable patients (Tomes, 1984). The Pennsylvania Hospital for the Insane, a public institution that began receiving patients in 1841, has been called by much of the literature one of the best American mental institutions of that era. Superintendents of corporate asylums welcomed public institutions as an alternative for poor inmates. The previous two-tier treatment system of the asylum versus the poorhouse or jail was evolving into one of the private versus the state institution.

Appropriate construction was a critical factor. Kirkbride thought "a properly constructed building . . . indispensable for such an effect [cure]" (Dain, 1964, p. 76). The building design was also important because it had to appeal to the public. The typical state hospital of the 19th century was constructed according to the Kirkbride Plan, which was officially endorsed by the Association of Medical Superintendents of American Institutions for the Insane. The Kirkbride Plan called for a large central administration building, from which extended several long, straight wings for housing patients. The design of the wings, with windows spaced evenly, embodied the belief that insanity could be cured by an ordered and rational environment (Rothman, 1971).

The internal structure of the asylum was considered as important to the ability to effect a cure as was the external structure. Classification of patients was an essential component of moral treatment and was incorporated into the building's internal structure. In the 19th century, physicians classified insane patients as manic, melancholic, or demented. These categories continued to form one basis for their classification in the asylum. Inmates were also separated according to sex, behaviors, and degree of illness (Tomes, 1984). At the private Friend's Asylum, for example, quiet convalescent inmates were separated from more acutely ill, violent, and noisy patients. Asylums that admitted more heterogeneous populations housed and grouped their inmates according to classes as well. Tomes described the rationale: "Since, in a non-institutional setting, patients would have expected to see class distinctions in housing and employment, the asylum replicated these features of everyday life" (p. 126).

Classification dictated various levels of care. Private asylums usually gave paying patients better treatment than they gave poor patients; this meant better accommodations and more attention. Moral treatment methods for individual patients, then, varied according to their socioeconomic status, sex, degree of illness, and ability to gain admission to an asylum.

Occupations Within the Asylum Context

Pinel (1806/1962) said that silence and tranquility prevailed in the Asylum de Bicetre when the Parisian tradesmen supplied the patients with employment that held their attention. He noted that even "the natural indolence and stupidity of *ideots* [sic] might in some degree be obviated, by engaging them in manual occupations, suitable to their respective capacities" (p. 203).

American superintendents made daily routine and occupation a central component of moral treatment. They claimed that the ultimate results of these two components outweighed the considerable initial cost of the arrangements necessary for their implementation. Labor, or occupation, judiciously used, contributed not only to patient comfort but also to health and recovery (Kirkbride, 1880/1973). Asylum staff went to exceptional lengths to engage patients in manual tasks. Kirkbride encouraged his patients to do any task; the critical thing was to keep busy. The therapeutic rationale was that occupation inculcated the regular habits necessary for recovery (Rothman, 1971). Throughout each carefully structured day, men engaged in agricultural pursuits, carpentry, painting, and general maintenance. Women performed domestic chores and manual crafts. The superintendents agreed that productive labor was the most important element in moral treatment (Grob, 1973). A precise schedule and regular work characterized the best private and public institutions.

The superintendents assigned occupations according to a patient's classification. Not all occupations were considered suitable at all stages of illness; superintendents were cautious about overtaxing patients or exposing them to potentially hazardous situations. Brigham felt that the members of the curable class benefitted most from the rational engagement of the mind through reading, writing, drawing, music, and various studies and recreational pursuits. Patients viewed as incurable benefitted more from manual labor to preserve whatever mind they still possessed (Brigham, 1847). In some cases, hardworking patients could reduce their board payments or earn placement on the free list (Tomes, 1984). Cooperative and industrious behaviors could also result in the acquisition of special privileges or "advancement to a better gallery" (Galt, 1846/1973, p. 497). In most asylums, occupation was supplemented by religious exercises, regular physical exercise, and group amusements organized by the staff. The use of occupations reflected an awareness of individual differences, of comfort level, and of degree of illness, but it also revealed a class and sex bias.

Dr. Lee, the superintendent at McLean Hospital, described the results of occupation: "Give a man constant employment, treat him with uniform kindness and respect, and, however insane he may be, very little may be feared from him, either of mischief or indolence" (Galt, 1846/1973, p. 50). He said that bodily labor proved immeasurably superior to all other aspects of treatment with a large class of male patients. The asylum staff encouraged patients to engage in energetic labor as a way to work off irritability. Perseverance and ceaseless efforts resulted in a patient's return to industrious habits, even with chronic cases. In these cases, attendants often helped patients initially with the motion required for a task until it was mastered. Asylum reports touted the successes at length and in great detail. Labor helped to inculcate moral habits in the patients; as a secondary benefit, labor often helped maintain the asylum.

Besides occupation, other treatment operatives were used in the early asylum. The superintendents in all institutions invoked the use of kindness. The patient population was kept low to facilitate individual care, and doctors met with individual patients daily. The Hartford Retreat, for example, housed only 40 patients (Deutsch, 1949). The staff used restraints minimally, appealing instead to patients' rationality. A system of rewards and privileges replaced a system of punishments. Cooperative patients could be promoted in classification, which encouraged self-control (Galt, 1846/1973). Radical medical treatments such as bleeding and the use of purgatives and emetics were replaced by the use of tonics and narcotics such as opium (Galt, 1846/1973). Family members were discouraged, but not forbidden, from visiting, because new associations were essential. The attendants became the patients' constant companions, and each attendant cared for one to six patients. The superintendents were diligent in obtaining attendants and nurses of the best character (Galt, 1846/1973). Families were encouraged to commit patients for a minimum of 3 to 6 months, time enough to demonstrate some progress. Confinement in a new environment and isolation from previous associations marked the beginning of a cure for environmentally caused insanity (Rothman, 1971).

Early Successes

In the small early asylum, success meant a cure. Statistics from the Worcester State Hospital between 1833 and 1842 show recoveries in 70% to 75% of the patients admitted, and improvements in 3% to 8% of the patients. Dr. Eli Todd of the Hartford Retreat reported recovery in 90% of the patients admitted with mental illness of less than 1 year's duration (Bockoven, 1963). Kirkbride (1880/1973) described his clinical observations of patients' behaviors both before and after the introduction of evening amusements. He said that a comparison of results "leaves no room to question the importance and great superiority of the last" (p. 273).

Countless case histories validated moral treatment's success. Many of these case histories appeared in Galt's The Treatment of Insanity (1846/1973) and in the asylum's annual reports. One man, for example, reportedly suffered violent fits at least once a month. After he took up gardening and became involved, he was subsequently free of attacks (Rothman, 1971).

Grob (1973) thought that the success of the early asylum rested on a series of circumstances: (a) the small number and homogeneous nature of patients, (b) the internal therapeutic atmosphere arising from the enthusiasm of the superintendent's personality, and (c) close interpersonal relationships. All this success resulted in a wild optimism that Deutsch called "the cult of curability" (Dain, 1964, p. 78).

The Demise of Moral Treatment

Moral treatment can perhaps be called a system. The systematization of moral treatment contributed in part to its own demise. Certain aspects of the practice and principles characterizing moral treatment made its survival incompatible with later 19th-century conditions.

Changes that led to the demise of moral treatment occurred first in 19th-century society, and second, in the medical community. While the providers of asylum care were touting its curative effects, a social reform movement was pushing to extend humane care to all insane persons. The push was successful; thousands of persons were crowded into existing asylums. A Civil War–taxed economy could not provide the rapid institutional growth that was needed to house this influx of patients. Asylum conditions deteriorated both from overcrowding and from a radical change in the types of patients treated. Because it was almost impossible to provide moral treatment, custodial care prevailed. Curative moral treatment was eliminated. Meanwhile, medicine was committing itself to more scientific inquiry and somatic treatments of all illnesses. A shift in thinking had occurred: insanity was caused by lesions in the brain. Therefore, consideration of environmental causes or treatments for what was essentially a physiological problem was unnecessary.

This course of events contributed to the demise of moral treatment partly because of certain characteristics inherent in the moral treatment system. For all its successes, moral treatment had its problems from the outset. One significant problem was the early superintendents' reluctance to deal with the poor, whether because of class bias or because of a genuine belief that the advanced condition of their disease precluded a cure. The early asylum experience tended to validate the assumption that poor persons presented hopeless cases. This validation occurred in the following manner. Superintendents sometimes labored under financial limitations. Public officials capable of providing funds were less concerned with effectiveness of treatment than with convenience of placement. These officials pressured superintendents to accept less curable cases to the asylum in greater proportions than had been recommended (Rothman, 1971). Additionally, it had been assumed that a therapeutic asylum would have a transient population because of a constant turnover of cured patients. In practice, a percentage of more chronic cases stayed at the asylum. This situation created a different type of institution from that originally envisioned (Grob, 1973). The poor and the chronically ill, because they stayed, validated physicians' assumptions about their hopelessness. This would create a major obstacle when larger numbers of poor persons were later admitted.

Given their original expectations, physicians embraced middle-class behaviors and values as the norm; their emphasis was on the order, moderation, and self-control inherent in a middle-class life-style (Rothman, 1971). The initial theoretical and practical groundwork of moral treatment (that insanity was curable and that moral treatment was the cure) could have inspired a vigorous progressive movement across all classes. Instead, asylums were small-scale experiments that reached only a select group. Moral treatment was isolated amid a scene of widespread stagnation begging for reform (Rothman, 1971). At the time, public provision for poor persons consisted of sending the "dangerous and violent" to prison; the harmless and mild "paupers" went to auction or the almshouse (Deutsch, 1949, p. 115). The asylum superintendents showed little desire to treat the very patients who were to dominate asylum populations after the reform movement.

Michel Foucault (1965), a harsh critic of institutions in any form, for any reason, described moral treatment of mentally ill patients as a gigantic moral imprisonment: a "structure that formed a kind of microcosm in which were symbolized the massive structure of bourgeois society and its values ... centered on the theme of social and moral order" (p. 274). Digby (1985) countered that any experience of moral imprisonment in the subjective estimation of patients would "turn on the extent to which they shared the moral values of the establishment" (p. 54). Real treatment successes would

come from inducing self-control in patients sharing the values, assumptions, and objectives of their therapists. Those not sharing institutional values would only conform superficially; problems would surface with discrepancies in values (Digby, 1985). In fact, as Bell (1980) wrote, "When poor people having different values formed the majority of the patient population, moral treatment ran into difficulties" (p. 14).

Another problem of the moral treatment system was its administration by physicians. The patients might have fared better had asylums been under the direction of lay superintendents (Bockoven, 1963). Physician-superintendents focused on the cure. When scientific theory was to later challenge moral treatment's curative potential, physicians rejected their recovery statistics and early successes. Eager to join the mainstream of scientific medicine, they increasingly distanced themselves from the moral care of the institutionalized mentally ill patients (Grob, 1983). Bockoven described the situation as one in which psychiatry did not have the courage to pursue its original course.

Moral Treatment in Crisis

Moral treatment in the asylum meant cure. Social reformers thought that all insane persons should have access to asylum cure. A widespread reform movement in the 1830s and 1840s worked to improve the lot of persons who were blind, deaf, slaves, alcoholics, convicts, or insane. Dorothea Dix, using superintendents' annual reports as testimony, led state after state to construct asylums. Her dream, however, soon turned into a nightmare (Bell, 1980). New state laws mandated that dangerously insane persons be sent to asylums. Those insane persons previously housed in jails and almshouses also went to asylums. This rapid admission of large numbers of patients taxed superintendents and facilities prepared for small homogeneous patient groups. Psychiatrist-superintendents were largely unsuccessful in their protest against the influx and their suggestion that violent or chronic patients be segregated (Bockoven, 1963).

Overcrowding restricted the practice of moral treatment. Rooms used for leisure activities and workshops became sleeping quarters. Individualized patient care was no longer possible in the congested asylum maze. Overcrowding stressed the sewage, ventilation, and water systems; the health of the patients was compromised. Epidemics struck at numerous institutions (Bell, 1980). The superintendents became increasingly concerned with order, regularity, and control among growing numbers of patients. They reinstituted the use of restraints among patients who were noisy or violent. The attendants assumed responsibility for larger groups of eight to 15 patients each. Inmates were often appointed as temporary nurses and attendants because of the staff shortage. The most critical personal quality sought in an attendant shifted from kindness to obedience (Grob, 1973). Overtaxed institutional facilities provided fewer patients with meaningful work; idleness further complicated behavioral problems. The superintendents recognized a growing gap between their original theory and their practices; their powers to close the gap were diminishing.

The wide range of persons admitted to the asylum jeopardized adequate care. Older patients with dementia accounted for 10% of the number of admissions from 1830 to 1875, thereby complicating hospital management considerably (Grob, 1973). Insane criminals often required maximum security. Alcoholic patients, mentally retarded patients, and patients suffering from general paresis (resulting from the advanced stage of a syphilitic infection) or other organic diseases often required individual care at a time when none was possible. Under these conditions, chronic patients failed to respond to treatment. They became troublesome, engaging in disruptive behaviors, escapes, and physical violence that perpetuated the need for restraint (Tomes, 1984).

Poverty-stricken immigrants joined this influx in the post-Civil War years. American physicians had difficulty empathizing with "foreign insane paupers" (Bockoven, 1963, p. 25). Admitted to already deteriorating institutions, foreign patients quickly became apathetic, leading physicians to believe them less capable, less motivated, and less curable. A vicious cycle developed, with predictable consequences. Because they were thought to be incurable, poor patients received less care. Without care, these patients showed little improvement—this confirmed their incurability.

New theories about mental illness dealt moral treatment yet another incapacitating blow. One school of thought linked mental illness with heredity; another linked mental illness with a somatic, mechanical defect. Both views led to a decline in optimism about a cure and to a total disillusionment about moral treatment in the 1850s. By the 1870s, pessimism was the trend; by 1900, moral treatment was reduced to a minor form of therapy even in the most affluent of corporate asylums (Dain, 1964).

Emphasis on hereditary predisposition began to fill the psychiatric literature. Heredity was thought to predispose the poor person to poverty and insanity (Bockoven, 1963). Inferior biological stock was thought to produce conditions leading to insanity. Some physicians debated the logic of heredity as an explanation for insanity; they argued against the heredity explanation in defense of a somatic view (Bell, 1980). Although earlier in the century it had been understood that a weakening of the body's vital forces could damage the brain, microscopic lesions now found in the central nervous system of mentally ill patients upset previous environmental theories and confirmed the somatic cause of insanity (Bockoven, 1963).

The early successes of moral treatment were challenged. In 1877, Dr. Pliny Earle published a critique of pre-Civil War curability statistics and accused early superintendents of having exaggerated their figures (Bockoven, 1963). Earle questioned the validity of the high cure rates cited because in the 1870s corporate asylums could no longer replicate these cure rates. Some physicians argued in response that insanity was becoming less curable because society was becoming more chaotic. Others claimed that insanity had become more complex in the late 19th century; it was less curable because the categories of insanity, such as general paralysis, senile dementia, and hereditary insanity, had multiplied. Many thought that the physiological causes of insanity were intensifying: Organic alterations in the nervous system were more involved in producing insanity than before (Bockoven, 1963).

Conversion toward a more somatic view seemed inevitable. From 1840 to 1860, three men had been responsible for most of the psychiatric research in the United States: Luther Bell, Amariah Brigham, and Isaac Ray. Their work had largely involved data gathering, certainly not serious research by 20th-century standards. Even the curability statistics gathered between 1833 and 1842 by superintendent Samuel Woodward at Worcester State Hospital had failed to delineate criteria used to determine the recovery or improvement of patients. Those succeeding the early superintendents were deeply discouraged by the apparent failure of moral treatment and by their inability to validate its effectiveness scientifically. Articles in the *American Journal of Insanity* supporting the mechanical defect theory exhorted a move toward somaticism. Scientific medicine was gaining respect and credibility; any psychological approach to the treatment of insanity seemed outdated, illogical, and irrelevant. In 1894, Dr. Weir

Mitchell, a neurologist, castigated physicians for having ever believed in some mysterious therapeutic influence (Bockoven, 1963).

Therapeutic regimens differed among asylums, depending on the superintendent's viewpoint. Moral treatment suffered in this respect as well. Bockoven (1963) attributed the demise of moral treatment to the lack of inspired and committed leadership after the death of its innovators. Only four of the original 13 founders of moral treatment survived the 1870s, and two of these founders had returned to private practice. Leaders seemed to have lacked foresight. They had failed to train moral therapists who might have been able to articulate or redefine moral treatment's efficacy in the face of social changes and scientific inquiry. This seemed a major failure.

The asylum, diverted from its original mission of treatment, and pressured into merely containing insane persons, sank into a mire of apathy and indifference (Bell, 1980). Moral treatment, once considered vital to the cure of persons with mental disorders, disappeared from psychiatric practice.

Conclusion

The complexity of moral treatment precludes the opposing views that it was a short-lived triumph of humanitarian zeal or that it was a rationalization of middle-class morality (Tomes, 1984). Moral treatment was neither of these stereotypes. One thing is clear: Moral treatment cannot be understood outside of the framework within which it developed and disappeared.

One can hope that occupational therapy practice today is free of the limitations that precluded the survival of moral treatment. One would hope to find, in this century, a freedom from class and economic bias, a freedom from a push for professional credibility that is blind to patient need, and a leadership committed to defend those humane aspects of practice only empirically validated.

One can also hope that occupational therapy practitioners understand the powerful forces that often define the character of occupational therapy practice. During the 19th century, the medical community and the society as a whole shaped several guiding principles and treatment concepts into the practice of moral treatment. These two communities cannot be underestimated in the 20th century; their demands shape the duration, direction, location, and quality of occupational therapy. Preventive care, accountability, and documentation of measurable progress are but a few of the trends grounded in challenges from these two sectors.

Moral treatment's decline relates closely to a lack of inspired and committed leadership willing to articulate and redefine the efficacy of occupation in the face of medical and societal challenges. The desire to embrace the most current trend of scientific thought led to the abandonment of moral treatment in spite of its established efficacy. The failure to identify and address the social and institutional changes that had gradually made the practice and success of moral treatment virtually impossible led to the erroneous conclusion that occupation was not an effective intervention. The responsivity to trends supplanted any reaffirmation of basic assumptions.

Occupational therapists need to recommit, in this century and in the next, to the assumptions about man and occupation that inform the practice of occupational therapy. In the face of changing trends, therapists must continually redefine and rearticulate the value of a humane practice that transcends scientific validation and bureaucratic understanding.

Acknowledgments

Special thanks to Ellen More, PhD, whose flexibility and encouragement enabled the integration of course material with occupational therapy issues. Thanks also to Lillian H. Parent, MA, OTR, FAOTA, for her supportive suggestions.

References

Bell, L. V. (1980). *Treating the mentally ill*. New York: Praeger.

Bing, R. K. (1981). Occupational therapy revisited: A paraphrastic journey. *American Journal of Occupational Therapy, 35*, 499–518. Reprinted as Chapter 2.

Bockoven, J. S. (1963). *Moral treatment in American psychiatry*. New York: Springs Publishing.

Bockoven, J. S. (1971). Legacy of moral treatment—1800s to 1910. *American Journal of Occupational Therapy, 25*, 223–225.

Brigham, A. (1844). Definition of insanity—Nature of the disease. *American Journal of Insanity, 1*, 107–108.

Brigham, A. (1847). The moral treatment of insanity. *American Journal of Insanity, 4*, 1.

Carlson, E. T., & Dain, N. (1960). The psychotherapy that was Moral Treatment. *American Journal of Psychiatry, 117*, 519–524.

Dain, N. (1964). *Concepts of insanity in the United States: 1789–1865*. New Brunswick, NJ: Rutgers University Press.

Dain, N., & Carlson, E. T. (1960). Milieu therapy in the 19th century: Patient care at the Friend's Asylum, Frankford, Pennsylvania, 1817–1861. *Journal of Nervous and Mental Disease, 131,* 277–290.

Deutsch, A. (1949). *The mentally ill in America: A history of their care and treatment from colonial times*. New York: Columbia University Press.

Digby, A. (1985). Moral treatment at the Retreat, 1796–1846. In W. F. Bynum, R. Porter, & M. Shepherd (Eds.), *The anatomy of madness. Essays in the history of psychiatry* (pp. 52–72). New York: Tavistock.

Engelhardt, H. T. Jr. (1977). Defining occupational therapy: The meaning of therapy and the virtues of occupation. *American Journal of Occupational Therapy, 31,* 666–672.

Foucault, M. (1965). *Madness and civilization: A history of insanity in the Age of Reason*. New York: Vintage Books.

Galt, J. M. (1973). *The treatment of insanity*. New York: Arno Press. Original work published 1846.

Grob, G. N. (1973). *Mental institutions in America: Social policy to 1875*. New York: Free Press.

Grob, G. N. (1983). *Mental illness and American society, 1875–1940*. Princeton, NJ: Princeton University Press.

Kirkbride, T. S. (1973). *On the construction, organization, and general arrangements of hospitals for the insane*. New York: Arno Press. Original work published 1880.

Pinel, P. H. (1962). *A treatise on insanity*. New York: Harper Publishing. Original work published 1806.

Ray, I. (1861). An examination of the objections to the doctrine of moral insanity. *American Journal of Insanity, 18,* 112–139.

Rothman, D. J. (1971). *The discovery of the asylum*. Boston: Little, Brown.

Scull, A. (Ed.). (1981). *Madhouses, mad-doctors, and madmen*. Philadelphia: University of Pennsylvania Press.

Tomes, N. (1984). *A generous confidence: Thomas Story Kirkbride and the art of asylum keeping*. New York: Cambridge University Press.

Related Readings

Beers, C. W. (1917). *A mind that found itself*. New York: Longmans, Green, & Co.

CHAPTER 2

Occupational Therapy Revisited: A Paraphrastic Journey

1981 ELEANOR CLARKE SLAGLE LECTURE

ROBERT K. BING

Try as one might, it is impossible to recount the evolution of occupational therapy so that it resembles the cliff-hanging biographies of Butch Cassidy and the Sundance Kid. Masters and Johnson, as well as Kinsey, who took years to amass their stories, had something going for them that does not exist for us. Somewhat puckishly I was tempted to entitle this paper *Everything You've Ever Wanted to Know About Occupational Therapy, But Were Afraid to Ask*. That would not have been altogether misleading. Because of my part-German heritage, and true to that cultural bias and tendency, I thought I should take us back to the Thirty Years' War and bring everyone up to date. After all, it is important territory occupational therapy has won and lost.

The title, *Occupational Therapy Revisited: A Paraphrastic Journey*, prevailed because this paper is a tour to what should be familiar historical landmarks and progenitors. For some of us, it will renew old friendships and acquaintances. For others, it will be a second-hand account of certain ancestors, not unlike those stories that emanate from grandmothers. For some, it will only be like an endurance of those pictures that inevitably get projected on the screen by vacationers returning home.

Because of the relative youthfulness of those of us in practice (most have entered within the past decade), now seems the time to critically examine our ancestral roots and subsequent grafts to determine the nature of the present and to offer some speculations about why we (and the profession) developed as we did through several generations. This is not *the* history of occupational therapy nor of the Association that supports our endeavors. Nor is it *a* history like someone else might well find it. It is *not* a detailed, definitive account of how we multiplied, divided, and invaded several areas of medicine and health care. It is *one person's* way of telling the story of who we are and citing some lessons to be learned. That is important! After several months of submergence just off the coast of Texas (as my colleagues in Galveston will attest), I have at long last come up for air and am ready to declare my findings.

This is a statement of how an idea, born in a philosophical movement, became activated through *the good works of men and women* who inalterably believed in the ideal that those who are sick and handicapped can regain, retain, and attain some semblance of function within the fundamental limitations of the human organism and the expectations of the society in which all must exist: that this may occur through the most obvious means of all—*one's reorganization through occupation, through activity, through leisure, and through rest.*

This journey about occupational therapy, its evolution and development, presents vexation: one must accept a fair number of ambiguities, something some today consider a fundamental problem in occupational therapy; a more than reasonable amount of astonishment; and a certain degree of messiness, closely akin to what is created by the beginner in fingerpainting. What can it all mean? What was taking place at the time? Will the patient recover? Most significantly, does it make any difference? To answer these and related questions I wanted to conduct some scholarly research that could be equally interesting, helpful, and valuable to students, occupational therapists, and others who are interested in our profession. This is how I interpret the intent of the originators of the Eleanor Clarke Slagle Lectureship.

Such an historical presentation should be long enough to say something, yet short enough to be tolerated.

To give you some idea of the continuing dilemma I encountered these past several months in preparing the lecture and in limiting its scope and length, I wrote:

There once was an historian named Dan,
Whose prose no one could scan,
When, once asked about it,

This chapter was previously published in the *American Journal of Occupational Therapy, 35*, 499–518. Copyright © 1981, American Occupational Therapy Association. Reprinted with permission. http://dx.doi.org/10.5014/ajot.35.8.499

He said, "I don't doubt it,
Because I try to cram as many facts and dates
into each sentence as I possibly can."

Significant Landmarks

Let us start this paraphrastic journey and take note of some significant landmarks along the way—those recurring patterns and themes of the past 200 years that give us today's relevance:

1. There is an inextricable union of the mind and the body; the employment of activity or occupation must be based on this precept, which is unique to occupational therapy.

2. Activity, inherently, contains modes the patient may employ to gain understanding of and ascendancy over one's feelings, actions, and thoughts: these modes include the habits of attention and interest; the perceived usefulness of occupation; creative expression; the processes of learning; the acquisition of skill; and evidence of accomplishment.

3. Activity provides a balance between the practical and intellectual components of experience; therefore, a wide variety of activities must be accessible to meet human objectives for work, leisure, and rest.

4. One's approach to the patient is as significant to treatment and rehabilitation as is the selection and utilization of an activity.

5. Essential elements of occupational therapy practice are continuous observation, experimentation, empiricism, and analysis.

6. An appreciation of the pain that accompanies any illness or disability; a strong desire to reduce or remove it; a gentle firmness; and a knowledge of the patient's needs are fundamental characteristics of the provider of therapeutic occupations.

7. Therapeutic processes and modes of treatment are synonymous with the processes of learning and methods of education.

8. The patient is the product of his or her own efforts, not the article made nor the activity accomplished.

A Theory of Experience

We could go back to the Garden of Eden to begin this story, if time permitted, since occupational therapy could well have started in that idyllic spot. Dr. Dunton, one of the founders of the 20th century movement, insisted that those fig leaves had to have been crocheted by Eve, who was trying to get over her troubles. They had something to do with her being beholden to Adam and his rib. We will unfortunately pass over all that and begin the modern epoch with a brief description of what was taking place in Europe approximately 200 years ago.

It was the *Age of Enlightenment,* or, as some prefer, the *Age of Reason.* The roots of 20th century occupational therapy are visible in the empiricism of John Locke, an English philosopher and physician, who fostered confidence in human reason and freedom; in Etienne de Condillac, a French philosopher, who advanced the dualism of body and mind; and Pierre Cabanis, a French physician and theorist, who offered an explanation of the importance of the moral and social sciences in perfecting the art of medicine. These three, together with others, popularized the new ideas. Indeed, it was the *best of times,* a clear demarcation in the emergence of the modern world.

If one were to combine the thoughts of these three, one would arrive at a *theory of experience.* John Locke, in his famous *Essay Concerning Human Understanding,* published in 1690,[1] examines the nature of the human mind and the processes by which it learns about and comes to know the world. When born, the human is a blank tablet (tabula rasa). Because of an innate ability to receive sensations from the outside world, the human can assimilate and organize impressions. As contact with the environment stimulates the senses and causes impressions, the mind receives and organizes these into ideas and concepts. Since the human mind does not already contain innate ideas, all must come from without.[2(p287)]

There is a second source for the accumulation of experience, according to Locke. It is the mind itself: ". . . the perception of the operations of our own mind . . . (such as) thinking, doubting, believing, reasoning, knowing . . . this source of ideas every man has wholly within himself."[3(p74)] Locke strongly held that the body and mind exist as real entities and they interact. He spent a great deal of time developing his perspective. He spoke of the aim of education as the process of knowing and learning through experience and in striving toward happiness. Ideally, he contended, one should work toward a sound mind in a healthy body. To achieve this ideal, Locke advocated physical exercise as a hardening process, and an exposure to a wide variety of sensations from the physical and social worlds.

Condillac was Locke's apologist. He tried to simplify Locke's fundamental theory by arguing that all conscious experiences are the result of passive sensations: these sensations are the raw materials from which one forms complex and interrelated ideas. Learning is the noting of incomplete ideas, considering each separately, combining them into relationships, and ordering them. This process results in retaining the strongest degrees of association. Condillac asserted: "Then we shall grasp (ideas) easily and clearly and shall understand their origins entirely."[3(p7)]

Elsewhere in his writings Condillac presented his thoughts on analysis. One cannot have the proper conception of a thing until one is in a position to analyze it. "To analyze," claimed Condillac, "is nothing more than to observe in successive order the qualities of an object . . . the simultaneous order in which they exist."[4(p17)]

The third philosopher, Pierre Cabanis, tended to apply medicine to philosophy and philosophy to medicine. Cabanis considered illness and its impact upon the formulation of values and ideas. Through the social sciences, which emerged in the *Age of Enlightenment,* he explained *moral* as a psychological phenomenon on a physiological base. He concluded that moral impressions can have both physiological and pathological results. At last, there was a rational explanation for the psychological production of disease in which the so-called moral (emotional) passions play a significant part.[5(p37–38)] Cabanis contributed a socially based theoretical explanation of human experience that became the cornerstone for the moral management of the insane.

Age of Enlightenment and Moral Treatment

Moral treatment of the insane was one result of the *Age of Enlightenment.* It sprang from the fundamental attitudes of the day: a set of principles that govern humanity and society; faith in the ability of the human to reason; and the supreme belief in the individual. The rapid changes caused by this new philosophy advanced the disappearance of the notion that the insane were possessed of the devil. Mental diseases became legitimate concerns of humanitarians and physicians. The discontinuance of the idea that crime, sin, and vice were at the core of insanity brought forth humane treatment. Up to this time the insane had been housed and handled no differently than were criminals or paupers—often in chains.

Two men of the 18th century working in different countries, and unknown to each other, initiated the moral treatment movement. "No two men could possibly have been chosen out of all Europe at that time of whom it could be said more truly that they were cradled, and nursed, and educated among widely differing social, political, religious influences . . ."[6(p24–25)] Philippe Pinel was a child of the French Revolution, a physician, a scholar, and a philosopher. He is described as ". . .far exceeding the bounds of pure humanitarianism . . . to encompass the goals of a naturalist, . . . a reformer, a clinician, . . . and, above all, a philosopher."[7(Intro)] William Tuke was a devout member of the Society of Friends (Quakers).

Philippe Pinel: Physician–Reformer

Whenever Philippe Pinel's name comes up in a conversation among health professionals, he is immediately mentioned as the striker of the chains at two French hospitals. His efforts and contributions go way beyond that reformational act. As a physician, he began his most serious work in 1792 as superintendent of Bicêtre, the asylum for incurable males in Paris.

As a natural scientist, Pinel achieved exceptional skill in the observation of human behavior and the bringing of ". . .some order into the chaos of . . . treatment methods by means of critical and objective investigations."[5(p42)] Pinel says this about himself: "Desirous of better information, I resolved for myself the facts that were presented to my attention; and forgetting the empty honors of my titular distinction as a physician, I viewed the scene that was opened to me with the eye of common sense and unprejudiced observation."[8(p109)] From his own experience, he urged that observations ". . .be the basis upon which (one) should decide what opinions to believe."[9(p74–75)] Throughout his work, he held constantly before him his own motto of independent thought: "Chercher à èviter toute illusion, toute prèvention, toute opinion adoptèe sur parole" (to seek to avoid all illusion, all prejudice, all opinion taken on authority).[10(p8–9)]

Pinel's descriptions of the mentally deranged provide insight into his own compassionate nature. For him, the loss of reason was the most calamitous of human afflictions. The ability to reason principally separates the human from other living forms. Because of mental illness, the human's ". . .character is always perverted, sometimes annihilated. His thoughts and actions are diverted. . . . His personal liberty is at length taken from him. . . . To this melancholy train of symptoms, if not early and judiciously treated . . . a state of the most abject degradation sooner or later succeeds."[8(p xv–xvii)]

What Pinel entitled *revolution morale,* or moral revolution, is the ultimate insight of the insane into the delusional and absurd nature of their experiences.[7(p256)] This, to him, was the basis for treatment. Some historians believe that he was stating that moral treatment is synonymous with the humane approach. His own writings do not bear this out. Pinel believed that each patient must be critically observed and analyzed; then treatment should commence. "To apply the principles of moral treatment, with undiscriminating uniformity, would be . . . ridiculous and unadvisable."[8(p66)] The moral method is well reasoned and carefully planned for the individual patient.

According to Pinel, moral management is a maintained continuity of approach; a predictable routine, infused with vigor by personnel who inspire confidence. Moreover, moral treatment calls for a constant, observed study of patient behavior and performance. It included a gentle, but firm approach. Each patient is given as much liberty within the institution as he or she can tolerate. The approach is designed to give the patient a feeling of security as well as a respect for authority. Pinel asserted: "The atmosphere should be the same as in a family where the parents are quite strict. To establish this relationship, the doctor must convince the patient that he wishes to help him and that recovery is a real possibility."[9(p76)]

Occupations figured prominently in Pinel's conception of moral treatment. He used activities to take the patients' thoughts away from their emotional problems and to develop their abilities. He considered literature and music as effective in altering patients' emotions. Physical exercise and work should be part of every institution's fundamental program and be employed in accord with individual tastes. He concluded: "The (occupations) method is primarily designed and intended to reach man at his best which . . . means human understanding, intelligence, and insight."[3(p63–64)]

The concept of *moral treatment* belongs solely to Philippe Pinel. His fundamental belief was that its purpose is to restore the patient to himself, ". . .to use the patient's own emotions to balance his emotional excesses."[9(p76)] Truly, Pinel and his efforts, rooted in the *Age of Enlightenment,* mark the beginning of the modern epoch in the care of the mentally ill.

William Tuke: Philanthropist– Humanitarian

Across the channel, in England, things were astir at the same time. King George III, who was giving the American colonies fits, was himself in similar trouble.

In 1788 it became public knowledge that the King was seized with mania. Questions arose about his fitness to continue ruling. Nevertheless, public sentiment was on his side. For the first time, insanity and its treatment formed a topic of public discussion: "The subject had been brought out of concealment in a way which defeated the conspiracy of silence."[11(p42)] This being the *Age of Enlightenment,* the public openly sympathized with the sufferer; there was no condemnation. No one suggested that the King was being visited by the Devil, or that he was being punished for his sins.

The Society of Friends, derisively called *Quakers,* originated in 17th century England and became one of the most distinctive movements of Puritanism: "They arose out of the religious unrest of England . . . and stood for a radical kind of reform within Christendom which contrasted sharply with Protestant, Anglican and Roman patterns alike."[12(p118)] George Fox, founder of the Society, discovered ". . .the spirit of the living Christ and knew that it was an experience open to all men. 'This was the true light that lighteth every man that cometh into the world!'"[13(p1)]

William Tuke, a devout Quaker, wealthy merchant, and renowned philanthropist, was made aware of the deplorable conditions in the insane asylum in York, England. There were tales of extreme neglect and possible cruelty. He was an unusual man, not given to listening to sensational reports and acting rashly.[14(p12)] In true Quaker fashion Tuke presented a concern at a Friend's Quarterly Meeting in the spring of 1792—that an institution for the insane be established in York under the direction of the Society. At first, he was met with considerable resistance by those who believed that there were too few mentally ill Quakers, and that no one would want them concentrated in such a lovely, quiet locale.[15(p58)]

The York Retreat

Initially, Tuke was disheartened; yet, he pressed on, and within 6 months *The Retreat for Persons* afflicted with *Disorders of the Mind,* or simply, *The Retreat* came into being. Up until then the term *Retreat* had never been applied to an asylum. Tuke's daughter-in-law suggested the term to convey the Quaker belief that such an institution may be ". . .a place in which the unhappy might obtain refuge; a quiet haven in which (one) . . . might find a means of reparation or of safety."[16(p20)] The cornerstone simply stated the purpose of the institution: "The charity or love of friends executed this work in the cause of humanity."[15(p19)]

William Tuke became the superintendent. Thomas Fowler, an unusually open-minded man, was appointed visiting physician. After a trial-and-error period, they came to believe that moral treatment methods were preferable to those involving restraint and use of harsh drugs. The new approach was a product of Tuke's humanitarianism and Fowler's empiricism.

Several fundamental principles became evident within a short time. The approach was primarily one of kindness and consideration. The patients were not thought to be devoid of reason, feeling, and honor. The social environment was to be as nearly like that of a family as possible, with an atmosphere of religious sentiment and moral feeling.[16(p35)]

Tuke and Fowler strongly believed that most insane people retain a considerable amount of self-command. Upon admission, the patient was informed that treatment depended largely upon one's own conduct. Employment in various occupations was expected as a way for the patient to maintain control over his or her disorder. As Tuke reported: ". . .regular employment is perhaps the most efficacious; and those kinds of employment . . . to be preferred . . . are accompanied by considerable bodily action."[16(p156)] The staff endeavored to gain the patient's confidence and esteem, to arrest the attention and fix it upon objects opposite to any illusion the patient might have. The fundamental purpose of employment and recreation was to facilitate the regaining of the *habit of attention,* as Tuke called it. Various learning exercises were used, such as mathematical problems, to help the patient gain ascendancy over faulty habits of attention.

Tuke and Fowler determined that "indolence has a natural tendency to weaken the mind, and to induce ennui and discontent. . ."[16(p180–181)] A wide range of occupations and amusements was available. Patients not engaged in useful occupations were allowed to read, draw, or play various games. Tea parties, walks, and visitations away from the institution were planned regularly in preparation for the patients' returning home. All activities were closely analyzed through observation in order to individualize patients' needs.

The pioneer work of William Tuke and his son, Samuel, who wrote the definitive treatise on *The Retreat,* opened a new chapter in the history of the care of the insane in England. Mild management methods, infused with kindness, and building self-esteem through the judicious use of occupations, resulted in the excitation and elicitation of superior, human motives. Patients recovered, left *The Retreat,* and rarely needed to return for further care. The entire regimen was carefully patterned

". . .to accord (patients) the dignity and status of sick human beings."[17(p687)]

Moral Treatment Expansion

As soon as Pinel's major work on moral treatment (1801) and Samuel Tuke's description of *The Retreat* were published (1813), there was a rush toward implementing many reforms in other hospitals, particularly in England and the United States. In both countries occupations were introduced as an integral part of moral treatment.[18(p83–84)] Some unusual experiments were undertaken by Sir William Charles Ellis, a physician, who became the superintendent of a pauper lunatic asylum. The mainstay of his asylum management was useful occupations. He moved well ahead of mere amusements and "introduced a gainful employment of patients on a large scale and even had them taught a trade."[19(p62)] Ellis and his wife undertook other reforms. She organized the women patients into groups under the supervision of a *workwoman* to make useful and fancy articles.

Another Ellis innovation was the development of what would eventually be called *halfway houses.* Keenly aware of environmental and social influences on insanity, Ellis suggested ". . .after-care houses and night hospitals as a stepping stone from the asylum to the world by which . . . the length of patients' stay would be reduced and in many cases the cure completed. . ."[17(p871)] He insisted that convalescing patients should go out and mix with the world before discharge. His proposals were made in the 1830s!

In the United States, few public and private asylums existed in the post-Revolutionary era; however, institutional reforms were needed. Any recounting of this period must include two very important individuals and their work: Benjamin Rush and Dorothea Lynde Dix. Their efforts did not overlap; they did not know one another; nor was one influenced by the other. Just as in the cases of Pinel and Tuke, no two individuals this side of the Atlantic could have been more unlike one another in background, education, or experience. Nevertheless, each recognized the hapless plights of the institutionalized insane and set out to alleviate dire conditions and the inauguration of moral treatment, including occupations and exercise.

Benjamin Rush: Father of American Psychiatry

Benjamin Rush, often referred to as the *father of American psychiatry,* was a Philadelphia physician in the latter half of the 1700s. Through his training in Europe and several visits there, he adopted many of Pinel's practices; however, Rush did not adopt moral principles until later. As a member of the staff of Pennsylvania Hospital, he was placed in charge of a separate section set aside for the insane, the first hospital in America to reserve such a section. He was appalled by the conditions and he appealed to the staff and the public for change. Change did come and humane treatment was instituted. Rush saw to it that "certain employments be devised for such of the deranged people as are capable of working. . ."[20(p257)] This approach was based upon his philosophical stance that man, by his very nature, is meant to be active; "Even in paradise (Garden of Eden) he was employed in the health and pleasant exercises of cultivating a garden. Happiness, consisting in folded arms, and in pensive contemplation . . . by the side of brooks, never had any existence, except in the brains of mad poets, and lovesick girls and boys."[21(p115–116)]

In his major writing, *Medical Inquiries and Observations Upon the Diseases of the Mind*, Rush clearly differentiates between goal-directed activity and aimless exercise: "Labour has several advantages over exercise, in being not only more stimulating, but more endurable in its effects; . . . it is calculated to arrest wrong habits of action, and to restore such as regular and natural. . ."[21(p224–225)]

Dorothea Lynde Dix: Humanitarian–Reformer

Dorothea Lynde Dix, a reform-minded humanitarian during the middle 1800s, vehemently pressed for improved conditions of the insane who were incarcerated in jails and almshouses. She presented a number of *Memorials* to state legislatures, believing that the public had an obligation to care for such individuals. By 1848 numerous states had responded to her efforts, and she decided to tackle a more formidable object—the federal government. Dix envisioned the sale of public lands to finance the building of a federal system of hospitals for the indigent blind, deaf, and mute, as well as the insane. For 6 years she wheedled and cajoled members of Congress. Finally, in 1854, the bill was ready for President Franklin Pierce's signature. He was a close friend of Miss Dix and she felt highly confident of the outcome. The President vetoed the bill claiming unconstitutionality: ". . .every human weakness or sorrow would take advantage of this bill if it became law. . . . It endangers states' rights."[22(p20)] Through her contacts with physicians in several states, Miss Dix embraced moral

treatment as the most humane method. She strongly advocated ". . .decent care, quiet, affection and normal activity (as) the only medicine for the insane."[22(p11)]

United States: Individual Treatment, Occupations, Education

The Quakers brought moral treatment to the United States as part of their intellectual and religious luggage. Through published accounts about *The Retreat* in York, some private asylums were established in which moral principles were practiced. A number of public institutions altered their programs to include individualized treatment, occupations, and education. Those patients who had remained for years unimproved and listless, even on the verge of apathy ". . .are seen in encouraging instances, when transferred to attendants who have more disposition to attend to them, . . . to waken (them) from their torpor, to become animated, active and even industrious. . . ."[23(p487–488)]

Moral management also was taking on a new facet: the influence of a sane mind upon the insane mind. Those who daily attended the sick were to impress upon the insane the influences of their own character, designed to specifically improve the patients' behavior. Personnel must possess a number of traits: observational skills to see the ". . .actual condition of the patient's mind . . . and a faculty of clear insight. . . ."[23(p489)] Other traits: ". . .seeing that which is passing in the minds of (patients). . . . Add to this a firm will, the faculty of self-control, a sympathizing distress at moral pain, a strong desire to remove it. . . ."[23(p489)]

Arguments appeared in the literature relative to the moral use of firmness and gentleness. Strong cases were made for both extremes; however, it took two alienists (the precursor to psychiatrist), John Bucknill and D. Hack Tuke, grandson of Samuel Tuke, in 1858 to settle the dispute: "The truth, as usual, lies between; and the (individual) who aims at success in the moral treatment of the insane must be ready to be all things to all men, if by any means he might save some."[23(p500)] They elaborate on their thesis by stating: "With self-reliance . . . it requires widely different manifestations, to repress excitement, to stimulate inertia, to check the vicious, to comfort the depressed, to direct the erring, to support the weak, to supplant every variety of erroneous opinion, to resist every kind of perverted feeling, and to check every form of pernicious conduct."[23(p500)]

Bucknill and Tuke also wrote that moral treatment included the gaining of the patient's confidence, fixing his or her attention on interesting and wholesome objects of thought, diverting the mind from introspection, and loosening the hold on concentrated emotion. They explain: "For (these) purposes useful occupation is far superior to any form of amusement. The higher the purpose, and the more appellant the nature of the occupation . . . the more likely it is to draw him from the contemplation of self-wretchedness, and effect the triumph of moral influences."[23(p493)]

The next step in institutional occupations emphasized education. Those occupations that require a process of learning and thought were determined far preferable, from a curative point of view, than those that require none. "Moral treatment is as wide as that of education; . . . it is education applied to the field of mental phenomena. . ."[23(p501)] Therefore, it was not unusual to find specific mental activities included with occupations. The purpose was to educate the individual in order to provide him or her with "the power of controlling his feelings, and his thoughts, and his actions."[24(p166–167)]

With continued experience, a number of alienists decided that occupations and amusements also could serve as a prophylactic against insanity. One interesting prescription for the return and maintenance of sanity was: ". . .rest in bed, occupation, exercise and amusements."[25(p14)] D. Hack Tuke declared: "If idleness is a curse to the sane, it is the parent of mischief and ennui to the insane, especially to the pubescent and adolescent."[26(p1315)] He urges that the same approach be taken with the sane and the insane: "Employment, Nature's universal law of health, alike for body and mind, is specially beneficial, . . . seeing that it displaces ideas by new and healthy thoughts, revives familiar habits of daily activity, restores (and maintains) self-respect while it promotes the general bodily health."[26(p1315)]

Decline of Moral Treatment

Moral management and treatment by occupations reached its zenith in the United States just before the outbreak of the War Between the States (Civil War). Corporate, private asylums continued to expand their efforts. Stateand public-supported institutions withdrew their programs, so that by the last quarter of the 19th century, virtually no moral treatment was taking place.

Several reasons for this decline and eventual disappearance can be identified, including a nation at war with itself. Bockhoven cites others: 1. the founders of the U.S. movement retired and died, leaving no disciples or successors; 2. the rapidly increasing influx of foreign-born and poor patients greatly overtaxed existing facilities and required more institutions to be built with diminished tax support; 3. racial and religious prejudices on the part of the alienists, beginning to be called *psychiatrists*, reduced interest in treatment and cure; and 4. state legislatures became increasingly more interested in less costly custodial care.[27(p20–25)]

Essentially, there was no place in the public institutions for moral treatment. "The inferior physical plants and facilities, poorly trained and insufficient staff, . . . and, worst of all, overcrowding, prohibited any attempts to practice moral management."[28(p128)] A belief emerged that many insane were incurable. One eminent psychiatrist stated: "I have come to the conclusion that when a man becomes insane, he is about used up for this world."[29(p155)] Such pessimism was predominant for a century in this country. Custodial care had come to stay for a very long time.

As we shall see next, moral principles and practices emerged in the early years of the 20th century through the efforts of individuals, then by a group who founded an organization dedicated to those principles. This group, in collaboration with others, established a definition and fundamental principles that have carried over through several generations of specifically educated practitioners of occupational therapy.

Once again, as with Pinel and Tuke, Rush and Dix, the individuals who founded and pioneered the 20th century occupational therapy movement could not have been more diverse in their backgrounds, experience, and education. They included a nurse, two architects, a physician, a social worker, and a teacher.

Susan Tracy: Occupational Nurse

Susan Tracy was this country's first proponent of occupations for invalids. A trained nurse, she initiated instruction in activities to student nurses as early as 1905 as part of their expanding responsibilities. She also developed the term *occupational nurses* to signify specialization.[30(p401)] By 1912 she decided to devote all her energies to patient activities and she distinguished herself by applying moral treatment principles to acute conditions. As Tracy stated, "The application of this most rational remedy to ordinary, everyday sick people, as found in the general hospital, is almost unknown."[31(p386)] She strongly claimed that remedial treatments "are classified according to their physiological effects as stimulants, sedatives, anesthetics . . . , etc. Certain occupations possess like properties."[31(p386)] The physician may select stimulating occupations, such as watercoloring and paper folding; or sedative occupations such as knitting, weaving, basketry.

Throughout Tracy's many years of work she employed experimentation and observation to enhance her practice. Her carefully worded writings provide ample evidence of her intense desire to bring scientific principles to the application of invalid occupations. In 1918 she published a remarkable research paper on 25 mental tests derived from occupations; for example, by instructing the patient in using a piece of leather and a pencil, "require him to make a line of dots at equal distances around the margin and at uniform distances from the edge. This constitutes a test of *Judgement* in estimating distances."[32(p15)] Continuing with the same piece of leather, the patient is instructed to punch a hole at each dot. "In order to do this he must consider the two sides of leather, the two parts of his tool and bring these together thus making a *Simple Coordination* test."[32(p16)] Other tests in the fabrication of the leather purse include *Aesthetic Coordination and Rhythm, Differentiation of Form and Size, Purposeful Relation*. In all 25 tests, she stressed a completed, useful and "not unbeautiful" object.

Tracy's other writings state the value and usefulness of discarded materials to successful ward work.[33(p62)] She also emphasized high quality workmanship: "It is now believed that what is worth doing at all is worth doing well, and that practical, well-made articles have a greater therapeutic value than a useless, poorly made article."[34(p198)] A premium is placed upon originality and the ". . . adoption of the occupation to the condition and natural tastes of the patient."[35(p63)] Further, she believes that ". . . the patient is the product, not the article that he makes."[33(p59)]

Tracy's major work, *Studies in Invalid Occupation*, published in 1918,[36] is a revealing compendium of her observations and experiences with different kinds of patients, for instance: "the child of poverty and the child of wealth, the impatient boy, grandmother, the business man."

By 1921, Susan Tracy had adopted the term *occupation therapy* originally coined by William Rush Dunton, Jr., and defined it and differentiated it from vocational training. She felt this was necessary because of the arising confusion between the two concepts following World War I. She wrote: "What is occupation? The treatment of disease by occupation. . . . The aim of occupation is to get the man well; that of vocational training is to provide him with a job. Any well man will look

for a job, but the sick man is looking for health."[37(p120)] Throughout all of her writings she stated that nothing is ". . .too small to be pressed into the service of resourceful mind and trained hands toward . . . the establishment of a healthy mind in a healthy body."[33(p57)]

George Barton: Re-education of Convalescents

George Edward Barton, by profession an architect, contracted tuberculosis in his adult life. This plagued him for the remainder of his years. His constant struggle led him into a life of service to the physically handicapped. Out of his own personal concerns came the establishment of Consolation House, an early prototype of a rehabilitation center. He was an effective speaker and writer, often given to hyperbole; he gained his point with the listening or reading public.

Barton's central themes were hospitals and their responsibility to the discharged patient; the conditions the discharged patient faces; the need to return to employment; occupations and re-education of convalescents. These were intense concerns to him because of his own health problems.

His first published article, derived from a speech given to a group of nurses, points out a weakness he perceived in hospitals: "We discharge from them not efficients, but inefficients. An individual leaves almost any of our institutions only to become a burden upon his family, his friends, the associated charities, or upon another institution."[38(p328)] In the same article, he warms to his subject: "I say to discharge a patient from the hospital, with his fracture healed, to be sure, but to a devastated home, to an empty desk and to no obvious sustaining employment, is to send him out to a world cold and bleak. . . ."[38(p329)] His solution: ". . .occupation would shorten convalescence and improve the condition of many patients."[38(p329)] He ended his oration with a rallying cry: ". . .it is time for humanity to cease regarding the hospital as a door closing upon a life which is past and to regard it henceforth as a door opening upon a life which is to come."[38(p330)]

Barton established Consolation House in Clifton Springs, New York. Those referred to his institution underwent a thorough review, including a social and medical history, and a consideration of one's education, training, experience, successes, and failures. Barton believed that "By considering these in relation to the condition (the patient) must presumably or inevitably be in for the remainder of his life, we can find some form of occupation for which he will be fitted. . . ."[39(p336)] He claimed that Consolation House was "getting down to our social difficulties."[39(p337)]

By 1915, Barton had adopted Dunton's term, *occupation* therapy, but preferred the adjectival form: occupational therapy. He declared: "If there is an occupational disease, why not an occupational therapy?"[40(p139)] He expansively stated: "The first thing to be done . . . is for occupational therapy to provide an occupation which will produce *a similar therapeutic effect to that of every drug in materia medica.* An exercise for each separate organ, joint, and muscle of the human body. An exercise? An occupation! An occupation? A useful occupation! Then (occupational therapy) can fill the doctor's prescriptions. . . written in the terms of materia medica."[40(p139)] He even advocated a laxative by *occupation.*

Re-education entered Barton's terminology with the aftermath of World War I. He viewed hospitals as taking on a mission different from that previously adopted. A hospital should become ". . .a re-educational institution through which to put the waste products of society *back and into the right place.*"[40(p139)] Using alliteration, he declared: ". . .by a catalystic concatenation of contiguous circumstances we were forced to realize that when all is said and done, what the sick man really needed and wanted most was the restoration of his ability to work, to live independently and to make money."[41(p320)]

Barton's major contribution to the re-emergence of moral treatment was the awakening of physical reconstruction and re-education through the employment of occupations. Convalescence, to him, was a critical time for the inclusion of something to do. Activity ". . .clarifies and strengthens the mind by increasing and maintaining interest in wholesome thought to the exclusion of morbid thought . . . and a proper occupation . . . during convalescence may be made the basis of the corollary of a new life upon recovery. . . . I mean *a job, a better job, or a job done better* than it was before."[42(p309)] With Susan Tracy, Barton held that the major consideration of occupations ". . .should be devoted to the therapeutic and education effects, not to the value of the possible product."[43(p36)]

William Rush Dunton, Jr.: Judicious Regimen of Activity

Of the founders of the 20th century movement, William Rush Dunton, Jr., was the most prolific writer and the most influential. He published in excess of 120 books and articles related to occupational therapy and rehabilitation; served as president of the National Society for the Promotion of Occupation Therapy; and, for 21 years, was editor of the official journal. As a physician, he spent his professional career treating psychiatric patients in an institutional setting. Key to his treatment methods is occupational therapy, a term he coined to differentiate aimless amusements from those occupations definitely prescribed for their therapeutic benefits. Before embarking on what he called *a judicious regimen of activity,* he read the works of Tuke and Pinel, as well as the efforts of significant alienists of the 19th century.

From his readings and from observations of patients in Sheppard Asylum, a Quaker institution in Towson, Maryland, Dunton concluded that the acutely ill are generally not amenable to occupations or recreation. The acutely ill exhibit a weakened power of attention. Occupations at this time would be fatiguing and harmful. The prevailing prescription is ". . .to let the patient alone, meanwhile improve (his) condition, restore and revivify exhausted mental and physical forces. . . ."[44(p19)] Later, activities should be selected that use energies not needed for physical restoration. Stimulating attention and directing the thoughts of the patient in regular and healthful paths would ensure an early release from the hospital. Dunton developed a wide variety of activities from knitting and crocheting to printing and the repair of dynamos, in order to gain the attention and interest, as well as to meet the needs, of all patients.

Dunton's proclivities for history and research led him to extensive readings and experimentations—all related to the human, his need for work, leisure, rest, and sleep; the causal factors of mental aberrations; various cures of mental illness. Each excursion brought him back to *a judicious regimen of activity* as the treatment of choice, regardless of whether the patient was mentally or physically ill. He became more and more convinced that attention and interest in one's work and play are as efficacious, if not more so, than the many and varied other medications available. He stated it this way: "It has been found that a patient makes more rapid progress if his attention is concentrated upon what he is making and he derives stimulating pleasure in its performance."[45(p19)]

At the second annual meeting of the National Society for the Promotion of Occupational Therapy (AOTA) in 1918, Dunton unveiled his nine cardinal rules to guide the emerging practice of occupational therapy, and to ensure that the new discipline would gain acceptance as a medical entity: 1. Any activity in which the patient engages should have as its objective a cure. 2. It should be interesting; 3. have a useful purpose other than merely to gain the patient's attention and interest; and 4. preferably lead to an increase in knowledge on the patient's part. 5. Curative activity should preferably be carried on with others, such as in a group. 6. The occupational therapist should make a careful study of the patient in order to know his or her needs and attempt to meet as many as possible through activity. 7. The therapist should stop the patient in his or her work before reaching a point of fatigue; and 8. encouragement should be genuinely given whenever indicated. Finally, 9. work is much to be preferred over idleness, even when the end product of the patient's labor is of a poor quality or is useless.[46(p26–27)]

The major purposes of occupation in the case of the mentally ill were outlined in Dunton's first book.[47(p24–26)] The primary objective is to divert the attention either from unpleasant subjects, as is true with the depressed patient; or from daydreaming or mental ruminations, as in the case of the patient suffering from dementia praecox (schizophrenia)—that is, to divert the attention to one main subject.

Another purpose of occupation is to re-educate— to train the patient in developing mental processes through ". . .educating the hands, eyes, muscles, just as is done in the developing child."[47(p25)] Fostering an interest in hobbies is a third purpose. Hobbies serve as present, as well as future, safety valves and render a recurrence of mental illness less likely. A final purpose may be to instruct the patient in a craft until he or she has enough proficiency to take pride in his or her work. However, Dunton did note that "While this is proper, I fear . . . specialism is apt to cause a narrowing of one's mental outlook. . . . The individual with a knowledge of many things has more interest in the world in general."[47(p26)]

Dunton continued to write and publish his observations, each one elaborating on a previous one. His texts became required reading for students preparing for practice. Even in his 90s, well beyond retirement from practice, he maintained an interest in our profession and continued to offer counsel.

Eleanor Clarke Slagle: Founder–Pioneer

Eleanor Clark Slagle qualifies as both a founder and a pioneer. She was at the birth of the Association in 1917. Before that time she had received part of her education in social work and had completed one of the early Spe-

cial Courses in Curative Occupations and Recreation at the Chicago School of Civics and Philanthropy. Following this, she taught in two courses for attendants of the insane; directed the occupations program at Henry Phipps Clinic, Johns Hopkins Hospital, Baltimore, under Dr. Adolf Meyer; returned to Chicago to become the Superintendent of Occupational Therapy at Hull House. Later, Mrs. Slagle moved to New York where she pioneered in developing occupational therapy in the State Department of Mental Hygiene. In addition, she served with high distinction in every elective office of the American Occupational Therapy Association, including President (1919–1920) and as a paid Executive Secretary for 14 years.[48(p122–125); 49(p473–474); 50(p18); 51]

She found occupational therapy to be ". . .an awkward term. . ." but felt ". . . it has been well defined as a form of remedial treatment consisting of various types of activities . . . which either contribute to or hasten recovery from disease or injury . . . carried on under medical supervision and that it be *consciously* motivated." Further, she emphasized that occupational therapy must be "a *consciously* planned progressive program of *rest, play, occupation and exercise*. . . ."[52(p289)] In addition, she explained it is ". . .an effort toward normalizing the lives of countless thousands who are mentally ill, . . . the normal mechanism of a fairly well balanced day."[53(p14)] She enjoyed quoting C. Charles Burlingame, a prominent psychiatrist of her day: "'What is an occupational therapist? She is that newer medical specialist who takes the joy out of invalidism. She is the medical specialist who carries us over the dangerous period between acute illness and return to the world of men and women as a useful member of society.'"[52(p290–291)]

Slagle placed considerable emphasis upon the personality factor of the therapist: ". . .the proper balance of qualities, proper physical expression, a kindly voice, gentleness, patience, ability and seeming vision, adaptability . . . to meet the particular needs of the individual patient in all things. . . . Personality plus character also covers an ability to be honest and firm, with infinite kindness. . . ."[54(p13)]

The issue would constantly arise about the use of handicrafts as a therapeutic measure in the machine age. Her response is a classic: ". . .handicrafts are so generally used, not only because they are so diverse, covering a field from the most elementary to the highest grade of ability; but also, and greatly to the point, because their development is based on primitive impulses. They offer the means of contact with the patient that no other medium does or can offer. Encouragement of creative impulses also may lead to the development of large interests outside oneself and certainly leads to social contact, an important consideration with any sick or convalescent patient."[52(p292-293)]

Habit training was first attempted at Rochester (New York) State Hospital in 1901. Slagle adopted the basic principles and developed a far greater perspective and use among mental patients who had been hospitalized from 5 to 20 years and who had steadily regressed. The fundamental plan was ". . .to arrange a twenty-four hour schedule . . . in which physicians, nurses, attendants, and occupational therapists play a part. . . ."[54(p13)] It was a re-education program designed to overcome some disorganized habits, to modify others and construct new ones, with the goal that habit reaction will lead toward the restoration and maintenance of health. "In habit training, we show clearly an academic philosophy factor . . . that is, the necessity of requiring attention, of building on the habit of attention—attention thus becomes application, voluntary and, in time, agreeable."[54(p14)]

The purposes of habit training were two-fold: the reclamation and rehabilitation of the patient, with the eventual goal of discharge or parole; and, if this was not reasonable, to assist the patient in becoming less of an institutional problem, that is, less destructive and untidy.

A typical habit training schedule called for the patient to arise in the morning at 6:00, wash, toilet, brush teeth, and air beds; then breakfast; return to ward and make beds, sweep; then classwork for 2 hours, which consisted of a variety of simple crafts and marching exercises. After lunch, there was a rest period; continued classwork and outdoor exercises, folk dancing, and lawn games. Following supper, there was music and dancing on the ward, followed by toileting, washing, brushing the teeth, and preparing for bed.[55(p29)]

Once the patient had received maximum benefit from habit training, he or she was ready to progress through three phases of occupational therapy. The first was what Slagle called *the kindergarten group*. "We must show the ways and means of stimulating the special senses. The employment of color, music, simple exercises, games and storytelling along with occupations, the gentle ways and means . . . (used) in educating the child are equally important in re-educating the adult. . . ."[54(p14)] Occupations were graded from the simple to the complex.

The next phase was *ward classes in occupational therapy*. ". . .graded to the limit of accomplishment of in-dividual patients."[56(p100)] When able to tolerate it, the patient joined in group activities. The third and final phase was the *occupational center*. "This promotes opportunities for the more advanced projects . . . (a) complete change in environment; . . . comparative freedom; . . . actual responsibilities placed upon patients; the stimulation of seeing work produced; . . . all these carry forward the readjustment of patients."[56(p102)]

This founder, this pioneer, this distinguished member of our profession provided a summary of her own accomplishments and philosophy by stating: "Of the highest value to patients is the psychological fact that the patient is working for himself. . . . Occupational Therapy recognizes the significance of the mental attitude which the sick person takes toward his illness and attempts to make that attitude more wholesome by providing activities adapted to the capacity of the individual patient and calculated to divert his attention from his own problems."[54(p290)] Further, she declared: "It is directed activity, and differs from all other forms of treatment in that it is given in increasing doses as the patient improves."[57(p3)]

Adolf Meyer: Philosophy of Occupation Therapy

Dr. Adolf Meyer is cited in this account of the evolution of occupational therapy because of his outstanding support and because his approach to clinical psychiatry was entirely consistent with the emerging occupational therapy movement.

Adolf Meyer, a Swiss physician, immigrated to the United States in 1892 and accepted a position initially as pathologist at the Eastern Illinois Hospital for the Insane in Kankakee. Over the next 14 years he held various positions in the United States and became professor of psychiatry at Johns Hopkins University in 1910. Throughout this period he developed the fundamentals of what was to become the psychobiological approach to psychiatry, a term he coined to indicate that the human is an indivisible unit of study, rather than a composite of symptoms. "Psychobiology starts not from a mind and a body or from elements, but from the fact that we deal with biologically organized units and groups and their functioning . . . the 'he's' and 'she's' of our experience—the bodies we find in action. . . ."[58(p263)] Meyer took strong issue with those in medicine: ". . .who wish to reduce everything to physics and chemistry, or to anatomy, or to physiology, and within that to neurology. . . ."[58(p262)] His enlightened point of view is that one can only be studied as a total being in action and that this ". . .whole person represents an integrate of hierarchically arranged functions."[59(p1317)]

His common sense approach to the problems of psychiatry was his keynote: "The main thing is that your point of reference should always be life itself. . . . I put my emphasis upon specificity. . . . As long as there is life there are positive assets—action, choice, hope, not in the imagination but in a clear understanding of the situation, goals and possibilities. . . . To see life as it is, to tend toward objectivity is one of the fundamentals of my philosophy, my attitude, my preference. It is something that I would recommend if it can be kept free of making itself a pest to self and to others."[60(p vi–xi)]

From the very beginning of his work in Illinois, he was concerned with meaningful activity. In time, it became the fundamental issue in treatment. "I thought primarily of occupation therapy," he stated, "of getting the patient to do things and getting things going which did not work but which could work with proper straightening out."[60(p45)] In a report to the Governor of the State of Illinois in 1895, Meyer wrote: "Occupation is, with good right, the most essential side of hygienic treatment of most insane patients."[60(p 59)]

By 1921, Meyer had become Professor of Psychiatry at Johns Hopkins University in Baltimore, and had extensive experiences with others, such as William Rush Dunton, Jr., Eleanor Clarke Slagle, and Henrietta Price, leaders in the occupational therapy movement. At the Fifth Annual Meeting of the National Society for the Promotion of Occupational Therapy in Baltimore, October 1921, Meyer brought together his fundamental concepts of psychobiology to produce his paper, *The Philosophy of Occupation Therapy* (see Chapter 4). Through time, this has become a classic in the occupational therapy literature. It bears study by all of us.

Psychobiology is clearly visible in his statement that ". . .the newer conceptions of *mental problems* (are) *problems of living,* and not merely diseases of a structural and toxic nature. . . ."[61(p4)] The indivisibility and integration of the human are cited in this manner: "Our conception of man is that of an organism that maintains and balances itself in the world of reality and actuality by being in active life and active use. . . ."[61(p5)]

Because of the nature of his paper, *The Philosophy of Occupational Therapy,* Meyer emphasized occupation, time, and the productive use of energy. Interwoven are the elements of psychobiology. He stated: "The whole of human organization has its shape in a kind of rhythm. . . . There are many . . . rhythms which we must be attuned to: the larger rhythms of night and day, of sleep and waking hours . . . and finally the big four—work and play and rest and sleep, which our organism must be able to balance even under difficulty. The only way to attain balance in all this is actual doing, actual practice, a program of wholesome living is the basis of wholesome feeling and thinking and fancy and interests."[61(p6)]

According to Meyer, a fundamental issue in the treatment of the mentally ill is ". . .the proper use of time in some helpful and gratifying activity. . . ."[61(p1)] He expands on this precept by stating: "There is in all this a development of the *valuation of time and work,* which is not accidental. It is part of the great espousal of the *values of reality and actuality* rather than of mere thinking and reasoning. . . ."[61(p4)] The introduction of activity is ". . . in giving opportunities rather than prescriptions. There must be opportunities to work, opportunities to do and to plan and create, and to learn to use material. . . . It is not a question of specific prescriptions, but of opportunities . . . to adapt opportunities."[61(p7)] He concluded his philosophic essay by returning once again to time and occupations: "The great feature of man is his new sense of time, with foresight built on a sound view of the past and present. Man learns to organize time and he does it in terms of doing things, and one of the many things he does between eating, drinking and . . . the flights fancy and aspiration, we call work and occupation."[61(p9–10)]

Near the end of his working life, Meyer summed up his major efforts. He wrote of dealing with individuals and groups from the viewpoints of *good sense; of science,* ". . .with the smallest numbers of assumptions for search and research. . ."; of *philosophy;* and of *religion,* ". . . as a way of trust and dependabilities in life."[62(p100)]

Occupational Therapy Definitions and Principles

As the founders and pioneers were experimenting with and writing their concepts, a definition of occupational therapy was emerging. It is remarkable that so early in the formation of the 20th century movement, a definition could be developed and stand for several decades and several generations of occupational therapists. Many of us were required in school to immortalize it through needlepoint, embroidery, and even printing.

H.A. Pattison, M.D., medical officer of the National Tuberculous Association, advanced his view at the annual conference of the National Society for the Promotion of Occupational Therapy in Chicago, September 1919. It was also adopted by the Federal Board of Vocational Education: "Occupational Therapy may be defined as any activity, mental or physical, definitely prescribed and guided for the distinct purpose of contributing to and hastening recovery from disease or injury."[63(p21)] Twenty-one years later, in 1931, John S. Coulter, M.D., and Henrietta McNary, OTR, added one phrase: ". . .and assisting the social and institutional adjustment of individuals requiring long and indefinite periods of hospitalization."[64(p19)] This was inserted in order to recognize occupational therapy's involvement in chronicity.

By 1925, a committee, made up of four physicians including William Rush Dunton, compiled an outline for lectures to medical students and physicians.[65(p277–292)] Though their document never received the official imprimatur of the AOTA, it nevertheless served for several years as a guide for practice.[66(p347)] Fifteen principles were enunciated: "Occupational therapy is a method of training the sick or injured by means of instruction and employment in productive occupation; . . . to arouse interest, courage, confidence; to exercise mind and body in . . . activity; to overcome disability; and to re-establish capacity for industrial and social usefulness."[65(p280)] Application called for as much system and precision as other forms of treatment; activity was to be prescribed, administered, and supervised under constant medical advice. Individual patient needs were paramount.

The outline stressed that "employment in groups is . . . advisable because it provides exercise in social adaptation and stimulating influence of example and comment. . . ."[65(p280)] In selecting an activity, the patient's interests and capabilities were to be considered and as strength and capability increased, the occupation was to be altered, regulated, and graded accordingly because "The only reliable measure of the treatment is the effect on the patient."[65(p280)]

Inferior workmanship could be tolerated, depending upon the patient's condition, but there should be consideration of ". . .standards worthy of entirely normal persons . . . for proper mental stimulation."[65(p281)] Articles made were to be useful and attractive, and meaningful tasks requiring healthful exercise of mind and body provided the greatest satisfaction. "Novelty, variety, individuality, and utility of the products enhance the value of an occupation as a treatment measure."[65(p281)] While quality, quantity, and the salability of articles made could be of benefit, these should not take precedence over the treatment objectives. As adjuncts to occupations, physical exercise, games, and music were considered beneficial and fell into two main categories: gymnastics and calisthenics, recreation and play.

One last principle spoke of the qualities of the occupational therapist: ". . .good craftsmanship, and ability to instruct are essential qualifications; . . . understanding, sincere interest in the patient, and an optimistic, cheerful outlook and manner are equally essential."[65(p281)]

Occupational Therapy's Second Generation

The die was cast. Practice rapidly expanded in a phenomenal number of settings following the establishment of the founders' principles and definition. A *second generation* of therapists emerged during the late 1920s and the 1930s. They were the practitioners and educators who elaborated, codified, and applied the initial theory upon which present-day practice is based. A chronicle of their efforts would offer a highly valuable and valued study in itself. The names of Louis Haas, Mary Alice Coombs, Winifred Kahmann, Henrietta McNary, Harriet Robeson, Marjorie Taylor, and Helen Willard would figure prominently in such an account.

For the purpose of *this history,* a composite of these and others is drawn into one individual who exemplifies the spirit and deeds of the *second generation* of occupational therapists—those whose efforts are lasting and ensure our present and future education and practice.

Understandably, it would be a woman. She would devote her professional career to either teaching, practicing, or administering. Quite possibly she would combine two or more of these. She would acquire an expertise in one area of practice, such as the mentally ill.

Her belief in the treatment of the total patient would guide her thoughts and actions. Occupational therapy, she would declare, "since its founding has concerned itself with the basic tenet—the treatment of the total patient. This approach is unique to occupational therapy among the . . . health disciplines. . . . There has always existed a strong component concerned with the behavior of the physically ill or disabled, as well as the mentally sick; with the entirety of man and his functioning as a patient. This occupational therapy concept," she would continue, "prevented (as has occurred in medical practice) an undesired separation of the psychiatric therapist from those who develop knowledge and skills centered in the treatment of the physically disabled."[67(p1)] Stated another way, "The major emphasis in occupational therapy is not the body *as such* but the individual *as such.* The therapist's background is strongly weighted in an understanding of personality adjustment and reactions to social situations; . . . and in the patients' attitudes toward an adjustment to acute and chronic disabilities."[68(p9)]

At some point in her work, she would be asked to serve as a consultant to one or more medical facilities, possibly a state hospital system. In time, she would produce a report and restate her definition of occupational therapy. It might well go this way: "The goal of all treatment in a modern mental hospital is the physical, social and economic rehabilitation of the patient. . . . The accepted function (of occupational therapy) . . . is the scientific utilization of mental and physical activities for the purpose of raising the patient to the highest level of integration; to assist him in making his initial adjustment to the hospital; to sustain him while his body responds to physical treatment and his mind to psychotherapy; or to assist him in making a satisfactory adjustment to chronic illness."[69(p24)]

In the report she would also call for an atmosphere as normal as possible, where a patient could be encouraged to respond in as normal a manner as possible: a balanced program of work and play, with flexibility to meet individual needs: "There must be organized a succession of steps through which the patient will be gradually led to his highest level of integration. . . . At each level . . . the patient experiences a feeling of success and self-respect. One cannot overemphasize the importance of careful planning . . . in order that there be a systematic progression up this ladder of integration."[69(p24)]

In another context, supportive care, as a vital concern to the therapist, would also be described, particularly in the care of the physically disabled: "To name only a few of its treatment objectives, occupational therapy may function as a diagnostic evaluative instrument; as corrective treatment; . . . or a design for effecting prevocational evaluation. Incorporated in each . . . is a treatment phase referred to as supportive care. This is a most fundamental and yet less definitive and indeed the least spectacular element of the total rehabilatory program. In supportive care, the occupational therapist (is concerned) with the behavioural factors which have and will affect the patient's response to the rehabilitation program. . . ." Convincingly, she would say: ". . .it can be said with conviction that successful rehabilitation can be effected only when the patient has attained a true state of rehabilitation 'readiness.'"[70]

Not just a woman of words, she would find one or more ways to activate her philosophy. She might well become active with a group of former patients and assist in organizing an association of and for individuals who have been hospitalized—for instance, the mentally ill. Such an endeavor would be the first of a kind. Through such an experience, she would conclude: "One difficulty which presented itself again and again was the need to instill in these (former) patients a philosophy toward their own rehabilitation: . . . an organized effort beyond the hospital which would offer special training, guidance and professional evaluation of their potentials."[71(p3)]

This would lead her to even greater endeavors on behalf of a whole category of patients. As an example, she would find that the 1920 Federal Vocational Rehabilitation Act excluded former psychiatric patients. In the manner of Dorothea Lynde Dix, whom she probably emulated, she would wage a relentless battle to right such a wrong. By enlisting the assistance of physicians' associations and veterans' groups she would see the legislation change. As part of her campaign she would write: "The former mental patient, in his struggle for economic rehabilitation, incurs the burden imposed on the physically handicapped 'plus' the stigmatization based on the popular misconception of mental disease. He must cast aside self-pity or the idea that the world owes him a living. The world does owe him understanding and guidance."[72(p114)] Finally, amendments to *Public Law 113* were passed and signed by President Franklin Roosevelt. Psychiatric patients could now qualify for the benefits of the vocational rehabilitation act.

With such efforts the therapist's personal beliefs about emotional illness become even more strongly felt: "The majority of mentally ill are (sick) through no fault of their own . . . any more than one who has contracted a physical illness. Persons suffering from mental disease are generally ill as a result of an accumulation of unsuccessful efforts . . . to adjust to his environment."[72(p83)]

Two continuing concerns of all occupational therapists would be commented upon: the qualifications of the therapist and the use of media. One is as significant as the other. "The personality of the therapist," she would say, "must command respect, admiration, hope and confidence, . . . for no therapy is better than the therapist who directs it."[72(p83)] Therapeutic media have a number of inherent qualities, such as providing a vehicle for objectively recording patient performance, and, for the patient, affording opportunities for ". . .creative expression and evidence of accomplishment. The therapist should have a wide variety of activities (available) in accordance with the interests, aptitudes, and mental state of the patient. A craft track mind had no place in preparing such a program," she would state.[72(p103)]

The accumulation of experiences as a clinician, and educator, or an administrator, or possibly a combination of these, would lead this *therapist of the second generation* to arrive at a new definition of occupational therapy. It would precede by several years an altered definition by the national organization. It would incorporate the social and behavioral sciences, with a diminished emphasis upon medicine. Human development would appear for the first time as a focus for the treatment of physical and psychosocial dysfunction. She would declare: "Occupational therapy's function is to provide skilled assistance in influencing human objectives; its approach is inextricably conjoined with the behavioral factors involved. It is interested in how the process of growth and development is modified by hospitalization, chronic illness or a permanent handicap."[73(p2)]

This re-focus was quite explainable and understandable to her since occupational therapy, and its ancestral emphasis, has always been the totality of the human organism. She would say, "It was inevitable, therefore, that there evolve an ever increasing emphasis in occupational therapy . . . a greater understanding of the part that the developmental process plays in the preventive and therapeutic factors of this form of treatment."[74(p3)]

The foregoing has been a descriptive composite of a whole generation of therapists and assistants. The composite is actually the story of one individual; her observations alone have been cited. That individual is *Miss Beatrice D. Wade, OTR, FAOTA.*

The story is far from finished. Without a doubt, someone sometime will chronicle the lives and works of those who are still making contributions from that era to the present generation. Among them are Marjorie Fish, Virginia Kilburn, Mary Reilly, Ruth Robinson, Clare Spackman, Ruth Brunyate Wiemer, Carlotta Welles, and Wilma West. Each one, together with many others, continues to serve us well as clarifiers and definers of reasonable and reasoned alternatives. As counselors, they confirm old values and clearly point out *new directions* as well as our faithfulness or infidelity to those timeless principles established by our professional ancestors.

Lessons From Our History

The history of occupational therapy is the most neglected aspect of our professional endeavors. Seemingly, *old values* are least considered when charting *new directions*. On occasion we have been accused of taking leave of our historical senses. More to the point is that we have no historical sense. The problem primarily lies in not taking the time to assiduously locate our profession's diggings, to excavate what is relevant, and, then, to learn from what has been unearthed.

Archival materials from the past 200 years have been abundantly used in the development of this paper. Location and excavation has been difficult at times; however, it is reassuring to note that records and accounts still exist that are extremely relevant to today's endeavors. Lessons can be learned and they must. May I encourage each of you to determine for yourself what you have learned from this paraphrastic journey to our profession's diggings. To assist in this endeavor, may I cite a few lessons I have gained.

Mind and Body Inextricably Conjoined

No less than our professional ancestors, we must refuse to accept any alternative to the belief in the wholeness of the human—that the mind and body are inextricably conjoined. Illness, treatment, and the return to a healthful state simultaneously affect the physiological and emotional processes. Indeed, should these processes ever become separated, then occupational therapy would be of no value. The patient has died!

The Natural Science of the Human

The inextricable union of the human leads to another lesson. The science fundamental to our practice is the natural science of the human. No amount of neurophysiology, psychology, sociology, or child development alone can determine the differential diagnosis, treatment, or prognosis of the patient undergoing occupational therapy. The current trend toward specialization, with its varying emphases upon one or another science, to the neglect of other human sciences, and indeed to the neglect of other nonscientific aspects of occupational therapy, borders on superstition and mythology. It is the continuous acquisition and scientific synthesis of the ingredients of the human organism and its surround that guarantees authentic occupational therapy.

The Human Organism's Involvement in Tasks

Occupational therapy is the only major health profession whose focus centers upon the *total* human organism's involvement in tasks—a making or doing. In spite of the many grafts we have effected, our roots remain in the subsoil of the *art*, the *craft*: a paradigm of the total activity of the human. Just as those who have come before us, we think of ourselves and others fundamentally as makers, as users, as doers, as tools. We look at: ". . .craft as a way in which man may create and cross a bridge within himself and center himself in his own essential unity."[75(p vii)] The procedures one goes through in rearranging and reassembling the basic elements in art or craft operate upon and within the doer: ". . . his material modifies him as he modifies it, in proportion to his openness, his awareness of the exchange that is taking place."[75(pvii)] The procedure one goes through in rearranging and reassembling the basic elements in art or craft operate upon and within the doer: ". . . his material modifies him as he modifies it, in proportion to his openess, his awareness of the exchange that is taking place."[75 (px)]

The Differentiation of Occupational Therapy

Any definition, any description, any differentiation between ourselves and other health providers must have as its major theme occupation and leisure. Without it, we become a blurred copy, a xerography of a host of others.

Without the dynamics of human motion inherent in purposeful activity, we become quasi-physical therapists. Without the interaction between human objects and the objects of work and leisure, we become quasi-social workers, psychologists, or nurses. Without the demonstrated and proven interrelationships between healthful, normal growth and development, activity, and the pathology of illness and disabling conditions, we become quasi-physicians and psychiatrists.

The more we intermingle our fundamental philosophy and our treatment techniques with others, the more likely we will become enfeebled, the more likely we will degenerate, the more likely we will eventually disappear.

A Refusal to Accept the Common Verdict

As Hugh Sidey has noted, "History is a marvelous collection of stories about men and women who refuse to accept the common verdict that certain achievements (are) impossible."[77(p18)] The history of occupational therapy is the story of the ideals, deeds, hopes, and works of *individuals.* Changes and advancements came from those who eliminated inhumaneness, which prevented or discouraged the sick and disabled from achieving their potential. These same individuals were willing to assume the care and responsibility for those *who were not highly valued by the society:* the mentally ill and retarded, the severely disabled—all those defined as "non-producing, . . . an economic burden."[65(p277)]

In numerous places and on countless occasions these same individuals were derided, hated, or, at best, ignored, because they pressed for change in the human condition. Yet, they persevered, knowing there was nothing innately unusual about themselves or what they wished to achieve. Few ever saw their names inscribed on monuments.

They were a *cast* quite diverse in character, and largely obscure because of the immensity of the saga being enacted. A few received *speaking parts,* primarily through reporting their own clinical findings. Only very few were singled out to be stars. None ever became members of the *audience,* passively observing events. All were *actors.*

The very same can be said of the present occupational therapy generation. We are actors, not observers. We continue to willingly strive on behalf of those who are not highly valued by the society. We refuse to see this as a burden. Rather, we perceive it as an obligation, as an opportunity, as a way of life.

Legacy of Experience

Too often we are disposed to think that those lessons another generation learned do not apply to the present generation. We should be mindful that there are two ways to learn: by our own experience and from those who have made discoveries, regardless of how long ago they were made. The experience of others is a magnificent heritage, and the more we learn from them, the less time we waste in the present, proving what already has been proved.

Those of us who are teachers and clinicians have a special obligation to pass on the legacy of experience, the knowledge of timeless principles and practices that do not change merely because times change.

Who They Were, What They Did

The legacy of experience suggests one more lesson. So often we are caught up in our daily activities we tend to forget what it is we owe those who came before us. All probably agree that each occupational therapy generation seemingly acquires a sense of self-sufficiency. It is true that we of the present occupy the positions that once were filled by others.

It is, however, of great import that we realize we are influenced by those who came before us more than we can truly know. Who they were and what they did has immeasurable bearing upon what we are and what we do. No generation is capable of isolating itself from its past. The past, plus what we are and what we do, greatly assists in fashioning our future.

The archives, the portraits and photographs, the published accounts, the personal memorabilia and scrapbooks are records of considerable moment. At the least, they are a profound reminder of the possibility that someday, someone may be looking back and may be wondering who we were and what we did.

Conclusion

It is altogether fitting and proper to conclude this lecture with the observations of two former Presidents of the Association, Mr. Thomas B. Kidner and Mrs. Eleanor Clarke Slagle. In 1930, Mr. Kidner offered a personal impression of the state of occupational therapy at the annual meeting of the Connecticut Occupational Therapy Society. In part, he said: "May we, therefore, look on occupational therapy—with the increased faith as the years go by—as a natural means of aiding in the restoration of the sick and disabled to health and working capacity (which means happiness) because it appeals to all our human attributes."[57(p11)]

Mrs. Slagle, a year after she retired in 1937, made this observation: "The story of the profession of occupational therapy will never be fully told, nor will that of the patients who have so abundantly appreciated the opportunities of the service. There has been no fanciful crusading 'for the cause'; it has meant that a few have perhaps borne many burdens, but in the slow process that make permanent things of great value, it can be said that there is a fine body of professional workers, experienced and well trained, coming forward and being welcomed to a really great human service, that of helping to show the way to the person with large disabilities to make the best of his incomplete self."[78(p382)] Finally, in an editorial "From the Heart," she concluded: "The integrity of your profession is in your hands. I bid you all Godspeed in your work."[79(p345)]

Acknowledgments

A study of this nature and scope is not possible without the valuable and valued assistance of numerous individuals and sources. I wish to recognize the incomparable services provided by the staffs of the Moody Medical Library, The University of Texas Medical Branch at Galveston; the Quine Library, University of Illinois at the Medical Center, Chicago; the McGoogan Library of Medicine, University of Nebraska Medical Center, Omaha; and the Archives, Shapiro Developmental Center (Eastern Illinois State Hospital), Kankakee.

Finally, I wish to recognize Frances Sawyer, COTA, and the Board of Directors, The Texas Occupational Therapy Association, Inc., who placed my name in nomination for this exalted honor. My gratitude to them is immeasurable.

Dedication

I wish to dedicate the 1981 Eleanor Clarke Slagle Lectureship to my parents, who provided me with those cumulative experiences and values that inevitably led me to the decision to become an occupational therapist; to a very great woman, Beatrice D. Wade, OTR, FAOTA, who has been my valued teacher and beloved mentor for more than 30 years; to my cherished colleagues, Lillian Hoyle Parent and Jay Cantwell, both occupational therapists, who constantly stimulate me and insist on a high level of constructive activity; to Charles H. Christiansen, OTR, FAOTA, whose personal and professional qualities and insistence on excellence from himself and others assure me of the future of occupational therapy.

Without the examples, teachings, guidance, counseling, and friendship of these individuals, I could never have achieved this exalted opportunity.

References

1. Locke J: *An Essay Concerning Human Understanding* (Two Volumes). New York: Dover Press, 1894F

2. Frost SE: *Basic Teachings of the Great Philosophers,* New York: Barnes and Noble, Inc., 1942

3. Riese W: *The Legacy of Philippe Pinel: An Inquiry into Thought on Mental Alienation,* New York: Springer Publishing Co., 1969

4. Condillac EB de: *Oeuvres Philosophiques de Condillac,* Paris: Presse Universataires de France, 1947

5. Ackerknecht EH: *A Short History of Psychiatry,* New York: Hafner Publishing Co., 1968

6. Tuke DH: *A Dictionary of Psychological Medicine* (Vol One). Philadelphia: P Blakinston, Son & Co., 1892

7. Pinel P: *Traité Médico-Philosophique sur 'Alienation Mentale,* Paris: Richard, Caille & Rover, 1801

8. Pinel P: *A Treatise on Insanity In Which Are Contained the Principles of a New and More Practical Nosology of Maniacal Disorders,* Translated by DD Davis. London: Cadell & Davis, 1806 (Facsimile published by Hafner Publishing Co., New York, 1962)

9. Mackler B: *Philippe Pinel: Unchainer of the Insane,* New York: Franklin Watts, Inc., 1968

10. Folsome CF: *Diseases of the Mind: Notes on the Early Management, European and American Progress,* Boston: A. Williams & Co., Publishers, 1877

11. Jones K: *Lunacy, Law, and Conscience: 1744–1845: The Social History of Care of the Insane,* London: Routledge & Kegan Paul, Ltd., 1955

12. Dillenberger J, Welch D: *Protestant Christianity: Interpreted Through Its Development,* New York: Charles Scribner's Sons, 1954

13. Philadelphia Yearly Meeting of the Religious Society of Friends: *Faith and Practice,* Philadelphia: Philadelphia Yearly Meeting, 1972

14. Tuke DH: *Reform in the Treatment of the Insane. Early History of the Retreat, York; Its Objects and Influence,* London: J & A Churchill, 1872

15. Tuke DH: *Reform in the Treatment of the Insane: An Early History of the Retreat, York: Its Objects and Influence,* London: J & A Churchill, 1892

16. Tuke S: *Description of The Retreat, An Institution Near York for Insane Persons of the Society of Friends: Containing an Account of Its Origins and Progress, The Modes of Treatment, and a Statement of Cases,* York, England: Alexander, 1813

17. Hunter R, Macalpine I: *Three Hundred Years of Psychiatry, 1535–1860: A History Presented in Selected English Texts,* London: Oxford University Press, 1963

18. Connolly J: *The Treatment of the Insane Without Mechanical Restraints,* London: Smith, Elder & Co., 1856 (Facsimile copy published by Dawson's of Pall Mall, London, 1973, with introduction by R Hunter and I Macalpine)

19. Ellis WC: *A Treatise on the Nature, Symptoms, Causes, and Treatment of Insanity,* London: Holdsworth, 1838

20. Goodman N: *Benjamin Rush: Physician and Citizen, 1746-1813,* Philadelphia: University of Pennsylvania Press, 1934

21. Rush B: *Medical Inquiries and Observations Upon the Diseases of the Mind* (4th Edition). Philadelphia: J Grigg, 1830

22. Buckmaster H: *Women Who Shaped History,* New York: Macmillian Pub. C., 1966

23. Bucknill JC, Tuke, DH: *A Manual of Psychological Medicine,* New York: Hafner Pub. Co., 1968 (Facsimile of 1858 Edition)

24. Barlow J: *Man's Power Over Himself to Prevent or Control Insanity,* London: William Pickering, 1843

25. Skultans V: *Madness and Morals: Ideas on Insanity in the Nineteenth Century,* London: Routledge & Kegan Paul, 1975

26. Tuke DH: *A Dictionary of Psychological Medicine: Volume Two,* Philadelphia: P Blakiston, Son & Co., 1892

27. Bockhoven JS: *Moral Treatment in American Psychiatry,* New York: Springer Publishing Co., Inc. 1963

28. Dain N: *Concepts of Insanity in the United States, 1789–1865,* New Brunswick, NJ: Rutgers University Press, 1964

29. Deutsch A: *The Mentally Ill in America: A History of Their Care and Treatment from Colonial Times* (2nd Edition). New York: Columbia University Press, 1949

30. Tracy SE: The development of occupational therapy in the Grace Hospital, Detroit, Michigan. *Trained Nurse Hosp Rev 66:*5, May 1921

31. Tracy SE: The place of invalid occupations in the general hospital. *Modern Hosp 2:*5, June 1914

32. Tracy SE: Twenty-five suggested mental tests derived from invalid occupations. *Maryland Psychiatr Q 8:* 1918

33. Barrows M: Susan E. Tracy, RN. *Maryland Psychiatric 16:* 1916–1917

34. Tracy SE: Treatment of disease by employment at St. Elizabeths Hospital. *Modern Hosp 20:*2, February 1923

35. Parsons SE: Miss Tracy's work in general hospitals. *Maryland Psychiatr Q 6:* 1916–1917

36. Tracy SE: *Studies in Invalid Occupation,* Boston: Witcomb and Barrows, 1918

37. Tracy SE: Power versus money in occupation therapy. *Trained Nurse Hosp Rev 66:*2, February 1921

38. Barton GE: A view of invalid occupation. *Trained Nurse Hosp Rev 52:*6, June 1914

39. Barton GE: Occupational nursing. *Trained Nurse Hosp Rev 54:*6, June 1915

40. Barton GE: *Occupational therapy. Trained Nurse Hosp Rev 54:*3, March 1915

41. Barton GE: The existing hospital system and reconstruction. *Trained Nurse Hosp Rev 69:*4, October 1922

42. Barton GE: What occupational therapy may mean to nursing. *Trained Nurse Hosp Rev 64:*4, April 1920

43. Barton GE: *Re-education: An Analysis of the Institutional System of the United States.* Boston: Houghton Mifflin Co., 1917

44. Sheppard Asylum: *Third Annual Report of the Sheppard Asylum,* Towson, MD: 1895

45. Dunton WR: The relationship of occupational therapy and physical therapy. *Arch Phys Ther 16:* January 1935

46. Dunton WR: *The Principles of Occupational Therapy. Proceedings of the National Society for the Promotion of Occupational Therapy: Second Annual Meeting,* Catonsville, MD: Spring Grove State Hospital, 1918

47. Dunton WR: *Occupational Therapy: A Manual for Nurses,* Philadelphia: WB Saunders, 1915

48. Komora PO: *Eleanor Clarke Slagle. Ment Hyg 27:*1, January 1943

49. Pollock HM: In memoriam: Eleanor Clarke Slagle, 1876–1942. *Am J Psychiatr 99:*3, November 1942

50. American Occupational Therapy Association: *Then and Now, 1917–1967,* New York: American Occupational Therapy Association, 1967

51. Loomis B, Wade BD: *Chicago. . .Occupational Therapy Beginnings: Hull House, The Henry B. Favill School of Occupations and Eleanor Clarke Slagle.*

52. Slagle EC: Occupational therapy: Recent methods and advances in the United States. *Occup Ther Rehab 13:*5, October 1934

53. Slagle EC: History of the development of occupation for the insane. *Maryland Psychiatr Q 4:* May 1914

54. Slagle EC: Training aids for mental patients. *Arch Occup There 1:*1, February 1922

55. Slagle EC, Robeson HA: *Syllabus for Training of Nurses in Occupational Therapy,* Utica, NY: State Hospital Press, date unknown

56. Slagle EC: A year's development of occupational therapy in New York State Hospitals. *Modern Hosp 22:*1, January 1924

57. Kidner TB: Occupational therapy, its development, scope and possibilities. *Occup Ther Rehab 10:*1, February 1931

58. Meyer A: The psychological point of view. In *Classics in American Psychiatry,* JP Brady, Editor. St. Louis: Warren H Green, Inc., 1975 (Also, In *The Problems of Mental Health,* M Bentley, EV Cowdey, Editors. New York: McGraw-Hill, 1934)

59. Arieti S: *American Handbook of Psychiatry* (Vol Two), New York: Basic Books, Inc., Publishers, 1959

60. Lief A: *The Commonsense Psychiatry of Dr. Adolf Meyer: Fifty-two Selected Papers, Edited with Biographical Narrative.* New York: McGrawHill Book Co., 1948

61. Meyer A: The philosophy of occupation therapy. *Arch Occup Ther 1:*1, February 1922. Also in Am J Occup Ther 31(10): 639–642, 1977. Reprinted as Chapter 2.

62. Meyer A: The rise to the person and the concept of wholes or integrates. *Am J Psychiatr 100:* April 1944

63. Pattison HA: The trend of occupational therapy for the tuberculous. *Arch Occup Ther 1*(1): February 1922

64. Coulter JS, McNarry H: Necessity of medical supervision in occupational therapy. *Occup Ther Rehab 10*(1): February 1931

65. An outline of lectures on occupational therapy to medical students and physicians. *Occup Ther Rehab 4*(4): August 1925

66. Elwood, ES: The National Board of Medical Examiners and medical education, and the possible effect of the Board's program on the spread of occupational therapy. *Occup Ther Rehab 6*(5): October 1927

67. Wade BD: Occupational Therapy: A History of Its Practice in the Psychiatric Field. Unpublished paper presented at 51st Annual Conference, American Occupational Therapy Association, Boston, October 19, 1967

68. Advisory Committee in Occupational Therapy: The Basic Philosophy and Function of Occupational Therapy. *University of Illinois Faculty—Alumni Newsletter of the Chicago Professional Colleges. 6:*4, January 1951

69. Wade BD: A survey of occupational and industrial therapy in the Illinois state hospitals. *Illinois Psychiatr 2*(1): March 1942

70. Wade BD: Supportive care. *Bull Rehab Inst Chicago,* date unknown

71. Wade BD: Supportive care. Bull Rehab Rehabilitation of the Mentally Ill. Unpublished paper presented to the Department of Public Welfare, State of Minnesota, June 26, 1958

72. Willard HS, Spackman CS: *Principles of Occupational Therapy* (First Edition). Philadelphia: JB Lippincott Co., 1947

73. Wade BD: The Development of Clinically Oriented Education in Occupational Therapy: The Illinois Plan. Unpublished paper presented at 49th Annual Conference, American Occupational Therapy Association, Miami, November 2, 1965

74. Wade BD: Introduction. *The Preparation of Occupational Therapy Students for Functioning with Aging Persons and in Comprehensive Health Care Programs: A Manual for Educators,* Chicago: University of Illinois at the Medical Center, 1969

75. Dooling EM: *A Way of Working,* Garden City, NY: Anchor Press/Doubleday, 1979

76. Sidey H: The presidency. *Time 116*(22):December 1, 1980

77. Slagle EC: Occupational therapy. *Trained Nurse Hosp Rev 100*(4): April 1938

78. Slagle EC: Editorial: From the heart. *Occup Ther Rehab 16*(5): October 1937

Occupational Therapy Service: Individual and Collective Understandings of the Founders

SUZANNE M. PELOQUIN

Florence Stattel (1977) pleaded for a comprehensive history of occupational therapy, because such a history would provide perspective for contemporary understanding and future growth. Her rationale was also that occupational therapists might, in formulating a history, seize the awareness that occupational therapy has "extended an idea" in the universe (p. 649). The present paper is an attempt to explore those beliefs held by occupational therapists in the earliest years of our history and to examine the personal understandings of service found in the occupational therapy literature between 1917 and 1930. This seems an apt place to start. Any idea, including the idea of service, rarely exists in the abstract, but emerges instead from the larger context of the understandings and experiences of the person who holds it.

Sutton wrote in 1925 that "service is, or should be, one of the stellar ideals of occupational therapy" (p. 54). In 1972, a special task force of the American Occupational Therapy Association (AOTA) issued a comprehensive definition of occupational therapy that included the statement, "occupational therapy provides service" (AOTA, 1972, p. 204). An early characterization of the occupational therapist was that "she must have a deep desire to serve" (Northrup, 1928, p. 267). Because service is an idea articulated by most professions, some unique character of service must account for occupational therapy's emergence as a profession distinct from others. The ideas held individually and collectively by our founders reflect contemporary values and norms, forces that shaped their understanding of how they might serve others in a unique manner.

This chapter was previously published as "Looking Back: Occupational Therapy Service: Individual and Collective Understandings of the Founders," Part 1. *American Journal of Occupational Therapy, 45,* 352–360, and as "Looking Back: Individual and Collective Understandings of the Founders," Part 2. *American Journal of Occupational Therapy, 45,* 733–744. Copyright © 1991, American Occupational Therapy Association. Reprinted with permission. Part 1: http://dx.doi.org/10.5014/ajot.45.4.352. Part 2: http://dx.doi.org/10.5014/ajot.45.8.733

An Idea Extended

The service particular to occupational therapy involves three primary agents: patient, therapist, and occupation. These agents interrelate; forces across time shape both their nature and their relationships. The character and quality of service provided to any person thus exist within a particular context shaped by contemporary trends. Our current understanding of practice acknowledges distinct patient-therapist-occupation interrelationships as well as the trends that shape them. If, for example, one considers a hand therapist in private practice, the image of service in this context differs from that of a therapist treating patients in an acute psychiatric setting, even though both situations include the patient, the occupational therapist, and some form of occupation. The characteristics of a therapist that shape the type of service provided include his or her personal traits, education and experiences, frame of reference regarding occupation and patient rapport, understanding of professional roles, position and authority held within the treatment environment, and degree of commitment to standards within the particular agency. Similarly, the particular patient and his or her occupational performance strengths and problems, expectations for service, goals for treatment, attitude toward therapy, and environmental circumstances shape the service received. The particular occupations selected from self-care, work, or play-related arenas, whether targeting functional increases in cognitive, psychological, neuromuscular, sensory integrative, or social interactional performances, also characterize the service provided. There can be many pictures of occupational therapy practice. Although no single picture of service exists, invariant features enable us to identify a practice as occupational therapy. The existence today of many forms of occupational service reflects the multifaceted yet singular understanding of our founders in 1917.

Historical inquiry discloses the invariant features of a service that may persist while also assuming different forms across time. A seminal idea can be extended while also being shaped in time. My particular inquiry aims to identify the founders' characterizations of the relationships among patient, therapist, and occupation, in order to better grasp their understanding of service in the earliest decades of occupational therapy practice. My search has constituted an attempt to "search out those unusual roots carefully planted and nurtured by our forebears" (Bing, 1983, p. 800). These roots intertwine with major forces that shaped early service: hospital treatment, industry, and war. Additional societal trends toward science, education, sex stereotyping, and professionalization nourished the subsoil that shaped our growth.

I hope that this inquiry will help therapists to estimate the value of our current reflections about caring. Yerxa (1980), for example, said that "caring means being true to our humanistic and functional heritage with its concern for the quality of daily living of our patients" (p. 534). She appealed for our allegiance to that heritage. Johnson (1981) (see Chapter 54) later cautioned against current forces that shape occupational therapy service into a form that might embarrass our forebears: "Part of the price we now pay is that our directions frequently seem to be predicated not upon the observations and concepts of our founders but upon external sources and influences" (p. 593). Many of us seem in this decade to regret the passing of a time in which we believe that it was somehow easier to care, to be humane, and to resist the forces that shape practice and service. The present inquiry aims to retrieve that time and to explore its influence in shaping the particular brand of caring that constituted occupational therapy.

Because the emphasis of this search is on the personal understandings that our founders had of the best way to serve in their time, a significant portion of the literature reviewed considers persons, personal stories, and personal philosophies. It seems apt to explore such narratives when researching a profession whose early aim was "not in the making of a product, but in the making of a MAN, of a man stronger physically, mentally, and spiritually than he was before" (Barton, 1920, p. 308). I also think it essential to consider, at least in broad strokes, what kind of world could want, shape, and nurture a service designed to reconstruct persons.

Crafting a New Service: Founders and Near Founders

In 1917, six persons gathered to found the National Society for the Promotion of Occupational Therapy: those attending the meeting at George Edward Barton and Dr. William Rush Dunton, Jr.'s, invitation were Thomas B. Kidner, Isabel G. Newton, Susan C. Johnson, and Eleanor Clarke Slagle. Because Susan Elizabeth Tracy was teaching a new course in occupation and could not attend, she was listed as an incorporator instead of a founder. Because Barton did not accept Dunton's nomination of Dr. Herbert Hall, Hall was not included as a member of the founding group, but became an early member and later president of the Society. Tracy and Hall might thus be called near founders. Johnson (1981) (see Chapter 54) described the group:

> Our founders were physicians, architects, social workers, secretaries, teachers of arts and crafts, nurses. . . . Each brought a different perspective and came from a unique background and orientation, yet each observed the effects of occupation in their individual environments and believed in its curative powers. (p. 592)

Johnson (1981) (see Chapter 54) characterized the group as a gathering of specialists who supported the wide use of occupation as a curative service. Each founder shared life in the world of 1917, a world quite different from that which we experience today. Dr. Sidney Licht (1967) permitted a colorful glimpse of contemporary self-care, work, and play in that era when writing about the founding of occupational therapy.

In 1917 there was neither television nor radio. For the first time that year, color movies ran in commercial theaters in New York. Admission to local movie houses was a dime for an adult and a nickel for a child. Children were not admitted unless accompanied by an adult. A loaf of bread cost a nickel; the annual cost of living for a family of four was $1,843. Dollar bills were longer and wider and obviously stretched farther. Homogenized milk had not been invented, but milk was delivered to homes 7 days a week by horse-drawn wagons. Neither electric refrigeration nor supermarkets existed. Oranges were prized Christmas stocking fillers, rare treats in winter. It cost a penny to send a postcard, a penny more to mail a letter. Most people who had telephones had party lines. There were no commercial flights. Ford's touring car sold for $360. There were no traffic lights and no parking meters; 729 people were killed in automobile accidents during that year. Street lamps were turned on each night by persons called *lamplighters*. In that year, Binet developed the IQ test; Dewey endorsed new educational techniques that proposed learning by doing. Sanitation was not particularly good. Most cities had a hospital for contagious diseases, and because antibiotics were nonexistent, a large part of medical practice was concerned with infection. A man with a bilateral inguinal herniorrhaphy was immobilized for 20 days. Houses were heated with wood or coal. The United States would enter its first world war, known then as the Great War. Though perhaps simpler because of fewer inventions and options, occupational tasks in 1917 were not easy by today's standards.

Beyond these daily exigencies, other societal concerns and trends greatly influenced the ideas of the founders of the National Society for the Promotion of Occupational Therapy. The major forces that shaped their perceptions of the need for occupational therapy emerge from their respective narratives; these forces include industry, war, educational reforms, and the nature of hospital care. A brief overview may prove helpful.

A recently industrialized society was increasingly aware of the adverse psychological and physical effects of mechanization. Arts-and-crafts societies emerged in a number of cities to restore pride in individual and quality workmanship against the increasing monotony and vanishing autonomy of factory work. Powerful machines maimed bodies at an alarming rate. Social workers such as Jane Addams of Chicago's Hull House recognized the negative effects of both industrialization and city living among poor persons and offered educational, recreational, and community-enhancing activities in neighborhood settlement houses. Advocates for reform in education, industry, and treatment of the ill used settlement houses as centers for generating changes in living and working conditions. Efficiency engineers such as Frank and Lillian Gilbreth promoted techniques to make persons and machines more effective on the job and at home. The crippling effects of war on neighboring countries and the ways in which their governments reconstructed their war heroes prompted a readiness in the United States to do the same. Hospital care was scrutinized. Inhumane conditions in state hospitals for "the insane" received public exposure, and the National Committee for Mental Hygiene sought to promote better treatment for institutionalized patients. Doctors, nurses, and patients increasingly criticized the failure of general hospitals to prepare patients for a society that valued effectiveness and productivity. Nurses and social workers strove for professional respect and credibility, often using contemporary pleas for reform as catalysts for changes in their practices. Each of our founder's conclusions about

the kind of service that would be most helpful connects back to personal experiences with and personal understanding of these broader issues.

Changes occurring within medical settings during these early years seem particularly important, because much of the expressed need for occupation as therapy came from hospital workers:

> This was a time of significant medical advance. Medicine moved from a discipline concerned solely with treatment to one involved with preventing the occurrence and the recurrence of disease. However, as such infectious and epidemic illnesses as typhoid and small pox were being eliminated, new medical problems, which were to result in an increased number of chronic patients, became apparent. These included heart disease, arteriosclerosis, and diabetes. The number of the institutionalized mentally ill increased five times. . . . As more people were able to survive illness and accident due to rapid medical advances, more were left with lasting impairments. The war, a severe polio epidemic in 1916, industrial accidents, and the widening use of the automobile all contributed to the need for new methods of treating residual disabilities. (Woodside, 1971, p. 226)

Each founder of the Society drew a common understanding from this larger context of 1917: the right occupation might in some way help. Exploration of each founder's unique view of patients, therapists, and occupations clarifies the manner in which occupational therapy became multifaceted yet rooted in one basic idea.

George Edward Barton

George Edward Barton was a successful architect who originated the idea of founding a society to promote occupation as therapy. Because his background included a year's work in nursing and some studies in medicine, he had a working knowledge of medical matters (Staff, 1923). He was also knowledgeable of the patient's point of view. He spent a year in a sanitarium for treatment of tuberculosis and had recurrent attacks of the disease. Two of his toes, which had frozen and become gangrenous, were amputated after a trip during which he was investigating famine among farmers for the governor of Colorado. After his surgery he developed a hysterical paralysis on the left side of his body. He was sent to Clifton Springs Sanitarium in New York, where he counseled with the Reverend Dr. Elwood Worcester and developed an interest in occupation as therapy. Aware that he could not return to architecture, he was determined to spend the rest of his life "devoted to the subject of reclamation of the sick and crippled" (Barton, 1968, p. 340). He bought a small old house and barn and named them Consolation House, where in 1914 he opened a school, a workshop, and a vocational bureau for convalescents (Barton, 1914; Licht, 1967). Barton hired a secretary, Isabel G. Newton, who helped him in his work and whom he later married. She described his early efforts: "Paralyzed in his left side, he could scarcely do more than stand. With no motion possible in his left hand and arm, he used his own body as a clinic to work out the problem of rehabilitation himself" (Barton, 1968, p. 342). She remembered that his medical friends, appreciating his results, sent patients to him for help. These referrals launched his "first experimental practice of occupational therapy" (p. 342). In 1917, Barton invited Newton to become one of the founders of the Society. She agreed and became its first secretary. She worked alongside her husband, teaching occupation to convalescents until his death in 1923.

Barton's early views on the subject of occupational therapy are of considerable interest. In his earliest writings he called the therapy "occupational nursing" (Barton, 1915a, p. 335). He regretted that the work was "unfortunately called Occupational Therapy . . . because the subject has so very many different sides that most people . . . have such difficulty in making out what it is all about anyhow" (Barton, 1920, p. 304). He viewed occupational therapy's goal as the making of a person, that is, a productive individual. He was critical of the hospital's restricted role in treatment:

> To get the patient well has been the aim and the end of it all. . . . But if the hospital world expands, as the public is demanding that it shall expand, so that to merely get the patient well is not the whole thing, but to get him well for something. (Barton, 1920, p. 305)

Barton (1920) argued that a man "is not a normal man just because his temperature is 98.6. A man is not a *normal* man until he is able to provide for himself" (p. 306). He believed that the hospital had lost a vital opportunity by becoming focused on the X ray and laboratory, thereby turning out "paupers instead of producers" (Barton, 1920, p. 307). He maintained that a patient fared better during the convalescent period with something to do (Barton, 1920). Occupying his or her mind with something worthwhile enabled that patient to sleep and heal at night. Barton thought that worthwhile activity meant activity with earning power. He reminded his audiences that concern over the inability to earn often impelled a patient to seize a nurse and say, "In God's Name, tell me what I'm going to do!" (Barton, 1915a, p. 335).

Barton (1920) believed that a "proper occupation" promoted physical improvement, "clarified and strengthened the mind," and could become "the basis or the corollary of a new life upon recovery" (p. 307). He believed that a person's spirit could resurrect in "greater strength and purity" to triumph over disability and despair (Barton, 1920, p. 308). He therefore chose a phoenix rising from the flames as the emblem for Consolation House. Barton recommended an extensive occupational diagnosis to include consideration of the patient's education and inclinations; present status, habits, and ambitions; and expectations. The diagnosis would suggest the prescription: the proper occupation in the proportion necessary to produce the desired physical, mental, and spiritual results. Barton believed that any prescription from *materia medica* (as cited by Barton, 1915b) could be translated into occupational terms. He explained that if medicine prescribed benzol to a patient as a leukotoxin for leukemia, occupational therapy would put the same patient to work in a canning factory where the fumes of hot benzine would "keep her in good health" while she supported herself (Barton, 1915b, p. 139). Each human activity could be associated with a physical effect. Barton's unique belief that every occupation had an effect analogous to that of a drug distanced some physicians and resulted in his being considered an extremist (Licht, 1948).

Barton thought that the teacher of the occupation must monitor its therapeutic effects. He called for scientific reeducation with an argument from Frank Gilbreth: "The teaching element is more important in this new phase of adequate placement than it has ever been before, because in every case a new or changed worker must be made useful, self-supporting, and interested" (as cited by Barton, 1920, p. 306). Gilbreth was himself elected to honorary membership in the Society at its founding meeting (Dunton, 1967).

Barton believed strongly that the teacher of occupation should be a nurse. He saw occupational work as an opportunity for the nursing profession to develop, expand, and become more important and useful (Barton, 1920). He exhorted nurses not to sit idly by while others took up this new line of work, leaving them to handle the "crescent basin" (Barton, 1915a, p. 338). Barton's commitment to occupational therapy's alliance with medicine is clear. He suggested that when Adam was cast from the Garden of Eden he was given a divine prescription to earn his bread by the sweat of his brow (Barton, 1915b). Barton used numerous medical analogies. One finds a now humorous medical reference in the paper entitled "Preparation of Patients for Inoculation [sic] of 'Bacillus of Work'" (as cited by Dunton, 1967, p. 287), which Barton read at the Society's founding meeting.

Barton was also the first secretary of the Boston Society of Arts and Crafts, a group allied with the arts-and-crafts movement against industrialization. He supported quality work crafted by conscientious persons. He was particularly fond of our Society's, if not our therapy's, name, including in his rationale a trait of the nonindustrialized worker:

> I am strongly in favor of the National Society for the Promotion of Occupational Therapy as a title. I know that it is long but it does tell the story and the S.P.O.T. suggests the ever alert "Johnnie." (as cited by Licht, 1967, p. 272)

Barton's understanding of occupational therapy was that the person providing occupation would be an advanced nurse who would be teaching scientifically from a medical and occupational knowledge base. This nurse-therapist would ensure harmony between occupational and medical treatments and use a frame of reference for treatment broader but parallel to that of medicine. The therapist would regard the patient as a mental, physical, and spiritual being and consider the patient's individual strengths, goals, and ambitions in these three realms when planning treatment. The addition of occupational therapy to hospital treatment would enable staff to remake a whole person who could lead a useful life.

Susan Elizabeth Tracy

Because Barton encouraged nurses to engage in occupational therapy, it seems fitting to next consider the legacy of one nurse who did: Susan Elizabeth Tracy. I refer to Tracy as a *near founder* because although not one of the founders, she was invited to the Society's founding

session. Licht (1967) believed that "no one did more in this country to resurrect and establish occupational therapy than did Miss Tracy" (p. 275). Moodie (1919), herself a nurse, argued that "Occupational Therapy, in other words, the application of various forms of handicraft to meet the individual limitations of invalids and the physically handicapped was first brought into being by Miss Susan E. Tracy" (p. 313). During her training, Tracy had noticed that those patients on surgical wards who kept occupied seemed happier than those who remained idle (Licht, 1967). After completing her course work she became director of the nurses' training school at the Adams Nervine Asylum, Boston, where she initiated a program of manual arts. Her program was the first course in the United States designed to prepare instructors for patients' activities (Licht, 1948). Tracy also taught nurses in practice in the Boston area, including those at the city's Massachusetts General Hospital. One indication of her positive relationships with others and her ability to share her convictions is that an early surgical patient published her *Studies in Invalid Occupations* (Licht, 1967).

Tracy's (1913) book communicates her values and her ideas about service. She valued the support of physicians. In the chapter that introduces Tracy's ideas, Dr. Daniel H. Fuller of the Adams Nervine Asylum noted that "suitable occupation is a valuable agent in the treatment of the sick . . . as an important adjunct to other forms of treatment, and sometimes it is quite all the treatment necessary" (Tracy, 1913, p. 1). Tracy no doubt perceived it important to include a physician's endorsement. She must have thought it also meritorious to include Fuller's characterizations of the quality of personal care required:

> Nurses are constantly being impressed with the fact that the technical and mechanical part of their work is but one aspect of their professional duty, that a broader conception must be attained—a sense of obligation to minister to the individual as well as to the disease. The value of wise human sympathy, of cheerfulness in work and mien, of tactful dealing with unreasonableness and irritability, of skillful diversion of thought from pessimistic channels . . . are essential parts of the trained nurse's equipment to do her work. (Tracy, 1913, pp. 9–10)

Although Fuller saw occupation as helpful in meeting a physician's goals, he did not believe that a nurse had to be the provider. He believed instead in possession of the proper character:

> Without the constant cooperation of the teacher or nurse, without the daily expression of interest and the stimulus of example, the work is either never begun, or if begun, is thrown aside. The personality of the teacher and nurse therefore becomes an important factor. Her real enthusiasm and love for the work react most powerfully on the patient. (Tracy, 1913, p. 3)

In subtitling her book *A Manual for Nurses and Attendants*, Tracy also extended the role of providing occupation to those competent persons who had not been trained to nurse.

Tracy (1913) believed that a physician could prescribe work for the patient "whose physical, nervous, mental and moral characteristics he had made the object of keen observation and study" (p. 5). The result of such broad prescription was "cure in the broadest sense, in that the mental attitude toward life has been changed" (Tracy, 1913, p. 3).

Tracy (1913) used Dewey's definition of occupation as it related to education: "A mode of activity on the part of the child which runs parallel to some form of work carried on in the social life" (p. 13). She felt challenged to identify parallel occupations for hospitalized patients:

> The real problem of the nurse is to find means whereby she may initiate and actually lead and cooperate in forms of occupation suited to every invalid condition and any natural temperament. (Tracy, 1913, p. 18)

Tracy (1913) pleaded for a certain dignity and quality to the work, for employment of time on worthy materials and purposeful productions. She believed that although a handicraft teacher was perhaps suited to the hospital shop or workroom, sicker patients required special care: "When the shop is a sickroom, and the bed the bench, it is almost a necessity that the nurse be the teacher" (Tracy, 1913, p. 10). Whatever their background or training, Tracy (1913) believed that teachers of occupation in hospitals must have similar traits:

> They must possess resourcefulness, unfailing patience, quick perception of capacities and limitations, an enthusiasm which can antic-

ipate for the patient the attractiveness of the finished product and the insight which substitutes a new piece of work or a new phase of the old before the patient is conscious of weariness or distaste. . . . The first requirement then in a teacher for this work is that she be able to understand abnormal conditions. (p. 18)

Tracy (1913) then proceeded to a chapter-by-chapter consideration of methods for the teaching of occupations to children and to patients in restricted positions, in quarantine, able to use only one hand, possessed of waning powers, without sight, and with clouded minds. Regardless of the patient's condition, Tracy believed that the teacher must be "thoughtful of the deeper needs of her patient" (Tracy, 1913, p. 10). She supported empathy because "in a large majority of the cases the trouble is local and the patient is like an animal caught in a trap" (as cited by Licht, 1948). Consideration of deeper needs would benefit patient and nurse alike:

> If a nurse can prove to the patient who chafes against his limitations that there is really a broad highway of usefulness opening before him of which he knew not, the mental friction is diminished and satisfaction steals in, while the whole physical organism prepares to respond by improved conditions. In this connection the effect upon the nurse herself must not be overlooked. She too will forget the tiresome routine. (Tracy, 1913, p. 171)

Almost a decade later, Tracy (1921) was calling occupational therapy a "healing force which should be used whenever possible" (p. 399). She personified occupational therapy:

> Suppose the door (to the hospital) is suddenly opened and Occupational Therapy is permitted to walk swiftly down the corridors to the wards. What is she looking for? If she is wise she is endeavoring to discover the human impulse for activity. It is certainly there. Here is a crowd of loafing, foot-swathed men on the veranda; no impulse to work visible. If work is proposed it may be, and often is, scouted. This is no signal for discouragement.
>
> Of what is this crowd composed? A young house-painter who has fallen hurt from a

staging and is pretty badly hurt. . . . Next a psychopathic patient in bed held in a restraining jacket. . . . Third a man who repairs furniture. Only one of his hands are [sic] available at present. . . . Then, a three-year-old baby with a new arm in place of the one crushed by an automobile. . . . Occupational Therapy sets down her basket.—There is always something interesting for each person. (Tracy, 1921, p. 398)

Tracy served as a nurse under the supervision of doctors and psychiatrists in hospital environments, and she was an instructor of other nurses. She had been exposed to multiple disabilities, she used occupation as a service provider rather than as a patient, and her training in occupations had been in the manual arts. These circumstances no doubt shaped her distinct perspective. She supported the use of occupation on wards with the more acutely ill and bedridden patients as a treatment well suited to a medical setting even in the earliest stages. She saw occupational treatment as a continuum along which the patient might move from bed to shop. She supported the physician's claim to authority in matters of the prescription for occupation, perhaps because the subordinate role in prescription writing was familiar or because the patients whom she wanted to treat were acutely ill. She must have recognized the slim chance of success for a hospital treatment that was not medically prescribed. Possibly, she also believed that her acknowledgment of their authority over occupation would enable physicians to admit, as did Fuller, that it was sometimes the only treatment required.

Tracy supported the employment of crafts teachers and attendants in hospital workshops. She valued occupation for the happiness and changed attitude that it produced and for that attitude's curative effect on disabilities. To Tracy, the *worthwhileness* of handicrafts referred to the quality and purposefulness of the end product, not to its earning power. She saw occupation as a means for the nursing profession to help and care for the whole patient. She emphasized interpersonal traits without which a nurse-teacher could not engage the patient successfully.

Barton and Tracy differed slightly in their understanding of how to provide occupations to patients; the differences relate largely to their respective life experiences. The narratives of other founders and near founders explain the additional facets of our heritage as reflections of their personal perspectives about how occupation might help.

William Rush Dunton, Jr.

Also concerned with the care of hospitalized patients, particularly with patients with mental illness, was William Rush Dunton, Jr., a psychiatrist whose contributions to the early Society can scarcely be enumerated. Dunton responded readily to Barton's suggestion that a national society be established. He was an organizer by nature, having himself founded both the Maryland Psychiatric Society and the Baltimore Physicians Orchestra (Licht, 1967). He was convinced of the merit of occupation in the treatment of persons with mental illness. Early in his 30-year career at Sheppard and Enoch Pratt Hospital, Towson, Maryland, he had discussed the value of occupation with its director, Dr. Edward Brush. In 1912, Brush appointed Dunton in charge of occupation; by 1915 Dunton had published a book on the subject.

Dunton described his early encounter with patients and occupation while he was an assistant physician. At that time, he organized dramatic performances for the patients, thus earning the "sobriquet of Charles Frohman Dunton" (Dunton, 1943, p. 245). He remembered an interaction with one patient:

> At this period we had a scene painter as a patient and I was able by much bossing to make him paint some attractive sets. Each morning he would say: "Won't you let me off today?" And I would harden my heart and refuse. . . . It is probable that in later years I would not have been so brutal in my treatment of my scene-painter patient and I would have drawn him back to his vocation by easy stages, but experientia docet and I wanted new scenery. (Dunton, 1943, p. 245)

Dunton described his concurrent activities: "In order to interest patients I sought various craftsmen, such as bookbinders, leather toolers, and others who were kind enough to show me the rudiments of their craft so that I could by a little practice start a patient on a craft which attracted his interest and helped him on the way to recovery" (Dunton, 1943, p. 246). Dunton's personal experience with occupation deepened his commitment to moral treatment, a treatment practice used by psychiatrists many years before.

Of all the founders, Dunton articulated more than most the belief that his use of occupation constituted an earlier form of treatment that he was simply extending into a new period of history. His practice in a psychiatric hospital enabled his ready access to articles in the *American Journal of Insanity* about moral treatment in the 19th century. As a psychiatrist, he was perhaps eager to claim occupational therapy's roots among his forebears. Much of Dunton's (1919) writing included references to moral treatment. He regretted the passing of moral treatment toward the end of the 19th century:

> It is a strange thing that the physician is so often willing, even anxious, to discard remedies which have proved efficacious in his practice and in that of others, for something new to him and perhaps hitherto untried, so that we have fashions in therapeutics, some of which seem quite as bizarre to us in after years as do those of costume. (p. 17)

Although Dunton accurately identified one factor that contributed to its discontinuance, there were multiple societal, professional, and institutional circumstances that contributed to the demise of moral treatment (Peloquin, 1989; see Chapter 1). Because moral treatment's particular form is not so much at issue here as is the core of its service, my discussion will be broad and brief.

Dunton (1919) cited Sir James Connolly, who in 1813 caught the essence of moral treatment when speaking of the York Retreat in Pennsylvania:

> The substitution of sympathy for gross unkindness, severity, and stripes; the diversion of the mind from its excitements and griefs by various occupations, and a wise confidence in the patients when they promised to control themselves led to the prevalence of order and neatness, and nearly banished furious mania from this wisely devised place of recovery. (p. 21)

Stories of interactions among therapist, patient, and occupation contribute to an understanding of moral treatment. Leuret (1948) shared one:

> I had one patient, an old fiddler, whom I had not been able to draw out. He believed that he was being trailed by the police and consequently did not dare or care to budge. In order to make him rise, walk, or feed himself, entreaty and even compulsion were necessary. I was unable to make further progress with him

until I thought of the violin. I led the patient into the bathing-room, turned on the shower, and at the same time gave him a violin. He had to choose between them. I greatly feared that he would choose the shower. He hesitated for quite some time but finally the memory of his calling returned; he took the violin and played a tune of his choice. . . . Two months after resuming his instrument he was discharged cured, to continue the practice of his calling and for his entire treatment I had used only music. (p. 30)

A more contemporary description of moral treatment is that it was "a grand scheme for activities of daily living, which placed the patient in a total program with the goal of arranging healthy living" (Kielhofner & Burke, 1977, p. 678). Bockoven (1971) indicated that the significant attitudinal features of moral treatment were "respect for human individuality and the rights of individuals. . . and respect for the need of every individual to be engaged in creative and recreational activity with his fellow citizens" (p. 223). Most recently, King (1980) argued that in moral treatment "caring for and caring about the patient was as implicit as occupation" (p. 523).

One must not unduly romanticize the practice of moral treatment. Asylum reports did verify that patients benefitted from individual attention, engagement in a wide variety of occupations, small patient–staff ratios, a family atmosphere, and a system that classified and treated patients according to severity of illness. But the patients' benefit was not the exclusive motivation for the practice. Moral treatment brought prestige to asylums and physicians alike. Systems for the classification of patients and for the involvement of patients in occupations reflected a class and sex bias: wealthy patients had carriage rides while poorer patients labored in the fields. Conceptualizations of the good life were those held by uppermiddle-class physicians who managed the asylums. Patient occupation was also a form of patient labor that helped to maintain the asylum. The particular form that moral treatment took lent itself to some distortions and to its eventual demise (Peloquin, 1989; see Chapter 1). Licht (1948) believed that "the disturbing element of this diminution is that it was world-wide, which points to a basic error in its conduct during that period" (p. 455).

Dunton warned always against repeating late-19th-century distortions of the use of occupation and in an issue of the *American Journal of Occupational Therapy* cited a cautionary segment written in 1892 by his former supervisor, Dr. Brush:

> Occupation is undoubtedly of very great importance in the treatment of the insane, but the idea of occupation which is satisfied by putting a row of twenty dements to picking hair or making fiber matts is as far short of the true aim of occupation as is the attempt to get labor out of cases of acute mania or melancholia already subject to exhaustive changes and waste . . . a misconception of its true value. (as cited by Dunton, 1955, p. 17)

The ideal of moral treatment was that occupations of all kinds be used for the benefit of persons with mental illness. Shaw (1929) reflected early-20th-century thinking about this ideal: "By a new name, an old idea has had rebirth, and is called occupational therapy" (p. 199). The structural invariants of patient, therapist, and occupation mutually acting to improve the patient's condition constitute those strands of the 19th-century idea that Dunton believed the Society had extended into the 20th century.

The extension was timely. Clifford Beers, himself a patient in three mental institutions in Connecticut between 1900 and 1905, had framed a plea for the reform of contemporary abuses. Inhumane conditions after the demise of moral treatment had led Beers to organize the National Committee for Mental Hygiene. Through this organization, Beers (1917) advocated numerous hospital reforms, including individualized care of patients, occupations, recreation, and a more home-like atmosphere.

In the personal chronicle of his experiences, Beers maintained that he had contributed to his own cure through his initiative in engaging himself in reading, writing, and drawing. He often struggled against the system to procure materials with which to occupy himself. When reflecting about the origins of the use of occupation in treatment, Dunton (1921) admitted that "possibly the credit belongs to a number of patients, each one of whom found a tranquilizing influence in work casually undertaken and so continued it in the form originally begun, or in other ways" (p. 11). Dunton thus credited persons such as Beers with having influenced the development of occupational therapy.

The appendix to the 1917 edition of Beers's book details his organizational efforts for institutional reform. He included a letter from Julia Lathrop of Hull House, who had agreed to become an honorary trustee. Lathrop wrote that she had "felt for some time that a national society for the study of insanity and its treatment, from the social as well as the merely medical standpoint, should be formed" (Beers, 1917, p. 326). Lathrop's name is significant in the history of occupational therapy also because of her association with another founder, Eleanor Clarke Slagle. Another letter supporting Beers came from Dr. Adolph Meyer, Director of the Phipps Clinic at Johns Hopkins Hospital in Baltimore. Beers (1917) thanked Meyer, "who, because of his profound knowledge of the scientific, medical and social problems involved, helped more than anyone else" (p. 322). Meyer also worked to support the growth of occupational therapy in substantial ways. He presented a paper entitled "The Philosophy of Occupational Therapy" at the Fifth Annual Meeting of the Society, in which he said:

> A pleasure in achievement, a real pleasure in the use and activity of one's hands and muscles, and a happy appreciation of time began to be used as incentives in the management of our patients, instead of abstract exhortations to cheer up and to behave according to rules. The main advance of the new scheme was the blending of work and pleasure. (Meyer, 1922, pp. 2–3) (See Chapter 4.)

One passage from Beers's (1917) book resembles other passages in which he decried the lack of activity, even in the better institutions:

> For one year no further was paid to me than to see that l had three meals a day, the requisite number of baths, and a sufficient amount of exercise. . . . As I shall have many hard things to say about attendants in general, I take pleasure in testifying that, so long as I remained in a passive condition, those at this institution were kind, and at times even thoughtful. (p. 68)

When Dunton read his paper at the founding meeting of the Society for the Promotion of Occupational Therapy, it consisted of a history filled with references to the use of occupation in antiquity and to the practice of moral treatment. He encouraged the use of work, recreation, and exercise among persons with mental illness by invoking the success of an earlier time (Licht, 1967). Dunton thus responded to the need and push for hospital reform from persons such as Beers by proposing occupational therapy as a viable solution.

The Shaping Force of World War I

William Rush Dunton, Jr., became president at the Second Annual Meeting of the Society in 1918. At that meeting, he outlined the effectiveness of occupational therapy in treating shell shock, and he addressed the need for occupational workers in the war effort. He thought it important to articulate fundamental therapeutic principles, because many persons entering military service erroneously equated skill in handicrafts with occupational therapy (Dunton, 1919). Dunton's contemporaries were divided on the type of training required to teach occupations. Some considered craftsmen suited for the job; others believed that some form of medical training was necessary and that those most qualified were nurses (Licht, 1948). Dunton expressed his personal preference by establishing the first occupational training course for nurses.

Before discussing principles, Dunton (1919) classified occupational work into three types: invalid occupation, occupational therapy, and vocational training. *Invalid occupation,* primarily diversional, was the simplest form of occupational work. It helped recovery by promoting cheerfulness, rest, and freedom from worry. *Occupational therapy* described occupation whose primary object was to restore the patient's mental or physical function. *Vocational training,* although not occupational therapy per se, became so when used to restore function to persons with disabilities (Dunton, 1919). In all cases, Dunton argued that "the primary purpose of occupational therapy [is] cure" (p. 317). He enumerated nine curative principles that he believed essential to each type of occupational work:

1. The work should be carried on with cure as the main object.
2. The work must be interesting.
3. The patient should be carefully studied.
4. One form of occupation should not be carried to the point of fatigue.
5. It should have some useful end.
6. It preferably should lead to an increase in the patient's knowledge.
7. It should be carried on with others.
8. All possible encouragement should be given the worker.
9. Work resulting in a poor or useless product is better than idleness. (p. 320)

Dunton continued to propose that there were different types of occupational work, saying "there are many facets to the gem of occupational therapy and one of them has been humorously expressed" (Dunton, 1930, p. 349). He then recited a poem titled "Decorative Therapeutics," which linked medicine with occupation while also identifying occupational work as a primary therapeutic agent:

Do you wish to lead a healthy, happy life?
Be particular what furnishings you choose.
For there isn't any question
That these things affect digestion
And have much to do with biliousness and blues.

Old candlesticks are excellent for colds,
And pewter is a panacea for pain;
While a pretty taste in china
Has been known to undermine a
Settled tendency to water on the brain.

A highboy is invaluable for hives,
Or a lowboy if you're feeling rather low.
Colonial reproductions
Will allay internal ructions
And are splendid for a case of vertigo.

Old Chippendale is warranted for coughs.
And Heppelwhite is very good for nerves.
If your stomach is unstable
There is nothing like a table,
If it have the proper therapeutic curves.

Decorative therapeutics are the thing
If you happen to be feeling out of whack
We are happy to assure you
That these things are bound to cure you,
For there's virtue in the smallest bric-a-brac.
(Dunton, 1930, p. 350)

Dunton communicated his belief in the power of occupation with a creed that introduced his book on wartime reconstruction therapy:

That occupation is as necessary to life as food and drink. That every human being should have both physical and mental occupation. That all should have occupations which they enjoy. These are more necessary when the vocation is dull or distasteful. Every individual should have at least two hobbies, one outdoor and one indoor. A greater number will create wider interests, a broader intelligence. That sick minds, sick bodies, sick souls, may be healed through occupation. (Dunton, 1919, p. 17)

The philosophical grounding of this creed supports the use of occupation with persons who are well. The concept of health maintenance through occupation constitutes yet another facet of the early legacy.

Dunton (1921a) identified war as a catalyst for clarifying the principles of occupational therapy. Within months of the Society's founding, the United States entered World War 1. This event was important in that (a) the wartime need for occupational workers prompted the founders to more clearly articulate the service that they were promoting, (b) the war actively engaged three of the founders (Dunton, Slagle, and Kidner), and (c) the war validated the successes of occupational therapy. Dunton described the effect: "I can well remember the thrill experienced at the second annual meeting of the National Society for the Promotion of Occupational Therapy, in September, 1918, when it was announced that General Pershing had cabled to send over two thousand more aides as soon as possible" (p. 17).

The war also influenced an early understanding of what type of person was best suited to provide occupation. The first few wartime aides to go overseas had achieved much success. The circumstances of their recruitment and early engagement are fascinating. Dr. Frankwood Williams, then Associate Director of the National Committee for Mental Hygiene, wanted to include occupational workers on his staff for Base Hospital 117. He had gathered a group of women who were ready to serve, but he could not get Washington officials to appoint them. He then noticed openings for civilian aides—scrubwomen with no official connection to the army. He proposed that he get the recruits overseas by identifying them as scrubwomen, and they agreed (Myers, 1948). One of the original aides wrote the following:

The Aides were small in number, but large in optimistic plans for the work ahead—of which we knew practically nothing. Our unit did attend two or three lectures at the Academy of Medicine. . . . There were only four of us to teach handicrafts. (Myers, 1948, p. 209)

Myers (1948) also confirmed the aides' scrubbing tasks on Ellis Island. The nature of the task is important in light of the aides' backgrounds. Cordelia Myers had graduated from Columbia University in New York and was working in the occupational therapy department at Bloomingdale Hospital. Her "scrubwoman" companions were Eleanor Johnson, a psychologist; Amy Drevenstedt, a history teacher at Hunter College; Corrine Dezeller, a Columbia graduate; and Laura LaForce, a graduate nurse (Myers, 1948). Spackman (1968) described these women as skilled teachers of crafts or commercial subjects with no medical background. The aides who followed these pioneers were required to obtain a general education from a secondary school; normal school and college graduates were preferred. The age preference was between 25 and 40 years. Personal qualifications sought were those held by good teachers: knowledge and skill in the particular occupation; attractive, forceful personalities; sympathy; tact; judgment; and industry (Spackman, 1968).

Many schools opened to meet the war emergency and gave basic medical instruction. A sample course of studies lasted 4 months and included lectures on psychology, blindness, hearing problems, orthopedics, subnormal mental conditions, disorders of the central nervous system, and hospital etiquette (Spackman, 1968). Hospital practice was required for half a day per week. Spackman (1968) observed that "the occupational therapists so trained were equipped as teachers of arts and crafts, and not as therapists" (p. 68). Although she did not elaborate, she seemed to regret, as did Dunton, the aides' lack of understanding of curative principles and the superficiality of their medical training. Some courses were more accelerated than the one that Spackman criticized. The Chicago chapter of the Red Cross, for example, gave a 6-week course directed by Eleanor Clarke Slagle at the Henry B. Favill School of Occupations, Illinois Society for Mental Hygiene, Chicago. Twenty young women, most with training in social services or special work in sociology, attended (Dunton, 1919).

A comment from Dunton (1921a), made 3 years after his cautionary note about wartime training, clarified his initial concern:

There not being enough cafeterias to accommodate all the silly society girls who wanted to do war work, and there being a call for occupational therapists, a number of them took emergency training courses and proved their earnestness by sticking through and getting certificates. Those of us concerned with the training of this group found that as a rule they were not silly society girls at all, but were fine, earnest women despite their veneering of silly society girlism. (p. 18)

This comment identifies another force that shaped the determination of who should be occupational therapists at the time: The feeling that occupational therapy was women's work. Aides recruited for the war effort were women. Dunton (1921a) attributed a measure of their success in the war to their sex: "It had been found that the presence of energetic women who went through the wards of hospitals stimulating the patients to occupy themselves making things had had a wonderful effect in keeping up the morale of the patients" (p. 17).

Dunton was not alone in this belief. A writer for *Carry On,* a war journal reporting reconstruction efforts, argued that women alone could have a powerful effect on the recovery of injured soldiers:

To prevent his losing hope, to keep his sense of responsibility is in the power of his womankind. . . . In every step the help of women is essential; not only in cheering him during the first stages, but in encouraging him to follow patiently and exactly the detail of his training. . . .The recovery of our disabled soldiers—their return to a useful life—is in the control of the women of this country. (Miller, 1918, pp. 17–18)

The rationale for this endorsement of women was the belief that a man's state of mind reflected that of his wife or his mother. The writer was a woman expressing a common view that women created a moral refuge for their men, sustaining their spirits so that they could return refreshed to the world of men. These female reconstruction aides returned to the United States to join the ranks of other occupational therapists.

Few studies in the literature that I reviewed for this inquiry suggested that nurses complained that this advanced form of nursing had been snatched from them. Reverby (1987) noted that the scarcity of nurses during the war "brought nursing more damnation than blessings" (p. 163). Her reference, however, was not to a loss of the use of occupation, but to the war's having contributed to an increase in the number of country girls training as "subnurses" (p. 163).

The wartime shift away from a conviction that nurses made the best occupational workers may well have

strengthened the belief that a physician should prescribe occupation; someone had to know medical conditions in depth. Dunton (1919) offered another reason for medical supervision:

If the [occupation] director has not had medical training it has been found that there will be a lack of sympathy between the medical staff and the occupational department so that this valuable therapeutic agent is not used so well as it should be. . . . For this reason alone, if for no other, it is believed that the director should be one of the senior physicians, who should at rounds, conferences, and elsewhere, instruct the juniors as to the value of occupation. (p. 55)

Dunton's argument for a physician's use and support of occupation reflected his role as the president of a society founded to promote occupation. His argument that the physiciandirector should train the staff and the teachers, arrange for the purchase of supplies, and supervise the shops seems consistent with a desire to replicate the managerial control held by physicians in the Moral Treatment era.

Dunton's (1919) estimation of the personal qualities required of the occupational director included tact, the "precious gift of inspiring others," knowledge of the psychology of everyday life, interest in occupation as therapy, "fertility of invention," and an artistic sense of form (pp. 43–45). These traits paralleled those thought necessary for occupational nurses and craft teachers. Physician-directors would provide a service centered on occupation and similar to that provided by nonphysicians.

The war also nurtured an idea of the kind of patient-therapist relationship that worked in occupational therapy. A soldier revealed the quality of the service that he as a patient experienced:

I got a new vision of life. . . . I saw that men made unfit for the work of the past must be equipped for work in the future . . . saw the dignity of labor made new and interesting, and even more powerful because of the handicap. (Cooper, 1918, p. 24)

The biography of Ora Ruggles, a reconstruction aide, chronicled this kind of service. Ruggles, a school teacher who had graduated from San Diego Normal School and had taken additional courses in the manual arts, responded to the war call for crafts experts. She quickly integrated the importance of engaging the interest and the heart of each patient. Physicians and administrators acknowledged her accomplishments. Ruggles's competence, warmth, and concern inspired awe, loyalty, and gratitude in her patients. She creatively adapted activities that allowed even patients with the most severe disabilities to succeed. Without having been trained to apply them, she understood many of the principles of occupational therapy:

> By now, Ora and the other reconstruction aides were keenly attuned to the word useful. It was a vital key to what they were trying to do. Whenever possible, they thought up projects that the patients could see had tangible use, particularly for the outside world, the world of the well. In this way they could literally work themselves to the level of the normal world. (Carlova & Ruggles, 1946, p. 81)

Ruggles summed up the essence of her view of service: "It is not enough to give a patient something to do with his hands. You must reach for the heart as well as the hands. It's the heart that really does the healing" (Carlova & Ruggles, 1946, pp. 249–250).

If the war shaped conceptualizations of the patient–therapist relationship, it acted similarly on the meaning of occupation. The founders' idea of prewar services was that occupation could be an effective treatment that would enable occupation after recovery. Occupation could serve both as the means and the goal of treatment. The wartime experience of occupational work affirmed this assumption while also emphasizing "the physical side of occupational therapy" (Dunton, 1919, p. 56). Wartime occupational therapy, often called *curative work*, was prescribed to "restore usefulness, overcome deformities or teach to the remaining portion of a limb or another member new functions" (Mock, 1919, p. 12). War injuries focused attention on the use of occupation to restore the patient to a functional condition.

During the war years, Frank Gilbreth had operationalized the efficiency principle of "fitting the machine to the man"; he designed numerous work adaptations that occupational therapists readily implemented as part of the goal of returning the patient to useful occupation (Dunton, 1919, p. 107). Dunton's (1919) book entitled *Reconstruction Therapy* contained several of Gilbreth's

photographs of men wearing prostheses (e.g., the Amar claw, the Carnes artificial arm, and the Hanger leg). The book also included photographs of men using self-help devices for dressing, doing farm work, and driving a car. If the disabled person could be equipped with some adaptive device that would facilitate accomplishing the task, the occupational therapist would modify the instructions accordingly. The idea seemed a logical extension of the founders' views. If the prosthetic device were considered part of the person, and occupational therapy taught the whole person, then teaching its use became part of teaching the person. Conversely, if the device were considered a tool required to get the job done, then teaching its use would be inherent in teaching the occupation. One is struck by photographs of men wearing hooks and gadgets, crude by today's standards. The devices permitted a restorative role for the machine that otherwise excelled at maiming, wounding, or dehumanizing. The machine advanced into treatment to touch the patient.

The language of science peppered the occupational therapy literature during the war years. It had been there before, both in the group's plea that occupations be taught with the best scientific methods and in the scientific aims articulated by the original Society. The war experience operationalized this philosophy with methods that appeared to be scientific. Dunton (1919) mused about the many terms describing occupational therapy at the time and thought the term *ergotherapy* the best and the most scientific. He thought it "a very simple matter to trace the development of occupational therapy from simple tasks and amusements to the more scientific occupational therapy or re-education applied to all forms of mental and physical disability" (p. 29). Dunton believed that a scientific evolution was evident in the growing number of studies on occupation, such as the one conducted by Kent at the Government Hospital in Washington, DC. Kent's study suggested that "definite practice effects can be obtained, by means of a short series of tests, from advanced cases of dementia praecox" among female patients (pp. 30–32).

The belief that occupational therapy's problems needed to be framed in a scientific manner appeared early in the literature. Dunton (1919) argued that much remained to be done before occupational therapy could be considered an exact science. He hoped that the task would attract the attention of the research worker:

> There are many difficulties to be encountered, chiefly centered about the emotional reaction

of the patient. Why does one form of work, say carpentry, appeal to one man and not to another, when they are apparently of similar mental caliber and from the same social level? . . . In all probability the answer lies somewhere in the associative activities, but how can we most quickly stimulate the association which will give us the best co-operation of the patient? (pp. 30–31)

Occupational therapists were interested in answers to questions about how people learned; they were teachers of occupations. They were also concerned with human motivation because so much of their service consisted of interesting the patient in occupation (Mock, 1919, p. 13). Not surprising]y, much of the early literature about occupational therapy included discussions of recent developments in education and psychology. The war experience directed the application of occupations within the context of the growing body of knowledge in arenas related to teaching occupations and in the increasing use of technology designed to enhance individual functioning. The war challenged the founders to examine their service within this context in terms of both immediate applications and unanswered questions.

Eleanor Clarke Slagle

Eleanor Clarke Slagle completed a course given by Julia Lathrop at the Chicago School of Civics and Philanthropy. Lathrop had pursued Beers's (1917) cause for reform in treating persons with mental illness by designing a course in curative occupations and recreations for attendants and nurses in institutions and by resigning from the State Board of Control in Illinois in 1908 to protest poor conditions in that state. Most patients in Illinois state hospitals at that time sat idly through each day, with an able few engaging in hospital industries that consisted of monotonous work designed to help the hospital (American Occupational Therapy Association, 1940). After completing Lathrop's course in 1911, Slagle taught a similar course in Michigan. She then went to the Phipps Psychiatric Clinic of the Johns Hopkins Hospital, Baltimore, to direct the occupational therapy department under the supervision of Dr. Adolph Meyer.

Meyer had experienced occupational conditions similar to those seen by Slagle and had also supported Beers in his reform efforts. He described "industrial shops and work in the laundry and kitchen and on the wards . . .

very largely planned to relieve the employees" (Meyer, 1922, p. 2 [see Chapter 4]). At the Phipps Clinic, he "secured the services of Mrs. Slagle," whose efforts he acknowledged as having positively contributed "to the level [then] represented at the Phipps Clinic" (Meyer, 1922, p. 4). While at the Phipps Clinic, Slagle gave 3week courses on occupation to groups of nurses in training at the Johns Hopkins Hospital. The instructions included both occupations and the principles underlying their use (Dunton, 1921b). She discussed with Dunton her ideas about their new form of therapy (Licht, 1967).

Slagle returned to Chicago in 1915 to establish the Henry B. Favill School of Occupations and directed the school from 1918 to 1922. She had taken courses in social work and had worked with Meyer, who advocated "the creation of an orderly rhythm in the atmosphere" of the hospital (Meyer, 1922, p. 6 [see Chapter 4]). These influences shaped Slagle's perspective: She taught habit training through occupation. She selected severely regressed and chronically ill patients for her training program. It is not surprising that she started habit training with this group, because Meyer had characterized the patient with dementia praecox as "suffering from disorganized habits" (Wilson, 1929, p. 189). An original principle of occupational therapy permeates the concept of habit training: Occupations could be useful and curative by fostering their habitual use among patients with mental illness.

In habit training, small groups of patients were given close supervision throughout the day. They followed a carefully designed schedule that included self-care and personal hygiene, occupational class, walks, meals in small groups, recreational activities, and physical exercise. Each patient was encouraged to get into a routine and then to assume responsibility for that routine. Excerpts from one care report on a patient convey a sense of the personal service that Slagle initiated:

May 3, 1926—Admitted to habit training. Will not dress or undress self. Clothing untidy and unbuttoned. Mute. Will not wash self. Wets and soils the bed. Eats excessively. Masturbation frequent.

June to June 30, 1926—Washes and dresses self. Wets and soils less frequently. Polishes floor when continuously supervised. Does lowgrade occupation.

July 10 to September 22, 1926—Speaks occasionally. Told superintendent that he was "slightly improved." Works on braid-weave rug. Helps attendant with cleaning and clears dishes from table at meals. Appetite more normal. (Wilson, 1929, pp. 196–197).

Physicians like Charles Vaux (1929) believed that habit training caused a "turning point that started [patients] on the road to recovery" (p. 329). He regretted that other physicians found it difficult to accept this "new viewpoint" and "work of reclamation" (p. 328). Slagle's reclamation work with occupation extended to those patients considered beyond the reach of contemporary treatments.

Slagle did not believe that the director of occupation had to be a physician, having herself assumed that role. She indicated that the "capability of such a person involved not only arts and crafts training, but, and most chiefly, personality and character" (Slagle, 1927, p. 126). Although she insisted on solid knowledge of materials and processes, she emphasized the personal element:

> For, if lacking in this—in understanding, in give and take, in spiritual vision of the "end problem" of all too many of the cases, the craftsman may make some initial showing, but the work will eventually flag and be largely a failure. (Slagle, 1927, p. 126)

Given her early training in social work, Slagle's belief in the therapist's personal influence made sense. An early conceptualization in social work held that the social worker's (or friendly visitor's) character and his or her relationship with the patient together constituted the agent of change.

Although she did not believe that the director of occupations should be a physician, Slagle sought medical authority in occupational prescriptions. She believed that the physician should prescribe at least the kind of occupation needed, "such as stimulating, sedative, mechanical, intellectual, academic or varied" (Slagle, 1927, p. 128). She argued that all therapeutic measures were the responsibility of the physician in charge. Her definition of occupational therapy included a medical metaphor: "It is directed activity and differs from all other forms of treatment in that it is given in increasing doses as the patient's condition improves" (Slagle as cited by Hull, 1931, p. 219).

Slagle regarded her 3-week training courses as an orientation to nurses about the merits of occupation rather than training in what they might themselves do. She believed that although some nurses completed a period of service in an occupational therapy department, "this did not mean that the nurse would become a specialist. . .but that she would become acquainted with the nature and possibilities" of the therapy (Slagle, 1927, p. 129). Slagle included attendants in habit training, much as Tracy (1913) had endorsed their direct involvement in invalid occupation with medically stable patients.

Slagle was a leader. She was described as "a woman whose presence was felt by all who were in her company. She was regally tall and there were those who found that some of her pronouncements were in keeping with her appearance and bearing" (Licht, 1967, p. 271). Ruggles remembered Slagle's inspiring words during a personally difficult time. Slagle had told Ruggles that the occupational therapy movement needed her to "get behind it and push!" (Carlova & Ruggles, 1946, p. 113). This urging prompted Ruggles to return to service. Elected vice-president at the first Society meeting, Slagle eventually held every office in the Association and did so for a longer period than anyone else (Licht, 1967). She also agreed to direct occupational therapy for the Illinois Department of Mental Hygiene (Smith, 1929).

Slagle's leadership was exceptional. Men held the highest positions of authority in those early years. In treatment, occupational therapists deferred to physicians, who were predominantly men; in promotional and organizational efforts, men were most often elected to the highest position. The view that women were most effective with patients shaped a leadership pattern that placed men in administrative and supervisory roles and made Slagle's leadership remarkable. (Editor's note: See Appendix I.B for Adolf Myer's address in honor of Eleanor Clark Slagle.)

Herbert J. Hall

Licht (1967) reported that although Dunton had nominated Dr. Herbert J. Hall for inclusion at the founding meeting, Barton rejected his nomination. Because Hall was nearly selected, because his involvement with occupation was widely cited by the other founders, and because he assumed leadership roles early in the Society's history, Hall's views can be considered, like Tracy's, to be those of a near founder.

As early as 1904, Hall was prescribing occupation as a means of regulating his patients' lives (Hopkins, 1978).

In 1906, Harvard University awarded him a grant to study the use of occupation in the treatment of neurasthenia. As a part of this grant project, Hall established an experimental workshop in Marblehead, Massachusetts. In a presidential address to the Society in 1921, he characterized the workshop as an experimental laboratory that addressed the technical problems of occupational therapy. The Society officially accepted his project as the Medical Workshop.

Hall's vision of service provided yet another understanding of the helping potential of occupation:

> The writer of these chapters undertook ten years ago to meet in a small way the needs of a class of people who were not in actual want but who from illness or the overstrain of modern life had been obliged to give up their usual occupations. (Hall & Buck, 1915)

Hall reached out to single young people, "nervous invalids" who had "gone to pieces" from a lack of "depth and substance in their lives" (p. 57). Hall believed that these persons learned something of the dignity and satisfaction of "work with the hands" when engaged in occupation (Hall & Buck, 1915, p. 58). His goal was to simplify life through occupations that could rest the mind. One recognizes Hall's concurrence with contemporary criticisms of the "strain of modern life" (Upham, 1917, p. 409). One can also recognize Hall's support of a popular view of "women's work." He believed that the absence of home-like occupations and nurturing functions caused problems among single women; these could be remedied with occupations that substituted one means of creative satisfaction for another.

Another of Hall's unique views was that industries should be established specifically for persons with disabilities. Although he urged the development of workshops within hospitals, he believed that a further step was necessary. Because "the regular industries could not change their rules and systems for the sake of giving him employment . . . the way out seems to lie in the establishing of special industries where the handicapped may be favored" (Hall & Buck, 1915, pp. xiii, xiv). Hall predicted a time when hospitals and sanatoriums would recognize the value of remunerative occupation for their patients and would conduct industries as adjunctive treatments (Hall & Buck, 1915). Hospital workshops and industries would help the patient take a first step toward later employment in special industries for disabled persons; there would be a continuum of restorative occupation. He described with deep feeling the patient who would otherwise face a life of idleness and dependence: "Put yourself in that man's place—imagine the despair and the final degeneration that must sap at last all that is brave and good in life" (Hall & Buck, 1915, p. viii).

Barton (1914) thought well of Hall's views because he thought that they represented a nonmedical orientation. Hall argued, however, for medical involvement in the use of occupations. He recommended the use of a prescription for occupation, providing illustrative models:

> May 1, 1914
> Occupation Work
> Mrs. X—Room 50
> Light occupation in bed
> Basketry or knitting
> Not more than 1 hour daily
> [Physician's name], MD (Hall & Buck, 1915, p. 76)

Hall (1921) called occupational therapy the "science of prescribed work" (p. 245). He believed that there had previously been a "fatal gap" in medicine that had released the patient cured but "totally unfit because of weakness or discouragement, to take his place immediately among competitive labor" (p. 245). He believed that nurses and social workers needed training in the use of work as treatment and in 1908 provided such training at the Devereaux Mansion, Marblehead, Massachusetts (Hopkins, 1978).

Hall differed from other founders in his belief that the medical diagnosis and the patient's problems should remain unknown to the teacher of occupations. He argued that "work was one of the few normal habits left to the patient, and the nearer he could approach to health in his relations with the teacher the better" (Hall & Buck, 1915, p. 77). Only an unbiased teacher could relate normally with the patient. He further believed that medical information might be easily misunderstood and misapplied by nonmedical personnel. He argued that the ideal teacher would be a nurse serving under a craftsman, because the doctor could then share information necessary for dealing with the "whole problem" (Hall & Buck, 1915, p. 55).

Hall sought teachers with traits that enabled a low-conflict interpersonal approach. He thought that individualized teaching was important (Hall & Buck, 1915). He reasoned that "praise for effort should be given ungrudgingly; but praise of results should not be too lavish" (Hall & Buck, 1915, p. 87). He thought it wise to allow the patient a "liberty of choice" (Hall & Buck, 1915, p. 88). He believed that special effort was the hallmark of caring. As an example, he discussed the case of a choreic boy, aged 11 years, who had at first been dull and discouraged in occupation. The boy had eventually recovered the use of his hands. Hall associated his recovery with the fact that "the teacher took pains to show him exactly how to use his hands, and he gradually became quite expert in fretsawing and other crafts" (Hall & Buck, 1915, pp. 138–139). Special, individualized effort had made the difference. If a teacher had to address a patient's symptoms directly, as in the case of a neurasthenic patient, Hall (Hall & Buck, 1915) hoped that she would "use tact as well as skill" (pp. 138–139). She should also be flexible, using "common sense in the application of all rules" (Hall & Buck, 1915, pp. 168–169). Hall (1921) believed that this profile created a new field for women:

> We are at the beginning of a new profession for educated women. The actual work must be done for the most part by women. Feminine tact and perseverance alone can be depended upon to break down the barriers of prejudice, and to secure the cooperation of difficult patients. (p. 246)

Hall (1921) elaborated on his meaning, while also qualifying the nature of the prejudice he described:

> The theory is so divertingly simple that we may fall easily into error, and fail to realize that we are concerned with the very sources of human power. . . . Occupational therapy is a means to an end. Some of its proceedings may seem trivial, but they gain in importance through the opportuneness of their application. Practice in this field is not so simple as it looks. All the ingenuity in the world may not be sufficient to overcome the shiftlessness, the hopelessness, the lack of ambition, the evasion, the prejudice which stands in the way. (p. 245)

Hall joined the other founders in recognizing occupation as one of the sources of human power.

Susan Cox Johnson

Susan Cox Johnson studied and taught high school arts and crafts in Berkeley, California. In 1912, she traveled in the Orient, eventually residing in the Philippines to teach crafts for 2 years. On her return, she accepted a position in the Hospital of New York City on Blackwell's Island and also agreed to direct the occupations committee for the Department of Public Charities of New York State. In this capacity, she aimed to prove that occupations could improve the mental and physical condition of patients and inmates in public hospitals and almshouses, that these persons could contribute to their selfsupport, and that occupation could be morally uplifting (Licht, 1967, p. 276). Her aim embodied her belief in the curative and restorative potential of occupation, a belief that was invariant among all the founders.

Johnson's work impressed Barton, who believed that she had "by all odds the most important job in the world, together with a very level head, a keen insight, good experience and a tremendous interest in the therapeutic side" (Reed & Sanderson, 1983, p. 196). Dunton had submitted Johnson's name for inclusion in the Society after Barton's rejection of Hall; Barton had readily agreed to her inclusion (Licht, 1967, p. 271). Shortly after the establishment of the Society and the United State's entrance into war, Columbia University in New York invited Johnson to teach occupational therapy in their nursing department. She accepted the position and soon directed the course (Licht, 1967). She simultaneously organized and directed an occupational therapy department at Montefiore Home and Hospitals, New York.

Five of Johnson's articles published in *Modern Hospital* addressed the training of personnel and the function of occupational therapy in the hospital (Reed & Sanderson, 1983). Her continued emphasis on the reeducational aspect of work and on the educational requirements for practitioners reflected her teaching background. Johnson shared the concerns of her cofounders about educational prerequisites. She regretted a "difference of opinion among those who are working with the same end in view" (Johnson, 1919, p. 221). She wrote:

> What seems to be a difference . . . is often not a real difference at all, but is a misunderstanding due to our failure to keep always before us the several natural divisions of our work and the different purposes of each, as well as the fact that each must overlap and merge one into the other instead of being separate and aloof. No standards for training teachers can be set with-

out the recognition of these different elements. (Johnson, 1919, p. 221)

Johnson (1919) believed that teaching occupations to invalids differed from other teaching; there was need to "plan with much greater consideration for the individual than is done in any system of instruction under normal conditions" (p. 221). She outlined various training programs suitable for working with specific populations. She reasoned that persons teaching invalid occupations in a hospital needed more understanding and training in handling sick people, whereas those teaching in curative workshops or outpatient shops needed more educational courses, because their teaching would "fall into more nearly normal lines" (p. 222).

Johnson's arguments resembled Tracy's. She believed strongly that the educational curriculum mattered; the "great field of occupation would never bear full fruit until the dignity and importance of the position of the teacher in this field is recognized" (Johnson, 1919, p. 223). She thought it "dangerous" that the pendulum might swing toward "losing sight of the nursing aspect of the work of the teacher" (Johnson, 1919, p. 223). She predicted that there would "always be a problem keeping a definite middle path between the nursing and teaching aspects of this work" (Johnson, 1919, p. 223).

Johnson (1919) recognized that the debate over suitable therapists' qualifications had escalated during the war:

> The idea that it was desirable to have teachers specially trained for this work and that they could well be nonmedical people was just coming to be accepted when the avalanche of war necessity descended upon us. The great demand for nurses and the need for numbers of teachers in this field swept occupations out of the hands of the nurse without further discussion and made necessary either the absorption of a foreign group into the hospital regime or the discard of the whole idea of using occupation for a therapeutic purpose. (p. 221)

Johnson (1919) urged occupational workers to resolve the conundrum of suitable training, and in so doing to balance the need for specialized skills against the need for skills required across all settings. She believed that all teachers of occupation needed "an understanding of the psychology of both normal and abnormal minds" and a grounding "in the principles and methods of teaching the sick," regardless of their practice settings (p. 222).

Johnson argued that the product of the patient's work should be of high quality. Her emphasis on "maintaining high standards in the products of occupation" seems reasonable after so many years teaching and learning crafts (Johnson, 1919, p. 223). Recognizing that the field was in a "formative period," she cautioned against any hasty standardization, but encouraged the Society to instead provide "practical aid to the teacher in maintaining the best standards in products" (Johnson, 1919, p. 223). She perhaps supported the Society's establishment in 1920 of an occupational therapy bureau in Boston to investigate the market and the wholesale purchase of staples to sell at a low price to occupational therapy departments everywhere (Hall, 1921).

Johnson's background distinguished her from many other founders. Her views and questions, born of her personal competencies, pushed for a balanced view of occupational therapy as a part-medical, part-teaching function.

Thomas Bessell Kidner

Barton invited Thomas Bessell Kidner to the founding meeting because Kidner resided in Canada and thus would give the Society an international flavor (Reed & Sanderson, 1983). Kidner's foreign status was not the exclusive criterion for his selection, however. In 1915, he had been appointed Vocational Secretary to the Canadian Military Hospitals to develop a vocational rehabilitation system. Before that, Kidner had established a number of technical educational programs in various Canadian provinces. Dunton described Kidner's chief aims in life as being "to prevent the convalescent soldier from falling into habits of idleness and self-indulgence, to educate the crippled soldier in some vocation by which he can support himself" (Dunton, 1967, p. 288).

Like Barton, Kidner had been trained as an architect. He included several architectural drawings in his journal articles that detailed the planning of occupational therapy departments. Kidner served as president of the Society for six terms (Licht, 1967). Barton (1968) described Kidner as "outgoing in expressing his enthusiasm about the use of occupation, a fascinating personality, so very British, even the tailoring of his morning coat, striped trousers, winged collar and tie" (p. 345).

During Kidner's presidency in 1923, the American Occupational Therapy Association (formerly known as the Society for the Promotion of Occupational Therapy) adopted an official insignia, which included a caduceus, and made this insignia available for use by Association members (Kidner, 1923; "Occupational Therapists Meet Again With A.H.A.," 1923). The pin symbolically fixed the affiliation of this new service to that of medicine.

Kidner (1923) spoke often about the progress of occupational therapy and the growing valuation of "curative work in practically every kind of disability" (p. 55). He reminded therapists that the Industrial Rehabilitation Act of 1920 had extended the use of occupation to many hospitals:

> Indeed, I think it is fair to say that many hospitals have had their attention drawn to the value of occupational therapy by the federal and state industrial rehabilitation authorities who are doing their best to place persons disabled by accident or disease in industry. (p. 500)

Kidner also credited the Act with introducing curative work into many new non-hospital-based service arenas. One new arena was the world of homebound persons, whom Kidner (1924) described as "the product of industrial accidents" (p. 500). Kidner (1923) estimated that the number of persons disabled by industrial and other accidents annually equaled the number of those who might be disabled in an army of 1.5 million men active in the field. He believed that the great number of disabled persons and the consequent "growth and development of occupational therapy naturally led to the evolution of standards" (Kidner, 1929b, p. 243).

In 1923, the year in which the standards were developed, the officers of the Association were mostly men; one of the three was a physician. Slagle was the only woman, reelected secretary–treasurer. Of the eight persons elected to the Board of Managers of the Association, five were physicians ("Occupational Therapists Meet Again With A.H.A.," 1923). In response to a growing interest in securing occupational therapists, "several doctors called the attention of the American Occupational Therapy Association" to the hurried wartime educational programs that gave "practically nothing more than instruction in simple manual arts" (Kidner, 1929b, p. 244). A committee that included physicians studied the problem of occupational therapy education; the membership then adopted a statement of

minimum standards at their annual meeting (Kidner, 1930). These first educational standards for training in occupational therapy further shaped the early characterization of the occupational therapist.

The standards outlined prerequisites for candidates and curriculum content. Admission to a training course required at least a high school education or its equivalent. A year's special training in some related field such as applied art, crafts, social service, or advanced academic work was desirable. Successful employment or experience could replace time spent in training school or some other educational institution (Kidner, 1924). The training course had to last a minimum of 12 months, with no less than 6 hours of work and lectures daily. The year's course had to include no less than 8 months of theoretical and practical work and no less than 3 months of hospital practice training and supervision. The official statement required that adequate instruction be given in (a) psychology, normal and abnormal; (b) anatomy, kinesiology, and orthopedics; (c) mental diseases; (d) tuberculosis; and (e) general medical cases, including cardiac diseases. At least 1,080 hours were required in practical handiwork such as "woodworking, weaving, basketry, metal work and jewelry, drawing and applied design" (Kidner, 1924, p. 55). The standards also required lectures on work in several types of hospitals, the principles of hospital management, hospital ethics, the history and development of curative occupations, arts and crafts in relation to the development of civilization, modern industry and the factory system, and the relation of occupational therapy to vocational rehabilitation (Kidner, 1929b).

Course titles and recommended lectures did not specifically include the principles for use of occupation that had been endorsed by Dunton, then serving on the Board of Managers. Neither did the listing include occupations such as habit training or recreational activities. These omissions are of interest because Kidner (1923) mentioned that "the original group of incorporators of the association [except Barton, who was deceased] continued active in its affairs" ("Occupational Therapists Meet Again With A.H.A.," 1923, p. 500). Among those persons with the greatest investment in the inclusion of their own perspectives, none disputed the minimum standards. Kidner (1924) did mention the existence of various views (p. 55) and suggested that the standards would warrant upcoming revisions, probably to increase their rigor. His summative statement that the standards "provided a fair and workable basis for the training of occupational therapists, and . . . represented the consensus of opinion on the subject of the great majority of those interested" (p. 55) suggests comfort with the standards. Kidner (1924) explained that "the board of managers endeavored to avoid the Scylla of placing the requirements so high that too few students would undertake the training, and, on the other hand, the Charybdis of lowering the standards of the work" (p. 55). Comprehensive requirements, although ideal, might stymie the development of a new group of therapists.

Whatever the rationale for the minimal curriculum, the standards purported to train the early therapist as both a medical worker and a crafts instructor, thereby resolving the question of which function, that of nurse or teacher, was more important. The occupational therapist had to be a bit of both. The therapist would understand the hospital world and the authority that the physician held in that world, and he or she would perform his or her service within that context. The therapist would be an instructor in crafts whose real end product would be a restored person.

Kidner (1924) detailed the end product of occupational therapy. He cautioned against misconstruing the value of occupation as the "making of a more or less useful and attractive object" for sale (p. 57). He reminded the membership that the "real value of curative work lay in the result obtained in the patient" (p. 57). He believed that to construe the "incidental products of occupational therapy to be the end and aim of treatment" was to not appreciate "the real meaning and significance of work" (Kidner, 1929b, p. 243). Although not acknowledged as such in the literature, Kidner's reminder might have constituted a redirection of members, trained primarily in handiwork, toward a valuation of the work process.

Kidner (1929a) spoke often of rehabilitation. When addressing graduating students, he shared his conception of the quality of service that they ought to provide:

> In your chosen field, a part of the noblest work of man—the care and relief of weak and suffering humanity—may you realize in increasing measure the value of certain spiritual things which are the real making of life, but which we call by many common names. Kindness, humanity, decency, honor, good faith—to give these up under any circumstances whatever would be a loss greater than any defeat, or even death itself. (p. 385)

Concern for the patient and for the quality of his or her personal relationship with the therapist wove

through Kidner's statements on standards, medical affiliation, and the curative goal of occupation. Kidner contributed much to legacy. In a memorial tribute, Dunton (1932) characterized Kidner's connection with occupational therapy as a "bond of interest in advancing a body of knowledge of occupational therapy" that "grew into a firm friendship which death has ended" (p. 195).

National Society for the Promotion of Occupational Therapy

Each of the founders contributed a unique perspective to the multifaceted service that constituted occupational therapy. The founders also shaped the early service when acting collectively as the Society. Early signs of this collective shaping appeared at the first meeting. The certificate of incorporation of the National Society for the Promotion of Occupational Therapy identified its objectives for "the advancement of occupation as a therapeutic measure; for the study of the effect of occupation upon the human being; and for the scientific dispensation of this knowledge" (Reed & Sanderson, 1983, p. 272). Concerns for science, for humanity, and for the advancement of this new therapy were clear. To operationalize their objectives and to recruit additional members to the Society, the founders appointed each other to chair six district committees: Barton, the Committee on Research and Efficiency; Slagle, the Committee on Installations and Advice; Dunton, the Committee on Finance, Publicity, and Publication; Johnson, the Committee on Admissions and Positions; Tracy, the Committee on Teaching Methods; and Kidner, the International Committee (Dunton, 1967). Barton outlined the plan:

> Let each member, that is, each chairman of a standing committee select from his own acquaintances four others who will become members of the committee and of the society at the next meeting. . . . Then for the next step—let special subjects be assigned to each member of the society, or rather to the 20 new members, according to the strength, interest, and ability of the individual member. Then let each of these members secure from his personal friends four others to be members of his subcommittee. . . . Thus the work will "pyramid." (Barton as cited by Licht, 1967, p. 272)

The plan virtually assured the perpetuation of the varied perspectives of the founders as well as the common objectives of the Society. It enabled the growth of special interest groups with a central interest in promoting occupation as therapy.

In 1921, Hall, then president, had suggested that the name of the Society be replaced by the "crisper and more descriptive" American Occupational Therapy Association (Reed & Sanderson, 1983, p. 182). Simultaneously, the larger membership generated by the pyramid plan adopted a new constitution that established two governing bodies—a Board of Managers and a House of Delegates. The House of Delegates voted in 1922 to hold the meetings of the American Occupational Therapy Association in conjunction with those of the American Hospital Association so that hospital executives might better understand occupational therapy (Reed & Sanderson, 1983). These joint meetings promoted occupational therapy while also sealing its affiliation with physicians and its practice in hospitals. The lectures on hospital management and ethics required by the 1923 standards affirmed this liaison.

In 1922, Hall articulated the goals of the Association and the service that it promoted:

> The association is a responsible, incorporated body with officers of large experience, and active committees encouraging research, collecting data and recommending standards. It seems reasonable to assert that here is a work of national importance, a human reclamation service touching vitally on matters of vast social and economic consequence. Mere encouragement, even placement in industry cannot restore men and women who have not learned through careful bedside training how to use their disabled bodies. The association is literally helping the helpless to help themselves. (pp. 164–165)

Much of the spirit and vitality of the individual founders permeates the statement.

When the official insignia was accepted in 1923, the House of Delegates also voted to establish a national registry, a measure that Kidner had promoted during his presidency. Numerous physicians had sought to secure the registration of occupational workers before 1921. The opinion of Dr. Salmon, a psychiatrist, is representative:

> We badly need a list of qualified workers in this field to which a hospital superintendent could refer with as much assurance in finding correct information with regard to an applicant for a position in an occupational therapy department as he could refer to the directory of the American Medical Association for the information regarding a doctor. (Salmon as cited by Kidner, 1929b, p. 245)

The Society's cooperation with physicians parallels that found in personal narratives of the founders. The early Association strived to cooperate with a number of groups. It endorsed a service that extended not only to the disabled patient and his or her family, but also to physicians, hospital managers, employers, and members of the scientific community. This accountability to many persons structured the Pledge and Creed for Occupational Therapists submitted by the Boston School and adopted by the Association in 1926:

> Reverently and earnestly do I pledge my wholehearted service in aiding those crippled in mind and body. To this end that my work for the sick may be successful, I will strive for greater knowledge, skill and understanding in the discharge of my duties in whatsoever position I may find myself.
>
> I solemnly declare that I will hold and keep whatever I may learn of the lives of the sick. I acknowledge the dignity of the cure of disease and the safeguarding of health in which no act is menial or inglorious.
>
> I will walk in upright faithfulness and obedience to those under whose guidance I am to work, and I pray for patience, kindliness and strength in the holy ministry to broken minds and bodies. (as cited by Welles, 1976, p. 45)

After an exploration of their personal understandings and stories, we can almost hear the voices of Barton, Tracy, Dunton, Slagle, Hall, Johnson, and Kidner reciting this creed.

Other than the writings of Barton, who was himself disabled, there was little written by patients about the early years of occupational therapy service. One article, "A Patient Looks at Occupational Therapy," written anonymously in 1930, is noteworthy. It coincides with what I consider the end of the early years. The patient wrote:

> It is hard when the rudiments of many crafts must be mastered . . . to keep the fuller vision of all that

occupational therapy does and must mean if we are to be really helpful to those who need us. . . . The broader and more inclusive our outlook as to the wholesome interest in real things the more helpful and effective our work. (p. 277)

Conclusion

This inquiry has supported a broad view of the nature of occupational therapy's early service: that the right occupation could resolve many problems, and that the patient, therapist, and occupation could interrelate therapeutically. These understandings of the founders reflect their sensitivity to the problems and issues of their times, that is, hospital care, industrialization, and war. Also reflected are the founders' responses to contemporary trends toward science, education, sexual stereotyping, and professionalization. Both individual narratives and the collective activities of the Society support Yerxa's (1980) claim that the heritage of occupational therapy includes a focus on care and function. To use occupation as a way of helping persons live their lives in a way that is meaningful to them is to care about persons and about function.

The heritage of occupational therapy was shaped by numerous societal forces and historical events that enabled each founder to visualize occupation as helpful. Events in the early years affirmed the merits of the vision. Had there not been a need created by war; discomfort with the depersonalization and machine-maiming of industry; a push for hospital and other societal reforms; growing knowledge about teaching, psychology, and efficiency; and advances in medicine sufficient to permit a focus on chronic illness, one wonders whether the outcome might have been the same.

To regret the passing of the early 20th century as a time during which the founders resisted forces that threatened to undermine their essential idea constitutes a misreading of the time and a romanticizing of the founders. The founders, visionary and caring people with varied backgrounds and life experiences, shaped the unique, multifaceted character of occupational therapy. Although the idea of the use of occupation was not new, having been used before by psychiatrists, attendants, nurses, and social workers, the founding of a Society to name and promote occupational therapy extended that idea in time and into many places. The multifaceted character of occupational therapy practice today, when centered on occupation and relationships, rooted in a concern for care and function, and sensitive

to broader societal issues and problems, extends the legacy into the 21st century.

References

American Occupational Therapy Association. (1940). History. *Occupational Therapy and Rehabilitation, 19,* 30.

American Occupational Therapy Association. (1972). Occupational therapy: Its definition and functions. *American Journal of Occupational Therapy, 26,* 204–205.

Barton, G. E. (1914). A view of invalid occupation. *Trained Nurse and Hospital Review, 52,* 327–330.

Barton, G. E. (1915a). Occupational nursing. *Trained Nurse and Hospital Review, 54,* 335–338.

Barton, G. E. (1915b). Occupational therapy. *Trained Nurse and Hospital Review, 54,* 138–140.

Barton, G, E. (1920). What occupational therapy may mean to nursing. *Trained Nurse and Hospital Review, 64,* 304–310.

Barton, I. G. (1968). Consolation house, fifty years ago. *American Journal of Occupational Therapy, 22,* 340–345.

Beers, C. W. (1917). *A mind that found itself.* New York: Longmans, Green.

Bing, R. K. (1983). Nationally Speaking—The industry, the art, and the philosophy of history. *American Journal of Occupational Therapy, 37,* 800–801.

Bockoven, J. S. (1971). Occupational therapy—A historical perspective: Legacy of moral treatment—1800s to 1910. *American Journal of Occupational Therapy, 25,* 223–225.

Carlova, J., & Ruggles, O. (1946). *The healing heart.* New York: Julian Messner.

Cooper, G. (1918). Re-weaving the web: A soldier tells what it means to begin all over again. *Carry On, 1*(4), 23–26.

Dunton, W. R. (1919). *Reconstruction therapy.* Philadelphia: Saunders.

Dunton, W. R. (1921a). The development of reconstruction therapy. *Trained Nurse and Hospital Review, 67,* 16–21.

Dunton, W. R. (1921b). *Occupational therapy: A manual for nurses.* Philadelphia: Saunders.

Dunton, W. R. (1930). Occupational therapy. *Occupational Therapy and Rehabilitation, 9,* 343–350.

Dunton, W. R. (1932). Thomas Bessell Kidner. *American Journal of Psychiatry, 89,* 194–196.

Dunton, W. R. (1943). How I got that way. *Occupational Therapy and Rehabilitation, 22,* 244–246.

Dunton, W. R. Jr. (1955). Today's principles reflected in early literature. *American Journal of Occupational Therapy, 9,* 17–18.

Dunton, W. R. Jr. (1967). Occupations and amusements: Organization of the National Society for Promotion of Occupational Therapy. *American Journal of Occupational Therapy, 21,* 287–289.

Hall, H. J. (1921). Forward steps in occupational therapy during 1920. *Modern Hospital, 16,* 245–247.

Hall, H. J. (1922). Editorial—American Occupational Therapy Association. *Archives of Occupational Therapy, 1,* 163–165.

Hall, H. J., & Buck, M. M. (1915). *The work of our hands.* New York: Moffat, Yard.

Hopkins, H. L. (1978). A historical perspective on occupational therapy. In H. L. Hopkins & H. D. Smith (Eds.), *Willard and Spackman's occupational therapy* (5th ed., pp. 3–23.) Philadelphia: Lippincott.

Hull, H. H. (1931). A survey of occupational therapy. *Occupational Therapy and Rehabilitation, 10,* 217–234.

Johnson, J. (1981). Old values—New directions: Competence, adaptation, integration. *American Journal of Occupational Therapy, 35,* 589–598. Reprinted as Chapter 54.

Johnson, S. C. (1919). Occupational therapy, vocational re-education, and industrial rehabilitation. *Modern Hospital, 12,* 221–223.

Kidner, T. B. (1923). Planning for occupational therapy. *Modern Hospital, 21,* 414–428.

Kidner, T. B. (1924). Occupational therapy in 1923. *Modern Hospital, 22,* 55–57.

Kidner, T. B. (1929a). Address to graduates. *Occupational Therapy and Rehabilitation, 8,* 379–385.

Kidner, T. B. (1929b). Standards of occupational therapy. *Occupational Therapy and Rehabilitation, 8,* 243–247.

Kidner, T. B. (1930). The progress of occupational therapy. *Occupational Therapy and Rehabilitation, 9,* 221–223.

Kielhofner, G., & Burke, J. P. (1977). Occupational therapy after 60 years: An account of changing identity and knowledge. *American Journal of Occupational Therapy, 31,* 675–689.

King, L. J. (1980). Creative caring. *American Journal of Occupational Therapy, 34,* 522–528.

Leuret, J. (1948). On the moral treatment of insanity. *Occupational Therapy and Rehabilitation, 27,* 27–33.

Licht, S. (1967). The founding and founders of the American Occupational Therapy Association. *American Journal of Occupational Therapy, 21,* 269–277.

Licht, S. L. (Ed.). (1948). *Occupational therapy source-book.* Baltimore: Williams & Wilkins.

Meyer, A. (1922). The philosophy of occupational therapy. *Archives of Occupational Therapy, 1,* 2–3. Reprinted as Chapter 4.

Miller, A. D. (1918). How can a woman best help? *Carry On, 1,* 17–18.

Mock, H. E. (1919). Curative work. *Carry On, 1*(9), 12–17.

Moodie, C. S. (1919). The value of occupational therapy to the nursing profession. *Hospital Social Service Quarterly, 1,* 313–315.

Myers, C. M. (1948). Pioneer occupational therapists in World War I. *American Journal of Occupational Therapy, 2,* 208–215.

Northrup, F. M. (1928). Work on wards: Methods, crafts and equipment. *Occupational Therapy and Rehabilitation, 7,* 267.

Occupational therapists meet again with A.H.A. (1923). *Modern Hospital, 21,* 499–502.

A patient looks at occupational therapy. (1930). *Occupational Therapy and Rehabilitation, 9,* 277–280.

Peloquin, S. M. (1989). Looking Back—Moral treatment: Contexts considered. *American Journal of Occupational Therapy, 43,* 537–544. Reprinted as Chapter 1.

Reed, K. L., & Sanderson, S. R. (1983). *Concepts of occupational therapy* (2nd ed.). Baltimore: Williams & Wilkins.

Reverby, S. M. (1987). *Ordered to care: The dilemma of American nursing, 1850–1945.* Cambridge, England; Cambridge University Press.

Shaw, C. N. (1929). Occupation as an aid to recovery. *Occupational Therapy and Rehabilitation, 8,* 199–206.

Slagle, E. C. (1927). To organize an "O.T." department. *Occupational Therapy and Rehabilitation, 6,* 125–130.

Smith, P. (1929). The value of occupational therapy from a medical inspector's standpoint. *Occupational Therapy and Rehabilitation, 8,* 331–334.

Spackman, C. S. (1968). A history of the practice of occupational therapy for restoration of physical function: 1917–1967. *American Journal of Occupational Therapy, 22,* 67–71.

Staff. (1923). Nurse's appreciation of George Edward Barton. *Modern Hospital, 21,* 658.

Stattel, F. M. (1977). Occupational therapy: Sense of the past— Focus on the present. *American Journal of Occupational Therapy, 31,* 649–650.

Sutton, B. (1925). Enthusiasm in occupational therapy. *Modern Hospital, 24,* 54.

Tracy, S. E. (1913). *Studies in invalid occupation: A manual for nurses and attendants.* Boston: Whitcomb & Barrows.

Tracy, S. E. (1921). Getting started in occupational therapy. *Trained Nurse and Hospital Review, 67,* 397–399.

Upham, E. G. (1917). Some principles of occupational therapy. *Modern Hospital, 8,* 409–413.

Vaux, C. L. (1929). Habit training. *Occupational Therapy and Rehabilitation, 8,* 327–329.

Welles, C. (1976). Ethics in conflict: Yesterday's standards—Outdated guide for tomorrow? *American Journal of Occupational Therapy, 30,* 44–47.

Wilson, S. C. (1929). Habit training for mental cases. *Occupational Therapy and Rehabilitation, 8,* 189–197.

Woodside, H. H. (1971). Occupational therapy—A historical perspective: The development of occupational therapy—1910–1929. *American Journal of Occupational Therapy. 25,* 226–230.

Yerxa, E. J. (1980). Occupational therapy's role in creating a future climate of caring. *American Journal of Occupational Therapy, 34,* 529–534.

Related Readings

Aims of the American Occupational Therapy Association. (1922). *Modern Hospital, 18,* 54.

Billings, F. (1919). Leaving too soon: The disabled soldier should remain in the hospital for full restoration, physical and mental. *Carry On, 1,* 8–10.

Boltz, O. H. (1927). The rationale of occupational therapy from the psychological standpoint. *Occupational Therapy and Rehabilitation, 6,* 277–282.

Bonner, C. A. (1929). Occupational therapy: Its contribution to the modern mental institution. *Occupational Therapy and Rehabilitation, 8,* 387–391.

Bowman, E. (1922). Psychology of occupational therapy. *Archives of Occupational Therapy, 1,* 171–178.

Brannan, J. W. (1922). Occupational therapy. *American Journal of Public Health, 12,* 367–376.

Carroll, R. S. (1910). The therapy of work. *Journal of the American Medical Association, 54,* 2032–2035.

Crane, B. T. (1919). Occupational therapy. *Boston Medical and Surgical Journal, 181,* 63–65.

Cromwell, F. S. (1977). Eleanor Clarke Slagle, the leader, the woman. *American Journal of Occupational Therapy, 31,* 645–648.

Cullimore, A. R. (1921). Objectives and motivation in occupational therapy. *Modern Hospital, 17,* 537–538.

Dunton, W. R. (1944). Some older occupational therapy literature. *Occupational Therapy and Rehabilitation, 23,* 138–141.

Dunton, W. R. Jr. (1913). Occupation as a therapeutic measure. *Medical Record, 83,* 388–389.

Durgin, D. D. (1923). The value of occupational therapy. *State Hospital Quarterly, 8,* 382.

Elton, F. G. (1924). Relationship of occupational therapy to rehabilitation. *Archives of Occupational Therapy, 3,* 101–108.

Gilfoyle, E. M. (1980). Caring: A philosophy of practice. *American Journal of Occupational Therapy, 34,* 517–521.

Gilligan, M. B. K. (1976). Developmental stages of occupational therapy and the feminist movement. *American Journal of Occupational Therapy, 30,* 560–567.

Grant, I. (1920). Practical side of occupational therapy. *Modern Hospital, 15,* 504–505.

Grant, I. (1928). Bedside, ward, porch, and shop methods. *Occupational Therapy and Rehabilitation, 7,* 95–98.

Gundersen, P. G. (1927). Dynamic occupational therapy. *Occupational Therapy and Rehabilitation, 6,* 131–135.

Haas, L. J. (1925). *Occupational therapy for the mentally and nervously ill.* Milwaukee: Bruce.

Hills, F. L. (1909). Work as an immediate and ultimate therapeutic factor. *Journal of the American Medical Association, 53,* 892.

Houston, I. B. (1928). Occupational therapy submerged. *Occupational Therapy and Rehabilitation, 7,* 413–415.

Kahmann, W. C. (1967). Fifty years in occupational therapy. *American Journal of Occupational Therapy, 21,* 281–283.

Kenna, W. M. (1927). Occupational therapy and hospital industries. *Occupational Therapy and Rehabilitation, 6,* 453–461.

Kielhofner, G., & Burke, J. P. (1983). The evolution of knowledge and practice in occupational therapy: Past, present, and future. In G. Kielhofner (Ed.), *Health through occupation: Theory and practice in occupational therapy* (pp. 3–54). Philadelphia: F. A. Davis.

Livingston, W. H. (1923). Useful occupational therapy vs. useless occupational therapy. *Modern Hospital, 21,* 51–52.

Mabie, H. R. (1919). A plea for occupational therapy. *Woman Citizen, 4,* 344.

Matthews, W. H. (1923). Work—The cure. *American Journal of Nursing, 24,* 164–167.

McNew, B. B. (1923). "Useless" versus useful occupational therapy. *Modern Hospital, 21,* 62–64.

Occupational therapy, vocational re-education and, industrial rehabilitation. (1919). *Modern Hospital, 12,* 221–223.

Occupational therapy. (1921). *Hospital Progress, 2,* 265.

Patients make attractive toys. (1921). *Modern Hospital, 16,* 42.

Patients to be trained. (1920). *Modern Hospital, 15,* 465.

Pennington, L. E. (1925). O.T. known for nearly 2,000 years. *Hospital Management, 19,* 37–38.

Reilly, M. (1962). Eleanor Clarke Slagle Lecture—Occupational therapy can be one of the great ideas of 20th century medicine. *American Journal of Occupational Therapy, 16,* 1–9. Reprinted as Chapter 7.

Robinson, G. C. (1919). Occupational therapy in civilian hospitals. *Modern Medicine, 1,* 159–162.

Sands, I. F. (1928). When is occupation curative? *Occupational Therapy and Rehabilitation, 7,* 115–122.

Second annual meeting of the National Society for the Promotion of Occupational Therapy. (1918). *Modern Hospital, 11,* 298.

Six "musts" for occupational therapy. (1921). *Modern Hospital, 16,* 169.

Slagle, E. C. (1921). To organize an "O.T." department. *Hospital Management, 12,* 43–45.

Spear, M. R. (1927). The value and limitations of attendants in occupational therapy departments in mental hospitals. *Occupational Therapy and Rehabilitation, 6,* 225–227.

Thayer, A. S. (1908). Work cure. *Journal of the American Medical Association, 51,* 1485–1487.

True occupational therapy. (1924). *Modern Hospital, 22,* 66.

Value of occupational therapy. (1921). *Hospital Progress, 2,* 316.

War brought wider recognition to O.T. (1923). *Modern Hospital, 20*(1).

What is occupational therapy? (1921). *Modern Hospital, 17,* 234.

Zamir, L. J. (1966). Editorial—Whither occupational therapy. *American Journal of Occupational Therapy, 20,* 195.

CHAPTER 4

The Philosophy of Occupation Therapy

ADOLF MEYER

There was a time when physicians and the public thought the art of medicine consisted mainly in diagnosing more or less mysterious diseases and "prescribing" for them. Each disease was supposed to have its program of treatment, and to this day the patient and the family expect a set of medicines and a diet, and a change of climate if necessary, or at least a restcure so as to fight and conquer "the disease." No branch of medicine has learned as clearly as psychiatry that, after all, many of these formidable diseases are largely problems of adaptation and not some mysterious devil in disguise to be exorcised by asfetida and other usually bitter and, if possible, alcoholic stuffs; and psychiatry has been among the first to recognize the need of adaptation and the value of work as a sovereign help in the problems of adaptation.

It so happened that in the first medical paper I ever presented, about December, 1892, or January, 1893—curiously enough before the Chicago Pathological Society, where one would least expect discussions of occupation—I asked my new neighbors and colleagues for suggestions as to the tastes and best lines of occupation of American patients. The proper use of time in some helpful and gratifying activity appeared to me a fundamental issue in the treatment of any neuropsychiatric patient. Soon after that, May 1, 1893, I went to Kankakee and found in that institution some ward work and shop work, and later, under the inspiration of Isabel Davenport, some gardening for the women in her convalescent cottages. But I also found there a little of a feeling which pervaded quite conspicuously much of the contemporary attitude toward this question.

This chapter was previously published in the *Archives of Occupational Therapy, 1*, 1–10.

This paper was originally read at "Fifth Annual Meeting of the National Society for the Promotion of Occupational Therapy" (now the American Occupational Therapy Association), held in Baltimore, MD, October 20–22, 1921.

Among a most interesting collection of abstracts from the history of American institutions put at my disposal by Dr. Wm. R. Dunton, I find a report on the employment of the insane by a committee from the Michigan institutions, dated 1822 and signed by Dr. Henry M. Hurd. The committee had visited European institutions and had been especially impressed by the use of occupation as a substitute for restraint. But they have a fear that the presence of *private* patients would interfere with the introduction of occupation. The conclusions contain the following statements:

> Employment of some sort should be made obligatory for all able-bodied patients. . . . (But) it would be feared that such measures would meet with much opposition from all quarters. . . . It might, consequently, be best to arrange at first for the employment of state patients and to procure legislative sanction of the step. If this works advantageously it will be comparatively easy to extend the system to other patients.

This represents the attitude of many hospital men of the time. Industrial shops and work in laundry and kitchen and on the wards were the achievements of that problem—very largely planned to relieve the employees.

A new step was to arise from a freer conception of work, from a concept of free and pleasant and profitable *occupation—including recreation and any form of helpful enjoyment as the leading principle.*

When in 1895 I was transplanted to Worcester, Mass., there was little in the atmosphere to foster interest in occupation: ward work and a few shops managed merely from the point of view of utility. Only the McLean hospital had the beginnings of some organized recreative occupations. From 1902 it was my good fortune to have to work on Ward's Island in a division which then was under the immediate direction of an unusually active and enterprising man, Dr. Emmett C. Dent, always eager for therapeutic results and untiring in his development of hospital principles in the face of very cramped opportunities. In this new atmosphere I was greatly assisted by the wholesome human understanding of my helpmate, Mrs. Meyer, who under these conditions may have been one of the first, if not the first, to introduce a new systematized type of activity into the wards of a state institution.

She had become a great help to my patients in visiting them in my ward and had started the visiting of the homes, as probably the first social worker with a systematic program of help to patient, family, and physician, just before Miss Louise Schuyler urged the introduction of a very eleemosynary type of aftercare in November 1906. When in 1907 a real social worker, Miss Horton, was appointed, Mrs. Meyer turned her attention to the occupation and organized recreations of the patients on the ward, not only in the shops and amusement hall, but in the employment of the available time on the ward.

Shortly after that, in 1909, Miss Lathrop and the Chicago School of Civics and Philanthropy undertook a course of training in play and occupation for nurses, and Miss Wright was chosen to attend it and she returned to organize the work throughout the institution—with a wise balance between organized shopwork and more individual work on the wards.

It had long been interesting to see how groups of a few excited patients can be seated in a corner in a small circle of two or three settees and kept wonderfully contented picking the hair off mattresses, or doing simple tasks not too readily arousing the desire for big movements and uncontrollable excitement and yet not too taxing to their patience. Groups of patients with raffia and basket work, or with various kinds of handwork and weaving and bookbinding and metal and leather work, took the place of the bored wall flowers and of mischief-makers. A pleasure in achievement, a real pleasure in the use and activity of one's hands and muscles and a happy *appreciation of time* began to be used as incentives in the management of our patients, instead of abstract exhortations to cheer up and to behave according to abstract or repressive rules. The main advance of the new scheme was the blending of work and pleasure—all made possible by a wise supplementing of centralization by individualization and a kind of redecentralization.

When the Phipps Clinic was opened, we were able to secure the services of Mrs. Slagle, who, with her succes-

sors—Mrs. Price and Miss DeHoff, and Mrs. Marion, Mr. Russell, and Mr. Cass—brought us to the level you find now represented at the Phipps Clinic.

This contact with the evolution of occupation therapy gave a good opportunity to see this movement grow to a position which we now want to consider more closely.

Somehow it represents to me a very important manifestation of a very general gain in human philosophy. There is in all this a development of the *valuation of time and work* which is not accidental. It is part of the great espousal of the *values of reality and actuality* rather than of mere thinking and reasoning and fancy as characteristic of the 19th century and the present day.

As I said in my brief abstract, we feel today that the culminating feature of evolution is man's capacity of imagination and *the use of time with foresight* based on a corresponding appreciation of the past and of the *present.* We know more definitely than ever that the 24 hours of the day are the problem of nursing and immediate therapy, and not the medicines taken *t. i. d.* Somehow something apparently *self-evident* has taken its *proper position* in our attention. Just as in the medical aspects we have come to value an appreciation of the exceedingly *simple* facts of basal metabolism (that is, the simple measure of the amount of CO_2 we produce), so the simple fact of employment of *time* has become an important measure and problem for physician and nurse. The most important factor in the progress lay *undoubtedly* in the newer conceptions of *mental problems* as *problems of living,* and not merely diseases of a structural and toxic nature on the one hand or of a final lasting constitutional disorder on the other. The formulation in terms of habit-deterioration of even those grave mental disorders presently the serious problem of *terminal dementia,* made *systematic engagement of interest, and concern about the actual use of TIME and work an obligation and necessity.*

It is very interesting that the progress of all the fundamental sciences has shown the same trend during the last 30 years. The 90s of the 19th and the first decade of the 20th century marked the rise of *energetics* (so effectively brought home to all scientists by Professor Ostwald in his lectures in this country some 15 years ago)—a determination to replace the interest in *inert matter* by a broad conception of the world of physics and chemistry in terms of *energies,* which means literally "applications of *work.*" Similarly, during this same period the study of human and of animal life gave birth to the concept of *behaviorism* with its emphasis on performance as the fundamental formulation of what had figured up to that time on the throne of an abstract timeless psychology, curiously enough, first invaded by science in the form of studies in reaction *time*. Direct *experience* and performance were everywhere acknowledged as the fullest type of life. Thought, reason, and fancy were more and more recognized as merely a *step* to *action*, and mental life in general as the integrator of *time*, giving us the fullest sense of past, present, and future, but after all the best type of reality and actuality only in real *performance*. We all know how fancy and abstract thought can go far afield—undisciplined and uncensured and uncorrected; while performance is its own judge and regulator and therefore the most dependable and influential part of life. Our body is not merely so many pounds of flesh and bone figuring as a machine, with an abstract mind or soul added to it. It is throughout a live organism pulsating with its rhythm of rest and activity, beating time (as we might say) in ever so many ways, most readily intelligible and in the full bloom of its nature when it feels itself as one of those great self-guiding *energy transformers* which constitute the real world of living beings. Our conception of man is that of an organism that maintains and balances itself in the world of reality and actuality by being in active life and active use, i.e., using and living and acting its *time* in harmony with its own nature and the nature about it. It is the use that we make of ourselves that gives the ultimate stamp to our every organ.

This growing conviction that personality is fundamentally determined by *performance* rather than by mere good-will and good intention rapidly became the backbone of our psychology and psychopathology. It became a fair task for our ingenuity to *obtain* performance wherever it had failed to come *spontaneously* and thereby to serve the organism in the task of keeping itself in good form.

This philosophy of reality, of work and time, seen in all the sciences appeals to me because it expresses, with respect for fact, the simple and yet most valuable experiences of real life.

The whole of human organization has its shape in a kind of rhythm. It is not enough that our hearts should beat in a useful rhythm, always kept up to a standard at which it can meet rest as well as wholesome *strain* without upset. There are many other rhythms which we must be attuned to: the *larger rhythms* of night and day, of sleep and waking hours, of hunger and its gratification, and finally the big four—work and play and rest and sleep, which our organism must be able to bal-

ance even under difficulty. The only way to attain balance in all this is *actual doing, actual practice,* a program of wholesome living as the *basis* of wholesome feeling and thinking and fancy and interests.

Thus, with our *patients,* we naturally begin with a simple regime of *pleasurable* ease, the creation of an orderly *rhythm* in the atmosphere (a wise rule of using all our natural rhythms), the sense of a day simply and naturally spent, perhaps with some music and restful dance and play, and with some glimpses of activities which any one can hope to achieve and derive satisfaction from.

In this frame of rhythm and order of time, we naturally heed also the other factors—the personal interests and personal fitness. A large proportion of our patients present inferiority feelings, often over a sense of awkwardness and inability to use the hands to produce things worthwhile, i.e., respected by themselves or others. To get the pleasure and pride of achievement and use of one's hands and muscles, the feeling of worthwhileness of a little effort and of a well fitted use of time, is the basic remedy for the blase tedium that characterizes the indifference or the hopeless depression (that stands in the way of rallying thwarted personalities). I am convinced that a premium should be put on the production of things that are finished in one or a few sittings and yet have an independent emotional value. They must give the satisfaction of completion and achievement, and that in the eye of the maker and of those for whom he has tried to work. Performance and completion form also the backbone and essence of what Pierre Janet has so well described as the "fonction du real"—the *realization* of reality, bringing the very soul of man out of dreams of eternity to the full sense and appreciation of actuality.

Our role consists in giving *opportunities* rather than prescriptions. There must be opportunities to work, opportunities to do and to plan and create, and to learn to use material. There are bound to be valuable opportunities for timely and actually deserved approval and encouragement. It is not a question of specific *prescriptions,* but of opportunities, except perhaps where suggestions can be derived from the history of the patient and a minute study of the trends of fancy and even delusions reveals the lines of predilections and native longings—yet even here the physician would only exert his ingenuity to adapt *opportunities*.

In a meeting like this, the personal contact of many practical inspirers brings out an interchange of experiences and resources from the side of the instructors and helpers.

It takes rare gifts and talents and rare personalities to be real pathfinders in this work. There are no royal roads; it is all a problem of being true to one's nature and opportunities and of teaching others to do the same with themselves. I went through the occupation departments of a large institution the other day and was profoundly impressed by the wide differences of the personnel and the manifold ways of approach leading to success with the work. It takes, above all, resourcefulness and ability to respect at the same time the native *capacities and interests* of the patient. Freedom from premature meddling, and tact in avoiding false comparisons or undue expectations fostering disappointment, orderliness without pedantry, cheer and praise without sloppiness and without surrender of standard—these may be the rewards of a good use of personal gifts and of good training.

Somehow I see in all this profound importance extending far beyond our special field. Our efforts seem to me destined to be the soil for helps of much wider applicability. Present day humanity seems to suffer from a deluded craze for finding substitutes for actual work. It seems more difficult than ever to guide with the traditional preachments.

Our industrialism has created the false, because one-sided, idea of success in *production* to the point of overproduction, bringing with it a kind of nausea to the worker and a delirium of the trader living on advertisement and salesmanship, instead of sound economics of a fair and sane distribution of the goods of this world according to need, and an education of the public as to where and how to find the best and worthiest.

The man of today has lost the capacity and pride of workmanship and has substituted for it a measure in terms of money; and now his money proves to be of uncertain value. A great deal of activity, to be individually and socially acceptable and exciting enough and mentionable for social exhibition of one's worth, has to be of the nature of conspicuous waste, a class performance like athletics and golf and racing about the country, and a display of rapidly changing fashions. Work and play, ambition and satisfaction, are apt to lose their natural contact with the natural rhythms of appetite and gratification, vision and performance, and finishable cycles of completion—of work and play and rest and sleep.

Our special work, which tries to do justice to special human needs, I feel is destined to serve again as the center of a great gain for the normal as well. It will work like the Montessori system of education. Grown out of the needs of defective children, it has become the source of inspiration and methods for a freer education for *all* children.

What satisfactions you may develop in the guidance in difficult conditions may bring out the best principles and philosophy for the ordinary walks of life.

We are often told, and I suppose it is largely true, that the world cannot and will not move back. A new sense of *uses of time,* new satisfactions from that inexhaustible fountain, that one thing, time, that will come and come, and only waits to become an opportunity used—that seems to me the gospel and salvation of the day. Human ideals have unfortunately and usually been steeped in dreams of timeless *eternity,* and they have never included an equally religious valuation of *actual time* and its meaning in wholesome rhythms. The awakening to a full meaning of time as the biggest wonder and asset of our lives and the valuation of opportunity and performance as the greatest *measure* of time; those are the beacon lights of the philosophy of the occupation worker. I have often felt that Dr. Herbert James Hall represents the true *religion* of work, leading us to a new sense of the sacredness of the moment—when fitted rightly into the rhythms of individual and social and cosmic nature. Another apostle of the Gospel is announced by Prof. Cassimir J. Keyser in his Phi Beta Kappa address in Science (September 9, 1921)—Count Alfred Korzybski's "Manhood of Humanity,"—the science and art of human engineering.

We might well sum up our philosophy in this way:

> In the great process of evolution there is a great law of unfolding which shows in every new and higher step what we call the *integration* of the simpler phases into new entities. Thus the inorganic world continues itself into the plant and animal world. The laws of physics and chemistry expand into laws of growth and laws of function, still physical and chemical, but physical and chemical in terms of plans and in terms of the active animal, and finally in terms of more or less highly gifted man, with all that capacity to enjoy and to suffer, to succeed and to fail, to fulfill the life-cycle of the human individual happily and effectively or more or less falteringly. The great feature of man is his new sense of time, with foresight built on a sound view of the past and present. Man learns to organize time and he does it in terms of *doing* things, and one of the many

good things he does between eating, drinking and wholesome nutrition generally and the flights of fancy and aspiration, we call *work and occupation*—we might call it the ingestion and digestion and proper use, and we may say a religious *conscience,* of *time* with its successions of *opportunities*.

With this type of background, we may well be able to shape for ourselves and our patients an outlook of sound idealism, furnishing a setting in which many otherwise apparently insurmountable difficulties will be conquered—and in which our new generations will find a world full of ever new opportunity and achievement in healthy harmony with human nature.

CHAPTER 5

Pragmatism and Structuralism in Occupational Therapy: The Long Conversation

BARB HOOPER AND WENDY WOOD

The history of occupational therapy may be understood as a continual transaction between two cultural discourses: pragmatism and structuralism. *Pragmatism* is a way of thinking that presupposes humans are agentic by nature and knowledge is tentative and created within particular contexts. *Structuralism* is a way of thinking that assumes humans are composites of recurring general frameworks and that knowledge is objective and can be generalized to multiple contexts. Early in the field's history, both pragmatist and structuralist assumptions about the human and knowledge produced different readings, or interpretations, of what constituted the appropriate tools, methods, and outcomes for occupational therapy. Consequently, occupational therapy adopted an interesting mix of pragmatist language regarding the human and structuralist approaches to knowledge, resulting in professional identity problems still experienced today. However, recent developments offer an opportunity for occupational therapists to correct old identity problems through critically evaluating incompatible assumptions and carefully reading the prevailing cultural ethos.

That occupational therapists have historically struggled with issues of professional identity is clear. Why occupational therapists have struggled and the consequences of that struggle for the profession's future viability are matters of much murkiness, complexity, and debate. This article enters into occupational therapy's long-standing foray into its identity by focusing on the role that discourse has played in the profession's evolution. A discourse is composed of a recurrent pattern of language that both shapes and reflects a profession's intellectual commitments by being the medium through which its practices are constituted (Tinning, 1991). In other words, how practitioners "read" the problems, tools, and desired outcomes of their services—and, consequently, the particular ways they eventually come to practice and the particular professional identity they eventually hone—are shaped partly by the discourses in which they participate. As Mattingly and Fleming (1994) observed in their landmark study of clinical reasoning, occupational therapy practitioners often work within "two different discourses" (p. 302): one that concentrates on restoring persons to satisfying lives and another that concentrates on fixing body parts. We propose herein that these discourses reflect those of pragmatism and structuralism, respectively; moreover, they have coexisted in various ways since occupational therapy's inception. Additional discourses, such as moral, humanist, feminist, and performance-dominated, have helped to pattern occupational therapy's practices and language and deserve historical analysis. However, we make a case that the profession's intellectual history may be conceived as one long conversation, at times conflictual, between the two divergent discourses of pragmatism and structuralism.

The basic purpose of this article is to analyze how pragmatist and structuralist discourses emerged and came to be expressed in occupational therapy. The larger purpose is to develop implications of this analysis for the profession's future. Our first consideration addresses the historical background of pragmatist and structuralist discourse and their guiding assumptions about the human and about knowledge. We targeted these assumptions because they represent the core intellectual commitments of a professional discourse (Kielhofner & Barrett, 1998; Tinning, 1991); consequently, they have been used in occupational therapy to show how pretheoretical assumptions influence clinical reasoning (Hooper, 1997), in occupational science to construct an occupational theory of health (Wilcock,

1998), and in philosophy as elements of theories of human nature (Stevenson & Haberman, 1998). Our second consideration pertains to how each discourse "reads" occupational therapy. As used here, reading refers to the interpretations or meanings that people attach to things. We propose that pragmatism engenders a particular reading of practice largely discordant with that of structuralism; that is, the two discourses highlight different phenomena as well as relegate different phenomena to the background of concern or edit them out altogether. Our analysis then proceeds to how these discourses have been negotiated and shaped, not as dichotomies, but as ratios and conjoined assumptions. Lastly, we pose ways in which this long conversation offers guidance to the future.

The method for this analysis included both historical and discourse analysis. Discourse analysis seeks to reveal the realities individuals or groups have forged, and continue to forge, through language and practice (Denzin & Lincoln, 2000). Accordingly, original historical texts of early and contemporary pragmatists were coded for theories of human nature (Stevenson & Haberman, 1998). After these theories were constructed, we used them as conceptual grids for analyzing language patterns in occupational therapy texts. Our emphasis throughout is on prominent works, as we presume that they have been especially influential in shaping the profession's discourses. Our analysis is also situated in the United States and, thus, although most likely germane to occupational therapy in other countries, is not intended as a broad generalization about the field's evolution on multinational levels.

Pragmatism: Historical and Conceptual Overview

In the late 19th century, America faced an intellectual crisis due to the impact of new scientific discoveries, Darwinism, new biblical criticism, and the emergence of the social sciences. Taken-for-granted religious explanations of knowledge, human nature, and reality were being vigorously debated, with pragmatism posed as one alternative to traditional religious views (Hodge, 1872/1997; Peirce, 1878/1995; Sumner, 1881/1997; Ward, 1884/1997). As a dominant intellectual discourse in the early 20th century, pragmatist tenets were adopted by many disciplines, such as law (Holmes, 1920/1997), anthropology (Mead, 1928/1997), sociology (Ward, 1884/1997), and business (Lippman, 1914). Core intellectual commitments of occupational ther-

apy were likewise being constructed from a pragmatist perspective at that time (Breines, 1986; Serrett, 1985).

Pragmatist Views of the Human

The philosophy of pragmatism promoted particular assumptions about human beings that these disciplines embodied. Fundamentally, the pragmatist view of the human was holistic given its rejection of anything that sublimated people to anything less than their total experiences. Early pragmatists thus rejected dichotomies like mind–body, thought–action, rational–practical, and function–structure that presumed people could be divided into parts (Dewey, 1908/1995; Leys, 1990). Additionally, because people were seen as agentic and in possession of potentials to cultivate their environs (Emerson, 1883/1995), the individual occupied the foreground of pragmatic discourse. Thus did Dewey (1915/1944) write that children are endowed with "native tendencies to explore, to manipulate tools and materials, to construct, to give expression to joyous emotion" (p. 195). Also conveying pragmatism's celebration of human agency, James (1907/1995b) observed that because every department of life bears the stamp of human power and imagination, "the trail of the human serpent is thus over everything" (p. 60).

Early pragmatists also delimited human agency in three ways having to do with other qualities of being human. First, humans were seen as teleological, meaning that they envisioned desired futures and directed action toward realizing those futures (Leys, 1990). Hence, part of human nature is to apply tools, technology, art, and knowledge toward a telos or vision of "the good." Yet because human activity also could be confined by what was seen as desirable, one "telos" could occlude views of other equally desirable or beneficial futures. Second, inextricable ties with biology, the physical environment, and society were seen to delimit human agency (Dewey, 1930; James, 1892/1985, 1907/1995a). Humans were seen as so interwoven into the fabric of their social and physical environs that Dewey (1939/1973) described this connection as "intercourse with our surroundings" (p. 571). Biology, environment, and society thus worked in tandem to both direct and constrain human activity in particular ways. Third, human agency was delimited by the sensory-reliant nature of people. Human understandings of the world (i.e., opinions, ideas, conceptions of "fact") were seen as molded from direct sensory experiences that shaped particular habits of mind and, in turn, guided future perceptions and actions (James,

1892/1985). Experiences that were novel to established habits of mind were thus difficult to assimilate and often ignored, even when potentially positive.

Pragmatist Views of Knowledge

The pragmatist view of the human not only is congruent with, but also informs and is informed by its view of knowledge. Because pragmatists believed that experiences undertaken with forethought and intentionality were needed to reveal the fluid truths of phenomena, they were skeptical of discourses that presumed absolutes and certainty in knowledge. Pragmatists instead promoted a view of knowledge as flexible, fallible, and contingent (Cherryholmes, 1999). Knowledge was flexible because it was determined in the making and doing of direct experience and, therefore, could not be "found" or become fixed. Knowledge was fallible because it was always being overturned by better ways of explaining or understanding things. As Emerson (1883/1995) expressed, "There is not a piece of science but that its flank may be turned tomorrow" (p. 28). Knowledge was likewise contingent because it issued from an iterative process between action and particular contexts. As Dewey (1908/1995) noted, "All knowledge issues in some action which changes things to some extent" (p. 82). Given these suppositions, pragmatic method was experimental in nature on the basis of critical inquiry into practical consequences. Emerson (1883/1995) captured this spirit of inquiry by proclaiming, "No facts are to me sacred; none are profane; I simply experiment, an endless seeker" (p. 31). James (1907/1995b) later stipulated that the key to pragmatic inquiry was its dedication to ascertaining, "What difference would it practically make to anyone if this notion rather than that notion were true?" (p. 54).

The pragmatist view of knowledge has mistakenly been interpreted as doing what works. Yet pragmatism stresses active inquiry far beyond mere expediency. Such inquiry scrutinizes not only the practicality of an action and its main or intended consequence, but also all of its effects (Dewey, 1939/1964; Peirce, 1878/1995). Knowledge is seen as continually being made through habits of reflection and inquiry regarding the consequences of chosen actions in light of a coveted future. Thus, pragmatist discourse recently has been associated with a nonfoundational approach to knowledge, the aim of which is to "arrive temporarily at warranted assertions" via continual engagement in a rich critical inquiry (Cherryholmes, 1999, p. 34). Such inquiry presumes that because ideas and theories (and other human creations) are socially embedded in the present and products of past discourses, they cannot be held to be theoretically neutral, timeless, or independent of particular historical or political contexts.

Pragmatist Readings of Occupational Therapy

One of the primary routes by which occupational therapy inherited its pragmatist discourse was from John Dewey and William James via their friend and colleague Adolf Meyer (Serrett, 1985). James's and Dewey's pragmatism played a large role in shaping Meyer's practice of psychobiology. This practice highlighted pragmatist themes by stressing the indispensability of understanding people in context of their environs, life histories, and ways of acting in the world (Leys, 1990; Meyer, 1933/1948; Muncie, 1939/1985). Meyer (1922) relied heavily on his psychobiology in writing *The Philosophy of Occupation Therapy*, possibly the most cited work in occupational therapy literature ever (see Chapter 4). The following classic quote from this work reveals how Meyer's view of the human accentuated certain clinical problems as critical, certain therapeutic tools as most helpful, and certain outcomes as most desirable:

> Our body is not so many pounds of flesh and bone figuring as a machine with an abstract mind or soul added to it. It is throughout a living organism pulsating with its rhythm of rest and activity, beating time (as we might say) in ever so many ways, most readily intelligible and in the full bloom of its nature when it feels itself as one of those great self-guiding energy-transformers which constitute the real world of living beings. Our conception of man is that of an organism that maintains and balances itself in the world of reality and actuality by being in active life and active use, i.e., using and living and acting its time in harmony with its own nature and the nature about it. (p. 5). (See Chapter 4.)

Meyer's (1922) reading of occupational therapy may be one of the field's cleanest examples of pragmatic discourse (see Chapter 4). His reading highlighted problems related to the suppression of natural experiences in total life contexts and to disturbances in self-efficacy and natural rhythms of time; it elaborated on tools of practice that dealt with the particularities of each case, such as providing opportunities to plan, do, and create according to patients' skills and interests; and it elaborated on outcomes that restored temporal rhythms and natural connections among work and play, ambition and satisfaction, and desires and performance. Conversely, Meyer's reading edited out clinical problems that were not problems of action, clinical tools that were generic or prescriptive, and clinical outcomes that did less than empower "the individual to face his or her own deficiencies and deploy his or her own resources" (Leys, 1990, p. 50). Also edited out were ideas that did not situate people in their environs or that divided them into physical–psychological or function–structure dichotomies.

Yerxa's 1966 Eleanor Clarke Slagle lecture, another frequently cited work, points out the agreement between occupational therapy and existential thinkers who see humans as agents involved in the process of becoming more authentically their true selves (Yerxa, 1967). Congruent with this view of the human, Yerxa (1967) used strong pragmatist themes to depict how occupational therapists help people become more authentic. That is, because occupational therapy clients needed to act in the world of reality as their own agents, her reading of practice highlighted problems of action, methods that supported patients' self-initiation, and outcomes pertaining to patients' self-actualization and realistic perceptions of themselves and their environs. This reading also highlighted knowledge as being constructed from within professional experience and supported by continuous inquiry. More recently, Clark's 1993 Slagle lecture promoted a pragmatist reading by emphasizing the individual case over general principles and the importance of nurturing "the human spirit to act" by empowering persons to define and solve their problems through a healing process of occupational storytelling and storymaking (Clark, 1993, p. 1076).

Pragmatic discourse regarding the human has more than endured in occupational therapy across the 20th century, but perhaps pragmatic discourse regarding knowledge has not—a situation that we traced to the field's earliest educational practices. Although herself educated in England, Wilcock (1998) characterized occupational therapy's educational practices in the late 1950s and early 1960s as "didactic and authoritarian" (p. 4). She further posed that such educational practices did not prepare practitioners to "defend the value of occupation to health when medicine adopted an increasingly reductionistic, scientific and technological stance from the late 1960s onward" (p. 4). Similarly, Reilly (1962) (see Chapter 7) and West (1992) vehemently argued, 30 years apart from one another, that

occupational therapists needed to develop far greater comfort and capacity for critical analysis if the field was to evolve into legitimate professionalism. Ultimately, the degree to which pragmatist views both of the human and of knowledge were adopted may have been thwarted by the early challenge of structuralism (Serrett, 1985), another powerful discourse with views of the human and knowledge that are largely discordant to those of pragmatism.

Structuralism: Historical and Conceptual Overview

Like pragmatism, structuralism was an interdisciplinary movement that sought new ways to establish truth following the rise of science and the secularization of society. Structuralists shared pragmatists' concerns with meaningful connections and, thus, rejected the disconnected and atomistic ideas produced by radical empirical science (Merquior, 1986; Sturrock, 1986). But unlike pragmatism, structuralism rejected Enlightenment liberal–rational values that privileged nature, natural experiences, and the rational individual over society (Harland, 1987). Guided by linguistics, structuralism instead treated underlying structures as ultimate. Thus, the analogy of a kaleidoscope has been used to describe the structuralist perspective. Although a kaleidoscope seems to consist of many different forms, it is actually only "a matrix composed of just a few recurring elements" (Merquior, 1986, p. 191). Likewise, how the structure of a whole building can be explained by its parts was seen as analogous to the anatomical, psychological, and social structures of people (Dosse, 1997). Given its explanatory power, structuralism was adopted by most social sciences by the mid 20th century and went on to produce "a veritable revolution" held akin to a powerful "scientific baptism" (Dosse, 1997, p. xxii).

Structuralist Views of the Human

As suggested by the analogy of the kaleidoscope, a structuralist perspective was one in which humans were viewed as composites of recurring general frameworks, thus placing emphasis on static parts rather than on dynamically assembled action that is contextual, volitional, and self-transforming. Structuralism, consequently, was far less preoccupied with human agency than pragmatism (Sturrock, 1986). Rather, the quality of being human derived from general frameworks that precede experience and to which experience conformed (Andi, 1999; Harland, 1987). Structuralist discourse thus downplayed the agentic and holistic individual, stressing instead general systems in which people act, general structures common to all people, and general internal systems of all people.

Structuralist Views of Knowledge

As in pragmatism, the structuralist view of the human both informed and was informed by its view of knowledge. Hence, structuralist discourse minimized the relevance of context, subjectivity, or case-specific particulars to the development of knowledge. Instead, knowledge was seen as being composed of various timeless, universal, and objectively verifiable structures and mechanisms, be they biological, sociological, or anthropological (among other possibilities) in nature (Harland, 1987). Moreover, because such structures and mechanisms were divorced from experience, they could be applied to most episodes of human behavior; likewise, their deliberate manipulation or unmasking was precisely what generated new knowledge. This allure of scientificity attracted numerous social sciences to structuralism in the 20th century (Dosse, 1997). Accordingly, structuralist discourse has been viewed as being consistent with a foundational approach to knowledge. This foundational approach presumes that various phenomena possess independent essences that can be objectively secured (Cherryholmes, 1999). Assuming that knowledge is foundational, structuralist inquiry seeks to represent a phenomenon as it "truly" is according to its fixed essence. Deciphering whether something represents a particular phenomenon is then accomplished by referring to that phenomenon's "objectively" established structure.

Structuralist Readings of Occupational Therapy

Because structuralism conveys very different intellectual commitments about the human and knowledge than does pragmatism, its produces very different readings of practice. The following quote from Fiorentino's 1974 Slagle lecture reflects a rather pure structuralist reading of practice; significantly, it also manifests a developmental model that has dominated pediatric practice in occupational therapy for many years (Coster, 1998):

> In the areas of gross and fine motor development, we cannot accept, as a goal of treatment, functional use of the hands without first attaining stability of everything to which the hand is attached. Development is cephalo–caudal, proximal–distal, medial–lateral, gross to fine. This is how treatment should progress if we are to give children their maximal functional potential. Also, we should place our emphasis on normal developmental sequences of CNS [central nervous system] development: for example, learning on a subcortical basis, followed by cortical, voluntary learning, finally reaching the stage of spontaneous automatic movements. (Fiorentino, 1975, p. 20)

Fiorentino's (1975) reading of practice relegated to the background of clinical consideration concern with the historical particularities of each case as well as with persons' subjective experiences and whole performances of doing. Conversely, highlighted were clinical problems related to disturbances in structures underlying performance, clinical tools that sequentially applied universal procedures, and clinical outcomes that could verify that children with disabilities were developing "on time" with and in the same ways and sequences as their peers without disabilities. Fiorentino's view of the human focused on internal systems that were presumed to be universal; likewise, she understood knowledge to derive from general and timeless principles of human development.

Similar themes in other structuralist readings of practice include using decontextualized clinical techniques as prerequisites for doing things "naturally" in ordinary rhythms of time and applying general cases to individuals. For example, Reed traced in her 1986 Slagle lecture the evolution of crafts as clinical media in occupational therapy (see Chapter 47). Reed's (1986) research suggested that practitioners gradually shifted from seeing bilateral sanding blocks as woodworking tools to seeing them as tools for facilitating upper-extremity integration and strength. Once a "therapist-reader" brought the motion of sanding out in the foreground, the next step was easy to have patients sand "without sand paper on an incline plane made of Formica" (p. 602) as a prerequisite to complex occupational engagement. This clinical strategy is rooted in a historic reliance on a priori, fixed knowledge of human movement in an ideal general case. Licht (1957), a mid-century physician and influential writer in occupational therapy, detailed a kinesiologic approach to craft analysis that was predicated on how a skilled crafter would work, including exact types of muscle contraction, amounts of joint movement, and total energy used by each joint. Paisley

(1929), an early occupational therapist, similarly executed very tight control over how children with cerebral palsy did craftwork, assuming that they ought to strive for "normal" movement as determined by the standard of children without disabilities.

Because a structuralist reading of practice views client problems as problems of underlying structures or mechanisms, such as muscle strength, muscle tone, or developmental age, it elaborates on clinical tools that address such structures and mechanisms as progressive resistive exercise, neurodevelopmental techniques, or linear sequences of developmental tasks. Although such a reading of practice can use activity as a therapeutic tool, it presumes that activity "works" by changing underlying structures and processes. Thus, a structuralist reading places into its background of concern persons' subjective experiences as they do things, their unique ways of doing things, and contextual influences on what they do and how.

Foundations of the Pragmatist–Structuralist Conversation

If both pragmatist and structuralist readings of practice have coexisted throughout occupational therapy's history, then on what bases have these discourses been negotiated and shaped? To answer this question, we examined the pragmatist–structuralist conversation in two ways that we believe shed some light on the field's persistent struggles over professional identity: (a) parallels in the shifting discourses of occupational therapy and the culture at large and (b) an internal incongruence between a pragmatist view of the human and a structuralist view of knowledge.

The Larger Cultural Ethos

Whereas pragmatism was a widely recognized and valued discourse in American society in the early 20th century, structuralism asserted its dominance by mid-century. Today, however, scholars argue that a revival of pragmatism and a shift to a poststructural discourse has occurred in the culture at large (Merquior, 1986; Putnam, 1990/1995; Rorty, 1992/1995). Therefore, nonfoundational knowledge, a critical stance toward language and power, and inquiries into the efficacy of actions to produce desired futures are once again prevalent in contemporary society (Cherryholmes, 1999; Kloppenberg, 1996). These reciprocating shifts in the culture at large have their parallel shift within occupational therapy, not in discrete phases, but in alternat-

ing ratios. Configuring the discourses as a ratio suggests that both remain present but in alternating proportions of dominance and influence.

The Early-20th-Century Conversation

Attesting to the early influence of pragmatism on occupational therapy, Slagle and Robinson (1941) described the field as a service that sought to "arouse interest, courage, and confidence; to exercise body and mind in healthful activity; to overcome disability; and to re-establish capacity for industrial and social usefulness" (p. 5). Habit training, a specific practice endorsed by Slagle, was described in words borrowed directly from James's work on habits: "There is no *general* habit, no *general* memory, that is common to all mankind. It is *individual* habit and memory. Everyone builds his or her own" (p. 33). The use of such pragmatist discourse that highlighted, like Meyer (1922) (see Chapter 4), the human capacity to restore oneself to usefulness and health through occupation was pervasive in the field's literature from about 1900 to 1940 (Kielhofner & Burke, 1983). Yet, on closer inspection of how some early practitioners actually provided services, structuralist approaches to clinical problems and methods are evident. Indeed, Slagle's habit training program consisted of a highly prescriptive regime of daily activity that a group of patients, after having been assigned to the program by a physician, were meticulously made to follow from the time they rose until just before bedtime (Slagle & Robinson, 1941). Thus, though described in bold pragmatist terms and certainly built around a balance of activity and rest at its core, the program concurrently evidenced structuralist themes of generalized procedures, standardization, and uniformity. Although infrequent, these structuralist themes and the idea that therapy "worked" by changing presumably universal internal structures or processes are evident in how other early occupational therapists provided services to other clinical populations in the 1920s and 1930s (e.g., Hurt, 1934; McNary, 1934; Paisley, 1929).

The Mid-Century Conversation

By mid-century, this ratio of pragmatist-to-structuralist discourses in occupational therapy was well under way to reversing itself along with the larger cultural shift toward structuralism. Thus, by the 1960s and 1970s, practitioners had mostly come to represent their profession and to base their methods on a view of humans that highlighted the ultimate importance of internal neurologic, psychic, or kinesiologic workings (Kielhofner &

Burke, 1983; see also Ayres, 1963; Huss, 1977; Moore, 1976). Nevertheless, some strong pragmatist readings of practice were evident, such as Yerxa's (1967) as already noted. Additionally, pragmatist themes kept repeatedly "popping up" in what were otherwise strong structuralist readings of practice. For example, Rood's 1958 Slagle lecture promoted the structuralist practice of applying a priori knowledge of presumably universal developmental patterns to all persons' "emotional, intellectual, and professional development as well as physical growth" (Rood, 1958, p. 328). Yet, by titling her lecture, "Every One Counts," and by stressing that people, whether patients or occupational therapists or their students, ought to be supported in setting their own goals, Rood (1958) simultaneously showed that she, like the pragmatists, valued human agency.

The Late-20th-Century Conversation

By century's end and, again, consistent with the general culture, the ratio of pragmatist-to-structuralist discourses in occupational therapy was reversing itself once again, and pragmatist readings of practice were ascending in dominance. Contemporary constructs of lifestyle redesign, conditional and narrative reasoning, and client-centered practice advanced a view of the human as agentic, teleological, and socially interdependent (Jackson, Carlson, Mandel, Zemke, & Clark, 1998; Law, 1998; Mattingly & Fleming, 1994). Likewise, new assessments urge continual evaluation of whether or how therapy helps persons do what they want and need to do given the particular circumstances of their lives, thus advancing a view of knowledge as flexible, fallible, and contingent (e.g., Coster, 1998; Law, 1998). Moreover, not only Clark's (1993), but also every other Eleanor Clarke Slagle lecture of the 1990s has placed pragmatist themes in the foreground: how resilience and a unique inner life can "transform…traumas into varying degrees of triumph" (Fine, 1991, p. 493 [see Chapter 32]); why "meaningfulness and purposefulness are key therapeutic qualities of occupation" (Trombly, 1995, p. 960 [see Chapter 11]); why "occupation…is so basic to human health yet so flexible" (Nelson, 1997, p. 11 [see Chapter 8]); how occupation enables "people to seize, take possession of, or occupy the spaces, time, and roles of their lives" (Fisher, 1998, p. 509 [see Chapter 9]); or how occupation is "the principal means through which people develop and express their personal identities" (Christiansen, 1999, p. 547 [see Chapter 34]). Perhaps Grady's 1994 Slagle lecture is the most telling of the field's shifting discourses given her correction of her own past practice theory for

wrongly emphasizing "ways therapists could influence the child's development rather than ways in which the environment could be prepared to accommodate the child's function" (Grady, 1995, p. 305 [see Chapter 25]).

Even as pragmatist discourse is again being loudly spoken in occupational therapy, structuralist discourse is far from mute. At times, the conversation between the two has been loud and impassioned. For example, the American Occupational Therapy Association's (AOTA's) 1991 debate over practitioners' use of physical agent modalities manifested a heated clash between pragmatist and structuralist readings of practice, unfolding just as a renewed pragmatist discourse was ascending in the field and eclipsing some of the esteem once reflexively attributed to structuralist practices (e.g., Ahlschwede, 1992; West & Wiemer, 1991). At other times in the conversation, structuralism has remained the louder voice of the two, especially when practitioners work within a biomedical culture. It was within this culture that Mattingly and Fleming (1994) found that practitioners straddle two discourses: one that concentrated on restoring persons to satisfying lives and another that concentrated on fixing body parts. Of considerable significance, many practitioners in their study experienced "an unease at the heart of their practice" as related to the field's self-portrayal as a service that treats "the whole person" (p. 296). That is, pragmatist values about holism, action, and natural experiences in the everyday world went "underground" (p. 296), meaning that practitioners did not speak too loudly of these values, if at all, during formal professional communications. Rather, to gain credibility in a culture that saw patients, their problems, and treatments in biomedical terms, the chart-talk, body-as-biomechanicalmachine language of medicine predominated.

A Pragmatist View of the Human but a Structuralist Approach to Knowledge

With the parallels between cultural and professional discourses duly noted, the pragmatist–structuralist conversation within occupational therapy did not, however, unfold in such equal exchanges. Indeed, a pragmatist view of the human was promoted early on in the field, but in tandem with a structuralist view of knowledge as objectively fixed, theoretically neutral, context free, universal, and derived from external authority. Hence, occupational therapy started cultivating at its inception a basic and problematic incompatibility between its oft-stated pragmatist view of the human and its structuralist approach toward knowledge.

The Evolution of Discordant Assumptions

We date these incompatible views of the human and knowledge at least to the start of World War I when early occupational therapists had a moral philosophy and a moral imperative to train more practitioners but no knowledge base of their own with which to educate them or much of any status or expertise with which to argue for particular educational practices. This vacuum was largely filled by deference to medical authorities. As Presseller (1984) noted in a historical study of the field's educational practices and policies, emergency war courses taught anatomy and kinesiology as core subjects to prepare reconstruction aides for their work with wounded soldiers. Also under the strong influence of physicians, basic medical sciences and applied medical lectures occupied more and more of the field's core curricula over ensuing decades. Of more significance than this core content per se (which is significant in and of itself), early pedagogical practices simultaneously embodied structuralist views of knowledge.

The Effects of Discordant Assumptions

Specifically, in approaching knowledge of the human body and disease as "core" professional knowledge received from medical authorities, occupational therapists were socialized early on into passively accepting knowledge as objectively "true" and inviolable. One cannot help but note the irony that as Meyer and Dewey were actively promoting richly experiential, self-exploratory, critically evaluative, and process-oriented pedagogic approaches for medical students and young children alike (Dewey, 1915; Muncie, 1939/1985), occupational therapy was being built on an educational foundation that all but forbade challenging medical authority and made virtually no room for critical inquiry (e.g., Quiroga, 1995; Serrett, 1985). This foundation presumed—contrary to the pragmatic method but in accord with the role of women at the time— that because male physicians would tightly control the work of female occupational therapists, the latter did not need to learn to evaluate and question received content for its coherence, implied actions, or the varying consequences of those actions across different life contexts. Hence, according to Presseller (1984), medical sciences, theory, and techniques were taught as subjects disconnected from one another and from their applications to practice in early educational programs. This lack of integration furthermore promulgated an immediate rupture between theory and clinical methods. Presseller blamed this rupture for many of the profession's identity issues and, therefore, for why practitioners could express "a commitment to activity" but could not connect theory to practice and would "use whatever technique was at hand" (p. iv). In our view, long-standing disconnections among basic academic content, theory, and techniques coupled with pedagogic methods that discouraged critical inquiry allowed a view of the human as a decontextualized biological system of presumably universal structures and functions to take root in occupational therapy and later thrive.

Beyond formal educational practices, structuralist approaches to knowledge are also evident in various clinical tools and ways of describing practice. In the 1930s and 1940s, occupational therapy faced increasing pressure to house its holistic conception of occupation in a container that could satisfy medicine's questions of efficacy and scientificity according to medical epistemology (Rogers, 1982). Licht's (1957) approach to activity analysis, a core clinical tool throughout the field's history, responded to and promoted this pressure by its kinesiologic formula of how movement ought ideally occur. As noted previously, by the 1960s and 1970s, practitioners commonly appropriated the language of kinesiology, neurology, and psychoanalysis to describe their methods and outcomes. In all cases, the structuralist analogy of a kaleidoscope as a matrix of a few recurring parts was advanced; that is, occupational behavior, a seemingly complex phenomenon, consisted "truly" of relatively few parts and mechanisms that could be fully enumerated.

Structuralist assumptions about how complex behavior is conceptualized continue to be evident today. *Uniform Terminology*, an influential document in practice and education, dates to 1979 when the field made an effort to define its domain of concern, clinical methods, and outcomes in standardized and theoretically neutral terms that captured "typical" practices irrespective of context (AOTA, 1979). By emphasizing performance components, all editions of the document have analogized, however tacitly, occupational performance to the structuralist kaleidoscope (AOTA, 1979, 1989, 1994). Moreover, although theory and context are acknowledged in the most recent edition, practice and occupational performance are still depicted with relatively few uniformly defined constructs that are presumably theoretically "neutral." It is furthermore presumed that these concepts can be readily interrelated using a preestablished grid with little regard to how various contingencies might influence or possibly even contradict implied relationships.

The Conversation Continues: Guideposts for the Future

Viewed as a whole, the intellectual history of occupational therapy may, in some important respects, be understood as a long conversation between pragmatist and structuralist discourses: Pragmatist readings of practice were first privileged over but did not silence structuralist readings, then the ratio of that privileging reversed itself, then reversed itself again, all in accord with the most compelling cultural ethos at hand. Moreover, this conversation has been characterized by numerous tensions, many of which remain unreconciled partly because of dynamics that took root early on and remain viable today. Specifically, a pragmatist view of the human was being spoken and clinically applied even as a structuralist approach to knowledge was instantiated in the earliest educational programs to legitimize the fledgling field. This incompatibility laid the groundwork, albeit not alone, for structuralist readings of practice to rise into eventual dominance. Structuralist views of knowledge as foundational, universal, and objectively securable contributed to an unease over critical evaluation of discordant professional practices. These dynamics speak to the profession's identity conundrum that has persisted for almost 100 years. Although its practitioners have portrayed their work as dedicated to treating patients holistically in accord with their personal interests and goals, they have struggled greatly in how best to realize and to match their clinical approaches to that portrayal.

If our interpretation of the profession's evolution is reasonably sound, then guideposts for navigating onward are suggested. These guideposts resonate with the more recent shift toward pragmatism in the larger culture: a state of affairs that we think is conducive to occupational therapy's best interests and offers practitioners great opportunities to author the profession's future. To exploit these opportunities, we propose that two new forms of literacy be cultivated.

Reading and Speaking the Language of Assumptions

One form of literacy concerns occupational therapists' capacities to apprehend the assumptions about humans and knowledge embodied in their readings of practice and, hence, how they interpret clinical problems, select media and methods, and conceive outcomes. With direct implications for the profession's internal and public identity, this form of literacy would allow occupational therapists to examine how the view of humans embedded in our shared language—"treating the whole person," "functional," or "meaningful occupation"—aligns with the view of humans embedded in actual professional methods. In complementary fashion, the capacity to examine assumptions about knowledge would raise occupational therapists' consciousness about what knowledge claims and whose knowledge claims inhabit their practice and on what bases they habitually grant legitimacy to claims of what is "core" or "truth" or "fact" in their practice. This consciousness would stimulate occupational therapists to adopt an appropriate skepticism toward categorical assertions about media and methods until the multifold consequences of those media or methods on persons' lives were credibly traced.

In effect, we are arguing on behalf of occupational therapists developing disciplined habits of mind that will spur their own conversations with themselves, ones that recurrently ask such questions as: What assumptions about the human are embedded in my therapy? What assumptions about knowledge dominate the criteria I use to legitimate my practice? On what evidence, on whose evidence, do I decide that my therapy actually helps persons do what they want and need to do given the particular hopes and challenges of their lives? Finally, do my clinical actions consequentially carry my patients to results that support the viability of occupational therapy?

Reading, Entering, and Shaping the Cultural Discourse

The second form of literacy has to do with cultural literacy. We refer specifically to occupational therapists' abilities to read the cultural ethos in which their practices (clinical, educational, research) are situated with respect to what values and ways of doing things are most privileged therein. Such cultural literacy would allow occupational therapists to discern when a particular ethos is in accord with the profession's best interests (as we believe is now the case with the pragmatist discourse) or significantly foil those interests (as we believe occurred during structuralism's dominance). Discernment of such matches and mismatches will be necessary to avoid passive absorption of cultural discourses and, instead, to decide proactively which forces to join, which to support or try to influence, and which to reject and resist outright.

These two forms of literacy would allow for the possibility of rich conversations not just within individual occupational therapists, but also among occupational therapists and the entire profession. Such literacy would help occupational therapists ensure that both disciplinary and interdisciplinary discourses are critically examined according to their capacity to deliver a particular coveted future: one that has transcended occupational therapy's identity confusions even as its eclectic array of media and methods have at times scattered in a helter-skelter of directions. We speak of the profession's dedication to helping people do what they want and need to do each day in ways that maximize their occupational capacities and health: key domains of the contemporary interdisciplinary construct of quality of life to which we believe occupational therapists can contribute enormously (Albert & Logsdon, 2000; Wilson & Cleary, 1995). In calling for these conversations, we stand in agreement with Kloppenberg (1996), a contemporary pragmatist, and Dewey who each regarded critical inquiry in social communication as the indispensable medium for clarifying and resolving disputes and instilling cooperation.

Were occupational therapists individually and collectively to resume a conversation started by Meyer and his pragmatist colleagues in which discordant views of humans and knowledge are understood to engender fundamentally different calls to action and ends, we believe that a number of desired outcomes would be facilitated. Consistent with the philosophy of pragmatism, a multiplicity of theories, viewpoints, and practices would be not only tolerated, but also generated by the communal process of anticipating how specific ideas and actions help usher in occupational therapy's particular coveted future: helping people do what they want and need to do each day in ways that maximize quality of life. Uncritical, unreflective, and uninformed practices would be explicitly eschewed because occupational therapists would skillfully draw crucial distinctions among divergent theories, assumptions, and practices with respect to whether and how well each serves this coveted future. Also with respect to this future, incompatibilities among a wide array of professional practices would be carefully scrutinized to ferret out those that were obstructive and to advance those that were progressive. Likewise, discussion and debate would be deliberately carried forward so that questions of great consequence to the profession's identity, and hence distinctive service to society, could be clarified and resolved. Three such questions in our view are these: What academic content and pedagogical practices best empower occupational therapists to ascertain

discourses and their corresponding claims about human nature and knowledge that shape professional practices? How do educators avoid the historical reliance on foundational knowledge and instead design curricula consistent with nonfoundational approaches to knowledge? What research questions and methods are relevant and conducive to a future where occupational therapists expertly address the occupational capacities of people and societies? If occupational therapists were to engage passionately and astutely in critical inquiry of present professional practices, and if they were to develop the kinds of literacy needed to identify influential discourses, the profession may begin to resolve its identity issues internally and within the culture at large and thrive as an autonomous academic profession whose value to society is both clear and great.

Acknowledgments

We thank Charles Cooper, PhD, Professor of History, University of North Carolina at Chapel Hill, for his review of an earlier draft of this article.

This article grew from Barb Hooper's original research into the core assumptions of occupational therapy that she completed in partial fulfillment of requirements for a doctoral cognate in occupational science undertaken in the Division of Occupational Science, University of North Carolina at Chapel Hill. Because both authors contributed equally to the article, order of authorship was determined alphabetically.

References

Ahlschwede, K. (1992). The Issue Is—Views on physical agent modalities and specialization within occupational therapy: A rebuttal. *American Journal of Occupational Therapy, 46,* 650–652. http://dx.doi.org/10.5014/ajot.46.7.650

Albert, S., & Logsdon, R. (Eds). (2000). *Assessing quality of life in Alzheimer's disease.* New York: Springer.

American Occupational Therapy Association. (1979). *Occupational therapy product output reporting system and uniform terminology for reporting occupational therapy services.* Rockville, MD: Author.

American Occupational Therapy Association. (1989). Uniform terminology for occupational therapy (2nd edition). *American Journal of Occupational Therapy, 43,* 808–815.

American Occupational Therapy Association. (1994). Uniform terminology for occupational therapy—Third edition. *American Journal of Occupational Therapy, 48,* 1047–1054.

Andi, R. (Ed.). (1999). *The Cambridge dictionary of philosophy* (2nd ed.). Cambridge, MA: Cambridge University Press.

Ayres, A. J. (1963). The development of perceptual–motor abilities: A theoretical basis for treatment of dysfunction, 1963 Eleanor Clarke Slagle lecture. *American Journal of Occupational Therapy, 17,* 221–225.

Breines, E. (1986). *Origins and adaptations: A philosophy of practice.* Lebanon, NJ: Geri-Rehab.

Cherryholmes, C. H. (1999). *Reading pragmatism* (Vol. 24). New York: Teachers College Press.

Christiansen, C. H. (1999). Defining lives: Occupation as identity: An essay on competence, coherence, and the creation of meaning, 1999 Eleanor Clarke Slagle lecture. *American Journal of Occupational Therapy, 53,* 547–558. Reprinted as Chapter 34. http://dx.doi.org/10.5014/ajot.53.6.547

Clark, F. (1993). Occupation embedded in a real life: Interweaving occupational science and occupational therapy, 1993 Eleanor Clarke Slagle lecture. *American Journal of Occupational Therapy, 47,* 1067–1078.

Coster, W. (1998). Occupation-centered assessment of children. *American Journal of Occupational Therapy, 52,* 337–344. http://dx.doi.org/10.5014/ajot.52.5.337

Denzin, N. K., & Lincoln, Y. S. (Eds.). (2000). *Handbook of qualitative research.* Thousand Oaks, CA: Sage.

Dewey, J. (1915). *Democracy and education: An introduction to the philosophy of education.* New York: Macmillan.

Dewey, J. (1930). *Human nature and conduct: An introduction to social thought.* New York: Modern Library.

Dewey, J. (1964). The continuum of ends–means. In R. D. Archambault (Ed.), *John Dewey on education: Selected writings* (pp. 97–107). Chicago: University of Chicago Press. Original work published 1939.

Dewey, J. (1973). Having an experience. In J. J. McDermott (Ed.), *The philosophy of John Dewey* (pp. 554–573). Chicago: University of Chicago Press. Original work published 1939.

Dewey, J. (1995). Does reality possess practical character? In R. B. Goodman (Ed.), *Pragmatism: A contemporary reader* (pp. 79–93). New York: Routledge. Original work published 1908.

Dosse, F. (1997). *History of structuralism* (D. Glassman, Trans.). Minneapolis, MN: University of Minnesota Press.

Emerson, R. W. (1995). Circles. In R. B. Goodman (Ed.), *Pragmatism: A contemporary reader* (pp. 22–34). New York: Routledge. Original work published 1883.

Fine, S. B. (1991). Resilience and human adaptability: Who rises above adversity? 1990 Eleanor Clarke Slagle lecture. *American Journal of Occupational Therapy, 45,* 493–503. http://dx.doi.org/10.5014/ajot.45.6.493 Reprinted as Chapter 32.

Fiorentino, M. R. (1975). Occupational therapy: Realization to activation, 1974 Eleanor Clarke Slagle lecture. *American Journal of Occupational Therapy, 29,* 15–21.

Fisher, A. G. (1998). Uniting practice and theory in an occupational therapy framework, 1998 Eleanor Clarke Slagle lecture. *American Journal of Occupational Therapy, 52,* 509–521. http://dx.doi.org/10.5014/ajot.52.7.509 Reprinted as Chapter 9.

Grady, A. P. (1995). Building inclusive community: A challenge for occupational therapy, 1994 Eleanor Clarke Slagle lecture. *American Journal of Occupational Therapy, 49,* 300–310. http://dx.doi.org/10.5014/ajot.49.4.300 Reprinted as Chapter 25.

Harland, R. (1987). *Superstructuralism: The philosophy of structuralism and post-structuralism.* New York: Methuen.

Hodge, C. (1997). Selection from systematic theology. In D. Hollinger & C. Capper (Eds.), *The American intellectual tradition* (Vol. II, pp. 6–12). New York: Oxford University Press. Original work published 1872.

Holmes, O. W. (1997). Natural law. In D. Hollinger & C. Capper (Eds.), *The American intellectual tradition* (Vol. II, pp. 123–126). New York: Oxford University Press. Original work published 1920.

Hooper, B. (1997). The relationship between pretheoretical assumptions and clinical reasoning. *American Journal of Occupational Therapy, 51,* 328–338. http://dx.doi.org/10.5014/ajot.51.5.328

Hurt, S. (1934). Occupational therapy in traumatic conditions. *Archives of Physical Therapy, X-ray, and Radium, 15,* 673–675.

Huss, A. J. (1977). Touch with care or a caring touch? 1976 Eleanor Clarke Slagle lecture. *American Journal of Occupational Therapy, 31,* 11–18.

Jackson, J., Carlson, M., Mandel, D., Zemke, R., & Clark, F. (1998). Occupation in lifestyle redesign: The well elderly study occupational therapy program. *American Journal of Occupational Therapy, 52,* 326–336. http://dx.doi.org/10.5014/ajot.52.5.326

James, W. (1985). Habit. *Occupational Therapy in Mental Health, 5*(3), 55–67. Original work published 1892.

James, W. (1995a). Pragmatism and humanism. In R. B. Goodman (Ed.), *Pragmatism: A contemporary reader* (pp. 65–75). New York: Routledge. Original work published 1907.

James, W. (1995b). What pragmatism means. In R. B. Goodman (Ed.), *Pragmatism: A contemporary reader* (pp. 53–64). New York: Routledge. Original work published 1907.

Kielhofner, G., & Barrett, L. (1998). Meaning and misunderstanding in occupational forms: A study in therapeutic goal setting. *American Journal of Occupational Therapy, 52,* 345–353. http://dx.doi.org/10.5014/ajot.52.5.345

Kielhofner, G., & Burke, J. P. (1983). The evolution of knowledge and practice in occupational therapy: Past, present, and future. In G. Kielhofner (Ed.), *Health through occupation: Theory and practice in occupational therapy* (pp. 3–54). Philadelphia: F. A. Davis.

Kloppenberg, J. T. (1996). Pragmatism: An old name for some new ways of thinking? *Journal of American History, 83*(1), 100–138.

Law, M. (1998). Client centered occupational therapy. Thorofare, NJ: Slack.

Leys, R. (1990). Adolf Meyer: A biographical note. In R. Leys & R. B. Evans (Eds.), *The correspondence between Adolf Meyer and Edward Bradford Titchener* (pp. 39–57). Baltimore: Johns Hopkins University Press.

Licht, S. (1957). Kinetic occupational therapy. In W. R. Dunton & S. Licht (Eds.), *Occupational therapy: Principles and practice* (pp. 53–83). Springfield, IL: Charles C Thomas.

Lippman, W. (1914). *Drift and mastery: An attempt to diagnose the current unrest.* New York: M. Kennerly.

Mattingly, C., & Fleming, M. H. (1994). *Clinical reasoning: Forms of inquiry in a therapeutic practice.* Philadelphia: F. A. Davis.

McNary, H. (1934). Anatomical considerations and technique in using occupations as exercise for orthopedic disabilities: Part III—Wrist and fingers. *Occupational Therapy and Rehabilitation, 13*(4), 24–29.

Mead, M. (1997). Selection from coming of age in Samoa. In D. A. Hollinger & C. Capper (Eds.), *The American intellectual tradition* (Vol. II, pp. 197–204). New York: Oxford University Press. Original work published 1928.

Merquior, J. G. (1986). *From Prague to Paris.* London: Verso.

Meyer, A. (1922). The philosophy of occupation therapy. *Archives of Occupational Therapy, 1,* 1–10. Reprinted as Chapter 2.

Meyer, A. (1948). Spontaneity. In A. Lief (Ed.), *The commonsense psychiatry of Dr. Adolph Meyer: Fifty-two selected papers* (pp. 576–589). New York: McGraw-Hill. Original work published 1933.

Moore, J. C. (1976). Behavior, bias, and the limbic system, 1975 Eleanor Clarke Slagle lecture. *American Journal of Occupational Therapy, 30,* 11–19.

Muncie, W. (1985). Historical and philosophical bases of psychobiology. *Occupational Therapy in Mental Health, 5*(3), 77–100. Original work published 1939.

Nelson, D. L. (1997). Why the profession of occupational therapy will flourish in the 21st century, 1996 Eleanor Clarke Slagle lecture. *American Journal of Occupational Therapy, 51,* 11–24. Reprinted as Chapter 8.

Paisley, A. (1929). Occupational therapy treatment for a group of spastic cases: Children under twelve years of age. *Occupational Therapy and Rehabilitation, 8*(2), 83–94.

Peirce, C. S. (1995). How to make our ideas clear. In R. B. Goodman (Ed.), *Pragmatism: A contemporary reader* (pp. 34–49). New York: Routledge. Original work published 1878.

Presseller, S. R. (1984). Occupational therapy education: Yesterday, today, and tomorrow (Doctoral dissertation, Boston University, 1984). *Dissertation Abstracts International, 45*(12B), 3777.

Putnam, H. (1995). A reconsideration of Deweyian democracy. In R. B. Goodman (Ed.), *Pragmatism: A contemporary reader* (pp. 183–205). New York: Routledge. Original work published 1990.

Quiroga, V. A. M. (1995). *Occupational therapy: The first thirty years, 1900–1930.* Bethesda, MD: American Occupational Therapy Association.

Reed, K. (1986). Tools of practice: Heritage or baggage? 1986 Eleanor Clarke Slagle lecture. *American Journal of Occupational Therapy, 40,* 597–605. Reprinted as Chapter 47.

Reilly, M. (1962). Occupational therapy can be one of the great ideas of 20th century medicine, 1961 Eleanor Clarke Slagle lecture. *American Journal of Occupational Therapy, 16,* 1–9. Reprinted as Chapter 7.

Rogers, J. C. (1982). The spirit of independence: The evolution of philosophy. *American Journal of Occupational Therapy, 36,* 709–715.

Rood, M. S. (1958). Every one counts, 1958 Eleanor Clarke Slagle lecture. *American Journal of Occupational Therapy, 12,* 326–329.

Rorty, R. (1995). Feminism and pragmatism. In R. B. Goodman (Ed.), *Pragmatism: A contemporary reader* (pp. 125–149). New York: Routledge. Original work published 1992.

Serrett, K. D. (1985). Another look at occupational therapy's history: Paradigm or pair-of-hands? *Occupational Therapy in Mental Health, 5*(3), 1–31.

Slagle, E. C., & Robinson, H. A. (1941). *Syllabus for training of nurses in occupational therapy* (2nd ed.). Utica, NY: State Hospital Press.

Stevenson, L., & Haberman, D. L. (1998). *Ten theories of human nature.* New York: Oxford University Press.

Sturrock, J. (1986). *Structuralism.* London: Paladin.

Sumner, W. G. (1997). Sociology. In D. Hollinger & C. Capper (Eds.), *The American intellectual tradition* (Vol. II, pp. 29–38). New York: Oxford University Press. Original work published 1881.

Tinning, R. (1991). Teacher education and pedagogy: Dominant discourses and the process of problem setting. *Journal of Teaching in Physical Education, 11*(1), 1–20.

Trombly, C. A. (1995). Occupation: Purposefulness and meaningfulness as therapeutic mechanisms, 1995 Eleanor Clarke Slagle Lecture. *American Journal of Occupational Therapy, 49,* 960–972. Reprinted as Chapter 11.

Ward, L. F. (1997). Mind as social factor. In D. Hollinger & C. Capper (Eds.), *The American intellectual tradition* (Vol. II, pp. 39–47). New York: Oxford University Press. Original work published 1884.

West, W. (1992). Ten milestone issues in AOTA history. *American Journal of Occupational Therapy, 46,* 1066–1074.

West, W. L., & Wiemer, R. B. (1991). The Issue Is—Should the Representative Assembly have voted as it did, when it did, on occupational therapists' use of physical agent modalities? *American Journal of Occupational Therapy, 45,* 1143–1147.

Wilcock, A. A. (1998). *An occupational perspective of health.* Thorofare, NJ: Slack.

Wilson, I. B., & Cleary, P. D. (1995). Linking clinical variables with health-related quality of life. *Journal of the American Medical Association, 273,* 59–65.

Yerxa, E. J. (1967). Authentic occupational therapy, 1966 Eleanor Clarke Slagle lecture. *American Journal of Occupational Therapy, 21,* 1–9.

CHAPTER 6

Occupational Therapy and Rehabilitation: An Awkward Alliance

JUDITH FRIEDLAND

In the preface to his book *Rehabilitation Medicine: A Textbook on Physical Medicine and Rehabilitation,* Rusk (1958) noted the objectives of the newly founded field of rehabilitation medicine. The first was:

> to eliminate the physical disability if that is possible; the second, to reduce or alleviate the disability to the greatest extent possible; and the third, to retrain the person with a residual physical disability to live and work within the limits of the disability but to the hilt of his capabilities. (p. 7)

Rusk went on to say that, although effective rehabilitation depended on the skills and services of members of many professions, "the physician, however, *by the very nature of the problem* [italics added], must be the leader of the team" (p. 7).

The phrase "by the very nature of the problem" provides the clue to the difficulty for occupational therapists in rehabilitation as well as the theme for this article. If the very nature of the problem *is the disability itself* and efforts are directed at eliminating it, then occupational therapists are at a disadvantage, because for us, the very nature of the problem *is not the disability but the occupational performance of the person with the disability.* We must then consider the possibility that some of the difficulties we have with our roles and with the content of our curricula are a result of there being more in the paradigm of rehabilitation that *conflicts* with occupational therapy than complements it.

In this article, I argue that rehabilitation is only a part of occupational therapy; that it *is an aspect but not the essence of occupational therapy,* that embracing

rehabilitation in the way that we have has contributed to our identity problems; and that, although occupational therapy has enhanced the field of rehabilitation, rehabilitation has not helped the profession of occupational therapy to the same extent. I briefly review early influences on occupational therapy and reflect on some philosophical ideas about activity and occupation. I examine the role of occupational therapy as treatment both in Canada and in the United States during the first part of this century and then trace the incorporation of occupational therapy into rehabilitation. Finally, I reflect on the influence that rehabilitation has had on our core values and note recent changes that hold some promise for our future directions.

Early Influences in Occupational Therapy

Articles that describe the use of occupation to promote or restore health (e.g., Bing, 1981 [see Chapter 2]; Engelhardt, 1977; Haas, 1944; Kielhofner & Burke, 1977; Peloquin, 1991a, 1991b [see Chapter 3]) often begin with ancient Egypt and work through biblical times to Greece and Rome, where the virtues of activities and pastimes (e.g., art, music, exercise, dance) were extolled. These chronicles tend to skip several centuries to reach the Moral Treatment Era of the early 1800s, where a caring environment and the notion of work were added to activities as a means of promoting health (Bockhoven, 1972). With World War I (WWI), the arts-and-crafts movement became well established (Levine, 1987), as did curative workshops (Robinson, 1981), and occupational therapy as we know it began to unfold. No longer do we see the profession as embedded in other movements; rather, it has become a separate entity (Peloquin, 1991a, 1991b [see Chapter 3]). In the late 1930s and early 1940s, the profession began to take a biomedical turn and pretty much stayed there for the next four decades, with periodic visits back to core concepts through contributions from, among others, Reilly (1962 [see Chapter 7]), Kielhofner and Burke (1977), Fidler and Fidler (1978), Gilfoyle (1984), and West (1984). It is as though the core concept of occupation as a means of promoting health and well-being was somehow elusive and, in not being well enough articulated, became dissipated.

Philosophical Ideas About Activity and Occupation[1]

For all the histories of the profession that have traced the idea of occupation, very few have grappled with what it is that is so therapeutic about occupation and why its value has persisted over the centuries. Philosophical ideas have contributed to the importance we attach to the concept of activity while also fostering its elusiveness. Plato came closest to noting what we consider the inherent need for activity when he suggested that "in every man and woman there is born the instinct to make and to do" (as cited in Bruce, 1933, p. 6).[2] The implication for occupational therapy is that although injured or ill in some way, people still need to make and to do. This idea is probably the closest we come in philosophical terms to the essence of occupational therapy.

Plato also spoke about *therapeutic arts,* which could be considered to include rehabilitation, and noted their different components:

> In the state of all [such] therapeutic arts, the corrective portion is more apparent but less important, while the regulative portion is largely hidden but far more essential. [Hence] there is grave danger lest "prevention" and "maintenance," the real work of the art, be overlooked, and attention exclusively be devoted to the correction of diseases already there, a mere by-product of the art. (Wild, 1946, p. 65)

Thus, in Plato's terms, because occupational therapy's role in rehabilitation does not cure disease or remove disability (i.e., the corrective portion of therapeutic arts) but, instead, works to develop or maintain occupational performance *despite* disease or disability (i.e.,

the regulative and essential portion of therapeutic arts), its importance is often overlooked.

Aristotle (trans. 1925) wrote about pursuing well-being. He saw well-being of the soul *(eudaimonia)* as the end result of desirable and satisfying activity or action *(praxis).* In *The Nicomachean Ethics,* he expounded on the notion that "of all things that come to us by nature, we first acquire the potentiality and later exhibit the activity." He said that "the things we have to learn before we can do them, we learn by doing them," and although his comment that "states of character arise out of like activities" (p. 28) refers to how man becomes virtuous, it also reflects the notion that only by doing can one become. Adler (1991) commented on Aristotle's view that both practical thinking and productive thinking are required to carry out purposeful activity and noted that Aristotle believed that "until making and doing actually begin, productive thinking and practical thinking bear no fruit" (p. 71).

In distinguishing between basic needs and wants, Aristotle noted that everyone has the same basic needs. These "needs" (for food, for shelter, for love, etc.) were called the "external goods," and like Maslow, Aristotle said that they must be met in order to approach the fulfillment of all our human capacities. The "wants" in life can also be met as long as they do not interfere with our abilities to satisfy our needs or fulfill our capacities. Occupational therapists facilitate their patients' abilities to meet their needs and wants and recognize the necessity of enacting thinking to achieve those ends.

Aristotle also examined the meaning of happiness and the ways in which it could be achieved. For him, happiness was in and of itself an activity; more specifically, happiness existed when one was engaged in "virtuous" activity. It was Aristotle, perhaps, who started the debate on the relationship between work and leisure when he stated that "happiness is thought to depend on leisure; for we are busy that we may have leisure." His ideas about reaching a sense of self through activity that develops our capacity and makes us happy and fulfilled in the process are certainly echoed within occupational therapy (e.g., Reilly, 1962 [see Chapter 7]; Yerxa, 1993) and psychology (Csikszentmihalyi, 1991; White, 1971).

Voltaire, whose works appeared in the middle and late 1700s, also thought about the meaning of occupation. For Voltaire, activity was a means of bringing relief to much of the unhappiness that life brought: "Man is born for action...not to be occupied and not to exist amount to the same thing" (as cited in Waterman, 1942, p. 40).

---

[1]Philosophical discussions refer primarily to activity but seem to use the term to mean what we would call occupations (e.g., "groups of activities and tasks of everyday life" [Townsend, 1997, p. 34]).

[2]A primary source for this quote by Bruce (1933) has not been found despite an extensive search; it may not have originated with Plato.

Thus, at the very least, to support existence, one must be occupied so as to see evidence of existing. Occupational therapists who have worked with persons who are severely depressed know the glimmer of hope that comes to one who has been occupied and has seen that something qualitatively different can be experienced that is outside of despair. Indeed, labeling such engagement as positive is a cornerstone of cognitive therapy for depression (Beck, Rush, Shaw, & Emery, 1979).

John Stuart Mill (1859/1947) wrote in *On Liberty* about the importance of encouraging and celebrating individuality in the activities that people undertake. Provided no harm was done to others, individuality could bring human beings nearer to the best thing they could be and could have a cumulative effect on the whole human race. Mill said, "In proportion to the development of his individuality each person becomes more valuable to himself, and is therefore capable of being more valuable to others" (p. 63). Therapists who assume a client-centered approach to enabling occupation help their clients to develop their individuality and increase their opportunities for self-fulfillment.

Philosophical ideas about occupation seem to have centered on, at the very least, making life bearable (Voltaire); maintaining health (Plato); being responsible for happiness (Aristotle); and at the highest level, being self-actualized (Mill, 1859/1947). These ideas can readily be seen in the roots of our profession (Friedland, 1988; Peloquin, 1991a, 1991b [see Chapter 3]) where it was believed that occupation could relieve despair (e.g., of persons who were mentally ill) and could contribute to overall well-being (e.g., of soldiers during WWI). It was also thought that lack of meaningful activity could make one more ill or dysfunctional (e.g., as with persons recovering from tuberculosis) and that the right type and level of activity could bring one to a state of mastery. Johnson (1996) noted the importance of these ideas remaining central to our profession: "The greater our understanding of occupations and how they maintain, enhance, and promote health and well-being, the greater will be our ability to link this knowledge with practice and education of future therapists" (p. 393).

Occupation as Treatment: The United States and Canada (1900–1940)

In the United States, an early rationale for occupation as treatment was simply that patients did better and were less restless if they were engaged in activity. Nurse Susan Tracy started using occupations as treatment in 1905 and is credited with providing the first course in occupations in 1906 (Reed & Sanderson, 1983). Other early courses in occupational therapy were prompted by similar reasoning; for example, the course at the Chicago School of Civics and Philanthropy in 1908 was instigated by two members of the State Board of Control in protest against the idleness they saw on the wards of the state hospitals (Dunton, 1918). Indeed the formation of the National Society for the Promotion of Occupational Therapy (NSPOT) was itself prompted by George Barton's experience of being ill with tuberculosis and finding that manual activities hastened his recovery. It is interesting to note the professions of the founders of NSPOT and to consider their perspectives on occupations. For psychiatrist William Rush Dunton, architects Thomas Kidner and George Barton, social worker Eleanor Clarke Slagle, teacher Susan Johnston, secretary Isabel Newton, and nurse Susan Tracy, the key idea was that the right occupation could help persons in need (Peloquin, 1991b [see Chapter 3]). Although they spoke of occupation as curative, it was not in relation to medical or psychiatric conditions but rather to the human condition, to harnessing occupation for what Hall called one of the "sources of human power" (as cited in Peloquin, 1991b, p. 739 [see Chapter 3]). Schwartz (1992) emphasized the similarities between Dewey's ideas on the importance of occupations in education and occupational therapy's use of occupations to facilitate healthy development in patients. Similarly, Schemm (1994) noted that the arts-and-crafts movement, which greatly influenced early practice in occupational therapy, saw activity as a means of improving society; it was a way "to socialize less accepted members of society such as disabled, mentally ill, impoverished, and underachieving persons in insane asylums and manual training programs" (p. 1083).

Although Adolph Meyer was not considered an official founder of occupational therapy, his influence in psychiatric circles of the day meant that his ideas on the importance of occupation carried considerable weight. Meyer (1922/1977 [see Chapter 4]) promoted the value of occupation, including work-like activities, and his words on the subject have become very familiar to occupational therapists: "The proper use of time in some helpful and gratifying activity appeared [to me] a fundamental issue in the treatment of any neuropsychiatric patient" (p. 639). Meyer stressed the need for "giving opportunities rather than prescriptions. . . opportunities to work, opportunities to do and to plan and create, and to learn to use material" (p. 641).

In Canada at the turn of the century, C. K. Clarke was prominent among those advocating occupation in the Ontario Hospitals for the Insane. Clarke, who was a noted psychiatrist, wrote of his experiences at the Rockwood Asylum in Kingston, Ontario, where he incorporated a wide range of activities (e.g., painting, carpentry, music, work, sports) into the daily regime. At that time, there was great concern over the need to restrain patients. Clarke noted that nonrestraint had become an established practice at Rockwood, and he (like Meyer) credited this fact to the use of occupation. Clarke (1922) stated:

> No one comforted himself with the belief that occupation was a panacea for all the ills that the mind is heir to, but we did realize that intelligently supervised occupation was a tremendous factor not only in aiding cure in recent cases, but in making happy and improving the most unfortunate class in our community. (p. 13)

In 1918, the University of Toronto offered the first course in occupations in Canada (Robinson, 1981). These short courses were established in the faculty of applied science at the request of Herbert Haultain, a professor of engineering, and Norman Burnette, the head of a workshop at a military hospital. Both men saw the need for occupations for soldiers who, on returning from WWI, were confined to bed. Professor C. H. C. Wright of the department of architecture was in charge, and Winifred Brainerd, an American occupational therapist, was brought from New York to teach. Kidner, the Canadian architect who had also been a founder of NSPOT, was then vocational secretary of the Canadian Military Hospitals Commission, and he helped to organize the venture. Within the year, some 350 women had graduated from one of these short courses, and most of them went on to work with soldiers returning from the war (Robinson, 1981).

C. B. Farrar (1940b), a noted psychiatrist who was later to become the first superintendent of the Toronto Psychiatric Hospital, wrote about occupation as treatment for war neuroses and psychoses during WWI. He stated that "congenital and systematic occupation should be given foremost place in any scheme of treatment. Idleness... should be reduced to the uttermost minimum" (p. 16). He elaborated on this idea, noting that:

> there is the benefit of occupation as such, common to practically all cases; and there is the pos-

sible benefit of an awakened and sustained interest in an employment which is new, and which affords a pleasing relief from a former distasteful or humdrum occupation. Here we have occupation-therapy passing over into vocational re-training, with the latter perhaps completing the cure begun by the former. (Farrar, 1940a, p. 23)

At Government House in Ottawa in 1925, Farrar was among those who spoke at an open meeting of the newly formed Ontario Society of Occupational Therapists. A prominent newspaper of the time reported his comments as follows:

> Next to proper housing and proper feeding, occupational therapy is the most important factor in the cure of nervous patients. The rest cure, so long ordered for these patients, has been supplanted by work, and occupational therapy provides this most necessary employment and effects the cure. ("Is Practical Christianity," 1925)

This link between occupations and work had been important since the Moral Treatment Era and has continued throughout our history.

In summary, the main focus of occupational therapy in the early part of the century, both in the United States and in Canada, was on the person and on the activity. The approach did not address pathology, which at the time was primarily mental illness; rather, it focused on interests and abilities and worked around the pathology to engage the person in occupations. It was engagement in occupation that could have an effect on the person and could, over time, be transformative. Engagement in occupation was made possible by the therapist's knowledge and understanding of the patient's condition and came from within the therapeutic relationship that had been established. As the profession continued to develop, occupational therapists began to work with persons with physical disabilities, for example, those who were injured in industrial accidents. The goal of therapy was to return them to productive lives, economic independence, and social usefulness (Ambrosi & Schwartz, 1995a). By the early 1920s, curative workshops were established in both the United States (Baldwin, 1919) and Canada (LeVesconte, 1935) where work-like activities were designed to prepare patients for employment.

The largest population of persons with physical injuries had been the soldiers returning from WWI, and, with them, began a gradual shift in occupational therapy toward a focus on medical outcomes and away from earlier humanitarian and social benefits (Ambrosi & Schwartz, 1995b). During this early period, different philosophies of occupational therapy for persons with physical disabilities began to be seen. In the United States, Wilson H. Henderson was one of the first physicians to apply occupational therapy to physical disabilities. He thought that occupational therapy for men with war-time injuries should require technical rather than physical strength, more mental than physical activity, and enough general exercise to stimulate recovery (Reed & Sanderson, 1983). Referring to Canadian war-time experience, Goldwin Howland (1944/1986), physician and first president of the Canadian Association of Occupational Therapists, delineated five forms of occupational therapy: diversional, physical, recreational, psychological, and preventive. All but the second of these (physical) were directed at maintaining interest and morale.

Graded activity, which had been widely used with patients with tuberculosis in both countries to improve overall physical endurance and maintain morale, soon became more focused and was directed to improving range of motion and strengthening muscle groups (Creigton, 1993). The psychologist Baldwin tried to use both a holistic approach and the scientific method in designing activities for WWI veterans attending his occupational therapy department at Walter Reed Hospital (Wish-Baratz, 1989). He stated that the purpose of occupational therapy was to "help each patient find himself and function again as a complete man, physically, socially, educationally and economically" (Baldwin, 1919, p. 447). However, the means of achieving that purpose was through remedial exercises that required "a series of specific voluntary movements involved in the ordinary trades or occupations, physical training, play, or the daily routine activities of life" (p. 448). By the 1940s, Sidney Licht, a physician and editor of the journal *Occupational Therapy and Rehabilitation* was promoting "kinetic" and "metric" occupational therapy (i.e., muscle strengthening, joint mobilization, coordination training) and increasing the amount of work completed in a unit of time or the number of times an activity was completed in a calendar unit (Reed & Sanderson, 1983).

Occupational Therapy and Rehabilitation

By 1937, occupational therapy practice patterns, as reported by the American Medical Association (AMA), which registered all American occupational therapists at that time, showed that 36 occupational therapists worked in orthopedics, 456 in general hospitals, and 1,809 in mental hospitals (Reed & Sanderson, 1983). These numbers reflect the state of health care at the time, that is, the high numbers of persons with mental illness who were institutionalized and the fact that people were not surviving the serious illnesses and injuries that were later to be seen with the development of modern medicine. However, the numbers also reflect the fact that the profession was still strongly focused in mental health.

It was not until after WWII that the shift in focus for occupational therapy from occupation as a means of developing or maintaining health to occupation as a means of enhancing medical outcomes became firmly established. The change came with the development of the new specialty of "physical therapy physicians" and the subsequent development of departments of physical medicine and rehabilitation. This medical specialty area, which had been developing since the turn of the century, had been based primarily on an interest in the use of "medical electricity," later called electrotherapy (Gritzer & Arluke, 1985).

Rusk, who was a major figure in the development of this new medical specialty, recalled that he had created programs in air force hospitals for making good use of convalescent time. He said that "gradually, the concept of rehabilitation came to me as I found out how much really could be done for these men" (as cited in Gritzer & Arluke, 1985, p. 91). After several years of battling with the AMA, orthopedic surgeons, the Department of Veterans Affairs, and the Office of Vocational Rehabilitation, physical therapy physicians were finally allowed to call themselves physiatrists and to call their field physical medicine and rehabilitation. One of their early acts was to bring physical therapy and occupational therapy training programs, such as those at Columbia University and the University of Illinois, under their authority (Gritzer & Arluke, 1985). At the University of Toronto, a department of physical medicine and rehabilitation was created in 1950 that actually combined the educational programs for physical therapists and occupational therapists into one and brought the new program, for "P&OTs," under the control of physiatry. During this same period, many hospitals in the United States and Canada developed departments of physical medicine and rehabilitation. As Brintnell, Cardwell, Robinson, and Madill (1986) pointed out, "The development of physical medicine was to influence the services provided by occupational therapy for years to come" (p. 27). (See also Colman [1992] for a description of occupational therapy's struggle to maintain its roots and autonomy as physical therapists and physiatrists came to dominate the field.)

In his chapter on the role of occupational therapy in rehabilitation, Rusk (1958) had delineated three areas of therapy: supportive (psychologic), prevocational (vocational), and functional (physical). Supportive therapy was intended to maintain morale by helping the patient to realize his or her abilities and was to be closely coordinated with the psychiatrist and psychologist. Prevocational therapy was designed to assess and train the patient in preparation for a return to work and was to be a joint effort with the vocational counselor. The functional component of occupational therapy was directed to exercise in which the patient used his or her disabled part in the course of some constructive procedure, such as woodworking. Principles of therapeutic exercise were followed, starting with active-assistive exercises for those muscles that had a muscle-testing grade of poor plus or better and working toward active and active-resistive activities. For Rusk, the activity had become the means, and improving joint range, muscle strength, and motor skill the end. Brintnell et al. (1986) summed up the period during which these practices were followed in Canada, stating that "the fifties and sixties saw the emergence of the rehabilitation movement and with it, mixed blessings for occupational therapy. The physical aspects of treatment gained prominence over psychological concerns" (p. 33).

Gradually, the role of occupation as central to maintaining health and well-being began to erode. The pressure for occupational therapists to be a part of rehabilitation as it was conceived and practiced was too hard to resist. To modify the concept and practice of rehabilitation to better suit occupational therapy was too difficult, given the small size of the profession and its perceived lack of power and credibility (Froehlich, 1992). Equally important was the fact that *rehabilitation* was a glamorous term. The medical model, complete with its uniforms and jargon, gave occupational therapists what was considered a loftier status. Rehabilitation was more respected and better understood than occupational therapy, and it caught the public eye. Persons with physical disabilities had the public's sympathy (certainly more so than persons who were mentally ill), and if we were helping them in such obvious and concrete ways as getting stronger, moving faster, or gaining a fuller range of motion, well, then we must be good too.

Another pressure away from the meaning and value attributed to occupation came in work with children with cerebral palsy and persons with polio. During this period, occupational therapists became fixated on the value of independence (Froehlich, 1992) and worked with their patients to achieve it despite the time away from occupations that might have been more meaningful, such as being a student. The focus on dressing as an end in and of itself rather than as the means to an end continues to this day in many settings. Of course, there were exceptions, and many facilities still engaged their patients in occupations. One interesting example of where meaningful activity continued to be important was in the craft work that occupational therapists did with Native North American populations with tuberculosis (Staples & McConnell, 1993).

So for many years we have devoted a large part of our energies to fitting in with the medical model, where occupational therapists were never intended to be (West, 1984). As occupational therapists continued to compete in the reductionist environment of medicine, we found that our qualifications were generally not as good as others who could fix broken parts. And although *no one else* could do what we did, no one, including ourselves, seemed to value that. No one, including ourselves, seemed to notice that we had abdicated our role in developing and maintaining health and well-being through occupation in order to join the ranks of the reductionists. Meanwhile, physical therapists, who most of us would agree are the better "fixers," grew in number and stature so that, today, in North America, there are twice as many physical therapists as occupational therapists. Some would support Yerxa (1992) in saying that in our efforts to align ourselves more closely with medical values and medical thinking, we have become more like physical therapy in the role we play in rehabilitation. It is ironic that we should be competing with physical therapists when, on the basis of the backgrounds of those who created our profession, one would have predicted that we would be competing with nurses, engineers, architects, social workers, or teachers.

Newer Models of Rehabilitation

Over the years since Rusk's initial description of rehabilitation, the concept of rehabilitation has broadened, and its definition is now somewhat more in tune with the foundations of occupational therapy. Instead of focusing only on restoring function, the field now recognizes other important outcomes. For example, the World Health Organization's 1981 definition stated that:

> rehabilitation includes all measures aimed at reducing the impact of disabling and handicapping conditions, and at enabling the disabled and handicapped to achieve social integration. Rehabilitation aims not only at training disabled and handicapped persons to adapt to their environment, but also intervening in the immediate environment and society as a whole in order to facilitate their social integration. (p. 9)

Such a definition recognized the end result of social integration, a broad category that could be considered to subsume occupations. It sharpened the focus of rehabilitation on reducing the impact of disability and handicap, thus opening the door to interventions in the environment.

More recently, the *Research Plan for the National Center for Medical Rehabilitation Research* (U.S. Department of Health and Human Services, 1993) has suggested that "the successful process of rehabilitation restores the individual to maximal functioning *and provides a foundation for a fulfilling, productive life following rehabilitation* [italics added]" (p. 29). Note that the definition is still tied to function, and rehabilitation needs only to provide the foundation for a fulfilling, productive life. It is as though somehow after rehabilitation these attributes of life will magically occur. However, the document further stated:

> Activities which enhance productivity and give a sense of purpose and enjoyment to life must be possible; these may include employment, education, recreation, family, and community involvement. This participation should provide meaning and dignity to life so that people with disability have a reason to live, not merely to exist. (p. 29)

So perhaps at last, we are beginning to see some of our occupational therapy values coming to the forefront in rehabilitation and that the field is richer for the role that we can play. Moreover, in this role, we can use our understanding of medical thinking without adopting the medical paradigm (Yerxa, 1992). And from a pragmatic point of view, if "social integration and fulfillment" become outcome measures in rehabilitation—as indeed they should—then our special skills and core values could become very important in this era of evidencebased practice. But how do we go from the *ifs, shoulds,* and *coulds* to the (re)enactment of our core values?

Friedson (1994) suggested that:

> the competition between professions for jurisdiction over a particular area may be analyzed as conflicting definitions of the *nature of the problem or activity* [italics added] each is seeking to control, and claims about the way they can best be solved or carried out. (p. 70)

Rusk and the founders of rehabilitation thought that the very nature of the problem was the disability itself, and in practice, they focused their efforts on restoring function to the person with the disability where our role was helpful, though limited. The founders of occupational therapy incorporated philosophical views about the importance of activity and determined that the very nature of the problem was a person's intrinsic need for occupation that was thwarted by illness or disability. Social integration, productivity, meaning, and dignity in life are outcomes of rehabilitation that are consonant with the core values of occupational therapy. Knowing how to enable persons with disabilities to achieve these outcomes is the special knowledge and skill that, in sociological terms, make occupational therapy a profession (Friedson, 1994).

Future Directions

Our profession has its own view of what the issue in rehabilitation is and how it is solvable; that is, we have our own paradigm within which to operate. Both in the United States and in Canada, there appears to be a growing consensus in occupational therapy that a return to our core values is needed (e.g., Kielhofner & Burke, 1977; Polatajko, 1992; Townsend, 1997; West, 1984; Yerxa, 1992). As a profession, occupational therapy must now be prepared to champion that cause and to advance its aims.

However, there is a deep concern that as a profession we may not be up to the task. In 1966, Thelma Cardwell, the first occupational therapist to hold the position of president of the Canadian Association of Occupational Therapists (which since its inception in 1926 had a male physician as president) stated:

> We are too diffident a group, both individually and collectively. We are much too timid in bring-

ing our work to the attention of others. In short, we are ineffective in selling our profession. It is time we learned to be vocal, to be enthusiastic, to be competent, in representing the professional point of view of our discipline and in interpreting our aims and functions. These, with an added degree of confidence, can do an immeasurable amount in establishing the personal and professional reputation and respect that our profession warrants. (Cardwell, 1966, p. 139)

Others have made this plea before (Reilly, 1962 [see Chapter 7]) and since (Johnson, 1996). We know what to do; the question is will we do it? Will we undertake the research needed to study occupation and expand our understanding of the concept? Will we develop a core body of knowledge regarding occupation? Will we redesign our curricula to reflect our focus on the centrality of occupation? Will we demand the liberal arts background for entry to our programs that this focus requires? Will we instill confidence in our students about the value of our focus, and can we establish the competence to underpin that confidence? Finally, can we move on from the education of our students to the reeducation of practicing therapists who for too long have supported narrow views of our role in rehabilitation? Only then will we have a strong enough voice to undertake the social and political activity that is required. For as Friedson (1994) noted:

> The maintenance and improvement of the profession's position in the market-place, and in the division of labour surrounding it, requires continuous political activity. The profession must become an interest group to at once advance its aims and to protect itself from those with competing aims. (p. 68)

Conclusion

We are the only health profession that can focus on occupation; others can focus on function but not on occupation. As philosophers noted centuries ago, activity is what defines the lives of human beings. With illness or disability, this route to meaning is often threatened. It is the mission of occupational therapists, alone among health professionals, to keep that route open. When we define ourselves exclusively as "rehab professionals"—even with the most modern of definitions—we limit our ability to make that unique contribution.

There is clearly a common denominator, a unifying theme, in all that we do, and as has been said in many

different ways, occupation is it. Occupation is what explains the "jack of all trades" epithet that makes us so uncomfortable. It is why we can help persons with all kinds of disabilities and at all ages. In occupation, we have had, and do have, a unique and powerful tool not to cure, but to positively influence health and well-being. However, we must get on with it and not continue to be lured away. For to paraphrase that great contemporary philosopher Will Rogers, we may be on the right track, but if we just sit on it, we will be run over by the train.

Acknowledgments

This article was originally prepared for the 1995 spring institute at the Department of Occupational Therapy, Dalhousie University, Nova Scotia, Canada. I thank the faculty members for inviting me to speak and the participants for their stimulating discussion. I also thank two students: Joanne Brady, whose final year major paper in this area added further insight, and Mary Liang, who assisted in the preparation of the final manuscript.

References

Adler, M. (1991). *Aristotle for everybody*. New York: Collier.

Ambrosi, E., & Schwartz, K. B. (1995a). Looking Back—The profession's image, 1917–1925, part 1: Occupational therapy as represented in the media. *American Journal of Occupational Therapy, 49*, 715–719. http://dx.doi.org/10.5014/ajot.49.7.715

Ambrosi, E., & Schwartz, K. B. (1995b). Looking Back—The profession's image, 1917–1925, part 2: Occupational therapy as represented by the profession. *American Journal of Occupational Therapy, 49*, 828–832. http://dx.doi.org/10.5014/ajot.49.8.828

Aristotle. (trans. 1925). *The Nicomachean ethics*. Oxford, U.K.: Oxford University Press.

Baldwin, B. T. (1919). Occupational therapy. *American Journal of Care for Cripples, 8*, 447–451.

Beck, A. T., Rush, J., Shaw, B., & Emery, G. (1979). *Cognitive therapy of depression*. New York: Guilford.

Bing, R. K. (1981). Occupational therapy revisited: A paraphrastic journey, 1981 Eleanor Clarke Slagle lecture. American Journal of *Occupational Therapy, 35*, 499–518. Reprinted as Chapter 2.

Bockhoven, J. S. (1972) *Moral treatment in community mental health*. New York: Springer.

Brintnell, S., Cardwell, T., Robinson, I., & Madill, H. (1986). The fifties and sixties: The rehabilitation era: Friend or foe. *Canadian Journal of Occupational Therapy, 53*, 27–33.

Bruce, H. (1933). An address. Third Annual Convention of the Canadian and Ontario Occupational Therapy Associations. *Canadian Journal of Occupational Therapy, 2*, 6–9.

Cardwell, T. (1966). President's address. *Canadian Journal of Occupational Therapy, 33*, 139–140.

Clarke, C. K. (1922). *Statement of Dr. C. K. Clarke re: occupational therapy in Ontario Hospitals for the Insane.* Unpublished manuscript.

Colman, W. (1992). Maintaining autonomy: The struggle between occupational therapy and physical medicine. *American Journal of Occupational Therapy, 46*, 63–70. http://dx.doi.org/10.5014/ajot.46.1.63

Creighton, C. (1993). Looking Back—Graded activity: Legacy of the sanatorium. *American Journal of Occupational Therapy, 47*, 745–748. http://dx.doi.org/10.5014/ajot.47.8.745

Csikszentmihalyi, M. (1991). *The psychology of optimal experience.* New York: Harper & Row.

Dunton, W. R. (1918). *Occupation therapy: A manual for nurses.* Philadelphia: Saunders.

Engelhardt, H. T., Jr. (1977). Defining occupational therapy: The meaning of therapy and the virtues of occupation. *American Journal of Occupational Therapy, 31*, 666–672.

Farrar, C. B. (1940a). Rehabilitation in nervous and mental cases among exsoldiers. *Canadian Journal of Occupational Therapy, 7*, 17–25.

Farrar, C. B. (1940b). War neuroses and psychoses. *Canadian Journal of Occupational Therapy, 7*, 5–16.

Fidler, G. S., & Fidler, J. W. (1978). Doing and becoming: Purposeful action and self-actualization. *American Journal of Occupational Therapy, 32*, 305–310.

Friedland, J. (1988). The Issue Is—Diversional activity: Does it deserve its bad name? *American Journal of Occupational Therapy, 42*, 603–608. http://dx.doi.org/10.5014/ajot.42.9.603

Friedson, E. (1994). Professions and the occupational principle. In E. Friedson (Ed.), *Professionalism reborn: Theory, prophecy, and policy* (pp. 61–74). Chicago: University of Chicago Press.

Froehlich, J. (1992). The Issue Is—Proud and visible as occupational therapists. *American Journal of Occupational Therapy, 46*, 1042–1044. http://dx.doi.org/10.5014/ajot.46.11.1042

Gilfoyle, E. M. (1984). The transformation of a profession, 1984 Eleanor Clarke Slagle lecture. *American Journal of Occupational Therapy, 38*, 575–584.

Gritzer, G., & Arluke, A. (1985). *The making of rehabilitation: A political economy of medical specialization, 1890–1980.* Berkeley: University of California Press.

Haas, L. J. (1944). *Practical occupational therapy.* Milwaukee, WI: Bruce.

Howland, G. (1986). Occupational therapy across Canada. *Canadian Journal of Occupational Therapy, 53*, 18–26. Original work published 1944.

"Is Practical Christianity" Occupational Therapy Praised. (1925, May 1) *The Evening Telegram* (Toronto), p. 14.

Johnson, J. (1996). Occupational science and occupational therapy: An emphasis in meaning. In R. Zemke & F. Clark (Eds.), *Occupational science: The evolving discipline* (pp. 393–397). Philadelphia: F. A. Davis.

Kielhofner, G., & Burke, J. P. (1977). Occupational therapy after 60 years: An account of changing identity and knowledge. *American Journal of Occupational Therapy, 31*, 675–689.

LeVesconte, H. (1935). Expanding fields of occupational therapy. *Canadian Journal of Occupational Therapy, 3*, 4–12.

Levine, R. E. (1987). Looking Back—The influence of the arts-and-crafts movement on the professional status of occupational therapy. *American Journal of Occupational Therapy, 41*, 248–254.

Meyer, A. (1977). The philosophy of occupation therapy. *American Journal of Occupational Therapy, 31*, 639–642. Original work published 1922. Reprinted as Chapter 4.

Mill, J S. (1947). *On liberty.* New York: Appleton-Century Crofts. Original work published 1859.

Peloquin, S. M. (1991a). Looking Back—Occupational therapy service: Individual and collective understandings of the founders, part 1. *American Journal of Occupational Therapy, 45*, 352–360. http://dx.doi.org/10.5014/ajot.45.4.352 Reprinted as Chapter 3.

Peloquin, S. M. (1991b). Looking Back—Occupational therapy service: Individual and collective understandings of the founders, part 2. *American Journal of Occupational Therapy, 45*, 733–744. http://dx.doi.org/10.5014/ajot.45.8.733 Reprinted as Chapter 3.

Polatajko, H. (1992). Naming and framing occupational therapy: A lecture dedicated to the life of Nancy B. *Canadian Journal of Occupational Therapy, 59*, 189–199.

Reed, K., & Sanderson, S. (1983). *Concepts of occupational therapy.* Baltimore: Williams & Wilkins.

Reilly, M. (1962). Occupational therapy can be one of the great ideas of 20th-century medicine, 1961 Eleanor Clarke Slagle lecture. *American Journal of Occupational Therapy, 16*, 1–9. Reprinted as Chapter 7.

Robinson, I. (1981). The mists of time, 1981 Muriel Driver memorial lecture. *Canadian Journal of Occupational Therapy, 48*, 145–152.

Rusk, H. (1958). *Rehabilitation medicine: A textbook on physical medicine and rehabilitation.* St. Louis, MO: Mosby.

Schemm, R. L. (1994). Bridging conflicting ideologies: The origins of American and British occupational therapy. *American Journal of Occupational Therapy, 48,* 1082–1088. http://dx.doi.org/10.5014/ajot.48.11.1082

Schwartz, K. (1992). Looking Back—Occupational therapy and education: A shared vision. *American Journal of Occupational Therapy, 46,* 12–18. http://dx.doi.org/10.5014/ajot.46.1.12

Staples, A. R., & McConnell, R. L. (1993). *Soapstone and seed beads: Arts and crafts at the Charles Camswell Hospital, a tuberculosis sanatorium* (Special publications no. 7). Alberta: Provincial Museum of Alberta.

Townsend, E. (Ed.). (1997). *Enabling occupation: An occupational therapy perspective.* Ottawa, Ontario: CAOT Publications ACE.

U.S. Department of Health and Human Services. (1993). *Research plan for the National Center for Medical Rehabilitation Research* (NIH Publication No. 93-3509). Washington, DC: Author.

Waterman, M. (1942). *Voltaire, Pascal, and human destiny.* New York: King's Crown Press.

West, W. L. (1984). A reaffirmed philosophy and practice of occupational therapy for the 1980s. *American Journal of Occupational Therapy, 38,* 15–23.

White, R. W. (1971). The urge toward competence. *American Journal of Occupational Therapy, 25,* 271–274.

Wild, J. (1946). *Plato theory of man.* New York: Octagon.

Wish-Baratz, S. (1989). Looking Back—Bird T. Baldwin: A holistic scientist in occupational therapy's history. *American Journal of Occupational Therapy, 43,* 257–260. http://dx.doi.org/10.5014/ajot.43.4.257

World Health Organization. (1981). *Disability, prevention, and rehabilitation* (Technical report series 668). Geneva, Switzerland: Author.

Yerxa, E. J. (1992). Some implications of occupational therapy's history for its epistemology, values, and relation to medicine. *American Journal of Occupational Therapy, 46,* 79–83. http://dx.doi.org/10.5014/ajot.46.1.79

Yerxa, E. J. (1993). Occupational science: A new source of power for participants in occupational therapy. *Occupational Science, 1,* 3–10.

CHAPTER 7

Occupational Therapy Can Be One of the Great Ideas of 20th-Century Medicine

1961 ELEANOR CLARKE SLAGLE LECTURE

MARY REILLY

Specifying the Theme

As an occupational therapist honored by her peers, I join my Eleanor Clarke Slagle predecessors in feeling the awesome responsibility of the award. The occasion, it seems to me, makes it obligatory for an awardee to objectify a lifetime experience and then speak of an issue of concern to all. With this in mind, I have elected to present an issue which impinges upon the very root meaning of our existence. In developing the idea I have sought to reflect it against the changing background of the world in which we live. My hope is that its exploration will add to an understanding of the profession which we practice.

The question I would like to speak to is one which each one of us has asked at some time or other in our professional lives. Some of us have asked it many times. It has been raised in different ways and expressed in different words, both within and outside our field. In all probability, it will continue to be asked by those who follow us. I am referring to an anxiety about our value as a service to sick people. This theme I have identified by the question: *Is occupational therapy a sufficiently vital and unique service for medicine to support and society to reward?*

The anxiety begins in a primitive form when we stand before our first patient and sense the enormous demands that a treatment problem makes upon the occupational therapy brush, hammer or needle. The wide and gaping chasm which exists between the complexity of illness and the commonplaceness of our treatment tools is, and always will be, both the pride and the anguish of our profession. Anxiety accumulates as we become increasingly involved in treatment, teach-

ing and research, and even more sophisticated questions tend to arise from that same source to plague us.

The theme of today's presentation is focused, therefore, on the critical appraisal of the essential worth of occupational therapy. I say critical because the technique of criticism will be the method by which the issue will be explored. The subject was selected because I found from my experience that the value of occupational therapy exists in a controversial state. Among any group of my colleagues who have practiced long and well, I found that this question of value constituted a continuous and almost lifelong dialogue.

The Theme Converted to an Hypothesis Test

Where and how does one begin to make dependable and hence usable judgments about value? Taking full advantage of the freedom inherent in the Slagle lectureship, I reasoned that the idea most basic to our practice ought to be searched out and then converted into a kind of a question which might be answerable to some degree. This search, I further reasoned, should begin in the time of our earliest days. I began there and found that there was a single root idea embedded deep in our foundation and this deeply embedded belief is what we call occupational therapy. In the stormy years between then and now, I found that there were few opportunities given to examine the roots of our foundation and to consider the growth which sprang from it.

My re-examination of our early history revealed that our profession emerged from a common belief held by a small group of people. This common belief is the hypothesis upon which our profession was founded. It was, and indeed still is, one of the truly great and even magnificent hypotheses of medicine today. I have dared to state this hypothesis as: *That man, through the use of his hands as they are energized by mind and will, can influence the state of his own health.* This is the inherited occupational therapy hypothesis passed on for proof by the early founders.

The splendor of its vision goes far beyond rating it as an idea conceived once in a lifetime or even once in a century. Rather, it falls in the class of one of those great beliefs which has advanced civilization. Its magnificence lies in the optimistic vote of confidence it gives to human nature. It implies that there is a reservoir of sensitivity and skill in the hands of man which can be tapped for his health. It implies the rich adaptability and durability of the central nervous system which can be influenced by experiences. And more than all this, it implies that man, through the use of his hands, can creatively deploy his thinking, feelings and purposes to make himself at home in the world and to make the world his home.

For a profession organized around this hypothesis it sets few limits to its growth. It merely endows a group with the obligation to acquire reliable knowledge leading to a competency to serve the belief. Because this is an hypothesis about health, it requires that this knowledge be made available for the guidance of physicians and that it be made applicable to a wide range of medical problems.

The Role of Criticism

Before preparing a brief for its validation I would like to make a detour into a description of the method whereby the issue will be explored. The method is in harmony with my temperament because, by choice, I am neither a conservative nor am I a conformist. I am a devout and practicing, card-carrying critic. Since criticism as a technique of public discussion has yet to emerge in our association affairs, I feel a need to define and describe it. Its philosophy, techniques and tactics will constitute the point of view from which I will speak.

The public use of criticism by a profession has been spelled out best by Merton[1] who sees it as a prevailing spirit within a group necessary to maintain a group's progress. Its greatest usefulness is that it acts to repudiate a smugness which assumes that everything possible has already been attained. Its presence commits an association to keeping its members from resting easily on their oars when they are so inclined. In general, Merton finds that criticism stings a profession into a new and more demanding formulation of purpose and maintains a policy position of divine discontent with the state of affairs as they are.

A disciplined person in either the sciences or the professions uses critical thinking as a personal tool of reality testing and problem solving. When a professional organization as a whole accepts criticism as the dominating mode of thought, then indeed, theorizing flourishes and the intellectual atmosphere of their gatherings is characterized by sweeping controversies. In this atmosphere of controversy, progress becomes somewhat assured.

But a card-carrying critic must do more than merely engage in critical thinking. Judgments made by a critic must emerge from a discreet use of techniques which are difficult to master and dangerous to apply. Basically, the skill is dependent upon an ability to analyze, interpret and synthesize. A critic must have a sharply developed capacity to see deficiencies in data and fallacies in interpretation. The best stock in trade that any critic has is a discerning eye for trends and an ability to pattern and verbalize them. Whether a critic is worth listening to is usually decided by an ability to use language well, by a creativeness in synthesizing new relations and by courage to propose provocative hypotheses. Ultimately, however, a good critic rests his case upon how well he has been able to restructure the issue so that the necessary powers for its resolution can be freed. These idealistic but difficult standards are the ones I hope to follow in restructuring the issue of how valuable is occupational therapy.

Design of the Presentation

Having discussed the point of view from which I will speak, it is now necessary to describe the plan of attack which will be made on this global theme. For the sake of this presentation let us suppose that the hypothesis I have proposed is the wellspring of our profession and that it is worth proving. It would not follow necessarily from this that it is provable. A large part of the power to act on the hypothesis, of course, resides with us, the members of the American Occupational Therapy Association. But the society in which our profession lives holds power too and can rule on its growth. Even before we begin the validation, we must look at the probability that this idea may not be capable of proof in this century. I plan to ask first whether the American culture can tolerate such an hypothesis. Next I shall question whether the 20th Century is the right time for the test. The most crucial aspect of the presentation will be an attempt to identify the point at which the process of proof ought to begin. This will be followed by an attempt to identify the basic pattern of our service by which the hypothesis will be proven. Finally, I shall comment on some ongoing crises which the hypothesis is undergoing and then leave for history its continuing proof.

Is America the Place to Test the Hypothesis?

Let us first consider the tolerance in America for the occupational therapy idea. In his social history, Max Lerner[2] identified certain dynamic forces which impelled the greatness of this country. He cited in the American mind two crucial images present since the beginning. One was the self-reliant craftsman, whether pioneer, farmer or mechanic. He was the man who could make something of the American resources, apply his strength and skill to nature's abundance, fashion new tools and machines, imagine and carry through new constructions. Without taking himself overseriously, Max Lerner's American has generally regarded the great engineering, business, government and medical tasks as jobs to be done. Progress in technology was seen simply as agenda for the craftsman.

The second image Lerner drew was from the American environment. It was that of a vast continent on earth, as in space, waiting to be discovered, explored, cleared, built-up, populated and energized. Lerner contends that our culture is dominated by an American spirit which hates to be confined. A drive toward action, he postulated, is a part of the American character.

This drive towards action seems to me to make reasonable the American idea of a patient. Our cultural concept of the man of action suffers little change when an American moves into a hospital community. It has been supported by a series of principles which merged and fused into what we now call rehabilitation. Early in this century, there emerged the principle in medical management that patients were easier to handle when they were occupied with mild tasks. Later when it was found that an active patient tended to recover faster, early ambulation became an acceptable principle of physiology and blended well with the principle of patient occupation. Concern for the psychological nature of patients brought forth the widespread acceptance of craft, recreation and work programs in hospitals. The need to train patients in self-care became almost a crusade to insure the rights of patients to be independent. Within the community, laymen cooperated in ventures to assure the handicapped's right to return to work.

Now we are implementing in full swing the socio-economic principle that it is good business for society to support such programs with public monies.

There are some obvious things which can be concluded about America's tolerance for the occupational therapy hypothesis. It would seem almost axiomatic that the American society in general, and medicine in particular, has need of a profession which has as its unique concern the nurturing of the spirit in man for action. In every way it knows how, America has said that this spirit must be served and served in a special kind of way when it has been blocked by physical or emotional ills. That this need will be persistent in American culture seems fairly certain. That occupational therapy will persist is not quite so certain. It is true, however, that if we fail to serve society's need for action, we will most assuredly die out as a health profession. It is also most assuredly true that if we did dissolve from the scene, in a decade or so, another group similarly purposed and similarly organized and prepared would have to be invented. I believe, therefore, that the occupational therapy hypothesis is a natural one to be advanced in America.

Is the 20th Century the Time?

The timeliness of the hypothesis is the next question I should like to raise. Are we the people and these the times for the test? We are all deeply entangled in the forces and events of the century in which we live. But if this entanglement commits our energies to the endless treadmill of survival, then the hypothesis cannot get off the ground. The social scientists tell us that the world we live in is in a state of indigestion from too much change. We have yet to absorb the disorganizations brought on by a depression, two wars and an ongoing massive technological revolution. This change is being reflected by society into all its component institutions. It follows naturally that we feel its reflection in our professional lives.

But our state of turmoil was not always so, because occupational therapy was born in the quieter times of this century. In the first several decades of our existence, medicine offered us a tranquil and supportive setting. Our literature reveals that physicians tended to nurture the development of our schools and clinics. In these earlier times we were helped to meet the challenges of contributing to the ongoing medical scene. The last several decades, however, have put excessive stress for expansion upon a profession whose role had been barely defined. We have seen our practice organized into specialty fields by the demands of World War II. Our clinicians have only recently been systematized into team behavior by the pressures of rehabilitation. Now in the sixties we are confessing to a mounting sense of confusion and voicing a need for direction. We are keenly aware of the conflicting demands being made upon our practice. The problems that our schools face in digesting the accumulating technical knowledge which practice demands is a matter of growing distress. Caught up in these forces, how free can we be to control our growth?

If we are anxious today, the social scientist offers the explanation that it is because we are now aware that the hopes we had cultivated in gentler times of the past are being threatened by the pace of the world around us. Historians, however, are quick to counter that when times of great change appear, they are forecasting a death to the old and a birth to a new way of life. It is inconceivable that we or any other group with organized intelligence would stand idly by and permit the random destruction of the old and encourage blind birth to the new. Fortunately, most institutions have centralized their action for controlling change through planning groups variously called the Task Force, Master Plan Committee or the Role Definition Study. Our national association has not remained aloof from such efforts and is currently involved in three change controlling studies. As many of us know well, the studies involve professional curriculum and clinical practice, the functions of the organization and the future development of the profession.

We may conclude that we have shown by our action that we have felt the buffeting of great change and are attempting to control it. But how can we know whether the efforts we are making are sufficient and are of the right kind? This difficult question has some partial answers. One common sense answer is that we must recognize the fact that we have grown and have changed as we grew. In our forty years of existence our sense of purpose, our anchorage points have shifted. It is only logical to reason that we will not rediscover a sense of purpose by merely reflecting within our professions the problems of the larger society in which we exist. Few rewards are granted to those who are content to reflect problems. Society demands that its problems be answered. Therefore, to any group which aspires to be a profession, there is placed before it a clear-cut mandate. This mandate says that if we wish to exist as a profession we must identify the vital need of man which we serve and the manner in which we serve it.

I contend that this is the point at which the proof of the occupational therapy hypothesis begins. The reality of our profession depends upon an identification of the vital need of mankind that we serve. How free we are in these troubled times to reconstruct our thinking at this basic level I do not know. But I do know that the crucial nature of our service cannot be spelled out in the loosely constructed way that it is today. I personally have little trust that we can continue to exist as an arts and crafts group which serves muscle dysfunction or as an activity group which serves the emotionally disabled. Society requires of us a much sharper focus on its needs. As the next step in the development of the theme it becomes necessary to make a critical examination of what, if any, vital need we serve.

What Vital Need Is Served?

As the first order of the business at hand we ought to have it clearly in mind what constitutes a vital need. Of all the descriptions of the need states of man which I have heard I like Eric Fromm's[3] the best. He says that needs are an indispensable part of human nature and imperatively demand satisfaction. The need we serve must fall within this category. He says further that they are rooted in the physiological organization of man and consist of hunger, thirst and sleep and that in general they all belong to self-preservation. He proposes a simple, forthright formula of self-preservation which is directly applicable to occupational therapy. According to Fromm, when man is born the stage is set for him. He has to eat, drink, sleep and protect himself from his enemies. Therefore, for his self-preservation he must work and produce. Work, in the Eric Fromm sense, is a physiologically conditioned need and therefore a need to work is postulated as an imperative part of man's nature.

In our 40 years of practice we have accumulated some fascinating odds and ends of understanding about the need to work. For example, early in my training I was taught that work was good for people. All people needed to work and sick people even more so. This kind of justification of service reminds me of the old story about the man who died and woke up surrounded by all kinds of delights which were his for the mere bend of the finger. After he had satiated himself well, he called for the headman, expressed his appreciation for the manner in which he was treated and then said, "Now that I have pleasured myself well, it is my wish to do something. My good man, what is there for me to do in this paradise?" The answer given to him was, "You are doing it now." "But," replied our man, "I must do something or else my stay in heaven will be intolerable." "Who" replied the headman firmly, "said that you were in heaven?" In the past I have been guilty of believing and having my patients persuaded that work was good and heaven would prove me right. The rationale that man works because it is good for him, regardless of its comfort to us, makes little contribution to our understanding of work as a basic need.

During the 30s, the economic depression gave us an unparalleled opportunity to learn that when able people could not find work, certain psychological disorganization occurred. These changes were deemed to be over and above the changes which could reasonably result from economic loss. We are able to generalize from the depression that human nature does not thrive in idleness. In the last several decades we have accumulated a few more broad generalizations. One is that the stress of work produces psychosomatic conditions in modern businessmen. Another generalization which is now being formulated is that when people retire from their work, they retire from life itself.

A vital need to be occupied however, is not to be inferred from such global generalizations. It is being left to the more rigorously controlled experimentations to do this. Now under laboratory conditions man's need-state for action is being rigorously investigated. In the United States and Canada basic research is going on in an area called sensory deprivation. The work began in reaction to the Russian brainwashing attempts. The research was designed on the principle of restricting man's interaction with the ongoing world of reality. Under controlled conditions of isolation man was found to suffer profound disturbances of his thought processes. In isolation men regressed to unrealistic and prelogical modes of behavior. The sensory deprivation findings suggest strongly that the concepts of man's response to his environment must be sharply revised. The behavioral aberrations which were observed in the idleness of depression and retirement, and the stress of overwork, appear to have been confirmed by the laboratory induced sensory deprivations. The data were checked out by neurologists, psychiatrists, biochemists, pharmacologists, mathematicians and engineers.

The final sensory-deprivation report sums up to a concept that the mind cannot continue to function efficiently without constant stimuli from the external world. The central nervous system is now seen as a complex guessing machine oriented outward for the testing of ideas. The experimenters postulate that each individual constructs a different development pattern with respect to strategies for dealing with reality. Jerome Brauner,[4] as one of the researchers, concluded that early sensory deprivation prevents the formation of adequate models and strategies for dealing with the environment. Later sensory deprivation in normal adults, he suggests, disrupts the vital evaluation process by which one constantly monitors and corrects the strategies one has learned to employ in dealing with the environment.

To summarize at this point, it seems to me that the American drive toward action as identified by Max Lerner and the human drive toward work as identified by Fromm have been verified in the laboratories. I believe that we are on safe ground right now to say that man has a vital need for occupation and that his central nervous system demands the rich and varied stimuli that solving life problems provides him and that this is the basic need that occupational therapy ought to be serving.

What Is the Unique Service?

A profession, however, must do more than identify the need it serves. There is a twin obligation to spell out its unique pattern of service. The next gigantic task which this presentation faces and with some trepidation, because of the limitation of time, is an attempt to identify the basic pattern of our service by which the hypothesis may be proven. The charge is gigantic because it makes it obligatory to define the occupational therapy body of knowledge, its treatment process and techniques.

A search for valid content, process and methods has been my preoccupation in the past 10 years of reading, study and practice. If I had the ability to do all this with any degree of clarity, I would not be here talking about it. I would be in a clinic doing it. However, I am now admitting to a rising sense of satisfaction in the project and a receding sense of frustration. At no time in technological history have the behavioral scientists been producing so much knowledge directly applicable to our field as they are now. The material is emerging from sources as divergent as neurological theory, animal psychology, developmental and personality theory and from psychologists as diverse as Allport, Murphy, Harlow, Hebb, Goldstein, Piaget and Schlachtel.

In order to plunge directly into this material I am going to have to make use of a device in logic known as a First Principle. For if we were to have a First Principle in occupational therapy it would provide us with a way to specify our knowledge. To those who may not be familiar with the meaning of First Principle, it is a device in reasoning to account for all that follows. For instance, the idea of God is a First Principle which accounts for the Universe. There has been a First Principle postulated to explain the nature of man. We are told that the first duty of an organism is to be alive. Medical science derives its premise from this first law of life. If it were not desirable to cure disease and prolong life, the rules of science and the skills and practice of medicine would be irrelevant. The second duty of an organism is to grow and be productive. Occupational therapy ought to derive its premise from the second law of life. If it were not desirable to be productive, the skills and practices of occupational therapy would be irrelevant.

These two laws merge into a concept of function which asserts that both the existence and the unfolding of the specific powers of an organism are one and the same thing. This concept of function is expressed as: the power to act creates a need to use the power, and the failure to use power results in dysfunction and unhappiness. The validity of the First Principle is easily recognizable in the physiological functions of man. Man has the power to talk and move, therefore, if he were prevented from using the power, severe physical discomfort would result. Freud utilized this First Principle to build a powerful theoretical position from which emotional illness was so successfully attacked. He accepted man's biological necessity to produce and generalized that when sexual energy was blocked, neurotic disturbances resulted. He endowed sexual satisfaction with all-encompassing significance. He developed his theory of sexual satisfaction into a profound symbolic expression of the fact that man's failure to use and spend what he has is the cause of sickness and unhappiness. The Freudian theory that human action is primarily sexually based has thrown a strong but restrictive shadow over other behavioral fields. It has been only lately that attention has been given to human productivity in non-sexual areas. Occupational therapy's focus, it is asserted here, lies in the nonsexual area of human productivity and creativity.

In Gardner Murphy's[5] brilliant defense of human productivity he makes us aware that there is a distinct path which leads to becoming human. This path is not seen as being sexually directed. The direction lies largely in the enrichment and elaboration of the sensory and motor experience and the life of symbolism which depends upon them. He maintains that the

sheer fact that we have a nervous system, the sheer fact that we can learn, means that we can prolong and complicate sensory and motor satisfactions, can make them richer, can give them more connections, can avoid boredom, can recombine them, can feed upon them, can become immersed in them and make them a part of ourselves. In all these respects, Murphy says man is most completely human. His primary thesis is that man achieves satisfaction in using what he has, in using the equipment that makes him human; and this entails not only the sensory and motor equipment but that central nervous system upon which the learning and thinking processes depend.

Murphy's spirited description of the conditions necessary for being human can provide the basis for an occupational therapy First Principle. This logic constitutes our mandate to discover and organize our body of knowledge; to develop a treatment process; and to devise techniques for its application to the health of man. The logic of occupational therapy rests upon the principle that man has a need to master his environment, to alter and improve it. When this need is blocked by disease or injury, severe dysfunction and unhappiness result. Man must develop and exercise the powers of his central nervous system through open encounter with life around him. Failure to spend and to use what he has in the performance of the tasks that belong to his role in life makes him less human than he could be. With this principle in mind I would like to summarize my thoughts of the last several years of work on our body of knowledge, our treatment process and techniques.

Regarding the Body of Knowledge

Because our profession is focused on influencing the health of people there will always be a need to include in our body of knowledge the fundamental material of anatomy, neurophysiology, personality theory, social processes and the pathological states to which these functional areas are subject. However, I do not feel this is our unique content. We should have as a special contribution a profound understanding of the nature of work.

Knowledge of work capacity lies scattered over many behavioral fields. We do know, for instance, that man's ability to work has been developed in the long evolutionary process. It began when man hunted and fished for his food and continued as he grew his food and fabricated objects for his comfort. The lot of man was considerably improved when he freed himself from arduous labor through tools and machinery. His comfort was immeasurably assured by the social institutions he built and operated with increasing skill over the centuries. It is my contention that this evolutionary process, plus a bit more, is present, symbolically expressed in today's culture. The concept of work capacity as being an outgrowth of an evolutionary process I call the phylogenesis of work. I believe that cultural history of work ought to be deeply embedded in the occupational therapy body of knowledge and its phylogenetic nature considered particularly in program building.

We know that as a child grows, he recapitulates the history of his race in the stages through which he himself must pass enroute to maturity. The need to pass through phylogenetic experiences in work is necessary for mature work capacity to be developed. There is historical evidence that a child's ability to play, to explore his environment, to exercise his motor skills are the foundation for his later school experiences. The problem-solving processes and the creativity exercised in school work, craft and hobby experiences are the necessary preparations for the later demands of the work world. Because we know that the random movements of the infant progress in developmental sequence toward the job competencies of the mature adult, I postulate an ontogenesis of work. I believe that the ontogenetic nature of work ought to be considered in the case study approach to each treatment problem.

The occupational therapy body of knowledge should include therefore, an understanding of the developmental nature of the sensory-motor systems, the patterning of aptitudes, abilities and interests, the nature of the learning process involved in the acquisition of skills. It should include also an understanding of the developmental nature of the problem-solving process and process of creativity. My epistemological conclusion is that the biological, psychological or social knowledge we select as part of our thinking content must be intermeshed deliberately with the knowledge of work–phylogenesis and work–ontogenesis.

Regarding the Treatment Process

The capacity to work develops in the long socialization process through which a child becomes an adult. It proceeds along the path of growth as man learns to intermesh his motor with his intellectual functions and adapt this integration to the tasks of his life which satisfy his need to control his environment. Work capacity, in this sense, can be said to develop out of the struggle with gravity for motor control, the struggle with

learning for manual and mental skills and the struggle with people and people purpose for economic and social control. When the struggle is great, the personal involvement is high; although conflict and frustration are high, so, too, is work satisfaction high. It follows, too, that when involvement is low, work satisfaction is low. The occupational therapy process becomes primarily concerned with that special aspect of the socialization process called work satisfaction. Its approach in treatment is biographical because work satisfaction is, by its nature, the result of past experiences expressed in the present ability to cope with the environment. Its focus is on the meaningful involvement in problem solving tasks or creative performances. The parameters of its concern are the ability to experience pleasure in achievement, to tolerate the frustrations of struggle, to sustain the burden of routine tasks and to maintain the level of aspiration within the reality level of work skills. The goal of the process is to encourage active, open encounter with the tasks which would reasonably belong to his role in life. The process is paced and guided by the supervision of the prescribing physician.

Regarding Treatment Techniques

Techniques which would emerge from the body of knowledge and the professional process as just described would be concerned with program and treatment execution. Methods would include all those administrative techniques of program building which would provide a laboratory setting for human productivity. The treatment technique would be all those procedures associated with modifying sensory-motor dysfunctions, perceptual difficulties and the difficulties inherent in coping with the world of play, work and school. It is suggested in terms of today's thesis that in the merging of our content, process and methods, the unique pattern of our function will be spelled out. If this pattern is focused strongly on man's need to be occupied productively and creatively, the hypothesis will grow stronger.

Major Tests of the Hypothesis

Of all the ongoing tests of the occupational therapy hypothesis, I have selected a few major ones upon which to comment. The first and obvious one is whether a need to accumulate substantial knowledge about human productivity and creativity will be recognized and acted upon in our schools and clinics. The problem of balancing our knowledge has been with us for some time. Until now our attention has been preoccupied with the medical science which supports the application of our craft knowledge to medical conditions. But medical science knowledge is a means for the application of our service and not an end in itself. A profound knowledge of human dynamics of productivity and creativity is the end to which our knowledge ought to be designed. As far as our practice today is concerned, we have more medical science knowledge than we know how to apply and we are applying more knowledge about human productivity than we actually have on hand.

The second, and not so obvious test, is the delimiting effect that psychoanalytical practice has on the promotion of a non-sexual concept of human productivity. The fundamental doctrine of the Freudian pleasure principle is that the essential movement of a living organism is to return to a state of quiescence and that primary pleasure is sought in sensual gratification. A fundamental principle of work is that primary pleasure can be sought through efficient use of the central nervous system for the performance of those ego integrating tasks which enable man to alter and control his environment. In this sense psychoanalytical theory is seen to focus on subjective reality while work theory becomes largely concerned with objective problem-solving reality. It is not that these points of view run counter to each other. They simply do not meet or interact except under very special conditions of intimate supervision by a psychoanalyst.

In 1943 Hendrick[6] raised this issue in the *Psychoanalytic Quarterly.* He argued that the psychosocial activities of the total organism are not adequately accounted for by the pleasure and reality principles when these are defined, in accordance with Freudian tradition, as immediate or delayed response, respectively, to the need for sensual gratification. He suggests that work is not primarily motivated by sexual need or associated aggressions, but by the need for efficient use of the muscular and intellectual tools, regardless of what secondary needs (self-preservation, aggressive, or sexual) a work performance may also satisfy. Hendrick postulated a need for a work principle which asserts that primary pleasure is sought by efficient use of the central nervous system for the performance of well integrated ego functions which enable the individual to control or alter his environment.

In psychoanalytic practice today sexual satisfaction is seen as being influenced by ontogenetic, phylogenetic and biographical considerations while no such con-

siderations are seen needed for work satisfaction. Although many analysts have agreed that sexual capacity correlates highly with work capacity, the idea has not been developed much beyond the statement. Work is seen as a kind of experience a patient ought to have and whatever satisfaction he derives from it will be dependent upon his subjective state. As a result, extensive activity programs have grown up around psychiatric treatment which have been designed for participation, but not specifically for ego involvement. These programs are now being called activity programs and those implementing them are called activity therapists.

Such activity programs encourage the participation of large groups and usually appeal to the automatic, learned patterns of behavior. However, activity programs so designed deny the dignity of a human being to struggle, to control his environment as witness the fact that they tend to make man quiescent within the hospital community. They tend to depersonalize, institutionalize and, in general, debase human nature. The occupational therapy hypothesis makes the assumption that the mind and will of man are occupied through central nervous system action and that man can and should be involved consciously in problem solving and creative activity. It is believed that psychoanalytical theory and the occupational therapy hypothesis can profitably co-exist if a work principle is postulated and executed. This will be even more true if occupational therapy deepens its understanding of the phylogenetic and ontogenetic nature of work and make a case study approach to ego involvement of patients. It is not so possible, however, that activity therapy and occupational therapy can co-exist. It is believed that the major crisis in the proof of our hypothesis will not be how to co-exist with psychoanalytical theory but to know the difference between activity and occupation and to act on the knowledge of this difference.

The last major test which I will discuss has to do with the physical disability field. In this specialty we have been placing heavy emphasis upon muscle efficiency and enabling devices. There is a long, perilous and complex ladder to be scaled between neuro-muscular efficiency and work satisfaction. The ontogenetic reconstitution of motor behavior is a tedious process and must be done step by step. It begins at the reflex muscle action stage and proceeds to the development of complex patterns of motor skills which are utilized in a rich variety of work skills. These, in turn, must be disciplined to a sustaining level of tolerance for routine labors. It is upon this broad pattern that human tolerance for working with people in people affairs is built. If any of these steps are missing, they must be re-fashioned and the whole pattern re-shaped accordingly. The proof of the occupational therapy hypothesis in the physical disability field will depend upon how much we know about the process of restoring work capacity. It cannot be done from prescriptions based upon a narrow understanding of human productivity. It cannot be done in cramped clinics dependent upon scrap material. Nor can it be done from our present ignorance of the world of industry for which we believe we are preparing patients. The challenge to the hypothesis in this area is severe, yet provocative. The technical literature of our profession is indicating that this challenge is not being ignored.

Summary and Conclusion

In summarizing the many ideas I have touched or expanded upon in this thesis, I once again return to my original question: *Is occupational therapy a service vital and unique enough for medicine to support and society to reward?* In answering it, I have said that we have had a magnificent hypothesis to prove and if it could be proven, even to some degree, the answer would be that we are valuable to medicine and to society. The hypothesis that I presented for evidence of proof was that *man, through the use of his hands as they are energized by mind and will, can influence the state of his own health.* I asked if this were a kind of idea that America could subscribe to and to that I replied with a resounding yes. I wondered about the stress that the terrible 20th Century was putting on this idea and worried some about the energy left to us to advance it. I suggested the hypothesis would begin its proof when we identified the drive in man for occupation and would continue as we shaped our services to fill that need. I speculated on some of the crises the hypothesis was now undergoing and left the decision not in the lap of the gods but in our own laps for us to think and act upon in our daily practice.

I have said that our profession has a magnificent medical purpose. Whether we shall fulfill it or whether it shall ever be fulfilled I have not said because I do not know. But this I can say from personal experience, that we belong to a profession that requires the mind to look at the history of man's achievements throughout civilization. It requires the spirit to respond to the wonders of what man has accomplished with his hands. It gives us a mandate to apply this knowledge and more to help man influence the state of his own health.

References

1. Merton, Robert K. "The Search for Professional Status." *American Journal of Nursing*, March, 1959.
2. Lerner, Max. *America as a Civilization*. New York: Simon and Schuster, 1957.
3. Fromm, Eric. *The Fear of Freedom*. London, England: Routledge and Kegan Paul Ltd., 1960.
4. Solomon, Philip, & etc. *Sensory Deprivation*. Cambridge, Massachusetts: Harvard University Press, 1961.
5. Murphy, Gardner. *Human Potentialities*. New York: Basic Books, 1958.
6. Hendrick, Ives. "Work and the Pleasure Principle." *Psychoanalytic Quarterly*, Vol. VII:3, 1943.

Bibliographical Notes

Work has been studied from the viewpoint of economics, philosophy, sociology and psychology, and although the literature is considerable, and is being added to constantly, it is a comparatively recent focus for scholars. So far no general study of work has been written, but to some extent a student in this field need not be left entirely without guidance. He needs to remember, however, that the literature is too extensive for one individual to investigate thoroughly. This bibliography noting is designed to serve as an introductory guide. Many of the recommended writings also include full bibliographies of the topic with which they are concerned.

Anyone who seeks to be a student of human occupation should attempt first to build a historical perspective of the field. *A History of Technology*, edited by Charles Singer, E. J. Holmyard and A. R. Hall, is a massive fivevolume series published by Clarendon Press in Oxford from 1954 to 1958 and provides a general historical background as far as science, economics and technology is concerned. An account of the effect of labor and technology on the culture of the west is set forth in another series titled *The History of Civilization*, edited by C. K. Ogden and published in New York by Alfred A. Knopf, 1926 to 1929.

The sociological nature of work may be approached through a study of the socialization process and the field of industrial social psychology. This aspect of study is excellently covered in *The Handbook of Social Psychology*, edited by Gardner Murphy and published in two volumes by Addison-Wesley Company in 1952. A recent perceptive and illuminating view of the social and economic nature of work and the worker is presented by *Theories of Society*, Vol. I and II, edited by

Parsons, Stills, Naegele and Pitts published by the Free Press of Glencoe, Inc., in 1961.

The specific classics regarding human occupations are exemplified by: Theodore Caplow's *The Sociology of Work* (Minneapolis: The University of Minnesota Press, 1954); Eli Ginzberg's *Occupational Choice: An Approach to a General Theory* (New York: Columbia University Press, 1951); Anne Roe's *The Psychology of Occupations* (New York: John Wiley and Sons, 1956); Donald Super's *The Psychology of Careers: An Introduction to Vocational Development* (New York: Harper and Brothers, 1957) and John Darley and Theda Hagenah's *Vocational Interest and Measurement: Theory and Practice* (Minneapolis: The University of Minnesota Press, 1955).

The classics concerned with human creativity are: Viktor Lowenfeld's *Creative and Mental Growth*, revised edition (New York: The Macmillan Company, 1952); Edwin Ziegfeld's *Education and Art: A Symposium* (Paris: 19 Avenue Kleber, United Nations Educational, Scientific and Cultural Organization, 1953) and Harold Anderson's *Creativity and its Cultivation* (New York: Harper and Brothers, 1958).

The author further recommends: Robert Gagne and Edwin Fleishman's *Psychology and Human Performance* (New York: Henry Holt and Company, 1959); Ernest Schachtel's Metamorphosis (New York: Basic Books, 1959); Gordon Allport's *Personality and Social Encounter* (Boston: Beacon Press, 1960); Hannah Arendt's *The Human Condition* (New York: Doubleday Anchor Books, 1959); Erich Fromm's *Man for Himself* (New York: Rinehart and Company, 1945); Gerald Gurin, Joseph Veroff and Sheila Feld's *Americans View Their Mental Health: Number Four* (New York: Basic Books, 1960); and Frederick Herzberg, Bernard Mausner and Barbara Snyderman's *The Motivation to Work* (New York: John Wiley and Sons, 1959).

APPENDIX I.A.

The Philosophical Base of Occupational Therapy

Occupations are activities that bring meaning to the daily lives of individuals, families, and communities and enable them to participate in society. All individuals have an innate need and right to engage in meaningful occupations throughout their lives. Participation in these occupations influences their development, health, and well-being across the lifespan. As such, participation in meaningful occupation is a determinant of health.

Occupations occur within diverse social, physical, cultural, personal, temporal, or virtual contexts. The quality of occupational performance and the experience of each occupation are unique in each situation due to the dynamic relationship between factors intrinsic to the individual, the contexts in which the occupation occurs, and the characteristics of the activity.

The focus and outcome of occupational therapy are individuals' engagement in meaningful occupations that support their participation in life situations. Occupational therapy practitioners conceptualize occupations as both a means and an end to therapy. That is, there is therapeutic value in occupational engagement as a change agent, and engagement in occupations is also the ultimate goal of therapy.

Occupational therapy is based on the belief that occupations may be used for health promotion and wellness, remediation or restoration, health maintenance, disease and injury prevention, and compensation/adaptation. The use of occupation to promote individual, community, and population health is the core of occupational therapy practice, education, research, and advocacy.

Authors

The Commission on Education:

Jyothi Gupta, PhD, OTR/L, OT(C), *Chairperson*
Andrea R. Bilics, PhD, OTR/L, FAOTA
Donna M. Costa, DHS, OTR/L, FAOTA
Debra J. Hanson, PhD, OTR
Mallory Duncan, *ASD Liaison* (ASD)
Susan M. Higgins, MA, OTR/L
Linda Orr, MPA, OTR/L
Diane Parham, PhD, OTR/L, FAOTA
Jeff Snodgrass, PhD, MPH, OTR, CWCE
Neil Harvison, PhD, OTR/L, FAOTA, *AOTA Staff Liaison*

Adopted by the Representative Assembly

Revised by the Commission on Education, 2011

This revision replaces the 1979 *The Philosophical Base of Occupational Therapy* (previously published and copyrighted in 1995 by the American Occupational Therapy Association in the *American Journal of Occupational Therapy, 49,* 1026). Reviewed by COE and COP in 2004.

Setting the Stage—Address in Honor of Eleanor Clarke Slagle

ADOLF MEYER

It is a great privilege to have an opportunity to speak on this occasion, which honors a friend and long-time co-worker, our Mrs. Eleanor Clarke Slagle, as a person and as the personification of occupational therapy. Presidents and officers have come and gone, but for 20 years Mrs. Slagle has brought into the field just that kind of personality which proved highly fruitful and auspicious: she has been, not a dictator, not a boss, but a leader by example, a human being and human factor among human beings, a cultivator of human relationships, in gathering around herself co-workers and in making co-workers of the patients. Such is the human being Mrs. Slagle and what she means to us and to the thousands of patients who have been and are still reached by her and her pupils. And inseparable from this personal human side, there stands before us the nature and character of the product of her work and the spirit and philosophy her life and life-work exemplify, that which brings us together in this assembly and in this large and impressive organization.

This gathering and the work achieved by this body with Mrs. Slagle as the head worker are enough of a testimonial for a cause and its leading and stabilizing captain. Obviously Mrs. Slagle has had her ideal not only in perpetuating herself in a special role but in training a rank and file ever able to furnish timber for leadership from the ranks and in the ranks, and growth from the ranks.

For 20 years, from the beginning of our organization, Mrs. Slagle has, as treasurer and secretary, done that work of continuity which with changing presidents and changing topics represents the very constitution of this growing force in the ranks of dealing with those who, for a time and sometimes for good, are forced into that army that needs shelter and protection and among whom the work of restoring health and better ways of prevention and achievement of the handicapped brings care and cure.

In these days in which we are perhaps too much inclined to look upon leadership as a profession, and upon professional agitators as the reapers of honor and power, it is a tremendous satisfaction to see one of the chief workers completing 20 years in that office which personifies the very constitution of this body. Mrs. Slagle and Dr. Dunton have been the spirits in the ranks and from the ranks and for the ranks, not imposed managers, but the souls of the essence of the work, giving freely of their time and experience while carrying on the work itself.

In the great division of labor we need continuity and examples that survive the changes and are embodiments of the very essentials which only the best workers can perpetuate in steady growth, in stability of motion and promotion, those who see that ever new deals are fair deals, deals embodying the wisdom of those who do and actually work and never cease to grow and to create.

Growth and work and achievement and attainment are all a function of that one virtual commodity—time, that steady rhythm of day and night, of seasons and years, not a mere eternal return but eternal progression. No 2 days can be quite the same, and no 2 years; but there has to be an element of continuity and cohesion; and for this it takes those starting with enough personality, capable of maintaining themselves and of remaining forces and centers of growth. And as in the nature of humanity, generation follows generation, the young work beside the old and the old work beside the young, those capable of being the bearers of continuity are few and rare and, we are glad to see, honored and sought as the very essence of progress.

Mrs. Slagle comes from the same source and soil that gave me my first opportunities and encouragement: the

Originally delivered on September 14, 1937, in Atlantic City at a testimonial banquet to honor Eleanor Clarke Slagle. Published 1985 in *Occupational Therapy in Mental Health*, 5(3), 109–113. Copyright © 1985, Taylor & Francis. Reprinted with permission.

opportunity to realize the need for more, the need for growth, the opportunity to find similarly minded forces and the spirit of action that has to go with knowledge and vision to make it both fertile and practical: Illinois, large needs and large enterprises, a whole group of aspiring forces and engaging problems, needs in practice and needs in hospitals, close to Missouri, wanting to be shown and shown by actual work and performances. The educator, the social worker, and the physician were bound to get together. Miss Lathrop was one of the great links. As the great gardener Froebel in education and his pupil Grossman in the therapeutic training of psychopaths by work recognized the need of a setting for work and for therapy in sound use of time, so there was the shaping of an atmosphere of work and action at Kankakee, encouraged by the social spirit about Hull House, all working for the training by action and not only by word. The old ideal of the Middle Ages, pray and work, took real form in the union of one's best thought and work, and when we opened the Phipps Clinic for action, Miss Lathrop was able to lend us Mrs. Slagle as the model and instigator of workmanship in the service of therapy. That the greatest benefit for the sufferer was to come from the philosophy of time and its use and from the right person to exemplify it was natural in the pragmatic atmosphere of the middle west and Mrs. Slagle brought the fruit of experience to our new center. She started us and, like all good workers, inspired others, so that, when she was needed for more and more training of new forces, she left with us the workers who carried on while she was drawn into that field of training and teaching and organizing, that did so much in the emergencies of that international madness called war and again for the needs arising from the madness and the immaturity and blunderings even in peace. As a contributor to the philosophy of time and life, as a cultivator of life and health in activity, Mrs. Slagle has become a guide, philosopher, and friend of hundreds and hundreds, and as I said, the embodiment of example and principle. What she has added in the nearly 25 years since she came to help us is a proud record, a rare fulfillment of a life still growing and still progressing.

The demands of actual life and work where it is most needed have wrought a wonderful change in turning psychology from esoteric contemplation into the service of actual life. Real needs and real opportunities have led us into modern psychobiology and a science of human nature and behavior. And the basis of this modern psychobiology is not mere analysis and preaching of license, but a study and cultivation of the person

and action. This is how the old principle of engaging patients in activity has become the basic setting of all modern therapy. Pathology is no longer a kind of gloating over what can be found at autopsy. It is the study of the mistakes and maladjustments, the failures of man to use his best sense and opportunities. Mistakes become damage and damage becomes disease and disease in turn has to be brought back to where it is treated as "poor work" to be replaced by good and helpful work. This is the role of occupational therapy, not merely making a lot of stereotyped articles but releasing or implanting and fostering action with the reward and joy of achievement. I heard Mrs. Slagle quote from a passage in the first paper I ever wrote on the treatment of nervous and mental disorders, addressed to the Chicago Pathological Society in February, 1893, nearly 45 years ago, in which I asked my colleagues for the discussion of the kind of work which could be expected from and recommended to American ladies. I do not know why I picked on the ladies; I suppose because the doctors present were all men and I felt I knew them. I said: 'Experience alone can give suggestions in this line.' I called it mental hygiene, foreshadowing what I now mean by "mind," the person in action, good or bad, helpful and effective or mere restlessness, often overactive only as the result of fatigue and mismanagement.

I should like to be able to voice adequately what so many of my patients have gained through Mrs. Slagle and her pupils and what it all means not only for the sufferer but also for the healthy of our time. When the development of machinery supersedes the driving power of necessity in the development of habits and possibilities of work, we turn to the ingenuity of those who know the creative possibilities available not only for the sick but for the rank and file of those with "time on their hands."

From reveling in thoughts of eternity, we now have the great task to inject again the joys of activity of the day so that we may make a return of the pleasure of the day's work an efficient competitor with the mere pleasure and glamour of night life. We are grateful to Mrs. Slagle and her pupils and co-workers for their devotion and skill and creative zeal and achievements in the furtherance of the joy and rewards of work and creation.

It must be a great satisfaction to Mrs. Slagle to see the onward march of what had but slender beginnings. There is a need of leisure for the spreading of the wisdom that has come from the wide experience under difficult conditions. As wisdom grows there comes the demand for a spreading into wider usefulness. Today we have come into a period of prostitution of the capacity and love for work to the service of the something and the somebody else of mere wages. We have more and more cause to search for the natural inducements to work and the opportunities for new creative principles. We have to study work for its own rewards and to honor and cherish it and to cultivate it so as to make it deserve the honor and joy. Working under the difficulties met by the psychiatric occupational worker should and will give us much material for a usable knowledge of the relation of person and work, worker and work, and worker and leadership.

What is the work one can love and live with and live on? What are the conditions of work that are needed if the worker is to love the work and to live on and through it?

I shall never forget the deplorable words of a Secretary of Labor in a discussion of immigration. He told us we needed some immigration to get labor to do the dirty work which no American parent would want his children to do.

We occupational workers know that there is no work that cannot be shaped so as to find its worker able to get satisfaction from the doing and the result.

In these days in which continuity of purpose seems overshadowed by doctrines of change and where leadership in a democratic sense threatens to be belittled and to degenerate in other lands into high-power dictatorships, it is a matter of great joy and cheer to see respect and honor brought to a leader of unusual modesty and gentleness.

In the midst of talk and reality of change we see careers of continuity of progress, of action and creativeness in the ranks, and as part of the ranks.

We see those natural and inspiring instances in which a rare individual becomes a live and effective example of ideas and ideals as the living and active person, and persons expressive of ideals.

And we are glad to see those persons who become living symbols of great movements and realizations, in the midst of the younger and the budding generations, sharing with them the experience of a lifetime and the spirit of everbudding youth.

It is the pride of democracy to cherish its leaders as parts of the ranks, as influence by example, and as recipients of recognition and of fellowship in the rank and file.

We like to see it brought home that a lifetime of work and service and devotion and leadership in a cause also finds its recognition, and recognition and esteem its expression.

Part II. Theoretical and Conceptual Frameworks to Guide Occupation-Based Practice

The old, unproductive controversy over what is "mental" and what is "physical" is ending . . . only an approach broad enough to permit . . . the psychobiological point of view throws light upon their nature.

—Salmon (1924, as cited in Dunton, 1928, pp. 9–10)

The importance of developing and then using an integrated theoretical framework to guide occupational therapy practice was strongly emphasized during the founding years of the profession. Since then, many leaders have underscored the importance of using theory-based interventions (Bruce & Borg, 2002; Christiansen, Baum, & Bass-Haugen, 2005; Dunn, Brown, & McGuigan, 1994; Fidler, 1996; Kielhofner, 2009; King, 1978; Kramer & Hinojosa, 2009; Llorens, 1970; Miller & Walker, 1993; Mosey, 1996; Schkade & Schultz, 1992a, 1992b).

Consistent with the *Centennial Vision's* (American Occupational Therapy Association [AOTA], 2007) call for occupational therapy to be science-driven, Hinojosa (2007) emphasized the criticality of ensuring that occupational therapy interventions are based on valid theories that provide practitioners with "the knowledge they need to make educated predictions" (p. 634). To ensure that occupational therapy practice is founded on science, the *Occupational Therapy Practice Framework: Domain and Process* (AOTA, 2014) includes the caveat that practitioners must apply the document "in conjunction with the knowledge and evidence relevant to occupation and occupational therapy" (p. S3). Because the *Framework* does not include conceptual models or theories, it is a practitioner's ethical responsibility to provide interventions based on established theories (Hinojosa, 2007). Theories that have been developed within the occupational therapy profession and outside of the field must be integrated to support the field's scope of practice and provide guidelines for intervention (Gutman, Mortera, Hinojosa, & Kramer, 2007).

In her 1978 Eleanor Clarke Slagle Lecture, King called for a unifying theory to ensure cohesiveness within the profession. King's appeal was based on her valid concern that increased specialization within occupational therapy would lead to fragmentation and a lack of consumer understanding about the value of occupation.

King acknowledged that her adaptive process theory was not the only tenable model to address these concerns. She expressed hope that her presentation would spur others to explore occupational therapy's philosophical foundations and professional practices to develop additional coherent models of practice. In the years since King put forth this challenge, several of the profession's best scholars have responded. Many influential works have been published that meet King's criteria for theory that is "based on a straightforward structure that can be widely understood and is clearly related to the client's life functioning" (King, 1978, p. 14).

Part II provides readers with several of the leading theoretical frameworks proposed by prominent occupational therapy scholars to clarify the link between theory and practice. Although these models differ in content, structure, and format, all emphasize the use of occupation and a client-centered approach throughout the occupational therapy process. Because all practice models (no matter how well developed) are considered works in progress, further conceptual development may have transpired since these original writings were published, and additional modifications may occur in the future.

It is important to note that a complete presentation of practice models and frames of reference is beyond the scope of this text. However, a thoughtful review of select practice models that reflect the occupational therapy profession's core commitment to occupation can help readers develop a theoretical mindset for client-centered, occupation-based practice. These frameworks can be particularly helpful in the assessment of a person's occupational profile, the analysis of his or her occupational performance, and the design of an intervention plan based on the concepts and principles identified in the *Framework* (AOTA, 2014). The use of a clear, well-developed practice model can ensure that the profession's philosophical foundations and core values are actualized in practice and that occupational therapy intervention facilitates the person's engagement in occupation to support life participation in context (see Active Reflections II.1 and II.2).

Active Reflection II.1. Commonalities in Theoretical and Conceptual Frameworks

Review this part's frames of reference and practice models.
- What core concepts and fundamental principles are consistently presented to help link theory to practice?
- What key theoretical guidelines are regularly provided for the therapeutic use of occupation throughout the occupational therapy process?

Theory and its application must be integrated with enough time for studying, thinking, and thoughtful application.

—Rood, 1958, p. 329

This part begins with Nelson's exploration of key concepts related to occupation and its therapeutic application in Chapter 8. In his 1996 Eleanor Clarke Slagle Lecture, Nelson reviews his lifework of seeking to adequately define occupation, which has culminated in the development of the Conceptual Framework for Therapeutic Occupation (CFTO). In this framework, Nelson defines *occupation* as a relationship between occupational form and occupational performance. The multidimensional nature of occupational form and its relationship with occupational performance is presented. The meaningfulness and purposefulness of occupation to the individual is examined.

Nelson explores the dynamics of occupation and the impact of occupational performance on the environment, the individual, and his or her occupational adaptation. He proposes that the power of therapeutic occupation is elicited when practitioners use their understanding of different occupational forms' possibilities to collaborate with each individual. This synthesis results in interventions that are purposeful and meaningful to the person. Nelson emphasizes that occupational therapy's specialized skills in occupation synthesis is the reason occupational therapy will thrive in the 21st century.

The significance of the use of occupation synthesis to elicit meaningful and purposeful occupational performance is supported by Nelson's analysis of past, current, and potential future models of practice. As he notes, these models have differing viewpoints, but they all share an emphasis on essential occupation-based princi-

ples, validating the importance of occupation synthesis to society. Key principles of the CFTO are presented. Several examples are provided throughout Nelson's treatise to illustrate the practical application of these concepts and support the profession's unique contribution to human health. Nelson concludes with a call for research to examine the power of therapeutic occupation. He advocates that all occupational therapy practitioners embrace and use the term *occupation* in the literature and public interactions to ensure that society recognizes the profession's ownership of occupation as therapy.

Another practice model that provides a conceptual framework that embraces the therapeutic use of occupation is elucidated in Chapter 9, which presents Fisher's 1998 Eleanor Clarke Slagle Lecture. Fisher begins her presentation by contrasting reductionistic, therapist-directed practice to occupation-based, person-driven practice and reflecting on her personal development as a practitioner and scholar with a strong belief in the value of occupation as a therapeutic agent. Fisher defines *occupation* as a noun of action, because it conveys the powerful essence of the profession and enables people to seize, take possession of, or occupy the space, time, and roles of their lives. She reflects that the profession's uniqueness lies in the use of occupation as a therapeutic agent. However, this unique focus on occupation is not always evident in practice.

In response to this gap, Fisher developed the Occupational Therapy Intervention Process Model to guide clinical reasoning so that occupational therapy intervention is based on a client-centered performance context. She presents four continua—ecological relevance, source of purpose, source of meaning, and focus of intervention—that can be used to evaluate the characteristics of activities used in occupational therapy intervention. On the basis of an analysis of occupational therapy practice according to these continua, she identifies four main activities (e.g., exercise, contrived occupation, therapeutic occupation, adaptive occupation) that are typically used in intervention.

Of these, Fisher argues that therapeutic occupation and adaptive occupation are the legitimate activities of occupational therapy. She describes the interrelated dimensions of context and provides clear guidelines for using a top-down approach to evaluation and for implementing intervention. A case example supports the clinical application of each step in this model.

Fisher's emphasis on a top-down approach to the occupational therapy process that focuses on occupation and collaboration is upheld in Chapter 10 by Gray,

Active Reflection II.2. Relevance of Theory to the *Occupational Therapy Practice Framework*

Consider each of this part's frames of reference and practice models using the lens of the *Occupational Therapy Practice Framework*.
- What are the commonalities in language between the *Framework* and the different theoretical models?
- Which models seem most congruent with the domain and process of occupational therapy as defined and described in the *Framework*?
- How can each model be used to develop a person's occupational profile and design an intervention plan that is in accordance with the *Framework*?
- Are there gaps in these models that would require the use of another theoretical framework to adequately complete an occupational profile and provide person-centered and occupation-based interventions?

who begins by exploring the disconnect that can occur when holistic practice models are not used to plan intervention. Gray openly discusses the difficulty many occupational therapy practitioners experience when they emphasize client factors and performance skills rather than occupation as the core of their therapeutic intervention. She reflects that this reductionism results from, and contributes to, the profession's identity crisis. She proposes that embracing the concepts of *occupation as ends* and *occupation as means* provides a guide to intervention planning. Gray defines each concept and analyzes its historical significance and applicability to current therapeutic problems. She gives useful guidelines to assist occupational therapy practitioners in their clinical decision-making and to facilitate their understanding and expression of the profession's unique occupational expertise.

Gray ends with a case example that includes realistic complexities faced by individuals who receive occupational therapy services. Her analysis supports the application of occupation as ends and occupation as means in evaluation and intervention.

> *Health must be established through the proper co-ordination of the whole man—body, mind, and will. The physical health of the man can be furthered by keeping up his morale and preserving a healthy mental balance.*
> —Wilson (1936/2002, p. 4)

Gray's chapter provides a clear overview of Trombly's 1995 Eleanor Clarke Slagle Lecture in Chapter 11. In this influential work, Trombly put forth her Model of Occupational Functioning, which conceptualizes occu-

pational performance as a descending hierarchy of roles, tasks, activities, abilities, and capacities. She clearly defines each component of her model and supports these with pertinent examples and relevant research.

Trombly distinguishes occupation as a treatment end-goal from occupation as a means to remedial impairment. She emphasizes that *both* are therapeutic *if* purposeful and meaningful. She hypothesizes that purposefulness *organizes* behavior, and meaningfulness *motivates* behavior. Trombly then analyzes the therapeutic impact of purposefulness and meaningfulness on both forms of therapeutic occupation. She recognizes that these aspects of occupation require exploration, clarification, and interpretation through research and proposes several highly relevant research questions. She presents a comprehensive literature review of research related to the use of occupation in the motor domain; however, it is apparent that more definitive research is needed. Trombly expresses her hope that her model will spark an explosion of research to further clarify and strengthen the link between occupation and therapeutic outcomes.

Chapter 12 explores the purposefulness and meaningfulness of occupational engagement according to the theoretical concepts of mindfulness and flow. In this work, Reid defines the construct of *flow* and presents Csikszentmihalyi's two-dimensional model of flow. According to this model, flow is experienced when the person's abilities and the activity challenges are both high. The resulting challenge–skill balance provides the person with the holistic sensation of being fully engaged. The moment-to-moment process of mindfulness, which is simultaneously comprised of intention, attention, and attitude, is also described.

Reid provides relevant conceptual links between the theoretical perspectives put forth in the literature on mindfulness and flow and different modes of occupational engagement. She highlights the philosophical and psychological theories that support the application of mindfulness and flow to occupational therapy practice, supporting her analysis with practice examples. Given the various conceptualizations of mindfulness and flow and the lack of standardized measurement tools, the empirical research on the application of these concepts in practice is limited. Despite these limitations, Reid hopes that an increased understanding of how mindfulness and flow can influence subjective well-being and foster occupational engagement will inform occupational therapy practice and inspire new research.

The relationship between subjective well-being and occupational engagement is explored in Chapter 13, which presents Doble and Santha's occupational well-being framework. Doble and Santha were motivated to develop this conceptual model on the basis of their observation that occupational therapy outcomes were too focused on people's occupational performance, with minimal attention to the subjectivity of their occupational experiences. To develop their descriptive framework, the authors reviewed the occupational therapy and occupational science literature along with personal narratives to determine factors that influence the satisfaction and fulfillment people derive from their occupational experiences. Doble and Santha examine how these critical issues can be applied to challenge the profession's traditional focus on performance-based outcomes and support practitioners' consideration of occupational well-being.

Doble and Santha contend that occupational well-being is enhanced when people's individual occupational needs are consistently met. These needs are described as accomplishment, affirmation, agency, coherence, companionship, pleasure, and renewal. The authors define each and provide relevant practice examples to support how these needs may be evident in people's daily lives. According to Doble and Santha, occupational therapy practitioners can assist people in the composition or re-orchestration of their occupational lives, enabling their attainment of occupational well-being. They explain the inherent congruence between their conceptualization of occupational well-being and established occupational therapy practice models.

Doble and Santha acknowledge the realistic and often inevitable systemic and personal barriers that can limit choice and hinder the fulfillment of a person's occupational needs. Therefore, they stress that occupational therapy practitioners must move beyond the sole provision of direct interventions to advocate for change at environmental, societal, organizational, and personal levels, as needed.

The importance of Doble and Santha's call to occupational therapy practitioners to consider people's unique subjective experiences of their occupations, adopt non-performance-based goals to enable occupational well-being, and confront systemic barriers that limit choice becomes clearly evident in this part's next chapter. In Chapter 14, Hammell confronts the underlying assumptions of established occupational therapy practice models and theoretical frameworks. She critically examines the evidence supporting long-held foundational beliefs of the profession and concludes that they are not supported by solid evidence.

Hammell provides a persuasive argument that these assumptions have been retained for decades due to the profession's allegiance to perspectives put forth by revered leaders in the field. She contends that to attain professional integrity, the profession must adopt a healthy skepticism and question the validity of its enculturation process that presents the field's founding views as universal truths. We must recognize that the value system on which occupational therapy's core tenets are based does not represent worldwide beliefs. Instead, these tenets are ableist and economically and culturally biased toward a middle-class, Western perspective (see Active Reflection II.3).

Active Reflection II.3. Challenges to Traditional Theoretical Conceptualizations

Review the theoretical and conceptual models presented in this part using the skeptical approach advocated for by Hammell.
- Are there any sacred texts evident in these works?
- What are the implications of universal acceptance of published frames of reference and models of practice?
- Which theoretical and conceptual frameworks presented in this part broaden the concept of *independence*?
- Which ones would you use to enable flow and occupational well-being?

Hammell's stance that occupational therapy's core tenets (and even one of the field's most beloved quotes) reflect ethnocentrism and theoretical imperialism may be disconcerting to readers not comfortable with critical discourse. However, it is a perspective that is worth serious consideration as the field moves to become more globally connected. As Hammell argues, the assumptions that *all* people can use their hands, exercise free will and autonomy, find positive meaning in occupation, and be driven to master their environment are all invalid because they ignore the realities of the majority of people in the world. In addition, the typical categorization of meaningful occupation into self-care, productivity, and leisure in most of the field's conceptual frameworks do not accurately reflect more global perspectives on the nature of occupation and the potential role of occupational therapy in enabling health and well-being. Because the marginalization of populations knows no geographic boundaries, Hammell's call to develop occupational therapy theories based on divergent cultural viewpoints to inform more inclusive practice is highly relevant, regardless of one's country of origin or dominant culture.

Hammell's view that interdependence, not independence, should be the prime construct included in occupational therapy's theoretical frameworks is supported by the AOTA Position Paper *Broadening the Construct of Independence*. This work, included in Appendix II.A, provides a relevant expanded definition of *independence* that emphasizes a self-directed state of being that enables participation in a life of one's choice. Most important, this definition recognizes society's responsibility to ensure that all citizens have the rights and access to full societal participation.

This part of the text concludes with another controversial work that challenges allegiance to occupational therapy's history as the foundation for the profession's identity and practice. In her landmark Eleanor Clarke Slagle Lecture in Chapter 15, Mosey confronts the field's tendency to use history to substantiate its current and envisioned identity. Specifically, she questions the wisdom of adopting a monistic approach to occupational therapy based on historical justifications. Rather than seek one basic principle to unify all aspects of the profession of occupational therapy, Mosey proposes the adoption of a pluralistic approach for a professional identity. According to Mosey, pluralism recognizes the reality that a profession is too rich, diverse, and complex to be reduced to a singularity. Thus, a pluralistic approach provides a broad perspective that considers all elements of a profession (see Active Reflection II.4).

Active Reflection II.4. Monism or Pluralism in Occupational Therapy Practice

Consider an area of practice that most interests you.
- Which practice models or frames of reference are most commonly used in this area?
- Do these conceptual frameworks represent a monistic or pluralistic perspective?
- Are they inclusive of the qualitative aspects of occupation, and do they promote occupational well-being?

In her treatise, Mosey clearly outlines and defines the multiple elements of a profession. She describes how the adoption of a monistic view to develop a comprehensive theory based on only one of a profession's elements (or a part of an element) can be rigid, exclusionary, and laden with philosophical overtones. The result is a constriction of creativity, independence, and diversity in thought and an oversimplification that provides limited guidelines for practice. Conversely, if a compre-

hensive theory attempts to be inclusionary, Mosey believes the resulting intricacies and complexities will put off most practitioners who are seeking clear guidance for their practice. In contrast, a pluralistic approach, which articulates a straightforward structure based on the elements of a profession, recognizes all facets of a profession as important, enables flexibility, promotes discourse, and allows for growth. Mosey contends that the mastery of the totality of a profession's elements is what makes a profession unique, and this is best obtained through the adoption of a pluralistic approach to the professional identity. Most important, pluralism embraces the inherent dynamic nature of a profession, rejects stagnation, and ensures progress, outcomes that are highly consistent with the profession's vision for its next century (AOTA, 2007).

References

American Occupational Therapy Association. (2007). AOTA's *Centennial Vision* and executive summary. *American Journal of Occupational Therapy, 61*, 613–614. http://dx.doi:10.5014/ajot.61.6.613

American Occupational Therapy Association. (2014). Occupational therapy practice framework: Domain and process (3rd ed.). *American Journal of Occupational Therapy, 68*(Suppl. 1), S1–S48. http://dx.doi.org/10.5014/ajot.2014.682006

Bruce, M. A., & Borg, B. (2002). *Psychosocial frames of reference: Core for occupation-based practice* (3rd ed.). Thorofare, NJ: Slack.

Christiansen, C., Baum, C., & Bass-Haugen, J. (2005). *Occupational therapy: Performance, participation, and well-being.* Thorofare, NJ: Slack.

Dunn, W., Brown, C., & McGuigan, A. (1994). The Ecology of Human Performance: A framework for considering the effect of context. *American Journal of Occupational Therapy, 48*, 595–607. http://dx.doi.org/10.5014/ajot.48.7.595

Dunton, W. R. (1928). *Prescribing occupational therapy.* Baltimore: Charles C Thomas.

Fidler, G. (1996). Lifestyle performance: From profile to conceptual model. *American Journal of Occupational Therapy, 50*, 139–147. http://dx.doi.org/10.5014/ajot.50.2.139

Gutman, S., Mortera, M., Hinojosa, J., & Kramer, P. (2007). The Issue Is—Revision of the *Occupational Therapy Practice Framework. American Journal of Occupational Therapy, 61*, 119–126. http://dx.doi.org/10.5014/ajot.61.1.119

Hinojosa, J. (2007). Becoming innovators in an era of hyperchange [2007 Eleanor Clarke Slagle Lecture]. *American Journal of Occupational Therapy, 61,* 629–637. http://dx.doi.org/10.5014/ajot.61.6.629

Kielhofner, G. (2009). *Conceptual foundations of occupational therapy* (4th ed.). Baltimore: Lippincott Williams & Wilkins.

King, L. J. (1978). Toward a science of adaptive responses. *American Journal of Occupational Therapy, 32,* 429–437.

Kramer, P., & Hinojosa, J. (Eds.). (2009). *Frames of reference for pediatric occupational therapy.* New York: Lippincott Williams & Wilkins.

Llorens, L. A. (1970). Facilitating growth and development: The promise of occupational therapy. *American Journal of Occupational Therapy, 24,* 93–101.

Miller, R., & Walker, K. (1993). *Perspectives on theory for the practice of occupational therapy* (2nd ed.). Rockville, MD: Aspen.

Mosey, A. C. (1996). *Psychosocial components of occupational therapy.* New York: Raven Press.

Rood, M. S. (1958). Every one counts [Eleanor Clarke Slagle Lecture]. *American Journal of Occupational Therapy, 12,* 326–329.

Salmon, T. W. (1924). *Mind and medicine.* New York: Columbia University Press.

Schkade, J., & Schultz, S. (1992a). Occupational adaptation: Toward a holistic approach for contemporary practice, Part 1. *American Journal of Occupational Therapy, 46,* 829–837. http://dx.doi.org/10.5014/ajot.46.9.829

Schkade, J., & Schultz, S. (1992b). Occupational adaptation: Toward a holistic approach for contemporary practice, Part 2. *American Journal of Occupational Therapy, 46,* 917–925. http://dx.doi.org/10.5014/ajot.46.10.917

Wilson, W. (2002). Recent developments in occupational therapy. In A. Wilcock (Ed.), *Occupation for health: A journey from prescription to self-health.* London: British Association and College of Occupational Therapists. Original work published 1936

CHAPTER 8

Why the Profession of Occupational Therapy Will Flourish in the 21st Century

1996 ELEANOR CLARKE SLAGLE LECTURE

DAVID L. NELSON

Welcome to this celebration of our profession! Eighty-eight years ago, a young woman named Eleanor Clarke Slagle attended a course that explored the potentials of occupation as a therapeutic medium (Quiroga, 1995, chap. 1). Convinced of the power of occupation to enhance human life, Slagle went on to help found our profession. In her name, I am honored to present the 35th Eleanor Clarke Slagle Lecture.

Occupational therapy as a profession will flourish over the next century for the same reason that it has flourished over the past century. Real human beings needed therapeutic occupation in the days of Eleanor Clarke Slagle; they need therapeutic occupation in our times; and they will continue to need it beyond our days. Our service of occupational therapy is so sound because the idea of therapeutic occupation is so basic: The human being can attain enhanced health and quality of life by actively doing things that are personally meaningful and purposeful, in other words, through occupation. We are the profession uniquely devoted to helping persons help themselves through their own active efforts.

The Need for a Historical Perspective

To appreciate the core of occupational therapy and its importance for human health and quality of life over the next century, we need a macroscopic point of view. I am not referring to the immediate time frame of next year's health legislation in Congress, the year 2000, or even the year 2050. My time frame is approximately the year 2096, a good time for someone, certainly not me, to be summing up the second century of organized

occupational therapy just as we are now in a position to sum up its first century.

What the 20th century teaches us is that apparently reliable trends on which people make predictions break down categorically in totally unforeseeable ways. Who in the progressive early 1900s could have predicted the horrors of World War I, the beginning of which was marked by soldiers on horseback and the end of which marked by mechanized trench warfare where combatants were at risk for instant death from distant unseen forces? Who could have predicted the Russian revolution; the worldwide economic depression; or the rise of fascism, genocide, and World War II with its unprecedented millions of dead, including civilians? Who could have predicted the nuclear terror of my generation or the rise of Pax Americana amidst the sudden, implosive collapse of the Soviet empire?

It will be at least as hard for us to predict the 21st century as it was for the first occupational therapists to predict the 20th century. We can do our best to extrapolate current trends into the future, but the trends that are visible now will break down categorically just as the optimistically progressive trends of 1900 broke down over the past century. We will be surprised. Our descendants will be surprised. I put it this way because this is the larger context from which we should view the profession. Only those things will endure that are both fundamental to human nature and adaptable to a changing world. I believe that one of those things is occupational therapy.

The profession of occupational therapy was founded for one reason: To use occupation as a therapeutic method. The original articles of incorporation of the National Society for the Promotion of Occupational Therapy (1917) clearly stated the purposes of this new organization: "the advancement of occupation as a therapeutic measure," "the study of the effect of occupation on the human being," and "the scientific

This chapter was previously published in the *American Journal of Occupational Therapy, 51*, 11–24. Copyright © 1997, American Occupational Therapy Association. Reprinted with permission. http://dx.doi.org/10.5014/ajot.51.1.11

dispensation of this knowledge" (p. 1). It is important to note that the founders thought of occupation as a method, not just a goal. They believed that occupation could have therapeutic effects on the human being, and they wanted to document these effects through scientific research.

Mores have changed dramatically since the founding of our profession, and they will change in the future in ways that are unimaginable to us now. When we look at photographs of early occupational therapy (e.g., Howe & Schwartzberg, 1986), we see starched uniforms, serious and even stern facial expressions, military-like decorum, and highly structured crafts that required many sessions to complete. Those early photographs reflect a different era of America and of occupational therapy. It was a different culture, and the therapeutic occupations of those times reflected that culture. In like manner, occupational therapists 100 years from now will look back at the archives documenting today's occupational therapy and see quaintness in our dress, our mannerisms, and our speech. Yet, they will recognize their essential connectedness to us. Therapeutic occupations change with the times and with the culture, but the underlying idea of occupation as therapy remains constant.

Defining Occupation

Given our title as *occupational* therapists and given our reason for being, it is ironic that we have not spent much effort in defining occupation. This curious omission has been pointed out by advocates of occupation as therapy (e.g., Christiansen, 1990; Gilfoyle, 1984). Much of my work has focused on the definition of the term *occupation* (Nelson, 1988, 1994, 1996). Occupation is defined as the relationship between an *occupational form* and an *occupational performance* (see Figure 8.1). Occupational performance means the doing. Occupational form means the thing, or the format, that is done. For example, consider the occupation of a boy

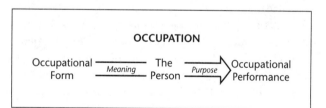

Figure 8.1. Occupation as the meaningful, purposeful occupational performance of a person in the context of an occupational form.

making potato pancakes (latkes) in December during the Jewish holiday of Hanukkah. His occupational form has physical features, such as the way those potatoes soak up oil and fry crispy on the outside, yet a little soggy on the inside. His occupational form also has sociocultural features, including its connection to his religious heritage and that the chef's hat he wears once belonged to his grandfather. The handle of the frying pan (part of the occupational form) elicits the occupational performance of grasping. Other aspects of his occupational performance include his speech, gaze, smile, and posture.

Occupational form and performance are objectively observable; we can see and analyze the boy's environment and movement patterns. But occupation also has subjective, experiential elements that are not directly observable. These subjective aspects of occupation are *meaning* and *purpose*. Meaning is the person's active interpretation of the occupational form. Meaning has to do with making sense of things perceptually; for example, the boy has a basic awareness that he is not too close to the fire. Meaning also has to do with interpreting the symbols in his occupational form, for example, the words of others and the idea of Hanukkah as a playful holiday. Meaning is also affective: The boy is having fun.

After meaning is present (i.e., the person makes sense of the occupational form), then purpose is possible. Purpose is the person's goal orientation; it is what the person wants or intends. For example, what does the boy making latkes want? Does he want to make his sister laugh? Does he want to make tasty latkes that he can douse with applesauce and eat or share with his family? Does he want to participate in a family tradition? At any given moment, a human being typically has multiple purposes—some immediate, such as wanting to hold onto the spatula, and some long term, such as wanting to belong within a family. It is characteristic of an occupational approach to consider both the immediate and the ultimate purposes of the person engaged in occupation.

Occupation influences the world around the person (see Figure 8.2). This influence is called *impact*. The human being is not just a passive respondent who is always under environmental control. The person can affect his or her own future occupational forms. The boy in the example actively changes his occupational form: The latkes are cooked and the kitchen is somewhat of a mess. The cooking occupation sets up the next occupation—eating.

Another dynamic of occupation is that a person can literally change his or her own nature by engaging in oc-

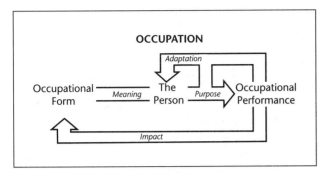

Figure 8.2. Occupation depicted with the occupational dynamics of impact and adaptation.

cupation. This is called occupational *adaptation*. Active doing, or occupation, can lead to changes in sensorimotor abilities, cognitive abilities, and psychosocial abilities. As we do, so we become. For example, consider the occupation of a healthy 8-month-old boy playing peek-a-boo with his mother. The boy's occupational form includes a piece of cloth first placed over his face and later over his mother's face. By putting the cloth over her own face, the mother gives the boy an opportunity to have an impact through active occupational performance. He is rewarded by her smiling face and her animated talk when the cloth is removed. There is an established game that is present in the occupational form: Our culture makes available to us the game of peek-a-boo. The boy's occupational performance involves complex patterns of reaching, grasping, trunk rotation, posture, laughing, facial expression, and prespeech sounds. This occupational form is meaningful to the boy perceptually, symbolically, and affectively. He is full of purpose as he tries to reestablish eye contact with his mother by attempting to remove the cloth from her face. We can infer multiple sensorimotor adaptations, such as posture, reach, and grasp, but perhaps more importantly, there are cognitive and psychosocial adaptations. For example, the boy is learning the rules of reciprocal play. Additionally, object permanence is being established, and the boy is learning that important things, like mother, do not go away just because they cannot be seen temporarily.

Brief occupations such as these are the dynamics that while interacting with physiological maturation power human development. These brief occupations are nested within higher level occupations. Indeed, large roles in life are occupations that consist of thousands of brief occupations. For example, consider the reciprocal occupations of a father and daughter on a roller coaster at an amusement park. The man is smiling, however terrified. The girl raises her hands in adolescent bravado. For the girl, the roller-coaster ride is nested within a series of amusement park occupations over many years from the merry-go-round of her toddlerhood to the ultimate goal of going to the amusement park with friends, including boys (no parents needed, thank you). The ride on the roller coaster is also nested within all the summer and family vacations of the girl's life. Given past adaptations, she is ready to go on to new occupations and adventures. From the father's point of view, his daughter is an immediate part of his occupational form, but he would not be there on that screaming roller coaster with his 48-year-old vestibular system if it were not because this occupation is integrally connected to all the occupations of fatherhood. The artful interlocking of successive levels of a person's occupations, bound together by corresponding levels of purpose, connects the present moment to the life span. It would be just as reductionistic to ignore brief moments of occupation as it would be to ignore occupational roles that span decades. We cannot really understand the long-term occupations without understanding the short-term occupations that make them up and vice versa.

Occupational adaptation marks every age of the developing person. Consider the occupations of happy elderly newlyweds singing at a microphone. Their occupational form is the small town wedding celebration. In the basement hall of the American Legion with Old Glory in the background and long wooden tables decorated with balloons and banners, the newlyweds take their turn at the microphone. More than 200 people are present, including new in-laws getting to know each other, townspeople discussing their views on local events, young children racing through the aisles, and teenagers trying to sneak off to the parking lot. The occupational form of marriage means something profound to each marriage partner. Their purposes are both to sing a pretty good tune (pertaining to the immediate occupation) and to start a life together (pertaining to their long-term occupations). Growing beyond their recent roles as widow and widower, they adapt to new occupational roles. Occupational forms, the gifts of nature and of culture, not only sustain us, but also challenge us to engage in the continuous adaptations that constitute life.

A Conceptual Framework for Therapeutic Occupation

Given the power of occupation in healthy human development, it makes great sense to have founded a profession on the idea of occupation as therapy. We as a

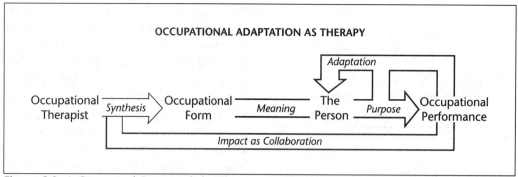

Figure 8.3. A Conceptual Framework for Therapeutic Occupation (for therapeutic adaptation). The occupational therapist collaboratively synthesizes an occupational form and makes a prediction concerning the person's meaning, purpose, occupational performance, and adaptation.

profession believe that a person can affect the quality of his or her life through occupation. We also believe that the person can be helped through this process by another person—an occupational therapist.

At the Medical College of Ohio, we advocate a Conceptual Framework for Therapeutic Occupation (CFTO; see Figure 8.3). The occupational therapist understands the potentials of various occupational forms and is willing to collaborate in synthesizing occupational forms that are meaningful and purposeful to the person. The occupational therapist hopes and predicts that the occupational form will be perceptually, symbolically, and emotionally meaningful to the person; that the occupational form and the meanings the person actively assigns to it will result in a multidimensional set of purposes (when therapy is best, the person is full of purpose); and that the person will engage in a voluntary occupational performance.

Consider the occupation of an older man who has had a stroke on the right side of his brain that led to left hemiparesis, perceptual problems, and left neglect. In the rehabilitation hospital, he was continuously told to do things with his left hand—"Use your left hand." "Look at your left hand." "Watch out for your left hand."—but he did not understand why until he hurt it in the spokes of his wheelchair. The man's therapeutic occupational adaptation occurs in the occupational therapy bathroom where he is given a comb in front of a mirror. Here the occupational form is full of salient cues for what is expected. Though there are many cues, the situation as a whole suggests a unified response: It is time to comb hair. The occupational form is immediately meaningful to him, words are really not necessary. He knows that the water should be turned on, so he independently does so. He combs his hair in his accustomed way; that is, his left arm rises in synchrony

and coordination with his right hand as he straightens his hair. Embedded in this occupation are left shoulder flexion and external rotation accompanied by elbow flexion with wrist, hand, and finger control. This coordinated pattern of movement takes place outside his visual range, hence guided by proprioceptive input. This occupation is an excellent intervention for his motor control, left neglect, and problems of body scheme. Of course, a single occupation does not result in dramatic gains, yet dramatic gains are impossible without a series of therapeutic occupations like this one.

Sometimes the person's problem is resistant to occupational adaptation. Hence, compensatory occupation is the goal (see Figure 8.4). In compensation, the therapist collaborates with the person in synthesizing an atypical or alternative occupational form. As always, the therapist hopes and predicts that the occupational form will be meaningful and purposeful. However, in compensation, the goal is to have a successful impact as a result of a substitute occupational performance or as a way around the problem.

Consider an older man who is holding his cafeteria tray with a myoelectric prosthesis. The prosthesis is an atypical part of an otherwise typical occupational form. However, the prosthesis has meaning to the man (he knows how to operate it), and it has purpose to him (he wants to operate it). The substitute occupational performance is that he contracts or relaxes the remaining segments of his upper arm muscles to control the device. The comparable impact is that the tray is held while he uses his dominant right hand to scoop the food. This is successful occupational compensation. Frequently, compensation depends on prior adaptations or learning how to use the compensatory device. In this example, the role of the occupational therapist was to help the man learn how to manipulate the prosthetic elbow

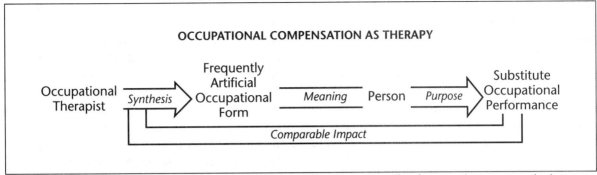

Figure 8.4. A Conceptual Framework for Therapeutic Occupation (for therapeutic compensation). The occupational therapist collaboratively synthesizes an occupational form (often somewhat atypical socioculturally). The resulting occupational performance substitutes for the typical way of doing things but leads to a comparable impact.

and wrist joints and how to match his muscle contractions to the electronics of the prosthesis so that objects could be picked up without dropping or crushing them. Hence, adaptations led to successful compensations.

Occupational adaptation and adaptational compensation are different but dynamically interacting processes. Both depend on *occupational synthesis,* or design, of forms that are meaningful and purposeful to the person. Occupational synthesis is what we occupational therapists do for a living. Our specialty is to know about occupational forms in all their variety and to perceive the special capabilities of persons so that a therapeutic match can be made. Sometimes this involves highly naturalistic, everyday forms. But often, there is an element of simulation involved. Consider a boy with cerebral palsy whose occupational form involves virtual reality equipment and a new power wheelchair with an unfamiliar joystick. The meaningfulness and purposefulness of the occupational form to him can be inferred from his occupational performance: He manipulates the joystick in a sustained way and his gaze is set on the feedback device. His occupational adaptation is his learning how to operate the joystick that will control his wheelchair. This will provide him with compensatory mobility in the future.

The virtual reality in this example is "high tech," but we occupational therapists have always used virtual reality, or simulation, whether high tech or low. For example, the occupational therapy kitchen is a treatment area that simulates the homes of many patients while providing the possibility of special safety features and assistive devices. In some cases, the occupational therapy kitchen provides the ideal location; in others, a home visit would be more therapeutic. Much of occupational therapy clinical reasoning and program de-

velopment depend on judgments about the suitability or unsuitability of simulated versus naturalistic occupational forms. Simulation can involve great creativity and technology, as with virtual reality or electronic work simulators. But the naturalistic occupational forms provided by our culture are the starting points for our ingenuity.

The Flexibility of Therapeutic Occupation: Diverse Models of Practice

Therapeutic occupation, the common core of occupational therapy, is a robust construct capable of accommodating many different approaches to intervention. Mosey (1970) introduced the term *theoretical frame of reference* to describe systematic guidelines for occupational therapy practice that are grounded in theoretical statements about the nature of the person and his or her relations to the world. Others, including Kielhofner (1992), have used the term *conceptual model of practice* to denote the diversity of theory-based approaches to occupational therapy.

My idea of model of practice has two main parts: (a) a theoretical base describing healthy and unhealthy occupation and (b) principles and techniques for occupational syntheses. The theoretical base draws from one or more disciplines. It is a coherent description of the potentials and pitfalls of human occupation, including the nature of the person, the role of occupational forms, the types of meanings and purposes experienced by the person, and the dynamics of successful and unsuccessful occupational performances. Basic research is cited as available. The second part of a model of practice provides principled yet practical guidelines for occupational syntheses that are consistent with the theoretical base.

How does the therapist conduct occupational syntheses in the evaluation process? How does the therapist use occupational analysis in the goal-setting process? How does the therapist collaborate with the person in synthesizing occupational forms for adaptation or compensation? Applied research is cited as available.

There currently are many models of practice in occupational therapy. Some are more carefully worked out than others; all are works in progress. Consideration of selected occupational therapy models of practice from the past can enhance appreciation of today's diverse models of practice. In discussing these models, I will apply the same occupational terminology introduced earlier in this article (e.g., *occupational form, occupational performance*) to the diverse ideas expressed by various authors. I believe that this terminology provides a systematic way to compare and contrast occupational therapy models of practice.

Slagle's Habit Training Model of Practice

Slagle (1922) was a proponent of one of the first models of practice in occupational therapy. She drew from many different theoretical sources, including John Dewey's Chicago-school philosophy of pragmatism; William James's psychology of attention; Ruskin's arts-and-crafts movement; the Society of Friends's moral treatment; and Adolph Meyer's ideas about holism, mental hygiene, and use of time. Slagle theorized that habit reactions largely constitute the lives of most people. The healthy person engages each day in a rich succession of habit occupations—a balance of productive work, self-reliance, rest, and activation of what Slagle called the "play spirit" (p. 16). Underlying all habits is the necessity for attention; indeed attention itself is a habit that can be built.

Unlike the well-organized habits of healthy persons, the habits of persons with mental disorders are deteriorated and disorganized. Attention drifts restlessly and irrelevantly. Neither the joy of productivity nor the joy of play is experienced. Grandiosity on the one hand and passivity on the other are poor substitutes for actual occupation. Given this theoretical base of healthy and unhealthy occupation, what kinds of occupational syntheses are called for in the Slagle model of practice? The main occupational form that Slagle described was a 24-hour perday schedule that provided a balance of self-care, physical exercises, work, and play (Kidner, 1930). Specifically noted were instructional periods for self-care (e.g., shoe lacing, teeth cleaning, toileting). Work occupations were to be individually graded from

simple to complex. Stimulating music with clearly evident rhythm was recommended to accompany the physical exercises. Moving pictures, folk dancing, storytelling, and simple competitive games rounded out the day. After the basic habit occupations were attained, the patient could progress to the *occupational center,* also called the *curative workshop.* Here patients engaged daily in major crafts or preindustrial groups that required sustained attention over many sessions. The developmental structure of the discharged patient was enhanced by adaptations in the attentional mechanisms and habit reactions.

Baldwin's Model of Practice for the Restoration of Movement

Another early model of practice focused on different aspects of the developmental structure from those focused on by Slagle. Baldwin's (1919) model of practice was designed to restore movement abilities in young soldiers wounded in World War I and drew into occupational therapy concepts from kinesiology, biomechanics, and psychology. He detailed the relationships between various occupational forms and joint range of motion, strength, and endurance. He saw coordination as a high-level skill involving complex series of movements across several joints, and he believed that this high-level skill is inextricably linked to everyday occupations. Movement skill was viewed not just in terms of immediate learning but also in terms of what can be "transferred to another occasion or to other types of movements" (p. 7). Although he focused on the patient's motor abilities, Baldwin also cited "interest," "attention," "initiative," "inspiration," "optimism," and "cheerfulness" (pp. 6–9) as factors that affect the overall quality of the patient's occupations. Baldwin specifically identified social factors that typically inhibited the development of self-responsibility among disabled veterans, including the military's discouragement of the initiative typical of civilian life and the public's misdirected sympathy. Baldwin also considered the patient's intelligence and vocational aptitude when synthesizing therapeutic occupational forms.

Given this view of the person's developmental structure, the main guideline for occupational synthesis was to provide occupational forms that naturalistically challenge the identified problems of range, strength, endurance, and coordination. In Baldwin's (1919) own terms:

> Occupational therapy is based on the principle that the best type of remedial exercise is that

which requires a series of specific voluntary movements involved in the ordinary trades and occupations, physical training, play, and the daily routine activities of life. (p. 5)

Occupational forms were analyzed in terms of their typical challenges for the purposes of grading from easy to hard and providing options to different patients, depending on their interests. The end-products, or the impacts, of the work were thought to enhance meaning and purpose; impact also provided direct feedback about the patient's progress. Baldwin favored the use of everyday occupational forms, including, but not restricted to, crafts. The advantages of naturalistic occupational forms were (a) the allowance for personal initiative, (b) the incentives provided for sustained effort, (c) the development of coordination, (d) the transfer of skills, and (e) the opportunity for membership in a social group of fellows working on parallel projects. Baldwin was a strong proponent of research that documented the effects of everyday occupational forms on motor abilities. Much of my research today (e.g., Nelson et al., 1996) investigates principles identified in Baldwin's model of practice that was described more than 75 years ago.

Other Early Models of Practice

It is important to realize that those who helped found the profession espoused different approaches to the use of therapeutic occupation. Each model of practice had its own conceptualization of healthy and unhealthy occupation, and each had its guidelines for synthesizing occupational forms. For example, Tracy (1910) presented a model for bedside occupations for hospitalized patients. The focus was on preventing the negative psychosocial consequences of bedrest so that the patient could be a full partner in his or her medical treatment. Synthesized occupational forms varied depending on the age of the patient, the nature of the disability, and interest. It is interesting to note that all three of the authors cited so far included calisthenics as a potentially valuable type of therapeutic occupation.

A fourth example of an early model of practice in occupational therapy is Hall's work cure for persons with what was then called neurasthenia. In a letter from Hall (1917) to William Rush Dunton, Hall expressed expertise in only one area of what he called therapeutic occupations. Is this not an early expression of specialization by model of practice while remaining cognizant of one's integral link to other models through the organizing framework of therapeutic occupations? Another early letter, however, makes clear that proponents of different models did not always accept or appreciate each other's differences. In a letter to Dunton, Barton (1916), the first president of the National Society for the Promotion of Occupational Therapy and an opponent of Hall's model of practice, expressed the hope that Hall "not put cyanide in our tea" (p. 2) to avenge his exclusion from the deliberations of the charter officers of the society. This facetious remark reflects an ongoing struggle among adherents of different approaches to the use of therapeutic occupation.

The Psychodynamic Model of Practice

How flexible is the concept of therapeutic occupation? Let us consider the change that accompanied American psychology and psychiatry in the 1930s and 1940s when the Freudians advocated a new and controversial view of the person. At that time, Fidler (1948), who has become one of the most influential leaders in the history of the profession, proposed the adoption of a psychodynamic approach in occupational therapy. How do dynamic theorists view the person and occupation, and given this viewpoint, what kinds of occupational forms are synthesized for therapy? In this model of practice, the most important meanings and purposes underlying occupation are unconscious reflections of biological drives. These powerful libidinal and aggressive impulses are theorized to be the products of psychosexual development in early childhood. With maturation, the ego defends itself against anxiety via a variety of unconscious mechanisms, some of which are relatively adaptive and some maladaptive.

Given this view of the occupational structure of the person, the early stages of occupational therapy involved a close, nonthreatening match between carefully selected occupational forms and individual personality. For example, the patient who is unconsciously aggressive is provided with clay to pound or with wood to cut, and the person who is compulsively neat is provided with an occupational form such as weaving, which requires much repetition and involves little waste. Over time, the therapist gradually introduces occupational forms that facilitate relatively mature defense mechanisms.

Humanistic Models of Practice

An illustration of how the profession can accommodate new models of practice can be seen in Fidler's ongoing developments. We can compare and contrast the Fidler and Fidler (1978) article, "Doing and Becoming: Purposeful Action and Self-Actualization," with the Fidler (1948) psychodynamically inspired article we have just discussed. The title of Fidler and Fidler's article indicates the sweeping changes occurring in the 1970s in American psychology and psychiatry. Humanism and existentialism were discovered and adopted as philosophical positions. Instead of conceptualizing the person as conflict laden due to unconscious drives, as in Freudianism, the humanist views the person as a consciously choosing, self-determining being with created values and interests. The person is looked on optimistically in terms of his or her ability to change self or to adapt via occupational performance. Self-actualization is viewed as a person's highest achievement.

The ideas of humanism have strongly influenced many leaders within the profession, including Reilly (1962), Yerxa (1967), and Kielhofner (1995). Kielhofner's Model of Human Occupation conceptualizes the person's occupations in terms of personal causation, values, interests, internalized roles, and habit patterns in addition to many different skills. Recently influenced by dynamic systems theory, Kielhofner currently emphasizes the volitional processes of attending, experiencing, and choosing, as well as the processes underlying changes in roles and habits. The person is the creator of a life story, a narrative. Given this viewpoint of the person, Kielhofner's occupational forms emphasize naturalistic options and the opportunity for success. Naturalistic options in the occupational form make choices with high levels of symbolic meaning possible. Intrinsic purpose in occupation is most highly valued. The occupational therapist's verbal responsiveness is also a critical aspect of the occupational form because the client and therapist collaboratively synthesize occupational forms. This model of practice has an optimistic viewpoint of the person's ability to adapt and take control of his or her own life, regardless of residual impairments.

The Sensory Integrative Model of Practice

Humanism was not the only great idea influencing Western civilization in the 1960s and 1970s. Another set of ideas with a profound effect on the development of occupational therapy models of practice has come through the advent of neuroscience. Consider Ayres's (1972) sensory integrative model. As with all the other occupational therapy models of practice we have and will discuss, most of the foundational ideas for sensory integration were taken from sources outside occupational therapy. Ayres conceptualized the person in neurological terms. The first words of her classic book were: "Learning is a function of the brain; learning disorders are assumed to reflect some deviation in neural function" (p. 1). In Ayres's original work, the brain is conceptualized phylogenetically and hierarchically, with higher level cognitive centers in the cerebrum that depend on lower level centers, especially those governing somatosensory input, including vestibular, tactile, and proprioceptive sensation. Ayres hypothesized that many children with learning disorders do not integrate somatosensory input with visual and auditory processing. She also hypothesized that children have an inner drive for mastery in occupation.

Given this conceptualization of the developmental structure, Ayres (1972) created some of the most fascinating occupational forms in the history of our profession: rolling and tumbling forms such as scooter boards and carpeted barrels that support or envelop the child while eliciting somatosensory meanings and bolsters, nets, and swings that hang from the ceiling and provide vestibular input in the occupational context of a game. These occupational forms that elicit whole-body occupational performances are prerequisites to the highly structured occupational forms of education, which assume adequate visual and auditory comprehension necessary for advanced cognition. Like humanistic models of practice, this neurologically based model of practice is optimistic about the person's ability to adapt via occupational performance.

Allen's Model of Cognitive Disabilities

A very different model of practice is also rooted in a neuroscientific conceptualization of the person. In Allen's (1985) model of cognitive disabilities, certain neurological disorders are considered intractable. Although the person's interests and sensorimotor abilities are considered, the focus of this model is on cognitive levels, which are viewed hierarchically from an unresponsive coma state to an advanced level of deductive reasoning. Given that progress from one cognitive level to the next cannot occur through occupation (but might occur in some disorders through the physiological healing of the brain), the emphasis in this model of practice is on evaluation and compensation. What kinds of occupational forms are used? The Allen Cognitive Levels test uses selected crafts (e.g., various forms of leather lacing) to challenge cognition. Crafts are readily recognizable in our society yet are not threatening in the way that many tests are. The materials provide definite structure across space and time, and the craft product (an impact) is an objective indicator of the quality of occupational performance. Hence, the occupational therapist can monitor changes along the cognitive dimension tested as the brain heals. In addition, the occupational therapist can synthesize compensatory occupational forms designed to match the patient's cognitive level. For example, the person who learns only by trial and error will need supervision for safety's sake in everyday occupational forms.

Toglia's Multicontext Approach to Perceptual Cognitive Impairments

An emerging model of practice that posits the adaptational capacity of persons with neurological impairment has been put forward by Toglia (1991). Drawing on knowledge from modern neuropsychology, Toglia hypothesized that metacognition and cognitive processing strategies can be enhanced through a variety of naturalistic occupational forms—a multicontext approach that uses everyday situations as the crux of therapy. Everyday situations from the supermarket to the bus line provide similar cognitive challenges yet provide sufficient variations for generalized learning to occur. Consistent with occupational therapy history, Toglia suggested that the everyday world of our communities can be the occupational therapist's clinic. As we encounter our everyday occupational forms, so we become.

Motor Control and Motor Learning Models of Practice

One of the fascinating events of the past 10 years has been the change in focus within the motor control models of practice. One way of describing this revolution is that theorists and therapists are focusing more on occupational synthesis. In the past, the emphasis was on the patient's physiology and movements (e.g., muscle tone, symmetry, isolation of movement patterns). While remaining sophisticated about the patient's physiology, therapists today are also becoming more sophisticated about the other half of the therapeutic equation: the occupational forms that the patient needs in order to engage in active occupational performance. Symbolic of this revolution is Trombly's (1995 [see Chapter 11]) Eleanor Clarke Slagle Lecture in which she cited research, theory, and practical experience in favor of occupational forms that are meaningful and purposeful to the person. Whether guided by the neurodevelopmental model of practice (Levit, 1995) or

a contemporary approach drawing from dynamic systems theory (Mathiowetz & Haugen, 1995), therapists today are synthesizing naturalistic occupational forms of work, play, and self-care, with the active collaboration of the patient in the choice of those forms.

Selected Other Models of Practice

To suggest the tremendous range of potential applications of our core concept of therapeutic occupation, I will briefly mention a few of the many other occupational therapy models of practice. Occupational models of practice are being refined for persons with Alzheimer's disease and their caregivers (American Occupational Therapy Association [AOTA], 1994), and some models are being developed for the handwriting problems of schoolchildren (Amundson, 1992). Als's conceptualization of the premature infant is compatible with an occupational therapy model of practice geared toward both the emerging occupations of the infant and the occupations of parents (Vergara, 1993). A fourth area in which the special skills of occupational therapists are needed is hospice care (Pizzi, 1993), where meaningful and purposeful occupation is a reflection of the value placed on human life. Although these are but a few samples of the many areas in which therapeutic occupation is contributing to quality of life, my experience tells me that creative occupational therapy practitioners will continue to develop new models of practice that meet the real needs of real persons for therapeutic occupations—therapy by doing.

Beyond Direct Service Models

A commitment to the use of occupation as the method of occupational therapy does not commit us to direct service models as opposed to educational models or consultative models. The occupational therapist can play an essential and cost-effective role in the collaborative synthesis of occupational forms, even though the therapist will not be physically present when the person engages in the occupational form. Because the therapist has expertise in occupational forms—their physical and sociocultural complexity—he or she can advise the daughter of a woman with Alzheimer's disease about least restrictive environments (AOTA, 1994), a teacher or nurse about proper positioning (Dunn & Campbell, 1991), or the foreman of a workstation with a high rate of carpal tunnel syndrome about repetitive trauma disorders (AOTA, 1992). Such advice is a collaborative occupational synthesis. For the same reason, a truly occupational model of practice is used when the therapist advises patients with diseases of the hand about occupations in the home, at work, and at play (Kasch, 1990).

Occupational Therapy Models of Practice in the Future

What future roles will the occupational therapist play in the health care system? Readers 100 years from now will no doubt be aware of occupational therapy practice that we cannot dream of today. And I am sure that there will be an occupational therapy reader 100 years from today because of the fundamental power of occupation and its adaptability to new circumstances.

Independent Living Movement

One current trend that may well grow in the future is the independent living movement in which persons with disabilities see themselves as consumers of health care services. As consumers, they make decisions about their lives and rehabilitation with professional help but without the authoritarianism that sometimes accompanies the medical model. This approach is in tune with the principles of occupational therapy (AOTA, 1993; Yerxa, 1994). The problem is not to be thought of as lying in the consumers (their developmental structures), but in the everyday occupational forms they encounter, such as barriers to restaurants, workstations, and fields of play. Given this philosophy, the occupational therapist emphasizes collaborative occupational synthesis and compensatory strategies from ramps to robots and from social acceptance to political power. The consumer who takes control of his or her life within an insensitive society could not do better than to have an occupational therapist as an advocate.

Technology

The independent living movement dovetails nicely with another identifiable trend for the future: new technologies that promote successful and personally satisfying occupation. As Mann and Lane (1991) pointed out, the occupational therapist "can—and should—be the professional who takes responsibility for assembling the appropriate assistive technology team" (p. 26). The occupational therapist has the knowledge and experience to take a leadership role in working with the consumer in making the best possible match between the multiple factors in technologically oriented occupational forms and the multiple capacities of the consumer's developmental structure. We need to think of assistive devices as parts of the occupational forms

that have meaning and purpose to the person, not as mechanical extensions of a mechanical person.

Wellness Models of Practice

Another trend is the move toward an increased emphasis on wellness, health promotion, and disease prevention. With the brave new world of capitation, managed care, primary care, efficacy, and efficiency, the health care system may at last get serious about wellness. Wellness pays. Nothing could be more positive for the profession of occupational therapy. Theorists within the profession have been preparing us for the advent of a health care system that emphasizes health as opposed to illness (Johnson, 1986; Rosenfeld, 1993). Occupational therapists working with persons who already have disabilities have long emphasized the importance of healthy occupational profiles and disease prevention to their patients, even though those efforts have not always been reimbursable. The wellness models of practice are in place and only await general funding.

Models for Public Health

Another role for the future of occupational therapy is in the solution of some of our society's chronic social and public health problems, such as drugs, violence, unprepared motherhood, unemployment, and homelessness. A problem of special interest for me is the development of an occupational therapy model of practice for the prevention of childhood obesity. Obesity has devastating lifelong consequences, with sensorimotor, cognitive, and psychosocial impairments and impoverished occupational patterns. A comprehensive model of therapeutic occupation needs to be tested for this major problem of public health. Occupational therapy leaders, such as Baum (1991), have found ways to fund occupational models of practice, even in a pessimistic sociopolitical environment where social programs are mistrusted. I call this America's 1990s regression to the social Darwinism of the 1890s. But sooner or later, the profession of Eleanor Clarke Slagle will provide occupational models of practice for homeless people with schizophrenia and occupational models of practice for persons in so-called nursing homes. (Let us call them homes for therapeutic occupation!) The mark of a great civilization is not its store of consumer goods but the meaningfulness and purposefulness of the everyday occupations of all its citizens.

Hospital-Based Models

I believe that occupational therapy will continue to play an essential role in the acute care hospital and in other medically related facilities from the rehabilitation hospital, to subacute sites, to extended care facilities, to the facilities of the future. It is true that hospitals are downsizing, and patients are being discharged more and more quickly. It is also true that the ideal health care system of the future will promote wellness as its highest goal. Nevertheless, people will continue to become ill; they will continue to go to the hospital, however downsized, for acute care. Many of these people will continue to need an occupational approach at one or more stages of their illness and recovery (Torrance, 1993). With increasing technology and quicker discharge, the need for therapeutic occupation increases, not decreases. Occupational therapists will be needed to work with patients in problem solving self-care occupations amidst the constraints of the tubes, monitors, and fixators; to activate patients at risk because of the deleterious effects of bedrest; to help patients and caregivers plan realistically for what the patients will do and for how the patients will live and care for themselves after discharge but before healing; and to assess patients' quality of life before and after hospitalization.

For an example of the importance of therapeutic occupation in an acute care setting, consider a 5-month-old girl born with a neuromuscular disease of unknown etiology. The disease is characterized by the total absence of many of the proximal muscles, including those responsible for respiration. Picture her with multiple intubations for respiration and nutrition and with life-support monitors. The occupational therapist carefully removes her from the crib and bounces her gently while talking to her in high-pitched, rhythmical tones. In response to this occupational form, the infant's adaptations are to learn to use the muscles controlling her vocal cords as she imitates the therapist; to learn to use the remaining muscles in her left arm as she grabs the therapist's keys; and most of all, to begin to learn that she too has a legitimate place in the human family. The therapist next places a piece of cloth playfully over the child's face, as in our prior example of the importance of peek-a-boo in healthy development. Like the healthy infant, this baby also removes the cloth and laughs. Despite the high technology setting, this baby also needs to encounter the occupational form of peek-a-boo in order to develop a sense of self and a sense of other. I believe that occupational models of practice will be needed for the acute care hospital for patients at all points on the life span as much as they are needed for community-based care.

Models of Practice and the Great Ideas of the 20th Century

Therapeutic occupation is a remarkably powerful yet flexible idea. Consider all the different philosophies and branches of science that have washed across the 20th century and that have become the theoretical bases of occupational therapy models of practice: the moral treatment initiated by members of the Society of Friends; the arts-and-crafts movement initiated by the British socialist Ruskin as an antidote to the negative effects of industrialism; the philosophy of pragmatism; the holistic medicine of Meyer; James's psychology of attention; principles of kinesiology and biomechanics; the dynamic theories of the Freudians, neo-Freudians, and ego psychologists; behaviorism and learning theory; developmental theory; humanism and existentialism; neuroscience and neuropsychology and their many schools; efficacy and competency theory; systems theory and dynamic systems theory; the social psychology of groups; ecological psychology; motor learning and motor control theories; cultural anthropology and ethnography; and narrative analysis. (For discussions of these topics and their influences on occupational therapy models of practice, see Breines, 1995; Christiansen & Baum, 1991; Kielhofner, 1992.) These schools of thought reflect many of the majestic ideas in the intellectual history of the 20th century. Even though every one of them originated from outside the occupational therapy profession, each has contributed essential theory to our models of practice. Across every model of practice, the core of therapeutic occupational synthesis can be identified: form, meaning, purpose, performance, evaluation, adaptation, and compensation. This robust flexibility at the core of our profession is the basis for my saying that therapeutic occupation will flourish in the 21st century.

Two Recommendations

Research

My first recommendation is research—research for occupational therapists conducted by occupational therapists and those who understand occupation as therapy. Our primary focus should be to examine the power of occupation as therapy. My vision for the 21st century is that occupational therapy will take its rightful place among the major professions in our society. The powers and complexities of occupation justify the sanctioning of a major profession. This will be especially true if the society of our descendants devotes increased attention to the actual occupations of daily life, to the meanings of life, and to the qualities of existence. Should there not be a Nobel prize for occupational therapy?

But to be a major force in research, we must examine our basic principles in highly systematic ways—ways that are accepted by the larger research community. If we do not examine the great ideas of occupational therapy, some other group will. For decades, occupational therapists have used common, everyday occupational forms and hands-on doing to enhance what Dunton (1945) called the "mental processes of reasoning or judgment or remembering" (p. 11). Recently, cognitive researchers, mainly psychologists, have developed a body of knowledge about the effects of subject-performed tasks (SPTs) on human cognition (e.g., Backman, 1985). The basic idea of SPTs is that handson doing, with its added sensory input and opportunity for feedback, is a greater cognitive stimulant than demonstration or other teaching techniques that do not involve hands-on experience. The problem is that the cognitive psychologists pursuing this line of research have not cited occupational therapy authors, who have advocated this principle since the beginning of the profession. Our problem here is that we have not done the research necessary to establish our special expertise in the area of hands-on doing, or occupation.

In like manner, we are only beginning to do the research that establishes our expertise in the area of occupationally embedded movement. Carr and Shepherd (1987) have written eloquently and at length about how everyday situations, such as a glass of water, can elicit therapeutic patterns of movement, such as a good hand path, in patients with neuromuscular disorders. However, these authors, neither of whom are occupational therapists, do not once cite occupational therapy or its history of using everyday occupational forms to promote therapeutic patterns of movement.

My point is that persons from other professions are coming late to the table and claiming credit for some of the great ideas of occupational therapy. These ideas deserve the most careful philosophical and scientific scrutiny. As occupational therapists, we need to own these ideas while enlightening other disciplines as to their usefulness.

Equally needed are basic research examining the nature of occupation and applied research examining models of practice. Academically respected quantitative and qualitative research methodologies should be used. One approach to research in occupational ther-

apy is what I have called the experimental analysis of therapeutic occupation (Nelson, 1993). Here, occupational forms are contrasted to each other in terms of participants' occupational performances, impacts, adaptations, or reported meanings and purposes. A different approach, termed *occupational science,* has been proposed by Clark et al. (1991). These authors have recommended qualitative methods for studying the multiple dimensions of naturally occurring occupations. It is critical that the profession encourage different types of inquiry, at least until there is a broad consensus that a single type of inquiry satisfactorily deals with all the research problems of the profession. I predict that no such consensus will ever develop.

To support the research enterprise, funding will be essential. A specific goal of the AOTA should be the establishment of study sections specifically devoted to occupational therapy research in federal grants management agencies, as is the case with nursing. Only those with considerable knowledge of the profession of occupational therapy can appreciate and nurture the full potential of occupational therapy knowledge. In the interim, the AOTA and the American Occupational Therapy Foundation, which is to say all of us, should make special efforts to support research that is specifically occupational. A priority is the further development of doctoral programs devoted to the development of occupational therapy knowledge. More than anything else, a sound doctoral program is a socialization experience toward a new identity as a scholar in a particular field. Although scholars of diverse backgrounds have made great contributions to knowledge in occupational therapy, a true profession requires the intense engagement at its core, which is expected in doctoral programs devoted to the development of occupational therapy knowledge.

Occupation, Not the *A* Word

My second recommendation is for all of us to embrace and own the idea of occupation as therapy. Wilma West (1984) not only urged us to use the term *occupation* with pride, but also wrote that the term *occupation* "is infinitely more expressive and encompassing than 'purposeful activity' " (p. 22). Nothing is more important to this profession. We are called *occupational* therapists, and the essence of our profession is the use of occupation as a therapeutic method. In contrast, the term *activity* lacks the connotation of intentionality. The term *activity* denotes motion, for example, *volcanic activity, molecular activity,* and *gastric activity,* not occupation that is replete with meaning and purpose.

Another major problem with the use of the word *activity* is that we confuse the public. Slagle (1922) wrote about her "system of occupational analysis" (p. 16). Neither she nor we need to say activity analysis. If the essence of our profession is activity, then why are we not called activity therapists (Darnell & Heater, 1994)? We need to be able to explain occupation and things occupational to many different audiences from fellow professionals to payers, from persons with immaturities to persons with various disabilities, from journalists to the arts media, and from our students to ourselves. If we explain clearly that occupational therapy involves the active doing of things (occupations) for the sake of enhanced health, our public relations problem and our socalled identity problem will disappear immediately. We have the power to influence standard usage. There are more than 50,000 of us in this country and tens of thousands more in other English-speaking countries. If we are clear and forthright about the essential nature of our service—the use of occupation as method—then society will accommodate us. New words and new professions come into the language system all the time. This problem is entirely within our control.

Over time—keep in mind that we are talking about the next century—society and fellow health care professionals will adopt new terms that are related to what we call occupation. For example, since the founding of occupational therapy the terms *rehabilitation, allied health, deinstitutionalization, function, functional outcomes,* and *inclusion* have come into favor for very good reasons. As occupational therapists, we need to promote the good that is represented in these terms. Yet, we need to resist the temptation to redefine ourselves with every new trend in health care. We are not rehabilitation professionals—we are occupational therapists whose mission is much more basic and enduring than even the rehabilitation movement. Nor are we functional therapists or functional outcomes therapists. The term *function* is reflective of the mechanistic, business-oriented climate of these times. Automobiles function, toasters function, and livers function. Human occupation is far richer than the term *function* can possibly connote. In our era, every health professional from the surgeon to the dietitian must document so-called functional outcomes if they are going to be paid. What makes us unique is not that we document functional outcomes but that we use occupation as the method to achieve positive outcomes.

We are *occupational* therapists, and we are aptly named. Indeed we are named more aptly than many of the professions with which we work. We need to explain this

clearly and assertively to the world, but a good starting point will be to explain this clearly and assertively to each other. Occupation as therapy is inclusive enough for all the occupational therapy models of practice. There is no reason to be afraid of cyanide in the tea.

Conclusion

To summarize, occupation is a powerful force in the development of the human being. The essence of our profession is the use of occupation as therapy whose core flexibly accommodates various past, present, and future models of practice drawn from historically important theories that originated outside the profession. I proposed a CFTO, including definitions of occupational form, occupational performance, developmental structure, meaning, purpose, impact, adaptation, compensation, and occupational synthesis. The CFTO highlights the core of therapeutic occupation across diverse models of practice and provides an analytical method for comparing and contrasting different models of practice.

Basic and applied research that investigate principles of occupation are necessary not only for the standing of the profession among other disciplines, but also for the sake of our own integrity. The ultimate statement of pride and confidence in the profession will be the full adoption of the term *occupation* in the language of the profession, with each occupational therapist taking personal responsibility for explaining to the world why we are called occupational therapists.

Acknowledgments

I thank all the colleagues, students, and loved ones who have contributed so much to the content and spirit of this lecture. My children, my sisters, and my mother say that they enjoyed being with us at the lecture.

This lecture included audiovisual themes that cannot be reproduced in article format; therefore, this article makes use of examples and explanations suited for the printed page as opposed to the lecture stage.

References

Allen, C. K. (1985). *Occupational therapy for psychiatric diseases: Measurement and management of cognitive disabilities.* Boston: Little, Brown.

American Occupational Therapy Association. (1992). Statement: Occupational therapy services in work practice. *American Journal of Occupational Therapy, 46,* 1086–1088.

American Occupational Therapy Association. (1993). Statement: The role of occupational therapy in the independent living movement. *American Journal of Occupational Therapy, 47,* 1079–1080. http://dx.doi.org/10.5014/ajot.47.12.1079

American Occupational Therapy Association. (1994). Statement: Occupational therapy services for persons with Alzheimer's disease and other dementias. *American Journal of Occupational Therapy, 48,* 1029–1031. http://dx.doi.org/10.5014/ajot.48.11.1029

Amundson, S. J. C. (1992). Handwriting: Evaluation and intervention in school settings. In J. Case-Smith & C. Pehoski (Eds.), *Development of hand skills in the child* (pp. 63–78). Rockville, MD: American Occupational Therapy Association.

Ayres, A. J. (1972). *Sensory integration and learning disorders.* Los Angeles: Western Psychological Services.

Backman, L. (1985). Further evidence for the lack of adult age differences on free recall of subject-performed tasks: The importance of motor action. *Human Learning, 3*(1), 53–69.

Baldwin, B. T. (1919). *Occupational therapy applied to restoration of movement.* Washington, DC: Commanding Officer and Surgeon General of the Army, Walter Reed General Hospital.

Barton, G. E. (1916, December 20). *Letter to W. R. Dunton, Jr.* (Available from the American Occupational Therapy Archives, Box 1, File 12, Wilma L. West Library, 4720 Montgomery Lane, Bethesda, MD 20814)

Baum, C. (1991). Professional issues in a changing environment. In C. Christiansen & C. Baum (Eds.), *Occupational therapy: Overcoming human performance deficits* (pp. 804–817). Thorofare, NJ: Slack.

Breines, E. B. (1995). Understanding 'occupation' as the founders did. *British Journal of Occupational Therapy, 58,* 458–460.

Carr, J. H., & Shepherd, R. B. (1987). A motor learning model for rehabilitation. In J. H. Carr & R. B. Shepherd (Eds.), *Movement science: Foundations for physical therapy in rehabilitation.* Rockville, MD: Aspen.

Christiansen, C. (1990). The perils of plurality. *Occupational Therapy Journal of Research, 10,* 259–265.

Christiansen, C., & Baum, C. (Eds.). (1991). *Occupational therapy: Overcoming human performance deficits.* Thorofare, NJ: Slack.

Clark, F. A., Parham, D., Carlson, M. E., Frank, G., Jackson, J., Pierce, D., Wolfe, R. J., & Zemke, R. (1991). Occupational science: Academic innovation in the service of occupational therapy's future. *American Journal of Occupational Therapy, 45,* 300–310.

Darnell, J. L., & Heater, S. L. (1994). The Issue Is—Occupational therapist or activity therapist—Which do you choose to be? *American Journal of Occupational Therapy, 48,* 467–468.

Dunn, W., & Campbell, P. H. (1991). Designing pediatric service provision. In W. Dunn (Ed.), *Pediatric occupational therapy* (pp. 139–159). Thorofare, NJ: Slack.

Dunton, W. R., Jr. (1945). *Prescribing occupational therapy* (2nd ed.). Springfield, IL: Charles C Thomas.

Fidler, G. S. (1948). Psychological evaluation of occupational therapy activities. *American Journal of Occupational Therapy, 2,* 284–287.

Fidler, G. S., & Fidler, J. W. (1978). Doing and becoming: Purposeful action and self-actualization. *American Journal of Occupational Therapy, 32,* 305–310.

Gilfoyle, E. M. (1984). Eleanor Clarke Slagle Lectureship, 1984: Transformation of a profession. *American Journal of Occupational Therapy, 38,* 575–584.

Hall, H. J. (1917, February 23). *Letter to W. R. Dunton, Jr.* (Available from the American Occupational Therapy Archives, Box 2, File 15, Wilma L. West Library, 4720 Montgomery Lane, Bethesda, MD 20814)

Howe, M. C., & Schwartzberg, S. L. (1986). *A functional approach to group work in occupational therapy.* Philadelphia: Lippincott.

Johnson, J. A. (1986). *Wellness: A context for living.* Thorofare, NJ: Slack.

Kasch, M. (1990). Acute hand injuries. In L. W. Pedretti & B. Zoltan (Eds.), *Occupational therapy practice skills for physical dysfunction* (pp. 477–506). St. Louis, MO: Mosby.

Kidner, T. B. (1930). *Occupational therapy: The science of prescribed work for invalids.* Stuttgart, Germany: Kohlhammer.

Kielhofner, G. (1992). *Conceptual foundations of occupational therapy.* Philadelphia: F. A. Davis.

Kielhofner, G. (1995). *A model of human occupation: Theory and application* (2nd ed.). Baltimore: Williams & Wilkins.

Levit, K. (1995). Neurodevelopmental (Bobath) treatment. In C. A. Trombly (Ed.), *Occupational therapy for physical dysfunction* (4th ed., pp. 446–462). Baltimore: Williams & Wilkins.

Mann, W. C., & Lane, J. P. (1991). *Assistive technology for persons with disabilities: The role of occupational therapy.* Rockville, MD: American Occupational Therapy Association.

Mathiowetz, V., & Haugen, J. B. (1995). Evaluation of motor behavior: Traditional and contemporary views. In C. A. Trombly (Ed.), *Occupational therapy for physical dysfunction* (4th ed., pp. 157–185). Baltimore: Williams & Wilkins.

Mosey, A. C. (1970). *Three frames of reference for mental health*. Thorofare, NJ: Slack.

National Society for the Promotion of Occupational Therapy. (1917, March 15). *Certificate of Incorporation of the National Society for the Promotion of Occupational Therapy.* (Incorporated in the District of Columbia and notarized by James A. Rolfe in Clifton Springs, New York)

Nelson, D. L. (1988). Occupation: Form and performance. *American Journal of Occupational Therapy, 42*, 633–641.

Nelson, D. L. (1993, June). The experimental analysis of therapeutic occupation. *Developmental Disabilities Special Interest Section Newsletter, 16*(2), 7–8.

Nelson, D. L. (1994). Occupational form, occupational performance, and therapeutic occupation. In C. B. Royeen (Ed.), *AOTA self-study series: The practice of the future: Putting occupation back into therapy, lesson 2* (pp. 9–48). Rockville, MD: American Occupational Therapy Association.

Nelson, D. L. (1996). Therapeutic occupation: A definition. *American Journal of Occupational Therapy, 50*, 775–782. http://dx.doi.org/10.5014/ajot.50.10.775

Nelson, D. L., Konosky, K., Fleharty, K., Webb, R., Newer, K., Hazboun, V. P., Fontane, C., & Licht, B. (1996). The effects of an occupationally embedded exercise on bilaterally assisted supination in persons with hemiplegia. *American Journal of Occupational Therapy, 50*, 639–646. http://dx.doi.org/10.5014/ajot.50.8.639

Pizzi, M. (1993). Environments of care: Hospice. In H. L. Hopkins & H. D. Smith (Eds.), *Willard and Spackman's occupational therapy* (8th ed., pp. 853–864). Philadelphia: Lippincott.

Quiroga, V. A. M. (1995). *Occupational therapy: The first 30 years, 1900–1930*. Bethesda, MD: American Occupational Therapy Association.

Reilly, M. (1962). Occupational therapy can be one of the great ideas of 20th century medicine. Eleanor Clarke Slagle Lecture. *American Journal of Occupational Therapy, 16*, 1–9. Reprinted as Chapter 7.

Rosenfeld, M. S. (1993). *Wellness and lifestyle renewal*. Rockville, MD: American Occupational Therapy Association.

Slagle, E. C. (1922). Training aides for mental patients. *Archives of Occupational Therapy, 1*, 11–17.

Toglia, J. P. (1991). Generalization of treatment: A multicontext approach to cognitive perceptual impairment in adults with brain injury. *American Journal of Occupational Therapy, 45*, 505–516. http://dx.doi.org/10.5014/ajot.45.6.505

Torrance, M. (1993). Acute care occupational therapy. In H. L. Hopkins & H. D. Smith (Eds.), *Willard and Spackman's occupational therapy* (8th ed., pp. 771–783). Philadelphia: Lippincott.

Tracy, S. E. (1910). *Studies in invalid occupation: A manual for nurses and attendants*. Boston: Whitcomb & Barrows.

Trombly, C. A. (1995). Occupation: Purposefulness and meaningfulness as therapeutic mechanisms. 1995 Eleanor Clarke Slagle Lecture. *American Journal of Occupational Therapy, 49*, 960–972. Reprinted as Chapter 11.

Vergara, E. (1993). *Foundations for practice in the neonatal intensive care unit and early intervention: A self-guided practice manual*. Rockville, MD: American Occupational Therapy Association.

West, W. L. (1984). A reaffirmed philosophy and practice of occupational therapy for the 1980s. *American Journal of Occupational Therapy, 38*, 15–23.

Yerxa, E. J. (1967). Authentic occupational therapy. 1966 Eleanor Clark Slagle Lecture. *American Journal of Occupational Therapy, 21*, 1–9.

Yerxa, E. J. (1994). Dreams, dilemmas, and decisions for occupational therapy practice in a new millennium: An American perspective. *American Journal of Occupational Therapy, 48*, 586–589. Reprinted as Chapter 56.

CHAPTER 9

Uniting Practice and Theory in an Occupational Framework
1998 ELEANOR CLARKE SLAGLE LECTURE

ANNE G. FISHER

The roots of this lecture began years ago in the late 1960s, when I was an occupational therapy student. Occupational therapy was in the midst of what Kielhofner (1997) has termed the *mechanistic paradigm*. My physical dysfunction theory courses had a heavy focus on exercise and the neurophysiologic approaches of the Bobaths (Semans, 1967), Brunnstrom (1970), and especially Margaret Rood (as interpreted by Stockmeyer, 1967). While on my affiliations, I was guided by some of my supervisors to use weight lifting to strengthen the wrist extensors of clients with spinal cord injury. During my psychiatric affiliation, I was encouraged to give clients with unconscious hostility opportunities to act out their emotions through metal hammering. All of these clients did these activities whether they wanted to or not.

But there was another side to my early experiences. I remember vividly working with a young man who had quadriplegia as a result of a spinal cord injury. He was fascinated with electronics, and he wanted to explore the possibilities of being able to build electronic devices. I went to the local electronics store and bought a do-it-yourself radio kit filled with resistors, capacitors, circuit boards, and tiny nuts and bolts. I also bought solder and a soldering iron. Together, we worked on developing strategies he could use to manage the tools and materials. He had no active movement in his fingers, but because he wore wrist-driven flexor hinge splints, he was able to hold on to many of the objects. When he had difficulty, we worked together to create alternative strategies.

He built the radio, not I. And in the end, he had a radio he could listen to; he had the satisfaction that comes from accomplishment; and he had learned that he could develop for himself compensatory strategies

when confronted with challenging circumstances. But that is not all he gained. As an indirect consequence of his participation in meaningful and purposeful activity, the muscles in his upper limbs became stronger, and his fine motor coordination improved. Although I regret that I do not remember this young man's name, I am grateful that he was included among the clients I worked with who have taught me the value of occupation as a therapeutic agent.

A few years later, I began working on a project with Lyla Spelbring. I remember Spelbring telling me about her philosophy of when occupational therapy practitioners should be involved with clients during the continuum of care that begins in the acute-care phase and extends through discharge and into the community. Spelbring proposed that occupational therapy practitioners have an initial role in the early part of the acute-care phase, addressing issues of self-care and the provision of assistive devices. Then, she said, we should let physical therapy take over to develop the clients' physical capacity. Only when the clients are strong enough to engage in occupation should we re-enter and work with them during the latter part of their rehabilitation stays and as they transition back into the community.

Spelbring seemed to be saying that, throughout our involvement, our focus should be on enhancing occupational performance and not the remediation of underlying impairments. Her ideas felt radical, and with my own interest in neurophysiological techniques designed to remediate neuromotor impairments, I was not at all ready to hear the intent of her message. But still, I remember it, and now I realize she may have been right.

Soon thereafter, I went to graduate school. My master's thesis had to do with the effects of the inverted head position on alpha and gamma motor neuron activity in the upper extremity. Obviously, the mechanistic paradigm remained alive and well.

This chapter was previously published in the *American Journal of Occupational Therapy, 52,* 509–521. Copyright © 1998, American Occupational Therapy Association. Reprinted with permission. http://dx.doi.org/10.5014/ajot.52.7.509

Catherine Trombly was my major advisor. Under her mentorship, I learned about, and came to value, the need for research that supports (and fails to support) the theories and intervention methods we use in occupational therapy. I also observed in her someone who has always valued the use of purposeful activity as a therapeutic mechanism.

Still later, after completing my doctorate, I began teaching with Gary Kielhofner. We worked together on a number of projects. With some resistance, I learned about, and ultimately became immersed in, the Model of Human Occupation. At the time, I was editing a textbook on sensory integration (Fisher, Murray, & Bundy, 1991). Kielhofner drew a figure of how he visualized the interrelationship between sensory integration and the Model of Human Occupation (see Figure 9.1). The figure was like an hourglass constructed of two overlapping triangles. The top triangle was inverted to show that the Model of Human Occupation stressed occupation and barely acknowledged the role of the brain in occupational behavior (Kielhofner, 1985). The lower triangle was upright to show that sensory integration theory stressed brain functioning, with minimal discussion of the occupational nature of humans (Ayres, 1972). About this figure, Kielhofner said that if we can bridge the gap and fill in the void so as to construct a rectangle, we will have a richer view of occupational therapy.

I believed strongly in the value of occupation as a therapeutic agent. I had not forgotten the man with the spinal cord injury who wanted to build a radio. And I had not forgotten Spelbring's view that we should return physical restoration to the physical therapists. No doubt, she would also have us return remediation of psychiatric impairments to the psychiatrists, the psychologists, and the social workers. Trombly helped me to recognize the importance of implementing research to validate occupational therapy theory and practice. But, even with all that, I still lacked a vocabulary to explain to others what I did, how what I did was unique, and how my role could be clearly differentiated from that of the physical therapist, the nurse, the social worker, and so on. My work with Kielhofner on the Model of Human Occupation paved the way for me to finally conceptualize the unique contribution of occupational therapy within the health-care arena and to articulate the important role of occupation as a therapeutic agent (Fisher, 1994, 1995, 1997d).

Occupation: A Noun of Action

I came to realize the incredible power of the term *occupation*. The term occupation is a noun of action. Occupation is defined as *the* action of seizing, taking possession of, or occupying space or time. It is also defined as *the* holding of an office or position, such as one's role. Finally, in the sense of action, occupation refers to *the* being engaged in something *(The Oxford English Dictionary,* 1989).

As I have argued elsewhere, occupational therapy practitioners enable their clients to seize, take possession of, or occupy the spaces, time, and roles of their lives (Fisher, 1994). When we speak of the action of seizing, taking possession of, or occupying space, we can think of the actions our clients must perform to occupy their homes, their schools, their workplaces, and the places where they engage in recreation or leisure. Similarly, when we speak of the action of seizing, taking possession of, or occupying time—and being engaged in something—we can think that as our clients engage in task performances, they engage in a course of action that unfolds over time. We can also think about our client's need to occupy time, not just in the sense of "being busy" but also in a sense that

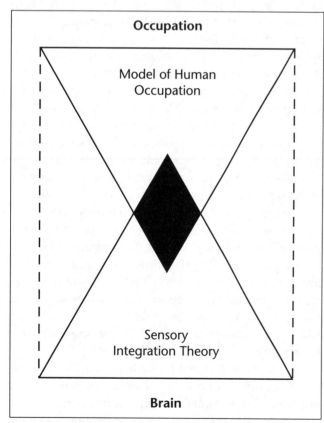

Figure 9.1. Schematic relationship between the Model of Human Occupation and sensory integration theory.

connotes the action of doing a mental, physical, or social task that is meaningful to the person. Lastly, when we speak of the action of seizing, taking possession of, or occupying roles, we can think about the performances our clients must enact in order to assume their life roles.

Occupation is a wonderful word. Think of it—a noun of action—it is about "doing!" It conveys the powerful essence of our profession—enabling people to perform the actions they need and want to perform so that they can engage in and "do" the familiar, ordinary, goal-directed activities of every day in a manner that brings meaning and personal satisfaction (American Occupational Therapy Association [AOTA], 1993, 1995; Clark et al., 1991; Evans, 1987; Kielhofner, 1997; Rudman, Cook, & Polatajko, 1997).

Occupation: Purposeful and Meaningful Activity

I believe that we must view occupation as not just any activity, not even just any purposeful activity but as activity that is both meaningful and purposeful to the person engaged in it. As I use the term here, *meaning* pertains to the personal significance of the activity to the client (see Figure 9.2). Meaningfulness is important as it provides a source of motivation for performance (Trombly, 1995a [see Chapter 11]). As I use the term *purpose,* it pertains to the client's personal aim, reason for doing, or intended goal. Purposefulness is important as it helps organize the client's performance (Trombly, 1995a).

I believe that purpose can be derived from the meaning one makes of a situation (Nelson, 1988), but I also believe that meaning can be derived from one's purpose for engaging in the activity (Fisher, 1994). Mean-

ing and purpose, when considered in relation to occupation, are inextricably interrelated.

Consider the following example. Ken is a minister. Each Sunday, he puts on slacks and dress shoes instead of his usual jeans and tennis shoes. Over that he dons his vestments and a cross. He does this for "appearance"—to be socially appropriate and to wear the "correct" attire. But he also wears them to make a statement about who he is and what he believes. For Ken, they are tied to tradition, and they are symbolic of his Christian faith. Ken's purpose and Ken's meanings are virtually inseparable.

But why does Ken wear the particular cross he does? Ken wears the cross he does because of the symbolism embedded within its design. The design is that of a desert rose. Imagine a rose blooming in the desert—a rose growing out of nothing. For Ken, this is a symbol of the Resurrection—in the darkest part of our lives we can bloom; we can heal and grow. This is a belief tied to his Christian faith, but the significance of Ken's wearing of this cross is also very personal.

Ken was very ill. He had to give up his position as senior pastor and discontinue all physical activity. He went on disability. He had excruciating pain and was heavily medicated. He says, "I was like a zombie." He could not talk, and he could only eat through a straw. He became even more ill and had to be hospitalized. There was concern that Ken might not live. But then he was given a new medication. He went into remission. With guidance from others, he developed strategies to deal with his residual disability. Six months ago, Ken resumed his ministry. Last week he went skiing. He has plans to begin rollerblading once again this spring.

Ken wears the cross he does as a symbol of his own life transition:

> I went from being a responsible professional, working 70 hours a week, to basically nothing. I went from 7 days a week being busy to having no purpose or meaning in life. I went from that to getting it all back.

The point is: Purposefulness is important, but it is not enough. Occupation is both purposeful and meaningful. If we can identify activities that have potential to be meaningful to the person, we can use them to increase motivation and a sense of purpose. In this process, we cannot confuse our purposes or meanings with those of our clients.

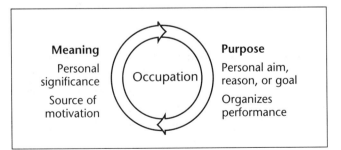

Figure 9.2. Interrelationship between meaning and purpose when applied to occupation.

Note. Copyright © 1998 by Anne G. Fisher. Reprinted with permission.

Defining Occupation Within a Practice Context

As I have traveled internationally, I have continued to be confronted with an apparent paradox—occupational therapy practitioners who know, implicitly, that they possess unique and important expertise but who have difficulty, just as I have had, articulating their uniqueness. Moreover, they often use evaluation and intervention methods that are so similar to those of their colleagues in physical therapy, neuropsychology, social work, and nursing that any distinctions between occupational therapy and these professions become blurred and even abolished.

Since the beginning of our profession, occupation has been viewed as both a means and an end (Clark, 1917; Dunton, 1928; Gritzer & Arluke, 1985; "Occupational Therapy in the General Hospital," 1917; Quiroga, 1995; Upham, 1917). Our uniqueness has been in the use of occupation as a curative or restorative force as well as in the view that enhanced occupational performance is the desired goal of therapy. These beliefs continue to be reflected in current official statements from within our profession. According to the AOTA (1997), occupational therapy practitioners use purposeful and meaningful activities in two ways: to restore underlying capacities and to develop meaningful occupations.

As I have talked with occupational therapy practitioners both here in North America and abroad, I have found that we indeed share an understanding of occupation, but that understanding often seems to be detached from what I observe in their daily practice. Our unique focus on occupation is not always obvious in practice.

Common Intervention Methods

To clarify what I mean, I will describe the intervention methods occupational therapy practitioners currently use in their everyday practice. The focal point here will be the characteristics of the activities in which clients are engaged. As I introduce the general activity types, the astute reader will no doubt think of activities that do not fall neatly within one of these groups. It may help, therefore, to begin by thinking of four continua (see Figure 9.3).

The first continuum indicates that an activity may be more contrived or offered as exercise, or the activity may be more naturalistic and offered as occupation. The second and third continua indicate that the purpose and the meaning of the activity, respectively, may be

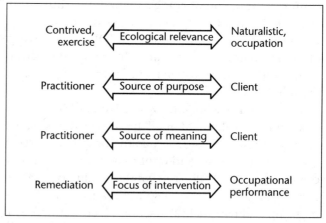

Figure 9.3. Four continua that can be used to evaluate the characteristics of any activity used as occupational therapy intervention.

Note. Copyright © 1998 by Anne G. Fisher. Reprinted with permission.

generated more by the practitioner or generated more from within the client. Finally, the focus of the intervention may be more on remediation of impairments or more on enhanced occupational performance. These four continua can be used to evaluate the characteristics of any activity we might use as intervention. As I proceed to describe each of the major activity groups, certain key characteristics of the activities will move from left to right along one or more of the continua.

The first group of activities I have termed *exercise*. The most salient feature of this type of activity is that the client is engaged in rote exercise or practice. The activity may have a purpose or goal, but more often than not, the purpose originated with the practitioner and not the client. In all probability, therefore, the exercise has little or no meaning to the client. Finally, the focus of the exercise is on the remediation of impairments. Examples of exercise include having the client draw a series of straight vertical lines on lined paper to develop eye-hand coordination, stretch Thera-Band®[1] or lift weights to develop strength, or stack cones to develop reach.

The second group of activities I have termed *contrived occupation*. Contrived occupation includes exercise with "added purpose" and occupation with a "contrived" component. Again, there may be a purpose or a goal, but if there is, the purpose most likely originated with the practitioner and not the client. Because the purpose originates with the practitioner, the meaning-

---

[1]Thera-Band Products, The Hygenic Corporation, 1245 Home Avenue, Akron, OH 44310.

fulness of the activity to the client remains minimal. Finally, as with exercise, the focus is on the remediation of impairments.

Exercise with added purpose is exercise embedded in an activity in which both task objects and any potential meanings or purposes are contrived. One example would be to have a woman practice picking up golf balls from the floor with a reacher and placing them in a nearby bucket. Another example would be to have a man place cones on a shelf, telling him that he should pretend that they are glasses and that he is putting the dishes away. The key element is that golf balls and cones have little relevance to the actual tasks that are being simulated.

In *occupation with a contrived component,* the objects are real and not simulated. Having a boy pound nails into a board, encouraging him to pretend that he is going to build a birdhouse, is one example. The objects are real and relevant to the *practitioner-specified* purpose, but there is to be no real birdhouse. Asking a girl to throw bean bags at a target without her engagement in a game is another example. In both of these examples, the purpose and the meaning have been contrived; they are more those of the practitioner than they are those of the children.

The third group of activities I have termed *therapeutic occupation.* A critical characteristic of therapeutic occupation is that the client actively participates in occupation. They are activities the client identifies as purposeful and meaningful. And, to the greatest extent possible, the occupational performance is naturalistic and contextual. The client performs the activities using real objects in natural environments. The focus of therapeutic occupation remains on the remediation of impairments.

An example of therapeutic occupation would be to use *graded occupation* to treat impairments of balance or reach. For example, Lillian loves to read. She has expressed concern that she is experiencing difficulty maintaining her balance while reaching for objects, including books, from shelves. Together, we decide to go to her library and work on her problem areas. By progressively grading the task in terms of the challenges to her balance or the extent of reach required, engagement in an activity that has purpose and meaning to the client can be used to remediate her underlying impairments that are limiting her occupational performance. As her underlying abilities improve, she can begin to retrieve from or return to higher shelves books that are heavier.

Another example of therapeutic occupation involves *direct intervention* of impairments in the context of occupation. Here, the occupational therapy practitioner might work on social abilities while a group of adolescents makes a cake for one of their mothers. Or the practitioner might attempt to remediate attentional deficits as the person engages in a favored card game.

The final group of activities I have termed *adaptive or compensatory occupation.* As with therapeutic occupation, a critical characteristic is the client's active participation in occupations that are chosen by the client. Again, the activities are purposeful and meaningful to the client, and the occupational performance is naturalistic and contextual. In fact, the major distinction between adaptive occupation and therapeutic occupation is that adaptive occupation is focused on improved occupational performance and not on the remediation of impairments. When we use adaptive occupation, we provide assistive devices, teach alternative or compensatory strategies, or modify physical or social environments. No attempt is made to remediate the underlying impairments.

An example of adaptive occupation might involve engaging Roy, who has lung cancer and resultant low endurance, in a desired grocery shopping task. While he is shopping for his needed groceries, the occupational therapy practitioner would use education to teach him alternative ways to manage his shopping. One strategy might be to teach him to put only a limited number of items into a bag. Another might be to teach him to use a cart to transport his groceries. The key characteristic of adaptive occupation is the use of adaptation to alter or change the activity so that the client can perform it successfully (Mosey, 1986). The goal is not to improve Roy's endurance.

Legitimate Activities for Occupational Therapy

What then are the legitimate activities for occupational therapy? Kielhofner (1997) has argued that the emerging paradigm of occupational therapy requires that we recognize occupation as the level of intervention. I believe that this should be true whether the intervention involves engaging the person in therapeutic occupation for purposes of remediation or engaging the person in adaptive occupation to directly enhance occupational performance. Certainly, if we tie current practice to our philosophical base, then the clear *emphasis* must be therapeutic occupation and adaptive occupation. At the same time, we must heed Spelbring's advice and return exercise and most of our use of contrived occupation to their legitimate "owners."[2]

We do not like to think that what we are doing is not legitimate occupational therapy. But, whether we want to admit it to ourselves or not, there are still many occupational therapy practitioners here in the United States and internationally who continue to *emphasize* the use of exercise or contrived occupation to remediate impairments, justifying their programs to themselves and others by stating that their *ultimate* goal is improved occupational performance. We are challenged to ask ourselves, how are these programs any different from those of physical therapy, neuropsychology, and others?

Conceptualizing an Occupational Therapy Intervention Process Model

How can we make the philosophical foundations of our profession a reality of everyday practice? I believe that we do that by uniting practice and theory in an occupational framework. That is, we must conceptualize and implement practice in a manner that explicitly ties what we do to our unique focus on occupation as a therapeutic tool. If we are to remain a viable profession and avoid the risk of being viewed as redundant, we must continue the move away from the mechanistic paradigm and reconnect to our philosophical foundations.

In the remainder of this lecture, I will propose the Occupational Therapy Intervention Process Model as a structure for realizing this objective (see Figure 9.4). This model stresses the use of a top-down approach to evaluation. It also provides a framework to guide professional reasoning that leads to implementation of adaptive occupation for purposes of compensation as well as therapeutic occupation for purposes of remediation.

Establish the Client-Centered Performance Context

The first step of the Occupational Therapy Intervention Process Model is to establish the client-centered performance context. The client-centered performance context provides the framework for understanding, evaluating, and interpreting the person's occupational performance. Occupational performance unfolds as a transaction between the person and the environment as he or she enacts a task (see Figure 9.5). Therefore, the person's motivational characteristics, roles, and capacities are just as critical as the task and the features of the environment for providing the framework that is needed to understand why, and how, a person performs the tasks he or she does and why certain aspects or the task performance may result in the person experiencing difficulty or dissatisfaction. This view is in contrast to the view that defines the context as being limited to the environment or all that is external to the person (Christiansen & Baum, 1997; Dunn, Brown, & McGuigan, 1994; Haugen & Mathiowetz, 1995).

The following interrelated dimensions define the *client-centered performance context:*[3]

1. The *temporal dimension* places the client's occupational performance within context of his or her past; present; and possibilities, priorities, and hopes for the future.

2. The *environmental dimension* includes the persons who are present, the objects that are present, and the physical spaces where the task performances occur.

3. The *cultural dimension* pertains to the shared beliefs, values, and customs of one's cultural group that influence where one performs tasks, what tasks one performs, how one performs them, and what tools and materials are used.

4. The *societal (institutional) dimension* includes one's available community resources, relevant economic factors, and implicit or explicit rules and regulations, including medical precautions.

---

[2]I believe that there is some justification for the *occasional* use of contrived occupation, especially with clients who lack motivation or who are too fearful to engage in activities that we might believe are more relevant to their daily life needs. In this case, group, craft, or play and leisure activities may be used early in the intervention in an attempt to facilitate the client's active participation and to increase motivation. The client may initially "go through the motions" of implementing the task performance, but his or her sense of purpose and meaning in relation to the activity likely is minimal. The hope is that purpose and meaning will emerge. If, however, the use of such activities has no apparent therapeutic benefit, and the client remains unwilling to engage in occupation, then perhaps we should turn the intervention over to other professionals whose methods and focus may be more appropriate.

---

[3]The dimensions included within the client-centered performance context may be likened to what Christiansen and Baum (1997) termed *performance enablers*. In fact, their term, *performance enablers*, is preferred to the term *performance components* (AOTA, 1994b). The use of the term *performance components* tends to imply small (component) units of the enactment of a task performance rather than the intended underlying supporting framework. The small, goal-directed units of a task performance are *actions*, not the person's underlying capacities. For that reason, I have deliberately avoided referring to performance components during this lecture, substituting instead terms such as *capacities, abilities, limitations*, and *impairments*.

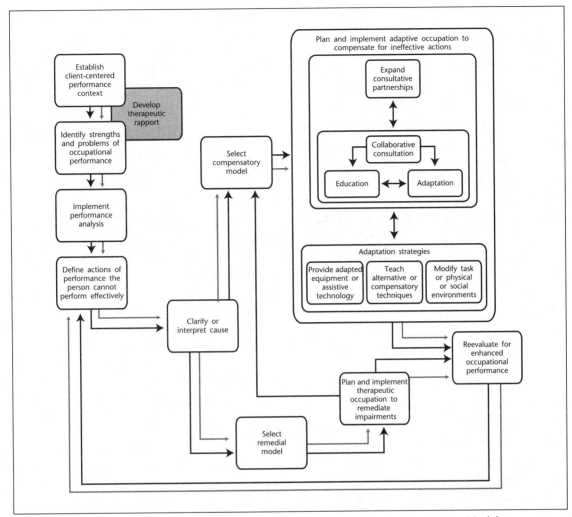

Figure 9.4. Schematic representation of the Occupational Therapy Intervention Process Model.

Note. Copyright © 1998 by Anne G. Fisher Reprinted with permission.

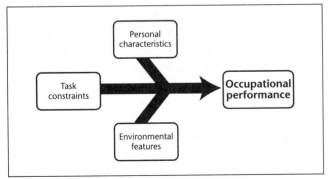

Figure 9.5. Schematic representation of occupational performance unfolding as a transaction between the person and the environment as he or she enacts a task.

Note. Copyright © 1998 by Anne G. Fisher. Reprinted with permission.

5. The *social dimension* includes one's connections and relationships with others as well as the extent of collaboration that occurs between the client and others during occupational performance.

6. The *role dimension* pertains to the relationship between one's roles and the related collection of task performances that must unfold in a logical, timely, and socially appropriate manner. We must understand the person's perceived roles and any incongruities between his or her role behavior and the role behavior that is expected by society or desired by the person.

7. The *motivational dimension* pertains to one's values, interests, and goals that give meaning to activity and provide a source of motivation.

8. The *capacity dimension* pertains to the clients' diagnosed condition and the broad clinical picture of his or her neurologic, musculoskeletal, cognitive, and psychosocial capacities and impairments we gain through our initial observations and interview with the client. These are the *initial* impressions we have of a client that *begin* to inform us about the client's potentials for change, delimiters to progress, and precautions we might need to consider during intervention.

9. The *task dimension* includes both the task to be performed and the constraints that define that task. The task constraints are a set of culturally defined task characteristics that result in shared recognition that "this" person is performing "this" task (Fisher, 1997c). These culturally defined task characteristics specify the appropriate context, the tools and materials to be used, the norms or rules for the performance, and the necessary temporal order of the task actions. They are a component of what Nelson (1988) has called *occupational form*. When a person does not enact the specified occupational form, we recognize such deviations as errors. Such errors may reflect inefficiencies in organizing time or space, inappropriate or unsafe object use, inappropriate actions that are irrelevant to the specified form, unsafe actions that place the person at risk, and so on. The important point here is that within the context of occupational therapy, we recognize "problems of performance" through the recognition that some aspect of what we observe the client doing is "out of form."

Establishing the context begins with an initial referral and perhaps a chart review. Then we meet the client. Through interview, observation, and the use of life stories (Clark, 1993; Kielhofner, 1995; Spencer, Davidson, & White, 1996), we begin to construct the client-centered performance context. The use of structured interviews, such as the Occupational Performance History Interview (Kielhofner & Henry, 1988) or the Canadian Occupational Performance Measure (Law et al., 1994), provides a structure to gathering information and identifying the client's goals.

The meaningfulness and relevance of specific task performances to the client are of critical importance in the evaluation and intervention process. Learning about the tasks that are most important to the person,

the meaning of those tasks, and the nature of the contexts within which those task performances are likely to be enacted requires taking the time and effort to establish the client-centered performance context. This step is critical, and it must occur, even under the pressures of cost containment, reduced duration of care, staff cuts, and increased accountability. In fact, there is some evidence that taking more time, initially, to establish the client-centered performance context will result in overall outcomes being enhanced and overall costs reduced (Bowen, 1996; Neistadt, 1995).

Consistent with a top-down approach, it is important to point out that we do not begin to formally assess the person's underlying capacities and abilities until later (Fisher & ShortDeGraff, 1993; Trombly, 1993). Rather, at this stage in the evaluation process, we consider only the person's diagnosed condition and what we learn through informal observation and interview.

For example, before I actually met Jim, I was aware that he had sustained a brain injury several years ago and that he was experiencing difficulty finding satisfying employment. This information led me to suspect that he might have either physical or cognitive limitations, but if he did, they were unlikely to change. My first contact with him was by telephone. During our conversation, I became aware that he has expressive aphasia but that he is able to communicate most of his ideas in a manner that I could understand.

Later, when I met Jim, I noticed that he does not use his right arm. He allows it to hang at this side. As Jim and I began to talk, I quickly learned that he is bilingual—he knows both American Sign Language and English. Jim cues himself visually, using sign language, when he has difficulty verbalizing what he wants to say. During our conversation, I sensed that Jim has good comprehension and no major memory deficits. He is outgoing and appears to have good social skills. Things he said also led me to infer that he likely has good self-awareness and problem-solving abilities. But a critical feature here is that I did not formally test any of Jim's capacities. I did not ask him to move his right arm. I did not ask him to tell me the meaning of a saying like "a rolling stone gathers no moss." I did not ask him to remember and repeat number sequences or count backward from 100 by 7s.

Instead, I learned about his history, his interests, his values, and his goals. Jim is 28 years old. He sustained a brain injury in an automobile accident 12 years ago as he was driving to diving practice. He had been a champion diver in state competition. He has had occupational therapy and speech therapy. He learned how to use a variety of assistive devices. He loves music and has taught himself to play both acoustic and electric guitar one-handed. When I asked him how he did it, he said, "Practice, practice, practice." He writes music, paints, and composes poetry. He is currently working on an album where his poetry will be set against his music. He speaks poignantly through his poetry:

> I am angry...
>> Where is the blame.
> I am alive...
>> If I find the treasure of life.
> I am alone...
>> Communications breakdown. (Cacciatore, 1994)

Jim is highly motivated to work and earn an income so that he can live on his own, but all of his past jobs have been low paying. He has worked as a companion for another young man with a brain injury. He tried working as a cashier, but found the work too stressful. He currently has a job gathering carts from the parking lot of a large warehouse department store. He has good work skills; he is friendly, on time, and able to carry out routine sequences. He has a small Tshirt company. He uses a computer to design the graphics and adds his own words. Jim wants to be a graphic designer, but he lacks the needed skills. He went to a local community college to study graphic design but did not complete the final course in English as it was too difficult. He did not earn the degree.

He says about himself, "I've adapted—I take a 'don't worry, be happy' attitude." He has maintained hope, but still he is concerned about work and wants very much to move out of his parents' home and live independently in his own apartment.

Develop Therapeutic Rapport

As I talk with Jim, I not only establish the client-centered performance context, but also begin the critical step of developing therapeutic rapport (Tickle-Degnen, 1995). "Rapport is the process of establishing and maintaining a comfortable, unconstrained relationship of mutual confidence and respect between a practitioner and client" (Mosey, 1981, p. 96). This is the beginning of a collaborative (consultative) partnership between Jim and myself that will continue to develop throughout the time we work together (depicted by the lighter gray line in Figure 9.4). Collaboration with the client *throughout the intervention process* is required by

the AOTA's (1994a) *Code of Ethics*. Effective goal setting and treatment planning demands the development of a collaborative partnership between the practitioner and the client. The practitioner brings to this partnership expertise related to available intervention strategies and knowledge related to potential outcomes. The client brings his or her values, interests, goals, and priorities. If the collaborative partnership is to be effective, there must be open sharing of each other's motivations and rationales (Bowen, 1996).

Identify Strengths and Problems of Occupational Performance

As I progress downward and narrow the focus of the evaluation, I identify tasks that are currently supporting or hindering Jim's role behavior. Task performances that support Jim's role behavior are Jim's strengths. Those that he experiences as problematic or that hinder his role behavior are his problems of occupational performance. In the process of narrowing the focus of the evaluation, I remain alert to potential discrepancies between my estimation of Jim's potential problem areas and those actually identified by him. I will include those tasks among those I will observe Jim performing. For example, Jim indicated that playing guitar is a strength; I wanted to verify his ability. I suspected that preparing meals that are not ready made may pose a problem, even though Jim did not identify cooking as a problem area. I also wanted to know more about his computer and graphic design skills.

Develop a Performance Analysis

As I proceed downward to the next step of the evaluation process, I implement a performance analysis (Fisher, 1997a, 1997d). Performance analysis is defined as the observational evaluation of a person's task performance to identify discrepancies between the demands of a task and of the person. The person's problems and strengths are described in terms of the quality of the goal-directed actions that comprise the occupational performance, not the client's underlying capacities and impairments. Perforce analyses should not be confused with task or activity analyses, which are intended for purposes of identifying the underlying impairments that limit occupational performance or the inherent therapeutic value of a task for remediating those impairments (AOTA, 1993; Hagedorn, 1995, 1997; Llorens, 1993; Trombly, 1995b; Watson, 1997).

Implementing a performance analysis requires that we observe the quality of the transaction between the client and the environment as the client performs a task that is similar, meaningful, purposeful, and relevant. The Assessment of Motor and Process Skills (AMPS) (Fisher, 1997b) is a standardized performance analysis. The performance analysis also can be accomplished through informal observation of a person's occupational performance.

Because I used the AMPS to evaluate Jim, I will describe a few of its key features. The AMPS skill actions are small units of the enactment of a daily life task. An important feature of the skill actions is that they are goal directed. Most frequently, the goal of the AMPS skill action pertains to an action or step embedded within the overall task performance—*reaching* for and *lifting* the jar from the shelf or *gathering* the lettuce to the table. For other AMPS skill actions, the goal pertains more to the overall task performance—*heeding* the client-specified goal (i.e., the client's doing what the client said he or she would do) or *sequencing* the steps of the task in a logical manner such that the person-environment transaction unfolds as a coherent and recognizable routine.

An important feature of scoring an AMPS observation is that no judgment is made regarding the person's underlying capacities. That is, a person may be assigned a low score on the AMPS skill action *Sequences* for reasons other than decreased sequencing capacity. Similarly, a high score on the AMPS skill action *Lifts* would not necessarily mean that the person has good lifting capacity. Because the AMPS is a test of the quality and effectiveness of a person's occupational performance (and not underlying capacities), the person is scored on the basis of what was observed—the transaction of the person with the environment as he or she performs a familiar and chosen task. More specifically, the quality of the performance is what is graded, not the "quality" of the person's underlying capacities nor the "quality" of the environment or task objects with which the person interacts. Those judgments are deferred to the interpretation stage (i.e., Clarify or Interpret Cause), where the practitioner uses professional reasoning and perhaps further assessment to determine person, environmental, task, or sociocultural factors that may be limiting performance.

Define Actions of Performance That the Person Cannot Perform Effectively

Having observed Jim perform tasks, I proceed to define the actions that he can and cannot perform effectively.

When I implemented an informal performance analysis and observed Jim set up and play his guitars, I learned that he is able to do so and, indeed, he is able to play very well using a hammer and "draw" method. When I used the AMPS and observed him prepare toast and coffee, I learned that he is able to lift, transport, and grip task objects effectively. He chose and used appropriate tools and materials, and he heeded the goal of the client-specified task. He had moderate difficulty, however, with effectively stabilizing the toast while buttering it, organizing his workspace, and adapting to problems he encountered during his task performance. Plans are under way to evaluate Jim's computer and graphic skills.

Clarify or Interpret Cause

Having identified the actions that Jim cannot perform effectively, I proceed to clarify or interpret the underlying cause of his ineffective performance. In Jim's case, the underlying cause was obvious. He has hemiplegia, and, during his task performance, he did not use any of the many assistive devices he had received earlier in his rehabilitation. Part of clarifying the cause of Jim's ineffective performance, however, will be to inquire as to why he did not use any assistive devices.

In other cases, as we seek to understand the underlying cause of a person's ineffective occupational performance, we can think in terms of impairments (e.g., John cannot put his arm into the sleeve of his shirt because of limitations in range of motion at the shoulder). We can think in terms of physical environments (e.g., Mary cannot reach the glasses from the cupboard shelf because they are too high). We can think in terms of social environments (e.g., Steven does not finish his school work tasks because the classroom environment is noisy and chaotic). We can consider societal constraints (e.g., Lillian must not bend her hip beyond 90 degrees and reach to put on her shoes because of total hip precautions). And finally, we can consider societal expectations (e.g., Bill's work performance is not acceptable because his low productivity affects company profits).

When the underlying cause is not clear, the occupational therapy practitioner may choose to implement further assessment. Selected practice models, such as the Model of Human Occupation (Kielhofner, 1995) or the Ecology of Human Performance framework (Dunn et al., 1994), provide conceptual structures for assessing characteristics of the person or the environment that limit and support occupational performance. Occupational therapy practitioners are never at a loss for tests of the person's underlying neurologic, musculoskeletal, cognitive, or psychosocial capacities. Finally, a wide range of environmental assessments also are available (Letts et al., 1994).

Select Compensatory Model

Now that I have clarified Jim's problems and the reasons for his limitations, I am ready to select one or more intervention models. I select the remedial model when I believe that restoration of underlying capacities will result in improved occupational performance. I select the compensatory model when I believe that remediation is unlikely to affect occupational performance significantly; when remediation will be "too costly in terms of time, energy or money" (Trombly, 1993, p. 255); or when I am directed by legislation to focus on occupational performance and role behavior. I also can implement both model types simultaneously. Because I suspect that remediation will not benefit Jim, I select the compensatory model.

Plan and Implement Adaptive Occupation to Compensate for Ineffective Actions

Once the compensatory model is chosen, the next step is to plan and implement adaptive occupation. The desired outcome is the design of adaptive occupation to compensate for the client's ineffective actions. Specific details have been published elsewhere (Duran & Fisher, in press; Fisher, 1997a; Trombly, 1995c), but I will present an overview here so as to demonstrate the process of implementing the compensatory model.[4]

Consultative partnerships. When we first meet a client and begin to develop therapeutic rapport, we develop a collaborative (consultative) partnership with the client. Once we know that we will be implementing adaptive occupation, we also must enter into shared *consultative partnerships* with those persons who have access to needed information or who will be affected by the proposed changes. For example, members of the cli-

ent's family who are living with him or her, or persons who will be providing the client with assistance, are important members of the consultative partnership.

Collaborative consultation, education, and adaptation. Once the members of the consultative partnership are identified, the practitioner implements methods of collaborative consultation (Fisher, 1997a), education (teaching-learning) (Mosey, 1986; Trombly, 1995c), and adaptation (Fisher, 1997a; Trombly 1995c). Through collaboration with the client and his or her family, client-centered goals are established. Then, building on the development of collaborative relationships, the members of the consultative partnership work together to propose and develop strategies for intervention that are based on the principles of adaptation. Finally, the members of the consultative partnership responsible for implementing the interventions are trained in how to do so on the basis of the principles of education. These persons may include the client, caregiver, service extender, or another professional.

Adaptation strategies. As I noted earlier, adaptation includes providing adapted equipment or assistive technology, teaching the client alternative strategies or compensatory techniques, and modifying the task or the physical or social environment. Maria uses a special keyboard and mouse to lessen the effects of repetitive motion. Jim has learned to tie his shoes one-handed. He has also taught himself how to play his guitar, using a one-handed hammer and "draw" method. Ken was taught to use lists to remember which of his many medications to take when. He use a stool to sit and preach because one of his medications has caused peripheral neuropathy in his feet. Because of continued safety risk, Lillian requires standby assistance when standing and transferring to and from her wheelchair: For occupational therapists, who are experts in adaptation, the list of possibilities is endless.

Re-evaluate for Enhanced Occupational Performance

Once the adaptations have been implemented, the client's occupational performance is re-evaluated. We again use performance analyses to verify whether the client has met his or her goals. Finally, documentation of the effectiveness of our occupational therapy interventions is a critical step toward communicating the unique role of occupational therapy as well as justifying payment of occupational therapy services by health-care payers.

---

[4]The compensatory model has been called the *rehabilitation* (compensatory) model by Trombly (1995c) and the *expanded rehabilitation* model by Fisher (1997a). In this lecture, I have chosen to call it the compensatory model as the term *rehabilitation* implies physical restoration and remediation of impairments. When the compensatory model is used in isolation of the Occupational Therapy Intervention Process Model, it includes all steps included in Figure 9.4, except Select Remedial Model and Plan and Implement Therapeutic Occupation to Remediate Impairments (Duran & Fisher, in press; Fisher, 1997a).

Redefine Actions of Performance That the Person Cannot Perform Effectively

If the performance analysis implemented during the re-evaluation results in the identification of additional problems, the actions the person cannot perform effectively must be redefined, and the cycle of clarifying the cause, selecting a model, and so on, is repeated.

Select Remedial Model—Plan and Implement Therapeutic Occupation to Remediate Impairments

In the event that the occupational therapy practitioner judges the client to be a good candidate for remediation, the practitioner can select one of many remedial models (e.g., biomechanical, sensory integration). Activity analysis and synthesis (Mosey, 1986) are then used to design therapeutic occupations to remediate the person's impairments that are limiting occupational performance. Ideally, the practitioner re-evaluates for enhanced occupational performance, documents changes in performance, and re-enters the cycle if further intervention is indicated. If the remediation not effective, or if recovery plateaus, the practitioner can abandon the use of therapeutic occupation and select the compensatory model.

Conclusions

I realize that we all face the ongoing challenges of changing health care. Many of you, especially those of you affected by managed care and prospective payment, will view what I say as idealistic. I disagree. I believe that my view is the more realistic one. As Karen Selley DeLorenzo (personal communication, March 15, 1998) has so clearly articulated, there will be reduced monies available for rehabilitation services. We will no longer have the luxury of providing intervention for as long as functional gains can be documented. Therefore, we must make every effort to enable our clients to achieve maximum gains within the limited time available. The only way to do this is to introduce adaptive occupation and consultation from day one. Remediation is time consuming, and there is growing evidence that remediation may have limited effects on functional outcomes.[5]

These challenges also provide us with opportunities. In an environment where we are expected to provide quality service in less time, we face a critical need to communicate who we are, why we are important, and that what we do is unique. Case managers and teachers should be the primary targets of these educational efforts. We need to make a philosophical shift. We may need to let go of the type of thinking that is *driven* by a focus on remediation of impairments. Instead, we need to focus on what the person wants and needs to do and work with the person to enable him or her to perform tasks that are meaningful to the person and in a manner that brings satisfaction. This means that we need to rethink what is really important from the perspective of the person—occupational performance or his or her impairments. We need to rethink the evaluation process, using a top-down approach that focuses on occupation. We need to revise our intervention strategies and focus more on adaptation, education, and collaborative consultation and less on remediation. Focusing on occupational performance instead of remediation does not mean that remediation will not occur. The man who built the radio developed better strength and coordination even though that was neither his goal nor mine. Restoration of self-esteem, interests, and values also can, and should, occur through participation in adaptive occupation. When we do focus on remediation, we need to tie our interventions to our philosophical base through the application of therapeutic occupation. And, although I have said little about it during this lecture, I will add that we need to recognize the need to set goals and document efficacy in terms of occupational performance and not impairments or performance components.

---

[5]I base this assertion on research that has not demonstrated a strong enough relationship between underlying impairments and occupational performance to support the basic assumption that if the underlying cause (i.e., neuromuscular, biomechanical, cognitive, or psychosocial impairments) of limitations in occupational performance can be identified and treated, then the effects will generalize to improved occupational performance (Bernspång, Asplund, Eriksson, & Fugl-Meyer, 1987; Jongbloed, Brighton, & Stacey, 1988; Lichtenberg & Nanna, 1994; Pincus et al., 1989; Reed, Jagust, & Scab, 1989; Skurla, Rogers, & Sunderland, 1988; Teri, Borson, Kiyak, & Yamagishi, 1989). I also make this assertion despite the fact that some researchers (Judge, Schechtman, Cress, & the FICSIT Group, 1996) continue to claim strong relationships between discrete physical performance measures and instrumental activities of daily living performance even though 75 percent of their observed relationships were $r < .50$ (<25 percent explained variance) and 100 percent of their observed relationships were $r < .60$ (<36 percent explained variance). Additional evidence to support my assertion lies in studies that indicate that the effectiveness of remedial approaches may be limited (Benedict et al., 1994; Fetters & Kluzik, 1996; Hutzler, Chacham, Bergman, & Szeinberg, 1998; Kaplan, Polatajko, Wilson, & Faris, 1993; Law et al., 1997; Nakayama, Jørgensen, Raaschou, & Olsen, 1994; Neistadt, 1992).

Are you prepared to heed Jim's final words?

I will accept and go on.
It is my problem, not you.
What are you going to do about it? (Cacciatore, 1994)

Acknowledgments

I thank my many colleagues and students, here and abroad, who have contributed so much to the development of this lecture through their support and assistance. Many of them have also provided constructive feedback either in the context of the classroom or through ongoing dialogues that, in some cases, have gone on for years. This feedback has played a critical role in the evolution of my thinking about occupation and occupational therapy. I also thank Carol Wassell, Coordinator, Instructional Services, Colorado State University, for her preparation of the figures included in this lecture.

References

American Occupational Therapy Association. (1993). Position paper: Purposeful activity. *American Journal of Occupational Therapy, 47,* 1081–1082.

American Occupational Therapy Association. (1994a). Occupational therapy code of ethics. *American Journal of Occupational Therapy, 48,* 1037–1038.

American Occupational Therapy Association. (1994b). Uniform terminology for occupational therapy—Third edition. *American Journal of Occupational Therapy, 48,* 1047–1054.

American Occupational Therapy Association. (1995). Position paper: Occupation. *American Journal of Occupational Therapy, 49,* 1015–1018.

American Occupational Therapy Association. (1997). Statement—Fundamental concepts of occupational therapy: Occupation, purposeful activity, and function. *American Journal of Occupational Therapy, 51,* 864–866. http://dx.doi.org/10.5014/ajot.51.10.864

Ayres, A. J. (1972). *Sensory integration and learning disorders.* Los Angeles: Western Psychological Services.

Benedict, R. H. B., Harris, A. E., Markow, T., McCormick, J. A., Nuechterlein, K. H., & Asarnow, R. F. (1994). Effects of attention training on information processing in schizophrenia. *Schizophrenia Bulletin, 20,* 537–546.

Bernspång, B., Asplund, K., Eriksson, S., & Fugl-Meyer, A. R. (1987). Motor and perceptual impairments in acute stroke patients: Effects on self-care ability. *Stroke, 18,* 1081–1087.

Bowen, R. E. (1996). The Issue Is—Should occupational therapy adopt a consumer-based model of service delivery? *American Journal of Occupational Therapy, 50,* 899–902.

Brunnstrom, S. (1970). *Movement therapy in hemiplegia: A neurophysiological approach.* New York: Harper & Row.

Cacciatore, J. (1994). *Head injury aggression.* Unpublished poem.

Christiansen, C., & Baum, C. (1997). Person–environment occupational performance: A conceptual model for practice. In C. H. Christiansen & C. M. Baum (Eds.), *Occupational therapy: Enabling function and well-being* (2nd ed., pp. 47–70). Thorofare, NJ: Slack.

Clark, F. (1993). Occupation embedded in a real life: Interweaving occupational science and occupational therapy (1993 Eleanor Clarke Slagle Lecture). *American Journal of Occupational Therapy, 47,* 1067–1078. http://dx.doi.org/10.5014/ajot.47.12.1067

Clark, F. A., Parham, D., Carlson, M. E., Frank, G., Jackson, J., Pierce, D., Wolfe, R. J., & Zemke, R. (1991). Occupational science: Academic innovation in the service of occupational therapy's future. *American Journal of Occupational Therapy 45,* 300–310. http://dx.doi.org/10.5014/ajot.45.4.300

Clark, F. P. (1917). The beneficial effects of work therapy for the insane. *Modern Hospital, 8,* 392–393.

Dunn, W., Brown, C., & McGuigan, A. (1994). The ecology of human performance: A framework for considering the effect of context. *American Journal of Occupational Therapy 48,* 595–607.

Dunton, W. R. (1928). *Prescribing occupational therapy* Springfield, IL: Charles C Thomas.

Duran, L., & Fisher, A. G. (in press). Occupational therapy assessment and treatment of a client with disorder of executive abilities. In C. Unsworth (Ed.), *Cognitive and perceptual dysfunction: A clinical reasoning approach to assessment and treatment.* Philadelphia: F A. Davis.

Evans, K. A. (1987). Nationally Speaking—Definition of occupation as the core concept of occupational therapy. *American Journal of Occupational Therapy, 41,* 627–628.

Fetters, L., & Kiuzik, J. (1996). The effects of neurodevelopmental treatment versus practice on the reaching of children with spastic cerebral palsy. *Physical Therapy, 76,* 346–358.

Fisher, A. G. (1994). Functional assessment and occupation: Critical issues for occupational therapy. *New Zealand Journal of Occupational Therapy 45(2),* 13–19.

Fisher, A. G. (1995). *Assessment of Motor and Process Skills.* Fort Collins, CO: Three Star Press.

Fisher, A. G. (1997a). An expanded rehabilitative model of practice. In A. G. Fisher, *Assessment of Motor and Process Skills* (2nd ed., pp. 73–86). Fort Collins, CO: Three Star Press.

Fisher, A. G. (1997b). *Assessment of Motor and Process Skills* (2nd ed). Fort Collins, CO: Three Star Press.

Fisher, A. G. (1997c). Background information. In A. G. Fisher, *Assessment of Motor and Process Skills* (2nd ed., pp. 11–34). Fort Collins, CO: Three Star Press.

Fisher, A. G. (1997d). Introduction. In A. G. Fisher, *Assessment of Motor and Process Skills* (2nd ed., pp. 1–9). Fort Collins, CO: Three Star Press.

Fisher, A. G., Murray, E. A., & Bundy, A. C. (1991). *Sensory integration: Theory and practice*. Philadelphia: F. A. Davis.

Fisher, A. G., & Short-DeGraff, M. (1993). Nationally Speaking—Improving functional assessment in occupational therapy: Recommendations and philosophy for change. *American Journal of Occupational Therapy, 47*, 199–202.

Gritzer, G., & Arluke, A. (1985). *The making of rehabilitation*. Berkeley: University of California Press.

Hagedorn, R. (1995). *Occupational therapy: Perspectives and processes*. Edinburgh, Scotland: Churchill Livingstone.

Hagedorn, R. (1997). *Foundations for practice in occupational therapy* (2nd ed.). New York: Churchill Livingstone.

Haugen, J. B., & Mathiowetz, V. (1995). Contemporary task-oriented approach. In C. A. Trombly (Ed.), *Occupational therapy for physical dysfunction* (4th ed., pp. 510–527). Baltimore: Williams & Wilkins.

Hutzler, Y., Chacham, A., Bergman, U., & Szeinberg, A. (1998 Effects of a movement and swimming program on vital capacity and water orientation skills of children with cerebral palsy. *Developmental Medicine and Child Neurology, 40*, 176–181.

Jongbloed, L., Brighton, C., & Stacey, S. (1988). Factors associated with independent meal preparation, self-care and mobility in CVA clients. *Canadian Journal of Occupational Therapy, 55*, 259–263.

Judge, J. O., Schechtman, K., Cress, E., & FICSIT Group (1996). The relationship between physical performance measures and independence in instrumental activities of daily living. *Journal of the American Geriatrics Society, 44*, 1332–1341.

Kaplan, B. J., Polatajko, H. J., Wilson, B. N., & Faris, P. D. (1993). Re-examination of sensory integration treatment: A combination of two efficacy studies. *Journal of Learning Disabilities, 26*, 342–347.

Kielhofner, G. (1985). *A model of human occupation: Theory and application*. Baltimore: Williams & Wilkins.

Kielhofner, G. (1995). *A model of human occupation: Theory and application* (2nd ed.). Baltimore: Williams & Wilkins.

Kielhofner, G. (1997). *Conceptual foundations of occupational therapy* (2nd ed.). Philadelphia: F. A. Davis.

Kielhofner, G., & Henry, A. D. (1988). Development and investigation of the Occupational Performance History Interview. *American Journal of Occupational Therapy, 42*, 489–498.

Law, M., Baptiste, S., Carswell, A., McColl, M. A., Polatajko, H., & Pollock, N. (1994). *Canadian Occupational Performance Measure* (2nd ed). Toronto, Ontario: CAOT Publications.

Law, M., Russell, D., Pollock, N., Rosenbaum, P., Walter, S., & King, G. (1997). A comparison of intensive neuro-developmental therapy plus casting and a regular occupational therapy program for children with cerebral palsy. *Developmental Medicine and Child Neurology 39*, 664–670.

Letts, S., Law, M., Rigby, P., Cooper, B., Stewart, S., & Strong S. (1994). Person–environment assessments in occupational therapy. *American Journal of Occupational Therapy, 48*, 608–618. http://dx.doi.org/10.5014/ajot.48.7.608

Lichtenberg, P. A., & Nanna, M. (1994). The role of cognition in predicting activities of daily living and ambulation functioning in the oldest-old rehabilitation patients. *Rehabilitation Psychology, 39*, 251–262

Llorens, L. A. (1993). Activity analysis: Agreement between participants and observers on perceived factors in occupation components. *Occupational Therapy Journal of Research, 13*, 198–211.

Mosey, A. C. (1981). *Occupational therapy: Configuration of a profession*. New York: Raven.

Mosey, A. C. (1986). *Psychosocial components of occupational therapy*. New York: Raven.

Nakayama, H., Jorgensen, H. S, Raaschou, H. O., & Olsen, T. S. (1994). Compensation in recovery of upper extremity function after stroke: The Copenhagen Stroke Study. *Archives of Physical Medicine and Rehabilitation, 75*, 852–857.

Neistadt, M. E. (1992). Occupational therapy treatments for constructional deficits. *American Journal of Occupational Therapy, 46*, 141–148. http://dx.doi.org/10.5014/ajot.46.2.141

Neistadt, M. E. (1995). Methods of assessing clients' priorities: A survey of adult physical dysfunction settings.

American Journal of Occupational Therapy, 49, 428–436. http://dx.doi.org/10.5014/ajot.49.5.428

Nelson, D. L. (1988). Occupation: Form and performance *American Journal of Occupational Therapy 42,* 633–641.

Occupational therapy in the general hospital. (1917). *Modern Hospital, 8,* 425–427.

Pincus, T., Callahan, L. F., Brooks, R. H., Fuchs, H. A., Olsen, N. J., & Kaye, J. J. (1989). Self-report questionnaire scores in rheumatoid arthritis compared with traditional physical, radiographic, and laboratory measures. *Annals of Internal Medicine, 110,* 259–266.

Quiroga, V. A. M. (1995). *Occupational therapy: The first1, years, 1900 to 1930.* Bethesda, MD: American Occupational Therapy Association.

Reed, B. R., Jagust, W. J., & Seab, J. P. (1989). Mental status as a predictor of daily function in progressive dementia. *Gerontologist, 29,* 804–807.

Rudman, D. L., Cook, J. V., & Polatajko, H. (1997). Understanding the potential of occupation: A qualitative exploration of seniors' perspectives on activity. *American Journal of Occupational Therapy, 51,* 640–650. http://dx.doi.org/10.5014/ajot.51.8.640

Semans, S. (1967). The Bobath concept in treatment of neurological disorders. *American Journal of Physical Medicine, 46,* 732–785.

Skurla, E., Rogers, J. C., & Sunderland, T. (1988). Direct assessment of activities of daily living in Alzheimer's disease: A controlled study. *Journal of the American Geriatrics Society, 36,* 97–103.

Spencer, J. C., Davidson, H. A., & White, V. K. (1996). Continuity and change: Past experiences as adaptive repertoire in occupational adaptation. *American Journal of Occupational Therapy, 50,* 526–534.

Stockmeyer, S. A. (1967). An interpretation of the approach of Rood to the treatment of neuromuscular dysfunction. *American Journal of Physical Medicine, 46,* 900–956.

Teri, L., Borson, S., Kiyak, H. A., & Yamagishi, M. (1989). Behavioral disturbance, cognitive dysfunction, and functional skill: Prevalence and relationship in Alzheimer's disease. *Journal of the American Geriatrics Society, 37,* 109–116.

The Oxford English dictionary (2nd ed.). (1989). Oxford, UK: Clarendon.

Tickle-Degnen, L. (1995). Therapeutic rapport. In C. A. Trombly (Ed.), *Occupational therapy for physical dysfunction* (4th ed., pp. 277–285). Baltimore: Williams & Wilkins.

Trombly, C. (1993). The Issue Is—Anticipating the future: Assessment of occupational function. *American Journal of Occupational Therapy, 47,* 253–257.

Trombly, C. A. (1995a). Occupation: Purposefulness and meaningfulness as therapeutic mechanisms, 1995. Eleanor Clarke Slagle Lecture. *American Journal of Occupational Therapy; 49,* 960–972. Reprinted as Chapter 11.

Trombly, C. A. (1995b). Purposeful activity. In C. A. Trombly (Ed.), *Occupational therapy for physical dysfunction* (4th ed., pp. 237–253). Baltimore: Williams & Wilkins.

Trombly, C. A. (1995c). Retraining basic and instrumental activities of daily living. In C. A. Trombly (Ed.), *Occupational therapy for physical dysfunction* (4th ed., pp. 289–318). Baltimore: Williams & Wilkins.

Upham, E. G. (1917). Some principles of occupational therapy. *Modern Hospital, 8,* 409–413.

Watson, D. E. (1997). *Task analysis. An occupational performance approach.* Bethesda, MD: American Occupational Therapy Association.

CHAPTER 10

Putting Occupation Into Practice: Occupation as Ends, Occupation as Means

JULIE MCLAUGHLIN GRAY

A recent conversation with a client yielded the following description of his past experiences with occupational therapy: "Pick that up there and put it over here." It was clear from the client's description that he was referring to some type of upper-extremity retraining. I found this conversation disheartening—this description of occupational therapy—yet very poignant. It struck me as a powerful example of how sometimes occupational therapy so heavily emphasizes performance components that it ceases to be occupational in terms of the client's perceptions and the overall emphasis of treatment planning. By *occupational* I mean interventions that have the following characteristics to varying degrees: purposefulness, or goal-directedness; meaningfulness to the individual; wholeness or finiteness, an inherent beginning, middle, and end; and the multidimensionality possessed by an activity in context, the human and his or her multiple systems—emotional, cognitive, perceptual, physical—interacting with the environment.

The client's portrait of occupational therapy seems a sad but honest reflection of the struggle faced by many occupational therapists and the profession as a whole—the struggle to provide occupation-centered treatment. I have prescribed similar activities with the intent of improving upper-extremity function. These activities provided structured, repetitive practice but seemed void of characteristics I had been taught to associate with occupational therapy, such as purposefulness, meaning, and holism. At times, I left these sessions questioning my unique role in the client's recovery, as well as whether or not I was meeting his or her occupational needs.

Despite a professional commitment to occupation-centered treatment, I have not found it an easy task either in the experiences described by my colleagues and students, nor in my own practice. Recent discussions with students returning from Level I fieldwork revealed observations by several that "no one is doing occupation out there." Worse, some received feedback from clinical preceptors that they were "trying to be too creative." One student was discouraged from participating in an outdoor gardening activity with a client who was very interested in "getting out" and gardening, because of role delineations at the facility. I have also observed interns and new therapists who leave the classroom with wonderful ideas of how to organize treatment around occupation, but limit themselves to the use of self-care, pure exercise, or purposeful activities that have no relevance to the client's interests or developmental level.

My own career path has involved a great deal of time and energy pondering the uniqueness of occupational therapy as well as how to incorporate occupation into treatment with adults with neurological disorders. I am a practicing clinician of 13 years, and I continue to work with clients, therapists, and interns in a hospital-based rehabilitation setting. My strong sense of dedication to our profession has been coupled with a strong sense of frustration about inadequate professional identity and recognition. In addition to clinical work, I have spent the last several years studying two areas in depth: neurodevelopmental treatment (NDT) and occupational science. Despite my concurrent interest in both of these areas and a sense of needing more information in both to work effectively with clients, I have often felt internal pressure to limit my focus to one or the other and have been unclear about how to integrate the two approaches effectively. Nevertheless, my solution has been to spend many hours reflecting on how they might best fit together in practice and how we as occupational therapy practitioners might best communicate to our clients and other health-care

This chapter was previously published in the *American Journal of Occupational Therapy, 52,* 354–364. Copyright © 1998, American Occupational Therapy Association. Reprinted with permission. http://dx.doi.org/10.5014/ajot.52.5.354

professionals the purpose of our services. Making the leap from classroom learning to working with adults with physical disabilities, from exercise and remedial training to the use of occupation as the therapeutic medium, is difficult for many therapists in many settings.

In this article, based upon my struggle, readings, observations, and conversations with colleagues, I will propose and analyze some problems that occupational therapists experience in upholding occupation-centered approaches to treatment, describe a possible solution to these difficulties by expanding upon the concepts of occupation as ends and occupation as means presented by Trombly (1995a) in her Slagle lecture, and apply that solution to an authentic case. In doing so, I hope to provide a framework that encourages and assists occupational therapists to become more occupational in our respective approaches. (See Chapter 11.)

The Nature of the Problem

The history of occupational therapy has been discussed by several scholars and is a helpful adjunct to an analysis of current difficulties in keeping occupation at the center of practice. In Kielhofner and Burke's (1983) overview of paradigms and paradigm shifts within occupational therapy, they described the early paradigm of occupational therapy as one that strongly emphasized occupation as central to practice. Beginning circa the late 1930s, however, occupational therapists were influenced by the medical model to shift away from this paradigm to an emphasis on "inner mechanisms" (p. 30), manifested in several approaches, such as the neurologic, kinesiologic, and psychodynamic approaches, that addressed the dysfunction treatment of components underlying occupation. This emphasis on inner mechanisms offered the benefit of an intensified scientific foundation for practice in occupational therapy, but brought the simultaneous detriment of a shift away from occupation as the central, unifying focus within theory and treatment (Kielhofner & Burke, 1983).

Component-Driven Practice

This shift away from occupation persists today (Wood, 1998). The client's comment quoted above represents the most common deterrent to occupation-centered treatment with physically disabled adults: the reduction of treatment goals to components. That is, clients' underlying problems are identified and therapists select exercises and purposeful or nonpurposeful activities specifically geared toward improving strength, range of

motion, coordination, visual perception, problem solving, balance, attention, and so forth. Often the "activities" are chosen on the basis of what is typically available in the occupational therapy clinic or within the facility. Materials (e.g., pegs, cones, parquetry boards) are chosen for their potential to provide repetitive, structured practice of a specific component. Although therapists may improve underlying performance components, a number of problems may nevertheless persist.

One problem is that component-driven approaches bear the assumption that changing underlying components will automatically create changes in occupational performance. This is especially problematic when these approaches are imported without correlation to a larger, occupational framework. The goal of treatment becomes improvement of the underlying neurologic, kinesiologic, or psychodynamic components without analysis of their relationships to the client's occupational health and recovery. This approach has facilitated a "bottom-up" approach to treatment, described by Trombly (1995b) as "treatment to enable the person to accomplish the tasks of his life. . . preceded by treatment to increase strength and other capacities and abilities that contribute" (pp. 15–16). It is established knowledge that improvement of underlying performance components may not lead to desired changes in engagement in occupation (Trombly, 1995b). The client may leave occupational therapy with unaddressed occupational problems. To assume that changing performance components will automatically yield occupational outcomes represents adherence to a hierarchical view of order, disorder, and change. According to dynamic systems theory, change in complex organisms interacting with the environment is nonhierarchical in nature (Prigogine & Stengers, 1984). Occupation can be viewed as the output of a complex system interacting with the environment in which change cannot always be predicted by a hierarchical arrangement of multiple variables. Approaches based on remediation of component deficits have limited value in achieving occupational outcomes (Gray, Kennedy, & Zemke, 1996; Trombly, 1995b).

A second problem is that the client may be learning decontextualized skills that do not easily or readily transfer to his or her daily activities. This type of learning emphasizes the distinction between remediative and adaptive approaches that warrants scrutiny. The influence of the rehabilitation movement, in combination with the emphasis on inner mechanisms, has led to the categorization of treatment as either remediative, that is, geared toward improving components of performance, or adaptive, focused on changing the task or the environment to enable performance of occupations within current limitations. Quintana (1995a, 1995b) discussed remediation and adaptation in terms of cognitive and perceptual treatment and outlined some of the problems associated with the approaches, particularly remediative, that must be addressed in today's treatment strategies. Parallels can be drawn between her analyses and the remediation of neurologic, kinesiologic, and psychodynamic mechanisms interfering with occupation.

A recognized problem with the traditional remediative approaches is lack of generalizability (Quintana, 1995a, 1995b). Although clients may demonstrate progress in the performance of a given subskill, there is no substantial research that shows these skills are transferred to their daily occupations. Quintana summarized, "The results of much of the research presented seem to indicate that there is little generalization from one treatment task to another or from more remedial tasks to function" (p. 536). Motor learning research has revealed similar characteristics in the acquisition of motor skills (Mathiowetz & Haugen, 1995). Quintana (1995a, 1995b) and others (Toglia, 1991) recommended a different form of remediative approach, namely methods that help to bridge the gap between the skill being learned, whether cognitive, perceptual, or motor, and its incorporation into function. Occupation as a treatment modality, when given careful activity analysis and therapeutic structuring by an occupational therapist, can be the perfect venue for establishing more generalizable skills. More research is needed on the application of occupation as a treatment modality in this way (Trombly, 1995a; see Chapter 11).

Experience with persons with disabilities has also informed us that the choice between remediative and adaptive approaches is often much more ambiguous than it seems. People are not always ready to just "accept" that their physical bodies are not going to improve and therefore do not always readily accept or express interest in adaptive approaches, particularly early on in treatment. For many clients, adaptation seems to symbolize finality in terms of progress. People often want to be able to perform occupations in ways they previously performed them. The adaptation involved in occupational recovery takes time and is a process about which we, as occupational therapists, need more research. If occupational goals, developed in conjunction with the client, are at the center of treatment planning, decisions about how to integrate adaptation and remediation might become more clear.

A third problem with component-driven practice is that the client has been deprived of the other beneficial outcomes of an occupational treatment. Namely, occupation, when it is applied as activity with wholeness, purpose, and meaning to the person, can also affect him or her psychologically, emotionally, and socially in ways that purposeful activity unrelated to the person cannot. As Wood (1995) stated, "Engagement in meaningful occupations has a kind of multiplicative impact, not merely an additive one, upon a person's state of health" (p. 47). And finally, the client may still not have a clear understanding of the expertise of occupational therapy, which could lead to a lack of future inquiries or referrals should occupational problems ensue.

Narrowing of Occupation to Basic Activities of Daily Living (ADL)

In many rehabilitation facilities, occupational therapists are encouraged by team members and standardized outcome assessments to focus treatment planning on feeding, bathing, toileting, grooming, hygiene, and dressing. Although these self-care occupations are familiar and can be important to the client, they are often reflexively used without analysis of their therapeutic impact. Self-care occupations are therapeutically applied only when they have been identified as activities of importance and value to the client, are incorporated as personal rituals approximating the normalized context as much as possible, emphasize not only independence but also active engagement and possibilities for interdependence, and are structured to provide the "just-right challenge" in light of underlying physical and psychosocial impairments. Moreover, because self-care occupations can be uninteresting to many clients and overly threatening to others, they should not be the *only* occupations considered in occupational therapy at any time. Occupational therapists should feel free to use other occupations from the client's history, such as home and leisure occupations, to address the client's needs and should feel compelled to address all domains of the occupational person (Baum, 1997).

The above discussions of component-driven practice and the narrowing of occupation outline the primary difficulties occupational therapists have in maintaining an occupational perspective in treatment, particularly with adults with physical disabilities. Several treatment approaches exist, both remediative and adaptive, some conflicting, which therapists are compelled to apply in rehabilitation facilities without an overarching theoretical perspective that relates those approaches to occupation. As one solution, therapists may choose one treatment approach and apply it solely, focusing exclusively on components or basic ADL. In the meantime, research is exposing the limitations of these traditional hierarchical approaches. The climate is ripe for new perspectives; however, integrating occupation with the traditional approaches is not easy! Guidance on how to place occupation at the center of treatment may be needed.

The Solution: Occupation as Ends, Occupation as Means

In her Eleanor Clarke Slagle lecture, Trombly (1995a) (see Chapter 11) discussed *occupation as ends* and *occupation as means* as two ways we "consider" occupation or two "uses" of occupation. Her descriptions parallel the adaptive and remediative approaches. Trombly's discussion has value for occupational therapy. In extending her discussion, I offer below a slightly different analysis of the two concepts, using the work of several theorists within occupational therapy and occupational science. I believe that occupation as ends and occupation as means are not only ways in which occupational therapists use occupation in treatment, but also represent the unique realm of occupational therapy's expertise.

Occupation as Ends

Trombly (1995a) described *occupation as ends* as situations in which "occupation (is) the goal to be learned" (p. 963; see Chapter 11). She linked *occupation as ends* with the performance of activities, tasks, and roles toward a functional goal within the individual's capacities and abilities and likened it to the adaptive or rehabilitative approach. It is similar to *performing functional daily tasks* in the bottom-up treatment approach (Trombly, 1995b). According to Trombly, *occupation as ends* does *not* involve the use of occupation or purposeful and meaningful activity to improve performance components.

I believe occupation as ends need not be limited to the goal or desired outcome of an occupation-centered treatment, but rather can be the over-arching goal of all occupational therapy interventions. In the current health-care arena, it is difficult at times to establish any one rehabilitation professional as the expert in functional outcomes. Insurance companies are requesting results in the form of functional gains, and all disci-

plines must be concerned with the effect of their interventions on a client's ability to function. Nevertheless, I believe that occupational therapists have the strongest backgrounds of all rehabilitation specialists for analyzing, from a multidimensional perspective, an individual's ability to perform functional activities in context. Relative to occupation as ends, in other words, occupational therapists are experts in analyzing a person's ability to function in his or her environment, and thus to participate in personally satisfying, organized daily routines of culturally and developmentally relevant activities: occupation. Maintaining a focus on occupation as ends directs our concern toward a client's occupational health and requires that our assessments and treatment modalities reflect that overarching purpose.

What can occupational therapists draw upon to assert and reinforce our expertise in the area of occupation as ends? The literature within the profession, and specifically within occupational science (Zemke & Clark, 1996), provides a knowledge base for occupational therapy's concern with occupation as ends. A helpful conceptual resource is Rogers' (1982) analysis of the differences between medicine's and occupational therapy's determination of a state of order or disorder in an individual. Rogers contended that occupational therapists must recognize that the phenomena they analyze and treat are different from the phenomena addressed by many other health-care professionals. She proposed the "occupational therapy diagnosis" (p. 33), which reflects the occupational therapist's perspective on states of order and disorder in the human, and how to bring about change from disorder to order. She described the state of order, or "ends," toward which occupational therapy is directed as occupational performance or engagement. Occupational performance includes competence in self-care, work, and play "activities" (p. 30) and involves "integration of the biopsychosocial dimensions" (p. 30) of the human. Kielhofner and Burke (1983) also encompassed a reference to occupation as an intended outcome of treatment, in terms of occupational roles, in their discussion of the goals of early occupational therapy. They presented the first paradigm of occupational therapy as having a strong emphasis on occupation as ends and occupation as means without categorizing it as such. In applying this perspective to occupational therapy today, Burke (1983) described occupation as ends as follows:

> The issues to be confronted in the occupational
> therapy clinic are no longer just those related

to increasing functional abilities, but are more precisely defined according to the goals and objectives that will serve the client in reestablishing and selecting new methods for continuing their chosen occupational lives. (pp. 126–127)

Under this analysis of occupation as ends, everything that is done in occupational therapy evaluation and treatment should be directed toward the ultimate outcome of restoring client's "occupational lives." Therapists are called upon to analyze not only a client's performance of given occupations, but also his or her overall use of time, daily habits and routines, activities in relation to the developmental continuum, and need as an occupational being for creativity, competence, and challenge. A complex arrangement of any number of variables, including the environment, may be reinforcing or interfering with that person's ability to engage. It is the occupational therapist's charge to analyze that complexity and determine which variables must be altered to effect a change in the entire system. Once those variables are identified, the occupational therapist structures intervention to achieve the goal of occupation as ends. Many times, ideally, an occupation or an aspect of an occupation is used as the means to that ends.

Occupation as Means

Occupation as means, according to Trombly's (1995a) analysis, "refers to occupation acting as the therapeutic change agent to remediate impaired abilities or capacities" (p. 964; see Chapter 11). She described occupation as means as "limited to simple behaviors" (p. 963) and gave examples of purposeful, repetitive activity designed to enhance a particular motor component of performance, such as muscle imbalance or incoordination. The question arises: If the occupation as means is "limited to simple behaviors," is it still occupation; or might these simple behaviors be viewed instead as exercise or physical modalities to be used as adjuncts to occupation? I would suggest that often they are precursors to occupation, necessary for the enhancement of underlying components interfering with occupation, but are *not* occupation. Similar to physical agent modalities, these "simple behaviors" should not replace occupation, but should be used in preparation for and in conjunction with occupation (American Occupational Therapy Association, 1994).

I propose that *occupation as means* refers to the use of therapeutic occupation as the treatment modality to advance someone toward an occupational outcome. This may include the adaptation and practice of the intended occupation or the employment of thoughtfully structured occupation to alter relevant performance components. The critical difference between my analysis and Trombly's analysis concerns the definition of occupation and results in the observation that once you apply occupation as redefined, occupation as ends and occupation as means begin to merge together in the therapeutic context. Occupation as means, in my analysis, is not limited to simple behaviors, but rather refers to using activities that have the following criteria—perceived as "doing"; pertaining to the client's sense of self; goal-directed, personally meaningful; and culturally and developmentally relevant (Christiansen, 1994; Clark et al., 1991; Gray, 1997)—to "treat" physical, cognitive, and psychosocial components of performance. Occupation, in this sense, cannot be effectively used as treatment without completion of a thorough occupational history to determine what activities fit these criteria for a given individual, as well as to gain some perspective on the typical physical, temporal, and social context of the person's occupations.

As with occupation as ends, there are numerous accounts of the notion of occupation as means within occupational therapy literature, often with different terminology. Reilly (1958) described a curriculum for occupational therapy that would isolate and focus upon the unique contributions of the profession as "occupational therapy is treatment with activity" (p. 296). Trombly (1995a; see Chapter 11) referred to the work of Cynkin and Robinson (1990) in her discussion of occupation as means. Cynkin (1979) discussed the emphasis within occupational therapy on activities as "occupational therapy undertakes remedy by means of activities" (p. 6), and she discussed the question of "what makes activities therapeutic" (p. 29). According to her analysis, the profession of occupational therapy began with the use of activities as a therapeutic tool, initially with arts and crafts and then, influenced by the rehabilitation movement, with ADL in the areas of self-care, work, and leisure.

Using occupation as the therapeutic modality to affect performance components interfering with engagement in occupation and to enhance a person's recovery from any type of disabling condition may steer us away from what I have described in this paper as component-driven practice. It is not that occupational therapists should ignore components. An important aspect of the occupational therapist's evaluation is careful examination of all of the elements that may be interfering with occupational performance to ensure outcomes that endure and relate to the individual's life. Occupational therapists also need, however, to reconsider the power of occupation to treat those components. Rather than completing an assessment and using problem areas (components) to decide which activities to use for treatment (e.g., macrame is great for coordination, parquetry puzzles are assumed to help visual perceptual deficits), the occupational therapist has the added challenge of looking into the client's occupational history and selecting activities related to the client's occupations and interests that can be modified and structured to improve coordination and visual perception. Perhaps that particular client enjoyed waxing the car, making fried chicken, or playing with his or her nieces. The occupational therapist could, with a little creativity and ingenuity, tailor those occupations to treat the very same coordination or visual perceptual deficits.

When occupation is used in this way, it has more relevance to the person's life, it more clearly emphasizes the expertise of occupational therapy to clients and health-care team members, and it has the benefit of overlapping cognitive, perceptual, kinetic, and psychosocial dimensions that a puzzle or purely motor task may not offer. Instead of being two distinct conditions as Trombly (1995a) described, occupation as ends and occupation as means exist simultaneously within the above treatment examples (see Chapter 11). Perspectives that separate "treating underlying components" and "performing functional daily tasks" as mutually exclusive categories seem to neglect this essential element of treatment and to suggest that occupation is incapable of affecting performance components; I propose a use of occupation as means that recognizes the powerful impact of therapeutic occupation on both component and occupational recovery.

Occupation, applied in this manner, is a unique contribution to a client's recovery. It is not, however, easy to do. Clients sometimes resist engaging in activities that may actually illuminate their weaknesses. Other health-care professionals often do not see the value of and scientific expertise behind the everyday tasks involved in therapeutic occupation. Clients and family members may subscribe to the widely held belief that if the body is healed, everything else will fall into place. Trombly (1995a; see Chapter 11) also identified the problem of the inconsistencies that arise among different therapists in analyzing the components of occupation for their therapeutic potential. All of these observations have some truth, but ignore the reality that occupation can be a valuable tool in a person's recovery that does not have to take the place of the healing of the body, but can actually supplement and enhance it, or even be the catalyst for healing. That using occupation in this way might present problems in terms of quantifying performance and progress should not be seen as a reason for not using occupation, but rather an area requiring more investigation by occupational therapists and occupational scientists. Using occupation to affect performance components is generally supported by current motor learning research, which suggests the need to practice skills with more variety in a more natural context (Mathiowetz & Haugen, 1995). The need for more research is clear. To apply occupation as means effectively, the occupational therapist must understand the complexity of action in the environment and the involvement of a number of systems in normal action.

Case Application: Alejandro

Top-Down Approach to Evaluation

As in all my cases, an initial outpatient occupational therapy evaluation was completed for the case of Alejandro to determine the occupational therapy diagnosis and to outline, in terms of long and short-term goals, the desired occupational outcomes (occupation as ends). The occupational evaluation followed a top-down approach (Trombly, 1993), beginning with a thorough occupational history, followed by evaluation of occupational performance, then relevant performance components. The occupational history reflected the work of Mattingly and Fleming (1994) on the narrative nature of clinical reasoning in occupational therapy and Clark's (1993) occupational storytelling and story making and revealed Alejandro's occupations and interests before and since his injuries. The key areas of occupation addressed included selfcare, home management, community activities and involvement, avocations and leisure, work, and daily routine and use of time. Alejandro's goals were discussed and incorporated into his treatment plan.

Occupational and Medical History

Alejandro is 50 years old and has been living with his parents in a house in South Central Los Angeles after rehabilitation from an assault in 1982. Before that assault, Alejandro was living alone. He is divorced. He was married for approximately 20 years and has four grown children. Before his injuries, Alejandro worked full-time for several years for a sign-making company as a factory mechanic. During his free time, often spent with his son, he played soccer and pool and enjoyed watching sports with his children.

Alejandro's initial injury occurred on his way home from work. He took the bus to and from work, and his usual shift ended in the middle of the night. Alejandro was waiting for the bus when he was mugged and attacked by a couple of men, who hit him over the head with a baseball bat. He was immediately hospitalized and underwent brain surgery, then subsequently transferred to another hospital for additional surgery and rehabilitation. He was discharged from inpatient rehabilitation to live with his parents and, in his words, it "works well for everyone" because they are older and benefit from having him around.

Alejandro indicated that he was in a wheelchair for a year after his injury and that his recovery had been taking a long time. He reported becoming very depressed at the reality of spending all that time in the wheelchair and not being able to do many things he did before the assault. It took Alejandro a long time to get to the point where he was able to leave the house to participate in activities with family members again. He still experienced a great deal of fear related to the incident. Family relations were strained at times, and he could not always rely on family members for transportation or other assistance.

In 1995, 13 years after his original accident, Alejandro was hit by a car as he was crossing the street. He suffered multiple injuries, including a possible closed-head injury, and was hospitalized again. His right upper and lower extremities were in casts, and his physical mobility was significantly limited. After hospitalization, Alejandro was again discharged to live at home with his parents, but described that everything was much more difficult than the first time. He was no longer able to get around, and he experienced significant pain and difficulty using his right side. He did not leave the house for any activities and, in addition to the decline in his overall ability to move and to do things for himself, the anxiety and depression that he had been experiencing since his initial assault had become nearly overwhelming for him. Once he was able get around a little, he resumed appointments at a county medical clinic for psychiatric consults and medications for anxiety and depression. It was via these appointments that the rehabilitation medical director encountered Alejandro and noted that he had significant restrictions in terms of his mobility and

had not overcome the decline in functional status resulting from the second accident. He admitted Alejandro for another course of inpatient rehabilitation from August 9 to September 6, 1996, which included occupational, physical, and speech therapies.

When Alejandro left the rehabilitation unit, he was able to walk with an assistive device and was able to do his personal care and some simple homemaking activities. He had made many friends on the inpatient unit and enjoyed spending time straightening the rehabilitation day room when he was not in therapy. He was discharged home with outpatient physical therapy. The physical therapist realized that Alejandro was experiencing difficulties in a number of areas and recommended outpatient speech therapy and occupational therapy as well.

During the occupational therapy evaluation, Alejandro expressed difficulty in various occupational areas. He was performing all self-care without problems. He sometimes participated in the home management, preparing meals or portions of meals, and especially liked to be involved in housecleaning. It was eventually disclosed that he did have some difficulties, however, in the kitchen, particularly with leaving a burner on and burning himself or food on occasion. He described consistent criticism that he received from his parents about his errors and his slowness at home. They did not seem to understand the nature of his mistakes and their relation to his brain injury. When questioned, Alejandro was certain that they would not be available for or interested in any type of family training or education.

In terms of community occupations, Alejandro's primary involvement was at a county hospital, where he attended numerous medical appointments, and at our facility, where he had become well-known during his inpatient stay and seemed to feel comfortable and attached. He did some errands on foot in his neighborhood but revealed that he would often make errors, such as buying two of one item at the market and none of something else that his mother had listed. He avoided all family gatherings. He did not drive or participate in any leisure or work activities. He was taking the bus to therapy, which took 2 hours each way, and reported incidents of extreme anxiety and fear about interactions with other passengers. At times, Alejandro would come to therapy and barely speak. When we attempted to discuss what was going on with him, he would describe a situation in which he had been scolded by his parents for making a mistake, had left a burner on, or had accidentally bumped someone on the bus with his cane and they had made a nasty remark to him. He seemed to live in almost constant, often disabling fear. When we discussed Alejandro's goals and the occupations he had enjoyed in the past, he would frequently comment on being extremely depressed.

Establishing Alejandro's Goals

Alejandro wanted to be able to "do everything" for himself, without problems, and was very interested in doing things for others. His ultimate goal was some sort of work, but initially he frequently discussed the idea of becoming a volunteer, preferably at the hospital, to "give back" what he had received. The "occupational end" toward which Alejandro's occupational therapy program was structured incorporated these long-term goals:

1. Independent and safe participation in home management tasks

2. Independent management of his daily schedule, incorporating use of a day planner and memory tool (in coordination with speech therapy)

3. Independent involvement in some type of support group addressing the psychosocial and emotional needs of individuals recovering from brain injury

4. Identification of leisure interests and beginning participation in one or two leisure activities as identified by the client

5. Exploration of and involvement in alternate transportation, preferably the county-provided transportation for people with disabilities

6. Involvement in a volunteer position, preferably closer to his home and community, providing some variation among his community outlets

I felt that all of these occupations, if engaged in on I regular basis with success, could have a positive impact on Alejandro's overall state of fearfulness and perception of himself.

Identifying Performance Assets and Impairments

Subsequent to the occupational history, performance components were evaluated to determine which variables were most *limiting* Alejandro's ability to participate in desired occupations and which variables were *contributing* in a positive way to his overall engagement. Physical, cognitive, and emotional components of performance were addressed.

Motor Control and Upper-Extremity Functional Use

Evaluations of range of motion and motor control were performed after observation of Alejandro's functional use of his upper extremities. He presented with limited shoulder range of motion, pain in his right upper extremity, and difficulty with rapid control. He was, however, able to use the right upper extremity functionally in any activity that did not require reaching overhead. He was receiving physical therapy and, after conference with occupational therapy, it was decided that physical therapy would address his right upperextremity range and pain problems. This way, the occupational therapy time could be spent on issues more directly related to his occupations, because his upper-extremity status was not a major limiting variable. Alejandro's physical mobility was generally functional for his desired home, community, and work-related occupations, and was considered an asset.

Cognition and Visual Perception

Cognition and visual perception were evaluated during observation of functional performance. Alejandro presented with moderate difficulties in his new learning and short-term memory, including recall of daily events. He had a memory book that he was beginning to use in speech therapy, and he required maximum cuing to incorporate the information into his daily routine and activities. He demonstrated good selective attention to structured tasks but difficulty with alternating or divided attention (hence the frequent accidents while cooking). He also demonstrated the ability to learn new tasks, starting at two to three steps at a time, but required maximum assistance with organization, planning, and problem solving. Alejandro's ability to learn new tasks with repetition and to recall global daily events were assets; however, cognition overall, in terms of memory for specific details and higherlevel attentional and organizational skills, was significantly limiting his ability to participate in desired occupations. Vision and visual processing were functional for reading and other daily activities.

Psychosocial and Emotional Factors

An absolutely essential discovery during Alejandro's evaluation was the realization that his anxiety, depression, and negative images of himself were playing a large part in his ability or inability to function on a daily basis. From Alejandro's accounts, these emotions were often debilitating. He would, in his words, "close down," unable to be around people or talk to anyone, if he had an awkward encounter with a stranger or became lost or confused in any way. Consequently he would miss appointments, remain lost, and so forth.

He was seeing a psychiatrist monthly and receiving medications; however, he had no daily or weekly support for these issues.

On the positive side, when he was not emotionally distressed about something, Alejandro was and is an extremely well-liked, polite, and considerate person. He made several acquaintances on the rehabilitation unit, and everyone had nothing but positive comments to make about him. He was somewhat reserved, but he demonstrated a high level of concern for others. This led to the sense that most difficulties Alejandro might have in social situations might be due to his inner life rather than his interactions with other people.

Alejandro's Occupational Therapy Program

I have seen Alejandro two to three times weekly in outpatient occupational therapy for approximately 9 months. The team worked together to establish a comprehensive and consistent program for Alejandro. He has been seen for an extraordinary length of time, but it has been justified based upon continued progress and remaining functional goals. Treatment included occupations or related activities that were either part of Alejandro's life or his occupational goals. The occupations were structured to influence the above performance components. In other words, every occupation was graded to challenge Alejandro's memory, planning, and organizational skills, as well as to provide a successful outcome to promote feelings of competence, mastery, and self-esteem. The following examples of occupation used in treatment with Alejandro are organized around the above long-term goals as well as chronologically.

Home Management

Alejandro planned a cooking activity of preparing a Mexican soup, an occupation that related to his environment and interests, which led to the discovery of difficulties he was having with his memory book. He planned to bring items for the soup and left them twice, once by the door at home and once on the bus. When all items were available, Alejandro performed well with this cooking activity, and the level of challenge was increased.

Next, Alejandro planned to make taquitos and guacamole. This occupation took several sessions to complete and involved opportunities for problem solving, practicing organizational skills, and using the memory book. Alejandro wanted to bring the chicken and gua-

camole from home so that we would not have to make both items in our 1-hour session. Within treatment, he made a menu and grocery list then went to a nearby market. We incorporated compensatory strategies, and Alejandro successfully purchased all but one item on the list without assistance. In the following session we made taquitos, incorporating a timer as another memory tool. An important goal of this occupation as the means of intervention was to influence the emotional components of Alejandro's performance. Alejandro was teaching me during these sessions. I had never made taquitos before, and he was obviously an expert. We spent a few sessions practicing the same tasks until Alejandro needed only occasional cuing for safety or use of the timer. The taquitos and guacamole were a hit! Everyone wanted his recipe for the guacamole. He spent additional sessions writing down the recipe and demonstrating, for several clients and staff members, how to make the guacamole. Again, all of these tasks required Alejandro to plan and organize; thus the occupation was used as a treatment for cognitive and emotional components.

Daily Schedule and Memory Book

As we attempted to expand his occupational repertoire, Alejandro had difficulty keeping track of changes and new activities that required action away from the hospital. A system was developed by the speech therapist, Alejandro, and myself that simplified his memory book and added space for daily "to do" lists. It was incorporated in treatment each visit to assist Alejandro in planning ahead for activities that could not be accomplished in the same day, such as recalling items he needed to bring for therapy or phone calls he needed to make. Alejandro was also involved in the tasks of making the new book, many of which were similar to work-related occupations. He photocopied the pages to go in the book and dated the new pages, again addressing cognitive components.

Community Support Group

Alejandro agreed that a brain injury support group might be helpful in dealing with his emotional and interpersonal difficulties. We looked at the list of local groups, and Alejandro chose one close to his home. We planned to attend the group together. Alejandro made the telephone calls to inquire regarding details of the group and arranged his own transportation. I was unable to attend the first session, and Alejandro decided to go on his own, which was a big step. Alejandro came to his next therapy session raving about the group. He had spent a long time in front of the group telling his story and everyone had clapped at the end. It was a very positive experience for him, and he has continued to attend independently.

Leisure

Alejandro explored his leisure interests in occupational therapy through discussion and completion of the Interest Check List (Matsutsuyu, 1969). There may not be enough therapy time (in terms of reimbursement) to pursue this area further, but I speculate that if other occupational areas are intact and Alejandro has good community support and reliable transportation, he may eventually pursue this on his own.

Transportation

Alejandro was involved in all of the steps of applying for county-provided transportation for individuals with disabilities. He completed, addressed, and mailed the application, partly in therapy and partly on his own, and I added information on Alejandro's cognitive and emotional difficulties, with his approval. Alejandro then called for a personal interview, recording necessary information into his memory book. He attended the interview on his own and was granted services. We reviewed the criteria for use of the services, including how and when to call for a pickup. He initially used the service to attend the brain injury support group because he did not want to take the bus in the evening. He was dropped off at the group on time, but unfortunately waited a couple of hours after the group for his ride home, which instilled some fear about using the service. He has used it again, with hesitance, to attend the support group, but not to attend therapy due to fear he will be late.

Vocational or Volunteer Work

Occupations performed in the above areas addressed performance components necessary for success in a volunteer position, such as organizational skills and effective use of a memory tool in daily tasks. Alejandro was also given prevolunteer activities, specifically two-to-three-step repetitive tasks that involved new learning and could be completed within one session. He was encouraged to evaluate his own performance at the end of each session. The tasks were graded for more difficulty and either additional steps were added, unfamiliar tasks were used, or Alejandro was assigned responsibility for task set-up and organization as well

as completion. Examples of tasks are assembly of soft charts for outpatient therapies, photocopying, collating, filing, and making deliveries.

Alejandro demonstrated the ability to learn new activities of up to three to four steps with a significant amount of repetition but consistently required a moderate amount of assistance to set up and organize those tasks He could not switch among different activities without assistance. He also had a difficult time evaluating his performance in a balanced way. If he made no errors, his performance was good; otherwise he focused on mistakes and could not evaluate in detail his problems and improvements. Toward the end of this process, Alejandro worked on these tasks with only distant supervision and was responsible for contacting the therapist when he became confused or had a problem or question about his work. He needed to become accustomed to gauging his own performance and working without constant monitoring by someone else.

Alejandro remained insistent upon volunteering at our facility. I contacted the director of volunteers and made an appointment for Alejandro and me to meet her during one of his sessions. We discussed the general requirements of volunteering as well as Alejandro's goals, abilities, and limitations. I proposed a transition to volunteering that would include the occupational therapist as a "job coach." We decided that Alejandro would begin at the front desk with the tasks of delivering mail, packages, and flowers. He was given instructions regarding the necessary steps of application, most of which he completed outside of therapy time. Alejandro began volunteering during his occupational therapy sessions, and continues his volunteering as this article is being written. At his suggestion, he is now doing 1 of 3 days without coaching and is progressing toward being discharged from occupational therapy.

The above outlines the primary occupations used in treatment with Alejandro. These included planning a snack, cooking Mexican soup and taquitos, grocery shopping, making a memory book, photocopying, making telephone calls, making deliveries within the hospital, attending a brain injury support group, and applying for public transportation. Of course, as sessions progressed, there were also opportunities for troubleshooting in relation to Alejandro's daily activities. He asked the therapist to make phone calls for him (e.g., to his dentist when his tooth was bothering him, the front desk regarding transportation) and he was required and assisted in therapy to make those arrangements himself. He had to make a decision about a shower chair because he had bought a used one that was unsafe. Modifications were made to his backpack strapping because it exacerbated his right shoulder pain. He worked with speech therapy on organizing and labeling his medications. The emphasis remained, in any activity, on Alejandro's ability to use memory tools, solve problems, and organize to ensure successful outcomes. and to promote feelings of competence and mastery. There were many times when all therapists working with Alejandro needed to discuss his psychosocial issues. I attempted to link those discussions to his performance in occupations and to the interpersonal and communication skills he would need for his goal of becoming a worker in the future.

Conclusion

The above discussion and case presentation are intended to provide occupational therapists with a practical solution to the difficulty many experience in keeping occupation at the center of treatment. I believe that recognizing and analyzing *occupation as ends* and *occupation as means* as the unique focus within occupational therapy can help guide treatment planning. The case of Alejandro provides an example. Alejandro's occupational goals—home management, community involvement, and work or volunteerism—guided treatment planning. We worked on the performance components that most strongly interfered with these goals, namely cognition and emotion, through the structuring and grading of several occupations, activities that were relevant to Alejandro's goals and interests. These sessions also provided opportunities for practice and adaptation toward Alejandro's occupational goals. When treatment is structured in this way, emphasizing the client's occupational goals and providing structured occupation to achieve those goals, remediation and adaptation, occupation as ends and occupation as means, begin to merge together in a single occupational therapy session. Treatment more closely relates to the client's life, providing greater opportunities for transference. The complexity of everyday occupation in context is recognized and addressed.

Such a grounding in occupation that is clearly manifested in treatment can, in turn, influence occupational therapy's reputation and collective spirit. The survival of the profession may seriously rest in each occupational therapist's ability to give coherent and attractive answers to the prevailing questions: "What is occupational therapy?" and "What do occupational therapists do that is different from other health care professionals?" Baum (1997) suggested that "the occupational therapy practitioner must see himself or herself as having expertise to address the self-care, productivity, and leisure needs of clients and their families" (p. 2). I would like to modify Baum's suggestion to include *the occupational therapy practitioner must see himself or herself as having expertise...* period. We know how to assess functional performance, how to communicate with clients to determine their interests and goals, and how to analyze activities and patterns of activity for problems and adaptive benefits. All these skills indicate occupational therapy's expertise in human engagement in purposeful and meaningful activity. Other health-care team members do not possess this occupational expertise.

Many people may not ascribe to the expanded definition of occupation that our profession uses but would rapidly begin to understand our focus if our treatment, documentation, and other reporting centered around the client as an occupational being and our concern for his or her ability to participate in meaningful, productive, and satisfying daily routines of self-care, work, rest, and play, at any stage of the developmental continuum. In this way, what we do and what we discuss with our clients would correspond to the name of our profession. Reilly's (1962) prediction (see Chapter 7) made over 35 years ago that "society will require that we occupational therapists grow up to our name" (p. 224) is most apt in the current health-care climate.

Acknowledgments

I thank Dr. Wendy Wood for her mentorship and support in the preparation of this article and Jaynee Taguchi for her encouragement and assistance via numerous conversations on the above ideas. The occupational science faculty at the University of Southern California have greatly influenced my ability to understand occupation and, therefore, my clinical practice, over the last several years. I also thank the individual, who shall remain anonymous, who willingly allowed me to share his story in order that others may benefit and learn.

References

American Occupational Therapy Association. (1994). *A guide for the preparation of occupational therapy practitioners for the use of physical agent modalities.* Rockville, MD: Author.

Baum, C. (1997). The managed-care system: The educator's opportunity. *Education Special Interest Section Quarterly, 7*(2), 1–3.

Burke, J. P. (1983). Defining occupation: Importing and organizing interdisciplinary knowledge. In G. Kielhofner (Ed.), *Health through occupation: Theory and practice in occupational therapy* (pp. 125–138). Philadelphia: F. A. Davis.

Christiansen, C. (1994). Classification and study in occupation: A review and discussion of taxonomies. *Journal of Occupational Science (Australia), 1(3),* 3–21.

Clark, F. (1993). Occupation embedded in real life: Interweaving occupational science and occupational therapy, 1993 Eleanor Clarke Slagle lecture. *American Journal of Occupational Therapy, 47,* 1067–1078. http://dx.doi.org/10.5014/ajot.47.12.1067

Clark, F. A., Parham, D., Carlson, M. E., Frank, G., Jackson, J., Pierce, D., Wolfe, R. J., & Zemke, R (1991). Occupational science: Academic innovation in the service of occupational therapy's future. *American Journal of Occupational Therapy, 45,* 300–310. http://dx.doi.org/10.5014/ajot.45.4.300

Cynkin, S. (1979). *Occupational therapy: Toward health through activities.* Boston: Little, Brown.

Cynkin, S., & Robinson, J. M. (1990). *Occupational therapy and activities health: Toward health through activities.* Boston: Little, Brown.

Gray, J. M. (1997). Application of the phenomenological method to the concept of occupation. *Journal of Occupational Science (Australia), 4(1),* 5–17.

Gray, J. M., Kennedy, B. L., & Zemke, R. (1996). Application of dynamic systems theory to occupation. In R. Zemke & F. Clark (Eds.), *Occupational science: The evolving discipline* (pp. 309–324). Philadelphia: F. A. Davis.

Kielhofner, G., & Burke, J. P. (1983). The evolution of knowledge and practice in occupational therapy: Past, present, and future. In G. Kielhofner (Ed.), *Health through occupation: Theory and practice in occupational therapy* (pp. 3–54). Philadelphia: F. A. Davis.

Mathiowetz, V., & Haugen, J. B. (1995). Evaluation of motor behavior: Traditional and contemporary views. In C. A. Trombly (Ed.) *Occupational therapy for physical dysfunction* (4th ed., pp. 157–186). Baltimore: Williams & Wilkins.

Matsutsuyu, J. S. (1969). The Interest Check List. *American Journal of Occupational Therapy, 23,* 323–328.

Mattingly, C., & Fleming, M. H. (1994). *Clinical reasoning. Forms of inquiry in a therapeutic practice.* Philadelphia: F. A. Davis.

Prigogine, I., & Stengers, I. (1984). *Order out of chaos: Man's new dialogue with nature.* New York: Bantam Books.

Quintana, L. A. (1995a). Remediating cognitive impairments. In C. A. Trombly (Ed.), *Occupational therapy for physical dysfunction* (4th ed., pp. 539–548). Baltimore: Williams & Wilkins.

Quintana, L. A. (1995b). Remediating perceptual impairments. In C. A. Trombly (Ed.), *Occupational therapy for physical dysfunction* (4th ed., pp. 529–537). Baltimore: Williams & Wilkins.

Reilly, M. (1958). An occupational therapy curriculum for 1965. *American Journal of Occupational Therapy, 12,* 293–299.

Reilly, M. (1962). Occupational therapy can be one of the great ideas of 20th century medicine. *American Journal of Occupational Therapy, 16,* 1–9. Reprinted as Chapter 7.

Rogers, J. C. (1982). Order and disorder in medicine and occupational therapy. *American Journal of Occupational Therapy, 36,* 29–35.

Toglia, J. P. (1991). Generalization of treatment: A multicontext approach to cognitive perceptual impairment in adults with brain injury. *American Journal of Occupational Therapy, 45,* 505–516. http://dx.doi.org/10.5014/ajot.45.6.505

Trombly, C. A. (1993). The Issue Is—Anticipating the future: Assessment of occupational function. *American Journal of Occupational Therapy, 47,* 253–257.

Trombly, C. A. (1995a). Occupation: Purposefulness and meaningfulness as therapeutic mechanisms, 1995 Eleanor Clarke Slagle lecture. *American Journal of Occupational Therapy, 49,* 960–972. Reprinted as Chapter 11.

Trombly, C. A. (1995b). Theoretical foundations for practice. In C. A. Trombly (Ed.), *Occupational therapy for physical dysfunction* (4th ed.). Baltimore: Williams & Wilkins.

Wood, W. (1995). Weaving the warp and weft of occupational therapy: An art and science for all times. *American Journal of Occupational Therapy, 49,* 44–52. http://dx.doi.org/10.5014/ajot.49.1.44

Wood, W. (1998). Nationally Speaking—It is jump time for occupational therapy. *American Journal of Occupational Therapy.* http://dx.doi.org/10.5014/ajot.52.6.403

Zemke, R., & Clark, F. (Eds.). (1996). *Occupational science: The evolving discipline.* Philadelphia: F. A. Davis.

CHAPTER 11

Occupation: Purposefulness and Meaningfulness as Therapeutic Mechanisms

1995 ELEANOR CLARKE SLAGLE LECTURE

CATHERINE A. TROMBLY

I chose the topic of therapeutic occupation because that was what attracted me to the profession, and it is the concept about which I have thought most. I became an occupational therapist because I liked arts and crafts and "medical things." When I was about 11 years old, my friend's sister came home with paintings and jewelry and other things she had made at college. She was enrolled in the occupational therapy program at the University of New Hampshire and told me she was preparing to work in a hospital using arts and crafts to help people get better. I decided then and there that that was the profession for me. So eventually I went to the university and enjoyed learning all those activities. Those were the days when a large proportion of the curriculum was devoted to developing knowledge and skill in crafts. We learned technique from artists and theory in our occupational therapy classes. We learned that activities were therapeutic because they were purposeful; that is, they demanded certain responses that might be deficient in people who had a disease or injury, and that by doing activities, people improved their skills and abilities. We learned how to adapt activities to change the demands as the person changed. We also learned that because the person got to choose from several activities that demanded similar responses, the chosen activity was meaningful and kept the person interested and working. These beliefs were based on anecdotal observations passed down from early occupational therapists.

These beliefs are still taught, but have hardly been researched. Current economic and scientific forces in our society require us to provide support for the hypothesis that engagement in purposeful and meaningful occupation improves impaired abilities or produces occupa-

tional functioning. It would be to our advantage also to discover *how* therapeutic occupation brings about those changes so that we can treat more effectively.

Because I have always felt the need to know more about what made occupation therapeutic, I took the opportunity of this lecture to attempt to sort out some concepts concerning therapeutic occupation for myself and to pull together evidence for whether and how occupation is therapeutic. My goal is to spark an explosion of research concerning therapeutic occupation.

If there is novelty in this lecture, to paraphrase White (1959), it lies in examining pieces that already lie before us, in seeing how to fit those pieces into a larger conceptual picture, and in determining what new pieces are needed to complete the picture.

Occupation

In the early days of occupational therapy, crafts were as diversions, as general methods of recovery from disease and injury (Llorens, 1993; Slagle, 1914), and for their utilitarian value because products were produced that could be sold (Haas, 1922). The purpose of the craft was to keep the patient occupied so that manic or depressive thoughts would be replaced (Dunton, 1914). Replacement happened because one cannot think about two things at once and occupation compelled attention. Believed prerequisite to the therapeutic value of the craft were the patient's feelings of interest and personal pride, which the instructor needed to instill if not evoked by the activity itself (Purdum, 1911). It was Susan Tracy who moved occupational therapy into the general hospital (Barrows, 1917; Editorial, 1929). She emphasized that the product was the patient, not the article he or she makes, and thereby changed the focus of occupation from a money-making enterprise to a specific therapeutic one (Barrows, 1917; Parsons, 1917). Occupation was primarily prescribed to remediate impairment (Barrows, 1917; Swaim, 1928), although there is a report that Tracy developed what we now call a *universal cuff* to enable persons to feed themselves (Cameron, 1917). By 1930, therapists were being invited to move beyond remediation to join the rehabilitation effort. The philosophy of rehabilitation is to focus not on what is lost, but on what capabilities remain, to prepare the person for return to the fullness of life's activities (Lowney, 1930). Occupation came to include activities of daily living (ADL) and prevocational training.

In the past several years papers have been written and several conferences held to discuss occupation, but consensus about what occupation is and is not continues to elude us. Nelson (1988) presented a detailed conceptualization of occupation in which he defined occupation as the relationship between occupational form and occupational performance. By *occupational form* he meant the task demands and environmental context. By *occupational performance* he meant the act of doing. According to his view, *therapeutic occupation* is the synthesis of an occupational form by the occupational therapist that either enables the patient to compensate to achieve a goal activity or produces an adaptive change in what Nelson called the person's developmental structure (1990). In this conceptualization, any voluntary activity a person does of *whatever complexity* is considered occupation as long as the occupational form of the activity has meaning from the person's point of view and the performance is based on a sense of purpose. According to this conceptualization, reaching for something of interest and preparing one's lunch are both occupations.

Occupation is limited to complex activity sequences by others. Clark and her colleagues (1991) defined occupation as "chunks of culturally and personally meaningful activity in which humans engage that can be named in the lexicon of the culture" (p. 301). By that they meant such things as doing one's job, dressing, cooking, and gardening. Christiansen and Baum, as reported by Christiansen (1991), defined *occupation* as all goal-oriented behavior related to daily living, including spiritual and sexual activities. In their view, the basic unit of occupation is activity. They defined *activity* as specific goal-oriented behavior directed toward the performance of a task. Bathing is an example of a task; filling the bathtub and washing one's self are examples of activities. They acknowledged that abilities are required to engage in activities and tasks, but did not seem to include this level in their characterization of occupation. *Occupation,* as defined by Clark and her colleagues

and by Christiansen and Baum, seems to assume ability to perform. For those who treat patients with physical impairments, occupation thus defined is problematic because most of our patients cannot perform.

A Model of Practice for Physical Dysfunction

I want to suggest a different way of considering therapeutic occupation, but first I need to tell you how I view the practice of occupational therapy for adults with physical dysfunction and define some terms. I am limiting my examples to physical dysfunction because that is what I know best, although the ideas apply to many areas of practice. The model I am presenting is not my original idea. I think it has been used since the inception of the application of occupational therapy to this population, but I have named it the model of occupational functioning (Trombly, 1993). This model of practice parallels a certain conceptualization of occupational performance. This conceptualization of occupational performance is a descending hierarchy of roles, tasks, activities, abilities, and capacities (see Figure 11.1).

In the model of occupational functioning, the goal of occupational therapy is to develop a sense of competency and selfesteem. A competent person has sufficient resources to interact effectively with the physical or social environments and to meet the demands of a situation (White, 1959). A sense of competency is highly associated with feelings of self-efficacy (Abler & Fretz, 1988; Bandura, 1977), a belief that one is capable of accomplishing a goal. To be competent means to be able to satisfactorily engage in one's life roles (or to voluntarily reassign a role to another). The American Occupational Therapy Association (AOTA) (1994) categorized roles into the three performance areas of work, play and leisure, and activities of daily living. However, I prefer to categorize roles from the point of view of the person (Trombly, 1993)—for example, roles that relate to self-achievement or productivity; roles that are essentially self-enhancing or that add pleasure or joy to one's life; and roles that maintain the self, which in my view includes family preservation and home maintenance.

Any categorization, however, is deceptive in that it implies that particular roles can be unequivocally classified into one category or another. They cannot. A particular person may categorize one role as an achievement–productivity role, whereas someone else

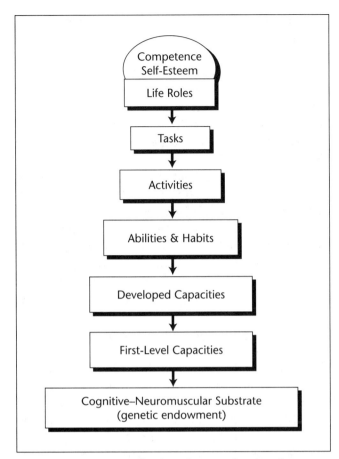

Figure 11.1. Conceptualization of occupational performance.

may classify the same role as an enhancement–recreational role. The example that comes quickest to mind is the role of shopper. For some persons shopping is recreation and adds joy to their lives; for others, shopping is a chore done simply to acquire the raw materials needed for living. The category depends upon the meaning that the role has for the person. This fact becomes readily apparent when we note the results of a study by Yerxa and Locker (1990). They examined how 15 subjects with spinal cord injury categorized their daily activities. They found that the same activity was often placed into different categories. For example, eating was categorized by different subjects as self-maintenance, rest, play, and "other."

In order to engage satisfactorily in a life role, a person must be able to do the tasks and activities that make up that role within the natural context. Some tasks are essential to the role and must be mastered by whoever chooses the role. For example, the role of bus driver requires that the person be able to do the activity of steering the bus on a city street. Other roles are defined by the person so that the same role may be constituted

in terms of different tasks by different persons. For example, one woman might consider the task of helping with homework an essential aspect of her mother role, whereas another, like the patient with chronic back pain interviewed by Nelson and Payton (1991), might consider roughhousing with her children as very important to that role. The patient, or a significant other, decides which roles the patient should work toward resuming. Furthermore, the person decides which tasks and activities constitute particular roles according to his or her values as well as sociocultural mores and expectations.

To go on with the description of the occupational functioning model, tasks are composed of *activities*, which are smaller units of behavior. For example, peeling a potato is an activity within the task of meal preparation. To continue further down the hierarchy, in order to be able to do a given activity, one has to have certain sensorimotor, cognitive, perceptual, emotional, and social abilities. *Abilities* are skills that one has developed through practice and that underlie many different activities—for example, eye-hand coordination. Abilities emanate from developed capacities that the person has gained through learning or maturation. *Developed capacities* are refinements, gained through maturation and learning, of biologically based capacities. Graded grasp to accommodate the size and shape of an object is an example of a developed capacity. Developed capacities depend upon first-level capacities. *First-level capacities* are reflex-based responses or subroutines that underlie voluntary movement and derive from a person's genetic endowment or spared organic substrate. For example, reflexive grasp and reflexive release, which underlie the higher capacity of graded grasp, are first-level capacities.

In this conceptualization, complex occupations, such as maintenance of one's clothes, have progressively simpler occupations nested within them (see Figure 11.2) (e.g., doing the laundry, hanging clothes on a clothesline, fastening the clothespin, grasping the clothespin). This nesting contributes to our quandary in characterizing what is, and what is not, occupation and in building a theory of therapeutic occupation. A second dimension that makes occupation difficult to define is time: occupations comprise a range of time from brief moments to the entire lifespan (Nelson, 1988; Yerxa et al., 1990). So not only does occupation have a vertical dimension, complexity, as I have just described, but it also has a horizontal dimension, time.

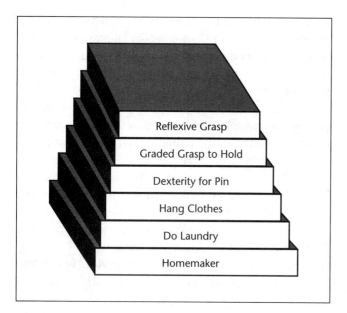

Figure 11.2. Nesting of levels of occupation.

Another Look at Occupation

For me, one way to begin the characterization of occupation was to notice, in the process of thinking about the occupational functioning model, that in some situations we consider occupation as the goal to be learned and in other situations we consider occupation as the change agent. I have termed these *occupation-as-end* and *occupation-as-means*. I suggest this distinction because I think the goals and therapeutic processes of these two forms of occupation are different. Furthermore, there is historical basis for this separation because these two uses of occupation came into occupational therapy practice at different times. I equate the idea of occupation-as-end to the levels of activities, tasks, and roles in the occupational functioning model. At each of these levels, the person has a functional goal and tries to accomplish it by using what abilities and capacities he or she has. I think this is close to how Clark and others (1991) and Christiansen and Baum (Christiansen, 1991) defined occupation. Occupation-as-means, on the other hand, is *the therapy* used to bring about changes in impaired performance components. Occupation at this level often is limited to simple behaviors. Both occupation-as-end and occupation-as-means garner their therapeutic impact from the qualities of purposefulness and meaningfulness.

Purposefulness in Occupation-as-End

Occupation-as-end is purposeful by definition. According to many occupational therapy writers, purposeful

occupation-asend organizes a person's behavior, day, and life (Kielhofner, 1985, 1992; Meyer, 1922/1977 [see Chapter 4]; Slagle, 1914; Yerxa & Baum, 1986; Yerxa & Locker, 1990; Yerxa et al., 1990). Early occupational "workers" imposed purposeful occupation on persons who could not choose it for themselves; they were then able to act in more healthy ways (Slagle, 1914). Time-use studies indicate that people who are mentally able to envision goals distribute their awake time among occupational tasks and activities. The studies also indicate that this distribution is affected by age (McKinnon, 1992) or disability (Yerxa & Baum, 1986; Yerxa & Locker, 1990). For example, Yerxa and Baum found that the number of hours that community-living subjects with spinal cord injury devoted to particular occupations differed significantly from the number of hours their friends without disabilities devoted to those occupations. The subjects with spinal cord injury worked fewer hours and devoted more hours to occupations categorized as "other," which for some subjects included shopping, going to church, eating, or watching television. The problem with this study, for our purposes, is that subject-designated categories were used as the data. Subjects categorized the same occupation (e.g., eating) differently. Further research is needed concerning purposefulness in occupation-as-end. Time-use studies inform us that persons fill their time with activities and tasks that they can name and categorize. However, I found no studies in our literature on how occupation-as-end organizes persons' lives. One paradigm that might be fruitful is to examine how persons without mental illness, who are recently retired, in extreme circumstances such as in prison or lost in the wilderness, or even on extended lazy vacations try to impose organization on their lives by planning and carrying out purposeful occupations of various complexities.

Meaningfulness in Occupation-as-End

Occupation-as-end is not only purposeful but also meaningful because it is the performance of activities or tasks that a person sees as important. Only meaningful occupation remains in a person's life repertoire. Meaningfulness as a therapeutic aspect of occupation derives from our belief in the mind-body connection. The actions of the body are guided by the meaning ascribed to them by the mind (Bruner, 1990). Meaningfulness of occupation-as-end is based on a person's values that derive from family and cultural experiences. Meaningfulness also derives from a person's sense of the importance of participating in certain occupations or performing in a particular manner; or from the person's estimate of reward in terms of success or pleasure; or perhaps from a threat of bad consequences if the occupation is not engaged in.

Meaning is individual (Bruner, 1990) and although the occupational therapist can guess what may be meaningful based on a person's life history, he or she must verify with each patient that the particular occupation is meaningful to that person *now* and verify that the person sees a value in relearning it. The therapist cannot substitute his or her own values in selecting appropriate occupational goals for the patient. Two studies concerning differences in valuing between therapist and patient come to mind. In 1974, Taylor reported that the values attached to goals by 19 occupational therapists differed significantly from those of 44 patients with spinal cord injuries. The patients valued development of work tolerance most, followed by bladder and bowel control. They did not value ADL skills highly. The therapists valued development of adapted devices and ADL skills most and bowel and bladder control least. Chiou and Burnett (1985) surveyed 26 patients living at home after stroke to determine the relative importance of 15 ADL tasks to each of them. Then the researchers paired each patient with one or more of 10 visiting occupational therapists and physical therapists who were treating these patients, to form 29 pairs. Patients and therapists, independently, ranked the 15 items from not at all important to very important for the particular patient. Scores for each patient and therapist pair were correlated. Only one of the 29 pairs yielded a significant correlation, and that was only of moderate strength [.57]. These results seem to indicate that therapists were not good judges of the value ascribed by patients to particular ADL tasks.

The meaningfulness of occupation-as-end is so profound that people at least partially define life satisfaction in terms of competent role performance. For example, in the study by Yerxa and Baum (1986) of 15 subjects with spinal cord injuries and their 12 friends without disabilities, a significant, moderate correlation of $r = .44$ was found between satisfaction with performance in home management and overall life satisfaction. A slightly higher correlation of $r = .62$ was found between satisfaction with performance of community skills and overall life satisfaction. Bränholm and Fugl-Meyer (1992) surveyed 201 randomly selected 25- to 55-year old northern Swedish persons without disabilities to determine what value they attached to certain roles in relation to their perceived level of life satisfaction. Roles associated with vocation, family life, leisure, and home maintenance correctly classified 62 percent to 78 percent of the subjects in terms of satisfaction with life. Smith, Kielhofner, and Watts (1986) studied 60 persons with a mean age of 78 years, half of whom were institutionalized, to determine the relationship between engagement in daily occupations and life satisfaction. They found that those subjects who were classified into the high-satisfaction category engaged in recreation and work significantly more and in ADL and rest significantly less than those classified in the low-satisfaction category.

Therapeutic Achievement of Occupation-as-End

I think that occupation-as-end is brought about by teaching the activity or task directly, using whatever abilities the patient has at his or her disposal or providing whatever adaptations are necessary. It is the Rehabilitative Approach (Trombly, 1995a) or skills training approach (Rogers, 1982). In this approach, occupations are analyzed to ensure that they are within the capabilities of the patient, but are not used to bring about change in those capabilities, per se. The patient learns, with the help of the therapist as teacher and as adaptor of the task demands and context. In the therapeutic encounter, the therapist organizes the subtasks to be learned so that the person will succeed, provides the feedback to ensure successful outcome, and structures the practice to promote improved performance and learning. The purpose of the activity or task is readily apparent to the patient and, if the therapist has allowed patient goals to guide treatment, it is meaningful. Therapeutic principles for this approach derive from cognitive information processing and learning theories.

Occupation-as-Means

Occupation-as-means refers to occupation acting as the therapeutic change agent to remediate impaired abilities or capacities. Various arts, crafts, games, sports, exercise routines, and daily activities that are systematically selected and tailored to each person (Cynkin & Robinson, 1990) are examples of occupations-as-means. Occupation in this sense is equivalent to what is called *purposeful activity* (AOTA, 1993). Purposeful activity demands particular, more circumscribed responses than occupation-as-end.

The therapist analyzes the occupation to determine that it demands particular responses from the person and that the responses demanded are slightly more challenging than what the person can currently easily produce. The therapist provides the opportunity to engage in the potentially therapeutic occupation (Meyer, 1922/1977 [see Chapter 4]), and as the person makes the effort and succeeds, the particular impairment that the occupation-as-means was chosen to remediate is reduced.

Although occupation is provided, therapy may be absent. What makes occupation-as-means therapeutic? First, the activity must have a purpose or goal that makes a challenging demand, yet has a prospect for success. Second, it must have meaning and relevance to the person who is to change so that it motivates the will to learn and improve (Cynkin & Robinson, 1990). The therapeutic aspects of occupation used as a means to change impairments, then, are purposefulness and meaningfulness.

Purposefulness in Occupation-as-Means

Occupation-as-means is based on the assumption that the activity holds within itself a healing property that will change organic or behavioral impairments. We have further assumed that those inherent therapeutic aspects can be reliably identified through the activity analysis process (Llorens, 1986, 1993). However if that assumption were true, therapists should fairly unanimously identify the inherent characteristic components of particular activities. But Tsai (1994), who surveyed 120 therapists experienced in the treatment of stroke, found poor consensus on the sensorimotor, cognitive-perceptual, or psychosocial components demanded by five particular activities that are commonly used in the treatment of patients who have had a stroke, such as stacking cones, putting on a shirt, and making a sandwich. Neistadt, McAuley, Zecha, and Shannon (1993) also reported discrepancies among therapists in identifying components required to do common activities.

Research Related to Purposefulness of Occupation-as-Means in the Motor Domain

When analyzing activities to remediate motor impairments, we have assumed that there are inherent aspects of an activity that elicit particular muscular responses. However, this assumption is not supported by electromyographic evidence. If the therapeutic benefit were inherent in the activity, then whenever any person did that activity, the effects should be similar from trial to trial and similar from person to person, especially in those with normal biomechanical and neuromuscular

systems. However, a colleague and I completed an electromyographical study some years ago that examined the responses of hand muscles of 15 persons without disabilities when they were doing 16 different occupational therapy hand activities (Trombly & Cole, 1979). I had assumed in designing this study that if the goal was the same (e.g., "open this lock with this key"), and placement of objects was the same from subject to subject, and if each subject was positioned the same in relation to the objects (i.e., if the task demands were the same), then the same muscles would be used at similar levels by the various subjects. However, the results indicated that each subject used his or her own muscle activation pattern and amount of muscle activity. This finding was contrary to my expectations, but fully in agreement with predictions of Bernstein (1967).

Bernstein theorized that neuromuscular variability between trials is due to the redundancies in the musculoskeletal systems. Such redundancies allow the same goal to be accomplished effectively by a wide variety of muscle combinations and movement patterns (Horak, 1991; Morasso & Zaccaria, 1986; Newell & Corcos, 1993). Bernstein's ideas, and the evidence that supports them, contributed to the paradigm shift to the dynamical systems theory of motor control. The term *dynamical systems* refers to any area of concern in which order and pattern emerge from the interaction and cooperation of many systems (Hawking, 1988). Applied to motor behavior, dynamical systems refers to movement patterns that emerge from the interaction of multiple systems of the person and performance contexts to achieve a functional goal (see Figure 11.3) (Mathiowetz & Haugen, 1994, 1995; Haugen & Mathiowetz, 1995).

According to Bernstein's hypothesis, the central nervous system temporarily yokes muscles together to constrain the number of degrees of freedom to within its capability of control at the moment, given the current resources of the person and the particular demands of the context. This synergic coupling, or coordinative structure, forms as needed at the moment and then dissolves. The next time the person does the same thing, his or her muscles may be more warmed up, or there may be a slight difference in placement of task object in relation to the active limb, so a new coordinative structure evolves. That is, different muscles may be recruited, or the same muscles used before may be more or less active in order to accomplish the movement goal in the most efficient way. The motor goal is constant or invariant and requires a constant, invariant response, but this response can be fulfilled by a vary-

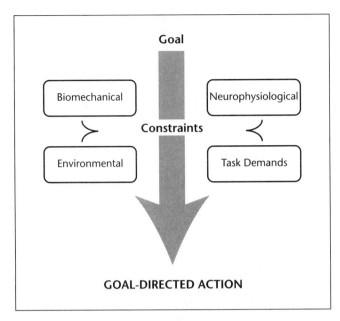

Figure 11.3. Dynamical systems theory of motor control hypothesizes that goal-directed action emerges from a synthesis of goal or purpose and personal and contextual constraints.

ing set of muscular contractions (Luria, 1973). The goal or purpose seems to organize the most efficient movement, given the constraints of person and context (see Figure 11.3).

What evidence is there that purpose organizes behavior? Motor commands issued to moving segments are not accessible to an experimenter and must be inferred from study of the limb trajectories that they ultimately produce (Jeannerod, 1988). Limb trajectories are recorded with instruments designed to track the spatial-temporal aspects of movement. Different spatial-temporal patterns, which are indicative of differences in movement organization, emerge for particular goals (Jeannerod, 1988). Movement organization can be detected from the shape of the velocity profile (Georgopoulos, 1986; Kamm, Thelen, & Jensen, 1990) that changes depending on goal (Nelson, 1983). The goal of reaching to a large target that does not demand accuracy produces a unimodal and bell-shaped velocity profile. The goal of reaching precisely to a target, which requires accurate, guided movement, on the other hand, has a left-shifted velocity profile because more time is spent in deceleration than in acceleration.

In 1987, Marteniuk, MacKenzie, Jeannerod, Athenes, and Dugas demonstrated for the first time the impact of goal on the organization of movement. They found that five university student subjects used a different movement organization when they reached for the same object for two different purposes. One goal was to pick up a 4-centimeter disk and place it in a slot; the other goal was to pick up the same disk and throw it into a basket. The task demands and the context were exactly the same. Only intent after the reach was different. The different purposes produced two different velocity profiles (see Figure 11.4), indicating different movement organizations, for the reaches to the disk. Reaches before placing the disk into a slot produced a left shift of velocity profile in which a significantly greater percentage of total reach time was spent in the deceleration phase and the acceleration phase was significantly shortened as compared to reaches before the throwing condition.

Mathiowetz (1991) tested whether the same motor organization was elicited when 20 subjects with multiple sclerosis performed functional tasks in natural, impoverished, partial, and simulated conditions. In one of the experiments, the subjects actually ate applesauce with a spoon in the natural condition; pretended to eat applesauce, with no applesauce, spoon, or dish present in the impoverished condition; pretended to eat applesauce with a dish and spoon, but no applesauce present in the partial condition; or did, in the simulated condition, the feeding subtest of the Jebsen-Taylor Hand Function Test (Jebsen, Taylor, Trieschmann, Trotter, & Howard, 1969) that requires the subject to pick up kidney beans with a spoon and transfer them to a can placed in front of him or her. The outcomes of each trial were described qualitatively in phase plane diagrams in which velocity is graphed against displacement. These should be replicable from trial to trial if the subject is using the same movement organization. However, the phase planes were judged, by experienced judges, to be different among the four conditions. Figure 11.5 depicts two trials of two conditions, the natural and the simulated, by one subject. The repeated trials are similar, but the two conditions are different. Because subjects produced unique phase planes for each condition, Mathiowetz concluded that subjects perceived each condition as a unique activity, having a different goal.

In another test of differences in goal situation, Van der Weel, van der Meer, and Lee (1991) tested nine children of average intelligence, aged 3 to 7 years, who had right hemiparesis. They measured the children's range of supination and pronation movement when moving a drumstick back and forth in the frontal plane with the instruction "to move as far as you can" (the abstract condition). The children had previously experienced

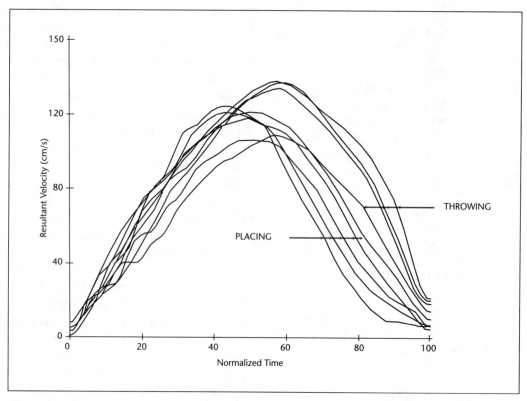

Figure 11.4. Velocity profiles for reaches to a 4-centimeter disk, after which the goal was to fit the disk into a slot or to throw it into a basket.

Note. From Marteniuk, R. G., MacKenzie, C. L., Jeannerod, M., Athenes, S., & Dugas, C. (1987). Constraints on human arm movement trajectories. *Canadian Journal of Psychology, 41*(3), 365–378. Used with permission.

the full range of movement passively. Range was also measured when the children were told to use the same drumstick to "bang the drums" which were placed to require full range of motion (the concrete condition). Movement range was significantly greater ($t_8 = 6.75$, $p < .0001$) for the concrete task of banging the drums than for the abstract task, which had a vague goal.

Wu (Wu, 1993; Wu, Trombly, & Lin, 1994) investigated whether actually reaching for a pencil to write one's name, reaching the same distance for an imagined pencil, or reaching forward in a biomechanically similar way would produce different outcomes in terms of the organization of movement. In the sample of 37 college-aged subjects without disabilities, the materials-based occupation of reaching for an actual pencil elicited significantly different and more efficient organization of movement than imagery-based occupation of reaching for a pretend pencil or exercise. The reach was faster ($F_{2,62} = 20.44$, $p < .001$) and straighter ($F_{2,62} = 23.25$, $p < .001$), was more preplanned ($F_{2,62} = 22.13$, $p < .001$), and used less force ($F_{1,62} = 6.13$, $p < .005$). The im-

agery-based occupation, on the other hand, produced a more guided, longer, and more convoluted path than did the exercise condition, probably because the goal was more vague in that condition.

Sietsema, Nelson, Mulder, Mervau-Scheidel, and White (1993) tested the effect of goal on overall active range of shoulder motion of 20 adults with brain injury. Each subject reached to a point 3 inches above the center of a table placed to require full forward reach. Each also reached the same distance to play a computer-controlled game of flashing lights and sounds. Overall active range of motion was significantly greater as a result of the game than simply reaching to the more vague target ($t_{19} = 5.77$, $p < .001$).

At least in terms of motor responses, then, purpose does appear to organize behavior. Of course, much more study is required to verify this finding.

Meaningfulness in Occupation-as-Means

Whereas a meaningful occupation has purposefulness, strictly speaking, a purposeful activity may or may not

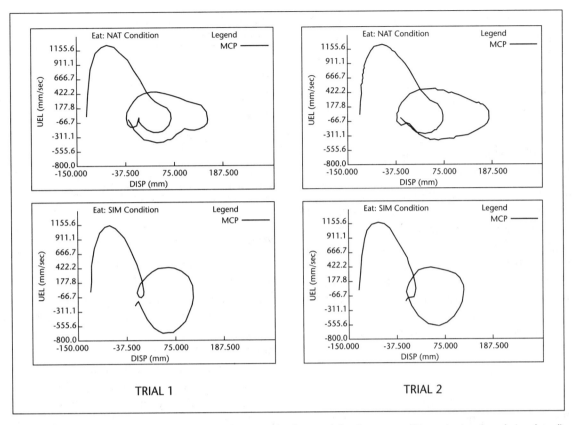

Figure 11.5. Phase planes (velocity × displacement) of two trials of two conditions (natural and simulated) by one normal subject.

Note. From Mathiowetz, V. G. (1991). *Informational support and functional motor performance.* Unpublished doctoral dissertation, University of Minnesota, Minneapolis. Used with permission.

be meaningful. Sharrott (1983) stated that the purpose of an action gives that action meaning. He may have been using *purpose* to denote the reason that a person does something, or the motive, rather than the goal of the action. I think that confounding these terms will impede research. The purpose is the goal, the expected end result. The meaning is the value that accomplishment of that goal has for the person. I have an anecdotal example of the separation between the two concepts. Some years back, my father had a right cerebrovascular accident with resultant hemi-inattention. The occupational therapist gave him parquetry blocks to do. There were two purposes. One was the goal of the activity—to place all the blocks on the diagram. He understood the goal and tried to do what he was told. However, it had no meaning to him; he viewed this activity as a children's game and found it degrading. The therapeutic purpose, of course, was to improve his hemi-inattention. That purpose had no meaning to him either; he did not think he had hemi-inattention and did not get the connection between the child's game and the therapeutic goal.

What do we mean by *meaningful* and how does that quality of occupation-as-means affect behavioral responses? Meaning related to occupation-as-means may relate to basic values held by the person—similar to the way meaning is derived for occupation-as-end. However, meaning is probably generated from a less profound source when it applies to particular, circumscribed, time-limited activities used to promote some performance component. The meaningful aspect of occupation-as-means may be the emotional value that an interesting and creative experience offers the patient (Ayres, 1958). Or meaningfulness may stem from familiarity with the occupation, or its power to arouse positive associations, or the likelihood that completion of it will elicit approval from others who are respected and admired (Cynkin & Robinson, 1990), or its potential to contribute to recovery.

Although we often count on meaningfulness to emanate from the activity, there is no inherent meaningfulness quality in a particular occupation. Meaningfulness is individual. Bruner (1990) said that "action is interpretable only by reference to what the actor says he or she is up to" (p. 20). In therapy, meaningfulness is developed through an exchange between the therapist and the person to construct the meaning of the activity within the context of culture, life experiences, disability (Fleming, 1990; Kielhofner, 1992), and present needs.

Research Related to Meaningfulness of Occupation-as-Means

The importance of meaningfulness to us as therapists is that we believe that it motivates. What evidence is there that meaning motivates behavior?

Meaningfulness has been operationalized in occupational therapy studies in one of three ways. One is to offer a choice, another is to provide a product, and the third is to enhance the context. The response, motivation, has been operationalized as the number of repetitions or length of time engaged in the occupation or as the effort expended.

Choice

Bakshi, Bhambhani, and Madill (1991) studied 20 female college students who chose their most preferred and least preferred activity from eight offered activities. They completed each under conditions of purpose and nonpurpose, defined respectively as working on a product or not. There were no differences in number of repetitions performed between the preferred and non-preferred occupation. Differences between product and no-product conditions were not significant due to high variability (see Table 11.1). On the other hand, LaMore and Nelson (1993), in a more controlled study, did find a significant increase in repetitions ($Z = 2.9$, $p < .01$) when 22 adult subjects with mental disabilities were given a limited choice of which ceramic object to paint as compared with when they were told to paint a particular one.

Table 11.1. Mean Number of Repetitions as a Result of Preference and Purpose in Assigned Tasks

Purpose	Task Assigned	
	Preferred	Nonpreferred
Yes	63	63
No	83	84

Note. Based on Bakshi, R., Bhambhani, Y., & Madill, H. (1991). The effects of task preference on performance during purposeful and nonpurposeful activities. *American Journal of Occupational Therapy, 45*, 912–916.

Table 11.2. Effects of Product-Oriented and Nonproduct-Oriented Activities

Measures	Product	
	Yes (Cutting Board)	No (Wood)
Preference	4.8	3.4*
Increased heart rate	13	17
Performance time	172	148

*$p = .001$.

Note. Based on Thibodeaux, C. S., & Ludwig, F. M. (1988). Intrinsic motivation in product-oriented and nonproduct-oriented activities. *American Journal of Occupational Therapy, 42*, 169–175.

Product

Thibodeaux and Ludwig (1988) tested whether performance time and heart rate (effort) would be significantly different when 15 occupational therapy students sanded a cutting board that they could keep as compared with when they sanded wood for no reason. Although the subjects reported enjoying the product-oriented activity significantly more and they worked longer at it, there was too much intersubject variability to detect significant differences between conditions (see Table 11.2).

Enhanced Context

Riccio, Nelson, and Bush (1990) studied the effects of enhanced context. They tested the effect of imagery-based activity and exercise on the number of repetitions of 27 elderly nursing home residents when they reached up to pretend to pick apples and reached down to pretend to pick up coins versus when they simply reached up or down for exercise. There was a significant difference between the two conditions for the up direction ($Z = 2.25$, $p = .012$), indicating that pretending to pick apples was more motivating than exercise. The outcome for reaching down was in the same direction, but nonsignificant ($Z = 1.60$, $p = .055$), possibly because of a confounding effect of fatigue.

Lang, Nelson, and Bush (1992) tested the responses of 15 elderly nursing home residents under three conditions: materials-based activity, imagery-based activity, and exercise. In the materials-based condition, subjects actually kicked a red balloon. In the imagery-based condition, they pretended to kick a described balloon. In the exercise condition, they kicked as demonstrated. The number of repetitions associated with really kicking the balloon (54) was significantly greater ($F_{2,28} = 6.62$, $p = .004$) than those associated with imagining kicking the balloon (26) or kicking for exercise (18). This study

Table 11.3. Average Effects of Materials-Based Occupation, Imagery-Based Occupation, and Rote Exercise

Measures	Type of Occupation and Exercise		
	Materials-Based	Imagery-Based	Rote
Repetitions to fatigue	127**	51	75
Distance foot lifted (cm)	29	31	26
Speed (cm/sec)	71	71	67

**$p < .001$

Note. Based on DeKuiper, W. P., Nelson, D. L., & White, B. E. (1993). Materials-based occupation versus imagery-based occupation versus rote exercise: A replication and extension. *Occupational Therapy Journal of Research, 13,* 183–197.

was later replicated by DeKuiper, Nelson, and White (1993) on 28 elderly nursing home residents. Materials-based occupation produced significantly more repetitions than imagery-based occupation or rote exercise ($F_{2,54} = 12.1$, $p < .001$). In this study they also measured effort in terms of distance the foot was raised and speed of kick. There were no significant differences among the various contextual conditions for these variables (see Table 11.3).

A number of other researchers (Bloch, Smith, & Nelson, 1989; Kircher, 1984; Miller & Nelson, 1987; Steinbeck, 1986; Yoder, Nelson, & Smith, 1989) all demonstrated significantly greater numbers of repetitions or duration for what they termed purposeful versus nonpurposeful activity. The differences in the activities were actually differences in meaning in terms of context, not differences in purpose—the motoric purpose was the same: jump up and down or jump rope, stir dough for exercise or stir dough that will be made into cookies that the subjects could smell baking, squeeze a bulb to keep a ping-pong ball suspended in air or squeeze the same bulb for exercise. Some demonstrated significantly greater effort (heart rate) expended for the enhanced condition, but this was not a consistent finding (Bloch et al., 1989; Kircher, 1984; Steinbeck, 1986).

Meaningfulness, as operationalized by enhanced context, and possibly by choice, appears to motivate continued performance. However, more definitive research is needed. Additionally, basic research on what makes occupation-asmeans meaningful and how best to operationalize this in both research and practice is needed.

Practice and Research

As occupational therapists we want our patients to achieve role competence. We use occupation-as-end

and occupationas-means now to achieve that. We need to document the successes of our current practices, but we also need to reconsider some of our practices. For example, practice based on an ascending hierarchical model has emphasized remediation of occupational components because it is assumed that lower-level skills and abilities are prerequisite to higher-level functioning. Although this assumption makes logical sense—persons who cannot lift their arms certainly cannot comb their hair in the usual way—practice has sometimes emphasized treatment to increase strength and other capacities and abilities to the exclusion of teaching functional skills. However, a thorough review of the literature on stroke rehabilitation (Wagenaar & Meijer, 1991a, 1991b) indicated that gains in component functions are small and do not automatically result in improved functional performance. When the results of several correlational studies were averaged together, the average correlation between motor impairment and ADL was .56 and between perceptual impairment and ADL was .58 (Trombly, 1995b). By squaring the *r*, the amount of variance of ADL accounted for by motor impairment was 31 percent (see Figure 11.6). Therefore, 69 percent of variance associated with ADL derives from other factors. Even if motor impairment were 100 percent remediated, would the patient be able to do ADL without specific training and adaptation? Studies are needed that compare skills training at the level of occupation-as-end with subskills training using occupation-as-means to effectively and efficiently achieve occupational functioning (Rogers, 1982).

How the purposefulness and meaningfulness aspects of both levels of occupation contribute to the therapeutic effect need explication to guide practice. We need to study in more detail how purposefulness organizes behavior and meaningfulness motivates performance. The literature reviewed here is a beginning in this regard. Some of the studies reviewed indicated that the organization of motor behavior is different when the

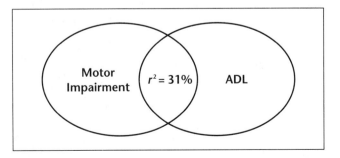

Figure 11.6. Pictorial description of r^2.

purposes or contexts are different, even if they are similar. This finding suggests that treatment in simulated contexts using simulated objects and simulated goals may not help a patient learn occupational performance for real life. Studies are needed to compare effectiveness of treatment with actual objects in natural contexts versus treatment with simulated objects in clinical settings. Follow-up studies of carryover of occupational performance from treatment center to home are also needed.

Those golden moments that we have all experienced as therapists probably came about when the patient succeeded in doing something that had great meaning to him or her. Sometimes we get complacent, though, and offer activities and occupations that we think ought to be meaningful to the person but are not really, or we offer a choice of activities from a selection in which none of the choices are meaningful. Much more attention needs to be applied to discovering the meaning of, or creating meaning for, therapeutic occupation. Methods to evaluate meaningfulness are needed both for research and practice. We need more well-controlled studies that test the effect of meaningfulness on perseverance and effort during therapy.

Conclusion

Occupational therapy was founded on the belief that engaging in occupation brought about mental and physical health. Over the years we have redefined health, for our purposes, as occupational performance having many levels of organization. In this context, occupation can be seen both as end and as means. In both dimensions, meaningfulness and purposefulness are key qualities. Purposefulness organizes and meaningfulness motivates. Purposeful occupation-as-end seems to organize time and a person's description of his life. Meaningful occupation-as-end motivates the person's participation in life. Purposeful occupation-as-means organizes behavioral responses, at least as far as motor responses are concerned. Meaningful occupation-as-means seems to motivate the person to persevere in his efforts long enough to achieve a therapeutic benefit. Research is needed to verify each of these hypotheses. I hope each occupational therapist will join me in taking responsibility to contribute to that effort.

Acknowledgments

Figures 11.1, 11.2, and 11.6, as well as all the slides in the original presentation, were prepared by Elizabeth (Boo) Murray, SCD, OTR, FAOTA, to whom I am very grateful.

I further want to acknowledge the support and constructive critique of my colleagues in the Neurobehavioral Rehabilitation Research Center (NRRC), which is the American Occupational Therapy Association and American Occupational Therapy Foundation Center for Scholarship and Research at Boston University: Sharon Cermak, EdD, OTR, FAOTA; Wendy Coster, PhD, OTR, FAOTA; Anne Henderson, PhD, OTR, FAOTA; Karen Jacobs, EdD, OTR, FAOTA; Noomi Katz, PhD, OTR; Boo Murray, SCD, OTR, FAOTA; and Elsie Vergara, ScD, OTR, FAOTA.

References

Abler, R. R., & Fretz, B. R. (1988). Self-efficacy and competence in independent living among oldest old persons. *Journal of Gerontology: Social Sciences, 43*, S138–S143.

American Occupational Therapy Association. (1993). Position Paper—Purposeful activity. *American Journal of Occupational Therapy, 47*, 1081–1082.

American Occupational Therapy Association. (1994). Uniform terminology for occupational therapy—Third edition. *American Journal of Occupational Therapy, 48*, 1047–1054.

Ayres, A. J. (1958). Basic concepts of clinical practice in physical disabilities. *American Journal of Occupational Therapy, 12*, 300–302, 311.

Bakshi, R., Bhambhani, Y., & Madill, H. (1991). The effects of task preference on performance during purposeful and nonpurposeful activities. *American Journal of Occupational Therapy, 45*, 912–916. http://dx.doi.org/10.5014/ajot.45.10.912

Bandura, A. (1977). Self-efficacy: Toward a unifying theory of behavior change. *Psychological Review, 84*, 191–215.

Barrows, M. (1917). Susan E. Tracy, R. N. *Maryland Psychiatric Quarterly, 6*, 57–62.

Bernstein, N. (1967). *The coordination and regulation of movements.* Elmsford, NY: Pergamon.

Bloch, M. W., Smith, D. A., & Nelson, D. L. (1989). Heart rate, activity, duration, and affect in added-purpose versus single-purpose jumping activities. *American Journal of Occupational Therapy, 43*, 25–30.

Bränholm, I. B., & Fugl-Meyer, A. R. (1992). Occupational role preferences and life satisfaction. *Occupational Therapy Journal of Research, 12*, 159–171.

Bruner, J. (1990). *Acts of meaning.* Cambridge, MA: Harvard University Press.

Cameron, R. G. (1917). An interview with Miss Susan Tracy. *Maryland Psychiatric Quarterly, 4*, 65–66.

Chiou, I. I. L., & Burnett, C. N. (1985). Values of activities of daily living: A survey of stroke patients and their home therapists. *Physical Therapy, 65*, 901–906.

Christiansen, C. (1991). Occupational therapy intervention for life performance (pp. 1–43). In C. Christiansen & C. Baum (Eds.), *Occupational therapy: Overcoming human performance deficits.* Thorofare, NJ: Slack.

Clark, F., Parham, D., Carlson, M. E., Frank, G., Jackson, J. Pierce, D., Wolfe, R. J., & Zemke, R. (1991). Occupational science: Academic innovation in the service of occupational therapy's future. *American Journal of Occupational Therapy, 45,* 300–310. http://dx.doi.org/10.5014/ajot.45.4.300

Cynkin, S., & Robinson, J. M. (1990). *Occupational therapy and activities health: Toward health through activities.* Boston: Little, Brown.

DeKuiper, W. P., Nelson, D. L., & White, B. E. (1993). Materials-based occupation versus imagery-based occupation versus rote exercise: A replication and extension. *Occupational Therapy Journal of Research, 13,* 183–197.

Dunton, W. R., Jr. (1914). Roundtable. *Maryland Psychiatric Quarterly, 4,* 20–32.

Editorial. (1929). Susan E. Tracy. *Occupational Therapy and Rehabilitation, 8,* 63–66.

Fleming, M. (1990). Untitled invited paper presented at the American Occupational Therapy Foundation planning meeting for the Occupation Symposium, Boston, MA.

Georgopoulos, A. P. (1986). On reaching. *Annual Review of Neurosciences, 9,* 147–170.

Haas, L. J. (1922). Crafts adaptable to occupational needs: Their relative importance. *Archives of Occupational Therapy, 1,* 443–455.

Haugen, J. B., & Mathiowetz, V. (1995). Contemporary task-oriented approach. In C. A. Trombly (Ed.), *Occupational therapy for physical dysfunction* (4th ed.) (pp. 510–528). Baltimore: Williams & Wilkins.

Hawking, S. W. (1988). *A brief history of time: From the big bang to black holes.* New York: Bantam.

Horak, F. B. (1991). Assumptions underlying motor control for neurologic rehabilitation. In M. Lister (Ed.), *Contemporary management of motor control problems. Proceedings of the II STEP Conference* (pp. 11–27). Alexandria, VA: Foundation for Physical Therapy.

Jeannerod, M. (1988). *The neural and behavioral organization of goal-directed movements.* Oxford: Clarendon.

Jebsen, R. H., Taylor, N., Trieschmann, R. B., Trotter, M., & Howard, L. A. (1969). An objective and standardized test of hand function. *Archives of Physical Medicine and Rehabilitation, 50,* 311–319.

Kamm, K., Thelen, E., & Jensen, J. L. (1990). A dynamical systems approach to motor development. *Physical Therapy, 70,* 763–775.

Kielhofner, G. (Ed.). (1985). *A Model of Human Occupation.* Baltimore: Williams & Wilkins.

Kielhofner, G. (1992). *Conceptual foundations of occupational therapy.* Philadelphia: F. A. Davis.

Kircher, M. A. (1984). Motivation as a factor of perceived exertion in purposeful versus nonpurposeful activity. *American Journal of Occupational Therapy, 38,* 165–170.

Lang, E. M., Nelson, D. L., & Bush, M. A. (1992). Comparison of performance in materials-based occupation, imagery-based occupation, and rote exercise in nursing home residents. *American Journal of Occupational Therapy, 46,* 607–611. http://dx.doi.org/10.5014/ajot.46.7.607

LaMore, K. L., & Nelson, D. L. (1993). The effects of options on performance of an art project in adults with mental disabilities. *American Journal of Occupational Therapy, 47,* 397–401.

Llorens, L. A. (1986). Activity analysis: Agreement among factors in a sensory processing model. *American Journal of Occupational Therapy, 40,* 103–110.

Llorens, L. A. (1993). Activity analysis: Agreement between participants and observers on perceived factors in occupation components. *Occupational Therapy Journal of Research, 13,* 198–211.

Lowney, M. E. P. (1930). The relationship between occupational therapy and rehabilitation. *Massachusetts Association for Occupational Therapy Bulletin, 4*(2).

Luria, A. R. (1973). *The working brain: An introduction to neuropsychology.* New York: Basic.

Mathiowetz, V. G. (1991). *Informational support and functional motor performance.* Unpublished doctoral dissertation, University of Minnesota.

Mathiowetz, V., & Haugen, J. B. (1994). Motor behavior research: Implications for therapeutic approaches to central nervous system dysfunction. *American Journal of Occupational Therapy, 48,* 733–745.

Mathiowetz, V., & Haugen, J. B. (1995). Evaluation of motor behavior: Traditional and contemporary views. In C. A. Trombly (Ed.), *Occupational therapy for physical dysfunction* (4th ed., pp. 157–186). Baltimore: Williams & Wilkins.

Marteniuk, R. G., MacKenzie, C. L., Jeannerod, M., Athenes, S., & Dugas, C. (1987). Constraints on human arm movement trajectories. *Canadian Journal of Psychology, 41,* 365–378.

McKinnon, A, L. (1992). Time use for self-care, productivity, and leisure among elderly Canadians. *Canadian Journal of Occupational Therapy, 59,* 102–110.

Meyer, A. (1977). The philosophy of occupational therapy. *American Journal of Occupational Therapy, 31,* 639–642. Originally published 1922. Reprinted as Chapter 4.

Miller, L., & Nelson, D. L. (1987). Dual-purpose activity versus single-purpose activity in terms of duration of task, exertion level, and affect. *Occupational Therapy in Mental Health, 1,* 55–67.

Morasso, P., & Zaccaria, R. (1986). Understanding human movement. *Experimental Brain Research, 15,* 145–157.

Neistadt, M. E., McAuley, D., Zecha, D., & Shannon, R. (1993). An analysis of a board game as a treatment activity. *American Journal of Occupational Therapy, 47,* 154–160. http://dx.doi.org/10.5014/ajot.47.2.154

Nelson, C. E., & Payton, 0. D. (1991). A system for involving patients in program planning. *American Journal of Occupational Therapy, 45,* 753–755.

Nelson, D. L. (1988). Occupation: Form and performance. *American Journal of Occupational Therapy, 42,* 633–641.

Nelson, D. L. (1990). Untitled invited paper presented at the American Occupational Therapy Foundation planning meeting for the Occupation Symposium, Boston, MA.

Nelson, W. L. (1983). Physical principles for economies of skilled movements. *Biological Cybernetics, 46,* 135–147.

Newell, K. M., & Corcos, D. M. (1993). Issues in variability and motor control. In K. M. Newell & D. M. Corcos (Eds.), *Variability and motor control* (pp. 1–12). Champaign, IL: Human Kinetics.

Parsons, S. E. (1917). Miss Tracy's work in general hospitals. *Maryland Psychiatric Quarterly, 6,* 63–64.

Purdum, H. D. (1911). The psycho-therapeutic value of occupation. *Maryland Psychiatric Quarterly, 1,* 35–36.

Riccio, C. M., Nelson, D. L., & Bush, M. A. (1990). Adding purpose to the repetitive exercise of elderly women through imagery. *American Journal of Occupational Therapy, 44,* 714–719. http://dx.doi.org/10.5014/ajot.44.8.714

Rogers, J. C. (1982). The spirit of independence: The evolution of a philosophy. *American Journal of Occupational Therapy, 36,* 709–715.

Sharrott, G. W. (1983). Occupational therapy's role in the client's creation and affirmation of meaning. In G. Kielhofner (Ed.), *Health through occupation: Theory and practice in occupational therapy.* Philadelphia: F. A. Davis.

Sietsema, J. M., Nelson, D. L., Mulder, R. M., Mervau-Scheidel, D., & White, B. E. (1993). The use of a game to promote arm reach in persons with traumatic brain injury. *American Journal of Occupational Therapy, 47,* 19–24.

Slagle, E. C. (1914). History of the development of occupation for the insane. *Maryland Psychiatric Quarterly, 4,* 14–20.

Smith, N. R., Kielhofner, G., & Watts, J. H. (1986). The relationships among volition, activity pattern, and life satisfaction in the elderly. *American Journal of Occupational Therapy, 40,* 278–283.

Steinbeck, T. M. (1986). Purposeful activity and performance. *American Journal of Occupational Therapy, 40,* 529–534.

Swaim, L. T. (1928). Does occupational work hasten recovery of the crippled? *Massachusetts Association of Occupational Therapy Bulletin, 2(3).*

Taylor, D. P. (1974). Treatment goals for quadriplegic and paraplegic patients. *American Journal of Occupational Therapy, 28,* 22–29.

Thibodeaux, C. S., & Ludwig, F. M. (1988). Intrinsic motivation in product-oriented and nonproduct-oriented activities. *American Journal of Occupational Therapy, 42,* 169–175.

Trombly, C. (1993). Anticipating the future: Assessment of occupational function. *American Journal of Occupational Therapy, 47,* 253–257. http://dx.doi.org/10.5014/ajot.47.3.253

Trombly, C. (Ed.). (1995a). *Occupational therapy for physical dysfunction* (4th ed.). Baltimore: Williams & Wilkins.

Trombly, C. A. (1995b). *Relationships between motor and perceptual performance components and activities of daily living.* Unpublished paper, Boston University.

Trombly, C. A., & Cole, J. M. (1979). Electromyographic study of four hand muscles during selected activities. *American Journal of Occupational Therapy, 33,* 440–449.

Tsai, P. L. (1994). *Activity analysis and activity selection among occupational therapists: A survey.* Unpublished master's thesis, Boston University, Boston.

Van der Weel, F. R., van der Meer, A. L. H., & Lee, D. N. (1991). Effect of task on movement control in cerebral palsy: Implications for assessment and therapy. *Developmental Medicine and Child Neurology, 33,* 419–426.

Wagenaar, R. C., & Meijer, O. G. (1991a). Effects of stroke rehabilitation (1): A critical review of the literature. *Journal of Rehabilitation Sciences, 4,* 61–73.

Wagenaar, R. C., & Meijer, O. G. (1991b). Effects of stroke rehabilitation (2): A critical review of the literature. *Journal of Rehabilitation Sciences, 4,* 97–109.

White, R. W. (1959). Motivation reconsidered: The concept of competence. *Psychological Review, 66,* 297–333.

Wu, C. Y. (1993). *The relationship between occupational form and occupational performance: A kinematic perspective.* Unpublished master's thesis, Boston University.

Wu, C. Y., Trombly, C. A., & Lin, K. C. (1994). The relationship between occupational form and occupational performance: A kinematic perspective. *American Journal of Occupational Therapy, 48,* 679–687.

Yerxa, E. J., & Baum, S. (1986). Engagement in daily occupations and life satisfaction among people with spinal cord injuries. *Occupational Therapy Journal of Research, 6,* 271–283.

Yerxa, E., & Locker, S. (1990). Quality of time use by adults with spinal cord injuries. *American Journal of Occupational Therapy, 44,* 318–326. http://dx.doi.org/10.5014/ajot.44.4.318

Yerxa, E. J., Clark, F., Frank, G., Jackson, J., Parham, D., Pierce, D., Stein, C., & Zemkè, R. (1990). An introduction to occupational science: A foundation for occupational therapy in the 21st century. *Occupational Therapy in Health Care, 6,* 1–32.

Yoder, R. M., Nelson, D. L., & Smith, D. A. (1989). Added purpose versus rote exercise in female nursing home residents. *American Journal of Occupational Therapy, 43,* 581–586.

CHAPTER 12

Mindfulness and Flow in Occupational Engagement: Presence in Doing

DENISE REID

Occupational engagement is a fundamental concept in the discipline of occupational therapy. The recently described Canadian Model of Occupational Performance and Engagement (CMOP–E) (Townsend & Polatajko, 2007) reflects the concerns that occupational therapists have regarding engagement in occupations. The interest in occupational engagement may include looking at outcomes of competence, contentment, satisfaction, and well-being in their clients when they are engaged. For example, feelings of satisfaction and pleasure may be significant factors that determine meaningful occupational engagement for persons with mental health problems (Mee & Sumsion, 2001). Occupational engagement has been linked to health and well-being (Jackson, Carlson, Mandel, Zemke, & Clark, 1998; Law, Steinwender, & Leclair, 1998; Reid, 2008; Wilcock, 1998, 2006; Yerxa, 1998). However, the mechanisms by which occupational engagement promotes health and well-being are still not fully understood. Mindfulness or flow may be ways for occupational engagement to contribute to a person's wellbeing (Bryce & Haworth, 2002; Carmody & Baer, 2007; Reid, 2008). Research is confirming that mindfulness improves the functioning of the brain and subjective mental well-being (Brown & Ryan, 2003; Farb, Segal, Mayberg, Bean, McKeon, Fatima, & Anderson, 2007). Fritz and Avsec (2007) studied the experience of flow and its relationship to subjective well-being in 84 music students. They concluded that the experience of flow was stronger when students were engaged in playing their instruments rather than other music-related activities, such as listening to music or composing music. They concluded that flow was related more to the emotional aspects of subjective well-being. In the field of occupational therapy, Jacobs (1994) studied flow experiences among occupational therapy practitioners in the work place, and found that those who experienced flow were working with a client in some type of intervention, which resulted in increased well-being.

This intention of this paper is first to discuss psychological and philosophical theoretical perspectives of flow and mindfulness and suggest how they are both relevant to the construct of occupational engagement. Second, methodological and conceptual limitations in research on flow and mindfulness will be reviewed. Third, case examples will illustrate how mindfulness or flow in occupational therapy practice affect the client as a way of being present in the world while engaged.

Conceptualizations of Flow and Mindfulness

Flow

Flow denotes the holistic sensation an individual has when he or she acts with total involvement with an occupation (Csikszentmihalyi, 1975). In flow people are usually so completely engaged in activity that they seem to forget their embodied being-in-the-world altogether. There is a sense of becoming one with the experience. Csikszentmihalyi (1990, 1996).The construct of flow that was introduced by Csikszentmihalyi in the late seventies (1975, 1990) shares many qualities with concepts of peak experience and self-actualization (Maslow, 1968; Privette, 1983). Maslow argued that few reach the highest level of self-actualization; however, such a peak level experience can be experienced by anyone. Flow can also be experienced by anyone while performing different activities, beginning from everyday ones to those that are extremely complex. According to Csikszentmihalyi (1990), the flow experience occurs in situations in which attention can be freely invested to achieve goals. The main idea of flow

This chapter was previously published in the *Canadian Journal of Occupational Therapy, 78*, 50–56. Copyright © 2011, Canadian Association of Occupational Therapists. Reprinted with permission. http://dx.doi.org/10.2182/cjot.2011.78.1.7

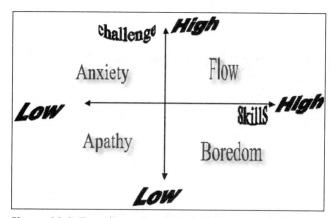

Figure 12.1. Two-dimensional model of flow.

Adapted, with permission, from "Flow in Sports", by S. A. Jackson and M. Csikszentmihalyi, 1999, Champaign, IL: Human Kinetics, p. 37. Originally adapted from "Optimal Experience: Psychological Studies of Flow in Consciousness," by M. Csikszentmihalyi and I. Csikszentmihalyi, 1988, Cambridge, UK: Cambridge University Press.

is Csikszentmihalyi's concept of challenge–skill balance. An activity should represent a challenge for an individual, but only the extent that he is able to realize it. Irrespective of the type of activity, it is the balance between the activity and the individual's abilities that is important. Jackson and Csikszentmihalyi (1999) put this idea into a two-dimensional model of flow (Figure 12.1). Flow is experienced when both the situational demand and the abilities are high. Other concepts are included in the model to explain cases of unequal situational demands and abilities. Whenever a person has much higher abilities than demanded by a situation, he or she gets bored, but when the demands are too high for his or her abilities, anxiety ensues. In the case of low situational demands and poor abilities, he or she becomes apathetic.

Mindfulness

Mindfulness has its roots in Eastern traditions and is most often associated with the formal practice of mindfulness meditation (Thera, 1996). Mindfulness is, however, more than meditation. It is "inherently a state of consciousness" that involves consciously attending to one's moment-to-moment experience (Brown & Ryan, 2003; Shapiro, Carlson, Astin, & Freedman, 2006). Meditation practice is simply a platform used to develop the state or skill of mindfulness (Kabat-Zinn, 2002).

Mindfulness has been discussed by many philosophers, psychologists, neuroscientists, educators, and healers over the years (Heidegger, 1996; Husserl, 1964;

Kabat-Zinn, 1994; Merleau-Ponty, 1962; Siegel, 2007). Kabat-Zinn defines mindfulness as "a means of paying attention in a particular way, on purpose, in the present moment, and in a non-judgmental way" (1994, p. 4). This definition suggests that being mindful is an active state, an intentional state, "paying attention on purpose." The essence of mindfulness is attending to intention, which embodies the sense of presence. The subjective feel of mindfulness is being aware of awareness, which embodies the sense of being present (Langer & Moldoveanu, 2000). This being in the now forces people to attend to intention, feel free of time, free of problems, and free of thinking (Tolle, 1999; Weick & Putnam, 2006). The intentionality in mindfulness is not purely cognitive (Heidegger, 1987/2001), but rather it is about engaging with and responding with a purpose (Dreyfus, 1991; Kabat-Zinn, 1994). Other characteristics of mindfulness that have been described by researchers (Brach, 2003; Epstein, 1999; Kabat-Zinn, 2002; Kornfield, 2008; Williams, Teasdale, Siegel, & Kabat-Zinn, 2007) include being open minded, curious, compassionate, a reflective thinker, and not holding onto preconceptions. When opportunities arise, being open allows one to put oneself out in the world in a way of being drawn into being there. S. Shapiro et al. (2006) have proposed a model of mindfulness that is relevant to occupational therapy and includes the core building blocks of intention, attention, and a mindful way attitude, which are the characteristics cited in the common definition of mindfulness by Kabat-Zinn (1994). The three building blocks of mindfulness—intention, attention, and attitude—are not separate stages but are seen as interwoven aspects of a cyclic process and occur simultaneously (S. Shapiro et al.). Mindfulness is this moment-to-moment process.

Intention

Kabat-Zinn (1990) says that it is our intentions that set the stage for what can happen. Research by D. Shapiro (1992) explored the role of intentions of meditation practitioners and found that intentions corresponded with goals that practitioners set for themselves, such as self-regulation and stress management. Another finding was that practitioners' intentions shifted and evolved over time, suggesting a dynamic quality that reflected that people change and develop deeper mindfulness characteristics, such as awareness, insight, and compassion.

Attention

In the context of mindfulness, paying attention involves observing the moment-to-moment processes, and the internal and external experience (S. Shapiro et al., 2006). Helminski (1992) says that whatever occupies attention, whether inwardly or outwardly, whether profound or trivial is what and where we are at that moment. S. Shapiro et al. predict that the self-regulation of attention most likely enhances the skills involved in attentional abilities as described in cognitive psychology, which include vigilance or sustained attention (Posner & Rothbart, 1992), switching, or the ability to shift, the focus (Posner, 1980), and cognitive inhibition, the ability to inhibit distracting mental events and sensations (Williams, Mathews, & MacLeod, 1996).

Attitude

How we attend is also critical. The qualities one brings to the act of paying attention are very important (Brach, 2003; KabatZinn, 2003; Kornfield, 2008). This is relevant to occupational therapy practice in that that there may be a more conscious commitment; for example, one might ask oneself, "Can I bring kindness, curiosity, and openness to my awareness without judgment?". These heart qualities brought into practice will help one to accept experiences and not continually strive for pleasant ones to push aversive experiences away (S. Shapiro et al., 2006)

Relevance of Flow and Mindfulness to Occupational Engagement

Occupational Engagement Modes: Flow and Mindfulness Experiences

Flow and mindfulness are associated with the concept of occupational engagement in terms of how they are experienced and practiced. There is a link between the critical aspects of mindfulness and flow that capture awareness and presence during occupational engagement. Both flow and mindfulness embody a presence to or attunement during modes of occupational engagement. Occupational engagement does not represent an absolute quality, and this is why individuals report having different experiences of being engaged in an occupation.

Sutton (2008) describes a continuum of engagement in the everyday world, from being disengaged, to being in an everyday engagement mode, to being fully engaged. Sutton's work with mental health survivors suggests that presence varies depending on what is being attuned to, such as the body, the immediate physical environment, or beyond to the social environment. In everyday modes of engagement, in which most individuals engage in occupations, there exist opportunities to experience presence to the requirements of the task, the outcomes, the body, and the immediate and social environment through conscious awareness. Mindfulness is a way of being attuned and consciously aware while engaged in an occupation in every day modes of engagement.

In contrast, in absorbed, or full, engagement modes, most of the everyday requirement, such as expectations, time, space, and the like, drift into the background, and one becomes attuned to and present with a deeper sense of connection, intuitiveness, naturalness and sheer enjoyment in the engagement (Sutton, 2008). It is during the absorbed engagement mode that flow experiences are more possible. Abdel-Hafez (2006) described the experience of one of her research participants who was engaged in an outdoor running race. He was so caught up in the process of pacing himself to run well that running appeared to take hold of his embodied being and kept him focused for the entire race time. He was so absorbed in what he was doing that it was as though all the other runners were not there. Another significant aspect of this participant's experience with running was that his perception of time also disappeared. This loss of awareness of time is an element of a flow experience according to Csikszentmihalyi (1990). Philosophically, the concept of an absorbed engagement mode, or being fully engaged, provides a form of transcendence that Heidegger (1927/1962) indicates is related to "being-in-the-world" and its possibilities of being. Heidegger says that transcendence is about being wholly occupied and absorbed within it, which is what flow is.

Environmental Contexts, Occupational Engagement

Occupational engagement occurs in environmental contexts, and these can open a space for accepting and understanding the possibility of the occupational engagement experience. In the occupational science and occupational therapy literature, there are some studies that demonstrate how the role of the social and physical environments have influenced occupational engagement and the experience of flow. Jacobs (1994) studied 90 occupational therapy practitioners in the work place in rehabilitation facilities in New England and found that most experienced flow an average of one to twelve times a day based on Csikszentmihalyi, Hektner, Hektner, and Schmidt's (2006) experience sampling method. Forty-three percent of therapists were interviewed and perceived their autonomy and self-esteem were higher during their flow experiences, and that they held such attitudes as being happy, positive, challenged, proud, and excited. Interestingly, subjects in flow also tended to describe their mood as "tense." Wright, Sadla, and Stew (2006) studied the processes of flow when one engage in art, music, and gardening. Three participants (artist, musician, horticulturist) maintained a written journal or a tape-recorded journal of their flow experiences during a two-week period. All participants were interviewed. Using a phenomenological data-analysis method based on Becker's (1992) method, each interview was analyzed separately. All three participants identified how the environment shaped what they did. An example included tidying up the work space in an art studio so that an environment with no distractions and worries could be had. Participants reported they were immersed in their activities and that perception of time was lost. They all reported having positive feelings after the activity.

In the fields of medicine and nursing, Irving, Dobkin, and Park (2009) and S. Shapiro, Schwartz, and Bonner (1998) investigated how an eight-week mindfulness training program helped reduce levels of stress and improved professional occupational effectiveness among medical and premedical students in a health care context. The core aspects of the program included developing awareness of body sensations, thoughts, and emotions.

Bruce and Davies (2005) conducted a study that explored how a hospice environment influenced caregiving. Mindfulness meditation was a practice engaged by hospice caregivers that was perceived to foster internal and external environments wherein ambiguous, uncertain, and paradoxical human experiences were supported. Findings indicated that among caregivers there was a "presence" that involved knowing patients phenomenologically and co-experiencing their worlds in the context of their health care. Mindfulness was one way that care providers could foster environments of spaciousness that supported whatever was required in a person's dying process. This study signifies the importance of conscious awareness and noting moment-to-moment experiences.

A Critical Look at Research on Flow and Mindfulness

Flow

In research work on flow, attention can be focused on the common characteristics of flow or to inter-individ-

ual differences. A major limitation in research focused on characteristics of flow is that many researchers have used different conceptualizations of flow for their investigations and measurements; thus, the concept of flow remains inconsistent. Thus, it remains unclear whether all the characteristics of flow suggested by Csikszentmihalyi (1996) need to be experienced to the same degree before it can be assumed that flow is experienced (Wright et al., 2006).

The characteristics suggested by Csikszentmihalyi (1990) for a flow experience are (1) clear goals, (2) immediate feedback, (3) balance between skills and challenges, (4) sense of control, (5) focus and concentration, (6) effortless action, (7) loss of self-consciousness, (8) distorted sense of time, and (9) merged action and awareness. In 1990, Csikszentmihalyi introduced the term "autotelic person," which refers to individuals who are highly capable of experiencing flow. These individuals are psychologically better equipped for experiencing flow. Little research has been conducted so far to investigate the characteristics of these individuals. Logan (1988) suggests that autotelic individuals desire more challenges, and Jackson and Roberts (1992) found that they are intrinsically motivated, have high self-esteem, and are less anxious.

Another limitation in flow research is that researchers have used varied methodologies when studying flow, including the experience sampling method and the use of questionnaires. Few researchers have investigated the concept of flow using phenomenological methods to investigate the personal experience. Wright et al. (2006) conducted a phenomenological study in which he conducted interviews to explore the experiences of individuals while they engaged in activities. The phenomena that were described in his study were related to either flow or mindfulness theory, which may have implications for our understanding of how occupational engagement can influence health and for occupational therapy practice. Researchers, including Wright et al., have suggested that more research is needed to examine how flow characteristics are related to states such as mindfulness (Brown & Ryan, 2003; Haybron, 2008).

Finally, researchers have approached the phenomenon of flow philosophically (Heidegger, 1927/1962), looking at being absorbed in an occupation to such an extent that one's way of being is revealed.

Mindfulness

Combining the results of studies on mindfulness is impossible because the interventions and outcomes are very different. Interventions range from the standard eight-week mindfulness-based stress reduction program developed through the University of Massachusetts with Dr. Jon Kabat-Zinn (Center for Mindfulness in Medicine, Health Care, and Society, 2009) to other related interventions, such as relaxation, body scan, yoga, sitting meditation. The small sample sizes and heterogeneous patient populations, lack of control groups, weak outcome measures, and limited description of the randomization process compromise the data of many studies (Shapiro, Bootzin, Figueredo, Lopez, & Schwartz, 2003; Smith, Richardson, Hoffman, & Pilkington, 2005), as well as a lack of reporting of recruitment methods and loss to follow-up information (Majumdar, Grossman, Dietz-Waschkowski, Kersig, & Walach, 2002), and compliance issues (Majumdar et al.; Saxe et al., ness interventions are multimodal; therefore, it is impossible to determine which aspect of the intervention has the therapeutic effect (Smith et al.).

Although many studies suffer from methodological limitations, the findings from other randomized controlled and uncontrolled studies suggest some positive outcomes. For example, mindfulness-based interventions help to alleviate a variety of mental health and physical problems (Smith et al., 2005; Walloch, 2006), improve awareness, enhance learning (Langer, 1989, 1997), improve psychological functioning (Baer, 2003), improve medical practice (Epstein, Siegel, & Silberman, 2008), and facilitate a heightened state of presence (Langer & Moldoveanu, 2000; Reid, 2009).

Despite the limitations in research and continued need to do more research, the two phenomena of flow and mindfulness have implications for how occupational engagement can influence well-being. The current knowledge about flow and mindfulness can assist occupational therapists when involving their clients in occupations for the purpose of experiencing flow or cultivating mindfulness. The following two scenarios illustrate how occupational engagement can be fully utilized by occupational therapists to achieve flow or to cultivate mindfulness for the benefit of their clients.

Scenario 1

A community occupational therapist has been asked by a group home for adolescents-at-risk to develop an activity group to provide flow opportunities for troubled youth. The youth spend little time engaged in active occupations, and spend most of their time watching TV or smoking outdoors at the group home where they live. The occupational therapist needs to decide what group activity will provide an experience that will enable youth to find the "just right challenge" and be fully engaged for a period of time. The occupational therapist decides that forming a running group could provide a goal—to run in an upcoming city wide 10k race. In addition, this activity is healthier than smoking or the passive pursuit of watching TV. After several weeks of organizing short practice run sessions, the occupational therapist notes that several of the youth have shown an interest and commitment towards realizing personal goals at running, and that running is viewed as challenging but possible. The occupational therapist gradually increases practice periods to organizing small 5k races with the youth. The 5k races allow the youth to become more attuned to their immediate world, their bodies (sensations), the physical environment (roads, hills, parks), and the social environment (other runners), and to be present as they engage in running. The occupational therapist notices that the youth begin to report that they feel freer and forget about their problems as the running appears to take hold of their embodied being and keeps them occupied for at least two hours a day. The occupational therapist concludes that many of the youth are possibly experiencing flow through their group running. This scenario illustrates that the youth were fully engaging in running and occupying their being-in-the-world in such a way that they transcended with the activity as discussed by Heidegger (1927/1962).

Scenario 2

The occupational therapist is working with Valerie, a 57-year-old woman in a mental health setting. Her goal is to enable Valerie to engage in everyday occupation and provide more possibilities for developing Valerie's state of being-in-theworld (Heidegger, 1927/1962). After several weeks of the occupational therapist's focusing on developing a relationship with Valerie, she notices that Valerie's attunement to her world has changed from being primarily preoccupied with her emotions to being more attuned to more of her immediate environment, and she was engaging more in everyday simple activities with her family when they visited. The occupational therapist is mindfully aware of her relationship with Valerie, and senses that being available and open with Valerie provides her with a more holistic and authentic view of her client. The occupational therapist reflects an awareness of Valerie's needs, expectations, fears, the like, and listens carefully to what Valerie says when she is with her. When Valerie reports her love of art to the occupational therapist, the occupational therapist readily supports Valerie by enabling her to engage in an art activity. The occupational therapist engages in the art activity alongside Valerie and at her pace. The activity that is chosen by the occupational therapist and agreed upon by Valerie is painting silk scarves. Engaging in this activity allows Valerie to be occupationally present and mindful (Reid, 2008) as she feels the texture of the silk, senses the texture of the paint on the silk while stroking the paint across the cloth, and takes in the colors of the paint on the silk. Engaging mindfully in this activity strengthens Valerie's sense of self as she tells the occupational therapist that she has decided to wear the scarf the next day. This scenario illustrates that with the support of the occupational therapist, Valerie can experience being more mindful of increasing her active engagement in her immediate world.

Conclusion

This paper discusses theoretical viewpoints and research on the concepts of mindfulness and flow, and explores how these concepts are relevant to occupational engagement. Different perspectives drawn from philosophy and psychology are used to bestow a broader understanding of mindfulness and flow as related to occupational engagement. While research on flow and mindfulness is limited by methodological and conceptual issues, a new understanding of these concepts will lead to more research. The intent of this paper is to suggest that mindfulness and flow have implications for how occupational engagement can influence well-being as a way of being present in the world. Flow and mindfulness embody a presence to, or attunement, during modes of occupational engagement. During everyday modes of engagement, most individuals engage in occupations; there exist more opportunities to experience presence to the requirements of the task, the outcomes, the body, and the immediate and social environment through conscious awareness.

Key Messages

- Occupational therapists should consider incorporating principles of mindfulness and flow in practice.
- Occupational therapists should consider how flow and mindfulness are influenced by the mode of occupational engagement.

- Mindfulness can be cultivated in occupational therapists so that they can be more present with their clients.

Acknowledgements

Thank you to my many colleagues and friends in Canada, New Zealand and Japan who engaged in discussions with me about my thoughts about mindfulness.

References

Abdel-Hafez, N. (2006). *Exploring presence through occupation* (Unpublished master's thesis). University of Toronto, Toronto, ON.

Baer, R. A. (2003). Mindfulness training as a clinical intervention: a conceptual and empirical review. *Clinical Psychology: Science and Practice, 10,* 125–143. http://dx.doi.org/10.1093/clipsy/bpg015

Becker, C. (1992). *Living and relating: An introduction to phenomenology.* Thousand Oaks, CA: Sage Publications.

Brach, T. (2003). *Radical acceptance.* New York: Bantam Dell, Random House.

Brown, K. W., & Ryan, R. M. (2003). The benefits of being present: Mindfulness and its role in psychological well-being. *Journal of Personality and Social Psychology, 84,* 822–848. http://dx.doi.org/10.1037/0022-3514.84.4.822

Bruce, A., & Davies, B. (2005). Mindfulness in hospice care: Practicing meditation-in-action. *Qualitative Health Research, 15,* 1329–1344. http://dx.doi.org/10.1177/1049732305281657

Bryce, J., & Haworth, J. (2002). Wellbeing and flow in sample of male and female office workers. *Leisure Studies, 21,* 249–263. http://dx.doi.org/10.1080/0261436021000030687

Carmody, J., & Baer, R. (2007). Relationships between mindfulness practice and levels of mindfulness, medical and psychological symptoms and well-being in a mindfulness-based stress reduction program. *Journal of Behavioral Medicine, 31,* 23-33. http://dx.doi.org/10.1007/s10865-007-9130-7

Center for Mindfulness in Medicine, Health Care and Society, University of Massachusetts. (2009). *The stress reduction program: An invitation to move toward greater balance, control, and participation in your life.* Retrieved from http://www.umassmed.edu/uploadedFiles/srp_brochure.pdf

Csikszentmihalyi, M. (1975). *Beyond boredom and anxiety.* San Francisco: Jossey-Bass.

Csikszentmihalyi, M. (1996). *Creativity: Flow and the psychology of discovery and invention.* New York: Harper Perennial.

Csikszentmihalyi, M. (1997). *Finding flow: The psychology of engagement with everyday life*. New York: Basic Books.

Csikszentmihalyi, M., Hektner, J., Hektner, M., & Schmidt, J. (2006). *Experience sampling method: Measuring the quality of everyday life*. Thousand Oaks, CA: Sage Publications.

Dreyfus, H. L. (1991). *Being-in-the-world: A commentary on Heidegger's Being and Time*. Cambridge, MA: MIT Press.

Epstein, R. (1999). Mindful practice. *Journal of the American Medical Association, 282*, 833–839.

Epstein, R., Siegel, D., & Silberman, J. (2008). Self-monitoring in clinical practice: A challenge for medical educators. *Journal of Continuing Education in the Health Professions, 28*, 5–13. http://dx.doi.org/10.1002/chp.149

Farb, N. A., Segal Z. V., Mayberg, H., Bean, J., McKeon, D., Fatima, Z., & Anderson, A. (2007). Attending to the present: Evidence for dissociable neural modes of self-reference. *Social Cognitive and Affective Neuroscience, 2*, 313–322. http://dx.doi.org/10.1093/scan/nsm030

Fritz, B., & Avsec, A. (2007). The experience of flow and subjective well-being of music students. *Horizons of Psychology, 16*(2), 5–17.

Haybron, D. (2008). *The pursuit of unhappiness: The elusive psychology of well-being*. New York: Oxford University Press, Inc.

Heidegger, M. (1962). *Being and time* (J. Macquarrie & E. Robinson, Trans.). New York: Harper and Row. (Original work published 1927)

Heidegger, M. (1996). *Being and time* (J. Stambaugh, Trans.). New York: New York State University Press.

Heidegger, M. (2001). *Zollikon seminars: Protocols, conversations, letters* (F. Mayr & R. Askay, Trans.). Evanston, IL: Northwestern University Press. (Original work published 1987)

Helminski, K. E. (1992). *Living presence*. New York: Penguin, Putnam.

Irving, J., Dobkin, P., & Park, J. (2009). Cultivating mindfulness in health care professionals: A review of empirical studies of mindfulness-based stress reduction (MBSR). *Complementary Therapies in Clinical Practice, 15*, 61–66.

Jackson, J., Carlson, M., Mandel, D., Zemke, R., & Clark, F. (1998). Occupation in lifestyle redesign: The well elderly study occupational therapy program. *American Journal of Occupational Therapy, 52*, 326–336.

Jackson, S., & Csikszentmihalyi, M. (1999). *Flow in sports: The keys to optimal experiences and performances*. Champaign, IL: Human Kinetices.

Jacobs, K. (1994). Flow and the occupational therapy practitioner. *American Journal of Occupational Therapy, 48*, 989–996. http://dx.doi.org/10.5014/ajot.48.11.989

Kabat-Zinn, J. (1990). *Full catastrophe living*. New York: Bantam Dell, Random House.

Kabat-Zinn, J. (1994). *Wherever you go you are there*. New York: Hyperion.

Kabat-Zinn, J. (2002). Meditation is about paying attention. *Reflection, 3*, 68–71.

Kabat-Zinn, J. (2003). Mindfulness based interventions in context: Past, present and future. *Clinical Psychology: Science and Practice, 10*, 144–156. http://dx.doi.org/10.1093/clipsy/bpg016

Kornfield, J. (2008). *The wise heart*. New York: Bantam Dell, Random House.

Langer, E. (1989). *Mindfulness*. Reading, MA: Addison-Wesley Publishing Co.

Langer, E. (1997). *The power of mindful learning*. New York: Perseus Publishing.

Langer, E., & Moldoveanu, M. (2000). Mindfulness research and the future. *Journal of Social Issues, 56*, 129–139. http://dx.doi.org/10.1111/0022-4537.00155

Law, M., Steinwender, S., & Leclair, L. (1998). Occupation, health, and well-being. *Canadian Journal of Occupational Therapy, 65*, 81–91.

Logan, R. (1988). Flow and solitary ordeals. In M. Csikszentmihalyi & I. Csikszentmihalyi (Eds.), *Optimal experience*. Cambridge, MA: Cambridge University Press.

Majumdar, M., Grossman, P., Dietz-Waschkowski, B., Kersig, S., & Walach, H. (2002). Does mindfulness meditation contribute to health? Outcome evaluation of a German sample. *The Journal of Alternative and Complementary Medicine, 8*, 719–730. http://dx.doi.org/10.1089/10755530260511720

Maslow, A. (1968). *Toward a psychology of being*. Oxford: D. Van Nostrand.

Mee, J., & Sumsion, T. (2001). Mental health clients confirm the motivating power of occupation. *British Journal of Occupational Therapy, 64*, 121–138.

Merleau-Ponty, M. (1962). *Phénomélogie de la pérception* [Phenomenology of perception]. Paris: Librairie Gallimard. (Original work published 1945)

Posner, M. (1980). Orienting of attention. *Quarterly Journal of Experimental Psychology, 32*, 3–25.

Posner, M., & Rothbart, M. (1992). Attentional mechanisms and conscious experience. In A.D. Milner & M.D. Rugg (Eds.), *The neuropsychology of consciousness* (pp. 91–111). Toronto: Academic Press.

Privette, G. (1983). Peak experience, peak performance, and flow: A comparative analysis of positive human experiences. *Journal of Personality and Social Psychology,*

45, 1361–1368. http://dx.doi.org/10.1037/0022-3514. 45.6.1361

Reid, D. T. (2008). Exploring the relationship between occupational presence, occupational engagement, and people's well-being. *Journal of Occupational Science, 15*, 43–47.

Reid, D. T. (2009). Capturing presence moments: The art of mindful practice in occupational therapy. *Canadian Journal of Occupational Therapy, 76*, 180–188.

Saxe, G., Hebert, J., Carmody, J., Kabat-Zinn, J., Rosensweig, P., Jarjobski, D., . . . Blute, R. (2001). Can diet in conjunction to stress reduction affect the rate of increase of prostate specific antigen after biochemical recurrence of prostate cancer? *The Journal of Urology, 166*, 2202–2207. http://dx.doi.org/10.1016/S0022-5347(05)65535-8

Shapiro, D. (1992). A preliminary study of long term meditators: Goals, effects, religious orientation, cognitions. *Journal of Transpersonal Psychology, 24*, 23–39.

Shapiro, S., Bootzin, R., Figueredo, A., Lopez, A., & Schwartz, G. (2003). The efficacy of mindfulness stress reduction in the treatment of sleep disturbance in women with breast cancer: An exploratory study. *Journal of Psychosomatic Research, 51*, 85–91.

Shapiro, S., Carlson, L., Astin, J., & Freedman, B. (2006). Mechanisms of mindfulness. *Journal of Clinical Psychology, 62*, 373–386. http://dx.doi.org/10.1002/jclp.20237

Shapiro, S., Schwartz, G., & Bonner, G. (1998). Effects of mindfulness-based stress reduction on medical and premedical students. *Journal of Behavioral Medicine, 21*, 581–599. http://dx.doi.org/10.1023/A:1018700829825

Siegel, D. (2007). *The mindful brain.* New York: W. W. Norton & Company.

Smith, J., Richardson, J., Hoffman, C., & Pilkington, K. (2005). Mindfulness stress reduction as supportive therapy in cancer care: A systematic review. *Journal of Advanced Nursing, 52*, 315–327. http://dx.doi.org/10.1111/j.1365-2648.2005.03592.x

Sutton, D. (2008). *Recovery as the refabrication of every day life: Exploring the meaning of doing for people re-covering from mental illness* (Unpublished doctoral thesis). Auckland University of Technology, Auckland, NZ.

Thera, N. (1996). *The heart of Buddhist meditation.* York Beach, MN: Samuel Weiser.

Tolle, E. (1999). *The power of now.* Vancouver, CA: Namaste Publishing.

Townsend, E., & Polatajko, H. (2007). *Enabling occupation II.* Ottawa, ON: CAOT Publications.

Walloch, C. (2006). Neuro-occupation and the management of chronic pain through mindfulness meditation. *Occupational Therapy International, 3*, 238–248. http://dx.doi.org/10.1002/oti.78

Weick, K., & Putnam, T. (2006). Organizing for mindfulness: Eastern wisdom and western knowledge. *Journal of Management Inquiry, 15*, 275–287. http://dx.doi.org/10.1177/1056492606291202

Wilcock, A. (1998). Reflections on doing, being and becoming. *Australian Occupational Therapy Journal, 46*, 1–11. http://dx.doi.org/10.1046/j.1440-1630.1999.00174.x

Wilcock, A. (2006). *An occupational perspective on health* (2nd ed.). Thorofare, NJ: Slack.

Williams, J., Mathews, A., & MacCleod, C. (1996). The emotional Stroop task and psychopathology. *Psychological Bulletin, 120*, 3–24. http://dx.doi.org/10.1037/0033-2909.120.1.3

Williams, M., Teasdale, J., Siegel, Z., & Kabat-Zinn (2007). *The mindful way through depression.* New York: The Guilford Press.

Wright, J., Sadla, G., & Stew, G. (2006). Challenge-skills and mindfulness: An exploration of the conundrum of flow process. *OTJR: Occupation, Participation and Health, 26*, 1–8.

Yerxa, E. (1998). Health and the spirit of occupation. *American Journal of Occupational Therapy, 52*, 412–418. http://dx.doi.org/10.5014/ajot.52.6.412

CHAPTER 13

Occupational Well-Being: Rethinking Occupational Therapy Outcomes

SUSAN E. DOBLE AND JOSIANE CARON SANTHA

The relative importance of individuals' abilities to derive satisfaction and fulfillment from their occupational experiences is often overshadowed by the central role that occupational performance plays within occupational therapy. This paper provides an initial introduction to the concept of occupational well-being and proposes a descriptive framework that occupational therapists can use to examine if and to what extent clients' occupational experiences are satisfying and fulfilling. Our intent is to challenge occupational therapists to rethink the focus of occupational therapy outcomes and consider the importance of individuals' subjective occupational experiences.

Background

Five critical issues have been discussed within occupational science and occupational therapy literature over the past two decades. These issues have influenced the development of the concept of occupational well-being and the framework we are proposing for practice in this paper. Separately and collectively, these five issues also challenge occupational therapists to re-evaluate the outcomes of occupational therapy.

First, when the *International Classification of Functioning, Disability and Health* (ICF) (World Health Organization [WHO], 2001) was introduced, the concept of participation was identified as an important outcome. Although the ICF does not specifically utilize the term occupation, it is based on the assumption that the health of individuals is influenced by their participation in life situations. This closely mirrors an assumption that grounds the profession of occupational therapy, which is that occupation affects individuals' health

and well-being (Wilcock, 1998, 2006). Within the ICF, participation is defined as observed performance, and therefore participation and occupational performance are often assumed to be comparable constructs. Consequently, participation has been adopted within the professional language of occupational therapy and considered to be a valid occupational therapy outcome. However, participation fails to capture the complexity of occupation (Borell, Asaba, Rosenberg, Schult, & Townsend, 2006; Hemmingsson & Jonsson, 2005). More specifically, it fails to reflect the variable nature of individuals' occupations (Polatajko et al., 2007), and acknowledge that individuals' subjective experiences of occupation influence their health. However, without a clearer framework that accounts for the idiosyncratic nature of individuals' occupations and acknowledges the importance of individuals' subjective occupational experiences, occupational therapists' ability to argue why participation alone is an insufficient occupational therapy outcome is constrained.

The second central issue is Wilcock's (1998) challenge for occupational therapists to broaden their understanding of occupation from 'doing' toward "a synthesis of doing, being and becoming" (p. 249). 'Doing' is captured within the traditional focus of practice models, that is, occupational performance. From this perspective, occupational therapy interventions are designed largely to enhance individuals' competent performance of occupations that they need or are expected to do. 'Being' refers to an introspective or meditative contemplation of the self. Thus, occupation does not simply refer to what is done but to the process of doing or the here and now of individuals' occupational experiences. The 'becoming' dimension of occupation refers to possibility, growth, and the ongoing evolution of individuals' occupational identities.

Building on this work, Rebeiro, Day, Semeniuk, O'Brien, and Wilson (2001) suggested that occupation

This chapter was previously published in the *Canadian Journal of Occupational Therapy, 75*, 184–190. Copyright © 2008, the Canadian Association of Occupational Therapists. Reprinted with permission. http://dx.doi.org/10.1177/000841740807500310

also provides opportunities to 'belong' by developing and maintaining connections with others. Hammell (2004) pushed thinking further by proposing that doing, being, belonging and becoming are fundamental sources of meaning experienced through occupation. Together, these ideas highlight the need for occupational therapists to enable their clients to meet their needs for doing, being, belonging, and becoming. The new Canadian Model of Occupational Performance and Engagement (CMOP–E) (Polatajko et al., 2007) continues to build on these ideas by challenging occupational therapists to expand their focus from occupational performance to also include engagement. As Polatajko and colleagues suggested, individuals are engaged in occupations whether they are actively, passively, sporadically or constantly involved, and even when they are barely attentive to what they are doing. Whether Evan fills the bird feeder, sketches the birds as they feed, or simply watches them feed, he is engaged in occupation.

The third central issue influencing the concept of occupational well-being is the need to recognize that individuals compose or orchestrate their occupational lives (Bateson, 1996). Zemke and Clark (1996) described people's lives as "progressive compositional art forms in which the next movement or phase, old strand or themes can be recycled and new ones simultaneously introduced" (p. 1). Over time, individuals' occupational lives continually change and evolve; occupations are added and eliminated; and level of engagement changes. The idea that individuals compose or orchestrate their occupational lives, shifts attention away from what individuals do to how individuals knit their occupations into patterns.

The fourth central issue relates to the idea that "a balance of occupation is beneficial to health and well-being" (Christiansen, 1996, p. 432). Balance has been defined in terms of the time spent in self-care, work/productivity, play/leisure occupations. Pierce (2001; see Chapter 61) argued that these occupational categories are "simplistic, value laden, decontextualized, and insufficiently descriptive of subjective experience" (p. 252). They focus attention on what is done rather than on why individuals choose the occupations they do, and what individuals hope to gain from engaging in these occupations. We contend that individuals experience balance when they are able to consistently meet their occupational needs. As such, each individual must determine when they experience a sense of balance.

The fifth and final issue that has shaped the development of the concept of occupational well-being is the construct of meaning (Christiansen, 1999; Hammell, 2004; Hasselkus, 2002; Wilcock, 1998, 2006). There is general acceptance within the literatures from occupational therapy and occupational science that individuals' health and well-being are enhanced when they engage in meaningful occupations. Meaning is shaped by personal, as well as cultural and societal values, beliefs, and attitudes. Current practice models guide occupational therapists to support clients to choose and engage in meaningful occupations that reflect their spirituality (Canadian Association of Occupational Therapists, 2002; Polatajko et al., 2007) or volition (i.e., their sense of their own capacities, values and interests) (Kielhofner, 2008). While these models clarify why individuals choose certain occupations, they do not shed light on how individuals' engagement in occupations generates meaning and satisfaction. It is our intent to propose a framework that occupational therapists can use with clients to examine their occupational lives, and determine the extent to which the occupations that they choose, engage in, and have orchestrated into their occupational lives generate meaning and satisfaction.

Occupational Well-Being

In keeping with Hasselkus' (2002) suggestion that occupational therapy should include the "goals of living with one's self and finding fulfillment in one's self " (p. 82), we propose that individuals' subjective experiences of their occupational lives are an important occupational therapy outcome. We refer to the meaning and satisfaction that individuals derive from their occupational lives as occupational well-being (Doble & Caron Santha, 2007). We contend that individuals are more likely to experience occupational well-being when they choose and engage in occupations, and orchestrate their occupational lives in ways that enable them to consistently meet their occupational needs. Within this paper, we will discuss seven occupational needs which include accomplishment, affirmation, agency, coherence, companionship, pleasure, and renewal.

These occupational needs were identified by examining propositions articulated within the occupational therapy literature suggesting that individuals are more likely to experience meaning and satisfaction when engaged in occupations that enable them to: (a) experience a sense of control, efficacy, value and worth; (b) demonstrate who they are and want to become as occupational beings (Christiansen, 1999; Kielhofner,

2008); (c) learn and master skills, (d) relate to others, and (e) make a connection with their pasts, presents, and futures (Polatajko et al., 2007). Although not specifically identified as occupational well-being, important elements of this concept were also gleaned from narratives presented in an array of qualitative studies in which individuals described their occupational experiences. In reading the literature, we noticed that various terms were used to refer to what appeared to be similar or related constructs. For example, accomplishment, achievement, and mastery refer to a similar construct. In developing this occupational well-being framework, we selected descriptors that we judged as most accurately reflecting the occupational needs individuals strive to meet.

We assert that individuals' need for accomplishment is addressed when individuals engage in occupations and thereby generate evidence that indicates they are learning and mastering skills, meeting performance expectations, and achieving goals (Hillman & Chapparo, 2002; Hvalsøe & Josephsson, 2003; Laliberte-Rudman, Yu, Scott, & Pajouhandeh, 2000; Öhman & Nygård, 2005; Piškur, Kinebanian, & Josephsson, 2002; Reynolds & Prior, 2006). Individuals may experience accomplishment when they master or perceive progress in their ability to perform components of an occupation (e.g., when Jordan learns to do a flip turn when swimming), produce a tangible outcome (e.g., when Callie frames a photograph), or help others (e.g., when Tony helps his mother during her doctor's appointment). Accomplishment may be experienced when individuals learn and utilize new skills (e.g., when James learns to use a new feature on his computer) or when their existing skills are challenged by changing demands of the occupation and/or environment (e.g., when Paul and Karen navigate their canoe across the lake despite high winds). A sense of accomplishment may be derived when adaptations to individuals' physical environments enable them to engage in occupations more easily or with greater competence and confidence (e.g., Ruth turns on the bathroom lights from her wheelchair after a new light switch is installed or Claire sets the table when she receives clear and simple directions). It is important to consider that individuals' need for accomplishment is not dependent on being physically engaged in an occupation. Accomplishment may be experienced when individuals plan occupations, share in the experiences of others, impart information or teach others how to do things, or even reflect on their own past accomplishments.

Affirmation refers to the need to recognize that individuals' occupational choices and occupational performances are important, worthwhile, and valued (Christiansen, 1999), and thus, contribute to their self-worth. We propose that when individuals do things with and for others, they are more likely to receive affirmation either from those people for whom they did something, or from others who are aware of what they did (Borell et al., 2006; Cipriani, Faig, Ayrer, Brown, & Johnson, 2006; Lyons, Orozovic, Davis, & Newman, 2002; Piškur et al., 2002). Pamela experiences affirmation when her teammate congratulates her for blocking a shot made by the opposing team. Ryan experiences affirmation when a passerby smiles after seeing him help someone who dropped some papers. Charlotte experiences affirmation when her neighbours thank her for advocating for a new playground at the local park. Affirmation, however, can also be self-generated. Using available evidence, individuals can recognize that they did something well, or permit themselves to feel proud of a task they completed, or acknowledge the value of their altruistic actions (e.g., Colin experiences affirmation when he prepares a meal for an ill friend).

We propose that individuals' need for agency is addressed when they perceive that they exert influence or control in important or valued aspects of their occupational lives. Agency may be experienced when individuals choose what occupations they do, and how, when, where, how often, and with whom they perform occupations (Borell et al., 2006; Hillman & Chapparo, 2002; Hvalsøe & Josephsson, 2003; Laliberte-Rudman et al., 2000; Piškur et al., 2002). Agency may be increased by setting priorities and by developing routine ways of performing occupations. These strategies in turn may enable individuals to predict what they will do at certain times of the day and ensure that they have enough occupation to fill their time. Agency may also be experienced when individuals choose to engage in occupations spontaneously (Laliberte-Rudman et al.; Leufstadius, Erlandsson, & Eklund, 2006; Nagle, Cook, & Polatajko, 2002).

Even when options are limited, agency may be experienced. Individuals may choose how they will use their skills. They may choose to spend more time engaged in personally rewarding occupations. They may even delegate necessary but less satisfying occupations to others (Hillman & Chapparo, 2002), or they may reframe or reinterpret their experiences. For example, even though Marc is unable to walk the long distances within airports because of arthritis in his hip, he experiences agency by making arrangements for airline staff to transport him in the airport, by directing them to his desired location, and by feeling confident that he will be able to work productively during a scheduled meeting.

Individuals' occupational identities develop as they engage in occupations and clarify their values, personal desires, and goals (Christiansen, 1999; Kielhofner, 2008). When individuals' occupational experiences generate evidence that confirms who they are and want to become, they will experience an increased sense of coherence. Coherence may be experienced when individuals orchestrate their occupational lives such that they engage in occupations that provide them with connections between their pasts, presents, and futures. For example, women with multiple sclerosis experienced a sense of "biographical continuity" (Reynolds & Prior, 2003, p. 1235) when they engaged in occupations that reflected lifelong passions, when they adapted former skills or occupations into their current lives, and when they drew on former interests or skills so they could participate in new occupations.

We suggest that individuals' need for companionship is met when they engage in occupations with others (Borell et al., 2006) who share common experiences, interests, values or goals. Such occupations enable individuals to feel a sense of belonging and sometimes even intimacy. Social relationships that support their engagement in social occupations (e.g., playing tennis, going to dinner with friends) may help individuals meet their companionship needs while also facilitating their ability to meet other occupational needs such as agency, coherence, and pleasure. When individuals meet their needs for companionship, they are less likely to experience feelings of loneliness and isolation (Laliberte-Rudman et al., 2000; Lyons et al., 2002; Piškur et al., 2002; Wilcock, 1998).

Individuals' need for pleasure may range from "the simple satisfaction derived from small daily rituals to the intense pleasure people feel in pursuing their driving passions" (Kielhofner, 2008, p. 43); and thus includes contentment, happiness, and joy. Pleasure may be derived from the anticipation of engaging in enjoyable or fun experiences. The magnitude of these experiences may be increased when individuals give themselves permission to redirect their attention away from stressors and distracters, and immerse themselves in the moment. Individuals may also enhance their opportunities to meet their needs for pleasure by making a conscious effort to savour the experience, squeeze as

much pleasurable occupation into their days as possible (Reynolds & Prior, 2003, 2006), and by focusing their attention on the here and now (Hammell, 2004). As noted above, opportunities to experience pleasure may also be increased when individuals engage in occupations with others (Lyons et al., 2002).

The occupational need for renewal is widely recognized and has been assigned many terms including minute acts of regression, timeouts, declarations of being, and acts of reclamation (Johnson, 1996). When individuals are physically and mentally renewed, they are rejuvenated and thus able to approach other occupations with a fresher perspective (Howell & Pierce, 2000; Pierce, 2001; Sellar & Boshoff, 2006; Watts & Teitelman, 2005). Renewal is experienced when individuals engage in occupations that provide a sense of inner peace, abandon, relief, and mental clarity, and leave them feeling refreshed, re-energized, and rejuvenated (Weinblatt & Avrech-Bar, 2003). The need for renewal may be met when individuals shut off the stresses and demands of everyday life, and become so engrossed in occupations that they lose track of time (Sellar & Boshoff, 2006; Weinblatt & Avrech-Bar).

As suggested above, several occupational needs may be met when even engaged in a single occupation. For example, to surprise his wife, Kevin decided to present his wife with a birthday cake. Rather than meet his need for accomplishment by buying a ready-made cake, he increased his chances of meeting more diverse occupational needs (e.g., companionship and pleasure) by making and decorating a cake with his young son. When Kevin's wife expressed her appreciation for the cake and Kevin's decision to include their son in the process, his need for affirmation was also addressed.

Influencing Factors

We recognize that several factors influence individuals' abilities to orchestrate their occupational lives to consistently meet their occupational needs. First, personal factors (e.g., expectations, competencies, mood, attitudes, and past experiences) and environmental factors will influence individuals' abilities to address their occupational needs. For example, Jill's needs for accomplishment, agency, pleasure, and renewal may be reduced when she sprains her ankle after slipping when hiking on a trail seriously damaged by heavy rains the previous week.

Second, individuals' potential to experience occupational well-being is dependent, in part, by the available occupational opportunities. Limited occupational choices may threaten individuals' abilities to meet their occupational needs. For example, despite completing a university degree, employment opportunities in Anna's community are limited. She views her current job in a fast-food restaurant as unchallenging and demeaning. Anna's occupational experiences at work severely threaten her ability to meet her occupational needs, particularly her needs for accomplishment, agency, coherence, and pleasure.

Third, although we propose that all individuals have these same occupational needs, we recognize that the relative importance of each need is highly individualized. For example, one person's need for companionship may be greater than someone else's. Moreover, an individual's need for companionship may vary across his lifetime. Thus we propose that occupational well-being is dependent on individuals' ability to orchestrate their lives in ways that will increase their chances to meet their diverse occupational needs.

Addressing Occupational Well-Being in Occupational Therapy Practice

We believe that occupational therapists should make a concerted effort to examine and address their clients' occupational well-being. The proposed framework for describing occupational well-being can be integrated into existing models of practice. For example, occupational therapists using the CMOP–E (Polatajko et al., 2007) would address their clients' occupational well-being, in addition to their occupational performance and engagement. Similarly, occupational therapists utilizing the Model of Human Occupation (Kielhofner, 2008) would support clients to choose and participate in occupations that enable them to construct a positive occupational identity and achieve occupational competence, while also ensuring that clients consistently and satisfactorily meet their occupational needs. Regardless of the model of practice used, the initial goal would be to determine the extent to which individuals' occupational lives are orchestrated to enable them to consistently meet their occupational needs.

If necessary, interventions would be designed and implemented with the target outcome of enhanced occupational well-being. Clients would be provided with opportunities to examine the extent to which their lives are currently orchestrated to consistently meet their occupational needs. Efforts might then be made to enable clients to enhance their performance

skills; clarify their values and interests; establish different standards against which they evaluate their own occupational lives; or even effect changes in their physical and social environments. Efforts may also be directed towards the broader environment in order to effect changes at an organizational or policy level. By advocating on behalf of individuals, occupational therapists may increase individuals' opportunities to access occupations that have the potential to enhance their occupational well-being. Finally, in order to determine if individuals derive greater satisfaction and fulfillment from their occupational lives following intervention, individuals' occupational well-being must be re-evaluated to determine if they are able to more consistently meet their occupational needs following intervention.

Case Example—Rob

Following amputations of both of his lower limbs above the knee, Rob underwent a period of rehabilitation. His occupational therapy intervention was designed to determine if he could effectively and safely perform his usual self-care and household activities, and safely move about his home and community. Following discharge from the rehabilitation centre, Rob returned to work as a computer analyst and thus continued to meet occupational needs formerly met through his engagement in work-related occupations. However, when Rob was seen for follow-up by a community-based occupational therapist, it was evident that Rob's re-orchestrated occupational life was not supporting his ability to meet his occupational needs. Although able to perform his job tasks, architectural barriers constrained Rob's ability to access the work lunch room and lounge. Unable to connect informally with his colleagues over coffee or lunch, or join departmental celebrations held in the lounge, Rob's needs for companionship and pleasure at work were not being met. His feelings of alienation from his co-workers also threatened his ability to meet other occupational needs within his work-related occupations (e.g., agency, accomplishment, and coherence). Rob's occupational therapist worked with him, his manager and other employees to increase their awareness of the impact of architectural barriers on Rob's occupational well-being. As a group, they identified several possible solutions, determined what financial and other resources could be accessed to help facilitate changes, and developed a plan of action that would benefit Rob.

A re-evaluation of Rob's occupational well-being enabled Rob and his occupational therapist to recognize that since his accident, Rob had withdrawn from former occupations such as downhill skiing. When he wasn't working, he watched television—a pattern of occupation that was incongruent with his former occupational life. Rob's occupational therapist encouraged him to recognize that he could still ski. Rob was unconvinced; he perceived adaptive equipment and reliance on others for assistance as threats to his need for agency. Rob's occupational therapist provided him with information about a national association organized to enable persons with disabilities to participate in downhill skiing, and arranged for him to speak with others with significant injuries whose use of adaptive equipment enabled them to ski again. These experiences, in turn, enabled Rob to recognize that he could exercise agency by using adaptive equipment and using available supports to engage in an occupation he loved.

Case Example—Home and School Association

A School Board implemented a 'hands-off' policy in an effort to reduce physical aggression between children on the school playground. Consequently, children were no longer permitted to engage in games such as tag and touch football. Parents at one school expressed concerns to their Home and School Association (H&SA). They complained that older children's physical activity levels had decreased and the level of verbal bullying among children had increased. When the H&SA presented their concerns to the school's principal, he argued that the policy enabled the teaching staff to reinstate discipline within the School. The H&SA approached their School Board member. Since the policy had been adopted before their School Board member took office, efforts made to raise the issue were cut short by the Chair of the School Board. However, the Board agreed to review the policy in two years.

Concerned about the students' well-being, the H&SA hired an occupational therapist to enable them to 'live with' the policy. Random observations were made to document children's level of physical activity and the actual occupations they did. The occupational therapist reviewed records in which the teachers and principal documented how often children were cautioned and disciplined in relation to the "hands-off" policy, the level of bullying experienced by children, and factors that appeared to contribute to bullying. The occupational therapist collaborated with students to identify ageappropriate games and activities that could be played at recess without contravening the "hands-off" policy. Students that were identified by teachers

as most likely to bully were included in this process. H&SA members developed an equipment list and raised monies to purchase necessary playground equipment. The occupational therapist chaired several discussions between the principal, teachers and members of the H&SA to ensure that reasonable discretion would be used when enforcing the 'hands-off' policy. During these discussions, all parties developed a greater respect and appreciation for the perspectives of the other people involved. Consequently, a situation that could have caused friction and divisiveness among members of the School community was averted. Recognizing that not all schools within the Board's jurisdiction were equally positioned to address this issue, the H&SA developed and disseminated a booklet in which they described a range of age-appropriate games and activities that did not contravene the "hands-off " policy to other schools within the School Board.

Conclusion

In this paper, we have taken an important first step in expanding the concept of occupational well-being and proposing a framework that can be used by occupational therapists to examine individuals' occupational lives. We began this paper by describing how five issues influenced our thinking about occupational therapy outcomes and led to the development of the concept of occupational well-being. First, the proposed framework reflects the complexity of occupation by embracing the idiosyncratic nature of individuals' occupations, and drawing attention to individuals' subjective experiences of their occupations. Second, references to occupational experiences within this framework include not only those ones where individuals are engaged in doing, but also being, belonging, and becoming. Third, individuals' occupational lives will be composed or orchestrated of different constellations of occupations; and it is their ability to orchestrate their occupational lives that will determine the extent to which they derive occupational well-being. Fourth, we believe that balance exists when individuals' occupational lives are orchestrated such that they perceive that they are able to meet their occupational needs. Finally, while the notion of meaning clearly shapes individuals' perceptions of their occupational lives and the satisfaction derived, we have not been able to understand how meaning is generated and thus, what steps can be taken to enhance meaning. The proposed framework, however, challenges occupational therapists to rethink occupational therapy outcomes and identify individuals' subjective occupational experiences as the central focus. We challenge occupational therapists to adopt the goal of enabling clients to choose, engage in, and orchestrate occupations into their lives that will enable them to consistently meet their occupational needs. While we are introducing another way of thinking about occupation, the concept of occupational well-being is congruent with and can effectively extend the focus of existing occupational therapy models. Moreover, this shift in focus will ensure that individuals' occupational lives are enriched.

Further development of the ideas presented in this paper will require empirical validation. Research designed to determine the validity and universality of the seven occupational needs identified in this paper with diverse populations is needed. Valid measures of occupational well-being are also needed that can be used to determine the effectiveness of interventions in enabling individuals to meet their occupational needs and experience greater satisfaction and fulfillment.

Key Messages

- Occupational therapists must extend their focus beyond occupational performance to examine how individuals compose their occupational lives and the extent to which they are able to meet their occupational needs.
- Occupational needs include: accomplishment, affirmation, agency, coherence, companionship, pleasure, and renewal.
- By working in collaboration with clients or advocating on their behalf, occupational therapists can ensure that clients have access to occupations that have the potential to meet their occupational needs.

References

Bateson, M. C. (1996). Enfolded activity and the concept of occupation. In R. Zemke & F. Clark (Eds.), *Occupational science: The evolving discipline* (pp. 5–12). Philadelphia: F. A. Davis Company.

Borell, L., Asaba, E., Rosenberg, L., Schult, M-L., & Townsend, E. (2006). Exploring perspectives of "participation" among individuals living with chronic pain. *Scandinavian Journal of Occupational Therapy, 13,* 76–85.

Canadian Association of Occupational Therapists. (2002). *Enabling occupation. An occupational therapy perspective* (rev. ed.). Ottawa, ON: CAOT Publications ACE.

Christiansen, C. H. (1996). Three perspectives on balance in occupation. In R. Zemke & F. Clark (Eds.), *Occupational science: The evolving discipline* (pp. 431–451). Philadelphia: F. A. Davis Company.

Christiansen, C. H. (1999). Defining lives: Occupation as identity: An essay on competence, coherence, and the creation of meaning. *American Journal of Occupational Therapy, 53,* 547–558. http://dx.doi.org/10.5014/ajot.53.6.547

Cipriani, J., Faig, S., Ayrer, K., Brown, L., & Johnson, N.C. (2006). Altruistic activity patterns among long-term nursing home residents. *Physical & Occupational Therapy in Geriatrics, 24,* 45–60.

Doble, S., & Caron Santha, J. (2007). Occupational well-being from the perspective of Susan Doble and Josiane Caron Santha. In E. A. Townsend & H. J. Polatajko (Eds.), *Enabling occupation II: Advancing an occupational therapy vision of health, well-being and justice through occupation* (pp. 69–71). Ottawa, ON: CAOT Publications ACE.

Hammell, K. W. (2004). Dimensions of meaning in the occupations of daily life. *Canadian Journal of Occupational Therapy, 71,* 298–305.

Hasselkus B. R. (2002). *The meaning of everyday occupation.* Thorofare, NJ: SLACK Incorporated.

Hemmingsson, H., & Jonsson, H. (2005). The Issue Is—An occupational perspective on the concept of participation in the *International Classification of Functioning, Disability and Health*—Some critical remarks. *American Journal of Occupational Therapy, 59,* 569–576. http://dx.doi.org/10.5014/ajot.59.5.569

Hillman, A., & Chapparo, C. J. (2002). The role of work in the lives of retired men following a stroke. *Work, 19,* 303–313.

Howell, D., & Pierce, D. (2000). Exploring the forgotten restorative dimension of occupation: Quilting and quilt use. *Journal of Occupational Science, 7,* 68–72.

Hvalsøe, B., & Josephsson, S. (2003). Characteristics of meaningful occupations from the perspective of mentally ill people. *Scandinavian Journal of Occupational Therapy, 10,* 61–71.

Johnson, J. S. (1996). Realistic expressions: Statements of being. In R. Zemke & F. Clark (Eds.), *Occupational science: The evolving discipline* (pp. 23–25). Philadelphia: F.A. Davis Company.

Kielhofner, G. (Ed.). (2008). *Model of Human Occupation: Theory and application* (4th ed.) Baltimore: Lippincott Williams & Wilkins.

Laliberte-Rudman, D., Yu, B., Scott, E., & Pajouhandeh, P. (2000). Exploration of the perspectives of persons with schizophrenia regarding quality of life. *American Journal of Occupational Therapy, 54,* 137–147. http://dx-.doi.org/10.5014/ajot.54.2.137

Leufstadius, C., Erlandsson, L-K., & Eklund, M. (2006). Time use and daily activities in people with persistent mental illness. *Occupational Therapy International, 13,* 123–141.

Lyons, M., Orozovic, N., Davis, J., & Newman, J. (2002). Doing–being–becoming: Occupational experiences of persons with lifethreatening illnesses. *American Journal of Occupational Therapy, 56,* 285–295. http://dx.doi.org/10.5014/ajot.56.3.285

Nagle, S., Cook, J. V., & Polatajko, H. J. (2002). I'm doing as much as I can: Occupational choices of persons with a severe and persistent mental illness. *Journal of Occupational Science, 9,* 72–81.

Öhman, A, & Nygård, L. (2005). Meanings and motives for engagement in self-chosen daily life occupations among individuals with Alzheimer's disease. *OTJR: Occupation, Participation and Health, 25,* 89–97.

Pierce, D. (2001). Occupation by design: Dimensions, therapeutic power, and creative process. *American Journal of Occupational Therapy, 55,* 249–259. http://dx.doi.org/10.5014/ajot.55.3.249 Reprinted as Chapter 61.

Piškur, B., Kinebanian, A., & Josephsson, S. (2002). Occupation and well-being: A study of some Slovenian people's experiences of engagement in occupation in relation to well-being. *Scandinavian Journal of Occupational Therapy, 9,* 63–70.

Polatajko, H. J., Davis, J., Stewart, D., Cantin, N., Amoroso, B., Purdie, L. et al. (2007). Specifying the domain of concern: Occupation as core. In E. A. Townsend & H.J. Polatajko (Eds.), *Enabling occupation II: Advancing an occupational therapy vision of health, well-being and justice through occupation* (pp. 13–26). Ottawa, ON: CAOT Publications ACE.

Rebeiro, K. L., Day, D., Semeniuk, B., O'Brien, M., & Wilson, B. (2001). Northern Initiative for Social Action: An occupational-based mental health program. *American Journal of Occupational Therapy, 55,* 493–500. http://dx.doi.org/10.5014/ajot.55.5.493

Reynolds, F., & Prior, S. (2003). Sticking jewels in your life: Exploring women's strategies for negotiating an acceptable quality of life with multiple sclerosis. *Qualitative Health Research, 13,* 1125–1251.

Reynolds, F., & Prior, S. (2006). Creative adventures and flow in artmaking: A qualitative study of women living with cancer. *British Journal of Occupational Therapy, 69,* 255–262.

Sellar, B., & Boshoff, K. (2006). Subjective leisure experiences of older Australians. *Australian Occupational Therapy Journal, 53,* 211–219.

Watts, J. H., & Teitelman, J. (2005). Achieving a restorative mental break for family caregivers of persons with Alzheimer's disease. *Australian Occupational Therapy Journal, 52,* 282–292.

Weinblatt, N., & Avrech-Bar, M. (2003). Rest: A qualitative exploration of the phenomenon. *Occupational Therapy International, 10,* 227–238.

Wilcock, A. A. (1998). Reflections on doing, being and becoming. *Canadian Journal of Occupational Therapy, 65,* 248–257.

Wilcock, A. A. (2006). *An occupational perspective of health* (2nd ed.). Thorofare, NJ: SLACK Incorporated.

World Health Organization. (2001). *International classification of functioning, disability and health.* Geneva: Author.

Zemke, R., & Clark, F. (1996). Importance of occupation. In R. Zemke & F. Clark (Eds.), *Occupational science: The evolving discipline* (pp. 1–3). Philadelphia: F. A. Davis Company.

CHAPTER 14

Sacred Texts: A Sceptical Exploration of the Assumptions Underpinning Theories of Occupation

KAREN WHALLEY HAMMELL

It is claimed that occupational therapists, like all professionals, "have some basic assumptions that, by definition, are not questioned, but rather are held to be true. They are challenged only when there is a large accumulation of prevailing evidence to suggest that the assumptions are no longer tenable" (Townsend & Polatajko, 2007, p. 20). But is such lack of intellectual rigour acceptable? How shall we find such evidence if we do not search for it? And, should our theoretical base be informed by unchallenged assumptions or by evidence?

Occupational therapy is self-portrayed as a scientific discipline (Townsend & Polatajko, 2007). A scientific discipline is defined as one that assures "a culture of healthy scepticism: a readiness to doubt claims and assumptions about the 'rightness' of any particular theory or intervention" (Brechin & Sidell, 2000, p. 12). In addition to the healthy scepticism demanded of a scientific discipline, professional integrity further requires that we challenge the beliefs and assumptions inherent in our field, continually raise questions, confront dogma, unmask conventional and accepted ideas, take nothing for granted, and be unwilling "to let half-truths or received ideas" (Said, 1996, p. 23) steer us along. In particular, professionals are exhorted to guard against the received ideas handed down in their own profession (Said, 1979) and to be unwilling to accept what the powerful or conventional have to say (Said, 1996). As a postcolonial theorist—one committed to critiquing all forms of colonial and imperialistic domination, such as the tendency to expound theories derived solely from the values and norms of a Western viewpoint (Young, 2003)—Said (1996) advocated a sceptical approach, to orthodoxy, proposing that: "The intellectual must be involved in a lifelong dispute with all the guardians of sacred vision or text" (pp. 88–89).

This paper probes some of the core assumptions that underpin current theories of occupation—our sacred texts—demonstrating that these are culturally specific, contestable, and lacking in supportive evidence.

Assumptions and Theory in Occupational Therapy

Assumptions are ideas that we assume to be right, or common sense, or that we take for granted. Occupational therapy is underpinned by shared assumptions concerning the nature of occupation and the role of occupation for human well-being. Although these taken-for-granted assumptions constitute the foundation on which the profession's theories and models are constructed, little regard has been paid to appraising their validity. Mocellin (1995, p. 503) observed that professional knowledge in occupational therapy consists "primarily of a collage of 'quotes' derived from distinguished and respected occupational therapists," as if these are somehow correct or true. Because of this habit of substituting authority for evidence, Mocellin argued that assumptions about occupational therapy's core knowledge have accumulated in the absence of supporting evidence. It is therefore unsurprising that recent efforts to enable a client-centred approach to theory building have exposed the culturally specific and ableist assumptions that underlie existing professional theories (Hammell, 2004a; Suto, 2004). Ableism refers to the discriminatory practices arising from the assumption that everyone's physical abilities conform to culturally valued norms.

Critics observe that the more powerful one's beliefs and assumptions become and the greater their longevity, the greater their ability to survive contact with contesting evidence (Childs & Williams, 1997; Taylor, 1999). Moreover, Mocellin (1996) claimed that instead of subjecting its core assumptions to critical scrutiny, occupational therapy has promoted specific language and models, not solely to advance the scientific basis of the profession, but as a defensive response by those who have invested heavily in the profession's conventional rhetoric. Mocellin (1995) therefore equates these beliefs and assumptions with the dogma of a fundamentalist faith. Occupational therapists' propensity for quasi-religious, theoretical fervour is also noted by Kelly and McFarlane (2007), who observe that the sort of hero worship accorded to respected theorists by their devoted followers cultivates the uncritical acceptance of specific beliefs and dogma. These are the guardians of the sacred texts (Said, 1996).

It has been argued that if occupational therapists are to live up to their espoused goal of enabling participation in meaningful occupations, they must think more critically and become aware of the value patterns and assumptions embedded in their theories and models (Kronenberg, Algado, & Pollard, 2005). Accordingly, this paper seeks to demonstrate that the assumptions shared by the occupational therapy profession in the minority (or Western) world are not universal, but culturally specific, and that the uncritical promulgation of these assumptions leads not solely to inadequate theories but constitutes both ethnocentrism (Iwama, 2003) and theoretical imperialism (Hammell, 2006). Ethnocentrism is the belief that one's own culture is superior to others and is the standard by which all other people should be judged (Leavitt, 1999). It is often manifested in the assumption that one's own values, priorities, and perspectives are universal rather than specific. Theoretical imperialism occurs when theorists develop and perpetuate theories that privilege their own perspectives while overlooking, ignoring, or silencing the perspectives of others (Mann, 1995). Theoretical imperialism is best understood as a form of intellectual colonialism.

The reality that few people now live in societies with a homogenous culture has led to an examination of ways in which occupational therapists might undertake their work in a culturally appropriate and respectful manner (Chiang & Carlson, 2003; Whiteford & Wilcock, 2000). However, before we can understand and respond appropriately as occupational therapists to the needs of those from other cultures, we need first to interrogate the assumptions, values, and beliefs of our own occupational therapy culture.

Culture and Occupational Therapy

The concept of culture is used to describe the knowledge, beliefs, attitudes, morals, norms, and customs that people acquire through membership in a particular society or group. Anthropologists identify two interlinked components of culture—mental and behavioural—demonstrating that learned attitudes, ideas, concepts, beliefs, assumptions, values, and perspectives inform particular actions and patterns of behaviour in everyday life (Ferraro, 1995; Peoples & Bailey, 1994). The transmission of cultural values and beliefs is so effective that certain ideas acquire the status of common sense, appearing both normal and natural. Indeed, it is claimed that "our culture entraps us in common sense" (Thomas, 1993, p. 3). This cultural common sense prescribes each person's system of meanings and values without the person having explicit awareness of this system (Charmé, 1984; Sartre, 1956). Occupational therapy is shaped by culture (Iwama, 2007), absorbing common sense from the social, political, economic, and legal environment.

As a profession, occupational therapy is also a culture. Its practitioners acquire specific knowledge, beliefs, concepts, perspectives, ideas, norms, assumptions, and values during prolonged periods of education, and these influence how they think and how they act. Indeed, many assumptions are transmitted so effectively that they acquire the status of common sense. This process of enculturation is particularly effective when initiates and insiders share personal traits. A particular alignment of traits constitutes one's *positioning*.

Positioning and Occupational Therapists

Contemporary theorists have noted that different social positions inevitably affect one's viewpoint on the world and it is therefore impossible for the development of knowledge to be either objective or value-free (Collins, 1991; Swigonski, 1993). Said (1979, p. 10) observed:

> No one has ever devised a method for detaching the scholar from the circumstances of life, from the fact of his [sic] involvement (conscious or unconscious) with a class, a set of beliefs, a social position, or from the mere activity of being a member of society.

The shared assumptions that underpin occupational therapy's theories reflect the specific value systems of theorists who share many dimensions of positioning by virtue of class, race, ethnicity, age, religious tradition, physical ability, economic status, language, education, professional status, and urban location. However, although shared positions tend to generate shared values, assumptions, and ways of thinking-as-usual (Collins, 1991), these assumptions are not universally shared by those whose positioning differs from these cultural norms. Thus, occupational therapy's shared assumptions should be understood to reflect unique perspectives rather than universal truths.

Further, while the most influential occupational therapy theories have been developed in urban areas of the English-speaking nations of the Western world, these reflect, by definition, minority viewpoints. That area of the world often labelled Western, first, or developed constitutes only about 17% of the global population and is thus appropriately termed the minority world. For the same reason, what is often termed the developing or third world constitutes approximately 83% of the global population and is more accurately termed the majority world (Penn, 1999). More than mere semantics, this acknowledges that as Western therapists and theorists we are members of a minority population, with values and assumptions that are specific to a minority of people. Some of these values and beliefs are revealed in our assumptions about occupation.

However, it is important to note that majority status is not the inevitable result of being a member of a statistical majority. Indeed, the majority of power can be wielded by a minority of people, both globally and nationally. In apartheid South Africa, for example, the white minority wielded the majority of power, while the statistical majority of the population was accorded minority status (Hammell, 2006).

Exploring Occupational Therapy's Assumptions

This section will briefly probe four of occupational therapy's core assumptions: that humans can positively influence their health using their hands and will power; that occupations contribute to life's meaning; that humans participate in occupations as autonomous agents; and that humans are compelled to master the environment. Next follows a sceptical analysis of the assumption that occupations can, or should, be divided into three categories—self-care, productivity, and leisure—highlighting the consequent neglect of occupations concerned with human interdependence and connectedness.

Humans Positively Affect Their Health Using Hands and Will-Power

One of occupational therapy's most frequently cited assumptions is Reilly's (1962, p. 2; see Chapter 7) belief that "man, through the use of his [sic] hands as energized by mind and will, can influence the state of his own health." This assumption, so central to occupational therapists' beliefs about the relationship between occupation and health, may appear to be common sense, but a sceptical interrogation suggests that this is a unique perspective. First, the assumption that all people can use their hands if they have the mind and will reflects ableism and the normative supposition that everyone has hands and the ability to use them if he or she so desires. Occupational therapists know that this is a false assumption.

Second, the assumption that all people have the opportunity to affect their own health positively through their occupations is problematic and betrays its origin in the comfortable middle class of the minority world. The majority of the world's population have little or no choice, control, or opportunity to exercise their will to affect their lives. Indeed, their own actions may make little or no difference to the circumstances of their lives, which are constrained by discriminatory practices arising from patriarchy, sexism, ableism, racism, or by factors such as factory closures, natural disasters, and wars, over which they have no control. Moreover, the daily occupations of the majority of the worlds' people—the uses of their hands—are associated with unremitting drudgery, grinding poverty, high risks of injury, illness, and premature death (Mocellin, 1995).

Occupations Contribute to Life's Meaning

Occupations are assumed to contribute to life's meaning (Townsend & Polatajko, 2007; Yerxa et al., 1989), and it is likely that such occupations as paid employment contribute to life's meaning for those people whose jobs are safe, rewarding, and well-paid. However, work that is rich in gratifying experiences such as self-fulfilment, meaning, pride, and self-esteem is "the privilege of the few, a distinctive mark of the elite" (Bauman, 1998, p. 34). There has been no search for evidence that the majority of people in the majority world, who live in desperate poverty, derive positive meaning from their daily occupations. Moreover, Eastern modes of thought (Kupperman, 2001) and research findings from the minority world (Clayton & Chubon, 1994; Kelly & Kelly, 1994; Ville & Ravaud, 1996) demonstrate that work is not universally perceived to be central to life's meaning or to contribute positively to life satisfaction.

It is stated that: "Occupations are meaningful to people when they fulfil a goal or purpose that is personally or culturally important" (Canadian Association of Occupational Therapists [CAOT], 2002, p. 36), which implies that meaningful is a positive term. However, "all occupations are meaningful: they all have some meaning for the individual engaged in them" (Hammell, 2004b, p. 297). The meaning given to and derived from occupations might be boredom, humiliation, or frustration.

Humans Participate in Occupations as Autonomous Agents

Another assumption that is demonstrably specific to privileged socio-economic groups in certain political and geographic places is Yerxa's (1992, p. 79) belief that each individual is "active, capable, free, self-directed, integrated, purposeful, and an agent who is the author of health-influencing activity." The belief that the capacity for personal causation resides in every person is central to the Model of Human Occupation (Kielhofner, 2002), which posits a universal capacity for mastery, control, and self-efficacy. The assumption that "humans participate in occupations as autonomous agents" is reiterated by Townsend and Wilcock (2003, pp. 253, 255) and may, indeed, be a reality for those humans whose occupations are not constrained on the basis of gender, class, caste, race, religion, education, poverty, ethnicity, age, culture, geographic location, sexual orientation, or other axes of difference or of access to power. This assumption is probably true for occupational therapists employed in the minority world, but it is challenged, for example, by women and girls incarcerated in brothels; by disabled people confined in institutions; by those whose caste dictates engagement in specific, degrading occupations; by refugees; or by those enduring conditions of slavery (Hammell, in press).

Humans Need to Master the Environment

Another assumption states that humans have an innate—indeed, universal—urge to achieve mastery over the environment (Kielhofner, 2002). Expanding this theme, Wilcock (1993, p. 20; see Chapter 30) claimed that one of the major functions of occupation is to "develop skills, social structures and technology aimed at superiority over . . . the environment." The assumption that humans are entitled to dominion and mastery over the environment—to control and rule over the planet—is specific to Judeo-Christian belief systems derived from Genesis 1:26–28 (Iwama, 2005a; Steger, 2003) and is alien to those cultures who value living in balance and harmony within the environment (Iwama, 2006; Kupperman, 2001). Because occupational therapists

assert that the environment has social, cultural, and institutional, as well as physical, dimensions (CAOT, 2002), we need to acknowledge the consequences of extolling superiority and mastery over one's environment. Domestic abuse, for example, reflects, in part, a perceived entitlement to exert mastery and superiority over one's domestic social environment (Hammell, in press). Indeed, mastery is a transparently patriarchal term, derived from "master": a man who has control over people or things. Moreover, human mastery over the physical environment has resulted in cataclysmic environmental degradation. The reality that 20% of the global population currently exploit (master and control) 86% of the planet's physical resources (Steger) is not only detrimental to the well-being and sustainability of the world's poorest people but is environmentally unsustainable (Steger). It is time that occupational therapists took a sceptical stance towards the assumption that an entitlement to superiority, mastery, and control over the environment is an innate human quality and one worthy of facilitation by occupational therapists. This is not a benign assumption, but one that reflects unchallenged patriarchal and Judeo-Christian values, and those of materialist capitalism and globalization, that are not only exploitative, but singularly unsustainable (Hammell, in press).

The Purposes of Occupation Are Self-Care, Productivity and Leisure

An assumption that has become firmly entrenched within occupational therapy's models is that occupations can be divided into three categories: self-care, work, and play (Kielhofner, 2002) or self-care, productivity, and leisure (Creek, 2003; Townsend & Polatajko, 2007). Indeed, it has been claimed that these three categories represent the "purposes" of occupation (CAOT, 2002, p. 37). However, Pierce (2001, p. 252; see Chapter 61) observed: "as occupational scientists have begun to examine these categories more closely . . . they appear to be simplistic, value-laden, decontextualized, and insufficiently descriptive of subjective experience." Those of us who have suggested that some of the most meaningful occupations of people's lives—for example, prayer or meditation; contemplating beauty in nature or art; caring for one's children, parents, or companion animals; making love; or sitting for days at the bedside of a dying friend—do not fit within this privileged triad have been told that any occupation can be made to fit one of the three categories. But can a theory be considered adequate if outlying data must be forced into preordained categories? Engel (1977, p. 130) observed that "in science, a model is revised or abandoned when it fails to fit all the data. A dogma, on the other hand, requires that discrepant data be forced to fit the model or be excluded."

Further, the assumption that leisure and work are divisible is culturally specific (Darnell, 2002; Primeau, 1996) and alien to members of simple societies (Horna, 1994; Storman, 1989) and farming communities. Moreover, there is little agreement on what constitutes leisure (Primeau) and evidence that the concept of leisure is an ableist (Aitchison, 2003) and class-bound concept (Suto, 2004), with many members of the global population lacking a word to name the concept of leisure (Kelly & Kelly, 1994). Suto (p. 30) observed that "there is an implicit assumption that leisure is a relevant concept to most, if not all, occupational therapy clients." Her research among immigrant women challenged this assumption. Because little research has been undertaken to inform occupational therapy's concept of leisure (Suto) and because there is little agreement on the parameters of this concept, the assumption that a balance of occupations that includes leisure is essential for well-being (Christiansen, 1996) would appear difficult to defend.

Perhaps most troubling is that the decision to prioritize and promote these three categories of occupation (self-care, productivity and leisure) reflects a specific, minority-world doctrine of individualism (Young, 2003) that specifically excludes those activities motivated by love and concern for the well-being of others. Clearly, the care of others does not fit comfortably within any of the three privileged categories because this is not concerned with care of the self, nor is it socially or economically productive or experienced as leisure. How might a man who dedicates the majority of his time and energy to caring for his wife (who has a severe neurological impairment) categorize his daily occupations: self-care? productivity? leisure? Or, perhaps, "none of the above"? Indeed, rather than positively influencing his health, his chosen occupations may instead diminish his physical health, although they may significantly enhance his wife's well-being and may contribute immeasurably to the quality and meaning of his own life. As Bunting (2004, p. 322) notes, paying attention to others' needs, or caring, "is the most deeply engaged experience of our lives." And how might this woman categorize her daily occupations: talking to her friends, children, and grandchildren; enjoying the radio, watching wild birds at their feeder;

listening to her husband reading aloud; and discussing issues with him? Though filling her days with occupations that provide meaning and purpose to her life, continuity of her valued role as family confidante and advisor, and a sense of connectedness to special people, these are not occupations she could easily label self-care, productivity, or leisure. Although the Canadian Association of Occupational Therapists (CAOT, 2002, p. 182) included a sense of "connectedness" as part of its definition of spirituality, and then placed spirituality at the very centre of the Canadian Model of Occupational Performance, occupations associated with connectedness are not manifested in the privileged triad.

It is significant that this core assumption—that occupations are divisible into these three specific categories—did not arise from research evidence so there is no way of determining whether these categories reflect universal human experiences. Moreover, because people define their occupations differently at different times, dependent upon such factors as their mood, goals, context, and the presence of other people (Primeau, 1996; Shaw, 1984), the validity of classifying occupations into three categories is contestable (Erlandsson & Eklund, 2001; Persson, Eklund, & Isacsson, 1999).

Individualism and Independence, or Interdependence and Connectedness?

Critical disability theorists claim that by prioritizing self-care and productive occupations, those that contribute to the social and economic fabric of communities (CAOT, 2002), occupational therapists denigrate those deemed dependent or unproductive and actively reinforce the economic and social status quo (French & Swain, 2001). They contend that productivity is an "irretrievably ableist discourse" (Devlin & Pothier, 2006, p. 18) and insist that "we need to argue against 'productivity' . . . as a measure of human value" (Finger, 1995, p. 15).

Although minority world culture extols individualism and applauds independence, many other cultures value reciprocal obligations and harmonious relationships, and in these societies "contentment derived from the well-being of others constitutes an especially salient aspect of quality of life" (Ryff & Singer, 1998, p. 8). Indeed, minority world values of independence and self-reliance are alien to those cultures that value social relationships, interdependence, reciprocity, mutual obligation, and belonging (Iwama, 2006; Lim, 2004). Within those cultures, people in seemingly dependent positions are not devalued (Katbamna, Bhakta, & Parker, 2000), yet within Western cultures occupational therapists tend to view dependence on others as "a state of being requiring amelioration" (Iwama, 2005b, p. 131).

Rather than extolling individualism and independence, Bunting (2004, p. 322) contends that we should acknowledge and assert "that we are all interdependent, and it is in that web of dependence that we find our deepest contentment." Contrary to Western egocentric ideology, research demonstrates that interdependence is "an indispensable feature of the human condition" (Reindal, 1999, p. 354). Indeed, even within minority world cultures, research evidence demonstrates that the ability to contribute to others is associated with lower levels of depression, higher self-esteem, and fewer health problems (e.g., Anson, Stanwyck, & Krause, 1993; Schwartz & Sendor, 1999; Stewart & Bhagwanjee 1999), suggesting that occupations that promote interdependence contribute positively to well-being. However, current theories of occupation provide little space for consideration of the importance of fostering interdependence or of contributing to the well-being of others.

Occupation Contributes to Health

The assumption that there is a positive relationship between occupation, well-being, and health is central to theories of occupation, despite the reality that there is little evidence in the occupational therapy literature to support it (Law, Steinwender, & Leclair, 1998; Piškur, Kinebanian, & Josephsson, 2002; Rebeiro, 1998). Perhaps, in part, this is because assumptions of what constitutes health, well-being, and occupation are, themselves, equivocal. There has been little research to determine what these concepts mean in the lives of people whose positioning bestows different experiences and perspectives. Kagawa-Singer (1993) found that people living with cancer redefined the conventional meaning of health and employed a definition "based upon their ability to maintain a sense of integrity as productive, able, and valued individuals within their social spheres, despite their physical condition" (p. 295). These study participants contributed a definition of health that incorporated their own experiences, one that appears to reflect the central tenets of occupational therapy. This prompts the question: What might occupational therapy's theories and models of occupation and well-being look like if they were informed by the perspectives not solely of middle-class, minority-world theorists, but by those of other cultural groups or ill and disabled people?

This section has briefly probed a few of the assumptions that underpin occupational therapy's theories of occupation. Although not intended to be exhaustive, it is hoped that the chosen examples will prompt occupational therapists to develop a healthy scepticism towards the assumptions perpetuated within our profession. When occupational therapists are told that a respected theorist has said x or y, intellectual integrity requires that we ask: What evidence supports the assertion? Whose evidence supports the assertion? Is this an evidence-based insight, or a value-laden opinion?

Conclusion

Despite the occupational therapy profession's declared allegiance to client-centredness, there has been little effort to enable the perspectives of diverse client groups to infiltrate theories of occupation, and there has also been little effort to critique existing assumptions to determine whether they are substantiated by evidence. Thus, for example, *Enabling Occupation II* "is *entrenched* in the values and beliefs" that informed its predecessor (Townsend & Polatajko, 2007, p. 3, emphasis added). Drawing from a diversity of perspectives, this paper has sought to demonstrate that some of occupational therapy's entrenched beliefs are specific rather than universal, contending for example, that occupations are not universally or usefully categorized as self-care, productivity, and leisure; that the concept of leisure is an ableist, classbound, and culturally specific concept; that current models of occupation leave little space for activities motivated by a sense of connection or care for others; that productivity is not universally perceived to be central to life's meaning nor universally experienced as a positive contributor to health; that independence is not universally prized; that mastery is a patriarchal concept; that human mastery of the environment has caused cataclysmic damage; and that humans do not all live in circumstances in which they can use their hands or exercise their will to positively influence their health.

Said (1979) argued that professionals must be on guard against the received ideas handed down in their profession; against being too smug, too insulated, too confident in ideological straightjackets and against colluding with cultural and political dogma. However, it has been noted that "robust academic argument is new to occupational therapy: to date, there has been a notable lack of scholarly articles presenting counter-arguments to theoretical ideas" (Duncan, Paley, & Eva,

2007, p. 200). Moreover, because many in the occupational therapy profession have invested heavily in re-iterating the received ideas and dogma handed down by the conventional and the powerful (Said, 1996), a more rigorous approach to the assumptions underpinning our profession is not inevitable. As Mocellin (1995, p. 502) observed: "When core assumptions, which are considered essential to the underpinning of occupational therapy, are perceived by some to be under threat, considerable efforts are made to enforce professional conformity."

Much of what we believe and assume about occupational therapy's theories may be justifiable. However, fostering a culture of healthy scepticism within our profession will enable us to challenge the veracity of our assumptions, contest the universality of their application, and insist on a supportive evidence base for our theories that is derived from a broad range of perspectives. This will inform more relevant and inclusive theory, and more relevant and inclusive practice.

Key Messages

- Occupational therapy's theories and models of human occupation are informed by unchallenged assumptions and the pronouncements of respected theorists rather than by research evidence.
- Many of occupational therapy's core assumptions are culturally specific, class-specific, or ableist.
- Scientific and professional integrity require a sceptical approach to occupational therapy's assumptions and dogma, and a sound evidence base with which to inform more relevant and inclusive theories of occupation.

References

Aitchison, C. (2003). From leisure and disability to disability leisure: Developing data, definitions and discourses. *Disability and Society, 18,* 955–969.

Anson, C. A., Stanwyck, D. J., & Krause, J. S. (1993). Social support and health status in spinal cord injury. *Paraplegia, 31,* 632–638.

Bauman, Z. (1998). *Work, consumerism, and the new poor.* Buckingham, UK: Open University Press.

Brechin, A., & Sidell, M. (2000). Ways of knowing. In R. Gomm & C. Davies (Eds.), *Using evidence in health and social care* (pp. 3–25). London: Sage.

Bunting, M. (2004). *Willing slaves: How the overwork culture is ruling our lives.* London: Harper-Collins.

Canadian Association of Occupational Therapists. (2002). *Enabling occupation. An occupational therapy perspective* (2nd ed.). Ottawa, ON: Author.

Charmé, S. L. (1984). *Meaning and myth in the study of lives. A Sartrean perspective.* Philadelphia: University of Pennsylvania Press.

Chiang, M., & Carlson, G. (2003). Occupational therapy in multicultural contexts: Issues and strategies. *British Journal of Occupational Therapy, 66,* 559–567.

Childs, P., & Williams, P. (1997). *An introduction to post-colonial theory.* London: Prentice-Hall.

Christiansen, C. (1996). Three perspectives on balance in occupation. In R. Zemke & F. Clark (Eds.), *Occupational science: The evolving discipline* (pp. 431–451). Philadelphia: F. A. Davis.

Clayton, K. S., & Chubon, R. A. (1994). Factors associated with the quality of life of long-term spinal cord injured persons. *Archives of Physical Medicine and Rehabilitation, 75,* 633–638.

Collins, P. H. (1991). Learning from the outsider within. The sociological significance of Black feminist thought. In M. M. Fonow & J. A. Cook (Eds.), *Beyond methodology: Feminist scholarship as lived research* (pp. 35–59). Bloomington: Indiana University Press.

Creek, J. (2003). *Occupational therapy defined as a complex intervention.* London: College of Occupational Therapists.

Darnell, R. (2002). Occupation is not a cross-cultural universal: Some reflections from an ethnographer. *Journal of Occupational Science, 9,* 5–11.

Devlin, R., & Pothier, D. (2006). Introduction: Toward a critical theory of dis-citizenship. In D. Pothier & R. Devlin (Eds.), *Critical disability theory: Essays in philosophy, politics, policy, and law* (pp. 1–22). Vancouver: University of British Columbia Press.

Duncan, E. A. S., Paley, J., & Eva, G. (2007). Complex interventions and complex systems in occupational therapy. *British Journal of Occupational Therapy, 70,* 199–206.

Engel, G. L. (1977). The need for a new medical model: A challenge for biomedicine. *Science, 196,* 129–136.

Erlandsson, L-K., & Eklund, M. (2001). Describing patterns of daily occupations: A methodological study comparing data from four different methods. *Scandinavian Journal of Occupational Therapy, 8,* 31–39.

Ferraro, G. (1995). *Cultural anthropology. An applied perspective* (2nd ed.). St. Paul, MN: West Publishing.

Finger, A. (1995). "Welfare reform" and us. *Ragged Edge, Nov/Dec,* 15 & 36.

French, S., & Swain, J. (2001). The relationship between disabled people and health and welfare professionals. In G. L. Albrecht, K. D. Seelman, & M. Bury (Eds.), *Handbook of disability studies* (pp. 734–753). London: Sage.

Hammell, K. W. (2004a). Using qualitative evidence to inform theories of occupation. In K. W. Hammell & C. Carpenter (Eds.), *Qualitative research in evidence-based rehabilitation* (pp. 14–26). Edinburgh, UK: Churchill Livingstone.

Hammell, K. W. (2004b). Dimensions of meaning in the occupations of daily life. *Canadian Journal of Occupational Therapy, 71,* 296–305.

Hammell, K. W. (2006). *Perspectives on disability and rehabilitation: Contesting assumptions, challenging practice.* Edinburgh, UK: Churchill Livingstone/Elsevier.

Hammell, K. W. (in press). Contesting assumptions in occupational therapy. In M. Curtin, M. Molineux, & J. Supyk (Eds.), *Occupational therapy and physical dysfunction* (6th ed.). Edinburgh, UK: Churchill Livingstone/Elsevier.

Horna, J. (1994). *The study of leisure.* Toronto, ON: Oxford University Press.

Iwama, M. (2003). Toward culturally relevant epistemologies in occupational therapy. *American Journal of Occupational Therapy, 57,* 582–588.

Iwama, M. (2005a). Occupation as a cross-cultural construct. In G. Whiteford & V. Wright-St. Clair (Eds.), *Occupation and practice in context* (pp. 242–253). Marrickville, NSW: Elsevier.

Iwama, M. (2005b). Situated meaning. An issue of culture, inclusion and occupational therapy. In F. Kronenberg, S. S. Algado, & N. Pollard (Eds.), *Occupational therapy without borders* (pp. 127–139). Edinburgh, UK: Churchill Livingstone/Elsevier.

Iwama, M. (2007). Culture and occupational therapy: Meeting the challenge of relevance in a global world. *Occupational Therapy International, 14,* 183–187.

Iwama, M. K. (2006). *The Kawa model. Culturally relevant occupational therapy.* Edinburgh, UK: Churchill Livingstone/Elsevier.

Kagawa-Singer, M. (1993). Redefining health: Living with cancer. *Social Science and Medicine, 37,* 295–304.

Katbamna, S., Bhakta, P., & Parker, G. (2000). Perceptions of disability and care-giving relationships in South Asian communities. In W. I. V. Ahmad (Ed.), *Ethnicity, disability and chronic illness* (pp. 12–27). Buckingham, UK: Open University Press.

Kelly, G., & McFarlane, H. (2007). Culture or cult? The mythological nature of occupational therapy. *Occupational Therapy International, 14,* 188–204.

Kelly, J. R., & Kelly, J. R. (1994). Multiple dimensions of meaning in the domains of work, family and leisure. *Journal of Leisure Research, 26,* 250–274.

Kielhofner, G. (2002). *A Model of Human Occupation: Theory and application* (3rd ed.). Baltimore: Williams & Wilkins.

Kronenberg, F., Algado, S. S., & Pollard, N. (2005). Preface. In F. Kronenberg, S. S. Algado, & N. Pollard (Eds.), *Occupational therapy without borders* (pp. xv–xvii). Edinburgh, UK: Churchill Livingstone/Elsevier.

Kupperman, J. J. (2001). *Classic Asian philosophy.* Oxford, UK: Oxford University Press.

Law, M., Steinwender, S., & Leclair, L. (1998). Occupation, health and well-being. *Canadian Journal of Occupational Therapy, 65,* 81–91.

Leavitt, R. L. (1999). Moving rehabilitation professionals toward cultural competence: Strategies for change. In R. L. Leavitt (Ed.), *Cross-cultural rehabilitation. An international perspective* (pp. 375–385). London: WB Saunders.

Lim, K. H. (2004). Occupational therapy in multicultural contexts. Letter to the editor. *British Journal of Occupational Therapy, 67,* 49–50.

Mann, H. S. (1995). Women's rights versus Feminism? Postcolonial perspectives. In G. Rajan & R. Mohanram (Eds.), *Postcolonial discourse and changing cultural contexts: Theory and criticism* (pp. 69–88). Westport, CT: Greenwood Press.

Mocellin, G. (1995). Occupational therapy: A critical overview. Part 1. *British Journal of Occupational Therapy, 58,* 502–506.

Mocellin, G. (1996). Occupational therapy: A critical overview. Part 2. *British Journal of Occupational Therapy, 59,* 11–16.

Penn, H. (1999). Children in the majority world: Is outer Mongolia really so far away? In S. Hood, B. Mayall, & S. Oliver (Eds.), *Critical issues in social research. Power and prejudice* (pp. 25–39). Buckingham, UK: Open University Press.

Peoples, J., & Bailey, G. (1994). *Humanity. An introduction to cultural anthropology* (3rd ed.). St Paul, MN: West.

Persson, D., Eklund, M., & Isacsson, Å. (1999). The experience of everyday occupations and its relation to sense of coherence: A methodological study. *Journal of Occupational Science, 6,* 13–26.

Pierce, D. (2001). Occupation by design: Dimensions, therapeutic power, and creative process. *American Journal of Occupational Therapy, 55,* 249–259. http://dx.doi.org/10.5014/ajot.55.3.249 Reprinted as Chapter 61.

Piškur, B., Kinebanian, A., & Josephsson, S. (2002). Occupation and well-being: A study of some Slovenian people's experiences of engagement in occupation in relation to well-being. *Scandinavian Journal of Occupational Therapy, 9,* 63–70.

Primeau, L. (1996). Work and leisure: Transcending the dichotomy. *American Journal of Occupational Therapy, 50,* 569–577. http://dx.doi.org/10.5014/ajot.50.7.569

Rebeiro, K. L. (1998). Occupation-as-means to mental health: A review of the literature and a call to research. *Canadian Journal of Occupational Therapy, 66,* 12–19.

Reilly, M. (1962). Occupational therapy can be one of the great ideas of 20th century medicine. *American Journal of Occupational Therapy, 26,* 1–9. Reprinted as Chapter 7.

Reindal, S. M. (1999). Independence, dependence, interdependence: Some reflections on the subject and personal autonomy. *Disability and Society, 14,* 353–367.

Ryff, C. D., & Singer, B. (1998). The contours of positive human health. *Psychological Inquiry, 9,* 1–28.

Said, E. W. (1979). *Orientalism.* London: Routledge.

Said, E. W. (1996). *Representations of the intellectual.* New York: Random House.

Sartre, J-P. (1956). *Being and nothingness* (H. Barnes, Trans). New York: Washington Square. (Original work published 1943)

Schwartz, C. E., & Sendor, M. (1999). Helping others helps oneself: Response shift effects in peer support. *Social Science and Medicine, 48,* 1563–1575.

Shaw, S. M. (1984). The measurement of leisure: A quality of life issue. *Society and Leisure, 7,* 91–107.

Steger, M. B. (2003). *Globalization.* Oxford, UK: Oxford University Press.

Stewart, R., & Bhagwanjee, A. (1999). Promoting group empowerment and self-reliance through participatory research: A case study of people with physical disability. *Disability and Rehabilitation, 21,* 338–345.

Storman, W. (1989). Work: True leisure's home? *Leisure Studies, 8,* 25–33.

Suto, M. (2004). Exploring leisure meanings that inform client-centred practice. In K. W. Hammell & C. Carpenter (Eds.), *Qualitative research in evidence-based re-*

habilitation (pp. 27–39). Edinburgh, UK: Churchill Livingstone.

Swigonski, M. E. (1993). Feminist standpoint theory and the questions of social work research. *Affilia, 8,* 171–183.

Taylor, G. (1999). Empowerment, identity and participatory research: Using social action research to challenge isolation for deaf and hard of hearing people from minority ethnic communities. *Disability and Society, 14,* 369–384.

Thomas, J. (1993). *Doing critical ethnography.* Newbury Park, CA: Sage.

Townsend, E. A., & Polatajko, H. (2007). *Enabling occupation II: Advancing an occupational therapy vision for health, well-being & justice through occupation.* Ottawa, ON: CAOT Publications ACE.

Townsend, E., & Wilcock, A. (2003). Occupational justice. In C. Christiansen & E. Townsend (Eds.), *Introduction to occupation: The art and science of living* (pp. 243–273). Thorofare, NJ: Prentice Hall.

Ville, I., & Ravaud, J-F. (1996). Work, non-work and consequent satisfaction after spinal cord injury. *International Journal of Rehabilitation Research, 19,* 241–252.

Whiteford, G. E., & Wilcock, A. A. (2000). Cultural relativism: Occupation and independence reconsidered. *Canadian Journal of Occupational Therapy, 67,* 324–336.

Wilcock, A. A. (1993). A theory of the human need for occupation. *Occupational Science, 1,* 17–24.

Yerxa, E. J. (1992). Some implications of occupational therapy's history for its epistemology, values and relation to medicine. *American Journal of Occupational Therapy, 46,* 79–83. http://dx.doi.org/10.5014/ajot.46.1.79

Yerxa, E. J., Clark, F., Frank, G., Jackson, J., Parham, D., Pierce, D., et al. (1989). An introduction to occupational science: A foundation for occupational therapy in the 21st century. *Occupational Therapy in Health Care, 6,* 1–17.

Young, R. J. C. (2003). *Postcolonialism.* Oxford: Oxford University Press.

CHAPTER 15

A Monistic or a Pluralistic Approach to Professional Identity?

ANNE CRONIN MOSEY

In my review of occupational therapy literature, professional identity seems to be one of our major areas of concern. Who are we, how do we define ourselves, what are we about? The issue of professional identity is important. Without a collective sense of self we cannot effectively deal with other factors, both internal and external, that do and will continue to influence our practice.

Professions can take one of two approaches to their identity: monistic or pluralistic (1, 2). Borrowing from philosophy and taking some liberties (3), these terms are defined as follows.

Monism is the belief that there is one basic principle that is the essence of reality: that all processes, structures, concepts, and theories can be reduced to one governing principle.

Pluralism is the belief that there is more than one basic principle: that everything cannot be reduced to a single principle.

Translated into a language more common to us, monism is the attempt to define occupational therapy by one of its elements or a facet of an element: for example, a philosophical statement, a legitimate tool, or a particular frame of reference. The element selected is viewed as the basic principle that governs all other elements. Because there is only one basic principle, a monistic approach to professional identity tends to be relatively static.

On the other hand, a pluralistic approach suggests a broader perspective. Pluralists feel that all elements of the profession must be taken into consideration. The whole can only be defined by all of its parts. Moreover, it should be defined in such a way that the ever-changing nature of the profession can be easily accommodated.

This chapter was previously published in *American Journal of Occupational Therapy, 39,* 504–509. Copyright © 1985, American Occupational Therapy Association. Reprinted with permission. http://dx.doi.org/10.5014/ajot.39.8.504

As a guide to where this presentation is going, I will
- Briefly outline the elements of a profession,
- Describe and assess a monistic approach to professional identity,
- Discuss some factors that lead to the consideration of a pluralistic approach, and
- Outline the rationale for the nature of a pluralistic identity.

My preference is pluralism, lest anyone think I intend to be totally unbiased here.

The Elements of a Profession

The term *elements* refers to those components that constitute the substance of a profession (4–8). Thus, any group that describes itself as a profession has the following elements.

A Set of Philosophical Assumptions

This is a collection of beliefs about the nature of the individual, the relationship of individuals with their environment, and the goals of the profession. Philosophical assumptions are identified, developed, and analyzed through philosophical inquiry, not, it should be noted, through empirical research.

A Code of Ethics

This is a statement of various principles of human conduct. This code outlines the responsibilities and privileges of members of a profession in relationship to society, their clients, and each other.

A Body of Knowledge

This is a collection of various theories that serve as the scientific foundation for practice. Theory, as used here, refers to a description of a set of events. It is concerned with predicting how and under what circumstances these events occur and how they relate to each other.

The body of knowledge of a profession is made up of theories that are a) selected from a variety of sources because they have specific relevance to practice and b) developed by the profession.

As mentioned, the goals of a profession are outlined in its philosophical assumptions, whereas a profession's body of knowledge describes the means for reaching these goals.

Domain of Concern

This is a statement of those areas of human experience in which a profession has expertise and offers assistance to others. In occupational therapy these areas are often described as being made up of occupational performances (e.g., activities of daily living, family interactions, play/recreation, and work) and of performance components (e.g., cognitive, psychological, and motor functions; sensory integration; and social interaction).

Aspects of Practice

This is a statement of the sequence of events whereby members of a profession assist clients in problem identification and resolution. In occupational therapy, these aspects include screening, formal evaluation, intervention, and termination. All of these interactions include communication and documentation.

Legitimate Tools

These are the vehicles that practitioners in a given profession use to assist clients. The legitimate tools of occupational therapy are not well defined. This issue is addressed later.

A Linking Structure

This is a framework whereby theories are restructured into a form that makes them applicable to practice (9–15). Professions need a linking structure because the only function of a theory is to predict relationships. No action is suggested or recommended. Theories do not answer the questions of how they should be applied, when they should be applied, relative to whom, and so forth. Linking structures answer these questions and thus provide the practitioner with a guide for action. The linking structure we have in occupational therapy is usually labeled a "frame of reference." We have a number of frames of reference, each of which addresses different components of our domain of concern. They help us identify what we should evaluate for and how to go about the process of evaluation, goal setting, and intervention.

Practice

This is the application of one or more linking structures (in our case, frames of reference) to meet the particular needs of each patient. This is what we do in the clinic, school, community, or wherever we choose to make use of our knowledge and skills.

Empirical Research

This is the study of people, things, and events through observation. It may be qualitative or quantitative in nature. The major types of empirical research in occupational therapy are a) evaluative, which determines the effectiveness of our various frames of reference, and b) theoretical, which develops and tests theories that are, or may become, part of our body of knowledge. These are two very different types of research that provide us with different kinds of information (16).

The elements outlined earlier are common to all professions. A profession without an ethical code, for example, would never be allowed to practice, at least not in our society; a profession without a set of philosophical assumptions, although a changing one, would be without direction.

Professions are complex and are made up of many elements. What is the best way, then, to go about the process of establishing professional identity? We are back to the major question raised earlier. Which is more prudent, a monistic or pluralistic approach?

A Monistic Approach

Some of the monistic approaches that have been suggested for occupational therapy are Human Growth and Development (17), Purposeful Activity (18, 19), Occupational Behavior (20), Adaptive Responses (21), the Ecological Systems Model (22), and Human Occupation (23). As mentioned, a monistic approach proposes that one of the profession's elements, or a facet of an element, serves, or ought to serve, as primary. This element becomes the principle that governs all other elements. Structurally, a monistic approach usually takes the form of a comprehensive theory. As used in the context of a profession, a comprehensive theory is a grand theory with broad parameters (24–26). One element, or a facet of an element, serves as the nucleus of the theory. A select number of concepts and postulates are derived from this nucleus and form the substance of the theory.

The following four assumptions are made about a theory: First, a comprehensive theory, when adequately stated, contains all the important content of the subordinate elements. Second, its structure allows it to serve as a guide to practice; no linking structure is necessary. The theory provides sufficient information for evaluation, goal setting, and intervention, regardless of a client's particular areas of function and dysfunction. Third, the theory is the sole valid focus of a profession's research endeavors. Fourth, a comprehensive theory gives a profession a unified identity.

Proponents of the various monistic approaches listed have each, in one way or another, recommended the development of a comprehensive theory. However, each has suggested a different theory, with a different element or concept as the nucleus.

Aside from the conflict inherent in so many different suggested monistic approaches, the idea of a single comprehensive theory raises the following critical issues.

1. A comprehensive theory tends to be exclusionary. Important aspects of a profession's practice may not be included. For example, if we decided that human growth and development should be the core concept of our comprehensive theory, how would we fit into that theory such things as dealing with diminished range of motion or edema? Moreover, who should decide what will be included and what will be excluded?

2. A comprehensive theory usually has a strong philosophical overtone (23, 27). The profession's body of knowledge and philosophical assumptions are often so intertwined that it is difficult to determine what is a theoretical statement and what is a statement of belief. Thus, scholarly activities may be difficult to pursue. For example, should one use the tools of empirical research or the tools of philosophical inquiry?

3. When a profession opts for a comprehensive theory, its members are placed in a constricted position. The comprehensive theory becomes so central and requires such a degree of loyalty that creative, divergent, and/or independent thinking may not be encouraged or even tolerated.

   To give a historical example, if we had decided that our comprehensive theory ought to be based on the nuclear concepts of play and work, would Ayres' ideas about sensory integration have been accepted, both as part of our body of knowledge and as one of our frames of reference? Research undertakings are usually considered appropriate only when they are concerned with the elaboration or refinement of the comprehensive theory or its ap-

plication in practice (28, 29). Research designed to test the validity of the theory is rarely suggested; in fact, it may not be considered.

4. A comprehensive theory, when well articulated, tends to be rigid; and by extension, the profession ascribing to that theory does also. The needs of society, new knowledge, and new ideas tend to be ignored. It is difficult to alter a comprehensive theory: if you add a new concept or postulate, the whole theory may need to be altered, which is a difficult task.

5. Occupational therapy is a diverse profession. We assist people in all age groups and who have difficulties in many areas of function. A comprehensive theory may simplify to the point that the diversity and the richness of our body of knowledge, domain of concern, and practice may be lost.

6. In simplification, a comprehensive theory may become so nebulous that it inhibits research. Global and ill-defined concepts (e.g., adaptive responses and purposeful activity) are difficult to operationalize. Only when a concept can be reduced to the level of a variable is the validity of a theory or the effectiveness of intervention based on that theory able to be determined.

7. Further, in simplification, a comprehensive theory may become so vague that it offers little guidance for practice. For example, the comprehensive theory of Human Occupation describes the individual as being an "open system," influencing and being influenced by external stimuli. The individual responds to external stimuli, receives feedback, alters his or her behavior, gets more feedback, and the cycle continues. When all goes well, the patient becomes a more functional individual. The problem here is what external stimuli? When a therapist assists an individual who has an eating disorder (as opposed to an individual with third-degree burns), what external stimuli should the therapist make available? Does Human Occupation provide this information? Does any proposed comprehensive theory provide this information?

8. A comprehensive theory that is not exclusionary, takes into consideration the diversity of the profession, and is not simplistic has to be complex. In its complexity, it may become so intricate and labyrinthine that it is incomprehensible to any but the most dedicated scholars. Unless we have a comprehensive theory that is easily understood by all therapists, theory may become disconnected from

practice. Not a happy situation to contemplate. We may indeed return to the time when it was acceptable to say, "My approach is eclectic." Such a statement is often an expression of considerable uncertainty about the theoretical bases for one's practice.

9. Finally, as mentioned, one of the major functions of a comprehensive theory is to give unity to a profession. If the deficits outlined earlier are not avoided, a comprehensive theory may provide an illusion of a unified identity but would serve no practical purpose.

A monistic identity, then, has many pitfalls. With that in mind, a pluralistic approach is another possibility. The following describes some of the factors that led me to consider such an approach. It is, if you will, a wandering in that direction.

Wanderings

The history of our profession has been used to substantiate most of the various monistic approaches identified earlier. That is a little hard to take. When history is used to support very disparate ideas, questions must be asked. We seem to have the idea that the original members of our profession were all of one mind about what occupational therapy ought to be. What their collective beliefs were, if there ever was such an agreement, differs according to who is writing the history. There are many individuals currently engaged in the study of our history. Hopefully, their efforts will provide more accurate information about our past.

The understanding and appreciation of our history is important. However, to use it to substantiate a number of different ideas of what we are or ought to be is a questionable practice. In addition, the year 1917 is a long time ago. The knowledge, beliefs, and issues of that time are not the same as those of 1985.

Another factor that leads me to consider a pluralistic approach is an issue raised by Rogers (30). She suggested that one of our major philosophical questions is whether the goal of the profession should be the enhancement of occupational performances or the development of performance components. She implied that it had to be one or the other; that a choice needed to be made. Why must we make such a choice? Multiple goals for the profession may provide needed flexibility.

A third reason to consider pluralism is related to our lack of a common vocabulary. Everyone has their own definition for a particular term, has no definition at all,

or uses the same term to label very different concepts. An example is the term *model*. It is used in several different ways in our literature. I have identified at least five, most of which are not clearly defined. In addition, the term is sometimes modified. Thus, we have conceptual models, theoretical models, practice models, and probably some I missed (22, 27, 31).

Let me give a few more examples. There are also no agreed-upon definitions for "theory," "frame of reference," or "taxonomy." Hypothesis may refer to a conjecture or a postulate stated in operational terms. Philosophical assumptions are rarely differentiated from theoretical statements. And I could continue . . . the lack of a common vocabulary could mean many things: a disregard for adequate definitions, an attempt to label each idea as new, or a lack of interest in communicating with each other.

Another factor in the consideration of a pluralistic identity was a review of other professions. Those who, in the past, embraced a monistic approach seemed to experience difficulties. The classical example is psychiatry. From approximately the early 1950s until the late 1960s, psychiatry on the whole had one comprehensive theory: psychoanalysis. This theory was used to explain all problems in mental health—from psychosis to marital discord. Every problem was made to fit into the theory. Psychoanalysis, with or without some modification, was the treatment of choice. However, many people were unable or unwilling to engage in this type of treatment. Also, for many of those who did, the treatment was not effective. Society turned to other sources for help: behaviorism, various types of self-help and encounter groups, and psychopharmacology. Thus, psychiatry lost a good deal of credibility, patients, and money.

The fifth situation that prompted me to consider a pluralistic approach is the difficulty we have in designating and defining our legitimate tools (32–35). "Purposeful activity" has received the most attention. Yet, it has been defined so broadly that it includes just about everything and so narrowly that it includes little that we actually do. Then there are those who suggest that we change the label of purposeful activity to "occupation." Our literature is replete both with attempts to define purposeful activity and documentation that we use other modalities for intervention (2, 36, 37). There are no criteria for determining what is and what is not a legitimate tool for occupational therapy.

Finally, I suggest a pluralistic approach based on the observation of everyday practice. What occupational therapists actually do is very diverse. There does not seem to be any one unifying element. It could be that we have had a pluralistic identity for some time; that such a decision was made long ago in action but was never recognized or clearly stated. Therefore, the limitations of a monistic approach and the factors just outlined seem to suggest consideration of pluralism.

A Pluralistic Approach

A pluralistic approach to professional identity is based on the belief that no one principle or element can define a profession, that each part is distinct and different. There are several characteristics of a profession that support a pluralistic approach. Some of the major ones follow.

First, all elements of a profession are of equal importance. One is in no way subordinate to another. The tools of a profession, for example, are of no greater or lesser importance than the theories that underlie their application.

Second, it is the content of each profession's elements that differentiates one from another (38). The collective content of each profession is unique in its totality, not in its parts. In illustration, we share part of our body of knowledge with other professions, such as human growth and development; we also share some of our philosophical assumptions, such as belief in the holistic nature of the individual. Early childhood educators use activities as one of their major tools. The content of a given profession, its beliefs, knowledge, and skills, is unique only because members of that profession have mastered it in its totality. Members of other professions and the average person may understand parts, but not the whole.

Third, the contents of elements change over time; there are both additions and deletions. And there will be change. Professions evolve to take advantage of new knowledge, new ideas, and beliefs and to meet society's ever-changing needs. For example, the original members of the profession did not fabricate splints. No one mentioned learning disabilities when I was in school. Our understanding of the brain is changing daily. This fluid and constant state of flux is good and necessary. Without such modifications, a profession would stagnate, wither, and become part of the past. We are not what we were ten years ago nor are we what we will be ten years from now.

Finally, and related to the last point, professions are rarely of one piece. Incompatibilities of elements and content of elements are legion. For example, our recognized body of knowledge does not include theories regarding the properties of heat. Yet, some occupational therapists use heat as one of their therapeutic modalities. Analytic frames of reference are not really congruent with frames of reference based on learning theories. A profession usually attempts to bring unity to the contents of its elements. But just as all of the elements are apparently in symmetry, another change comes along that must be integrated.

To reiterate, all elements of a profession are of equal importance, professions are unique only in their totality, they are in a continual state of change, and there is always likely to be incompatibility between elements and within elements. Because of these characteristics, a pluralistic approach to professional identity may be more in accord with reality.

The structure for articulation of a pluralistic identity must be loosely organized. Rather than the composition of theory, which by definition is closely knit, a taxonomy is proposed. As used here, taxonomy refers to schema for classifying and ordering a set of phenomena. There are, of course, many different kinds of taxonomies. I recommend a cluster taxonomy in which groupings are formed based on similarity of defined characteristics. The groupings suggested for a pluralistic identity are the elements of the profession. In other words, each element would be clearly defined, and under that major heading the content of each element would be outlined. Thus, for example, we would clearly define what we meant by a philosophical assumption and then list our various philosophical assumptions. The same would be done for our ethical code, frames of reference, and so forth. With such a schema, the content of each element is apparent. Incongruencies can be readily identified. Content can easily be added or deleted as circumstances dictate. Our identity would be all of our elements. And, as their content changes over time, our identity is modified.

The structure for articulation of a pluralistic identity may seem too simple, too plain. No mystery at all. But perhaps that is as it should be. There really is no need to pretend complexity and enigmas where there are none. A straightforward statement of who we are may serve us best.

A pluralistic identity gives us freedom to grow and progress. It gives us the opportunity to engage in practice and scholarly pursuits unencumbered by tradition, authority, or ideology. More specifically, it allows us to

- Analyze critically our philosophical assumptions,
- Select and/or develop new theories,
- Make changes in our domain of concern,
- Consider alternative legitimate tools, and

- Formulate more definitive and additional frames of reference.

A pluralistic identity may not be comfortable for everyone. It is certainly not a panacea, nor is it meant to be. But perhaps such an identity would prepare us to meet the needs of those who seek our help. Perhaps it can enable us to deal effectively with internal and external factors that will always influence our practice.

Acknowledgments

The author thanks Estelle Breines, MA, OTR, FAOTA; Wendy Colman, PhD, OTR; Francia de Beer, MA, OTR; and Brena Manoly, PhD, OTR, for providing assistance in the preparation of this paper.

References

1. Gilfoyle EM: Eleanor Clarke Slagle lectureship, 1984: Transformation of a profession. *Am J Occup Ther* 38:575–584, 1984

2. Llorens LA: Changing balance: Environment and individual. *Am J Occup Ther* 38:29–34, 1984

3. *The Random House Dictionary of the English Language,* J Stein, Editor. New York: Random House, 1966

4. *Education for the Profession of Medicine, Law, Theology and Social Work,* EC Hughes, Editor. New York: McGraw-Hill, 1973

5. McGlothlin W: *The Professional Schools.* New York: The Center for Applied Research in Education, 1964

6. Mosey AC: *Occupational Therapy: Configuration of a Profession.* New York: Raven, 1981

7. Popper KP: *Objective Knowledge: An Evolutionary Approach.* London: Oxford Univ Press, 1972

8. Schein EH: *Professional Education.* New York: McGraw-Hill, 1972

9. Cassidy HG: *The Sciences and the Arts: A New Alliance.* New York: Harper, 1962

10. Ford D, Urban H: *Systems Psychotherapy.* New York: Wiley, 1963

11. Hilgard E, Bower G: *Theories of Learning.* New York: Appleton-Century-Crofts, 1975

12. Marx M, Hillix W: *Systems and Theories in Psychology.* New York: McGraw-Hill, 1963

13. Nagel E: *The Structure of Science.* New York: Harcourt, Brace & World, 1961

14. Pittinger OE, Gooding CT: *Learning Theories in Educational Practice.* New York: Wiley, 1971

15. Snelbecher GE: *Learning Theory, Instructional Theory and Psycho-Educational Design.* New York: McGraw-Hill, 1974

16. Llorens LA, Gillette NP: Nationally speaking—The challenge for research in a practice profession. *Am J Occup Ther* 39:143–145, 1985

17. Llorens LA: *Application of Developmental Theory for Health and Rehabilitation.* Rockville, MD: AOTA, 1976

18. Fidler GS: From crafts to competency. *Am J Occup Ther* 35:567–573, 1981

19. Huss AJ: From kinesiology to adaptation. *Am J Occup Ther* 35:574–580, 1981

20. Reilly M: A psychiatric occupational therapy program as a teaching model. *Am J Occup Ther* 20:61–67, 1966

21. King LJ: Eleanor Clarke Slagle lectureship, 1978: Towards a science of adaptive responses. *Am J Occup Ther* 32:429–437, 1978

22. Howe MC, Briggs AK: Ecological systems model for occupational therapy. *Am J Occup Ther* 36:322–327, 1982

23. Kielhofner G: *Health Through Occupation: Theory and Practice in Occupational Therapy.* Philadelphia: Davis, 1983

24. Merton RK: *Social Theory and Social Structure.* Glencoe, IL: Free Press, 1968

25. Mills CE: *The Sociological Imagination.* New York: Oxford Univ Press, 1967

26. Williamson GG: A heritage of activity: Development of theory. *Am J Occup Ther* 36:716–722, 1982

27. Sundstrom C: In search of erudition: The evolution of a philosophical base for occupational practice in the army. *Occup Ther Ment Health* 3:7–13, 1983

28. Yerxa EJ: Research priorities. *Am J Occup Ther* 37:699, 1983

29. Christiansen CH: Editorial: Towards resolution of crises: Research requisites of occupational therapy. *Occup Ther J Res* 1:115–124, 1981

30. Rogers JC: The spirit of independence: The evolution of a philosophy. *Am J Occup Ther* 36:709–715, 1982

31. Reed KL: Understanding theory: The first step in learning about research. *Am J Occup Ther* 38:677–682, 1984

32. Breines E: The issue is—An attempt to define purposeful activities. *Am J Occup Ther* 38:543–544, 1984

33. Hinojosa J, Sabari J, Rosenfeld MS: Purposeful activities. *Am J Occup Ther* 37:805–806, 1983

34. Lyons BG: The issue is—Purposeful versus human activity. *Am J Occup Ther* 37:493–495, 1983

35. West WL: A reaffirmed philosophy and practice of occupational therapy for the 1980s. *Am J Occup Ther* 38:15–23, 1984

36. Bissell JC, Mailloux Z: The use of crafts in occupational therapy for the physically disabled. *Am J Occup Ther* 35:369–374, 1981

37. English C, Karch M, Silverman P, Walker S: The issue is—On the role of the occupational therapist in physical disabilities. *Am J Occup Ther* 36:199–202, 1982

38. *The Body of Knowledge Unique to the Profession of Education.* Washington, DC: Pi Lambda Theta, 1966

Position Paper
Broadening the Construct of Independence

We, the members of the occupational therapy profession, support the following expanded definition of independence: Independence is a self-directed state of being characterized by an individual's ability to participate in necessary and preferred occupations in a satisfying manner, irrespective of the amount or kind of external assistance desired or required.

We submit this Position Paper to embrace this broad definition and to support the view that

- self-determination is essential to achieving and maintaining independence;
- an individual's independence is unrelated to whether he or she performs the activities related to an occupation himself or herself, performs the activities in an adapted or modified environment, makes use of various devices or alternative strategies, or oversees activity completion by others;
- independence is defined by the individual's culture and values, support systems, and ability to direct his or her life; and
- an individual's independence should not be based on preestablished criteria, perception of outside observers, or how independence is accomplished.

The occupational therapy profession is committed to a broad definition of independence for all members of society. We believe that an individual's self-directed state of independence strengthens the inclusion of all people into society as functional members, regardless of how they perform their chosen endeavors. In support of this view, occupational therapy practitioners are committed to supporting and training individuals in the use of a variety of strategies to increase their independent participation in their chosen occupations. Occupational therapy practitioners support a society that embraces an expanded definition of independence and that provides reasonable accommodations that allow individuals to have access to social, educational, recreational, and vocational opportunities.

Author
Jim Hinojosa, PhD, OT, FAOTA
for
The Commission on Practice
Mary Jane Youngstrom, MS, OTR, FAOTA—*Chairperson*

Adopted by the Representative Assembly 2002M40

Note: This document replaces the 1995 Position Paper, *Broadening the Construct of Independence.*

Originally published in *American Journal of Occupational Therapy, 56*(6), 660. Copyright © 2002, American Occupational Therapy Association. Reprinted with permission. http://dx.doi.org/10.5014/ajot.56.6.660

Part III. Contextual Considerations for Engagement in Occupation and Participation

Occupational therapy should not be a thing too much apart from the rest of the world in which the patient lives. . . . The work will have much more vital interest for the patient if in some way it has immediate bearing upon his daily life.

—McMurtrie (1920, p. 326)

A basic philosophical premise of occupational therapy is that people and their occupations can be understood or worked with therapeutically only if their contexts and environments are considered. This fundamental belief is clearly evident in the above quote and Part I of this text. Consistent with the founders' emphasis on the environmental and contextual aspects of occupation, many of the profession's scholars have put forth frames of reference and practice models in which environmental factors and contextual influences are the primary foci (Letts, Rigby, & Stewart, 2003). Over the years, these have included (but are not limited to), the Model of Human Occupation (Kielhofner & Burke, 1980), Occupational Adaptation (Schkade & Schultz, 1992), Ecology of Human Performance (Dunn, Brown, & McGuigan, 1994), Lifestyle Performance (Fidler & Fidler, 1996), and the Person–Environment–Occupation model (Law et al., 1996). Application of these theoretical frameworks, and others that maintain environment and context as core to occupational therapy, can help practitioners systematically consider the complexities of people's multifaceted lives.

According to the *Occupational Therapy Practice Framework* (3rd ed.; *Framework;* American Occupational Therapy Association [AOTA], 2014a; see Appendix A of this volume), occupational engagement and participation take place within social and physical environments and are influenced by several interrelated contexts that are internal or external to the person. These contexts include the cultural, temporal, personal, and virtual aspects of performance and service delivery (AOTA, 2014a). Context's influence on people's occupational performance and the occupational therapy process cannot be underestimated. Context can enable or limit people's ability to engage in occupation and attain and maintain health and well-being (AOTA, 2014a). Thus, in all practice settings and throughout the occupational therapy process, practitioners must consider the individual's current and expected contexts to ensure a comprehensive evaluation and a relevant plan of intervention (AOTA, 2014a; Donovan, VanLeit, Crowe, & Keefe, 2005; Mosey, 1996).

Having a strong theoretical foundation for the inclusion of context throughout the occupational therapy process is essential. Part III presents several significant conceptualizations of key dimensions of context. It includes influential works by prominent national and international occupational therapy scholars and occupational scientists that critically examine temporal, cultural, sociopolitical, and personal contexts as they relate to occupation.

Temporal Contexts

My first experience of occupational therapy as a remedial help on a properly organized basis takes me back to 1908 at the Manhattan State Hospital, Ward's Island, New York. A small part of that hospital constituted the New York Psychiatric Clinic of which Adolf Meyer was director. Dr Meyer was tremendously interested in "the creation of an orderly rhythm in the hospital atmosphere" and constantly stressed the importance of creating balance between work and play, rest and sleep.

—Henderson (1957, p. 8)

The temporal context of occupation has a rich historical base in occupational therapy literature and practice, as is evident in the quote by Henderson, which reflects the founders' emphasis on the need for a balanced daily life. The continued importance of people's performance patterns to the profession is supported by the *Framework's* inclusion of habits, routines, roles, and rituals as key aspects of occupational therapy's domain. According to the *Framework*, performance patterns that are used in the process of occupational engagement can promote or hinder participation and health. Occupational performance is also influenced by the *temporal context*, which is "the experience of time as shaped by engagement in occupation" (AOTA, 2014a, p. S28). In Chapter 16, Pemberton and Cox critically examine the relevance of time to occupational therapy from the profession's roots to the present. They base their analysis on a comprehensive, multidisciplinary literature review that includes many seminal works on the temporal dimensions of occupation.

Perspectives on the reciprocal relationship time shares with occupation and how this interconnection has been embraced by leading theorists (but not actualized in practice) are explored by Pemberton and Cox. The centrality of the core constructs of tempo, temporality, and time use to the profession's philosophical foundations is described. They discuss diverse conceptualizations of time (i.e., occupation as a consumer of time, time as a context for occupation, the rhythm of life, occupation temporality, temporal dysfunction, temporal adaptation) and how these pragmatically apply to occupational therapy. Throughout this work, Pemberton and Cox strongly emphasize the need for practitioners to move beyond a one-dimensional perspective of time as a commodity. As they effectively argue, the relationship of time to occupation is far greater than measuring the temporal aspects of task performance.

> *Our modern world is time conscious and we are keyed to schedules and to a rapid pace, that we may accomplish the utmost immediately.*
> —Brunyate (1958, p.198)

Pemberton and Cox urge practitioners to broaden their understanding of time to include its social, cultural, and personal dimensions. They call for a return to the profession's core values and the integration of balance, rhythm, and time awareness into everyday practice. Capturing the unique meaning of time to each person is critical for understanding the complexities of daily patterns and the lived experience of time through occupation. Pemberton and Cox conclude with a thoughtful reflection on the future challenges the profession will face related to time. Humanity's changing relationship with time is presented as an opportunity for the profession to promote the essentiality of occupation to balance, harmony, and well-being.

The viewpoint that engagement in occupation over time contributes to a positive psychological state is strongly supported by the temporal concept of *flow*, which is presented in Chapter 17. Although much has been studied and written about flow since the original

publication of Emerson's work (Engeser, 2012; Jonsson, & Persson, 2006; Wright, Sadlo, & Stew, 2007), her clear and comprehensive discussion of flow and occupation remains relevant. Emerson proposes that the shift in the profession's scholarship to include qualitative examinations of the subjective experiences of people engaged in occupation can greatly benefit from knowledge acquired through flow research. According to Emerson, this research provides a wealth of information about the measurement of time spent in activity and the subjective experience of its pursuit.

As Emerson reviews, *flow* is a subjective psychological state that occurs when one is completely immersed in an activity. She describes the characteristics of the flow experience and the positive outcomes of this experience, which has been viewed to be the highest level of well-being. The postulate that a match between environmental demands and a person's perception of his or her skills is needed to achieve flow is particularly relevant to occupational therapy practitioners' knowledge and skills related to activity synthesis.

Emerson reviews the continuum used to study flow—the optimal state of flow, anxiety, boredom, and apathy. Flow activities and flow experiences across cultures, in adversity, and in everyday life are examined. The personality type that is inclined to experience flow is explained. From this literature review, the relevance of flow theory to the philosophy and practice of occupational therapy is clearly evident. Eight principles are provided for occupational therapy practitioners to use to help people engage in flow-inducing activities. As Emerson notes, flow "names and frames" (p. 242) a phenomenon that is highly congruent with the core values and fundamental beliefs of the occupational therapy profession (see Active Reflection III.1).

> *Our clinical director feels that weeks of wholesome routine and stimulating social contacts undoubtedly raised these patients to higher levels of existence.*
> —Wilson (1929, p. 192)

Typically, the relationship between occupation and well-being is examined via active doing. However, not doing is equally critical to life satisfaction. The need for rejuvenation is acknowledged in the *Framework*, which identifies rest and sleep as occupations and describes the activities related to restorative rest and sleep as supportive of "healthy, active engagement in other occupations" (AOTA, 2014a, p. S20). In Part III's next chapter, Chapter 18, Green examines sleep's critical role in

Active Reflection III.1. Balance, Harmony, and Flow

Think about your typical daily routine and the activities in which you engage throughout the day.
- Which activities reflect the use of time as a commodity vs. those that enable balance and harmony in your life?
- What are the key differences between these?

Reflect on an entire week of activities.
- Did engagement in any of these enable you to experience flow?
- Describe the characteristics of the activity or activities that resulted in flow.
- How do you think the transformation of humanity's relationship with time, as described by Pemberton and Cox, will affect people's ability to attain flow, balance, and harmony?
- How can you incorporate the relationship between occupation and time into the occupational therapy process to foster the attainment of flow for your clients?

occupational performance and the extent to which it has been addressed by the profession. He summarizes the coverage of sleep (or lack thereof) in occupational therapy publications. The contributions of leading occupational scientists who have increased our understanding of sleep and its role in time use are reviewed.

Green proposes that the reason sleep is not consistently or comprehensively considered in the literature is due to questions about its status as an occupation and its relevance to occupational therapy. He explores this controversy as reflected in key works on occupation and sleep and outlines several definitions of *occupation* and their relationship to sleep. Green analyzes the place for sleep within each respective definition and provides comments with related context. Although these definitions seem to only include sleep as an occupation because it uses time, Green proposes a broader view based on the science of sleep. Factors that enable people to initiate and maintain sleep and the importance of regulating the sleep–wake cycle are described. Consistent with the *Framework's* multidimensional view of sleep, Green advocates for occupational therapy practitioners and occupational scientists to consider sleep's vital role in the attainment and maintenance of a balanced lifestyle.

The importance of balance in lifestyle is explored in depth in Chapter 19 by Westhorp. Adopting the stance that lifestyle balance is synonymous with occupational balance, Westhorp supports her position by applying several definitions of balance to occupation. She briefly reviews historical and contemporary multidisciplinary perspectives on the value of leading a balanced life, highlighting the relationship between balance in oc-

cupations and health and well-being. The centrality of occupational balance to the founding philosophy of occupational therapy and the evolution of views as to what comprises a balanced lifestyle is presented. Westhorp's observation of the profession's abandonment of independence in activity performance as its primary aim, and its corresponding recognition that technology or personal assistance can enable self-directed occupations to attain a balanced lifestyle of choice, is important. Equally significant is the profession's adoption of broader sociocultural perspectives that do not universally believe that a balance among self-care, work, and play and leisure is necessary; balance in occupation encompasses far more than this triad.

> *By occupation is not meant any kind of "busy work" or exercise that may be given to a child to keep him out of mischief or idleness when seated at his desk. By occupation I mean a mode of activity on the part of the child which reproduces or runs parallel to some form of work carried on in the social life. . . . The fundamental point of the psychology of an occupation is that it maintains a balance between the intellectual and the practical phases of experience.*
> —Barton (1944, p. 282)

Westhorp analyzes contemporary perspectives on balance in occupation as put forth by leading scholars in occupational therapy, occupational science, and other fields. Although most of the literature focuses on individuals' lifestyle balance, the concept of a *balanced lifestyle* can be extended to groups, communities, states, and nations. Westhorp discusses key works that apply balance in occupation to these entities. The characteristics of balance in relationships and social change (i.e., holism, interconnectedness, dynamic state) and epidemiological perspectives are presented. Westhorp proposes an occupational perspective on balance that includes personal control. Hence, balance is evident when a person expresses and develops capabilities by engaging in self-selected, personally meaningful occupations that enable and maintain health and well-being.

This occupational and lifestyle balance is a dynamic process that resonates from individuals to their respective family, social groups, community, and wider society. In turn, these external forces and others influence the person's balance. On the basis of this interdependence, occupationally balanced and healthy people contribute to occupationally balanced and healthy systems, and vice versa. Westhorp advocates for the use of

211

a dynamic cycle of personal reflection (i.e., self-monitoring, values clarification, decision making, implementation) to achieve occupational balance. She urges the adoption of an attitude of inclusion to attain a desired balance in occupation and a healthy lifestyle.

Westhorp's advice to embrace a life perspective that includes the pursuit of "good things" in sufficient amounts in one's daily life is echoed in Chapter 20. In this Muriel Driver Lecture, Majnemer reflects on the value of doing things simply because one wants to rather than doing things because one must. Because leisure provides respite from the stresses of daily life and opportunities to reenergize, self-express, socially engage, pursue interests, develop capacities, attain aspirations, and simply enjoy oneself, engagement in leisure activities promotes well-being across the lifespan. Conversely, role strain and the increasing intrusion of technology into daily life can negatively affect work–life balance.

Majnemer urges occupational therapy practitioners to consider the adverse effects of lifestyle imbalance and recognize the importance of discretionary activities to health, life satisfaction, and community participation. If the purpose of occupational therapy is to enable engagement in occupation, practitioners must expand their focus beyond the person's functional impairments and limitations. By integrating the assessment of leisure into daily practice and directly asking clients which activities they want to do, occupational therapy practitioners can promote personal control and enable choice.

To actualize the profession's holistic view of occupation, practitioners must collaborate with clients to develop opportunities for personally meaningful leisure exploration and engagement. The essentiality of leisure to well-being is supported by Majnemer's discussion of leisure participation for children and youth with disabilities. Contextual barriers and facilitators to leisure participation are identified. Best practice requires consideration of the multidimensional and complex personal and environmental factors that may impede the pursuit of leisure. By partnering with individuals, families, schools, organizations, and communities, practitioners can proactively advocate for policies, practices, and resources that help people of all ages attain balanced and satisfying lives through engagement in desired leisure activities (see Active Reflection III.2).

Having no other interests, life becomes a dull routine . . . and they suffer an attack of depression.

Had they taken a broader view of life with wider interests the attack might have been avoided. Such individuals have to learn "how to live." That is an essential part of their treatment. Occupation by broadening their interests is naturally the best method of accomplishing this.

—Dunton (1919, p. 48)

The widely accepted view that lives comprised of certain configurations of occupations are healthier and more satisfying than lives without these patterns is explored in the next chapter by Matuska and Christiansen. They summarize their previously published literature review, which examined lifestyle balance according to early historical beliefs, occupational therapy's founding philosophy, and contemporary perspectives based on research (Christiansen & Matuska, 2006). Synthesizing this theoretical and empirical literature from the social, behavioral, and occupational sciences, Matuska, and Christiansen put forth a model of lifestyle balance. This framework builds on interdisciplinary research on time use, social roles, and biological rhythms and is informed by established theories of well-being, motivation, and self-determination.

Matuska and Christiansen propose five needs-based dimensions of occupation essential for well-being and a balanced life. These include the use of occupation to (1) meet biological health and safety needs; (2) have rewarding and self-affirming social relationships; (3) feel interested, engaged, challenged, and competent; (4) create meaning and a positive personal identity; and (5) organize time and energy to meet important personal goals and renew one's self. Individual and environmental factors influence how people configure their patterns of occupation each day to satisfy these dimensions.

Thus, *lifestyle balance* is viewed as a dynamic interaction between daily occupational patterns and the environment in which important needs are met at various levels of satisfaction and sustainability. When there is perceived congruence between desired participation in occupation across these five dimensions and their actual occupational patterns, a satisfying, healthy, and meaningful lifestyle is attained. Matuska and Christiansen acknowledge how physical, economic, political, social, and cultural barriers affect people's ability to participate in desired occupations to meet their needs, thereby hindering lifestyle balance. Subsequent chapters in this part will address these issues in more depth.

Active Reflection III.2. Life: A Balancing Act

Majnemer concluded her Muriel Driver Lecture by urging occupational therapy practitioners to take the time to balance their boat, while Westhorp encouraged the adoption of an attitude of inclusion (i.e., adding good things to one's life) to attain a healthy lifestyle.

- Reflect on your occupational patterns.
- Is your boat balanced, or are there more good things you can add to your life to attain a desired lifestyle?
- Does your daily pattern of occupation enable you to adequately meet the 5 needs-based dimensions of occupation Matuska and Christiansen proposed as essential for a balanced life?
- Describe the individual and environmental factors that influence how you configure your patterns of occupation each day to satisfy these dimensions.

A daily influence on a balanced and healthy lifestyle is sleep. Green reflected on the impact of modern life on the natural sleep–wake cycle.

- Are your sleep habits and patterns reflective of sleep deprivation, or are they more in tune with the restorative aspects of sleep as described in the *Framework* (AOTA, 2014a)?

Cultural Contexts

The occupational therapy worker . . . must have poise and common sense and a social sense to meet all kinds of patients, from the richest to the poorest, those with many interests and those with few, black and white, and of foreign birth.

—Shaw (1929, p. 200)

From the founding of occupational therapy in the early settlement houses, which served European immigrants in the United States (Quiroga, 1995), to the recent globalization of the profession (AOTA, 2007), the relevance of the cultural context to occupational therapy is evident. In diverse nations, such as the United States, occupational therapy practitioners work with people of multicultural backgrounds on a daily basis. In addition, many practitioners across the world are choosing to engage in international cross-cultural work (Bourke-Taylor & Hudson, 2005; Humbert, Burket, Deveney, & Kennedy, 2011). The value of the globalization of occupational therapy is supported by AOTA's (2007) *Centennial Vision,* which calls for occupational therapy to become widely recognized with a "globally connected and diverse workforce meeting society's occupational needs" (p. 613). To attain this goal, occupational therapy practitioners must be open to cultural diversity and responsive to the complex, dynamic, and multifaceted intricacies of cross-cultural work (Humbert et al., 2011; see Active Reflection III.3).

According to the *Framework,* culture is external to the person and determines beliefs, customs, behavioral norms, and expectations. However, the individual also internalizes these factors (AOTA, 2014). Thus, culture affects how people perceive health, illness, and disability; activities' purposefulness and occupation's meaningfulness; and relationships with care providers (Bickenbach, 2009; Bourke-Taylor & Hudson, 2005; Muñoz, 2007; Odawara, 2005). Consequently, the cultural context must be considered throughout the occupational therapy process. Because culture influences all aspects of occupation; that is, "what we do, how, when, where, for how long, and with whom we do it" (Cynkin, 1995, p. 151), practitioners must have a thorough understanding of a person's cultural context to ensure that the occupational experiences they provide are culturally appropriate (Odawara, 2005). The benefits of culturally relevant practice are many, including the simplification of "the work of occupational therapy personnel by adding individualized meaning to the interventions, thereby increasing motivation to participate in therapy" (Barney, 1991, p. 586).

The influence of culture on the person's engagement in occupational therapy is clearly evident in Chapter 22. Schemm begins this work with a realistic case vignette that highlights the undeniable impact culture has on the establishment of a therapeutic relationship (or lack thereof) and the occupational therapy process. She presents a historical overview of the beliefs about culture that were held by occupational therapy founders and theorists. Schemm defines *culture* and identifies its components, examining how they pertain to and affect occupational therapy practice. The influence of culture on a person's perception of illness, health, and therapy and a person's belief in the meaning of his or her own life and activities are explored. Schemm provides specific suggestions on how to increase cultural literacy and helpful guidelines for considering cultural factors during evaluation and treatment. Throughout her clear analysis, Schemm includes concrete examples to support the relevance of culture to the process and ultimate outcome of occupational therapy.

Although competent practitioners may be aware of the need to address culture throughout the occupational therapy process, the authors of Chapter 23 contend that unclear definitions of *culture* provide little guidance to practitioners about how to actualize this awareness in practice. In Chapter 23, Bonder, Martin, and Miracle review diverse definitions of *culture* and

---

Active Reflection III.3. Cross-Cultural Awareness

Dickie (2004) reminds us, "Attending to cultural moments, sensitivity to the possibility of difference, and awareness of the cultural in our own realities are strategies to help us achieve cultural competence in the moment" (p. 172).

Pair up with a peer or colleague from a different cultural background. Identify your respective culture's values, beliefs, and norms. Discuss each culture's view of health, illness, professional and personal interactions, and therapeutic interventions.

- What is similar?
- What is different?
- How will your cultural realities affect your professional roles, tasks and relationships?
- What strategies can you use to enhance your cultural competence?

---

examine the usefulness and limitations of description-based and rules-based approaches to defining it. To counter these constraints, Bonder and colleagues propose a third approach to examining culture, putting forth a pragmatic definition of *culture* as emergent in everyday interactions of individuals. This culture emergent view proposes that the symbolic aspects of culture and cultural identity develop through the interaction of individuals. Bonder and colleagues explore how this culture emergent perspective requires a reconsideration of the characteristics of culture.

The traditional conceptualization of culture as being learned, localized, patterned, evaluative, and persistent is challenged, with Bonder and colleagues concluding that these characteristics can change and adapt because of interaction. They propose that understanding culture as emerging from interaction (including the therapeutic relationship) has important implications for practitioners. Bonder and colleagues analyze how culture affects occupation patterns and choice. They provide suggestions for occupational therapy practitioners to use to frame effective intercultural therapeutic encounters. They emphasize that careful attention to the emergent nature of culture in each person, active curiosity about the cultural aspects of interactions, and self-reflection and self-evaluation of therapeutic interaction can enhance the occupational therapy process due.

There is no such thing as a man alone. An individual must be orientated not only as regards himself, but as regards his place in society. An understanding of this basic concept provides one of the corner stones of rehabilitation, and must be understood by all who do this work. A specialist in rehabilitation

is not a specialist at all. He considers himself a member of a team of workers, both lay and medical, directed towards the patient as a whole.

—Sommerville (1954, p. 37)

Bonder and colleagues provide a relevant contemporary model to facilitate culturally informed practice by focusing on the individual interactive components of occupational therapy. However, the reality that individual agency cannot be free of the collective culture, which may be resistant to change, cannot be ignored (Dickie, 2004). Occupational therapy practitioners in the United States must recognize that they largely share a Western perspective that may differ from the collective beliefs of non-Western cultures. For example, the *Framework* (AOTA, 2014a) strongly advocates that there is a positive correlation between health and occupational engagement. However, this relationship should not be unquestionably accepted. The reality is, many cultures do not share this view (Kelly & McFarlane, 2007).

Although ours is a multicultural world filled with immense diversity, most occupational therapy practice models are founded on Western, White, middle-class sociocultural norms. These models typically include concepts such as *autonomy, achievement, performance,* and *independence;* beliefs about self, health, illness, disability, and well-being; and values of temporality and activity. However, these perspectives are not universally held (Bourke-Taylor & Hudson, 2005; Muñoz, 2007). According to Muñoz (2007), developing occupational therapy models "in the area of cultural competence is in its infancy" (p. 258). One conceptual structure that has been recognized as bridging this theoretical gap by broadening the profession's view of culture is the Kawa model.

In Chapter 24, Iwama, Thomson, and MacDonald present the Kawa model, which is named for the Japanese word for *river* and is based on East Asian sociocultural perspectives. They describe how the Kawa model was developed as an alternative to practice models that reflected only Western beliefs and values, which are irrelevant when they are applied to persons of non-Western cultures. In contrast to Western models, which primarily focus on the individual, the Kawa model emphasizes contexts that shape and influence the realities and challenges of people's day-to-day lives. According to Iwama and colleagues, the use of the river as a metaphor provides the practitioner with a nonmechanistic way to explore the unique sociocultural contexts of a person's daily life. They describe the structure, define the concepts, and explain principles of the Kawa model.

By applying this model, the purpose of occupational therapy is redefined as the enablement of life flow (i.e., well-being), not the attainment of independence or individualism. Well-being is enabled by enhancing the harmony between the internal and external contextual elements of a person's life, which are represented metaphorically as various components of a river. Iwama and colleagues propose that applying the river metaphor can be an effective tool for generating cultural knowledge, developing cultural competence, and providing culturally responsive occupational therapy. They expose that practice that universally applies Western-centric models inevitably reflects the exercise of power and the propagation of inequities. They maintain that adopting a culturally responsive model that recognizes the complex sociocultural challenges that hinder equity is required in a contemporary, global practice environment.

> *An occupational therapist will always work with people from all walks of life. Frequently he is pulled far from his own native environment and thrown into the problems of varied standards of living . . . the ability to appreciate the commonplace, to note a touch of beauty in the midst of squalor or be aware of tenderness even in frugal living, this is the train that refreshes and strengthens the individual as he is introduced to the ways of others.*
> —Brunyate (1958, p. 197)

Sociopolitical Contexts

The social and economic divides that Brunyate identifies as needing to be forged by occupational therapy practitioners requires more than openness to differences. While this receptiveness is vital to culturally responsive practice, deep-rooted power differentials must also be confronted. Historically, the profession of occupational therapy has been largely apolitical with a few notable exceptions (Fleming-Castady, 2014; Pollard, Sakellariou, & Kronenberg, 2011). In Chapter 2, Bing described the tenacity of Beatrice Wade, who fought relentlessly for over a decade to amend the Smith–Fess Act of 1920 (now called the *Vocational Rehabilitation Act*) to extend coverage for persons with psychiatric disorders. This exemplary leader provides an excellent role model for those working to end entrenched inequities. Over the past decade, a call for the practitioners to commit to and advocate for social and political changes that empower people and enable participation has become more evident in the literature (Cottrell, 2005, 2007;

Galheigo, 2011; Kronenberg & Pollard, 2006; Lohman, Gabriel, & Furlong, 2004; Pollard et al., 2011).

Because the power of occupation is constrained when social, political, and legal systems exclude people and limit their access to resources, the *Framework* includes occupational justice as a desired outcome of occupational therapy. Infusing justice into the *Framework* empowers practitioners to work with people to transcend social and occupational barriers and "enhance their social participation, health, and well-being" (Gupta & Walloch, 2006, p. CE1). All occupational therapy practitioners have an ethical responsibility to confront abuses to human rights, including the right to occupation (Galheigo, 2011). We must advocate for the allocation of adequate resources that allow all people to access their rights, meet their needs, live in environments of choice, and fully participate in society. Occupational therapy evaluations and interventions are rendered meaningless if vulnerable and marginalized people are not participating members of their communities. A sociopolitical system that devalues people by providing insufficient resources renders full participation an elusive goal based on empty rhetoric rather than achievable reality.

> *An individual can be studied properly only in relation to his environment, and it therefore follows that the economic pressure of security or insecurity has a strong influence on the recovery of the patient.*
> —Association of Occupational Therapists (1951, p. 1)

Occupational therapy practitioners share a collective responsibility to use their knowledge and skills to transform words into actions and fight for sociopolitical change and legislative initiatives that support and finance participation (Cottrell, 2005, 2007; Galheigo, 2011; Kronenberg & Pollard, 2006; Lohman et al., 2004; Pollard et al., 2011). Major societal change is required globally to enable all people to assert their fundamental human right to participate in life. The irrefutable relationship among occupation, participation, and human rights throughout the world are clearly articulated in the World Federation of Occupational Therapists's *Position Statement on Human Rights* (see Appendix III.A). This important endorsement of the United Nations (n.d.) *Universal Declaration of Human Rights* provides key principles and action strategies to guide practitioners in their efforts to achieve an occupationally just society.

The sociopolitical contexts that affect people, institutions, communities, and societies and promote or constrain occupational justice and full participation are examined in Part III's next four chapters. In Chapter 25, Grady explores the role of occupational therapy practitioners in building inclusive communities. In her Eleanor Clarke Slagle Lecture, Grady describes challenges to inclusion and analyzes the nature and meaning of *community*. She examines the relationships among individuals, families, culture, environmental contexts, and community. Foundations for building personal communities of choice are identified. The interaction among a person's past experience, present situation, future aspirations, and ability to choose are explored as they affect the relationship between the practitioner and the consumer of occupational therapy services.

Grady provides a solid overview of the evolution of the disability rights movement and the paradigm shift from the medical model to an interactive model of disability. She discusses key ideas about the philosophy of inclusion, societal mandates, and legislative initiatives for inclusion. Grady emphasizes the need to recognize disability as a dimension of diversity and not as a limiting handicap. She proposes four key values for occupational therapy reflective of the interactive model of disability and supportive of inclusion and choice. Grady entreats practitioners to create opportunities for people with disabilities that develop capacities and enable choice, even if these choices reflect personal priorities that differ from "expert" opinion.

To foster people's ability to engage in meaningful activity within their chosen community, environmental barriers must be removed and supports and adaptations must be provided. Grady cautions that attitudinal and emotional barriers, supports, and adaptations must be considered along with the physical aspects of the environment. She proposes that applying spatiotemporal adaptation theory can provide a useful way to meet the challenges of building inclusive communities. Grady revisits this theory in light of the aforementioned paradigm shift to an interactive model of disability. She describes a spiraling continuum of environments that promote inclusion, independence, interdependence, and successful adaptation. Emphasizing the therapeutic communication process, Grady presents interactive strategies for practitioners to use to develop collaborative models of consumer-driven, community-based practice. Grady concludes with a call for occupational therapy practitioners to confront prevailing challenges to choice and participation and take the lead in developing inclusive communities (see Active Reflection III.4).

We must develop our ability to become leaders, to move with confidence into the community and collaborate in the creation of a healthier environment, contributing our knowledge of activities and human action. We need, therefore, to be able to problem-solve, to understand the factors involved in complex social systems and define the problems where we can make a contribution.

—Finn (1972, p. 66)

Active Reflection III.4. Inclusive Communities and Occupational Justice

Consider the contexts of your home community and imagine you acquired a serious, long-term disability.
- What contextual characteristics would support your occupational performance and full participation in community life?
- Describe how these contextual supports can facilitate the achievement of occupational justice for all.
- Are there contextual barriers or constraints in your community (e.g., stigmatizing attitudes, limited community resources) that would limit your occupational performance and full participation and contribute to occupational injustice?
- What recommendations would you make for additional services, adaptations, and modifications to enable your community to be occupationally just and one of full inclusion?

More than 20 years have passed since Grady's seminal lecture, but the challenges she identified remain. Although progress has been made toward enabling people with disabilities to live in environments of choice and fully participate in society, much more needs to be done for full equity to be attained. In recognition of this need, the AOTA has issued several official statements that are consistent with Grady's message: *Occupational Therapy's Commitment to Nondiscrimination and Inclusion* (AOTA, 2014b), *AOTA's Societal Statement on Livable Communities* (AOTA, 2009), and *Occupational Therapy's Perspective on the Use of Environment and Contexts to Support Health and Participation in Occupations* (AOTA, 2010). These works are provided as Appendixes III.B–III.D in this part. Appendix III.D contains an excellent outline of key legislative acts and judicial decisions that have mandated services for and expanded the rights of people with disabilities. The document also provides multiple case studies that describe environmental considerations for occupational therapy service delivery with diverse populations across the lifespan. All three of these documents affirm our profession's commitment and responsibility to apply our expertise and actualize our values to enable full societal participation for all.

As emphasized in Grady's discussion of inclusive community and highlighted in the *Framework,* political, social, and cultural barriers to the achievement of full participation often exist. Chapter 26 by Whiteford provides a thoughtful discussion about the effects of external restrictions on people. When these are beyond personal control and restrict the ability to engage in occupations of meaning, occupational deprivation results. As Whiteford emphasizes, deprivation is not the product of the person's internal limitations but the result of outer forces. She defines *occupational deprivation* and analyzes the related phenomena of occupational disruption and dysfunction to clarify their differences from deprivation.

Whiteford explores the conceptual origins of occupational deprivation, noting that, although this is a relatively new term, the phenomenon itself has been present throughout world history. Recent global trends such as advances in technology, the maldistribution of labor, the marginalization of people, and the experience of refugeeism are contributing to increased occupational deprivation. Whiteford reflects on the human costs of occupational deprivation and identifies ways that occupational therapy practitioners can address it. She suggests adopting a perspective that incorporates occupation with broader social, international, and cultural dimensions. Having a global viewpoint can help practitioners think and act in ways that are congruent with concerns for social and occupational justice. Most important, Whiteford presents a call to arms for practitioners to address deprivation through social and political action.

The relevance of occupational deprivation and justice to the profession is further explored by Townsend and Wilcock in Chapter 27. They analyze the phenomena of occupational justice and derive four types of injustice from their exploratory theory of occupational justice. The significance of these injustices (i.e., occupational alienation, occupational deprivation, occupational marginalization, occupational imbalance) is examined. Townsend and Wilcock contend that the naming of these suggests four occupational rights: (1) the right to experience meaning and enrichment in ones' occupation, (2) the right to participate in a range of occupations for health and social inclusion, (3) the right to make choices and share decision-making power in daily life, and (4) the right to receive equal privileges for diverse participation in occupations. Townsend and Wilcock's reflections on their ongoing international dialogue about the relationship between occupational justice and client-centered practice provide a stellar example for practitioners seeking to work for justice. They accurately state that, because silence implies compliance with the status quo, practitioners should develop their own dialogue about occupational injustices to bring these issues to the forefront of the profession.

Townsend and Wilcock remind us that discourse about occupational injustice is timely, as occupational therapy practitioners around the world focus on providing best practices that synthesize and apply our knowledge, skills, and attitudes about occupation, enabling, and justice. In their treatise, they present a persuasive argument that occupational therapy exists as a profession to address occupational injustice and that it is up to its members to make this explicit to the world. They describe specific actions occupational therapy clinicians, managers, educators, policymakers, and researchers can take to support client-centered activism for occupational justice to ensure that all individuals attain and maintain their rights to occupation.

> *Rehabilitation this is more than the dynamic process of rebuilding the physical lives of disabled individuals. It is a fierce belief in our individual responsibility for what happened to our fellow man. It is compounded of hope and freedom, hope to conquer every natural plague and every human mischief, and freedom from the shackles and bondage of human disability.*
>
> —Kreeger (1958, p. 53)

As emphasized by Townsend and Wilcock, occupational therapy practitioners must confront the externally imposed barriers and entrenched inequities that deprive people of their basic human rights, including occupational ones. To be effective advocates, practitioners must recognize that the shackles and bonds that disable are the result of social, political, and economic disparities. People with disabilities are handicapped by these, not their functional limitations. The imperative for occupational therapy practitioners to expand their professional responsibilities beyond direct care to include advocacy for societal change that respects human rights and promotes well-being is well-articulated in Chapter 28. In this work, Hammell and Iwama apply critical theory to occupational therapy practice and highlight the need for the profession to move beyond an individualized focus on improving function. Critical occupational therapy requires practitioners to commit to facilitating structural, social, and political change that enables equitable access to participation in occupations of choice.

Because engagement in occupation is essential for well-being, and the attainment of well-being is widely accepted as a basic human right, Hammell and Iwama conclude that occupational engagement is a fundamental human right. The relationships among human rights, well-being, occupation, occupational justice, and occupational rights are examined. Hammell and Iwama challenge practitioners to expand their view of occupation beyond the traditional triad of self-care, productivity, and leisure. Broadening the profession's theoretical frameworks to include personally meaningful occupations that promote interdependence, community development, and collective well-being is required. Hammell and Iwama contend the role of the environment in occupational therapy theories must move beyond Western perspectives to include ecological perspectives that describe the interconnections between humans and their environments. This is vital, because people are not inseparable from their environmental circumstances. Thus, occupational therapy practitioners must make a personal and professional commitment to address the multidimensional environmental conditions of people's lives which enable or constrain their occupational rights and well-being (see Active Reflection III.5).

Active Reflection III.5. Willpower, Occupation, and Well-Being

Hammell and Iwama maintain that Reilly's (1962) oft-quoted statement of "man, through the use of his hands as energized by mind and will, can influence the state of his own health" (Reilly, p. 2) is ableist and sexist because it ignores the reality that sheer willpower cannot surmount entrenched oppression, social inequities, sexism, racism, homophobia, relentless poverty, incapacitating illness or disability, natural disasters, famine, and wars. Review Reilly's Eleanor Clarke Slagle Lecture (see Chapter 7), which includes this famous quote.

- In what contexts (i.e., social, cultural, political, professional, personal) did Reilly make her declaration?
- How do these contextual considerations affect your view of Reilly's statement and Hammell and Iwama's critique of it?
- Do you agree or disagree with their assessment of Reilly's proclamation? Why?

In her lecture, Reilly asserts she is a "card-carrying critic" (p. 2) and advocates for the use of critical thinking. She proposes that the controversy that results from criticism ensures progress.

- How do you think Reilly may have responded to Hammell and Iwama?
- Are there any indications in her work that Reilly could have expanded her American perspective on the relationships among willpower, occupation, and well-being to include global perspectives inclusive of occupational rights?

Personal Contexts

We are dealing with persons, not cases, and with this firmly fixed in our minds we shall be more likely to find a solution. In reality these considerations should often have the first place in our minds.

—Varrier-Jones (1941, p. 368)

Hammell and Iwama's contention that engagement in occupation is essential for well-being and that the achievement of well-being is a fundamental human right is further analyzed in this part's section on the personal contexts of occupation. In Chapter 29, Hayward and Taylor begin this exploration by urging the profession to reconceptualize its desired outcome. They argue that occupational therapy's historic emphasis on *doing* as its purpose has negated the vitality of *being*. Hayward and Taylor examine the multiple dimensions of well-being and the conceptual congruence between eudaimonic well-being and spirituality, client-centeredness, and occupational integrity.

Because eudaimonic well-being occurs when people fully engage in life activities that are congruent with their beliefs and values, Hayward and Taylor question occupational therapy's relevance and efficacy that does not consider each person's subjective experience of occupation. They urge practitioners to not marginalize the power of occupation by focusing only on functional outcomes in accordance with mainstream practice models.

Hayward and Taylor advocate that eudaimonic well-being be adopted as a primary concept in occupational therapy models. This theoretical shift from a narrow focus on health and wellness to the consideration of the personal, spiritual, moral, sociocultural, and political dimensions that affect subjective well-being is critical for the profession to actualize its stated commitment to social justice. The value of reframing and promoting eudaimonic well-being as an expected, routine, and global outcome of occupational therapy is well-articulated by Hayward and Taylor. They contend that embracing eudaimonic well-being as central to the profession can contribute to a renaissance of authentic occupational therapy that views well-being through occupation as core to humanity.

The belief that occupation is innate to the human experience is further explored in Chapter 30, which presents Wilcock's theory of the human need for occupation. According to Wilcock, occupation is not just the purpose of human function but an integral component of each human being's relationship with the world. She explores the biological need to do and proposes that needs have a three-way role in maintaining the health and stability of the person. Wilcock relates these three functions to occupation, explaining how engagement in purposeful occupation contributes to the survival of the species. Occupation not only fulfills human biological needs but also develops the sociocultural capacities of the person, enabling the person to grow and adapt to environmental changes and challenges. Moreover, occupation provides the mechanism for people to socially interpret and form the foundation for community. Wilcock contends that occupation is the means by which humans demonstrate their value to their society and the world. She expresses concern that the centrality of occupation to the human experience is being threatened by sociocultural, economic, and political forces and that the occupational needs of people have become obscured by the increased complexities of a technological world.

> *The complexities of a rapidly expanding, industrialized society make it imperative for the health professional to attend to those factors that preclude or inhibit doing.*
> —Fidler & Fidler (1978, p. 309)

Wilcock's reflections on how changing occupational structures and technologies affect the human need for occupation warrant further discussion. In the decades that have passed since her theory was originally published, technology has exploded beyond anything envisioned at that time. Besides the physical and sociocultural world Wilcock examined, we now have a complete virtual world. In recognition of this, the *Framework* (AOTA, 2014a) identified the virtual context as relevant to the occupational therapy process. The virtual context and the use of technology offers many benefits to disenfranchised people, including those with disabilities (e.g., the use of electronic aids to daily living to master the environment, the use of social media to interact with others). The emerging delivery system of telehealth presents additional opportunities for practitioners to provide services which can develop people's capacities to meet their inherent need for occupation. Part V, "Tools of Practice that Enable Occupational Engagement," of this text will explore these practice advances in more depth.

The analysis of the personal context is continued by Yerxa in Chapter 31. She explores the relationship

---

Active Reflection III.6. Virtual and Personal Contexts: A Symbiotic or Parasitic Relationship?

As defined in the *Framework* (AOTA, 2014a), the *virtual context* is an "environment in which communication occurs by means of airwaves or computers and in the absence of *physical contact*" (p. S28, italics added).

- Given that our profession's core philosophy supports Wilcock's view that occupation is a fundamental human need that enables social participation, how does removing physical contact affect the person?
- How has society's increased emphasis on technology affected people with disabilities and other marginalized groups?
- Have technological advances furthered people's abilities to meet their human need for occupation, or have these created occupational structures and sociocultural expectations which hinder the capacity to attain occupational balance and subjective well-being?
- Has the explosion of the virtual context been at the expense of the personal context, or do these contexts share a mutually beneficial relationship?
- How can occupational therapy practitioners promote a symbiotic relationship between the virtual and personal context?

---

among occupation, health, and spirit and provides thoughtful reflections on Adolf Meyer's foundational work and his enduring legacy. She examines postindustrial societal forces that are endangering human's occupational being and balance. Yerxa describes her view of *health* as the possession of a repertoire of skills that enable individuals to attain well-being and achieve desired goals in their chosen environments, not as the absence of pathology. Adopting this perspective means that health is possible for all people, including those with chronic illnesses and disabilities.

Yerxa reviews the literature from occupational therapy and other disciplines to highlight the key influences of occupations on health, including interests, satisfaction in everyday doing, balance, the latent consequences of work, and transcendence. Yerxa continues her exploration of the literature by focusing on research about the "hardy" personality and mortality. She challenges occupational therapy practitioners to create environments that enable meaningful occupation and provide all people with just-right challenges to achieve participation in life. Yerxa concludes that both theory and research support a relationship among occupation, health, well-being, and survival (see Active Reflection III.6).

> *I got a new vision of life. I was made to realize it is intensely better to be unfit below the shoulders than above. . . . Now the vision . . . has become a vivid re-*

ality. Restless minds have become engaged and active; patients whose existence was a terrible monotony now hurry here and there in the pursuit of their daily studies and tasks; what was once inactivity and stagnation is now a constructive, enthusiastic organization.

—Cooper (1918, p. 24)

Yerxa calls on practitioners to end the marginalization of occupation by asking, "What could be less trivial than survival?" (p. 404). Survival and related experiences which threaten humanity are explored by Fine in Chapter 32. In this inspiring Eleanor Clarke Slagle Lecture, Fine examines the relationship between an individual's most personal characteristics and inner life as she answers the question, "Who rises above adversity?" She explores remarkable examples of human adaptability and resilience in the face of extraordinary hardships and major adversities. Fine reflects on the reality that occupational therapy practitioners often work in a world of incredible trauma and stunning triumph. She examines factors that influence resilience, the relationship between these internal qualities and the external world, and the person's emerging capabilities to adapt to adversity. Several theories on stress and various perspectives on coping are provided.

Fine's analysis of the social and personal meaning of trauma and resilience is interwoven with striking personal anecdotes and poetry from people who have experienced extreme life events. She proposes that an increased appreciation of the power of a person's inner psychological life can strengthen the occupational therapy process. Fine reminds us that many people occupational therapy practitioners work with have their capacities for resilience threatened by an often unresponsive health care system and the daily challenges of living with chronic illness and disability. Therefore, practitioners must use their expertise and compassion to provide timely and meaningful interventions that assist in the reintegration process and transforming hardships into possibilities, thereby facilitating the person's ability to attain an inner life that rises above adversity. Fine calls for occupational therapy practitioners to move beyond the maintenance of professional objectivity to connect to clients' deeper personal experiences and acquire an understanding of their inner state.

The increasing realization in the past few decades of the tripartite nature of man—mind, body, spirit—has had a most important effect in increasing the use of occupation.

—Kidner (1932 p. 233)

One intensely personal context that is a core component of many people's inner state and often related to resilience is spirituality. According to Moyers and Dale (2007), *spirituality* is "the personal quest for understanding answers about life, about meaning, and the sacred" (p. 28). The *Framework* categorizes spirituality as a client factor, not a context. Regardless of how it is classified or defined, spirituality is internal to the individual; influences his or her personal beliefs, perceptions, and expectations; and inspires and motivates the individual; thus, influencing service delivery. The relationships among spirituality, occupation, and occupational therapy are analyzed by Wilson in Chapter 33. In her opinion piece, Wilson examines the spiritual dimensions of occupation and reflects on the place occupation has in a spiritual life. She reviews major definitions of *spirituality* and its defining attributes while acknowledging that the attainment of a precise definition remains elusive.

Wilson proposes that the inability to define *spirituality* is inherent to its highly personal and nebulous nature. However, this should not prevent spirituality from being a primary consideration in occupational therapy practice. She describes the ongoing dialogue that questions whether spirituality is a legitimate domain of occupational therapy. Wilson advocates for practitioners to consider clients' capacity, willingness, and need to engage on a spiritual level and their own ability to use and elicit the spiritual potential of occupation in a client-centered manner. Given spirituality's established connection to well-being, the opportunity to engage clients on a spiritual level is one which should not be lost. However, as Wilson notes, all do not express comfort or have experience with the spiritual aspects of practice. Thus, active reflection and education on the relationships between spirituality, occupation, and occupational therapy is needed (McColl, 2000).

Exhibit III.1 contains a series of questions McColl asked of persons who recently acquired disabilities and occupational therapy practitioners during two research studies that examined spirit, occupation, and disability (see Active Reflection III.7). In her Muriel Driver Lecture, which included the findings of these studies, McColl provides helpful suggestions for integrating spirit into evaluation and intervention. Because space constraints preclude the inclusion of all relevant literature, I encourage readers to review McColl's lecture and other seminal works on spirit and spirituality to increase their knowledge of this important personal construct.

Exhibit III.1. McColl's Spirituality Research Questions

Questions Asked of Persons With Disabilities	Questions Asked of Occupational Therapists
1. Would you describe yourself as a spiritual person? 2. Has your understanding of yourself changed since you acquired your disability? 3. Have your relationships with others changed since your disability? 4. Has your way of viewing the world changed since your disability? 5. Have your beliefs changed since the onset of your disability? 6. Have your religious practices changed? 7. Has your soul or spirit been affected by your disability?	1. In your practice as an occupational therapist: • Do you see evidence of the spiritual aspect of your patients? • Have you seen people whose understanding of themselves has changed when they acquired a disability? • Have you seen people whose relationships with others have changed after the onset? • Have you seen people whose way of viewing the world had changed after the onset? • Have you seen people whose belief in a Supreme Being or higher power changed? • Have you seen people whose religious practices changed after the onset of a disability? 2. Do you feel adequately prepared to deal with these issues when they arise with your patients?

Source. From "Spirit, Occupation, and Disability," by M. McColl, 2000, *Canadian Journal of Occupational Therapy,* Vol. 67, p. 218. Copyright © 2000 by the Canadian Association of Occupational Therapists. Reprinted with permission.

Just as people's spirit is inherently personal, so too is their identity. In Chapter 34, Christiansen explores how people develop and express their personal identities. In his Eleanor Clarke Slagle Lecture, he asserts that occupation is the principal means through which each individual creates and maintains his or her own unique identity. Christiansen supports his proclamation on the basis of a review of theory and research from which he derived four key propositions about the human need to express a personal identity in a meaningful manner: (1) identity shapes and is shaped by interpersonal relationships; (2) identity is linked to doing, and these actions are interpreted in an interpersonal context; (3) identity is a central component a person's life story and provides meaning for his or her everyday doings and life itself; and (4) identity is essential for well-being and life satisfaction. These assumptions are viewed as tentative due to the need for research on the construction and maintenance of identity. However, Christiansen's discussion of each provides useful reflections for practitioners to consider about identity throughout the occupational therapy process. His elaboration on the roots of identity (i.e., reflexive consciousness, interpersonal aspects of selfhood, the agential aspects of the self) provide an additional framework for understanding the implications of identity for practice. The relationships among identity, people's life stories, how people make sense of these life stories, and how life experiences shape identities and create life meaning are explored (see Active Reflection III.8).

Active Reflection III.7. Personal Perspectives on Spirituality and Resilience

Review the questions posed by McColl in Exhibit 3.1.
• How would you respond to the first question asked of clients?
• Describe the influence of spirituality on your life, if any.
Consider the first series of questions McColl asks of occupational therapists.
• During your professional education or practice, did you learn about or observe any of the issues addressed by McColl?
• How would you answer her final question to occupational therapists?
• Have your beliefs and resilience ever been challenged by adversity?
• Describe how these personal experiences have shaped you and your ability to address issues of spirituality and adversity with your clients.

Active Reflection III.8. The Contexts of Personal Identity and Subjective Well-Being

Consider the characteristics of different practice settings (e.g., school, home, psychosocial clubhouse, hospital, skilled nursing facility).
• How do the temporal, cultural, sociopolitical, and personal contexts of each setting influence a person's identity and the attainment of subjective well-being?
• Given the many constraints presented in these practice settings, how can occupational therapy practitioners contribute to the formation and maintenance of a positive self-identity and eudaimonic well-being?
• Describe concrete actions practitioners can take to honor people's uniqueness and provide the just-right challenge to enable their meaningful and desired participation, development of an identity based on occupational competence, and attainment of subjective well-being.

The web is lengthening and broadening; the woof is welded with understanding; the broken threads have been skillfully pieced together, and life takes on a newer meaning daily.

—Cooper (1918, p. 26)

Christiansen proposes that identity is instrumental to social life, because it gives people a context that enables them to derive meaning from daily experiences and interpret their life story. He describes how identity provides a framework for goal setting and motivation when the person envisions a future "possible self" that includes images in action. Christiansen further asserts that these thoughts of actions are influenced by social approval and competent performance, thereby shaping identity. Because engagement in occupations provides opportunities to express the self and form identity, the development of an identity on the basis of competent performance can be threatened by limitations, impairments, illnesses, participation restrictions, and disability. In addition, Christiansen contends that stigma and bodily disfigurement can hinder the development of identity, because of the lack of social approval. Occupational therapy practitioners can help address the identity challenges faced by those with whom we work by enabling them to maintain or reclaim an identity acceptable to self and on the basis of occupational competence. Christiansen claims that the resulting identity will provide a sense of coherence and well-being for the person.

The positive influence occupation has on participation, identity, and well-being is strongly supported by the authors of this part. However, as several emphasize, the reality that participation can be blocked, identity diminished, and well-being compromised by temporal, cultural, sociopolitical, and personal contexts cannot be ignored. Thus, in accordance with the profession's recognition that the contexts of people's lives must be considered throughout the occupational therapy process, practitioners must partner with those they serve to confront ethnocentric viewpoints, entrenched biases, and systemic inequities that marginalize and disempower people. Only then can the profession's vision of being a powerful, widely recognized force that globally meets society's occupational needs be fully actualized (AOTA, 2007).

The occupational therapist must evaluate what people need under given circumstances and how these needs can be met within the confines of existing circumstances. He must be able to see himself and others in relation to community as well as world problems.

—McNay (1953, p. 221)

References

American Occupational Therapy Association. (AOTA). (2007). AOTA's *Centennial Vision* and executive summary. *American Journal of Occupational Therapy, 61,* 613–614. http://dx.doi.org/10.5014/ajot.61.6.613

American Occupational Therapy Association. (2009). AOTA's societal statement on livable communities. *American Journal of Occupational Therapy, 63,* 847–848. http://dx.doi.org/10.5014/ajot.63.6.847

American Occupational Therapy Association. (2010). Occupational therapy's perspective on the use of environments and contexts to support health and participation in occupations. *American Journal of Occupational Therapy, 64*(Suppl.), S57–S69. http://dx.doi.org/10.5014/ajot.2010.64S57

American Occupational Therapy Association. (2014a). Occupational therapy practice framework: Domain and process (3rd ed.). *American Journal of Occupational Therapy, 68*(Suppl. 1), S1–S48. http://dx.doi.org/10.5014/ajot.2014.682006

American Occupational Therapy Association. (2014b). Occupational therapy's commitment to nondiscrimination and inclusion. *American Journal of Occupational Therapy, 68.*

Association of Occupational Therapists. (1951). *Occupation for health: A journey from prescription to self-help.* London: College of Occupational Therapists.

Barney, K. (1991). From Ellis Island to assisted living: Meeting the needs of older adults from diverse cultures. *American Journal of Occupational Therapy, 45,* 586–593. http://dx.doi.org/10.5014/ajot.45.7.586

Barton, W. E. (1944). Training programs for occupational therapists in the US Army. *Occupational Therapy in Rehabilitation, 23,* 282.

Bickenbach, J. (2009). Disability, culture, and the UN convention. *Disability and Rehabilitation, 31,* 1111–1124. http://dx.doi.org/10.1080/09638280902773729

Bourke-Taylor, H., & Hudson, D. (2005). Cultural differences: The experience of establishing an occupational therapy service in a developing country. *Occupational Therapy International, 52,* 188–198.

Brunyate, R. (1958). Little common things [Eleanor Clarke Slagle Lecture]. *American Journal of Occupational Therapy, 12,* 193–202.

Christiansen, C., & Matuska, K. (2006). Lifestyle balance: A review of concepts and research. *Journal of Occupational Science, 13*(1), 49–61. http://dx.doi.org/10.1080/14427591.2006.9686570

Cooper, G. (1918). Reweaving the web: A soldier tells what it means to begin all over again. *Carry On, I,* 23–26.

Cottrell, R. P. (2005). The Olmstead decision: Landmark opportunity or platform for rhetoric? Our collective responsibility for full community participation. *American Journal of Occupational Therapy, 59,* 561–567. http://dx.doi.org/10.5014/ajot.59.5.561

Cottrell, R. P. (2007). The New Freedom Initiative: Transforming mental health care—Will OT be at the table? *Occupational Therapy in Mental Health, 23*(2), 1–24.

Cynkin, S. (1995). Activities. In C. B. Royeen (Ed.), *The practice of the future: Putting occupation back into therapy* (Lesson 7). Bethesda, MD: American Occupational Therapy Association.

Dickie, V. (2004). Culture is tricky: A commentary on culture emergent in occupation. *American Journal of Occupational Therapy, 58,* 169–173. http://dx.doi.org/10.5014/ajot.58.2.169

Donovan, J. M., VanLeit, B. J., Crowe, T. K., & Keefe, E. B. (2005). Occupational goals of mothers of children with disabilities: Influence of temporal, social, and emotional contexts. *American Journal of Occupational Therapy, 59,* 249–261. http://dx.doi.org/10.5014/ajot.59.3.249

Dunton, W. R. (1919) *Reconstruction therapy.* Philadelphia: W. B. Saunders.

Dunn, W., Brown, C., & McGuigan, A. (1994). Ecology of Human Performance: A framework for considering the effect of context. *American Journal of Occupational Therapy, 48,* 595–607. http://dx.doi.org/10.5014/ajot.48.7.595

Engeser, S. (2012). *Advances in flow research.* New York: Springer.

Fidler, G. S., & Fidler, J. W. (1978). Doing and becoming: Purposeful action and self-actualization. *American Journal of Occupational Therapy, 32,* 305–310.

Fidler, G. S., & Fidler, J. W. (1996). Lifestyle Performance Model: From profile to conceptual model. *American Journal of Occupational Therapy, 50,* 139–147.

Finn, G. (1972). The occupational therapist in prevention programs [Eleanor Clarke Slagle Lecture]. *American Journal of Occupational Therapy, 26,* 59–66.

Fleming-Castaldy, R. P. (2014). Activities, human occupation, participation, and empowerment. In J. Hinojosa & M. -L. Blount (Eds.), *The texture of life: Occupations and related activities* (4th ed., pp. 393–415). Bethesda, MD: AOTA Press.

Galheigo, S. M. (2011). What needs to be done? Occupational therapy responsibilities and challenges regarding human rights. *Australian Occupational Therapy Journal, 58*(2), 60–66.

Gupta, J., & Walloch, C. (2006). Process of infusing social justice into the practice framework: A case study. *OT Practice, 11,* CE1–CE7.

Henderson, D. K. (1957). Life and work. *Scottish Journal of Occupational Therapy, 30,* 7–10.

Humbert, T. K., Burket, A., Deveney, R., & Kennedy, K. (2011). Occupational therapy practitioners' perspectives regarding international cross-cultural work. *Australian Journal of Occupational Therapy, 58,* 300–309. http://dx.doi.org/10.1111/j.1440-1630.2010.00915.x

Jonsson, H., & Persson, D. (2006). Towards an experiential model of occupational balance: An alternative perspective on flow theory analysis. *Journal of Occupational Science, 13*(1), 62–73. http://dx.doi.org/10.1080/14427591.2006.9686571

Kidner, T. B. (1932). Occupational therapy: Its aims and developments. *Occupational Therapy and Rehabilitation, 11*(4), 233–240.

Kielhofner, G., & Burke, J. (1980). A Model of Human Occupation, Part 1: Conceptual framework and content. *American Journal of Occupational Therapy, 34,* 572–581.

Kelly, G., & McFarlane, H. (2007). Culture or cult? The mythological nature of occupational therapy. *Occupational Therapy International, 14*(4), 188–202. http://dx.doi.org/10.1002/oti.237

Kreeger, M. H. (1958). The middle ground between hospitals and home. *Hospitals, 32*(6), 52–55.

Kronenberg, F., & Pollard, N. (2006). Political dimensions of occupation and the roles of occupational therapy. *American Journal of Occupational Therapy, 60,* 617–625. http://dx.doi.org/10.5014/ajot.60.6.617

Law, M., Cooper, B., Strong, S., Stewart, D., Rigby, P., & Letts, L. (1996). The Person–Environment–Occupation model: A transactive approach to occupational performance *Canadian Journal of Occupational Therapy, 63,* 9–23. http://dx.doi.org/10.1177/000841749606300103

Letts, L., Rigby, P., & Stewart, D. (2003). *Using environments to enable occupational performance.* Thorofare, NJ: Slack.

Lohman, H., Gabriel, L., & Furlong, B. (2004). The Issue Is—The bridge from ethics to public policy: Implications for occupational therapy practitioners. *American Journal of Occupational Therapy, 58,* 109–112. http://dx.doi.org/10.5014/ajot.58.1.109

McColl, M. (2000). Spirit, occupation, and disability [Muriel Driver Lecture]. *Canadian Journal of Occupational Therapy, 67,* 217–228. http://dx.doi.org/10.1177/000841740006700403

McMurtrie, D. (1920). Occupational therapy, vocational reeducation and industrial rehabilitation. *The Modern Hospital, 14,* 326–327.

McNay, H. (1953). Nationally speaking. *American Journal of Occupational Therapy, 7,* 221–231.

Mosey, A. (1996). *Psychosocial components of occupational therapy.* New York: Raven Press.

Moyers, P. A., & Dale, L. M. (2007). *The guide to occupational therapy practice* (2nd ed.). Bethesda, MD: AOTA Press.

Muñoz, J. P., (2007). Culturally responsive caring in occupational therapy. *Occupational Therapy International, 14*(4), 256–280.

Odawara, E. (2005). Cultural competency in occupational therapy: Beyond a cross-cultural view of practice. *American Journal of Occupational Therapy, 59,* 325–334. http://dx.doi.org/10.5014/ajot.59.3.325

Pollard, N., Sakellariou, D., & Kronenberg, F. (2011). *A political practice of occupational therapy.* New York: Churchill Livingstone/Elsevier.

Reilly, M. (1962). Occupational therapy can be one of the great ideas of 20th-century medicine. *American Journal of Occupational Therapy, 16,* 1–9.

Quiroga, V. A. (1995). *Occupational therapy: The first 30 years—1900 to 1930.* Bethesda, MD: AOTA Press.

Schkade, J., & Schultz, S. (1992). Occupational adaptation: Toward a holistic approach for contemporary practice, Part 1. *American Journal of Occupational Therapy, 46,* 829–837. http://dx.doi.org/10.5014/ajot.46.9.829

Shaw, C. (1929). Occupation as an aid to recovery. *Occupational Therapy and Rehabilitation, 8*(3), 199–206.

Smith-Fess Act of 1920, Pub. L. 66–236, 41 Stat. 735.

Sommerville, J. (1954). Medical rehabilitation. *Scottish Journal of Occupational Therapy, 27,* 30–43.

United Nations. (n.d.). *The universal declaration of human rights.* Retrieved from http://www.un.org/en/documents/udhr/index.shtml

Varrier-Jones, P. J. (1941). The middle case: An unsolved problem in tuberculosis. *Lancet, 237,* 368.

Wilson, S. C. (1929, November 22). Habit training for mental cases. *Occupational Therapy and Rehabilitation, 8,* 189–198.

Wright, J., Sadlo, G., & Stew, G. (2007). Further explorations into the conundrum of flow process. *Journal of Occupational Science, 14*(3), 136–144. http://dx.doi.org/10.1080/14427591.2007.9686594

Part III.A. Temporal Contexts

CHAPTER 16

What Happened to the Time? The Relationship of Occupational Therapy to Time

SUE PEMBERTON AND DIANE COX

Introduction

The pace of life connected to our biological rhythms (tempo), our subjective perception of the past, present and future (temporality) and what we do with our time and why (time use) are central to philosophies of occupation (Farnworth and Fossey 2003). However, although Farnworth (2003) argued that these aspects of time are the essence of occupational therapy's business, she was critical that occupational therapists are not developing their expertise in this area, which would enable them to distinguish themselves from other professions. This paper seeks to explore this challenge by reviewing the presence of time conceptualisations within the professional literature and the relevance of time to occupational therapy practice.

Methodology

This paper synthesises a review of the literature encompassing the disciplines of occupational therapy, occupational science, physics, anthropology and sociology to identify different conceptualisations of *time* and their manifestations within occupational therapy paradigms. Literature searches used electronic databases, including Medline, CINAHL, AMED and Academic Search Complete, and key words, such as time, time use, tempo, temporality, temporal adaptation and time perception, from 1960 to January 2010. The review also included a hand search of academic texts.

The Past: A Historical Perspective on Time and Occupation

In the founding years of occupational therapy, Meyer (1922/1977 [see Chapter 4]) pioneered the role that oc-

cupation could play as an integrator of mind and body and the benefits it has on wellbeing. Importantly, he perceived that the value of occupation or work exists within a connected relationship with time, each having an interdependent relationship with the other. To Meyer (1922/1977), time included the concept of *rhythm*, with there being a natural balance in the body between activity and rest. He described rhythms related both to recurring cycles, such as night and day, sleep and waking, and hunger and eating, and to the need for harmony between the functions of work, play, rest and sleep. These existed within a cognitive framework that conveyed a full sense of past, present and future. Therefore, he proposed a vital correlation between time and occupation, advocating that:

> awakening to a full meaning of time as the biggest wonder and asset of our lives and the valuation of opportunity and performance as the greatest measure of time: those are the beacon lights of the philosophy of the occupation worker (Meyer 1922/1977, p642 [see Chapter 4]).

Definitions of occupational therapy have continued to reflect the role of occupation in "filling" time and the need for balance between work, rest and play (Wilcock 1998). However, Reed and Sanderson (1999) warned that many misinterpret Meyer's (1922/1977) emphasis on the balance of time as meaning that there should simply be an equal division of time between each element. Narrowing the focus onto the division of time helps to delineate forms of occupation, but loses the added temporal dimensions of harmony and rhythm between the elements of work, rest and play. Therefore, there is a need within practice to reflect on how occupational therapists both explore the division of time with their clients and understand the rhythms and tempo of their clients' lives.

This chapter was previously published in the *British Journal of Occupational Therapy, 74*, 78–85. Copyright © 2011, College of Occupational Therapists. Reprinted with permission.

The advance of industrialisation changed time from being tied to the rhythmic cycles of our natural environment to being a commodity that can be controlled (Adam 1995). Following World War II, concepts of *efficiency, task analysis* and *standardisation* spread from the factories to services and other activities (Menzies 2005). In this context, the focus changed to maximising the activity that could occur within a given period of time. This influence can be seen within practice models that emphasise the importance of task performance. Within task performance, time is a means for measuring occupation.

Reed and Sanderson (1999) provided a review of occupational therapy models, many of which illustrated the shift in western societies towards a focus on *clock time* or the measurement of time. The concept of *clock time* originates from Newton's hypothesis that it is possible to measure an interval of time that is independent of our existence, symbolised by a universal clock (Hawking 1988). This perspective complements the view of the human body as a machine, with time as a constant metronome against which the functions of human systems are measured.

Analysing the descriptors of each practice model given by Reed and Sanderson (1999) illustrates this influence. For example, the biomechanical model includes the concept of *endurance*, defined as exertion over time. Similarly, the model of cognitive disability refers to sustaining engagement in activity over time. Therefore, time acts as a means to assess and improve functional ability. Within these models, *time* is conceptualised purely as a measure of duration. In addition, a review of the indexes of occupational therapy textbooks demonstrated little reference to other concepts of time, such as tempo or temporality. Time appears to be mentioned only in the context of how the therapist manages his or her own time.

It could be argued that understanding time as a measure is sufficient for occupational therapists in their practice; however, there is knowledge across occupational science, sociology and other disciplines that is relevant to how occupational therapists use dimensions of time within their practice. This paper explores the opportunities for advancing practice through understanding other perspectives of time and its relationship to occupation.

Advancing Our Understanding of Time

Although Newton's theory of clock time complemented the mechanistic model of health and still has a significant influence over modern society's perception of time (Klein 2006), both physicists and philosophers over the past century have evolved the understanding of time. It is interesting that although Newton had abstracted time from the natural world, Einstein placed it back into the heart of our physical existence (Davies 1995). Einstein proposed that time is relative to the observer; therefore, it is experienced differently by all of us and is not the abstract phenomenon encapsulated by the universal clock (Einstein and Minkowski 1920).

Within practice, occupational therapists frequently ask clients about how time relates to a particular occupation, but what do they understand from the answers? If a client describes taking 30 minutes to complete a task, this could be interpreted as an objective measure of his or her ability or as his or her subjective perception of this experience, which may or may not correlate with the time that has passed on a clock. Ultimately, it has been suggested that, from a scientific perspective, time may not exist at all and is only an articifical mechanism that humanity has invented (Folger 2007).

Furthermore, human interest in time goes beyond the mere reckoning of time. Sociologists and anthropologists propose that time exists because we are social beings and it is defined by socially derived periodisations, often referred to as *social time* (Gell 1992). The recurrence of cultural rituals illustrates this, such as religious festivals. Often, clients describe their lives in relation to significant events that have happened to them; using the concept of *social time* would support the occupational therapist focusing on the sequence and order between life events, rather than the calendar point at which they occurred. This is supported by Levine (2006), who described the antithesis of clock time as being *event time*, which is defined by engagement in social and occupational tasks rather than the time on the clock. His research on the pace of life across different countries demonstrated that event time cultures predominate in non-industrialised societies, such as in South America where there is a slower pace of life. In these settings, time is valued as an integral part of activity and periods between tasks or 'waiting' are seen as enhancing the value of the occupation itself.

Within these philosophies, time transforms from an arbitrary measure to an aspect that defines our being, is lived through our experiences and is enacted through our social networks. Therefore, our occupations give definition and meaning to our experience of time, and both doing and time constitute aspects of being, converging occupation and time. This leads us to explore how this broader conceptualisation of time has an impact upon occupational therapy.

The Time of Occupation

As occupational therapy reasserted its heritage in occupation (Mosey 1986), the value of time and studying temporality within occupational therapy re-emerged in the literature. Kielhofner (1977) highlighted the need to reclaim and revitalise the profession, arguing that a lack of concern for temporal functioning had resulted in a substantial loss of content for the profession. Pierce (2001a) proposed that occupation had a non-repeatable nature, with a location within time, duration, pace and sequence, arguing that these temporal factors differentiated occupation from activity. This suggests that time brings definition and meaning to occupation.

The emergence of occupational science raised interest in ideas about power, diversity, situatedness and temporality (Whiteford et al 2000). The development of occupational science focused on the study of humans as occupational beings (Wilcock 2003) and led to re-engaging with broader temporal perspectives. Zemke and Clark (1996) viewed human occupation as occurring within a matrix of time and space. They reiterated Meyer's (1922/1997; see Chapter 4) position that it is important to gain a sense of how time, including temporal rhythms, influences occupation.

Despite the increasing evidence within occupational science literature of the theoretical importance of different aspects of time to occupation, occupational therapists have predominantly retained their concentration on quantifying time. The majority of studies focus on time use across different health conditions and age groups (Stanley 1995, Fricke and Unsworth 2001, Van-Leit and Crowe 2002, Krupa et al 2003, Bejerholm et al 2006, Kroksmark et al 2006, Leufstadius et al 2006, McKenna et al 2007, Stewart and Craik 2007, Lynch 2009). In these studies, time allocation is seen as a measure, which is often correlated with other factors such as life satisfaction.

Although Farnworth (2004) advocated the advantages of studying time use as a means to accessing an understanding of occupational beings, she admitted that this restricted us to the perspective of clock time. There are limitations to this approach if seeking to understand the complexities of lifestyle patterns and wellbeing (Christiansen and Matuska 2006). It has been suggested that occupational therapists need to enhance their understanding of the complexity of daily patterns of occupation and health (Erlandsson

et al 2004) or to combine time use studies with a number of other factors, such as perceived time pressure, life stress, physical and mental wellbeing, and life cycles (Zuzanek 1998). The challenge remains as to how to capture the meaning of time to the individual and his or her rhythm of life in a way that enables occupational therapists to understand time as a dimension of being, not just as a measure for the content of existence.

The Present: Finding Time in Occupational Therapy Practice

Although there is evidence within the occupational science literature of the importance of temporal conditions to the conceptualising of occupation, the absence of time within models of practice and educational texts raises the question of how this knowledge is influencing occupational therapists. This section discusses in more detail how different approaches to time as defined within the literature apply to clinical practice.

Occupation as a Consumer of Time

Wilcock (1998) stated that occupation is a natural user of time. In understanding how and why people use time, occupational therapists have an insight into different sociocultural and health issues. This transcends the individual's ability to perform a task and situates it within his or her reality. The economic metaphors of "spending time" and "saving time" equate time with being another resource or commodity and that we make consumer choices about how to distribute it (Peloquin 1991). However, our time choices are increasingly influenced by assimilating media-promoted cultural values.

Although there is consistency across western nations in the distribution of time between obligatory (such as work and self-care) and discretionary (such as leisure) tasks (Christiansen and Baum 1997), this gives little understanding of the intensity or value of this time allocation, or of the impact that this has upon our health (Christiansen 1996). Primeau (1995) warned that there is also danger in ascribing labels to forms of time consumption, as in postindustrial societies, for example, leisure activities have become as demanding as work. This demonstrates the increasing pressure within industrialised societies to maximise our occupational consumption of time, disrupting the balance and rhythm between elements of work, rest and play. The expectation that time is used constructively and not "wasted" within clock time societies (Levine

2006) can lead to negative cultural assumptions about rest and play. Therefore, occupational therapists need to be aware of how they and others perceive the value of these elements. For example, they cannot presume that activities that an individual defines as leisure are free of the elements of stress and demand, which are often associated with work tasks.

The ways in which people consume time will also be altered by factors such as gender (Zuzanek and Mannell 1993, Daly 2002), age (Szmigin and Carrigan 2001, McKenna et al 2007), illness or disability (Winkler et al 2005, Bejerholm et al 2006) and the enviroment (Stewart and Craik 2007). This may also change who has control over decisions regarding time use. Therefore, it is important that an occupational therapy assessment takes full account of how individuals allocate their time and their reasoning for this, being cognisant of any changes that have occurred and the influences upon these changes. It is not simply how time is divided but also the beliefs and judgements that inflence this, and the harmony or disharmony that this creates. This knowledge can be used to explore the opportunities to adjust time allocations so that they can support the individual's needs most effectively, such as increasing the time devoted to relaxation or pleasure.

Time as a Context for Occupation

To have purpose, an activity must have a temporal location. If people are given the skills to perform a task, but without a place for it either within their routines or as a priority for their time, it is less likely to be integrated into their daily life. Some models have incorporated temporal factors as an element of the context or environment in which the occupation takes place (Pierce 2001b, Dunn et al 2003, McHugh Pendleton and Schultz-Krohn 2006). However, even though temporal factors are recognised, these models still take the approach of encapsulating time as a measure. For example, in the Ecology of Human Performance Model (Dunn et al 2003), the temporal features of a person that are included are chronological age, development stage, life cycle and health status, which still measure the individual against a linear progression of time. It is not clear how this integrates with the person's own view of his or her time and its lived experience.

Velde and Fidler (2002) considered time within a variety of dimensions, with a framework that incorporated both inner models of time, including biological rhythms and self-perception, and external influences, such as cultural understanding and expectations. These

can be synthesised to enhance the meaning of the occupation to the individual.

It is important, however, to locate the occupation within both the internal and the external temporal context of the individual. This can be illustrated by, for example, considering the time of day people may choose to get dressed. If their biological rhythms mean that they wake late and take time to orientate themselves to the day, they may choose to dress later. Alternatively, if their social expectation is to be dressed and eat breakfast as part of a social group, it may be more temporally appropriate to dress early. The occupational therapist must consider both the requirements of the task and how it will need to adjust to fit its desired temporal location.

The Rhythm of Life

Human beings live to the tempo of internal biological clocks or cellular oscillating systems, part of our circadian rhythms (Christiansen and Baum 1997). These are believed to play an important role in regulating biological functions, such as blood pressure, body temperature, hormone cycles, and patterns of activity and rest. They naturally run on a 25-hour cycle, so they are kept synchronous with our environment through physical and social triggers (zeitgebers), such as light, heat, social interaction and patterns of daily activity. Therefore, occupation has an influence on our physiological sense of time, just as disturbances to our biological clocks can affect our ability to perform occupations, for example when experiencing jet lag.

Walker (2001) explored the impact that shift work has upon biological rhythms, such as increasing fatigue and disrupted sleep patterns, and the occupational strategies that shift workers use to adapt to this effect. This highlights the need to be cognisant of disruptive factors and to address these within routines, such as strategies for sleeping, eating properly and maintaining relationships. Living within a different time frame to others may also have an emotional impact, such as feelings of guilt (Gallew and Mu 2004), and the occupational therapist needs to understand how this affects both individuals' views of themselves and their relationships to others.

Occupatiotemporality

Zemke and Clark (1996) introduced the concept of *occupatiotemporality,* in which occupation shapes our experience of time. This encapsulates the lived experience of time through occupation, so we may experience time going slowly when we are waiting for an activity to start or a sense of timelessness while we are fully absorbed in a task, which Csikzentmihalyi (1988) described as flow. When Wright et al (2007) described the experience of flow during occupation for seven participants, they proposed that altering our time experience through flow could produce a positive psychological state and protect wellbeing. However, Menzies (2005) urged caution in her reflections on the impact that engrossment in some activities, particularly when accessing the virtual world, can have upon our experience of time:

> Something human has been lost in the coming-to-be of an advanced technology . . . a sense of time . . . Reflection on one's existence. An ability to really exist and have complex relationships with others (p116).

However, the loss of time may be preferable to the experience of boredom. Farnworth (1998) described how the use of the term "boredom" had become endemic in western industrialised nations. She proposed that boredom could be a consequence of the changing pace and imbalance of occupations within this technological age. This raises ethical considerations for occupational therapists because some people seek to escape boredom and the passing of time itself through engagement in the virtual worlds available through computer technology. Occupational therapists need to balance the increasing focus on a constant state of occupation or "filling time" and Meyer's (1922/1977) concept of balance and harmony.

Larson and Zemke (2003) further developed the concept of occupatiotemporality to incorporate a broader spectrum of temporal aspects of occupation, including its rhythm, tempo, synchronisation, duration and sequence and whether it is enfolded with other occupations. Larson (2004) used this to construct the Dynamic Occupation in Time Model to address the issues caused by six types of temporal variation that people can experience. These include variations between perceived time and clock time, that is, time feels protracted or compressed, or is in synchrony with the clock, or experiences of the movement of time, that is, feeling outside time (flow), the space between occupations (interstitial time) or where time is disrupted (temporal rupture). Although Larson and von Eye (2010) have used the model to research students' experiences of temporality, this remains an area for further research across the

health spectrum, both as a consequence of disability and as a precursor to ill-health.

These dynamic temporal factors need consideration when assisting an individual to achieve mastery in their occupations and are a legitimate focus for occupational therapists (Zemke 2004). For example, adjusting the pace or duration of an activity may enable someone with limited function to experience success. Conversely, there may be increased anxiety if someone perceives a high level of time pressure with insufficient time to complete all their intended tasks. Experiencing a life-changing event, such as bereavement, can disrupt someone's synchronicity with time and therefore needs considering within the process of adaptation and re-establishing a relationship with events in the present.

Temporal Dysfunction

Hagedorn (2001) outlined forms of occupational dysfunction, arising because of problems related to time, that are incorporated within Person-Environment Occupation Performance models. These include tasks taking longer to perform, difficulty with sequencing tasks within time and using time effectively. Temporal dysfunction can arise from both physical and psychosocial factors (Mosey 1986) and cause problems in the organisation of daily life (Kielhofner 1977). Nygård and Johansson (2001) examined how dementia can cause temporal problems, in this case demonstrating changes in temporal relationships and coherence, supporting the need to consider these within occupational therapy interventions.

Temporal Adaptation

Kielhofner (1977) proposed a perspective on temporal adaptation as a conceptual framework across all areas of occupational therapy practice, constructed around seven propositions. Four of the propositions relate to external influences on temporal consciousness, including culture, socialisation during development, social roles, and the balance of life spaces for self-maintenance, work and play. Internal factors then mediate these, including internal values, interests and goals, and habits, which organise our behaviours within time. He finally related temporal dysfunction as an aspect of mental illness or consequence of disability. This focused on the alteration to our time experience because of illness. However, there is still the question of whether our relationship with time can precipitate changes in our health.

Although Kielhofner's (1977) framework of temporal adaptation was explored in the context of psychiatric patients, demonstrating how time distortions can affect people's ability to cope and adjust to their environment (Neville 1980), this is not developed further within the literature. Kielhofner (1977) may have influenced this loss of focus by assimilating his perspective on time into the Model of Human Occupation (Kielhofner 1980). Farnworth (2003) expressed concern that although this evolution of the theory continued to highlight the importance of time within the context of habits and routines, by diffusing temporality within a comprehensive occupational paradigm the aspects of time become lost and less clearly defined.

Alternatively, Mosey (1986) used the construct of temporal adaptation to focus on the ability that a person has to organise his or her time to meet the responsibilities and enjoy the pleasures of social roles. She placed this within our experience of temporality, as our historical past acts as a source for planning future actions. Our awareness of the boundaries of our own existence influences this throughout our lifetime. Therefore, in our youth, time seems eternal, whilst as we grow through to our old age, time becomes scarce and our time perception more focused on the present. Mosey (1986) suggested that it was important within occupational therapy intervention to identify the client's current state of temporal adaptation, applying planning skills to gain control over future time, using future accomplishment goals, establishing a schedule to accommodate demands and pleasure, and following through implementation, so that adjustments are made to ensure maintenance.

In addition to the individual's experiences of time, temporal coordination is an important element in the creation and maintenance of social groups, such as the family. Larson and Zemke (2003) described that 'external social structuring of time, internalised biological rhythms and learned expectancies regiment temporality and synchrony of occupation' (p81). Consequently, it is important that occupational therapists investigate how temporal factors influence individuals, their social groups, and the broader culture in which they exist. For example, technology is enabling people to communicate with their social networks 24 hours a day, though the internet or mobile communication. This may increase accessibility to social contact for many people with health problems or disabilities, but may make it increasingly difficult to segregate time into different occupations, because activities can run concurrently and can occur across a broader time frame.

There is, therefore, current theory regarding the connected relationship between time and occupation, particularly related to how people allocate time to different types of occupation, the temporal demands of the occupation and the disruptions that can occur within our experience of temporality. Synthesising these dimensions can enhance the interventions of occupational therapists through increasing the quality and meaning of occupations (Persson and Erlandson 2002). However, although there are theoretical discussions, particularly within occupational science, there is limited evidence of the actual application of these theories to shaping occupational therapy practice, as championed by Farnworth (2003). Occupational therapists need to consider how a particular problem, such as pain, fatigue or depression, affects the client's relationship to not only time use but also experiences of tempo and temporality.

Knowing how people consume time provides us with only limited insight into the balance and rhythm of life. Just as the musical notes on a page require a tempo to transform them into music, occupations reveal their lived experience through understanding the rhythm of our life. Although Meyer (1922/1977) conceptualised that *doing* required *balance, rhythm* and *time awareness* to enable wellbeing, occupational therapy still needs to evolve and embrace a more complex temporal understanding to achieve this harmony.

The Future: Time Changes

There are transformations occurring within humanity's relationship with time that will have implications for the possible role of occupational therapists, strengthening the need to master this domain. The last section of this article discusses the future challenges for the profession.

Globalisation of Clock Time

Human beings have constantly sought to track time, with the invention of the clock allowing humanity to bring order to daily life (Aveni 1989). However, the clock now drives human endeavour rather than acting as a means to measure it. As technology has improved, our ties to the rhythms of the natural world have diminished (Clark 1997). For example, electrical light means we no longer require daylight to participate in many activities. There are consequences to humanity's pursuit of increased productivity and efficiency. Mirroring Levine's (2006) differentiation of event time and clock time cultures, Yalmambirra (2000) described his experience of *Koori time* and *white time*. The traditional conceptualisation of time in his aboriginal tribe was imbued with the features of the natural world and the traditions and events of his people, but was stopped by the invasive force of the regulated time of clocks. As the world shrinks through global communication systems and travel, the rule of clock time is spreading around the globe (Adam 1995).

Occupational therapy needs to consider how the increasing dominance of clock time and loss of event time may change practice. There is a danger that the value and meaning of occupations change as time becomes compressed and people operate within an environment in which the social elements of occupation are desynchronised in an increasingly virtual world.

Pace of Life

Since the Industrial Revolution, there has been an unprecedented speeding up of the pace of life (Robinson and Godbey 1997). People feel more rushed, with more intensity to their participation in all areas of life, including work, home maintenance and leisure time. The computer is increasingly becoming the new time-ordering device, changing our relationship to time, because we are always accessible, can hold conversations by email which are disjointed in time, and lose connections to the natural rhythms of night and day (Menzies 2005). We are experiencing increasing time pressure (Larson and Zemke 2003) as every moment of the day fills with constant activity. In this way, human beings are becoming closer to the ideal of the machine, constantly in motion and abstracted from the rhythms of nature (Persson and Erlandsson 2002). The growing dominance of clock time is leading people away from the concept of rhythm and harmony, the need for balance between work, rest and play.

There is a risk that the role of the occupational therapist becomes focused on enabling clients to keep up with the runaway pace of society. Alternatively, this presents an opportunity to shift the focus of occupational therapy from increasing function and efficiency, virtues of the machine and clock time, to introducing new occupational strategies that seek to slow the pace of life and focus on the harmony of our body's natural rhythms. As suggested by Clark (1997) and Persson and Erklandsson (2002) some years ago, occupational therapists have a key role in lifestyle redesign interventions and this remains an area for further development in practice.

A Time for Occupational Therapy

Occupational therapy needs to be proactive in meeting the challenges of time in our modern and global society

(Whiteford 2001). There is a need for research on temporal aspects of health (Larson 2004, Christiansen and Matuska 2006) to help us to understand more about how disruptions to time use, tempo and temporality can influence the development of health problems, as well as the changes that illness and disability can cause within temporal experiences. There is also the need to research how concepts of time, including addressing the pace of life or tempo, can be applied within the process of recovery or adaptation.

The connected relationship between occupation and time also highlights a role for occupational therapy within health promotion. As lifestyle factors become increasingly recognised in the understanding of health (Matuska and Christiansen 2008), occupational therapy must advocate the need to ensure balance, reduce the pace of activity and reestablish natural rhythms as a means to maintaining health.

Conclusion

The founders of occupational therapy recognised the connectivity between doing, being, rhythm and balance. Although theorists have explored the links between occupation and time, there is still little evidence that occupational therapy has heeded Farnworth's concerns (Farnworth 2003) and embraced temporal perspectives within practice. There remains a need to build upon the growing research evidence into how our individual relationship to time affects our health, the consequences of disability and illness on temporal experiences, and the role that temporal adaptation can play in recovery. There is a cultural need to understand more about the changing nature of occupation and time, as life speeds up and humanity increasingly races to the beat of the clock. Ironically, there is also the challenge of achieving this within a health care ethos that increasingly seeks to emulate the machine by emphasising increased outcomes, efficiency and productivity (Department of Health 2005). As occupational therapists themselves are asked to work to the speed of the clock, is it possible to embrace time within the profession before our time runs out?

Acknowledgements

We would like to thank Dr Gonzalo Araoz, Dr Carol Marrow, Leeds Partnerships NHS Foundation Trust and the University of Cumbria for supporting this research.

Conflict of interest: None declared.

Key Findings

- There is a connected relationship between time and occupation.
- Occupational therapists need to consider temporal factors, such as time use, tempo and temporality, in order to maximise the benefits of occupation.
- This is an important domain for further research and health promotion.

What the Study Has Added

The review demonstrates that time is an important consideration for occupational therapists and highlights the changing nature of time and occupation, which merits future investigation.

References

Adam B (1995) *Timewatch: the social analysis of time.* Cambridge: Polity Press.

Aveni A (1989) *Empires of time: calendars, clocks and cultures.* New York: Basic Books.

Bejerholm U, Hansson L, Eklund M (2006) Profiles of occupational engagement in people with schizophrenia (POES): the development of a new instrument based on time-use diaries. *British Journal of Occupational Therapy, 69(2),* 58–68.

Christiansen C (1996) Three perspectives on balance in occupation. In: R Zemke, F Clark, eds. *Occupational science: the evolving discipline.* Philadelphia: FA Davis, 431–51.

Christiansen C, Baum C (1997) *Occupational therapy—enabling function and well-being.* Thorofare, NJ: Slack.

Christiansen C, Matuska K (2006) Lifestyle balance: a review of concepts and research. *Journal of Occupational Science, 13(1),* 49–61.

Clark F (1997) Reflections on the human as an occupational being: biological need, tempo and temporality. *Journal of Occupational Science: Australia, 4(3),* 86–92.

Csikzentmihalyi M (1988) The flow of experience and its significance for human psychology. In: M Csikzentmihalyi, I Csikzentmihalyi, eds. *Optimal experience: psychological studies of flow in consciousness.* Cambridge: Cambridge University Press, 15–35.

Daly K (2002) Time, gender, and the negotiation of family schedules. *Symbolic Interaction, 25(3),* 323–42.

Davies P (1995) *About time.* London: Viking.

Department of Health (2005) *Health output and productivity: accounting for quality change.* London: DH.

Dunn W, Brown C, Youngstom M (2003) Ecological Model of Occupation. In: P Kramer, J Hinojosa, C Brasic Royeen. *Perspectives in human occupation: participation in*

life. Baltimore, MD: Lippincott Williams and Wilkins, 222–63.

Einstein A, Minkowski H (1920) *The principle of relativity.* (Saha and Bose, Trans.) Calcutta: University of Calcutta.

Erlandsson LK, Rognvaldsson T, Eklund M (2004) Recognition of similarities: a methodological approach to analysing and characterising patterns of daily occupations. *Journal of Occupational Science, 11(1),* 3–13.

Farnworth L (1998) Doing, being, and boredom. *Journal of Occupational Science, 5(3),* 140–46.

Farnworth L (2003) Time use, tempo and temporality: occupational therapy's core business or someone else's business? *Australian Occupational Therapy Journal, 50(3),* 116–26.

Farnworth L (2004) Time use and disability. In: M Molineux, ed. *Occupation for occupational therapists.* Oxford: Blackwell Publishing, 46–65.

Farnworth L, Fossey E (2003) Occupational terminology interactive dialogue: explaining the concepts of time use, tempo and temporality. *Journal of Occupational Science, 10(3),* 150–53.

Folger T (2007) In no time. *Discover, 28,* 78–83.

Fricke J, Unsworth C (2001) Time use and the importance of instrumental activities of daily living. *Australian Occupational Therapy Journal, 48(3),* 118–31.

Gallew H, Mu K (2004) An occupational look at temporal adaptation: night shift nurses. *Journal of Occupational Science, 11(1),* 23–30.

Gell A (1992) *The anthropology of time.* Oxford: Berg.

Hagedorn R (2001) *Foundations for practice in occupational therapy.* 3rd ed. London: Churchill Livingstone.

Hawking S (1988) *A brief history of time.* New York: Bantham.

Kielhofner G (1977) Temporal adaptation: a conceptual framework for occupational therapy. *American Journal of Occupational Therapy, 31(4),* 235–42.

Kielhofner G (1980) A Model of Human Occupation, Part 2. Ontogenesis from the perspective of temporal adaptation. *American Journal of Occupational Therapy, 34(10),* 657–64. http://dx.doi.org/10.5014/ajot.34.10.657

Klein S (2006) *Time: a user's guide.* London: Penguin.

Kroksmark U, Nordell K, Bendixen H, Magnus E, Jakobson K, Alsaker S (2006) Time geographic method: application to studying occupation in different contexts. *Journal of Occupational Science, 13(1),* 11–16.

Krupa T, McLean H, Eastabrook S, Bonham A, Baksh L (2003) Daily time use as a measure of community adjustment by person served by assertive community treatment teams. *American Journal of Occupational Therapy, 57(5),* 558–65. http://dx.doi.org/10.5014/ajot.57.5.558

Larson E (2004) The time of our lives: the experience of temporality in occupation. *Canadian Journal of Occupaitonal Therapy, 71(1),* 24–35.

Larson E, von Eye A (2010) Beyond flow: temporality and participation in everyday activities. *American Journal of Occupational Therapy, 64(1),* 152–163. http://dx.doi.org/10.5014/ajot.64.1.152

Larson E, Zemke R (2003) Shaping the temporal patterns of our lives: the social co-ordination of activity. *Journal of Occupational Science, 10(2),* 80–89.

Leufstadius C, Erlandsson L, Eklund M (2006) Time use and daily activities in people with persistent mental illness. *Occupational Therapy International, 13(3),* 123–41.

Levine R (2006) *A geography of time: the temporal misadventure of a social psychologist.* Oxford: Oneworld.

Lynch H (2009) Patterns of activity of Irish children aged five years to eight years living in Ireland today. *Journal of Occupational Science, 16(1),* 44–49.

Matuska K, Christiansen C (2008) A proposed model of lifestyle balance. *Journal of Occupational Science, 15(1),* 9–19. Reprinted as Chapter 21.

McHugh Pendleton H, Schultz-Krohn W (2006) *Pedretti's occupational therapy: practice skills for physical dysfunction.* 6th ed. St Louis, MO: Mosby Elsevier.

McKenna K, Broome K, Liddle J (2007) What older people do: time use and exploring the link between role participation and life satisfaction in people aged 65 years and older. *Australian Occupational Therapy Journal, 54(4),* 273–84.

Menzies H (2005) *No time: stress and the crisis of modern life.* Vancouver: Douglas and McIntyre.

Meyer A (1922) The philosophy of occupational therapy. *Archives of Occupational Therapy, 1,* 1–10. Reprinted in: *American Journal of Occupational Therapy* (1977), *31(10),* 639–42. Reprinted as Chapter 4.

Mosey AC (1986) *Psychosocial components of occupational therapy.* Philadelphia: Lippincott Williams and Wilkins.

Neville A (1980) Temporal adaptation: application with short-term psychiatric patients. *American Journal of Occupational Therapy, 34(5),* 328–31.

Nygård L, Johansson M (2001) The experience and management of temporality in five cases of dementia. *Scandinavian Journal of Occupational Therapy, 8(2),* 85–95.

Peloquin S (1991) Time as commodity: reflections and implications. *American Journal of Occupational Therapy, 45(2),* 147–54. http://dx.doi.org/10.5014/ajot.45.2.147

Persson D, Erklandsson LK (2002) Time to reevaluate the machine society: post-industrial ethics from an occupational perspective. *Journal of Occupational Science, 9(2),* 93–99.

Pierce D (2001a) Untangling occupation and activity. *American Journal of Occupational Therapy, 55(2),* 138–46. http://dx.doi.org/10.5014/ajot.55.2.138

Pierce D (2001b) Occupation by design: dimensions, therapeutic power and creative process. *American Journal of Occupational Therapy, 55(3),* 249–59. http://dx.doi.org/10.5014/ajot.55.3.249

Primeau L (1995) Work and leisure: transcending the dichotomy. *American Journal of Occupational Therapy, 50(7),* 569–77. http://dx.doi.org/10.5014/ajot.50.7.569

Reed R, Sanderson S (1999) *Concepts of occupational therapy.* 4th ed. Baltimore: Lippincott Williams and Wilkins.

Robinson J, Godbey G (1997) *Time for life: the surprising ways Americans use their time.* 2nd ed. Pennsylvania: Pennysylvania University Press.

Stanley M (1995) An investigation into the relationship between engagement in valued occupations and life satisfaction for elderly South Australians. *Journal of Occupational Science, 2(3),* 100–14.

Stewart P, Craik C (2007) Occupation, mental illness and medium security: exploring time-use in forensic regional secure units. *British Journal of Occupational Therapy, 70(10),* 416–25.

Szmigin I, Carrigan M (2001) Time, consumption and the older consumer: an interpretive study of the cognitively young. *Psychology and Marketing, 18(10),* 1091–116.

VanLeit B, Crowe T (2002) Outcomes of an occupational therapy program for mothers of children with disabilities: impact on satisfaction with time use and occupational performance. *American Journal of Occupational Therapy, 56(4),* 402–10. http://dx.doi.org/10.5014/ajot.56.4.402

Velde B, Fidler G (2002) *Lifestyle performance—a model for engaging the power of occupation.* Thorofare, NJ: Slack.

Walker C (2001) Occupational adatation in action: shift workers and their strategies. *Journal of Occupational Science, 8(1),* 17–24.

Whiteford G (2001) The occupational agenda of the future. *Journal of Occupational Science, 8(1),* 13–16.

Whiteford G, Townsend E, Hocking C (2000) Reflections on a renaissance of occupation. *Canadian Journal of Occupational Therapy, 67(1),* 61–69.

Wilcock A (1998) *An occupational perspective of health.* Thorofare, NJ: Slack.

Wilcock A (2003) Occupational science: the study of humans as occupational beings. In: P Kramer, J Hinojosa,

C Brasic Royeen, eds. *Perspectives in human occupation: participation in life.* Baltimore, MD: Lippincott Williams and Wilkins, 156–80.

Winkler D, Unsworth C, Sloan S (2005) Time use following a severe traumatic brain injury. *Journal of Occupational Science, 12(2),* 69–81.

Wright JJ, Sadio G, Stew G (2007) Further explorations into the conundrum of flow processes. *Journal of Occupational Science, 14(3),* 136–44.

Yalmambirra (2000) Black time . . . white time: my time . . . your time. *Journal of Occupational Science, 7(3),* 133–37.

Zemke R (2004) Time, space, and the kaleidoscopes of occupation. *American Journal of Occupational Therapy, 58(6),* 608–20. http://dx.doi.org/10.5014/ajot.58.6.608

Zemke R, Clark F, eds (1996) *Occupational science: the evolving discipline.* Philadelphia: FA Davis.

Zuzanek J (1998) Time use, time pressure, personal stress, mental health, and life satisfaction from a life cycle perspective. *Journal of Occupational Science, 5(1),* 26–39.

Zuzanek J, Mannell R (1993) Gender variations in the weekly rhythms of daily behaviour and experiences. *Journal of Occupational Science: Australia, 1(1),* 25–37.

CHAPTER 17

Flow and Occupation: A Review of the Literature

HEATHER EMERSON

For the past 75 years occupational therapists have claimed an interest in occupation and its impact on human beings (Weimer, 1979). We have identified conditions of occupational engagement that seem to influence the quality and outcome of these experiences. Only during the past 15 years, however, have we begun to focus our research on the subjective experiences of people engaged in occupation in their natural settings (Kielhofner, 1981; Kremer, Nelson, & Duncombe, 1984; Johnson & Yerxa, 1989). The literature on flow theory by Csikszentmihalyi has also been addressing the subjective experiences of persons engaged in occupation. Studies on flow can provide occupational therapy and occupational science with data on subjective occupational experience and the personal and activity properties that relate to it. In addition, this literature offers theoretical and methodological considerations for future research on occupation. The purpose of this paper is to introduce the construct of flow to occupational therapists who may not be familiar with this body of literature and to offer some principles for the application of this knowledge to clinical practice.

Occupation

Occupation refers to "the active or 'doing' process of a person engaged in goal-directed, intrinsically gratifying, and culturally appropriate activity" (Evans, 1987, p. 627). Occupational therapists have long recognized that occupation has a role in integrating the mind and body (Breines, 1984; Cynkin & Robinson, 1999), maintaining psychic order (Meyer, 1922/1982; see Chapter 4), motivating the individual (Kielhofner, 1992; Meyer, 1922/1982), and promoting a sense of

worth and competence (Fidler & Fidler, 1978); (Yerxa, 1980). Other benefits of occupational engagement identified in the literature include its ability to influence time perception (Meyer, 1922/1982; see Chapter 4), (Yerxa et al., 1990); reconnect the individual with his or her natural environment (Yerxa, 1980); and focus attention on a clear goal and away from one's self or one's worries (Friedland, 1988; Levine, 1987 [see Chapter 22]).

What is it about occupation or activity that promotes feelings of competence and well-being? The literature suggests that the answer pertains to the interplay between an individual and an activity, yet the nature of this relationship is not clearly understood (Breines, 1984; Meyer, 1922/1982; see Chapter 4).

An American Occupational Therapy Association Position Paper (1993) on purposeful activity discussed properties of activities that influence one's sense of competence and well-being. Beneficial aspects of activity that were recognized include their adaptability in that they can be graded to match the individual's abilities, structured to direct attention toward a goal rather than to the process, and altered to provide direct objective feedback on performance.

Breines (1984) viewed the process of bringing a person's attention beyond choice into "automaticity," where actions are elicited without conscious awareness, as a benefit of occupation. Others have claimed that the success of outcomes is an important aspect of occupation (Baum, 1985; Fidler & Fidler, 1978). Yerxa (1980) recognized the importance of choice and self-initiation. Fundamental to occupational therapy's philosophy are the beliefs that humans have an innate need to explore and master the environment, and that an important reward of occupation is in the process of doing (Kielhofner, 1992; Reilly, 1960).

These reflections can be found in the philosophical writings of occupational therapy. They are grounded in the opinions, experience, and observations of occupational therapists. Until recently, occupational therapists have focused their research on properties and responses to activity identified by clinicians. However, during the past 15 years occupational therapists have begun to study the subjective experiences of individuals while they are engaged in activity (Kielhofner, 1981; Kremer, Nelson, & Duncombe, 1984; Johnson & Yerxa, 1989; Laliberte, 1993; Merrill, 1985; Park, 1995; Steinmetz, 1995). They have begun to look outside the clinic at how people experience occupation in their daily lives (Kielhofner, 1981, 1982). Yerxa and colleagues reflected this focus when they wrote "To fully understand occupation it is necessary to comprehend the experience of engagement in it" (1990, p. 9). The shift toward an appreciation for subjective occupational experiences has been influenced by many factors. These factors include increased knowledge of qualitative research methods, increased interest in occupational science, and the recognition that the profession has much to learn from other disciplines besides medicine (Yerxa et al., 1990).

Subjective Occupational Experience

One source from which occupational therapists can learn about the subjective experience of activity and its measurement is the literature on flow by Csikszentmihalyi and his colleagues (Carlson & Clark, 1991). Csikszentmihalyi (1990, 1992) has spent three decades examining the question "What makes some action patterns worth pursuing for their own sake, even without any rational compensation?" He examined literature on intrinsic motivation by such authors as Hebb, Maslow, McClelland, Harlow, Bem, and DeCharms (Csikszentmihalyi, 1975). Through interviews, diaries, time logs, questionnaires, ethnography, and a technique he devised called "experience sampling method" (ESM), he collected data about the subjective experience of people engaged in activities and occupations in their natural settings during their everyday lives (Csikszentmihalyi, 1975). The ESM uses beeper technology to randomly signal participants several times a day to prompt them to fill out a form describing their most recent activity, its context, and their subjective experience at the time. Through these studies he developed a theory about a source of intrinsic motivation called "flow." This theory articulates and explores many beliefs about occupation that are fundamental to the philosophy of occupational therapy.

Flow

Flow is a subjective psychological state that occurs when one is totally involved in an activity (Csikszentmihalyi, 1975). It is "the state in which people are so involved in an activity that nothing else seems to matter; the experience itself is so enjoyable that people will do it even at great cost, for the sheer sake of doing it" (1990, p. 4).

The flow experience is characterized by the ability to concentrate on the activity, a sense of control over one's actions, and a clear sense of purpose or goals (Csikszentmihalyi, 1975, 1988a). During flow there is a removal from awareness of one's worries, a loss of self-consciousness, and a distorted sense of time (Csikszentmihalyi, 1990). Other conditions connected with flow include a choice of participation, a sense that the outcome of the activity is under one's control and is meaningful, immediate clear feedback, a merging of awareness with activity, and a sense that the activity is rewarding in and of itself (Csikszentmihalyi, 1975, 1990).

When a person is in flow, a positive affective state, high motivation, high cognitive efficiency, and high activation are experienced. This activation involves arousal, alertness, energy, and interest (Csikszentmihalyi & Larson, 1987; Csikszentmihalyi & Mei-Ha Wong, 1991). Flow involves an active use of skills which causes "enjoyment" and growth, in contrast to the more passive construct of "pleasure," which does not require effort and is based on genetically programmed drives for survival of the species, such as eating and sexual behavior (Massimini, Csikszentmihalyi, & Delle Fave, 1988).

Csikszentmihalyi believed that the unfocused mind is in a state of chaos, "entropy," and that psychic order, "negentropy," is achieved by learning to control consciousness through the focusing of one's energy, attention, and skills on the goals offered through engagement in challenging activities (Csikszentmihalyi, 1988b). Flow is sometimes called "optimal experience" or "autotelic enjoyment" and is considered by some to be the highest level of well-being (Csikszentmihalyi & Mel-Ha Wong, 1991).

The Flow Channel

A match between an individual's perceptions of his or her skills and of the environmental demands has been identified as a prerequisite to this type of optimal experience (Csikszentmihalyi, 1975, 1988b, 1988c; Massimini et al., 1988). Educators on flow believe that to sustain a combination of interest, enjoyment, and motivation, the dimensions of perceived skill and perceived challenge must be matched and considered above average for that individual (Csikszentmihalyi, 1988b). This balance between high skills and high challenges is referred to as "the flow channel" (Csikszentmihalyi & Csikszentmihalyi, 1988, p. 261).

In models of flow, this optimal state is contrasted with states of anxiety, boredom, and apathy (Csikszentmihalyi, 1975; Massimini, Csikszentmihalyi, & Carli, 1987). When environmental demands are perceived by the individual as exceeding his or her capacity, anxiety states are apt to occur (Csikszentmihalyi & Larson, 1984). When the demands of the environment do not tax the individual's perceived skills, boredom or apathy may occur (Csikszentmihalyi & Larson, 1984; Massimini et al., 1987). Csikszentmihalyi and Larson (1984) claim that, to remain in the flow channel with an activity, the person must believe that the demands are increasing as his or her skills improve.

ESM studies have measured time in flow using the high skill/high challenge criterion. There is variance in the amount of time spent in flow from person to person. Some studies use the four-channel model (anxiety, apathy, flow, and boredom) while others use eight or 16 channels. Using the four-channel model, LeFevre studied 107 adults who volunteered from five Chicago companies (1988). On average, they spent 33 percent of work time in flow, 34 percent in apathy; while leisure time was spent 19 percent in flow channel, and 42 percent in apathy (LeFevre, 1988). LeFevre found that managers had more flow at work than did blue collar workers, but that the opposite was true of leisure time. Wells' (1988) four-channel study of working mothers found that time in flow ranged from 4 to 40 percent and averaged 23 percent. Occupational therapy practitioners in physical rehabilitation settings spent about 23 percent of their work time in flow, and a surprising 44 percent of work time in the anxiety channel of this model (Jacobs, 1994).

An eight-channel model has also been used in some ESM studies (Csikszentmihalyi & Mei-Ha Wong, 1991). In addition to the states of flow, boredom, apathy, and anxiety, these studies measured time in the intermediate states of arousal, control, relaxation, and worry (Massimini, Carli, & Cikszentmihalyi, 1988). Because a person's time is divided among eight, rather than four channels, the proportion of time in each channel is expected to be less than on studies using four-channel

models. Studies using this model found that adolescents in Milan spent an average of 19 percent of their time in flow, while adolescents in Chicago spent 16 percent of their time in flow (Carli, Delle Fave, & Massimini, 1988; Massimini et al., 1988).

Flow Activities

Activities that bring about flow are called "autotelic activities" after the Latin *auto* meaning *self* and *teleos* meaning *goals* (Csikszentmihalyi, 1975). Csikszentmihalyi said of autotelic activities, "the most basic requirement is to provide a clear set of challenges" and the most basic challenge is that of "the unknown, which leads to discovery, exploration, and problem-solving" (1975, p. 30). Although these activities differ from person to person, they have some properties in common (Csikszentmihalyi, 1975, 1988b, 1990). They provide opportunities for action that match the person's skills. There are clear goals with adequate means for reaching them. Clear consistent feedback on performance is provided. The stimulus field is limited to decrease distraction. The activity is viewed by the person as having surmountable goals and outcomes that he or she can influence.

Often autotelic activities involve competition, rules, and risks. These activities are not necessarily virtuous or instrumental (Csikszentmihalyi & Larson, 1984). A youth who lacks prosocial skills may find flow in antisocial activities such as stealing. Sometimes flow activities are addictive in that they are so intriguing or appealing that the individual may neglect or fail to find enjoyment in other aspects of life (Csikszentmihalyi, 1975).

Autotelic activities occur in leisure, self-care, and work contexts. Examples include playing chess, rock climbing, ocean cruising, yoga, painting, performing surgery, playing with one's child, and doing sports (Csikszentmihalyi, 1975, 1988b, 1990; Jackson, 1994).

Flow Experience Across Cultures

The potential for flow is felt to be both universal and individualized. It exists across a variety of cultures, ages, and social classes (Carlson & Clark, 1991; Csikszentmihalyi & Larson, 1984; Massimini et al., 1988). Sato (1988) wrote about a collective of "group flow" experienced by Japanese youths on motorcycle runs. Delle Fave and Massimini (1988) studied flow in alpine villages in northern Italy and found that, while members of the traditional culture experienced flow through farm work, the modern generation experienced flow primarily in leisure contexts. Han (1988) found that life satisfaction for Korean immigrants was more closely tied to flow for women than men and suspected that women were more sensitive to the affective effects of flow. There have been studies of flow among Italian cave explorers, drug addicts, students from Bangkok, Navajo college students, white collar workers, dancers, and blind nuns (Csikszentmihalyi & Csikszentmihalyi, 1988; Massimini et al., 1988).

Flow theory has been applied in retrospect to some trends documented in history. Researchers who have reviewed historical documents and anthropological writings have found evidence to suggest that flow experiences may have occurred among pygmies, Shuswap Indians, fourth-century Japanese shrine builders, natives of New Guinea, Mayan ball players, Indian Brahmins, Athenian citizens, Chinese intellectuals, and violent warriors of the ancient Turkish and Tartar cultures (Csikszentmihalyi, 1990). It was hypothesized that the Jesuit order of St. Ignatius of Loyala in the 1500s attracted young missionaries because of the complex system of graded challenges that provided flow opportunities (Csikszentmihalyi, I., 1988).

The types of activities that promote flow differ based on gender, a finding that may relate to differing opportunities for skill development (Csikszentmihalyi, 1975). It seems that as age and socioeconomic status increase, people are more inclined to enjoy activity engagement for its own sake. The characteristics of flow are the same in all cultures, but the contexts and opportunities differ. Flow can be found in cultures where there are goals, rules, and challenges matched to the skills of the population (Csikszentmihalyi, 1990). Csikszentmihalyi viewed flow as a higher-level need, essential for happiness, but not necessarily for survival of an individual. Flow seems to only occur, and take precedence, in cultures and times where basic survival and safety needs are not threatened (Csikszentmihalyi, 1990).

The Autotelic Personality

There are differences from person to person in the inclination to experience flow (Adlai-Gail, 1994; Csikszentmihalyi & Mei-Ha Wong, 1991; Massimini et al., 1988). In LeFevre's (1988) sample of 107 workers, 40 percent seemed content to spend their time in the apathy channel, while another 40 percent sought situations that placed a higher demand on their skills. Studies of students have suggested that for some, the

desire to avoid anxiety-provoking situations is stronger than the desire to face challenges (Carli et al., 1988; Nakamura, 1988).

People who seek out flow opportunities have "autotelic personalities" (Csikszentmihalyi, 1988b). They welcome opportunities for action and are most content when involved in a challenging activity (Logan, 1988). These individuals seem to have reduced cortical activity when focused on tasks inducing the flow state (Hamilton Halcomb & Csikszentmihalyi, 1975). Kimiecik and Stein (1992) discovered that athletes with autotelic personalities were more task-oriented and less ego-oriented than those without autotelic traits. Although just about everyone has the potential for flow, individuals who are self-centered or self-conscious seem less inclined to experience flow (Csikszentmihalyi, 1988b, 1990; Logan, 1988). When people focus their thoughts on themselves, there is less energy left to devote to their activities. Csikszentmihalyi suggested that individuals with stimulus over-inclusion problems, such as schizophrenia and attention deficit disorder, lacked the ability to focus adequately on a task to experience flow (1990).

Some researchers claim that differences in the predisposition to flow are inherent (Csikszentmihalyi, 1993). The cause of these genetic differences is unclear but may relate to differences in ability to focus attention. In addition, certain conditions in a family seem to influence the child's development of "autotelic personality." These conditions may include choices; clarity of feedback; and a focus on activity, trust, and manageable challenges (Rathunde, 1988).

Flow in Adversity

Differences in the ability to achieve flow may account for differences in the ability to cope with conditions of chronic stress among people (Csikszentmihalyi, 1990; Logan, 1988). Massimini et al. (1988) studied flow among persons with visual and physical disabilities and persons who have survived extremely tragic human conditions. His team concluded that it was the ability to experience flow in everyday life that accounted for differences in the capacity to cope effectively in the face of adverse or disastrous conditions. Individuals who were able to cope most effectively transformed seemingly hopeless conditions into a series of manageable challenges with clear goals. They could report positive experiences in striving to meet these goals. They were able to find flow experiences in everyday living. When faced with adversity they followed a sequence of actions where they would scan the environment, set a goal, monitor progress, and increase the level of difficulty as they achieved success (Logan, 1988).

Flow in Everyday Life

Flow experiences can occur in everyday life when individuals engage in activities that match their skills with task demands. Flow is best seen on a continuum, rather than as an all-or-nothing phenomenon (Csikszentmihalyi, 1975). It is a subjective state that varies in intensity, depth, and strength of purpose. How often flow states occur for an individual depends on how flow is defined by the researcher (Csikszentmihalyi, 1992).

Graef (1975a) used the term '"microflow activities" for trivial, sometimes automatic behavior patterns that require less skill but are intrinsically rewarding, enjoyable, and may facilitate involvement with more structured activities. He suggested that people need to involve themselves in seemingly unnecessary activities that provide activation, structure, and goals to cope with gaps in daily routine. Examples of microflow activities include doodling, jokes, foot-tapping, word games, and other noninstrumental activities.

Individuals who have been deprived of flow or microflow activities experience negative effects (Graef, 1975b). Following a 48-hour flow-deprivation experiment, college students reported feeling dull and unreasonable (Graef, 1975b). Some individuals were disorganized and had a sense of no longer being actively in control of the environment. Graef pointed out similarities between the disorganized state brought on by flow deprivation and the cognitive disorganization reported by individuals with acute schizophrenia. He suggested that microflow activities help make reality manageable and that there may be a relationship between flow and psychopathology (1975b).

While microflow falls at one end of the flow continuum, intense memorable flow experiences that are difficult to interrupt fall at the opposite end. These "deep flow" or "macroflow" experiences share features with Maslow's "peak experience" and other spiritual experiences (Csikszentmihalyi, 1975). In deep flow there is a sense of transcendence and harmony with one's surroundings. The literature has reported such experiences during rock climbing, chess, and figure skating (Csikszentmihalyi, 1975; Jackson, 1992).

Significance of Flow

The flow experience is considered vital to adaptation and growth, while constant involvement with low challenge environments leads to regression and disorganization (Logan, 1988; Massimini et al., 1987). Research has related flow to happiness, self-esteem, work productivity, role satisfaction, and satisfaction with life (Carlson & Clark, 1991; Csikszentmihalyi, 1988b, 1990, 1993; Han, 1988; Jacobs, 1994; Kipper, 1992; Logan, 1988; Massimini et al., 1988). Applications of flow theory have influenced the design of school curriculums, museums, homes for the aged, work sites, leisure products, and rehabilitation programs for juvenile delinquents (Csikszentmihalyi, 1990).

Massimini and colleagues (1987) have suggested that monitoring the experience of flow in everyday contexts could provide information applicable to psychiatric rehabilitation. They noted emotional atrophy among people with psychiatric diseases. They hypothesized that if flow theory applies to this population, then the prescription for psychiatric patients would include involvement in activities that are challenging, but do not overwhelm the individual's skills. These comments echo the sentiments of Meyer, one of the early founders of occupational therapy:

> Thus, with our patients we naturally begin with a natural simple regime of pleasurable ease, the creation of an orderly rhythm in the atmosphere. . . . We naturally heed also the other factors—the personal interests and personal fitness. . . . To get the pleasure and pride of achievement and use of one's hands and muscles, the feeling of worthwhileness of a little effort and of a well fitted use of time is the basic remedy for the blase tedium that characterizes the indifference or hopeless depression that stands in the way of rallying thwarted personalities. (1921/1982, p. 84; see Chapter 4)

Limitations of Flow Research

When Csikszentmihalyi (1975) first began to identify elements of flow, his intention was to eventually operationalize flow with a standardized assessment, for fear its essence might be lost (1992). Researchers have differed in their opinions about whether all elements associated with flow must be present, and whether some of these are more important to the identification of flow than others (Kimiecik & Stein, 1992). While in some studies researchers have defined flow by the performer's account of the subjective experience (Csikszentmihalyi, 1975; Sato, 1988), in others flow is operationalized by the perceived presence of certain conditions, such as a balance between challenges and skills (Carli et al., 1988; Csikszentmihalyi, 1975; LeFevre, 1988; Massimini et al., 1988).

Another limitation of flow studies is that, although flow falls somewhere on the continuum between microflow and macroflow, different researchers have used different boundaries along this continuum (Csikszentmihalyi, 1992). In addition, while some researchers have used the four-channel model to study time in flow (Wells, 1988), others have used eight channel, and 16 channel models (Carli et al., 1988; Massimini et al., 1988). Therefore, cross comparisons among experience-sampling studies require caution. Also, Wernick (1992) found that the channels used in flow studies were not sufficient to encompass all of the diverse subjective experiences of work.

Because data collection is disruptive to flow experience, descriptions are based on retrospective recall. There are very few critiques of flow in the literature. The study of flow is less than 25 years old, and much of what is written is philosophical and exploratory, without empirical evidence to support it.

Flow and the Occupational Therapy Literature

The occupational therapy literature contains some references to this construct. Howe and Schwartzberg (1988) include flow in a list of considerations for running a group, and Jacobs (1994) studied job satisfaction and flow among occupational therapy practitioners at work in physical rehabilitation settings. Jackson (1989) referred to flow studies in describing considerations for designing an independent living skills program for adolescents. In her Muriel Driver Lecture, Law (1991) discussed the connection between flow and occupational satisfaction. Flow is seen as relevant to occupational science (Primeau, Clark, & Pierce, 1990; Yerxa et al., 1990). The ESM was described by Carlson and Clark (1991) as an innovative method for naturalistic research. Finally, do Rozario (1994) discussed flow in terms of changing societies and the belief that deep flow and spiritual experiences came more naturally through occupation in traditional societies than in modern technological societies. Although flow has been discussed as a useful construct, it has not been well examined in the occupational therapy literature.

Relevance of Flow to Occupational Therapy

The study of flow is important to occupational therapists because it "names and frames" a phenomenon consistent with the fundamental beliefs of the occupational therapy profession (Carlson & Clark, 1991; Schon, 1982; Yerxa et al., 1990). Naming and framing permit discussion and study of a phenomenon. The autotelic, or intrinsically motivating, nature of this experience is congruent with the conviction that activity is rewarding in itself and that "occupation gives meaning to life" (Polatajko, 1992, p. 1923). The philosophy underlying occupational therapy includes the belief that the experience of becoming absorbed in a "just-right challenge" is therapeutic and influential to one's overall sense of well-being (Yerxa et al., 1990). If occupational therapists can understand more about the properties and conditions of the flow experience, they can help in the client's discovery of occupations that are intrinsically motivating and that promote this sense of well-being and meaning.

The following principles, extracted from the literature on flow, may be useful to occupational therapy practitioners in helping clients engage in activities that may induce flow:

1. The client's own perception of his or her capabilities, and of the challenges inherent in the task, must be appreciated by the occupational therapy practitioner as indicators of the complexity which may provide the "just-right challenge."

2. The occupational therapy practitioner may solicit descriptions of experiences that the client found enjoyable in the past. Exploration and analysis of these accounts may clarify whether the constructs of enjoyment and flow are synonymous, and uncover information about the conditions that induce enjoyment and/or flow for the client.

3. The client should have a clear sense of the goals of the task and feel in control of these requirements. The practitioner should ensure that the requirements of the task are clear to the client and that the client is able to set his or her own standards for success.

4. The outcomes must be meaningful to the client. The practitioner may explore the client's values, needs, and interests for cues about what challenges may be meaningful to the individual.

5. Consistent feedback on performance of tasks must be available. The client must be able to see the connection between his or her performance and outcomes of these actions.

6. The practitioner must continually observe the client for signs of boredom or anxiety and adjust task demands to increase or decrease the level of challenge perceived by the client.

7. To induce flow, the client must have opportunities to focus deeply on the task. Thus, the environment may need to be adapted to eliminate other demands on his or her energy and attention.

8. The potential for flow varies from person to person, and for each person it varies across time. The practitioner should keep in mind that the individual may have more pressing concerns, for example, needs related to safety, security, and avoidance of anxiety.

Areas for Future Research

In 1960 Reilly said, "For us, in occupational therapy, the most fundamental area for research is, and probably will always be, the nature and meaning of activity" (p. 208). Several questions are crucial to the understanding of flow and its place in occupational science and occupational therapy: Can everybody experience flow? Is flow experienced differently by certain groups of people than by others? What conditions promote and inhibit flow for our clients? How do flow experiences affect rehabilitation outcomes? How do flow experiences affect health and well-being among persons with disabilities? Do people who frequently experience flow differ in occupational adaptation from those who do not? Are people with stimulus inclusion problems really unable to experience flow? If so, what are the consequences of genuine, long-term flow deprivation?

Given occupational therapy's concern for the impact of occupation on human beings, and the availability of innovative techniques for naturalistic data collection, the time is right for us to explore these questions. The answers may provide support for the philosophical foundation of our profession and lead us in directions that can improve the subjective occupational experience of our clients.

Acknowledgments

The author is indebted to Dr. Joanne Valiant Cook, Associate Professor in the School of Occupational Therapy at the University of Western Ontario, for her editorial and content suggestions for this paper.

References

Adlai-Gail, W. (1994). Exploring the autotelic personality (competence). DAI-B 55/4, p. 1684. [CD-ROM]. Abstract from: ProQuest File: Dissertation Abstracts Item: AAC 9425350.

American Occupational Therapy Association. (1993). Position paper: Purposeful activity. *American Journal of Occupational Therapy, 47*, 1081–1082.

Baum, C. (1985). Growth, renewal, and challenge: An important era for occupational therapy. *American Journal of Occupational Therapy, 39*, 778–784.

Breines, E. (1984). The Issue Is: An attempt to define purposeful activity. *American Journal of Occupational Therapy, 38*, 543–544.

Carli, M., Delle Fave, A., & Massimini, F. (1988). The quality of experience in the flow channels: Comparison of Italian and U.S. students. In M. Csikszentmihalyi & I. Csikszentmihalyi (Eds.), *Optimal experience: Psychological studies of flow in consciousness* (pp. 288–306). Cambridge, UK: Cambridge University Press.

Carlson, M., & Clark, F. (1991). The search for useful methodologies in occupational science. *American Journal of Occupational Therapy, 49*, 235–241. http://dx.doi.org/10.5014/ajot.45.3.235

Csikszentmihalyi, I. (1988). Flow in historical context: The case of the Jesuits. In M. Csikszentmihalyi & I. Csikszentmihalyi (Eds.), *Optimal experience: Psychological studies of flow in consciousness* (pp. 232–247). Cambridge, UK: Cambridge University Press.

Csikszentmihalyi, M. (Ed.). (1975). *Beyond boredom and anxiety: The experience of play in work and games.* San Francisco, CA: Jossey-Bass.

Csikszentmihalyi, M. (1988a). The flow experience and its significance for human psychology. In M. Csikszentmihalyi & I. Csikszentmihalyi (Eds.), *Optimal experience: Psychological studies of flow in consciousness* (pp. 15–35). Cambridge, UK: Cambridge University Press.

Csikszentmihalyi, M. (1988b). Introduction. In M. Csikszentmihalyi & I. Csikszentmihalyi (Eds.), *Optimal experience: Psychological studies of flow in consciousness* (pp. 3–14). Cambridge, UK: Cambridge University Press.

Csikszentmihalyi, M. (1988c). The future of flow. In M. Csikszentmihalyi & I. Csikszentmihalyi (Eds.), *Optimal experience: Psychological studies of flow in consciousness* (pp. 364–383). Cambridge, UK: Cambridge University Press.

Csikszentmihalyi, M. (1990). *Flow: The psychology of optimal experience.* New York: Harper & Row.

Csikszentmihalyi, M. (1992). A response to the Kimiecik & Stein and Jackson Papers. *Journal of Applied Sport Psychology, 4,* 181–183.

Csikszentmihalyi, M. (1993). Activity and happiness: Toward a science of occupation. *Australian Journal of Occupational Science, 1*(1), 38–42.

Csikszentmihalyi, M., & Csikszentmihalyi, I. (1988). Introduction to part IV. In M. Csikszentmihalyi & I. Csikszentmihalyi (Eds.), *Optimal experience: Psychological studies of flow in consciousness* (pp. 251–265). Cambridge, UK: Cambridge University Press.

Csikszentmihalyi, M., & Larson, R. (1984). *Being adolescent: Conflict and growth in the teenage years.* New York: Basic Books.

Csikszentmihalyi, M., & Larson, R. (1987). Validity and reliability of the experience-sampling method. *Journal of Nervous and Mental Disease, 1975,* 526–535.

Csikszentmihalyi, M., & Mei-Ha Wong, M. (1991). The situational and personal correlates of happiness: A cross-national comparison. In F. Strack, M. Argyle, & N. Schwartz (Eds.), *Subjective well-being* (pp. 193–212). Toronto, ON: Pergammon Press.

Cynkin, S., & Robinson, A. (1990). *Occupational therapy and activities health: Toward health through activities.* Boston, MA: Little, Brown.

Delle Fave, A., & Massimini, F. (1988). Modernization and the changing contexts of flow in work and leisure. In M. Csikszentmihalyi & I. Csikszentmihalyi (Eds.), *Optimal experience: Psychological studies of flow in consciousness* (pp. 193–213). Cambridge, UK: Cambridge University Press.

do Rozario, L. (1994). Ritual, meaning, and transcendence: The role of occupation in modern life. *Australian Journal of Occupational Science, 1,* 46–53.

Evans, K. (1987). Nationally speaking: Definition of occupation as the core concept of occupational therapy. *American Journal of Occupational Therapy, 41,* 627–628.

Fidler, G., & Fidler, J. (1978). Doing and becoming: Purposeful action and self-actualization. *American Journal of Occupational Therapy, 31,* 305–310.

Graef, R. (1975a). Flow patterns in everyday life. In M. Csikszentmihalyi (Ed.), *Beyond boredom and anxiety: The experience of play in work and games* (pp. 140–160). San Francisco, CA: Jossey-Bass.

Graef, R. (1975b). Effects of flow deprivation. In M. Csikszentmihalyi (Ed.), *Beyond boredom and anxiety: The experience of play in work and games* (pp. 161–178). San Francisco, CA: Jossey-Bass.

Hamilton Halcomb, J., & Csikszentmihalyi, M. (1975). Enjoying work: Surgery. In M. Csikszentmihalyi (Ed.), *Beyond boredom and anxiety: The experience of play in work and games* (pp. 123–139). San Francisco, CA: Jossey-Bass.

Han, S. (1988). The relationship between life satisfaction and flow in elderly Korean immigrants. In M. Csikszentmihalyi & I. Csikszentmihalyi (Eds.), *Optimal experience: Psychological studies of flow in consciousness* (pp. 138–171). Cambridge, UK: Cambridge University Press.

Howe, M., & Schwartzberg, S. (1988). Structure and process in designing a functional group. *Occupational Therapy in Mental Health, 8*(3), 1–8.

Jackson, J. (1989). En route to adulthood: A high school transition program for adolescents with disabilities. *Occupational Therapy in Health Care, 6*(4), 33–51.

Jackson, S. (1992). Athletes in flow: A qualitative investigation of flow states in elite figure skaters. *Journal of Applied Sport Psychology, 4,* 161–180.

Jacobs, K. (1994). Flow and the occupational therapy practitioner. *American Journal of Occupational Therapy, 48,* 989–996. http://dx.doi.org/10.5014/ajot.48.11.989

Johnson, J., & Yerxa, E. (Eds.) (1989). *Occupational science: The foundation for new models of practice.* Binghamton, NY: Haworth Press.

Kielhofner, G. (1981). An ethnographic study of deinstitutionalized adults: Their community settings and daily experience. *Occupational Therapy Journal of Research, 1,* 135–141.

Kielhofner, G. (1982). Qualitative research: Part two: Methodological approaches and relevance to occupational therapy. *Occupational Therapy Journal of Research, 2,* 150–164.

Kielhofner, G. (1992). *Conceptual foundations of occupational therapy.* Philadelphia, PA: F. A. Davis.

Kimiecik, I., & Stein, G. (1992). Examining flow experiences in sports context: Conceptual issues and methodological concerns. *Journal of Applied Sport Psychology, 4,* 141–160.

Kipper, D. (1992). The dynamics of role satisfaction: A theoretical model. *Group Psychotherapy, Psychodrama, and Sociometry, 44,* 71–86.

Kremer, E., Nelson, D., & Duncombe, L. (1984). Effects of selected activities on affective meaning in psychiatric patients. *American Journal of Occupational Therapy, 38,* 522–528.

Laliberte, D. (1993). *An exploration into the meaning seniors attach to activity.* Unpublished master's thesis. London, ON: University of Western Ontario.

Law, M. (1991). Muriel Driver Lecture. The environment: A focus for occupational therapy. *Canadian Journal of Occupational Therapy, 58,* 171–179.

LeFevre, J. (1988). Flow and the quality of experience during work and leisure. In M. Csikszentmihalyi & I. Csikszentmihalyi (Eds.), *Optimal experience: Psychological studies of flow in consciousness* (pp. 307–318). Cambridge, UK: Cambridge University Press.

Levine, R. (1987). The influence of the arts-and-crafts movement on the professional status of occupational therapy. *American Journal of Occupational Therapy, 45,* 248–254.

Logan, P. (1988). Flow in solitary ordeals. In M. Csikszentmihalyi & I. Csikszentmihalyi (Eds.). *Optimal experience: Psychological studies of flow in consciousness* (pp. 172–180). Cambridge, UK: Cambridge University Press.

Massimini, A., Carli, M., & Csikszentmihalyi, M. (1988). Systematic assessment of flow in daily experience. In M. Csikszentmihalyi & I. Csikszentmihalyi (Eds.), *Optimal experience: Psychological studies of flow in consciousness* (pp. 266–281). Cambridge, UK: Cambridge University Press.

Massimini, A., Csikszentmihalyi, M., & Carli, M. (1987). The monitoring of optimal experience, *Journal of Nervous and Mental Disease, 1975,* 545–549.

Massimini, F., Csikszentmihalyi, M., & Delle Fave, A. (1988). Flow and biocultural evolution. In M. Csikszentmihalyi & I. Csikszentmihalyi (Eds.), *Optimal experience: Psychological studies of flow in consciousness* (pp. 60–81). Cambridge, UK: Cambridge University Press.

Merrill, S. (1985). Qualitative methods in occupational therapy research: An application. *Occupational Therapy Journal of Research, 5,* 213–222.

Meyer, A. (1922/1982). Worth repeating: The philosophy of occupational therapy. *Occupational Therapy in Mental Health, 2,* 79–86. Reprinted as Chapter 4.

Nakamura, J. (1988). Optimal experience and the uses of talent. In M. Csikszentmihalyi & I. Csikszentmihalyi (Eds.), *Optimal experience: Psychological studies of flow in consciousness* (pp. 319–326). Cambridge, UK: Cambridge University Press.

Park, H. (1995). *Occupation, well-being, and women with rheumatoid arthritis.* Unpublished master's thesis. London, ON: University of Western Ontario.

Polatajko, H. (1992). Muriel Driver Lecture: Naming and framing occupational therapy: A lecture dedicated to the life of Nancy B. *Canadian Journal of Occupational Therapy, 59,* 189–192.

Primeau, L., Clark, F., & Pierce, D. (1989). Occupational therapy alone has looked upon occupation: Future applications of occupational science to pediatric occupational therapy. *Occupational Therapy in Health Care, 6*(4), 19–32.

Rathunde, K. (1988). Optimal experience and the family context. In M. Csikszentmihalyi & I. Csikszentmihalyi (Eds.), *Optimal experience: Psychological studies of flow in consciousness* (pp. 342–363). Cambridge, UK: Cambridge University Press.

Reilly, M. (1960). Research potentiality of occupational therapy. *American Journal of Occupational Therapy, 14,* 206–209.

Sato, I. (1988). Bosozoku: Flow in Japanese motorcycle gangs. In M. Csikszentmihalyi & I. Csikszentmihalyi. (Eds.), *Optimal experience: Psychological studies of flow in consciousness* (pp. 92–117). Cambridge, UK: Cambridge University Press.

Schon, D. (1982). *The reflective practitioner.* New York: Basic Books.

Steinmetz, H. (1995). *Occupational performance and life satisfaction among community-dwelling stroke clients: A pilot study.* Unpublished master's thesis. London, ON: University of Western Ontario.

Wells, A. (1988). Self-esteem and optimal experience. In M. Csikszentmihalyi & I. Csikszentmihalyi. (Eds.), *Optimal experience: Psychological studies of flow in consciousness* (pp. 327–341). Cambridge, UK: Cambridge University Press.

Wernick, R. (1990). Work: An analysis of subjective work experience utilizing Cikszentmihalyi's theory of play. [CD-ROM]. DAI-A 51/06, p. 2173, Dec. 1990. Abstract from ProQuest File: Dissertation Abstracts Item: AAC 9033369.

Wiemer, R. (1979). Traditional and nontraditional practice arenas. In American Occupational Therapy Association (Ed.), *Occupational therapy 2001* (pp. 43–53). Rockville, MD: author.

Yerxa, E. (1980). Occupational therapy's role in creating a future climate of caring. *American Journal of Occupational Therapy, 34,* 529–534.

Yerxa, E., Clark, F., Frank, G., Jackson, J., Parfiam, D., Pierce, D., Stein, C., & Zemke, R. (1990). An introduction to occupational science: A foundation for occupational therapy in the 21st century. In J. Johnson & E. Yerxa (Eds.), *Occupational science: The foundation for new models of practice.* Binghamton, NY: Haworth Press.

CHAPTER 18

Sleep, Occupation, and the Passage of Time

ANDREW GREEN

Introduction

In his early exposition of the philosophy of occupational therapy, Adolf Meyer named sleep as one of the 'Big Four' factors that a person should balance for the maintenance of health, along with work, play and rest (Meyer 1922, 1977, p641; see Chapter 4). Westhorp (2003) and Christiansen and Matuska (2006) have addressed the complexities of balance and Weinblatt and Avrech-Bar (2003) have examined the concept of rest but, as Christiansen and Baum (1997) observed, little attention has been paid by occupational therapists to sleep. Howell and Pierce (2000) suggested that Meyer's message might be ignored in western society because of beliefs that time spent sleeping is time wasted. Another possible reason is that influential writers have omitted it from definitions and classifications of occupation. For example, Kielhofner and Burke (1985) stated that 'occupational behaviour' is 'activity in which persons engage during most of their waking time' (p12), thereby appearing to exclude sleep from the domain of occupational therapy. More recently, Persson et al (2001) dismissed sleep from discussion about occupation, despite acknowledging its importance for daytime performance, because 'it is an unconscious process that cannot be influenced or directed' (p12). Similarly, Larson et al (2003) ruled out sleep by stating that occupations are 'consciously executed' (p16).

The main purposes of this article are to propose that the neglect of this interesting area is unjustified and to raise awareness among occupational therapists of issues relating to sleep. The article first reviews the existing information on sleep in the occupational therapy and occupational science literature. Secondly, the theoretical relationship between sleep and occupation (and the

nature of occupation itself) is explored in order to determine the relevance of sleep to occupational therapy. Lastly, it takes an overview of the current knowledge of sleep science insofar as it relates to occupation and to the promotion of good sleep.

Before proceeding, it is appropriate to define sleep and stress its importance by summarising the effects of poor sleep. Carskadon and Dement (2005) offered a behavioural definition of sleep:

> Sleep is a reversible behavioral state of perceptual disengagement from and unresponsiveness to the environment . . . typically (but not necessarily) accompanied by postural recumbence, behavioral quiescence, closed eyes and other indicators . . . (p13).

According to Alford and Wilson (2008), the varied consequences of poor sleep include:

> increased daytime sleepiness and fatigue leading to cognitive impairment and poor work performance and absenteeism in addition to increased accident risk including driving, increased risk of new or recurrent psychiatric disorder and increased substance use, poorer prognosis, increased healthcare-related financial burden, and poorer social functioning at work and at home (p51).

Sleep in the Occupational Therapy and Occupational Science Literature

The first difficulty in researching sleep and occupational therapy or occupational science is finding information. Electronic searches using broad terms such as 'occupation' or 'occupational therapy' and 'sleep' are largely unhelpful: the words are common and often co-located, but frequently unconnected. For example, a search on *Google Scholar* with the terms 'occupational therapy' and 'sleep' anywhere in the article yielded over 11,000 results; conversely, a search for those terms in the title yielded nothing.

Sleep and Occupational Therapy

A manual search of standard occupational therapy textbooks published since 1990, held in a university library, revealed only one substantial reference to sleep. Christiansen and Baum (1997) drew attention to the relationship of sleep and occupation, referred to the science of sleep, and offered sleep hygiene advice. Christiansen and Baum (2005) subsequently discussed sleep and occupation and sleep science but omitted sleep hygiene advice. (The work of Christiansen will be discussed in detail later.) The word 'sleep' does not appear in the index of several general textbooks on physical dysfunction; for example, McHugh Pendleton and Schultz-Krohn ['Pedretti'] (2006) and Blesedell Crepeau et al ['Willard and Spackman'] (2003). Where sleep is indexed in other standard textbooks, the reference relates

mostly to specific conditions and the material is often limited, however relevant to the condition concerned.

Exceptionally, wide-ranging and concise advice on sleep was provided by Yasuda (2008), in the context of fibromyalgia, and by Hammond and Jefferson (2002), in the context of rheumatoid arthritis. Other references in general occupational therapy textbooks are summarised in Table 18.1. Similarly, in some textbooks concerning mental health (Creek 1990, Finlay 2004), there is no indexed reference to sleep, but, where sleep is listed in the index of one book (Creek 2002), it turns out to be a brief reference connected to child and adolescent mental health (Lougher 2002). References to sleep in other mental health textbooks are also listed in Table 18.1.

Books relating to occupational therapy for single conditions provide some useful discussion of sleep. Although the word 'sleep' does not appear in the index of a book on multiple sclerosis (Silcox 2003), sleep is discussed in relation to fatigue. Energy conservation advice refers to 'well known rules' (p79) to which getting enough sleep is added, but there is no clear ad-

Table 18.1. References to (Adult) Sleep Found in Indexes of Occupational Therapy Textbooks

Author(s)	Country	Condition	Content	Page ref.
Beresford and Hill (1996) [in Turner et al]	UK	Motor neurone disease	Refer to cramp and spasms disturbing sleep.	p. 490
Cara and MacRae (2005)	USA	Serious mental illness	Observe that sleep-wake cycle is disrupted in serious mental illness and note relationship between sleep, medication and function.	pp. 128–29
Cooper (2002) [in Turner et al]	UK	Cancer	In a passing reference to sleep, recommends appropriate timing of medication and relaxation.	p. 577
Duncan (2005)	UK	Anxiety disorders	Mentions insomnia as a feature of anxiety disorders and recommends self-management skills.	pp. 445–46
Hammond and Jeffreson (2002) [in Turner et al]	UK	Rheumatoid arthritis	Provide useful advice on sleep hygiene, including the use of resting orthoses, and highlight the role of medication.	p. 557
Kelly (2002) [in Turner et al]	UK	Back pain	Refers to 'standard strategies' (unspecified) for tackling insomnia, position and use of medication.	pp. 537–38
King (1992) [in Turner et al]	UK	Cardiac rehabilitation	Notes wellbeing produced by sleep and offers sleep hygiene advice.	pp. 770–71
Levy (2005)	USA	Old age psychiatry	Notes problems caused by lack of sleep and recommends standard sleep hygiene.	p. 329
Wood and Hawkins (2002) [in Turner et al]	UK	HIV/AIDS	Stress the importance of regular routines where there is cognitive impairment.	p. 473
Yasuda (2008)	USA	Fibromyalgia	Notes some sleep hygiene measures with references to other sources.	p. 1236

vice about improving sleep. Although there was no reference to sleep by Strong (1996) in connection with chronic pain, nor by O'Hara (1996), there is more recent acknowledgement by Strong (2002) of the significant problems with sleep for people with chronic pain. She gave detailed advice to improve sleep, noting the importance, for example, of modifying the behaviours and environment that have an impact on sleep. Chronic fatigue syndrome (CFS) is another condition where input from occupational therapists is important and where sleep problems may also occur (Cox 2000). After examining evidence from the literature, Cox concluded that sleep disruption is a consequence of CFS rather than a causative factor, and provided advice on sleep first compiled in 1994 (Cox 2000). Like Strong's (2002) advice, it is comprehensive and, similarly, stressed the importance of a regular rising time, but, like Strong (2002), Cox (2000) did not explain the rationale for it.

Chapman (1924), a psychiatrist and contemporary of Meyer, stated that occupational therapy 'intelligently used' (p496) could help sleeplessness,[1] but there are few references to the contribution of occupational therapy to the resolution of sleep disorders. However, two teams involving occupational therapists have reported interventions specifically aimed at improving the sleep of people with insomnia. First, a group approach and course content, including information on sleep science, was described in detail by a Canadian team (Kupych-Woloshyn et al 1993); they stated that their philosophy emphasised balance in lifestyle, individuality and a focus on function. Unfortunately, they did not record outcomes, but did observe that the participants felt more accepted and welcomed opportunities to meet others in similar circumstances. Secondly, Green et al (2005) reported a group, based on the Canadian team's model, and presented preliminary outcome data that indicated modest improvements in total sleep time and decreased subjective levels of anxiety about sleep; similarly, there was perceived acceptance, and the support of other sufferers was also considered valuable. However, it is uncertain whether, or how much, either team could be said to have been practising oc-

cupational therapy, although Green et al (2005) argued that close attention to lifestyle factors that affect sleep is an appropriate concern for occupational therapists.

Sleep and Occupational Science

It is to the occupational science literature that one must turn to find discussion of the relationship between sleep and occupation. This has been led by Charles Christiansen (with others) and by Ann Wilcock. The contributions of Christiansen will be discussed later in debating whether sleep is an occupation. Wilcock (2003) did not classify sleep clearly as an occupation, but mentioned sleep (and rest) as part of the 'occupation cycle' (p171). However, she has investigated the science of sleep (Wilcock 1998) and observed that, because of the negative effects of sleep deprivation on occupation, 'sleep can be viewed as necessary to engagement in occupation' (p61). She cited evidence that deep sleep and total sleep time might increase after extreme exertion and suggested that there may, therefore, be 'a close relationship between sleep patterns and regular occupations' (p62). Wilcock (1998) also noted that whereas electroencephalograph (EEG) patterns seem to relate to when the person is best fitted for different types of occupation or rest, they are flexible and enable people to be nocturnal. She concluded:

> The sleep systems are therefore facilitatory to immense occupational flexibility, as well as servicing all systems so they can be used as required in occupational behaviour (p63).

By this, Wilcock (1998) appears to suggest that we can override natural rhythms. This is important because, as will be seen, human rhythms do not entirely accord with the patterns of modern life.

Howell and Pierce (2000) highlighted the conflict between natural rhythms and modern life. They observed that 'it has long been considered socially unacceptable in the United States to nap or even to be tired in the afternoon' and that electric lighting 'plunged humans into chronic and culture-wide sleep debt' (p68). This anticipates the discussion of sleep science (below), but Howell and Pierce (2000) suggested that occupational therapy and occupational science, being shaped by the cultural values from which they emerged, have 'largely ignored sleep and other restorative occupations' (p68). Howell and Pierce (2000) investigated quilting as a restorative occupation and dwelt on the association of quilts and sleep, suggesting that quilt use is unique be-

---

[1]Chapman (1924) recommended a programme of recreation and exercise, mass games and group singing, and considered occupational therapy an important part of the maintenance of 'the rational hospital régime'. He added: 'The value of the occupational department moreover is not confined to what it does for patients, but its influence as [sic] promoting industry extends throughout the hospital organization and is of inestimable value in the promotion of morale' (p. 496).

cause a quilt could help to enhance the sleep environment. Perhaps so, but they also implied that beneath a quilt is a good place to make a phone call or watch television, while failing to note that these are *waking* activities that 'may inhibit sleep or strengthen associations in the mind between being in bed and being awake' (Wilson and Nutt 2008, p34).

One area where there has been interest in sleep is in time use studies, especially those concerning people with a mental illness. Citing her research in forensic units, Farnworth (2004) suggested that, in unusual circumstances, sleep itself could be an activity or occupation: for forensic patients it could be an escape, allowing 'one to dream of other life possibilities' (p59). The reference to that page in the index of the book (Molineux 2004) posed the tantalising question, 'Sleep, "activity" or "occupation"?', which, unfortunately, is not addressed directly. It is an interesting possibility, nevertheless, that sleep could serve purposes other than restoration.

In a community-based study involving people with schizophrenia in Canada, Aubin et al (1999) found that their respondents slept for 9.06 hours out of 24 (37.75%). They also observed that sleeping was 'the activity that was found to be especially meaningful in the participants' daily life' (p58), being given the highest rating regarding perceived competence and pleasure and the second highest rating for importance. Similarly, in a study involving five respondents with schizophrenia detained in forensic units, Stewart and Craik (2007) found that, on average, they slept for 4% of the 'daytime' (unspecified duration), but for 39% of a 24-hour period. Neither of these studies suggested what constitutes a normal period of sleep in a day, but Christiansen (1996) cited a figure of 30% as the approximate average proportion of the 24-hour period that an average employed adult in the United States sleeps. This accords with the frequently cited figure of 7–8 hours' sleep for adults (Wilson and Nutt 2008). There is no indication in either study as to whether excessive sleep could relate to medication or how much it relates to mental illness or to incarceration. The Beirut hostage, Brian Keenan (1992), attempted unsuccessfully to sleep away time during his period in solitary confinement.

To summarise so far: there is evidence in the literature of occupational therapists giving advice for problems with sleep and of occupational scientists exploring both the science of sleep and sleep as an element of time use. Coverage has been neither consistent nor comprehensive and it is unclear why sleep has been considered by so few writers. A possible reason for this is the uncertainty about whether sleep is an occupation and, therefore, whether it is relevant to occupational therapists. However, establishing this is difficult because it has also not been established exactly what occupation is: a brief investigation is necessary.

Occupation and Sleep

The definition of occupation, including its relationship with activity, has been discussed at length over the years. Hagedorn (1995) and Reed and Sanderson (1999), for example, devoted chapters to occupation and its differentiation from activity. Hasselkus (2002) reviewed a number of definitions and concluded simply and wisely: 'The effort to reach consensus on the meaning and definition of occupation continues' (p16). Although this is not the place to review such effort in detail, Table 18.2 summarises a selection of definitions, with an assessment of whether sleep could be considered an occupation, or an activity, by the given criteria.

Few of the writers cited in Table 18.2 mention sleep in discussing occupation. Sleep appears to be largely excluded from occupation but, since Christiansen has written so much on sleep, it is appropriate to look more closely at his view on occupation. Christiansen and Baum (2005) cited several other authors' definitions and went on to note the common characteristics of occupations (see Table 18.2). By those criteria, it could be concluded that sleep is an occupation. It has a goal (rest and recuperation) and situations influence how and with whom it is done. It can be clearly identified by others, although not entirely by the doer while in the process of sleep. It might have meaning for the individual and shared meaning, even if the term 'sleeping together' has more than one connotation. Christiansen and Baum (2005) confirmed the conclusion by, first, observing that in any classification of categories of occupation in 'everyday discourse' the domain of sleep is included—with paid work, household work, leisure and self-care (p9). Secondly, citing a major, and substantial, textbook on sleep medicine (but without a page reference), they stated that sleep is a 'specific personal-care occupation that is necessary for health' (p10).

Previously, Christiansen and Townsend (2004) had suggested that classifying sleep as an occupation was controversial because 'occupations are usually equated with action' (p15). They thereby echoed the comments of Larson et al (2003), noted already, and Kielhofner (2002) who, citing a number of authors, stated that 'in the broadest sense, occupation denotes the action or

Table 18.2. Some Definitions of *Occupation* and Relationship of Sleep

Author(s)	Definition	Place of sleep	Comments
Clark et al (1991)	'Chunks of culturally and personally meaningful activity in which humans engage that can be named in the lexicon of our culture' (p301).	Definition does not exclude sleep if sleep can be considered a meaningful activity.	Definition of occupation by founders of occupational science.
Hagedorn (1995)	'An occupation is an organised form of human endeavour, having a name and associated role title . . . ' (p84).	Sleep is not an occupation but could be an activity in that it 'takes place on a specific occasion, during a finite period of time [and] for a particular purpose' and it 'results in a change in the previous state of objective reality or subjective experience' (p82).	According to Hagedorn (1995), a person *possesses* an occupation but *performs* activities (p79).
Christiansen et al (1995)	'Occupations are the ordinary and familiar things that people do every day' (p1015).	This definition could encompass sleep.	Position paper from AOTA. It states that 'while all occupations constitute purposeful activity, not all purposeful activities can be described as occupations' (p1016).
Golledge (1998)	'The daily living tasks that are part of an individual's lifestyle' (p102).	Terms are defined in the context of therapy and there is no place for sleep in this taxonomy.	Distinction between purposeful activity, activity and diversional activity.
Carlson and Clark (2001), cited in Larson et al (2003)	Occupations: – 'are units of action with identifiable start and end points' – 'are repeatable, intentional and consciously executed' – 'tend to be meaningful in the context of a person's life' – 'are intermediate in terms of scope' (between microbehaviours and global life concerns) – 'are labelled by members of a culture' (being customary rather than idiosyncratic) (p16).	'Sleep itself would not qualify as an occupation' (p16), not being consciously executed, although it appears to meet several other criteria.	It is suggested that it is crucial for occupational therapists to consider the place of sleep in a client's routine in order to achieve a balanced healthy lifestyle.
Pierce (2001)	'An occupation is a specific individual's personally constructed, nonrepeatable experience. [It is] a subjective event in perceived temporal, spatial, and sociocultural conditions that are unique to that one-time occurrence. [It] has a shape, a pace, a beginning and an ending, a shared or solitary aspect, a cultural meaning to the person, and an infinite number of other perceived contextual qualities. A person interprets his or her occupations before, during, and after they happen' (p139).	Sleep could not be considered an occupation by this definition, despite meeting some of the criteria, because a person cannot interpret the sleep during the experience.	An activity by contrast is a culturally defined and general class of human actions, for example, play or cooking.
Kielhofner (2002)	'Human occupation refers to the doing of work, play or activities of daily living within a temporal, physical and sociocultural context that characterizes much of human life' (p1).	Sleep appears not to be an occupation according to this definition or Kielhofner's earlier definitions of human occupation (for example, Kielhofner and Burke 1985).	Kielhofner (2002) notes that all humans exist in a framework of time and that we are moved to fill or occupy time with the things we do (p2).
Christiansen and Baum (2005)	'Occupations are human pursuits that: – are goal-directed or purposeful – are performed in situations or contexts that influence how and with whom they are done – can be identified by the doer and others – have individual meaning for the doer as well as shared meaning with others' (p5).	By these criteria, sleep can be considered an occupation and the authors describe it as such (p10).	

doing' (p1). Fisher (1998) went further in celebrating occupation: 'a wonderful word . . . a noun of action—it is about doing!' (p511). Christiansen and Baum (2005) added: 'occupations involve more than just doing' and 'all occupations require specific abilities and skills if they are going to be performed competently' (p7). However, it is difficult to make a case for a normal sleeper needing specific abilities or skills in order to sleep, although perhaps people who experience chronic insomnia lack the ability to calm the mind and body sufficiently to initiate sleep. It is also difficult to argue that sleep is normally 'more than just doing' or that it is doing at all, especially as Christiansen and Baum (2005) also observed that, when asleep, organisms are 'quiet and devoid of movement' (p10). It appears, therefore, that within one chapter Christiansen and Baum (2005) produced evidence both for and against the place of sleep among occupations.

The apparent contradiction by Christiansen and Baum (2005) is unsurprising, given the complexity of occupation, the diversity of opinion about it and the difficulty of its definition. Perhaps that difficulty is highlighted by the question: what is a person doing when not engaged in occupation? Someone who appears to be 'doing nothing' may be occupied with his or her thoughts. For example, a passer-by seeing Isaac Newton sitting under the apple tree in his garden might have noticed an absence of action, or doing, and considered him unoccupied: history indicates otherwise. A possible resolution to the difficulty of categorising activity that does not involve action was also provided by Christiansen and Baum (2005) in their comment that 'occupation and time use are two sides of the same coin' (p11). In that statement, they endorsed remarks by other writers. Finlay (2004) suggested that 'However we define and differentiate occupations, they are concerned with people's use of time' (emphasis in original) (p42) and Farnworth (2004) stated: 'Occupation describes time use at an individual level' (p47).

There appears to be no conclusive answer to the question: is sleep an occupation? This is partly because of the difficulty in defining occupation and its changing definition (Reed and Sanderson 1999). Many authorities suggest that it is not, directly or by default. On the other hand, if occupation is defined in terms of use of time, sleep could be categorised as an occupation by virtue of the time spent engaged in it; the consideration of sleep in a growing number of time use studies supports this view. However, it is not only the definition of occupation that has changed with the passage of years:

patterns of sleep and occupation have also changed. It is useful to understand this, and the rudiments of the science of sleep, before considering further the reciprocal relationship between sleep and occupation.

Historical Interlude

The modern expectation is that we should sleep in an unbroken stretch of 7 or 8 hours at night and, to achieve that, we are advised to avoid daytime sleep (Stepanski and Wyatt 2003). However, it was not always thus. The historian, Ekirch (2005), has shown how sleep has changed in Europe since preindustrial times. People would take a few hours of 'first sleep' and then wake to spend some hours of restful wakefulness, talking with their bedfellows, before taking their second sleep. Criminals might use the opportunity to get up and go about their business. However, from the 6th century the Church 'colonized' this time (p303) and monks would also rise after midnight to recite psalms and prayers. Ekirch (2005) cited numerous examples from literature (such as Chaucer and Smollett) and from other contemporary accounts; for example, a 17th century doctor advised students not to study by night until after their first sleep, as did Bishop Ward of Salisbury who read between his first and second sleeps. At the other end of the social scale, servants might get up and do some work in preparation for the day. According to Ekirch (2005), this pattern of sleep was also found in 20th century anthropological studies in Africa and he cited experiments by Thomas Wehr (see below) which suggested that, after several weeks deprived of artificial light, people revert to broken slumber 'practically identical to that of preindustrial households' (pp303–304).

It was not only in the night-time that habits were different; so it could be by day. In *The Return of the Native* (Hardy 1974)—published in 1878 but set in the 1840s—the protagonist, Yeobright, first tried to improve his prospects by reading 'far into the small hours during many nights' (p270) but, after suffering a problem with vision, he took up manual labour:

> His custom was to work from four o'clock in the morning till noon; then, when the heat of the day was its highest, to go home and sleep for an hour or two; afterwards coming out again and working till dusk at nine (p273).

Similarly, according to Cannon (2007), medieval stonemasons would work on cathedral construction from dawn until dusk during the summer but stopped to sleep at midday. In modern times, we are reminded by Wilcock (1998, p62) of Winston Churchill's comment: 'You must sleep sometime between lunch and dinner . . . that's what I always do.'

A look back over the years since Churchill's death will remind us how the timing of occupations has also changed. Leaving aside the dramatic changes in the things that we do and how we do them, consider *when* we do them. In the 1960s and 1970s, it was not possible in England and Wales to go shopping on Sundays or public holidays; some shops might remain open later on one evening a week. Sunday observance was stronger; for example, some people might have regarded it inappropriate to hang out laundry on a Sunday. Weekend football matches kicked off only at 3:00pm on a Saturday. Pubs closed at 10:30pm, or at 11:00pm if you were lucky. BBC radio was not a 24-hour service and television stations did not generally broadcast during the day and closed down before midnight (at 10:30pm in the 1973/74 UK energy crisis). On the whole, there was much less, except shift work, to keep people up into the night.

Taking the longer historical view, Wehr (1996) has noted how, by the gradual development of increasingly efficient lamps and energy sources and by moving activity from country to city and from outdoors to indoors where natural light does not penetrate, humans have insulated themselves from natural cycles of light and darkness. He observed that modern humans probably obtain less than their full quota of nightly sleep and in this he shared the view of others, such as Martin (2002), that we live in a sleep-deprived society. This prompts questions about natural sleep.

Aspects of Sleep Science

It has been seen that the 'social' night was longer in preindustrial times, but Wehr (1996) has also described a longer human biological night. With increased propensity for sleep, the night starts, in hormonal terms, with the abrupt onset of melatonin secretion, the doubling of prolactin secretion and a rise in cortisol secretion. The start of the biological day sees the reverse, starting with the abrupt offset of melatonin secretion (Wehr 1996). This human biological night is about 11 hours long, whereas modern people allocate only about 8 hours for sleep. Wehr (1996) cited his own research, which had shown that in long nights human sleep is not naturally 'consolidated into one continuous nocturnal bout' (p334). In experimental conditions, peo-

ple will typically lie awake for an hour or more before sleeping in spells of several hours, separated by periods of quiet wakefulness. Not only did Wehr (1996) suggest that modern people are sleep deprived, he also speculated that, because the periods of wakefulness tend to follow rapid eye movement (REM) sleep (when dreaming occurs), there was once a clearer channel of communication between dreams and wakeful life. He argued that with consolidated sleep, modern humans might therefore have lost touch with the 'wellspring of myths and fantasies' (p341).

Historical and scientific evidence indicates that modern humans might be swimming against the current when it comes to sleep. We now sleep less than we have for the greater part of human history and we probably sleep in different patterns. This is not to suggest that we should return to preindustrial sleep or activity patterns, but perhaps that we should pay more attention to the importance of sleep and how to maintain it despite the negative influences of modern life: shift work, intercontinental travel and the 24-hour society. To do this, it is helpful to understand the factors involved in initiating and maintaining sleep, of which there are three (Wilson 2003).

First, arousal levels must be low. Occupational therapists are likely to have observed a tendency for patients or clients to fall asleep in relaxation sessions. Although dependence on a relaxation tape or CD is inadvisable, physical relaxation is essential for sleep. It is also necessary to calm the mind before sleep. This is often a problem for people with insomnia, as found by Robertson et al (2007), and not so easily achieved as physical relaxation. For example, in clinical interviews people with insomnia often speak of 'racing thoughts' or their mind being 'in overdrive'.

The second factor is the homeostatic drive to sleep. The longer a person goes without sleep, the greater the drive; during sleep, the drive declines (Borbely and Achermann 1999). If a person usually rises at 7:00am, the maximum drive to sleep will be at around 11:00pm, but daytime sleep delays the maximum drive. This is the main reason that people with insomnia are advised to avoid daytime naps. Of course, in some cultures people take advantage of the slight circadian increase in sleepiness in the early afternoon and take a siesta: in that case, they should expect a later and shorter block of night-time sleep. Wilson (2003) made a further point of importance to nurses or therapists working with older people, or with others, who experience boredom or enforced inactivity: if arousal levels are reduced, a pattern of frequent short naps is more likely and the readiness for night-time sleep is reduced.

The third factor concerns the human body clock, or pacemaker, which is a group of cells in the hypothalamic suprachiasmic nucleus—above the crossing of the optic nerves (Roenneberg et al 2007). The clock regulates hormone secretion, among other things, but running freely it would not operate on quite a 24-hour cycle, hence the term *circadian rhythm* (about a day). Christiansen (1996) stated that the free-running cycle is approximately 25 hours, whereas just over 24 hours is most usually cited. An experiment by Middleton et al (1996), for example, found a period of 24.26 hours but, whatever the length of the cycle, it remains necessary to regulate the clock every day. As Christiansen (1996) noted, this is done by *zeitgebers* (time-givers) in a process known as entrainment (Roenneberg et al 2007).

Regulating the Sleep–Wake Cycle

The most important zeitgeber is light, detected exclusively by the eyes in mammals (Roenneberg et al 2007). Resetting of the pacemaker is therefore usually achieved by seeing daylight in the morning and, along with regulating the homeostatic drive to sleep, underlies the rationale for advice, as given by Cox (2000) and Strong (2002), to maintain a regular rising time. Importantly, as Wehr (1996) noted, the pacemaker accounts for seasonal changes in day length. Van Someren and Riemersma-Van Der Lek (2007) have suggested other ways of enhancing zeitgeber input, including melatonin supplements, which may be helpful for people experiencing jet lag. Some methods, such as regulation of temperature and cortisol levels, are complex but are, in any case, related to two crucial methods over which the individual has more control: regular feeding and regular rest–activity cycles. In their thorough review, Van Someren and Riemersma-Van Der Lek (2007) cited various studies suggesting that the regularisation of sleep–wake schedules can improve nocturnal sleep efficiency and increase daytime alertness in young adults and that 'prolonged and regular exercise is associated with better nocturnal sleep and less daytime tiredness' (p477). Exercise is more important for older people, in whom the circadian system is weaker and, whereas it may take some months of exercise for sleep to improve objectively, Benloucif et al (2004) showed that regular exercise, with social activity, could improve subjective sleep quality (and neuropsychological performance) among older people after just 2 weeks.

Given the importance of zeitgebers in regulating sleep, it becomes clear that the comments of Persson et al (2001), cited earlier, are only part of the story. Plainly, sleep cannot be influenced or directed during sleep, but there are things that a person can do to influence sleep and thereby enhance daytime performance. Most simply, as Christiansen and Townsend (2004) put it, actions are necessary to prepare for sleep, such as relaxing or creating an environment for sleep (for example, excluding light and noise). This is particularly important for poor sleepers.

Researchers who have studied the characteristics of poor sleepers have found higher relative physiological and psychological arousal during the day when compared with controls. By measuring air-flows and oxygen levels over the 24-hour period, Bonnet and Arand (1997) found that people with insomnia had an increased metabolic rate; they concluded that insomnia was 'perhaps more of a disorder of arousal than a disorder of sleep' (p587). Robertson et al (2007) used self-report scales to investigate de-arousal among people with insomnia and poor sleepers during the pre-sleep period. They found that, in people with insomnia, there was greater cognitive arousal and less sleepiness before bedtime and in the bedroom. It is therefore important for everyone, but especially for poor sleepers, to decrease arousal and to wind down during the evening. This is done by separating daytime activities involving exercise or intense intellectual or emotional effort from less demanding activities near bedtime. Similarly, it is advisable to create an environment conducive to sleep, and that usually excludes waking activities, except sex, from the bedroom (Wilson and Nutt 2008). Whether sex is an activity or an occupation is another matter.

Conclusion

Attention by occupational therapists to sleep has been variable and the question of whether or not sleep is an occupation is unanswered, unless occupation is defined in relation to time use. Nevertheless, the importance of sleep for the performance of occupations is undisputed. It is necessary to have sufficient sleep to maintain safety at work or on the road, to enhance cognitive function, and just to feel better. It has been seen that the modern sleep pattern may not be 'natural', but that the human system permits a marked degree of flexibility. To promote good sleep, individuals need to be aware of the demands of the body clock and to keep regular hours, to exercise but to wind down sufficiently before bedtime, and to keep waking activities separate from the sleeping environment.

Waking activities affect sleep, and sleep affects the performance of occupations, but the extent to which sleep problems should be the concern of occupational therapists remains open to debate. Sleep difficulties occur in a wide range of conditions commonly seen by occupational therapists and a greater knowledge of sleep science and of simple measures to improve sleep could be of great benefit to patients and clients. If occupational therapists consider it their role to advise on lifestyle, it would be essential to take account of the part that sleep plays in maintaining balance. From the point of view of occupational science, since it affects performance and occupies so much of our time, sleep appears to be an important and fascinating area for research.

Acknowledgements

Thanks are due to Dr Sue Wilson, Senior Research Fellow at the Psychopharmacology Unit of the University of Bristol, for technical advice.

References

Alford C, Wilson S (2008) Effects of hypnotics on sleep and quality of life in insomnia. In: JC Verster, SR Pandi-Perumal, D Streiner, eds. *Sleep and quality of life in medical illnesses.* Totowa, NJ: Humana Press, ch. 7.

Aubin G, Hachey R, Mercier C (1999) Meaning of daily activities and subjective quality of life in people with severe mental illness. *Scandinavian Journal of Occupational Therapy, 6*(2), 53–62.

Benloucif S, Orbeta L, Oritz R, Janssen I, Finkel SI, Bleiberg J, Zee PC (2004) Morning or evening activity improves neuropsychological performance and subjective sleep quality in older adults. *Sleep 27*(8), 1542–51.

Beresford S, Hill G (1996) Motor neurone disease. In: A Turner, M Foster, SE Johnson, eds. *Occupational therapy and physical dysfunction: principles, skills and practice.* 4th ed. Edinburgh: Churchill Livingstone, 481–96.

Blesedell Crepeau E, Cohn ES, Boyt Schell BA, eds (2003) *Willard and Spackman's occupational therapy.* 10th ed. Philadelphia, PA: Lippincott Williams and Wilkins.

Bonnet MH, Arand DL (1997) Hyperarousal and insomnia. *Sleep Medicine Reviews, 1*(2), 97–108.

Borbely AAF, Achermann P (1999) Sleep homeostasis and models of sleep regulation. *Journal of Biological Rhythms, 14*(6), 557–68.

Cannon J (2007) *Cathedral.* London: Constable.

Cara E, MacRae A (2005) *Psychosocial occupational therapy: a clinical practice.* 2nd ed. Clifton Park, NY: Thomson Delmar Learning.

Carskadon MA, Dement WC (2005) Normal human sleep: an overview. In: MH Kryger, T Roth, WC Dement, eds. *Principles and practice of sleep medicine.* 4th ed. Philadelphia, PA: Elsevier Saunders, 13–23.

Chapman RMcC (1924) The control of sleeplessness. *American Journal of Psychiatry, 3,* 491–502.

Christiansen CH (1996) Three perspectives on balance in occupation. In: R Zemke, F Clark, eds. *Occupational science: the evolving discipline.* Philadelphia, PA: FA Davis, 431–51.

Christiansen CH, Baum CM (1997) Understanding occupation: definitions and concepts. In: CH Christiansen, CM Baum, eds. *Occupational therapy: enabling function and wellbeing.* 2nd ed. Thorofare, NJ: Slack, 3–25.

Christiansen CH, Baum CM (2005) The complexity of human occupation. In: CH Christiansen, CM Baum, J Bass-Haugen, eds. *Occupational therapy: performance, participation and well being.* 3rd ed. Thorofare, NJ: Slack, 2–23.

Christiansen CH, Matuska KM (2006) Lifestyle balance: a review of concepts and research. *Journal of Occupational Science, 13*(1), 49–61.

Christiansen CH, Townsend EA (2004) An introduction to occupation. In: CH Christiansen, EA Townsend, eds. *An introduction to occupation: the art and science of living.* Upper Saddle River, NJ: Prentice Hall, 1–27.

Christiansen CH, Clark FA, Kielhofner G, Rogers J (1995) Position paper: Occupation. *American Journal of Occupational Therapy, 49*(10), 1015–18.

Clark EA, Parham D, Carlson ME, Frank G, Jackson J, Pierce D, Wolfe RJ, Zemke R (1991) Occupational science: academic innovation in the service of occupational therapy's future. *American Journal of Occupational Therapy, 45*(4), 300-310. http://dx.doi.org/10.5014/ajot/45.4.300

Cooper J (2002) Oncology. In: A Turner, M Foster, SE Johnson, eds. *Occupational therapy and physical dysfunction: principles, skills and practice.* 5th ed. Edinburgh: Churchill Livingstone, 565–80.

Cox DL (2000) *Occupational therapy and chronic fatigue syndrome.* London: Whurr.

Creek J (1990) *Occupational therapy and mental health: principles, skills and practice.* Edinburgh: Churchill Livingstone.

Duncan M (2005) Occupational therapy with anxiety and somatoform disorders. In: R Crouch, V Alers, eds. *Occupational therapy in psychiatry and mental health.* London: Whurr, 425–58.

Ekirch AR (2005) *At day's close: a history of nighttime.* London: Phoenix.

Farnworth L (2004) Time use and disability. In: M Molineux, ed. *Occupation for occupational therapists.* Oxford: Blackwell, 46–65.

Finlay L (2004) *The practice of psychosocial occupational therapy.* 3rd ed. Cheltenham: Nelson Thornes.

Fisher AG (1998) Uniting practice and theory in an occupational framework: 1998 Eleanor Clark Slagle Lecture. *American Journal of Occupational Therapy, 52*(7), 509–21. http://dx.doi.org/10.5014/ajot/52.7.509

Golledge J (1998) Distinguishing between occupation, purposeful activity and activity, part 1: review and explanation. *British Journal of Occupational Therapy, 61*(3), 100–105.

Green A, Hicks J, Weekes R, Wilson S (2005) A cognitive–behavioural group intervention for people with chronic insomnia: an initial evaluation. *British Journal of Occupational Therapy, 68*(11), 518–22.

Hagedorn R (1995) *Occupational therapy: perspectives and processes.* Edinburgh: Churchill Livingstone.

Hammond A, Jefferson P (2002) Rheumatoid arthritis. In: A Turner, M Foster, SE Johnson, eds. *Occupational therapy and physical dysfunction: principles, skills and practice.* 5th ed. Edinburgh: Churchill Livingstone, 543–64.

Hardy T (1974) *The return of the native.* London: Macmillan. (Originally published in 1878.)

Hasselkus BR (2002) *The meaning of everyday occupation.* Thorofare, NJ: Slack.

Howell D, Pierce D (2000) Exploring the forgotten restorative dimension of occupation: quilting and quilt use. *Journal of Occupational Science, 7*(2), 68–72.

Keenan B (1992) *An evil cradling.* London: Random House.

Kelly SJ (2002) Spinal disorder (back pain). In: A Turner, M Foster, SE Johnson, eds. *Occupational therapy and physical dysfunction: principles, skills and practice.* 5th ed. Edinburgh: Churchill Livingstone, 523–42.

Kielhofner G (1995) Introduction. In: G Kielhofner, ed. *A model of human occupation: theory and application.* 2nd ed. Baltimore, MD: Williams and Wilkins, 1–7.

Kielhofner G (2002) Introduction to the model of human occupation. In: G Kielhofner, ed. *A model of human occupation: theory and application.* 3rd ed. Baltimore, MD: Lippincott Williams and Wilkins, 1–12.

Kielhofner G, Burke JP (1985) Components and determinants of human occupation. In: G Kielhofner, ed. *A model of human occupation: theory and application.* Baltimore, MD: Williams and Wilkins, 12–36.

King JC (1992) Cardiac rehabilitation. In: A Turner, M Foster, SE Johnson, eds. *Occupational therapy and physical dysfunction: principles, skills and practice.* 3rd ed. Edinburgh: Churchill Livingstone, 763–78.

Kupych-Woloshyn N, MacFarlane J, Shapiro CM (1993) A group approach for the management of insomnia. *Journal of Psychosomatic Research, 37*(Suppl. 1), 39–44.

Larson E, Wood W, Clark F (2003) Occupational science: building the science and practice of occupation through an academic discipline. In: E Blesedell Crepeau, ES Cohn, BA Boyt Schell, eds. *Willard and Spackman's occupational therapy.* 10th ed. Philadelphia, PA: Lippincott Williams and Wilkins.

Levy LL (2005) Cognitive aging in perspective: implications for occupational therapy practitioners. In: N Katz, ed. *Cognition and occupation across the lifespan: models for intervention in occupational therapy.* Bethesda, MD: AOTA Press.

Lougher L (2002) Child and adolescent mental health services. In: J Creek, ed. *Occupational therapy and mental health.* 3rd ed. Edinburgh: Churchill Livingstone, 393–413.

Martin P (2002) *Counting sheep: the science and pleasures of sleep and dreams.* London: Harper Collins.

McHugh Pendleton H, Schultz-Krohn W (2006) *Pedretti's occupational therapy: practice skills for physical dysfunction.* St Louis, MO: Mosby.

Meyer A (1977) The philosophy of occupational therapy. *American Journal of Occupational Therapy, 31*(10), 639–42. (Originally published in 1922.) Reprinted in Chapter 4.

Middleton BF, Arendt JF, Stone BM (1996) Human circadian rhythms in constant light (8 lux) with knowledge of clock time. *Journal of Sleep Research, 5*(2), 69–76.

Molineux M, ed (2004) *Occupation for occupational therapists.* Oxford: Blackwell.

O'Hara P (1996) *Pain management for health professionals.* London: Chapman and Hall.

Persson D, Erlandsson L-K, Eklund M, Iwarsson S (2001) Value dimensions, meaning and complexity in human occupation—a tentative structure for analysis. *Scandinavian Journal of Occupational Therapy, 8*(1), 7–18.

Pierce D (2001) Untangling occupation and activity. *American Journal of Occupational Therapy, 55*(2), 138–46. http://dx.doi.org/10.5014/ajot.55.2.138

Reed KL, Sanderson SN (1999) *Concepts of occupational therapy.* 4th ed. Philadelphia, PA: Lippincott Williams and Wilkins.

Robertson JAF, Broomfield NMF, Espie CA (2007) Prospective comparison of subjective arousal during the pre-sleep period in primary sleep-onset insomnia and normal sleepers. *Journal of Sleep Research, 16*(2), 230–38.

Roenneberg T, Kuehnle T, Juda M, Kantermann T, Allebrandt K, Gordijn M, Merrow M (2007) Epidemiology of the human circadian clock. *Sleep Medicine Reviews, 11*(6), 429–38.

Silcox L (2003) *Occupational therapy and multiple sclerosis.* London: Whurr.

Stepanski EJ, Wyatt JK (2003) Use of sleep hygiene in the treatment of insomnia. *Sleep Medicine Reviews, 7*(3), 213–25.

Stewart P, Craik C (2007) Occupation, mental illness and medium security: exploring time-use in forensic regional secure units. *British Journal of Occupational Therapy, 70*(10), 416–25.

Strong J (1996) *Chronic pain: the occupational therapist's perspective.* Edinburgh: Churchill Livingstone.

Strong J (2002) Lifestyle management. In: J Strong, AM Unruh, A Wright, GD Baxter, eds. *Pain: a textbook for therapists.* Edinburgh: Churchill Livingstone, 289–306.

Van Someren EJW, Riemersma-Van Der Lek RF (2007) Live to the rhythm, slave to the rhythm. *Sleep Medicine Reviews, 11*(6), 465–84.

Weinblatt N, Avrech-Bar MA (2003) Rest: a qualitative exploration of the phenomenon. *Occupational Therapy International, 10*(4), 227–38.

Wehr TA (1996) A 'clock for all seasons' in the human brain. *Progress in Brain Research, 111,* 321–42.

Westhorp P (2003) Exploring balance as a concept in occupational science. *Journal of Occupational Science, 10*(2), 99–106.

Wilcock AA (1998) *An occupational perspective of health.* Thorofare, NJ: Slack.

Wilcock AA (2003) Occupational science: the study of humans as occupational beings. In: P Kramer, J Hinjosa, C Brasic Royeen, eds. *Perspectives in human occupation: participation in life.* Philadelphia, PA: Lippincott Williams and Wilkins, 156–80.

Wilson S (2003) The reasoning behind a good night's sleep. *Nursing and Residential Care, 5*(5), 230–33.

Wilson S, Nutt D (2008) *Sleep disorders.* Oxford: Oxford University Press.

Woods S, Hawkins C (2002) HIV AIDS. In: A Turner, M Foster, SE Johnson, eds. *Occupational therapy and physical dysfunction: principles, skills and practice.* 5th ed. Edinburgh: Churchill Livingstone, 445–75.

Yasuda YL (2008) Rheumatoid arthritis, osteoarthritis and fibromyalgia. In: M Vining Radomski, CA Trombly Latham, eds. *Occupational therapy for physical dysfunction.* 6th ed. Philadelphia, PA: Lippincott Williams and Wilkins, 1214–43.

CHAPTER 19

Exploring Balance as a Concept in Occupational Science

PENELOPE WESTHORP

The notion of balance in life and in occupations is one that continues to intrigue. One reason for this continued interest is the range of physical and mental health, social, relationship, and productivity benefits thought to ensue from a balance of occupations even in the presence of disability. Furthermore, individuals accruing these benefits are believed to have positive effects on others, whether these are life-partners, children, family, social and work associates, and ultimately like spreading ripples, the community and broader society. The notion of balance in occupation is of interest to occupational scientists who are concerned with the ways humans use a variety of occupations to meet the demands of their culture and society, develop skills, achieve satisfaction, and maintain health.

Throughout this article, the terms 'balance in lifestyle' and 'balance in occupations' are taken to be synonymous, referring to the relative importance of, and proportionate amounts of time and energy required by, a daily constellation of occupations. Here the term occupation refers to all activities that are meaningful to the individual, regardless of whether the meaning is positive or negative, or derived from the occupation itself or as a secondary outcome of the activity. For example, work tasks may be perceived as meaningless and unsatisfying, but the fact that one is paid for working gives the occupation meaning.

Developing a Definition of Balance

The Macquarie Dictionary (Delbridge, Bernard, Blair, Peters, & Butler, 1992), defines *balance* as, amongst other things:
- A state of equilibrium or equipoise; equal distribution of weight, amount etc.

This chapter was previously published in the *Journal of Occupational Science, 10*, 99–106. Copyright © 2003, Taylor and Francis. Reprinted with permission.

- Mental steadiness, habit of calm behaviour, judgement etc.
- Harmonious arrangement or adjustment.
- To estimate the relative weight or importance of; compare.
- To arrange adjust or proportion the parts symmetrically.
- To move in rhythm to and from (as in dancing).
- To waver or hesitate.
- To move forwards and backwards, or in opposite directions [as in dancing, to give the sense intended in the Dictionary).

These various definitions are selected purposely by this author, as having relevance to the notion of balancing occupations. (Other definitions in the Dictionary related mainly to financial balancing of accounts, etc.). When applied to occupation, these definitions suggest balance as equipoise, which involves estimating and proportioning all the inputs to, and importance of, components of occupations or complete occupations; achievement through consideration (and hesitation) about judgements to make change in the occupations undertaken; and achieving a harmonious arrangement from which might arise states of calmness, mental steadiness, and improved health and well-being. The conceptualisation of balance as equipoise does not amount to defining it in occupational terms. A working definition of *balance in occupations* still needs to be developed. To begin this process, an exploration of the perspective of various disciplines in relation to balance is presented below.

Perspectives on Balance

The importance of leading a balanced life has been advocated from a variety of perspectives. Primary amongst these are the many religions and philosophies, which, from earliest times to the present day, have recommended a balance of some sort to develop peace, a calm demeanour, a spiritual attitude, an open mind, or a pathway to the godhead. Both Christianity and Buddhism, for instance, advocate seeking a balanced awareness of self within the wider environment, including our relationship with humans, other beings, and the physical and spiritual world (Hanh, 1995). Notions of balance are also evident in early civilisations such as the ancient Greeks, who believed that "illness resulted from imbalance of the four humours, and that a physician's job was to advise on due proportion, to 'restore a healthy balance', and to aid 'the natural healing powers believed to exist in every human being'" (Wilcock, 1998, p. 137, citing Hippocrates). Balancing the humours remained a function of physicians and apothecaries throughout the Middle Ages and beyond, influencing even Machiavelli's world view and political thought in the 1600s (Parel, 1992).

In contemporary educational settings, the value of a balanced education that addresses all or most aspects of a student's life, rather than a focus on pure academics has been stressed. Here the emphasis is on producing a 'balanced person', possessing life skills to respond to a wide variety of occupations. Accordingly early childhood educators (Carter, 1997) and campus activity co-ordinators (Amy & Smith, 1996) have been urged to attend to their own professional development by examining their balance of personal and professional activities. A similar emphasis is found in sociology, focusing this time on the ways people balance the demands of work and family (e.g. Bielby & Bielby, 1989; Spearritt & Edgar, 1994). Key sociological concerns include individual responses to role overload, or role ease or strain (e.g. Marks & MacDermid, 1996); the effect of multiple roles on family and how demands are balanced; and how social structures (eg. institutions and businesses) respond to the competing demands of work and family such as parental leave, maximum working hours, and work overload.

Psychologists have also investigated notions of balance in occupations. Examples include the effect of occupations on affect in the aged (Chang & Dodder, 1985), on work stress and productivity in women (Bean & Wolfman, 1979), and in family power relationships (Maguire, 1999).

Finally, in anthropology, there is a growing interest in how cultures prescribe and constrain roles and occupations. For example, a training manual for early childhood educators working with the first peoples of America indicates that cultural understanding of the roles and balance of activities undertaken by both genders is essential to creating culturally sensitive education for young children of those cultures (Luera, 1994).

Occupational Perspective

An occupational perspective on balance starts from the perspective of humans as occupational beings (Wilcock, 1998) who experience and express their sense of self through occupation. An occupational perspective on balance looks at the effect of occupations and the *balance* of occupations as determinants of health, well-being, and satisfaction. This is complementary to previous perspectives, which have explored the components of occupations such as physical capacity, or mental or social skills as determinants of health. One source from which to investigate an occupational perspective on balance is the literature of occupational therapy, where balance was posited as a central tenet by some of the profession's founders.

Historical Development

Adolph Meyer, an early 20th century psychiatrist, was a member of the group of physicians, architects and social workers who came together in Hull House in Chicago to found a new profession, which later came to be called occupational therapy (Peloquin, 1991; see Chapter 3). Meyer, who had been strongly influenced by the Moral Treatment movement of the late 1800s (Serrett, 1985), advocated a balance between the "big four—work and rest and play and sleep, which our organism must be able to balance even under difficulty" (1922/1977, p. 641; see Chapter 4). Meyer strongly advocated a balance of time allocated to the major areas of occupation (Jonsson, Borrell, & Sadlo, 2000), but he did not stipulate whether this balance indicated equal amounts of time for each.

As the occupational therapy profession developed, the main occupations with which occupational therapists were concerned became work (or productivity), play/leisure and self-care activities (Reed & Sanderson, 1992). It was an early assumption of this predominantly white, Western profession that patients with illness or disability needed to have personal independence in each of these areas. For many patients, the goal of independence could not be reconciled with balanced use of time and energy. They struggled to achieve independence in one or two areas (often self-care) at the cost of their total reserves of time and energy. With improved technology and changes in social and health policy, that made paid assistance available, it became possible to purchase assistance and preserve time and energy for desired rather than obligatory activities. Thus, balance came to be seen as balance between occupations Reed and Sanderson's (1992) basic text in occupational therapy, illustrates this change in thinking:

> A balance of occupations is facilitatory to the maintenance of health and a satisfying life. A person who manages to perform or have performed those occupations that facilitate health maintenance, provide for basic needs and permit leisure pursuits is more likely to achieve a state of health than a person who does not. Balance does not imply an equal amount of time in self-maintenance, productivity and leisure, but does imply some time on a regularly occurring basis. (p. 75)

As occupational therapy moved to considering a wider range of both macro- and micro-cultures, it became apparent that the division of occupations into work, play/leisure, and self-care did not apply to all people. Some cultures do not discriminate between work and play/leisure, and even within Western culture, the divisions may not apply to children, or people who are unemployed, retired, ill, or disabled (Wilcock, 1998). In fact, even for those whose occupations do span work, play/leisure, and self-care, it could be argued that this is an incomplete coverage of the occupations between which balance may be sought. For instance, it is not clear how spiritual, social, relationship and sexual occupations might be included in the balance. Furthermore, the notion of occupational balance has not been well researched by occupational therapists. Indeed, one of the most respected texts in occupational therapy defines occupational balance as "a belief, not substantiated by research, that a general configuration of daily occupations can contribute to health and well being" (Christiansen & Baum, 1997, p. 592).

Contemporary Occupational Perspective of Balance

A more recent occupational perspective of balance in life specifies balance in the use and development of capabilities (Wilcock, 1998). That is, people need to exercise their physical, mental, social, emotional, and spiritual capabilities in proportions that are satisfying and health promoting, and entirely individual. In addi-

tion, Wilcock (1998) indicates that "a balance between and within intrinsic and extrinsic factors appears to be a key concept in achieving health and well-being" (p. 137). Intrinsic factors are those within the individual, such as drives, talents and motivations, while extrinsic factors are opportunities or barriers in the environment that affect the development of capacities. These may range from factors in the local environment right through to the kind of economy and social policies a region or country has.

This balance of capabilities perspective is perhaps related to psychologist Csikszentmihalyi's (1993) concept of flow. Flow is a highly engaging, pleasurable mental state which occurs when the person's capabilities are fully engaged in a challenging occupation. Occupations in which we experience flow are those that develop and engage a wide range of capacities, which psychologists in flow research and occupational scientists assert is health enhancing. It may be that one of the characteristics of a well-balanced life is when a broad range of capabilities are engaged and developed through occupation, and our choice of occupations provides sufficient experiences of flow to maximise good health and well-being (Csikszentmihalyi, 1993, p. 41), even in the presence of disability (Wilcock, 1998, p. 105).

This idea needs further development, as it is also possible for flow to be experienced in occupations usually deemed unhealthy, such as in war and delinquency. Such activities do not usually result in health and well-being, at least in the long term. My contention here is that while these activities can be fully engaging, they require the suspension of judgement that these occupations are likely to be dangerous or deleterious. That is, the capacity for judgement and self-preserving action based on judgement is not fully engaged in these occupations, which renders the individual fully vulnerable to their negative effects.

Sociological, Community, and Adult Education Perspectives

Sociologists Marks and MacDermid (1996) have applied the notion of balance to peoples' social roles, asserting that people experience role balance when they have "a set of *equally positive* commitments to all of their typical roles" (emphasis added). In their 1996 article, Marks reflected on some of his earlier works, where he had hypothesised that people exercising such role balance would experience salutary health and well-being consequences. He suggested that role balance might lead to a state of role ease, even when very busy, as compared to the role strain that might arise from hierarchically prioritised roles. This balanced state of equally positive and equally prioritised commitment to each role and its occupations was later described as giving rise to a state of mindfulness (Marks & MacDermid, 1996). Being fully present and committed to each role and its occupations as they occur does not, however, eliminate the necessity of choosing which competing demands can be met. However, once the decision to be fully present in carrying out that choice is made, it leads to a feeling of being focussed, aware, and relaxed, rather than carrying on the familiar debate about what one "should really" be doing or what is coming next. This leads to the state of inner balance and tranquillity, and can be thought of as a product of Marks and MacDermid's role balance.

So far, this discussion has considered balance in lifestyle to be the province of the individual. However, occupational scientists, sociologists and adult educators alike indicate that balance is a concept that applies equally well from the cellular level to the community, state and national level. At the cellular level, balanced nutrition contributes to being able to balance over time the demands for energy, and for repair and regeneration of tissues, as well as balancing the incursions of disease organisms with immune system responses (Wilcock, 1998).

The health of a group or community may be a product of its ability to support its members' involvement in a healthy balance of occupations. The balance involves not only the range of occupations, but also the level of demand in those occupations. Most of us are familiar with the poor health indices of communities with high levels of unemployment, which from an occupational perspective may be attributed to an imbalance in the opportunities to develop capabilities. In contrast, Wilcock (1988, p. 144) gives examples from several researchers of the deleterious health effects of overwork, that is work which that is too demanding, for which there is not compensatory rest and recreation, or that is carried out in harmful environments, both psychological and physical. From an occupational perspective, overwork is just as imbalanced as under-work. There are few opportunities to develop the full range of capabilities, and an over-reliance on the use of just a few. These negative work states exist across both economically advantaged and disadvantaged countries. Wilcock goes on to suggest that "community disease" (p. 145) is an outcome of "imbalances in health opportunities through occupation throughout the community, be-

tween the haves and the have nots, between the rich and the poor, between the informed and illiterate, and between the employed and the unemployed" (p. 144).

At the social level, Clements (2000), a community based adult educator, describes a theory of balance as a way of creating social change within a community education context. She describes how she attempted to use community education to create social change by working with the disempowered to challenge those who had control. However, this only left vacuums in which new controls emerged. A second approach attempted to make social change by pursuing freedom, but this only highlighted other areas of "unfreedom" (p. 6). Finally, she pursued a balanced approach to facilitating social change, which achieved the desired results. Her concept of balance is evident in her assertion that:

> When the people involved in these interactions (ones of oppression/s) respect the whole person, they can focus on bringing balance into the relationship in a way in which both sides benefit. The whole interaction moves into balance. The same dynamic occurs in the relationship between groups. (p. 16)

Clements (2000) has also acknowledged the need to be cognisant of the full range of human capacities, in a balanced manner, in order to achieve social change:

> When a holistic approach is adopted, the human ability to empathise, physical abilities and spiritual aspects are as important as intellectual abilities. The integration of parts within a focus on balance applies at all levels from the intercellular to the historical, global level. Whether the imbalance occurs over minutes or centuries, at an atomic or a global level, the dynamics are the same. Tension is created which creates oppression/s until released. It is in everyone's interest to correct imbalances. (p. 19)

Clements describes her concept of balance in relationships and social change by describing its three main characteristics: holism, interconnectedness and the dynamic day-to-day quality.

Holism

Holism is defined by Clements (2000) as non-dualistic. This can be understood to mean *not* attempting to find a balance between two extremes, as this would maintain dualism. Sociologist Ellen Galinsky, president of the Families and Work Institute in the USA, when addressing the same issue, is reported as saying "the term 'balancing' work and family life is part of the problem. 'Balancing implies an either/or situation—a scale where if one side is up, the other side is down. It is a win/lose seesaw'" (Gunn, 2001). Instead, Clements defines holism as inclusive, containing everything we already know, and all that we do not know as well.

Clements (2000) also discusses holism in relationships between those seeking change and those holding the power to change. She adds:

> Social change workers who focus on balance. do not establish an 'enemy' in the form of an oppressor and set out to take control of others. Rather they acknowledge common humanity and differences. They encourage the development of structures and relationships which do not acknowledge one side as superior to the other, or as being entitled to more resources or participation than the other. (p. 18)

Interconnectedness

Clements indicates this characteristic of balance is nearly inseparable from holism (p.19). Entering into interconnectedness and a sense of community requires us to understand and be tolerant of the many conflicting roles and demands that people juggle, which means being cognisant of the occupational load and state of balance under which others are working. A study of the role strain felt by adult women university students (Home, 1998) suggested that women with three major roles (home, work and study) are most at risk of role strain. The competing demands of the university (study) and the family were the most difficult to manage, as both were seen as "greedy institutions [which] demand constant availability, exclusive loyalty and high flexibility" (p.93). Work was less difficult to deal with, as its demands could be contained within the time at work. Single motherhood, having a pre-adolescent youngest child, and low income were the most statistically significant factors in predicting those with the greatest role strain.

The occupational perspective on interconnectedness would be highly compatible with the views of Home (1998). Interconnectedness also can be seen in the mesh and balance of our activities, which not only affect ourselves and our well-being but interact with the occupations of others around us and impact on the environment. For example, the materials we choose for our activities need to be considered not only for their cost-effectiveness, but also for their environmental cost, and impact on production and waste disposal.

Balance as a Dynamic Process

Clements' (2000) view of change achieved through a focus on balance sees change occurring in small incremental movements, as individuals seek a balanced harmony in everyday activities and choices. It is the dynamic state of balance that is being sought. It is important to remember that the only time when a balancing system is stable is when a state of total imbalance is achieved. Consider a lever balancing on a fulcrum or a spinning plate balancing on a stick; stability is only achieved when balance is totally lost. Balance on the other hand, is only achieved when the system is in dynamic interaction. Thus to achieve a balance in our lives we must seek dynamic interaction and change at all levels, attempting always to bring all elements into balance to produce an optimally health enhancing state. Any one component that changes will induce change in all other components as they adjust.

Many of us seek to establish stability by using routines and repetition—for example, in our diet, our daily workload, and our family commitments. However, we are all familiar with how easily one small change can have a cascade effect throughout our lives. It is the flexibility to respond to and manage these changes which leads to a state of healthy balance in occupations.

Epidemiological Perspective

Recent research in Western cultures has indicated that control over one's life is the single most significant factor in determining health and well-being (Bosma et al., 1997; Marmot, 1998; Marmot & Bosma, 1997; Syme & Balfour, 1997). The critical features seem to be:

- The balance between the demands made on the person (by work or home life etc) and their control over how they meet those demands, and
- The balance between the effort put into meeting demands and the rewards gained from the effort, in terms of financial reward, social status and self-esteem (Wilkinson & Marmot, 1998).

There is mounting evidence that these factors contribute significantly to the rates of illness and mortality in occupational groups when other contributing factors (age, height [as a marker of nutritional status), and known individual risk factors for disease) are accounted for (Mastering the control factor, 1998). These findings cut across governmental boundaries, influencing the social policy of countries in Europe in such diverse areas as health, education, ergonomics, social support, unemployment, workplace management, food production and distribution, transport, and civil design (Wilkinson & Marmot, 1998).

From an occupational perspective, this raises vital and interesting questions. At what level is control to be sought? Is it control over one's choice of actions within tasks within occupations; or the choice of tasks; or is control sought over the choice of occupational categories, such as between productivity/leisure/self care, or between desired and obligatory occupations? Or is control not only in the choice of action, but also in the sequencing, level of detail or speed of completion? Resolving these questions would help all disciplines interested in occupational science to more finely focus their efforts on determining their areas of interest, research, and intervention.

Synthesising an Occupational Perspective on Balance

To summarise then, I suggest that an occupational perspective indicates that a balanced lifestyle, which is more likely to be one in which health and well-being are experienced, may be one in which:

- Individuals can determine the range occupations in which they engage
- Individuals can determine the amounts of time, energy, and other resources that are put into these occupations
- Individual's determination of inputs and desired outcomes will vary from day to day in response to environmental demands, skill development and motivation
- Individuals have opportunities to engage and develop their full range of capabilities across their chosen meaningful occupations
- Individuals experience flow frequently enough to also experience its health giving consequences
- Understanding the issues of occupational load and role strain/ease leads to better management of self and tolerance of others who are having difficulty managing these issues
- Individuals can appreciate the effects of their occupations in a web of interconnectedness with others, including their effect on the environment, social policy and group dynamics

- A continuous process of dynamic balance, usually by small increments, is maintained in the face of continuous changes, and
- Individuals have appropriate levels of control over their actions and, for the effort made receive adequate recognition, such as financial reward, social status, and/or self-esteem.

What Are We Trying to Keep in Balance?

The discussion above indicates that the concept of balance is very broad. In this article, it is suggested that one way in which balance is be addressed is in the expression and development of our capabilities through engagement in a wide range of individually meaningful occupations that promote health and well-being. What exactly constitutes a balance of occupations will vary for each individual. The choices made by individuals in relation to such engagement impact on others around them and on the environment, eventually and collectively resonating throughout families, networks, groups, communities and the larger society. The concept implies having some control over apportioning our capabilities (mental, physical, social, emotional, and spiritual) and our resources (time, energy, money, and material) to engagement in occupations that will maintain and promote health and well-being for ourselves, others, and the environment.

The daily apportioning is a dynamic process, always open to influence by factors outside our control, and we respond to such changes by the application of our will and effort, to maintain the fluctuations within boundaries within which we are both comfortable and healthy. Each adjustment of the apportioning of capabilities and resources will resonate throughout our personal system, requiring other adjustments to maintain the dynamic balance.

The accretion of such balancing activities amongst individuals leads to a similar state of dynamic balance for families, groups, networks, communities, and society. Such systems are interdependent. Through their actions, occupationally balanced and healthy individuals give rise to occupationally balanced and healthy groups and societies, and vice versa.

The consequences of a balanced lifestyle are most often discussed in terms of the effects of long lasting imbalance. Wilcock (1998, pp. 137–145) discusses imbalance as a risk factor for ill health for both individuals and communities. Negative outcomes of imbalanced use of capabilities are postulated to effect all levels of functioning, including cellular activity, physical fitness, higher order mental functions, and the capacity to meet "high end" needs/drives for satisfaction, meaning and purpose in life in the individual. Wilcock, also postulates the circular effects of occupational structures in society (such as workplaces, schools and leisure resources) and the policies underpinning these. These create occupational environments that affect health and well-being on a continuum ranging from healthy to unhealthy. In these various environments, it is respectively either easier or harder for individuals to achieve and maintain occupational balance. In turn, individuals who are occupationally balanced strive to create occupationally balanced institutions and policies, whereas those who are unaware of balance will focus on only a few elements and reinforce an unbalanced society.

How Is Balance to Be Achieved?

This discussion of balance sounds ideal, in the sense of a goal for which we should all strive. It also sounds very idealistic, in the sense of naivety. In the world of ever increasing demand, how can we achieve and maintain that dynamic balanced state for ourselves and the groups to which we belong?

I propose that there is a cycle by which occupational balance may be achieved. Perhaps the first require-

ment for achieving balance is a state of watchfulness, of monitoring what is health-promoting and valuable in our lives and what is not (see Figure 19.1). Wilcock (1998) refers to *watchfulness* as a period of time in animal behaviour where physical activity is low, resting between other occupations, but alertness and monitoring of the environment is high (p. 142). She suggests that such watchful behaviour in humans may manifest as passive recreational activities such as television watching, which may be necessary time for reflection and learning about the world (although she cites Kubey and Csikszentmihalyi [1990] who found it rated as not very satisfying in itself).

Having monitored our occupations and the use of our capabilities and resources to determine what is best for achieving and continuing a healthy life, the next step is to decide on the balance required. I believe this can only be decided after reflection about our values, requiring judgement on a moment by moment basis about what is of most value—obligatory or desired activity, rest, recreation, work, self-care, or a change in the use of capabilities and resources. Reflecting and deciding upon our use of capabilities and resources requires the identification of values.

It seems to me that one of the greatest skills for achieving balance is in the fine determination of when to say *yes* or *no*. Sometimes the choice of whether to say *yes* or *no* to an occupational activity is easy, when what

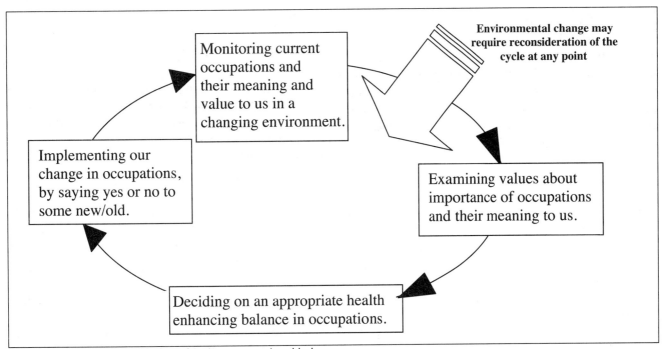

Figure 19.1. Proposed cycle for achieving occupational balance.

Text in figure:
- Monitoring current occupations and their meaning and value to us in a changing environment.
- Environmental change may require reconsideration of the cycle at any point
- Implementing our change in occupations, by saying yes or no to some new/old.
- Examining values about importance of occupations and their meaning to us.
- Deciding on an appropriate health enhancing balance in occupations.

is going to be given up in order to engage in a particular occupation is of little value to us. But sometimes the choice is very difficult, when the decision is between two occupations of equal value, or between two outcomes with very different natures. My own encapsulation of this dilemma is "there are no choices without losses". It is the decision about what one is prepared to lose or give up which is critical.

Saying no to something habitual, expected or highly valued by others can be extremely difficult. Saying no to these in order to make space for something else that may be valued by us and others as frivolous can be even more difficult, even though we know it may be more health promoting. Making the choice exposes some deeply held values. Is it more important to be working hard, or to be looking after ourselves by 'indulging' in rest or recreation? In Western culture, work is valued extraordinarily highly, and looking after ourselves may seem self-indulgent, which is generally viewed as a negative.

Equally, the challenge to say yes to some new activity or challenge also exposes values. Is it more health promoting to stay within the established safe routine of occupations, or is it more important to attempt growth and change in a previously under-challenged capability?

Further into the dynamic cycle of reflection, judgement and decision comes the hard work of implementation. Implementing our decisions may well require us to give up some of our established patterns of obligatory and desired occupations. For most of us, obligation is a powerful determinant of the use of capabilities in occupations. We are contracted to work, or obliged to render care or we accept responsibilities that have inherent timelines. It is all too easy to go on accepting obligations until there is no more flexibility in our occupational system, until we have lost all our discriminatory leeway in terms of our capacities and/or our resources.

The notion of implementing a balanced use of capabilities within occupations is inclusive. Very often when we think about balancing our lives, we think in terms of exclusion. What will we have to take away, to leave a balanced remainder? But an attitude of inclusion, "how many good things can I include, in sufficient degree to be good for me?" may be more health promoting. It will still require reflection on our most important values, and the necessity of saying no or losing some current occupations and their meaning for us. However, the attitude of inclusion opens us up to

a richness of experience and potential for well-being which our current pattern of occupations may not. Investigating the accuracy of this postulated cycle for achieving occupational balance, I propose, would contribute to our understanding of how humans may develop a balance in occupations. Having achieved such a balance would allow further exploration of the costs and benefits of the balanced state.

References

Amy, C., & Smith, B. F. (1996). Balancing our personal & professional lives. *Campus Activities Programming, 29*(1), 36–40.

Bean, J. P., & Wolfman, B. R. (1979). *Superwoman: Ms or myth: A study of role overload.* A Report to the National Institute of Education.

Bielby, W. T., & Bielby, D. D. (1989). Family ties: Balancing commitments to work and family in dual earner households. *American Sociological Review, 54*(5), 776–789.

Bosma H., Marmot M. G., Hemingway H., Nicholson A. C., Brunner E., & Stansfeld S. A. (1997). Low job control and risk of coronary heart disease in Whitehall II (prospective cohort) study. *British Medical Journal, 314*(7080), 558–65.

Carter, M. (1997). Nurturing our professional lives. *Child Care Information Exchange, 115*, 59–61.

Chang, R. H., & Dodder, R. A. (1985). Activity and affect among the aged. *Journal of Social Psychology, 125*(1), 127–128.

Christiansen, C. & Baum, C. (Eds.) (1997). *Occupational therapy: Enabling function and well-being.* Thorofare, NJ: Slack.

Clements, E. (2000). The politics of control. the politics of freedom. and the politics of balance: Three ways of creating social change. *New Zealand Journal of Adult Learning, 28*(1), 6–22.

Csikszentmihalyi, M. (1993). Activity and happiness: Towards a science of occupation. *Journal of Occupational Science: Australia, 1*(1) 38–42.

Delbridge, A., Bernard, J., Blair, D., Peters, P., & Butler, S. (1992). *The Macquarie dictionary (2nd ed).* The Macquarie Library, Macquarie University, Australia.

Gunn, M. (2001, May 2). Children reassure parents. *The Australian,* p. 5.

Hanh, T. N. (1995). *Living Buddha, living Christ.* London: Rider.

Home, A. (1998). Predicting role conflict, overload, and contagion in adult women university students with families and jobs. *Adult Education Quarterly, 48*(2), 85–98.

Jonnson, H., Borell, L., & Sadlo, G. (2000). Retirement: An occupational transition with consequences for temporality, balance and meaning of occupations. *Journal of Occupational Science, 7*(1), 29–37.

Luera, M. (1994). *Understanding family uniqueness through cultural diversity Project Ta-kos.* Publisher not given.

Maguire, M. C. (1999). Occupational self-direction, values and egalitarian relationships in dual-earner couples. *Dissertation Abstracts Jnternational: Section B: The Sciences & Engineering. Vol l0*(1-B).

Marks, S. R., & MacDermid, S. M. (1996). Multiple roles and the self: A theory of role balance. *Journal of Marriage & the Family, 58*(2), 417–433.

Marmot M. G. (1998, January 3). Improvement of social environment to improve health. *Lancet, 351*(9095), 57–60.

Marmot, M. G., & Bosma, H. (1997). Contribution of job control and other risk factors to social variations in coronary heart disease incidence. *Lancet, 350*(9073), 235–240.

Mastering the control factor. Parts 1–4. The Health Report with Norman Swan, Radio National, Monday 09–11–98 to 30–11–98. Accessed on line at: http://www.abc.net.au/rn/talks/8.30/helthrpt/stories/s10743.htm Part three on 5–12–98. http://www.abc.net.au/rn/talks/8.30/helthrpt/stories/s14314.htm Part one on 12–11–98. http://w w w.abc.net.au/rn/talks/8.30/helthrpt/stories/s17092.htm Part two on 5–12–98. http://www.abc.net.au/rn/talks/8.30/helthrpt/stories/s17549.htm Part four on 5–12–98.

Meyer, A. (1977). The philosophy of occupational therapy *American Journal of Occupational Therapy 31*(10), 639–642. (Originally published 1922) http://dx.doi.org/10.514/ajot.31.10.639

Parel, A. J. (1992). *The Machiavellian cosmos* New Haven: Yale University Press.

Peloquin, S. M. (1991). Occupational therapy service: Individual and collective understandings of the founders, Part 1. *American Journal of Occupational Therapy, 44*(4), 352–360. Reprinted as Chapter 3.

Reed, K., & Sanderson, S. (1992). *Concepts of occupational therapy (3rd ed.).* Baltimore: Williams & Wilkins.

Serrett, K. D. (1985). Another look at occupational therapy's history: Paradigm or pair of hands? *Occupational Therapy in Mental Health, 5*(3), 1–31.

Spearritt, K., & Edgar, D. (1994). *The family friendly front: A review of Australian and international work and family research.* Melbourne: National Key Centre for Industrial Relations, Monash University.

Syme, S. L., & Balfour, J. L. (1997). Explaining inequalities in coronary heart disease. *Lancet, 350*(9073), 231–233.

Wilcock, A. A. (1998). *An occupational perspective of health.* Thorofare, NJ: Slack.

Wilkinson, R., & Marmot, M. (1998). *Social determinants of health: The solid facts.* World Health Organisation. Accessed online at http://www.who.dk/document/e59555.pdf on 10–01–02.

CHAPTER 20

Balancing the Boat: Enabling an Ocean of Possibilities

ANNETTE MAJNEMER

This year's conference theme for the annual Canadian Association of Occupational Therapists [CAOT] meeting in Halifax (May 26–29, 2010) was "Meaningful occupation: Enabling an ocean of possibilities." As occupational therapists, we make it possible for individuals with functional challenges to choose, plan and perform the occupations that are most meaningful and relevant to them. The ocean is deep and vast; the possibilities are endless. Working in partnership with our clients, we consider the vast expanse of possibilities, weighing the options and providing solutions that will promote their personal autonomy and well-being. Intrinsic with our holistic approach, we must "balance their boat" to ensure that they are stable and can meet the challenges of their meaningful occupations, as they journey through life.

Balancing the Boat: Importance of Leisure

"A boat cannot move very well in the water if it's unbalanced, if it's not stable. If it's a sailboat, it may be leaning over in the wind, but to proceed, it still must somehow be in equilibrium. The same is true for us" (Sloman, 1997). Work–life balance is a broad concept that entails prioritization between work on one hand and other life experiences (e.g., leisure, family and spiritual) on the other. We take on many occupational roles and responsibilities, such as parent, spouse, caregiver of elderly relatives, friend, teacher, or community volunteer. These many different roles compete for our time and most adults experience overload. Over the last decade, this competition has been exacerbated by greater accessibility through technologies such as

This chapter was previously published in the *Canadian Journal of Occupational Therapy, 77*, 198–208. Copyright © 2010, Canadian Association of Occupational Therapists. Reprinted with permission.

email, cell phone, and teleconferencing. Although there is no "just right" proportion of work and play needed to achieve the right balance, it is important that we feel that our personal aspirations and interests in all life occupations are fulfilled. Achieving appropriate work-life balance implies having equilibrium among the many priorities in our life. Unfortunately, it is common to feel stressed and out of balance, particularly if we put most of our efforts and attention to the "must-do" activities (Canadian Mental Health Association, 2010).

Leisure activities provide freedom from the demands of work or duty, where we can rest, restore our energy, and enjoy particular hobbies or sports ("Leisure," n.d.). Leisure is the "free time" that we spend outside of work (or school) and essential domestic and self-care activities, and these activities can be differentiated as being discretionary ("would like to do") rather than compulsory ("must do"). Choice is an important defining attribute of leisure (Cassidy, 1996). As occupational therapists, we need to appreciate how meaningful and valuable these leisure activities are, and in particular, how these activities make individuals feel. Leisure activities provide us with opportunities for relaxation, enjoyment, amusement and self-expression (Jonsson & Persson, 2006; Turner, Chapman, McSherry, Krishnagiri, & Watts, 2000). Choosing and participating in leisure activities are health-promoting, enabling us to experience pleasure, rejuvenation, personal identity and autonomy (Imms, 2008). The key ingredients of leisure identified by adolescents include activities that are enjoyable and fun, and there is the freedom of choice and sense of control. Whether achieving new skills, socializing with friends or just relaxing, leisure activities provide adolescents with opportunities to enhance self-worth and self-efficacy, improve skill competencies and social acceptance, and offer time for reflection or escape from stressors (Passmore & French, 2003).

Leisure and Occupational Therapy Practice

Occupations include all the activities that we do in our daily lives. As occupational therapists, we focus on occupational engagement in self-care, work, study, volunteerism and leisure (CAOT, 2010; Townsend, 2002). Designation of occupations within the performance domains of productivity, self-care and leisure may be argued as overly simplistic, as these domains may not adequately capture all occupations important for our well-being (Hammell, 2009). Nonetheless, it highlights that leisure comprises one of the essential spheres of life experience and thus, is important for occupational therapists. As part of enabling engagement in everyday life through occupation, participation in leisure activities is critical in fostering health and well-being and community integration (Townsend & Polatajko, 2007). Therefore, leisure participation is, or at least should be, an integral part of occupational therapy practice.

In occupational therapy practice, there is a preoccupation with the necessary "must do" occupations to include promoting independence in personal care and domestic activities of daily living, and maximizing productivity at work or school. But applying a holistic approach, are we truly considering all the occupations that are important to the individual's well-being? Do individuals that we provide services to perceive that they have achieved an optimal balance in their life; given the challenges their health condition or disability imposes upon them? Do we actually "go there"?

Two recent studies suggest that practicing occupational therapists are not "going there." A survey was conducted in Quebec with occupational therapists and physical therapists that provide services to young children with cerebral palsy (CP). As part of a telephone interview, several case vignettes of preschoolers with different patterns and severity of motor impairment were presented and therapists were asked to indicate the assessment and treatment approaches they would use. Although most used at least one standardized assessment tool, the assessment focused predominantly on impairments and particular activity limitations (self-care, mobility). For assessment or intervention, little emphasis was placed on play and leisure, social integration, family or environmental factors (Saleh et al., 2008). A second study specifically determined leisure assessment practices of occupational therapists in different settings, with either an adolescent or adult clientele. This telephone survey included 105 therapists

from three states in the USA, with 15 also participating in face-to-face interviews. Only 5% used formal methods (12% used a mixture of formal and informal) to evaluate leisure performance which could have included checklists or other non-standardized tools. Formal assessment of the leisure domain was related to how much the therapist valued these occupations. When assessed, the information about leisure performance or preference was primarily used to guide selection of activities to work on component skills or as a motivator for therapy; only about 10% either adapted leisure activities to the client's functional status or prioritized goals to include leisure interests (Turner et al., 2000). Last fall (2009) in class at McGill University, I asked my occupational therapy students (Masters level) to estimate the percentage of clients that were formally evaluated in the leisure domain in their summer rotations, which included a wide range of practice settings and clientele. The estimation was done confidentially using "clickers," with the distribution appearing on the screen. Unfortunately, 65% indicated that none of their clients were formally evaluated in the leisure domain, 24% indicated that few (<10%) or some clients (10-25%) were, and only 12% specified that most (>75%) were.

A holistic approach to occupational therapy practice implies that we conscientiously consider all occupational performance domains relevant to the health and functioning of an individual. My concern is that for many practicing therapists, leisure activities are only superficially considered, if at all; the "tip of the iceberg" so to speak. If we are to be effective in "balancing the boat" of our clientele, we have the responsibility of ensuring that individuals we service have safe, successful and enjoyable voyages to the destinations of their choosing. Therefore, this process involves attention to maintaining the boat (self-care), getting the boat to its intended destination (productivity) and ensuring an enjoyable ride (leisure).

Promoting Health in Children and Youth: Role of Leisure Participation

Promoting healthy living, in spite of a chronic health condition or disability, is an emerging, important preoccupation of occupational therapists. The World Health Organization [WHO] defines *health* as a state of complete physical, mental and social well-being and not merely the absence of disease or illness. For children and youth, health-promoting activities and experiences have been strongly endorsed by the WHO Global Strategy on Diet, Physical Activity and Health (WHO, 2010), Canada's Healthy Living Strategy (Secretariat for the Intersectoral Healthy Living Network, 2005), and a variety of position papers by the Canadian Pediatric Society (Advisory Committee on Healthy Active Living for Children and Youth, 2002) and the American Academy of Pediatrics (n.d.). Participation in leisure activities is a component of health, as framed by the *International Classification of Functioning, Disability and Health (ICF)* and is incorporated within "community, social and civic life" (WHO, 2007).

Health promotion initiatives are meant to support physical health and mental health, and augment one's ability to enjoy life by facing challenges, interacting socially, regulating emotions and finding meaning and purpose in life (WHO, 2008). There is a burgeoning literature demonstrating that participation in physical activity is associated with substantial physical health benefits including decreasing risk for latent cardiovascular disease, obesity, diabetes, osteoporosis, and even cancers. Engagement in leisure activities, more broadly defined, also has important benefits for mental health and well-being. Leisure participation can relieve stress and anxiety and has a restorative ability on the body and mind, contributing to emotional well-being. Furthermore, the ability to pursue preferred leisure activities that are highly valued and meaningful contributes to identity formation, achievement motivation and the possibility of creative expression. For children and youth, these contributions are particularly valuable for their development of self-worth and self-efficacy. Involvement in different leisure activities provides opportunities to experience social connections with family, friends and the community at large (Calfas & Taylor, 1994; Cassidy, 1996; Giada et al., 2008; Groff, Lundberg, & Zabriskie, 2009; Hammell, 2004; Harrison & Narayan, 2003; Melzer, Kayser, & Pichard, 2004).

Participation in leisure activities is vital to the growth and development of children and youth. Engagement in preferred leisure activities enhances particular skill competencies, fosters friendships with peers, facilitates refinement of personal interests and identity, and provides opportunities to explore new roles. Leisure participation is particularly important at schoolage and adolescence, as children gain greater autonomy from their parents and make more choices (King et al., 2006; Majnemer, 2009; McConachie, Colver, Forsyth, Jarvis, & Parkinson, 2006). Children with disabilities are at greater risk for poor physical and mental health, and

concomitantly, for decreased involvement in leisure activities. For children and youth with physical disabilities, physical inactivity over time promotes a cycle of deconditioning, whereby there is a gradual decline in physical functioning. There are clear benefits of physical activity and other leisure activities in promoting physiological and psychological health in children and youth with disabilities, and therefore should be actively endorsed (Maher, Williams, Olds, & Lane, 2007; Rice & the Council on Sports Medicine and Fitness, 2008; Thorpe, 2009). These health benefits also extend to their whole family. Sharing leisure occupations helps balance other preoccupations with caregiving tasks, and provides shared meaning, cohesiveness and happiness. Family leisure routines can augment the positive effects of having a child with a disability (Downs, 2008; Mactavish et al., 2005; Mactavish & Schleien, 2004; Taanila, Jarvelin, & Kokkonen, 1999).

Leisure Participation in Children With Disabilities: Lessons Learned

On the surface, leisure participation appears to be a transparent and straightforward concept, much like the clear blue ocean. However, it is only when we gaze beyond the surface and we delve into the waters, that we begin to see the "ocean of possibilities," both in terms of the extent and nature of leisure opportunities, but also, the complexity and diversity of factors that can positively or negatively influence participation in leisure occupations. There is a growing body of evidence on participation in leisure activities in children and youth with disabilities. The preponderance of studies has focused on children with physical disabilities, especially cerebral palsy. However, there is a paucity of studies addressing this issue in children with other developmental disabilities or mental health conditions, and should be a focus of future research efforts. My comments below draw largely from this recent literature on leisure participation and from studies we are conducting on children (6–12 years) and adolescents (in progress) with cerebral palsy.

Lesson #1: It Is Really Important!

As part of a qualitative study, we asked adolescents with cerebral palsy about the factors that they felt were important in "making life good" for them. We anticipated that disability characteristics would play a key role as determinants of quality of life however the adolescents did not share this view. Indeed, the factors contributing to a good quality of life for them were comparable to what you would expect any adolescent to articulate. Being able to participate in age-appropriate leisure activities of their choosing was emphasized as critical in optimizing their well-being. Other factors, such as family and peer support, and personal strengths such as mastery motivation and ability to manage challenges, were also important determinants of quality of life (Shikako-Thomas et al., 2009). Therefore, the significance of engagement in meaningful leisure activities should not be underestimated by occupational therapists, and thus these activities should be prioritized in program planning.

Lesson #2: Leisure Participation Is a Challenge

Several recent descriptive studies have clearly demonstrated that participation in leisure activities is decreased for children with physical disabilities compared to peers without disabilities, and this extends into adulthood (Liptak, 2008). Overall, leisure activities for children and youth with disabilities are less varied (diversity) and less intense (frequency) than their peers, and activities are predominantly home-based and sedentary (Law et al., 2006; Maher et al., 2007; Majnemer et al., 2008). However, studies reveal that level of enjoyment of all types of leisure activities is high, comparable to typically developing peers. Diminished participation in active-physical activities has implications for health, whereas lack of involvement in more structured, formal skill-based activities decreases opportunities for social interactions and skill development (Imms, 2008; Law et al.; Maher et al.; Majnemer et al.; Michelsen et al., 2009). For these children and youth, it is as if they are observers in an aquarium, looking at the wide-ranging "ocean of possibilities" through the glass, but being unable to plunge in and participate. As occupational therapists with a holistic view of meaningful occupations, we have the capacity to enable participation in preferred activities. Our challenge is to find the best practice methods to make this happen.

More Lessons: Contextual Factors Are Key Determinants of Participation

The barriers and facilitators to involvement in leisure activities are multidimensional and complex, and thus, the *ICF* classification provides a useful framework in which to consider the "ocean of possibilities" within these murky waters. With respect to body functions, cognitive and motor deficits and behavior problems in particular, as well as developmental impairments more

broadly are associated with degree of participation in leisure activities (Fauconnier et al., 2009; Majnemer et al., 2008; Michelsen et al., 2009). Nonetheless, children's developmental abilities only partially explain (i.e., low percentage of variance explained) their level of engagement in leisure activities, but do not necessarily prevent participation (Morris, Kurinczuk, Fitzpatrick, & Rosenbaum, 2006). Severity of developmental deficits is likely overemphasized as barriers to "plunging into the water."

Not surprisingly, activity limitations and participation restrictions across domains are significantly associated with leisure participation. For example, for children with cerebral palsy, limitations in mobility, manual ability and communication can pose barriers to engagement in preferred leisure activities (Fauconnier et al., 2009; Law et al., 2006; Lepage, Noreau, Bernard, & Fougeyrollas, 1998; Maher et al., 2007; Majnemer et al., 2008; Morris et al., 2006; Shikako-Thomas, Majnemer, Law, & Lach, 2008). In our study, we found involvement in active-physical leisure activities was correlated to motor function whereas self-improvement activities were associated with motor function and communication skills (Majnemer et al.). Therefore, it remains important for occupational therapists to play a proactive role in maximizing functional potential at school-age and adolescence, not only in the early years of functional acquisitions.

Personal factors are important determinants of leisure participation for all children and youth. With increasing age, children with or without disabilities are more involved in self-improvement activities but less engaged in physical activities, with greater time allocated to sedentary activities, especially small screen recreation (e.g., computer, television, videogames). Gender differences are apparent in choice of activities, with males preferring active-physical activities and females more likely to engage in arts and social activities. Cultural differences are also apparent (Hardy, Bass, & Booth, 2007; Law et al., 2006; Maher et al., 2007; Shikako-Thomas et al., 2008; Telford, Salmon, Timperio, & Crawford, 2005). For example, Australian adolescents with Asian-speaking background or those in urban environments opt for more sedentary leisure activities. Within Israel, Israeli girls are more likely to prefer skill-based activities than their Druze counterparts, although girls from both cultures enjoy social activities more than boys (Engel-Yager & Jarus, 2008; Hardy, Dobbins, Booth, DenneyWilson, & Okley, 2006; Imms, 2008; Michelsen et al., 2009; Shikako-Thomas et al.).

In terms of personality traits and lifestyle predilections, personal preferences regarding leisure activities play an important role, although preferences may not always be realized (Law et al., 2006; Majnemer et al., 2010). We have found that mastery motivation and mastery pleasure are important determinants of participation in social and recreational activities (Majnemer et al., 2008). Mastery motivation is an intrinsic psychological force that encourages an individual to attempt to master a skill that is at least moderately challenging for them. The extent to which a child with a disability will persist in solving a problem or mastering an activity that requires physical or psychological effort can facilitate or limit engagement in leisure occupations. Occupational therapists must consider preferred leisure activities in the selection of activities for rehabilitation interventions, but more importantly, as part of goal-setting to ensure that children and youth participate optimally in the activities of their choosing. Self-efficacy, self-confidence and feelings of competency relate to intrinsic motivation and are areas that occupational therapists can specifically address to overcome fear of failure and enhance willingness and capacity to participate in preferred activities that are not as yet realized (Majnemer, Shevell, Law, Poulin, & Rosenbaum, in press). Potentially modifiable personal factors such as mastery motivation and self-efficacy are therefore critical to consider in planning programs that can promote successful participation.

The "ocean of possibilities" becomes much greater when one considers environmental factors, as they collectively play a vital role in influencing a child's level of involvement in leisure activities. Parents assume the primary responsibility of supporting and optimizing opportunities for participation for their child with a disability. The family's stress levels, leisure preferences, adaptive coping skills, financial and time constraints, and support from others can either facilitate or hinder their child's involvement in preferred leisure activities. Therefore, occupational therapists should pay close attention to evidence of suboptimal family functioning and need for resources and supports, given their important influence on their child's well-being (Law et al., 2006; Lawlor, Mihaylov, Welsh, Jarvis, & Colver, 2006; Majnemer et al., 2008; ShikakoThomas et al., 2008; Welsh, Jarvis, Hammal, & Colver, 2006). Segregated school environments often provide greater opportunities for skill-based leisure activities, both in terms of improving competencies and enhancing awareness of adapted recreation programs in the community. We

found that children who were receiving rehabilitation services were more likely to participate in skill-based activities and were also more likely to enjoy active-physical activities, possibly because services augmented their self-confidence and competence in more challenging skilled activities (Majnemer et al.). Therefore, we need to ensure those children who are in integrated school environments are more aware of adapted community programs and may need targeted direct interventions to enhance self-confidence and competencies to participate in active-physical and more structured leisure activities. The community a child lives in either may facilitate or hinder participation, due to contextual physical, social and attitudinal factors (Heah, Case, McGuire, & Law, 2007; Imms, 2008; Modell, Rider, & Menchetti, 1997). Indeed, the SPARCLE study across nine regions of Europe demonstrated that some environments (i.e., Denmark in particular) were more supportive in terms of attitudes, legislation, information and services (Fauconnier et al., 2009).

Once we look beyond the surface of the clear ocean waters, we can more readily appreciate the complex and captivating reefs that exist below. If we take the time to plunge into "leisure," we can comprehend the diversity and intricacy of the many "corals" that contribute to the complete picture. Taking the time to evaluate, intervene, inform and advocate on behalf of children and youth with disabilities is in our hands.

Survive or Thrive: Occupational Therapist's Role in "Balancing the Boat"

As occupational therapists, we are positioned optimally to actively promote participation in leisure activities. As navigator, the first step is to "go there" don't miss the boat! Leisure is essential for individuals of all ages and types of disability, providing life-enhancing meaning and pleasure. By taking the time to ask our clients about preferred leisure activities in which they would like to participate, we can promote choice and a sense of control (McConachie et al., 2006). Formal evaluation tools are lacking that provide a comprehensive understanding of involvement, importance and enjoyment of leisure activities, however use of existing measures offers the opportunity to probe further. For a paediatric clientele, global measures of participation exist such as Life Habits (Noreau et al., 2007), Child & Adolescent Scale of Participation (Bedell, 2009), Paediatric Activity Card Sort (Mandich et al., 2004) and Perceived Efficacy and Goal Setting Scale (Missiuna & Pollock, 2000);

each of which tap into selected leisure activities. The Children's Assessment of Participation and Enjoyment provides a more refined depiction of involvement and enjoyment of a range of leisure activities. The Canadian Occupational Performance Measure and Goal Attainment Scaling can also be used to focus on particular leisure activities that are problematic but important for the child (McConachie et al.; Sakzewski, Boyd, & Ziviani, 2007).

Older children and youth with developmental disabilities are less likely to benefit from direct interventions or group programs that focus on leisure participation. Indeed, direct contact with occupational therapists years after the initial diagnosis is often limited and primarily focused on providing aids and adaptations for the "must do" (self-care and school-related) activities. Leisure activities are particularly crucial at school-age and adolescence, when parents can no longer navigate these occupations. As occupational therapists, we need to find creative solutions to "bring the boats into the bay" and ensure that we can develop targeted services that are aimed at "balancing the boat." Using our clinical reasoning and expertise in interventions at the level of the child, task and environment, we can optimize the health and participation of these children as they mature. In particular, we can focus on potentially modifiable personal and environmental factors such as intrinsic drive, environmental opportunities and exposure to meaningful activities (Majnemer et al., in press; Poulsen, Ziviani, Cuskelly, & Smith, 2007; Wiseman, Davis, & Polatajko, 2005). Prioritizing the child's preferences and personal achievement goals, addressing fears and enhancing skill competencies and mastery motivation can facilitate leisure participation. Exploring options and providing adaptive strategies (e.g., new aids, assistive technologies and virtual reality) can ensure that the activities are feasible. Informing the children and their families about available resources and supports to include adapted programs, transport and community clubs is essential in empowering them to capitalize on opportunities. Finally, our advocacy role in removing physical and attitudinal barriers cannot be underestimated (Poulsen et al., 2007; Wiseman et al.).

By enabling ability, rather than focusing on disability, occupational therapists can maximize adaptive capacity and well-being. My challenge to occupational therapy practitioners and to university educators is to "rock the boat"! A World Federation of Occupational Thera-

pists [WFOT] position statement on human rights challenges us to raise "collective awareness of the broader view of occupation and participation in society as a right" (WFOT, 2009). Occupational therapists have the knowledge and expertise to minimize barriers to participation in occupations of one's choosing by working with individuals, communities and organizations and by advocating for policy and practice changes that will promote healthy living. My challenge to researchers is to address the paucity of evidence on leisure participation, so as to inform best practice.

Final Lesson: Balance Your Boat

As busy professionals, we are often consumed by our responsibilities at work as well as other life roles. It is important that we take the time to "balance our boat," and create the opportunities to enjoy life's ocean voyage. Establishing greater balance in our lives is likely to improve our energy and attitudes at work, and also ensure that we are satisfied with our journey and can weather the inevitable storms that lie ahead. Maintaining life balance requires constant attention, but is worth the effort!

Acknowledgements

I am indebted to Bernadette Nedelec, Laurie Snider and Mary Law for nominating me for this incredible honor, and to CAOT for selecting me as this year's recipient of the Muriel Driver Award. I am really overwhelmed and so touched by this level of recognition. There is no doubt that my academic accomplishments have been enhanced by my environmental context. The Occupational Therapy Faculty at McGill University is a remarkably creative, talented and cohesive group of individuals that value the unique contributions of each member of our team. I am truly privileged to be part of McGill occupational therapy. I am also very fortunate to have wonderful graduate students. Their curiosity and enthusiasm continues to inspire me. It is really a pleasure to work with and learn from both my graduate trainees and my occupational therapy students. Most especially, I want to thank my family; my daughters Meaghan and Allison and my husband Michael Shevell. They are my anchors, providing me with greater balance and stability in my life. I am so appreciative of my family's ongoing support as I try my best to juggle my tasks. I am enormously grateful to you.

References

Advisory Committee on Healthy Active Living for Children and Youth, Canadian Pediatric Society. (2002). *Healthy active living for children and youth*. Retrieved from http://www.cps.ca/english/statements/HAL/HAL02-01.htm

American Academy of Pediatrics. (n.d.). *Children's health topics. Health promotion*. Retrieved from http://www.aap.org/healthtopics/healthpromotion.cfm.

Bedell, G. M. (2009). Further validation of the Child and Adolescent Scale of Participation (CASP). *Developmental Neurorehabilitation, 12*, 342–351.

Calfas, K., & Taylor, W. (1994). Effects of physical activity on psychological variables in adolescents. *Pediatric Exercise Science, 6*, 406–423.

Canadian Association of Occupational Therapists. (2007). *Profile of occupational therapy practice in Canada*. Ottawa, ON: CAOT.

Canadian Association of Occupational Therapists [CAOT]. (2010). Occupational therapy: Definition. In *About CAOT* (Definition of OT). Retrieved from http://www.caot.ca/ default. asp?pageid=1344

Canadian Mental Health Association. (2010). Work/Life balance. In *Your Mental Health* (Work/Life balance). Retrieved from http://www.cmha.ca/bins/content_page.asp?cid=2-1841&lang=1

Cassidy, T. (1996). All work and no play: A focus on leisure time as a means for promoting health. *Counseling Psychology Quarterly, 9*, 77–90. http://dx.doi.org/10.1080/09515079608256354

Downs, M. L. (2008). Leisure routines: Parents and children with disability sharing occupation. *Journal of Occupational Science, 15*, 105–110.

Engel-Yager, B., & Jarus, T. (2008). Cultural and gender effects on Israeli children's preferences for activities. *Candian Journal of Occupational Therapy 75*, 139–48

Fauconnier, J., Dickinson, H. O., Beckung, E., Marcelli, M., McManus, V., Michelsen, S. I., . . . Colver, A. (2009). Participation in life situations of 8-12 year old children with cerebral palsy: Cross sectional European study. *British Medical Journal, 338*, b1458. http://dx.doi.org/10.1136/bmj.b1458

Giada, F., Biffi, A., Agostino, P., Anedda, A., Bellardinelli, R., Carlon, R., . . . Zeppilli, P. (2008). Exercise prescription for the prevention and treatment of cardiovascular diseases: Part II. *Journal of Cardiovascular Medicine, 9*, 641-652. http://dx.doi.org/10.2459/JCM.0b013e3282f7ca96

Groff, D. G., Lundberg, N. R., & Zabriskie, R. B. (2009). Influence of adapted sport on quality of life: Perceptions of athletes with cerebral palsy. *Disability and Rehabilitation, 31*, 318–326. http://dx.doi.org/10.1080/09638280801976233

Hammell, K. W. (2004). Dimensions of meaning in the occupations of daily life. *Canadian Journal of Occupational Therapy, 71*, 296–305.

Hammell, K. W. (2009). Self-care, productivity, and leisure, or dimensions of occupational experience? Rethinking occupational "categories." *Canadian Journal of Occupational Therapy, 76*, 107–114.

Hardy, L. L., Bass, S. L., & Booth, M. L. (2007). Changes in sedentary behavior among adolescent girls: A 2.5-year prospective cohort study. *Journal of Adolescent Health, 40*, 158–165. http://dx.doi.org/10.1016/j.jadohealth.2006.09.009

Hardy, L. L, Dobbins, T., Booth, M. L., Denney-Wilson, E., & Okely, A. D. (2006). Sedentary behaviours among Australian adolescents. *Australian and New Zeland Journal of Public Health, 30*, 534–540. http://dx.doi.org/10.1111/j.1467-842X.2006.tb00782.x

Harrison, P. A., & Narayan, G. (2003). Differences in behavior, psychological factors, and environmental factors associated with participation in school sports and other activities in adolescence. *Journal of School Health, 73*, 113–120.

Heah, T., Case, T., McGuire, B., & Law, M. (2007). Successful participation: The lived experience among children with disabilities. *Canadian Journal of Occupational Therapy, 74*, 38–47.

Imms, C. (2008). Children with cerebral palsy participate: A review of the literature. *Disability and Rehabilitation, 30*, 1867–1884. http://dx.doi.org/10.1080/09638280701673542

Jonsson, H., & Persson, H. (2006). Towards an experiential model of occupational balance: An alternative perspective on flow theory analysis. *Journal of Occupational Science, 13*, 62–73.

King, G., Law, M., Hanna, S., King, S., Hurley, P., Rosenbaum, P., . . . Petrenchik, T. (2006). Predictors of the leisure and recreation participation of children with physical disabilities: A structural equation modeling analysis. *Children's Health Care, 35*, 209–234. http://dx.doi.org/10.1207/s15326888chc3503_2

Law, M., King, G., Kertoy, S., Hurley, M., Rosenbaum, P., Young, N., & Hanna, S. (2006). Patterns of participation in recreational and leisure activities among children with complex physical disabilities. *Developmen-*

tal Medicine and Child Neurology, 48, 337–42. http://dx.doi.org/10.1017/S0012162206000740

Lawlor, K., Mihaylov, S., Welsh, B., Jarvis, S., & Colver, A. (2006). A qualitative study of the physical, social and attitudinal environments influencing the participation of children with cerebral palsy in northeast England. *Pediatric Rehabilitation, 9,* 219–228. http://dx.doi.org/10.1080/ 13638490500235649

Leisure (n.d.). In *Dictionary.com unabridged.* Retrieved from http://dictionary.reference.com/browse/leisure

Lepage, C., Noreau, L., Bernard, P. M., & Fougeyrollas, P. (1998). Profile of handicap situations in children with cerebral palsy. *Scandinavian Journal of Rehabilitation Medicine, 30,* 263–272.

Liptak, G. S. (2008). Health and well being of adults with cerebral palsy. *Current Opinion in Neurology, 21,* 136–142.

Mactavish, J. B., MacKay, K. J., Lutfiyya, Z. M., Mahon, M. J., Iwasaki, Y., Rodrigue, M. M., . . . Betteridge, D. (May, 2005). *Parents of children with intellectual disability: Perspectives on leisure, vacation patterns, and life quality.* Paper presented at the Eleventh Canadian Congress on Leisure Research, Nanaimo, BC. Retrieved from http://lin.ca/Uploads/cclr11/CCLR11-87.pdf

Mactavish, J. B., & Schleien, S. J. (2004). Re-injecting spontaneity and balance in family life: Parents' perspectives on recreation in families that include children with developmental disability. *Journal of Intellectual Disability Research, 48*(Pt 2), 123–41. http://dx.doi.org/10.1111/j.1365-2788.2004.00502.x

Maher, C. A., Williams, M. T., Olds, T., & Lane, A. E. (2007). Physical and sedentary activity in adolescents with cerebral palsy. *Developmental Medicine and Child Neurology, 49,* 450–7. http://dx.doi.org/10.1111/j.1469-8749.2007.00450.x

Majnemer, A. (2009). Promoting participation in leisure activities: Expanding role of pediatric therapists. *Physical & Occupational Therapy in Pediatrics, 29,* 1–5. http://dx.doi.org/ 10.1080/01942630802625163

Majnemer, A., Shevell, M., Law, M., Birnbaum, R., Chilingaryan, G., Rosenbaum, P., & Poulin, C. (2008). Participation and enjoyment of leisure activities in school-aged children with cerebral palsy. *Developmental Medicine and Child Neurology, 50,* 751–758. http://dx.doi.org/10.1111/ j.1469-8749.2008.03068.x

Majnemer, A., Shevell, M., Law, M., Poulin, C., & Rosenbaum, P. (in press). Level of motivation in mastering challenging tasks in children with cerebral palsy. *Developmental Medicine and Child Neurology.*

Majnemer, A., Shikako-Thomas, K., Chokron, N., Law, M., Shevell, M., Chilingaryan, G., . . . Rosenbaum, P. (2010). Leisure activity preferences for 6to 12-year-old children with cerebral palsy. *Developmental Medicine and Child Neurology, 52,* 167–173. http://dx.doi.org/10.1111/ j.1469-8749.2009.03393.x

Mandich A., Polatajko, H., Miller, L., & Baum, C. (2004). *The Pediatric Card Sort.* Ottawa, ON: CAOT Publications ACE.

McConachie, H., Colver, A. F., Forsyth, R. J., Jarvis, S. N., & Parkinson, K. N. (2006). Participation of disabled children: How should it be characterized and measured? *Disability & Rehabilitation, 28,* 1157–1164. http://dx.doi.org/10.1080/09638280500534507

Melzer, K., Kayser, B., & Pichard, C. (2004). Physical activity: The health benefits outweigh the risks. *Current Opinion in Clinical Nutrition and Metabolic Care, 7,* 641–647.

Michelsen, S. I., Flachs, E. M., Uldall, P., Eriksen, E. L., McManus, V., Parkes, J., ... Colver, A. (2009). Frequency of participation of 8-12-year-old children with cerebral palsy: A multi-centre cross-sectional European study. *European Journal of Paediatric Neurology, 13,* 165–177. http://dx.doi.org/10.1016/j.ejpn.2008.03.005

Missiuna, C., & Polloc, N. (2000). Perceived efficacy and goal setting in young children. *Canadian Journal of Occupational Therapy, 67,* 101–110.

Modell, S. J., Rider, R. A., & Menchetti, B. M. (1997). An exploration of the influence of educational placement on the community recreation and leisure patterns of children with developmental disabilities. *Perceptual & Motor Skills, 85,* 695–704.

Morris, C., Kurinczuk, J. J., Fitzpatrick, R., & Rosenbaum, P. L. (2006). Do the abilities of children with cerebral palsy explain their activities and participation? *Developmental Medicine and Child Neurology, 48,* 954–961. http://dx.doi.org/10.1017/S0012162206002106

Noreau, L., Lepage, C., Boissiere, L., Picard, R., Fougeyrollas, P., Mathieu, J., Desmarais, G., Nadeau, L. (2007). Measuring participation in children with disabilities using the Assessment of Life Habits. *Developmental Medicine & Child Neurology, 49,* 666–671.

Passmore, A., & French, D. (2003). The nature of leisure in adolescence: A focus group study. *British Journal of Occupational Therapy, 66,* 419–426.

Poulsen, A. A., Ziviani, J. M., Cuskelly, M., & Smith, R. (2007). Boys with developmental coordination disorder: Loneliness and team sports participation. *American Journal of Occupational Therapy, 61,* 451–62. http://dx.doi.org/10.5014/ajot.61.4.451

Rice, S. G., & the Council on Sports Medicine and Fitness. (2008). Medical conditions affecting sports participation. *Pediatrics, 21*, 841–848. http://dx.doi.org/10.1542/peds.2008-0080

Saleh, M. N., Korner-Bitensky, N., Snider, L., Malouin, F., Mazer, B., Kennedy, E., & Roy, M. A. (2008). Actual vs. best practices for young children with cerebral palsy: A survey of paediatric occupational therapists and physical therapists in Quebec, Canada. *Developmental Neurorehabiliation, 11*, 60–80. http://dx.doi.org/10.1080/17518420701544230

Sakzewski, L., Boyd, R., & Ziviani, J. (2007). Clinimetric properties of participation measures for 5to 23-year-old children with cerebral palsy: A systematic review. *Developmental Medicine and Child Neurology, 49*, 232–240. http://dx.doi.org/ 10.1111/j.1469-8749.2007.00232.x

Secretariat for the Intersectoral Healthy Living Network. (2005). *The integrated pan-Canadian healthy living strategy.* Retrieved from http://www.phac-aspc.gc.ca/hl-vs-strat/pdf/hls_e.pdf

Shikako-Thomas, K., Lach, L., Majnemer, A., Nimigon, J., Cameron, K., & Shevell, M. (2009). Quality of life from the perspective of adolescents with cerebral palsy: "I just think I'm a normal kid, I just happen to have a disability." *Quality of Life Research, 18*(7), 825–832. http://dx.doi.org/10.1007/s11136-009-9501-3

Shikako-Thomas, K., Majnemer, A., Law, M., & Lach, L. (2008). Determinants of participation in leisure activities in children and youth with cerebral palsy: Systematic review. *Physical and Occupational Therapy in Pediatrics, 29*(2), 155–169. http://dx.doi.org/10.1080/01942630802031834

Sloman, J. (1997). *Handbook for humans.* Retrieved from http://www. mayyoubehappy.com/61balyourboa.html

Taanila, A., Jarvelin, M. R., & Kokkonen, J. (1999). Cohesion and parents' social relations in families with a child with disability or chronic illness. *International Journal of Rehabilitation Research, 22*, 101–9.

Telford, A., Salmon, J., Timperio, A., & Crawford, D. (2005). Examining physical activity among 5- to 6- and 10- to 12-year-old children: The Children's Leisure Activities Study. *Pediatric Exercise Science, 17*, 266–280.

Thorpe, D. (2009). The role of fitness in health and disease: Status of adults with cerebral palsy. *Developmental Medicine and Child Neurology, 51*, 52–58. http://dx.doi.org/10.1111/j.1469-8749.2009.03433.x

Townsend, E. A. (Ed.). (2002). *Enabling occupation: An occupational therapy perspective.* Ottawa, ON: CAOT Publications ACE.

Turner, H., Chapman, S., McSherry, A., Krishnagiri, S., & Watts, J. (2000). Leisure assessment in occupational therapy: An exploratory study. *Occupational Therapy in Health Care, 12*, 73–85. http://dx.doi.org/10.1080/J003v12n02_05

Welsh, B., Jarvis, S., Hammal, D., & Colver, A. (2006). How might districts identify local barriers to participation for children with cerebral palsy? *Public Health, 120*, 157–175. http://dx.doi.org/10.1016/j.puhe.2005.04.006

Wiseman, J. O., Davis, J. A., & Polatajko, H. J. (2005). Occupational development: Towards an understanding of children's doing. *Journal of Occupational Science, 12*, 26–35.

World Federation of Occupational Therapists. (2009). WFOT position statement on human rights. *WFOT Bulletin, 59*, 5. Retrieved from http://www.wfot.org/wfot2010/docs/WI_04_ Elizabeth%20Townsend.pdf

World Health Organization. (2007). *ICF–CY International Classification of Functioning, Disability, and Health: Children and Youth Version.* Geneva, Switzerland: WHO Press. D910-d950.

World Health Organization. (2008). *WHO health policy for children and adolescents No.5. Inequalities in young people's health. Section 3: Health Behaviours.* Retrieved from www.euro.who.int/ pubrequest

World Health Organization. (2010). *Global strategy on diet, physical activity and health.* Retrieved from http://www.who.int/ dietphysicalactivity/en/

CHAPTER 21

A Proposed Model of Lifestyle Balance

KATHLEEN M. MATUSKA AND CHARLES H. CHRISTIANSEN

The belief that living a balanced life is important for well-being has ancient roots in Chinese, Native American and Ayurvedic Medicine and more recent support (from diverse perspectives) in the contemporary literature of the economic, social and behavioral sciences (Christiansen & Matuska, 2006; Sternberg, 1997). Nowhere, however, does the concept enjoy more widespread support than in the popular press.

The demands of modern life in developed nations have led to widespread public perceptions of increased stress and insufficient time available to engage in occupations viewed as fundamental to well-being (Bachmann, 2000; Bond, Galinsky, & Swanberg, 1998). American government reports are clear that perceived stress is increasing and a decade ago, epidemiologists predicted that stress-related diseases would be prominent among the most costly health conditions (Murray & Lopez, 1996). Changing practices associated with paid work, such as longer hours and increased shift work, have been at the heart of these concerns. It is commonly believed that modern work encroaches on nonwork occupations to create an undesirable and unhealthy imbalance. Over time, growing concern with this perceived imbalance has given rise to such concepts as *quality time, workaholism,* and *burnout* (Hochschild, 1997; Perlow, 1999; Robinson & Godbey, 1997).

Although it is widely accepted that certain occupations are more beneficial to health and quality of life than others, little theoretical and empirical work has been done to identify optimal lifestyle patterns. Investigators in the management sciences, sociology and family studies have reported studies related to negative consequences of spillover of work requirements into non-work domains (Frone, Russell & Cooper, 1992; Greenhaus, Collins, & Shaw, 2002; Marks & MacDermid, 1996). Meanwhile, scholars in psychology, leisure studies, nursing, public health and occupational therapy have studied patterns of human occupation in an attempt to identify characteristics that contribute to higher levels of life satisfaction, health and general well-being (Camporese, Freguja, & Sabbadini, 1998; Marino-Schorn, 1986; Walker, Sechrist, & Pender, 1987; Zuzanek, 1998). An implicit assumption underlying these studies is that lifestyles with certain configurations of occupation are more likely to promote health and well-being by virtue of meeting essential needs and/or reducing stressful circumstances over time than others.

Given the assumed relationships between lifestyle patterns and well-being, an understanding of the recurring lifestyle occupations that reduce stress and promote health would be of potential interest to social scientists and occupational scientists. Despite this, surprisingly little attention has been paid to patterns of occupation within the health sciences literature. Moreover, there exists no consensus definition of lifestyle balance, even though the concept appears regularly in the popular press and seems to be implicitly understood by the public.

In this paper we propose a model of a balanced lifestyle that is resilient and health promoting. We recognize the complexity of this topic and offer a beginning attempt to conceptualize lifestyle balance, realizing that the task is formidable and understandings will progress over time. Our aim is to stimulate dialogue and additional research on this topic.

Review of the Literature

This section summarizes a comprehensive review of the literature related to lifestyle balance published earlier

This chapter was previously published in the *Journal of Occupational Science*, 15, 9–19. Copyright © 2008, Taylor and Francis. Reprinted with permission.

(Christiansen & Matuska, 2006). That review included studies of time use, life roles, biological rhythms and need satisfaction. Those studies provided a context for identifying specific lifestyle characteristics related to health and well-being.

Ancient ideas of balance broadly focused on maintaining health through a balance among thoughts, actions and feelings, influenced by the physical and social environments in which people lived. In modern western cultures, new emphasis for balance was placed on time spent in work and home, and an increased focus on leisure as a valued activity for life balance (Pierce, 2003). Time use across these domains, then, became important in modern conceptualizations of balance with the assumption that a balance among them is optimal for health and well-being. However, studies examining time allocation alone have not proven very useful for understanding the broad complexities of lifestyle patterns and well-being because of methodological weaknesses and conflicting findings. Other approaches have provided richer time use data by supplementing diaries with event sampling procedures and/or interviews in order to gather more qualitative information on the meanings and feelings associated with different occupations (Erlandsson & Eklund, 2001; Erlandsson, Rögnvaldsson, & Eklund, 2004; Klumb & Perraz, 2004; Reis & Gable, 2000). Additionally, studies of time structure (Jonsson, Borell, & Sadlo, 2000; Zuzanek, 1998) have found that lower levels of mental health are associated with both high and low levels of time pressure (i.e., activity requirements within a specified timeframe), suggesting that a moderate amount of structured time may be beneficial to well-being. This finding was also supported in a study of retirement adjustment (Jonsson, Josephsson, & Kielhofner, 2001). Comparing health outcomes with the congruency of how people want to use their time and how they actually use their time may represent useful ways to conceptualize a balanced life. We conclude that enriched time use studies may have benefit, but that data on time use alone does not seem useful in formulating recommendations about balanced lifestyles.

Another way to understand what people actually do with their time is to study roles. Studies that explored roles, well-being, and quality of life have concluded consistently that participation in valued roles is related to life satisfaction and measures of well-being (Verbrugge, 1983). Too much conflict among multiple roles can be associated with stress (Goode, 1960); yet having more social roles typically has beneficial consequences, since it may enable the individual to have access to more social support, thus reducing a person's vulnerability to stress (Linville, 1987). Marks and MacDermid (1996) showed that finding a way to balance multiple demands on their time and role responsibilities correlated with peoples' perception of ease and satisfaction with adequately meeting daily role demands. They found that positive role balance was reflected in a person's "tendency to become fully engaged in the performance of every role in one's total role system, to approach every typical role and role partner with an attitude of attentiveness and care" (p. 421).

Although research on roles and time use has provided insight into factors that contribute to or alleviate the consequences of life stress, studies have generally failed to provide information about the patterns or types of specific occupations and practices that typify the roles of the most (or least) successful study participants. In other words, what is an optimal level of participation in various life occupations? Are people who have a balance among occupations better off than people who focus on only one or two primary occupations? These questions are keys to understanding lifestyle balance and have only begun to be explored.

There are only a few studies that have actually explored how a balance among different types of activities might influence positive states. Seleen (1982) found that for older adults, perceived congruence between desired and actual time use among 10 categories of activities was related to life satisfaction. Using Self Determination Theory (Deci & Ryan, 2000), Sheldon and Niemiec (2006) provided evidence that a balance of satisfaction in the three need areas of competence, autonomy, and relatedness is important for well-being. In four studies using multiple designs, they found that a balance of satisfaction in the three need areas had unique additive effects on psychological well-being. In other words, people who experienced balanced need satisfaction (similar scores across the three need areas) reported higher well-being than those with greater variability in need satisfaction, even when the sum of total scores was equal.

The most directly relevant work was a pilot study done in Australia, exploring the perceptions of occupational balance and its relationship to health from the viewpoint of physical, mental, social and rest occupations. It was found that for the respondents, ideal balance was represented by approximately equal involvement in each category and a significant relationship was found between the closeness of current occupational patterns to those perceived by the respondents to be ideal and his or her reported health (Wilcock et al, 1997). This finding was supported by Håkansson, DahlinIvanoff, and Sonn (2006), who found that women with stress-related disorders reported a sense of balance (that they felt was synonymous with well-being) when they had a harmonious repertoire of daily occupations that was meaningful and created a positive self image, and when they used strategies to manage and control everyday life.

According to current supposition, living a balanced life should yield positive states such as happiness, subjective well-being, resilience and quality of life. Cummins, Gullone, and Lau (2002) theorized that people who maintain a state of subjective well-being homeostasis are able to do so by having adequate core resources (such as healthy relationships, financial stability, etc.), thus faring better after stressful life events than people without such core resources. A similar argument can be made that people with balanced lives should have adequate core resources and thus should be better able to cope successfully with life's stressors and regain homeostasis.

Clearly, the idea of living a balanced life and the psychological and physiological outcomes is multidimensional and complex, and only beginning to be explored. The research summarized above highlighted different ideas related to dimensions such as time allocation, role demands, and need satisfaction and their relationship to well-being. In the following section, we describe a proposed model of lifestyle balance that synthesizes these concepts. Our intention is to stimulate research and dialogue that moves the idea of lifestyle balance beyond philosophical and lay formulations toward practical application based on evidence.

A Proposed Model of Lifestyle Balance

The proposed model builds on interdisciplinary research about the physiological and psychological attributes considered important for well-being. It is also influenced by research that has explored relationships between well-being and situational/contextual/ or environmental factors. The model's approach to conceptualizing life balance is based on how the configurations of everyday patterns of occupation meet essential human needs. We acknowledge that people can meet the same needs through participation in different daily occupations, and the model thus allows for variability in occupational configurations based on individual differences and cultural and environmental influences. Balance then, is construed as the extent to which an individual's unique patterns of occupation (in con-

text) enable needs essential to resilience, well-being and quality of life to be met. The focus on *occupational patterns* (i.e., doing things over time) and the combination of their perceived and actual states of balance (i.e., what people actually do relative to what they desire doing) differentiates this concept from other positive state constructs such as happiness and satisfaction with life. Definitions of those constructs typically focus more on global, subjective appraisals of well-being. The current model proposes that lifestyle balance is best represented by a continuum of occupational patterns over the life-course with a variable range of satisfactory states rather than a designated point on a fulcrum. Rather than prescribing a static or ideal state of balance, our model suggests a dynamic interaction between the environment and everyday patterns of occupation, with varying degrees of satisfaction and sustainability in how these occupations meet important needs and are congruent with people's values over time.

The model defines a *balanced lifestyle* as *a satisfying pattern of daily occupation that is healthful, meaningful, and sustainable to an individual within the context of his or her current life circumstances*. The term *satisfying* in this definition means congruence between actual participation in occupations and *desired* participation in occupations. This definition recognizes that individuals have different roles, role requirements, personalities, values and interests and that these change over time. It also recognizes that the opportunities and means for meeting needs vary according to the resources available within given physical, social, and cultural environments. It is conceivable, then, that resource limitations can influence the extent to which a person can meet needs and participate in valued activities, thus constraining the opportunity to attain a balanced lifestyle.

Furthermore, the need related aspects of the model suggests that lifestyle patterns must consist of a congruent array of occupations that enable people to: (1) meet basic instrumental needs necessary for sustained biological health and physical safety; (2) have rewarding and self-affirming relationships with others (3) feel engaged, challenged, and competent; (4) create meaning and a positive personal identity; (5) organize their time and energy in ways that enable them to meet important personal goals and renewal.

The model proposes that to the extent people are able to engage consistently in overall patterns of occupations that address these dimensions, they will perceive their lives as more satisfying, less stressful, and more meaningful, or *balanced*. The model also proposes that lifestyles with greater balance contribute to psychological well-being and overall health (i.e., people with greater balance will be less likely to become victims of illness, chronic disease or depression).

Support for a Need-Based Approach to Lifestyle Balance

Our concept of lifestyle balance implies a satisfactory congruence between an array of actual and desired occupational patterns; what people want to spend their time doing and what they actually do. Studies show that in addition to satisfaction with occupational congruency, the particular array of occupations chosen is an equal determinant of a balanced life. For example, an individual may consider himself balanced because of a satisfactory congruence between time spent at work and the time spent in leisure playing video games, yet have minimal personal relationships and poor health habits (e.g. excessive drinking, obesity, and a sedentary lifestyle). Intuitively, most individuals would agree that his perceived congruency does not represent a balanced life, although this individual may call it a satisfactory life. Studies suggest that a potentially useful approach for determining which types of occupational patterns need to be included in a balanced lifestyle involves determining the extent to which an individual's pattern of regular occupations enables a core set of psychological and physiological needs to be met. How these needs are met will vary with individuals in context. Thus it is not the particular occupational patterns that need to be balanced, but the way needs are met through occupation. For example, two of the dimensions in our model include the importance of practices that support physiological health and occupations that enable satisfactory interpersonal relationships. The occupations chosen to meet these needs may look very different for each individual and will change for individuals over time. Although the particular occupations change, the needs remain. Thus the individual in the example above may feel satisfied with his lifestyle because he is not recognizing the importance of these other needs, but over time may experience physical or psychological health consequences as a result. We propose that meeting core needs through a balanced and satisfactory repertoire of everyday occupations fosters health and well-being, and provides a buffer to stressors.

What is it that influences people to choose the particular occupational patterns that make up their lifestyles? The five need-based occupational dimensions identified in the model are supported by theories of motivation and well-being and provide some understanding about lifestyle choices. Maslow's theory (1943, 1970) recognizes the interrelatedness of the needs, drives, perceptions, and the environment and how these influence motivation. Maslow asserted that both *being needs* (cognitive, aesthetic and self-actualization) and *deficiency needs* (drives, safety and security, affiliation, and esteem) motivate everyday occupational choices and drive the behavior that makes up people's lifestyles. Although Maslow's theory has been criticized (Haymes & Green, 1982; Strong & Fiebert, 1987), a growing recent literature is finding support for the assumptions and motivational categories Maslow proposed, particularly as elaborated in his later writings (Cameron, Banko, & Pierce, 2001; Hagerty, 1999; Wicker, Brown, et al., 1993; Wicker & Wiehe, 1999; Wicker, Wiehe, Hagen, & Brown, 1994).

Recent research on positive psychological functioning has included studies of the protective features associated with well-being. These have shown that basic psychological needs associated with living a meaningful life must be satisfied if optimal functioning and wellbeing are to be achieved (Ryff, 1995). Ryff and Singer (1996) found similarities among many mental health, clinical and life-span developmental theories of well-being and converged the ideas into a theoretical model of positive psychological well-being. Their theory of psychological well-being contains six theory-guided dimensions that have been supported in numerous publications of empirical findings (Ryff, 1989, 1995; Ryff & Singer, 1998). The six dimensions considered core to well-being in their theory include: self-acceptance, positive relations with others, autonomy, environmental mastery, purpose in life, and personal growth.

In their Self Determination Theory (SDT), Deci and Ryan (2000) asserted that humans have innate needs that specify necessary conditions for psychological growth, well-being, and integrity. They identify competence, autonomy and relatedness as the fundamental psychological needs that must be satisfied for self-organization and effective social relations. Deci and Ryan proposed that satisfaction of these needs is associated with effective functioning and alternatively, negative consequences will result from their neglect. According to Self Determination Theory, well-being requires competence and flexibility to interact effectively with a changing environment; relatedness to connect meaningfully with others and integrate into society; and autonomy for self-regulation of actions and to be true to one's identity.

Considered together, Maslow's need hierarchy, Ryff's Psychological Well-being Theory, and Deci and Ryan's

Table 21.1. Comparison of Need-Based Theories Related to the Model of Lifestyle Balance

Maslow (1943, 1970) Hierarchy of Needs	Ryff (1989, 1996, 1998) Psychological Well-Being	Deci & Ryan (2000) Self Determination Theory	Matuska & Christiansen (2008) Lifestyle Balance Model Occupational Patterns
Self actualization	Self acceptance Purpose in life Autonomy	Autonomy	Create meaning and a positive personal identity through occupation
Aesthetics/cognition Esteem	Personal growth Environmental mastery	Competence	Feel engaged, challenged, and competent Organize their time and energy in ways that enable them to meet important personal goals and renewal
Affiliation	Positive relations with others	Relatedness	Have rewarding and self-affirming relationships with others
Safety/security	These appear to be treated as "givens" determined more by physiological drives and instincts than conscious thought. Therefore, they are so obvious and ubiquitous that the theorists accept them as deficiency needs and move on.		Meet basic needs Instrumental needs necessary for sustained biological health, security and physical safety

Self-Determination Theory propose need categories that support each of the five occupational dimensions proposed in the lifestyle balance model outlined in this paper. Table 21.1 shows a convergence of these theories with the lifestyle balance model.

If there are empirically strong theories of needs essential for well-being, one might ask what is new or different about the lifestyle balance model since it is based on meeting those essential needs. We assert that the need-based theories form the empirical foundation and the model focuses on how these needs are met through occupational choices and the satisfaction, congruence, and sustainability of the total configuration of occupations over time. Because life is complex, it is likely that a person's choices at any one instant will be motivated by a multitude of factors with changing valences of potency. Moreover, people often make choices that, in hindsight, are contrary to their best interests. What seems evident is that unmet needs influence human occupation, and that being satisfied with the balance of occupations that in totality meet biological needs, foster rewarding relationships with others, are interesting and challenging, are congruent with one's desired identity, and allow goals to be met constitute important dimensions of well-being and a balanced lifestyle.

Support for the Dimensions of the Model

Dimension 1: Biological Health and Physical Safety

Creating lifestyles that meet the needs of biological health, security and safety seem to be accepted as a given by most people. How to best meet these needs may still require research and dialogue, but the idea that they are essential is rarely disputed. Cumulative research is convincing on the beneficial effects on health of good nutrition, exercise, safety practices (seat belt use, safety equipment use), adequate sleep, and avoiding addictive substances. Although health and safety were clearly identified as important needs by Maslow (1943), they are not typically highlighted in positive psychology literature because of their general acceptance as health promoting. The model brings these basic needs to the forefront, asserting that one important part of a balanced lifestyle would be sustainable patterns of occupation that maintain physiological health and safety. Without good health, the likelihood of sustaining occupations to meet other critical needs is diminished.

One of the key influences to physiological health is managing stress, and it has direct relevance to the model of lifestyle balance because stress is related to lifestyle choices. Research has established that chronic stress can have serious health consequences (McEwen & Lasley, 2002), whether resulting from situations where people are feeling constantly pressed for time, or because people live in environments that do not enable them to pursue a satisfying pattern of occupations that support human flourishing. The negative physical effects of chronic stress on health can be measured as allostatic load, or the cumulative affect of 10 physiologic responses to stress. When allostatic load is elevated over a long period, the physiological responses are harmful to the body, and can contribute to cardiovascular disease and immune response suppression (McEwen & Lasley). Stress has also been associated with depression, disrupted sleep patterns, memory problems, obesity, and various other health conditions (Sapolsky, 2004).

Given the significant impact of stress on health and well-being, a balanced lifestyle would be one where stress is managed in a way that minimizes its long term negative effects. Considerable research has shown that there are certain lifestyle choices that buffer against stress and improve overall health. For example, regular exercise has been associated with decreased stress response (Skully, Kremer, Meade, Graham, & Dudgeon, 1998), improved sleep (Youngstedt, O'Connor, & Dishman, 1997), and decreased depression (Craft & Landers, 1998). Good nutrition and eating habits have also been associated with lower stress effects and better overall health (Baum & Posluszny, 1999). Reams of evidence support the idea that healthy lifestyle choices have long term beneficial effects on overall health and well-being. Therefore, this factor is considered one of the key dimensions in our model of a balanced life.

Dimension 2: Rewarding and Self-Affirming Relationships With Others

Having rewarding and self-affirming relationships with others is also well supported in the literature and for brevity, only a few studies are mentioned here. For example, socially supportive environments have been associated with psychological well-being (Thompson & Heller, 1990), quality of life (Achat, et al, 1998), higher cognitive performance (Seeman, Lusignolo, Albert, & Berckman, 2001), and healthy aging (Gurung, Taylor, & Seeman, 2003). Socially supportive family environments have long-term effects in children by reducing their risk for mental health disorders, chronic diseases, and early mortality (Repetti, Taylor, & Seeman, 2002). Even when people live in stressful situations such as in low socioeconomic conditions, social support seems to lower stress associated with living in impoverished environments (Taylor & Seemen, 1999).

The link of positive relationships to overall health status has growing evidence with strong associations found between social support and specific physiological functions, including the cardiovascular, immune and endocrine systems (Uchino, Cacioppo, & Kiecolt-Glaser, 1996). Social support also appears to be a buffer to stress because it has been linked to lower levels of allostatic load (Kiecolt-Glaser, McGuire, Robles, & Glaser, 2002; Seeman, Singer, Ryff, Love, & Levy-Storms, 2002; Seeman, et al., 2004). The positive physiological benefits of social support have also been shown to reduce worker sickness and absenteeism. In research of middle aged employees, workers with satisfactory social relations reported significantly less sickness and less absenteeism than workers who did not have satisfactory social support (Melchoir, Niedhammer, Berkman, & Goldberg, 2003). Additionally, studies show that even when people become ill, better recovery from the illness and less onset of disability in daily living occupations is fostered by social support (Mendes de Leon, et al., 1999).

One component of healthy relationships that requires more research involves understanding the balance between care for self and care for others. Healthy relationships involve both giving and receiving support, but little is known about a healthy balance between the two. Care giving can be deeply meaningful, but in excess it can be depleting as well. The Western focus on individualism is also contrasted by the Eastern values of collectivism, and these cultural differences can influence one's perception of optimal balance. The proposed model of lifestyle balance does not prescribe occupational patterns necessary for healthy relationships, but states that the meaning and satisfaction with their chosen occupational patterns in context influence perceived balance.

Dimension 3: Feel Interested, Engaged, Challenged, and Competent

An important component of a balanced lifestyle includes opportunities to feel competent and engaged through occupations that are interesting and challenging. Engagement in occupation is fundamental to life because it is through the active transactions with people, places and things in an environment that people develop a sense of competence and self-efficacy. This contributes to identity and creates meaning in lives (Christiansen, 1999; see Chapter 34). When people are successful in their actions to meet their needs and fulfill their roles, they develop mastery, which increases their sense of competence and self-efficacy. This leads to a willingness to try other novel or challenging things (Bandura, 1977, 2000, 2001). Since life is continually changing, people need to have the ability to respond to these challenges in new ways that allow them to continue to grow as individuals.

Competency and efficacy are not only important for continued adaptation to the demands of living; they also have been linked to well-being and quality of life (Deci & Ryan, 2000). A sense of control over one's personal environment relates to competency and efficacy and is fundamental to life and drives behavior. For example, the ability to make decisions and control many of the events in life has been linked to improved alertness, participation and well-being in nursing home residents (Langer & Rodin, 1976). In a study of personal project dimensions, Christiansen, Backman, Little, and Nguyen (1999) found that efficacy and stress were the factors explaining the most variation in well-being. Efficacy emerged as a central factor in explaining progress and outcome, and was significantly related to the dimension of project meaning. Britt and Bliese (2003) also found that being personally self-engaged in meaningful occupations was related to well-being of soldiers in stressful situations, through their effect as a stress-buffer.

The idea of an optimal person–environment match for a sense of well-being was researched extensively by Csikzentmihalyi (1990, 1997). He described a phenomenon termed flow that occurs when people have a sense of control over what they're doing, where they feel competent and efficacious in their ability to do the occupation, where they know the goal of the occupation and receive feedback from their efforts, and where time is suspended because they are deeply involved in the occupation for its own sake. This optimal state is achieved when there is a balance between high skill and high challenge resulting in enjoyment, interest and motivation. In contrast, occupations that provide low challenge and require low or medium skills results in apathy or boredom (Persson, Eklund, & Isacsson, 1999). The physical and psychological consequences of engagement and participation in occupations can range from emotional rewards (such as pleasure and satisfaction) to increased knowledge, wisdom, and a sense of life meaning and are important for a balanced lifestyle.

Dimension 4: Create Meaning and a Positive Personal Identity

Frankl (1984) and Antonovsky (1979, 1987) are among prominent clinical scientists who have asserted the importance of creating meaning (or life purpose) in human flourishing, suggesting that it may be the lifestyle characteristic that is most important for resilience under stressful conditions. Life is given meaning by what we do. The meaning dimension of occupations includes all of the subjective, emotional appraisals of the events in our life, the significance attributed to them in relation to our goals, and the underlying values, beliefs, and personal identity that are created and supported by them. Meaning is infused in the five occupational dimensions of the model and is stated explicitly in the dimension that people need to pursue occupations that

enable the development of a positive personal identity. To conceptualize meaning in the context of human lifestyles requires an integrative approach and fortunately, human occupation is an ideal framework to enable this synthesis to occur.

A growing body of research in the social and behavioral sciences demonstrates wide agreement on the importance of meaning to human flourishing (Christiansen, 1999; see Chapter 34; Deci & Ryan, 2000; Klinger, 1977, 1998; Little, 1988, 1998; Ryff, 1989; Taylor & Seeman, 1999; Zika & Chamberlain, 1992). We believe that in pursuing meaningful lifestyles and creating a positive identity, people engage in an array of occupations, some of which are related to understanding of their situations at the moment and others pertaining to evaluating purpose in their lives over the longer course. These occupations range from regular meditation and contemplation during walks in the forest to the more formal rituals and fellowship embodied in the activities and worship of organized religion. These spiritual occupations, and their meanings, must be fully considered if studies of lifestyle and health are to be complete.

We contend that a physically healthy lifestyle but with little meaning, is insufficient for a balanced lifestyle (Reker, Peacock, & Wong, 1987; Ryff, 1989; Wong, 2000). Maslow (1970) distinguished between people who are "merely healthy" and those who are "transcenders." The transcenders are those who live more at the level of being, who have more peak experiences and are motivated to a greater good beyond them. It is the meaningfulness of life that makes it worth living and supports well-being. Similarly, Victor Frankl (1984) believed that "man's search for meaning is the primary motivation in his life" (p. 121). Frankl considered finding meaning as fundamental to existence, that we accomplish by creating or doing, experiencing people or things, and by the attitude we take towards suffering. This ability to find meaningfulness in our everyday events, even in deplorable circumstances makes the difference between a life worth living and despair. Other theorists support the belief that a prolonged existence without meaning, values or ideals creates boredom and apathy, lack of personal fulfillment, personal distress, and illness (Frankl, 1984; Maslow, 1970; Yalom, 1980).

The inadequacy of defining health as the absence of symptoms is clear when one considers why two individuals given similar illnesses have remarkably different lifestyle outcomes or why individuals considered physically robust can be at the brink of despair. Certainly, some of these differences are related to how different actions are experienced and interpreted. Persson, Erlandsson, Eklund, and Iwarsson (2001) described value dimensions of occupations and related these to how people assign meaning to what they do. They concluded that personal meaning is based on the perceived value underlying action and that individuals, within the context of their lives and situations, interpret meanings uniquely. Yet, although they are highly individual, such meanings must also have coherence. Aaron Antonovsky (1979) proposed a salutogenic model of health that emphasized factors that keep people healthy. His clinical work revealed that a basic attitude of experiencing the world as manageable, meaningful and comprehensible seemed to contribute to a sense of coherence that was central to maintaining health. According to Antonovsky, this attitude reduced states of tension and was related to increased health promoting behaviors (Antonovsky, 1987).

Other researchers have found that living a meaningful existence or having a purpose in life is associated with well-being. Studies of personal projects have shown that having projects with personal meaning in and relating to one's identity are associated with greater well-being (Christiansen, 1999; see Chapter 34; Little, 1998; Little & Chambers, 2003). Of particular interest in these studies is the finding that people make time for those goal-related occupations that are viewed as important by themselves and others. In summary, there is abundant empirical evidence supporting the importance of having lifestyles that engender the creation of meaning and a positive identity.

Dimension 5: Organize Time and Energy to Meet Important Personal Goals and Personal Renewal

In order to meet needs, people must manage the multiple demands on their time sufficiently to accomplish their goals and create opportunities for energy renewal. This dimension is different from the others because it is a contextual dimension that influences all other aspects of occupational patterns in a lifestyle. Time and energy are viewed as key dimensions in the proposed model because they are central to lay understandings of lifestyle balance, play a pervasive role in the orchestration of social occupation, influence how and when occupations are undertaken and experienced, and perhaps most importantly, contribute in significant ways to the creation of meaning. Organizing time and energy is viewed in two distinct ways in our model; one view refers to the more immediate perception of time as in

the allocation of time in day-to-day occupations, while the other view recognizes that lifestyle choices and values change with the passage of time and context.

Lay understandings of lifestyle balance universally involve the perceived time-stress associated with social pressures to fit more occupations within a timeframe that cannot be expanded. In contemporary Western society, there is a growing perception that the routine demands of living exceed the time available for them, and that there is insufficient time to rest or participate in discretionary pursuits or to accomplish work-related tasks at desired performance levels (Robinson & Godfrey, 1997). Time is seen as a commodity that must be rationed (Peloquin, 1990) and stress results when there is a perceived press for time or multiple demands on time.

Time management can also be viewed as *occupation* management because it represents a planned and purposeful choice of which occupations will be engaged in over time. As the proposed model suggests, a balanced lifestyle would be one where there is satisfaction in the congruency between desired and actual use of time. One approach to finding congruency is using time management strategies that organize attention and energy for satisfactory completion of daily occupations. This was demonstrated in several studies of college students who typically have multiple demands on their time. Compared to college students who had poor time management, students who used effective time management strategies demonstrated less stress (Misra & McKean, 2000), and had better academic performance (Britton & Tesser, 1991). Employees who used effective time management strategies reported less role overload and greater work and life satisfaction, and had fewer job-induced and somatic tensions (Macan, Shahani, Dipboye, & Phillips, 1990).

Well-being and life satisfaction are compromised when time is perceived as inadequate to meet goals and fulfill roles. Satisfaction with how time is spent was one of the moderate predictors of life satisfaction in adults with spinal cord injuries (Pentland, Harvey, & Walker, 1998) and older adults (Seleen, 1982). People are also more satisfied and report a higher sense of well-being when they feel they are achieving the goals of their long- or short-term projects (Christiansen, Backman, Little, & Nguyen, 1999). Conversely, having too much time available with subsequent boredom and inactivity has been related to lower levels of mental health and life satisfaction (Jonsson, Borell, & Sadlo, 2000; Zuzanek 1998). Time allocation, then, is one factor in a balanced lifestyle, but partitioning certain amounts of time to various occupations does not adequately represent a well balanced life. Rather, it is the contextual influence of time relative to healthy habits, positive relationships, challenge, and meaning that contributes to lower stress and life satisfaction. In other words, we assert that, in balanced lifestyles, need-based occupations are engaged in through time in a manner that, at the end of the day, week, or year, people feel satisfied that their needs have been met and that their important roles have been fulfilled.

Time can also be viewed from a more biological perspective when considering the control exerted by nature, such as circadian rhythms that impose an internal structure and rhythm on occupation. People spend one-third of their lives sleeping, and regular routines (acting as zeitgebers) are necessary to help entrain people to their natural environments. Disentrainment interrupts customary occupational routines and can have deleterious health consequences (Monk, et al., 1997; Monk, Flaherty, Frank, Hoskinson, & Kupfer, 1990; Szuba, Yager, Guze, Allen, & Baxter, 1992). Research shows that biological rhythms and social occupations have a reciprocal relationship, and when loss of synchrony occurs, sleep and mood disturbances result (Brown, et al., 1996; Monk, Reynolds, Buysse, DeGrazia, & Kupfer, 2003).

There is also a temporal influence on the selection and subjective experience of occupations. The nature and timing of chosen occupational pursuits, while influenced by social expectations, seems also to be a function of stage of life. Early stage theories of development posited that as individuals move through stages of life chronologically, they are motivated by different primary tasks or issues (Erikson, 1982; Havighurst, 1972). As people age, they tend to pursue goals that are more meaningful and with more emphasis on the present, in recognition that time remaining is diminishing (Carstensen, 1998), and they choose personal projects that are more congruent with their values and identity (Christiansen, 2000; Little, 1998; McGregor & Little, 1998).

Finally, time is also a factor in the creation of meaning. The perspective of time as experienced in most Western cultures is that of a progressive, continuous, finite, and normatively sequential series of occupations marked typically by cultural milestones such as puberty, marriage, children, the completion of formal schooling, retirement and the end of life. This linear structure provides a means for understanding past, present and future occupations and events as part of an unfolding narrative or story, as described in the section on meaning. In anticipating the future in the context of their lives and personal stories, people are motivated to pursue occupations that shape positive identities and address unmet needs and potentials (Christiansen, 1999; see Chapter 34; Markus, 1986; McAdams, 1992, 1993, 1999). Thus time creates a contextual backdrop that influences the selection of occupations and their meanings both prospectively and retrospectively.

The Environment

The proposed model of lifestyle balance recognizes that lives are dynamic and that economic, social, political, physical, and cultural environmental influences have a profound effect on participation in daily occupations. Each of the primary motivational theorists whose work has influenced our thinking about lifestyle balance recognizes that an individual's choices, actions and success in goal attainment represent the product of their personality, experience, and the opportunities provided them within a given situation or environmental context. The interaction between the person and the environment is dynamic; where one's presence and actions influence the environment and alternatively, the physical and social characteristics of the environment influence the emotions and actions of the individual (Shaw, 2003; Wells, 2002).

Ideal situations provide just right levels of stimulation, challenge and support to elicit feelings of competence, comfort, support, growth and need fulfillment (Csikszentmihalyi, 1997; Deci & Ryan, 2000). Depending on their circumstances, however, people may be unable to participate regularly in the types of occupations that address needs considered essential for a balanced lifestyle. Terms such as occupational deprivation, alienation, and disruption have been used to describe situations when people are unable to engage in daily occupations that foster health, well-being and quality of life because of environmental constraints (Christiansen & Townsend, 2004; Whiteford, 2000; see Chapter 26; 2001, 2004). A convincing example of how social class privilege influenced role balance was found in research where financial strain was a robust predictor of lower levels of role balance for married women (Marks, Huston, Johnson, & MacDermid, 2001).

Environments may also encourage and support occupational patterns through the availability and character of physical and social resources (Gibson, 1979). For example, having family and friends who are physically active, or living in communities that have attractive parks and recreational facilities, represent helpful environmental features for maintaining an exercise regimen. There are also advantages to having stable living environments, since consistent and recurring features, such as social conventions, customs and rituals, can influence habits and routines that provide helpful rhythms to sustain occupational patterns (Clark, 2000; Zerubavel, 1981). Lawton, Nahemow, and Yeh (1980) contributed important research showing the associations between neighborhood environmental factors and well-being. For example, among 3000 older tenants in 153 planned housing units, living in safe, quiet, and small communities accounted for a significant proportion of variance in every index of well-being. The model recognizes the profound impact of the environment on occupational choices and opportunities and proposes that needs can be met in different ways given the context and conversely, in some contexts essential needs cannot be met.

Visual Model

Figure 21.1 shows a visual depiction of the model, which conveys the idea that perceived satisfaction in the five need based dimensions of the model will vary in a given time frame but that over the life course (measured in months, years, decades) a balanced life is one where adjustments and adaptations are made in occupational patterns when they feel imbalanced. The five dimensions are represented by the wavy lines showing various degrees of balance/imbalance over time. Balance or imbalance is related to perceived satisfaction in each of the five occupational areas. The line representing organizing time and energy is shown encircling the others because it is a contextual dimension influencing them. Satisfaction and sustainability in occupational patterns are highly influenced by the environmental constraints or affordances, thus the environment is shown as affecting and being affected by an individual's occupational patterns.

Implications for Research

Clearly, lifestyle balance is a broad concept that cuts a wide swath across many disciplines in the health and social sciences. Much research currently underway, including that related to understanding the role of emotions in cognition and motivation, the psychoneuroimmunology of lifestyle factors, sophisticated research in time-use, and efforts in positive psychology, are contributing important information to support this construct. The authors are currently developing a lifestyle-balance screening tool, which, in preliminary research, has demonstrated satisfactory psychometric properties and has shown evidence of concurrent and construct validity. Additional research is needed to identify life-stage related differences in wellness promoting occupations and research that provides insight into the occupational categories that, when neglected, place the individual at highest risk. Research is also needed to increase understanding of the impact of habits and routines (both healthful and maladaptive) and their relationship to a health and well-being (Yerxa, 2002).

Conclusion

This paper presented a proposed model of lifestyle balance, asserting that sustained patterns of occupation that meet biological and psychological needs within the unique environments of individuals can lead to reduced stress, improved health and well-being, and greater life satisfaction. Five dimensions regarding occupational areas necessary for well-being were identified and supported by brief reviews of empirical research. The concept of lifestyle balance, particularly as it may serve as an antidote to life stress, is worthy of more empirical research and conceptual development. The present model is proposed as a first step toward understanding how specific characteristics of lifestyles viewed as occupational patterns can positively influence overall health and well-being.

Editor's Note

Differences exist in the terminology employed in the interdisciplinary research into well-being and that

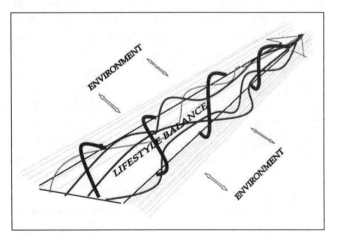

Figure 21.1. Visual depiction of the model of lifestyle balance.

used by occupational scientists. There is tension between being true to the scholarship that informs the discussion and promoting an occupational perspective of health. While both arguments have merit, occupational terms consistent with the *Journal of Occupational Science* are used in this discussion. The equivalence in meaning of the terms *activity, life activity* and *occupation; activity patterns* and *patterns of occupation;* and *need-based activity dimensions* and *need-based dimensions of occupation,* as used in this article, are nonetheless asserted.

References

Achat, H., Kawachi, I., Levine, S., Berkey, C., Coakle, E., & Colditz, G. (1998). Social networks, stress and health-related quality of life. *Quality of Life Research, 7,* 735–750.

Antonovsky, A. (1979). *Health, stress, and coping: New perspectives on mental and physical well-being.* San Francisco: Jossey-Bass.

Antonovsky, A. (1987). The salutogenic perspective: Toward a new view of health and illness. *Advances: Journal of Mind-Body Health, 4,* 47–55.

Bachmann, K. D. (2000). *Work–life balance: Measuring what matters.* Ottawa: Conference Board of Canada.

Bandura, A. (1977). Self-efficacy: Toward a unifying theory of behavioral change. *Psychological Review, 84,* 191–215.

Bandura, A. (2000). Exercise of human agency through collective efficacy. *Current Directions in Psychological Science, 9,* 75–78.

Bandura, A. (2001). Social cognitive theory: An agentic perspective. *Annual Review of Psychology, 52,* 1–26.

Baum, A., & Posluszny, D. (1999). Health psychology: Mapping biobehavioral contributions to health and illness. *Annual Review of Psychology [electronic version], 50,* 137–163.

Bond, J., Galinsky, E., & Swanberg, J. (1998). The national study of the changing workforce. New York: Families and Work Institute. *Journal of Personality, 71,* 245–266.

Britt, T., & Bliese, P. (2003). Testing the stress-buffering effects of self engagement among soldiers on a military operation. *Journal of Personality, 71,* 245–257.

Britton, B., & Tesser, A. (1991). Effects of time-management practices on college grades. *Journal of Educational Psychology, 83,* 405–410.

Brown, L., Reynolds, C., Monk, T., Prigerson, H., Dew, M., Houck, P., et al., (1996). Social rhythm stability following late-life spousal bereavement: Associations with depression and sleep impairment. *Psychiatry Research, 62,* 161–169.

Cameron, J., Banko, K., & Pierce, W. (2001). Pervasive negative effects of rewards on intrinsic motivation: The myth continues. *Behavior Analyst, 24,* 1–44.

Camporese, R., Freguja, C., & Sabbadini, L. L. (1998). Time use by gender and quality of life. *Social Indicators Research, 44,* 119–144.

Carstensen, L. L. (1998). A life span approach to social motivation. In J. Heckhausen, & C. Dweck (Eds.), *Motivation and selfregulation across the life-span* (pp. 341–364). New York: Cambridge University Press.

Christiansen, C. H. (1999). Occupation as identity. Competence, coherence and the creation of meaning. *American Journal of Occupational Therapy, 53,* 547–558. http://dx.doi.org/10.5014/ajot.53.6.547

Christiansen, C. H. (2000). Identity, personal projects and happiness: Self construction in everyday action. *Journal of Occupational Science, 7,* 98–107.

Christiansen, C. H., Backman, C., Little, B., & Nguyen, A. (1999). Occupations and well-being: A study of personal projects. *American Journal of Occupational Therapy, 53,* 91–100. http://dx.doi.org/10.5014/ajot.53.1.91 Reprinted as Chapter 34.

Christiansen, C., & Matuska, K. (2006). Lifestyle balance: A review of concepts and research. *Journal of Occupational Science, 13,* 49–61.

Christiansen, C., & Townsend, E. (2004). *Introduction to occupation: The art and science of living.* Thorofare, NJ: Prentice Hall.

Clark, F. A. (2000). The concepts of habit and routine: A preliminary theoretical synthesis. *Occupational Therapy Journal of Research, 20,* 123S–138S.

Craft, L., & Landers, D. (1998). The effects of exercise on clinical depression and depression resulting from mental illness: A metaanalysis. *Journal of Sport and Exercise Psychology* [electronic version], *20,* 339–357.

Csikszentmihalyi, M. (1990). *Flow: The psychology of optimal experience.* New York: Harper and Row.

Csikszentmihalyi, M. (1997). *Living well. The psychology of everyday life.* London: Phoenix Books.

Cummins, R. A., Gullone, E., & Lau, A. L. D. (2002). A model of subjective well-being homeostasis: The role of personality. In E. Gullone & R. A. Cummins (Eds.), *The universality of subjective well-being indicators* (pp. 7–46). Dordrecht, The Netherlands: Klewer Academic Publishers.

Deci, E. L., & Ryan, R. M. (2000). The "what" and "why" of goal pursuits: Human needs and the self-determination of behavior. *Psychological Inquiry, 11,* 227–268.

Erikson, E. H. (1982). *The life cycle completed*. New York: Norton.

Erlandsson, L. K., & Eklund, M. (2001). Describing patterns of daily occupations: A methodological study comparing data from four different methods. *Scandinavian Journal of Occupational Therapy, 8*, 31–39.

Erlandsson, L-K., Rögnvaldsson, T., & Eklund, M. (2004). Recognition of similarities (ROS): A methodological approach to analysing and characterising patterns of daily occupations. *Journal of Occupational Science, 11*, 3–13.

Frankl, V. (1984). *Man's search for meaning*. New York: Washington Square Press.

Frone, M., Russell, M., & Cooper, M. (1992). Antecedents and outcomes of work family conflict: Testing a model of the work–family interface. *Journal of Applied Psychology, 77*, 65–78.

Gibson, J. J. (1979). *The ecological approach to vision perception*. Boston: Houghlin-Mifflin.

Goode, W. J. (1960). A theory of role strain. *American Sociological Review, 25*, 483–496.

Greenhaus, J., Collins, K., & Shaw, J. (2002). The relation between work–family balance and quality of life. *Journal of Vocational Behavior, 63*, 510–531.

Gurung, R., Taylor, S., & Seeman, T. (2003). Accounting for changes in social support among married older adults: Insights from the MacArthur studies of successful aging. *Psychology and Aging, 18*, 487–496.

Hagerty, M. (1999). Testing Maslow's hierarchy of needs: National quality of life across time. *Social Indictors Research, 46*, 249–271.

Håkansson, C., Dahlin-Ivanoff, S., & Sonn, U. (2006). Achieving balance in everyday life. *Journal of Occupational Science, 13*, 74–82.

Havighurst, R. (1972). *Developmental tasks and education*. New York: D. McKay.

Haymes, M., & Green, L. (1982). An assessment of motivation within Maslow's framework. *Journal of Research in Personality, 16*, 179–192.

Hochschild, A. R. (1997). *The time bind: When work becomes home and home becomes work*. New York: Metropolitan.

Jonsson, H., Borell, L., & Sadlo, G. (2000). Retirement: An occupational transition with consequences for temporality, balance and meaning of occupations. *Journal of Occupational Science, 7*, 29–37.

Jonsson, H., Josephsson, S., & Kielhofner, G. (2001). Narratives and experience in an occupational transition: A longitudinal study. *American Journal of Occupational Therapy, 55*, 424–432. http://dx.doi.org/10.5014/ajot.55.4.424

Kiecolt-Glaser, J., McGuire, L., Robles, T., & Glaser, R. (2002). Emotions, morbidity, and mortality: New perspectives from psychoneuroimmunology. *Annual Review of Psychology, 53*, 83–107.

Klinger, E. (1977). *Meaning and void: Inner experience and the incentives in people's lives*. Minneapolis: University of Minnesota Press.

Klinger, E. (1998). The search for meaning in evolutionary perspective and its clinical implications. In P. S. Fry (Ed.), *The human quest for meaning* (pp. 27–50). Mahwah, NJ: Lawrence Erlbaum.

Klumb, P., & Perraz, M. (2004). Why time sampling studies can enrich work–leisure research. *Social Indicators Research, 67*, 1–20.

Langer, E. J., & Rodin, J. (1976). The effects of choice and enhanced personal responsibility for the aged: A field experiment in an institutional setting. *Journal of Personality and Social Psychology, 34*, 191–198.

Lawton, M. P., Nahemow, L. & Yeh, T. (1980). Neighborhood environment and the well-being of older tenants in planned housing. *International Journal of Aging and Human Development, 1*, 211–227.

Linville, P. (1987). Self-complexity as a cognitive buffer against stress-related illness and depression. *Journal of Personality and Social Psychology, 52*, 663–676.

Little, B. R. (1988). *Personal projects analysis: Theory, methods and research*. Ottawa: Carleton University.

Little, B. R. (1998). Personal project pursuit: Dimensions and dynamics of personal meaning. In P. T. P. Wong & P. Fry (Eds.), *The human quest for meaning: A handbook of theory, research and application* (pp. 193–212). Hillsdale, NJ: Lawrence Erlbaum Associates.

Little, B. R., & Chambers, N. (2003). Personal project pursuit: On human doings and well-beings. In M. Cox & E. Klinger (Eds.), *Handbook of motivational counseling: Concepts, approaches, and assessment* (pp. 65–82). Chichester, UK: Wiley.

Macan, T. H., Shahani, C., Dipboye, R. L, & Phillips, A. P. (1990). College students' time management: Correlations with academic performance and stress. *Journal of Educational Psychology, 82*, 760–768.

Marino-Schorn, J. A. (1986). Morale, work and leisure in retirement. *Physical and Occupational Therapy in Geriatrics, 4*, 49–59.

Marks, S. R., & MacDermid, S. M. (1996). Multiple roles and the self: A theory of role balance. *Journal of Marriage and Family, 58*, 417–432.

Marks, S., Huston, T., Johnson, E., & MacDermid, S. (2001). Role balance among white married couples. *Journal of Marriage and Family, 63,* 1083–1098.

Markus, H. (1986). Possible selves. *American Psychologist, 41,* 954–969.

Maslow, A. H. (1943). A theory of human motivation. *Psychological Review, 50,* 370–396.

Maslow, A. H. (1970). *Motivation and personality.* New York: Harper and Row.

McAdams, D. P. (1992). Unity and purpose in human lives: The emergence of identity as a life story. In R. A. Zuker (Ed.), *Personality structure in the life course* (pp. 323–376). New York: Springer.

McAdams, D. P. (1993). *The stories we live by: Personal myths and the making of the self.* New York: Guilford Press.

McAdams, D. P. (1999). Personal narratives and the life story. In O. P. John (Ed.), *Handbook of personality: Theory and research* (pp. 478–500). New York: Guilford Press.

McEwen, B., & Lasley, E. (2002). *The end of stress as we know it.* Washington, DC: National Academic Press.

McGregor, I., & Little, B. R. (1998). Personal projects, happiness, and meaning: On doing well and being yourself. *Journal of Personality and Social Psychology, 74,* 494–512.

Melchoir, M., Niedhammer, I., Berkman, L., & Goldberg, M. (2003). Do psychosocial work factors and social relations exert independent effects on sickness absence? A six-year prospective study of the GAZEL cohort. *Journal of Epidemiology and Community Health* [Electronic version], *57,* 285–293.

Mendes de Leon, C. Glass, T. Beckett, L. Seeman, T. Evans, D. & Berkman, L. (1999). Social networks and disability transitions across eight intervals of yearly data in New Haven EPESE. *Journals of Gerontology* [electronic version], *54B,* S162–S172.

Misra, R., & McKean, M. (2000). College students' academic stress and its relation to their anxiety, time management, and leisure satisfaction. *American Journal of Health Studies, 16,* 41–50.

Monk, T., Reynolds, C., Buysse, D., DeGrazia, J., & Kupfer, D. (2003). The relationship between lifestyle regularity and subjective sleep quality. *Chronobiology International, 20,* 97–107.

Monk, T., Reynolds, C., Kupfer, D., Hoch, C., Carrier, J., & Houck, P. (1997). Differences over the life span in daily life-style regularity. *Chronobiology International, 14,* 295–306.

Monk, T. H., Flaherty, J. F., Frank, E., Hoskinson, K., & Kupfer, D. J. (1990). The Social Rhythm Metric: An instrument to quantify the daily rhythms of life. *The Journal of Nervous and Mental Disease, 178,* 120–126.

Murray, C. J. L., & Lopez, A. D. (Eds.). (1996). *The global burden of disease: A comprehensive assessment of mortality and disability from diseases, injuries and risk factors in 1990 and projected to 2020* (Vol. 1). Cambridge, MA: Harvard School of Public Health.

Peloquin, S. (1990). Time as a commodity. *American Journal of Occupational Therapy, 43,* 775–782.

Perlow, L. A. (1999). The time famine: Toward a sociology of work time. *Administration Science Quarterly, 44,* 57–81.

Pentland, W., Harvey, A., & Walker, J. S. (1998). The relationship between time use and health and well-being in men with spinal cord injury. *Journal of Occupational Science, 5,* 14–25.

Persson, D., Eklund, M., & Isacsson, Å. (1999). The experience of everyday occupations and its relation to sense of coherence: A methodological study. *Journal of Occupational Science, 6,* 13–26.

Persson, D., Erlandsson, L., Eklund, M., & Iwarsson, S. (2001). Value dimensions, meaning, and complexity in human occupation: A tentative structure for analysis. *Scandinavian Journal of Occupational Therapy, 8,* 7–18.

Pierce, D. (2003). *Occupation by design: Building therapeutic power.* Philadelphia: F. A. Davis.

Reis, H. T., & Gable, S. L. (2000). Event sampling and other methods for studying daily experience. In H. Reis & M. Judd (Eds.), *Handbook of research methods in social and personality psychology* (pp. 190–222). New York: Cambridge University Press.

Reker, G. T., Peacock, E. J., & Wong, P. T. P. (1987). Meaning and purpose in life and well-being: A life-span perspective. *Journal of Gerontology, 42,* 44–49.

Repetti, R., Taylor, S., & Seeman, T. (2002). Risky families: Family social environments and the mental and physical health of offspring. *Psychological Bulletin* [electronic version], *128,* 330–366.

Robinson, J. P., & Godbey, G. (1997). *Time for life: The surprising ways Americans use their time.* University Park, PA: The Pennsylvania University Press.

Ryff, C. D. (1989). Happiness is everything, or is it? Explorations on the meaning of psychological well-being. *Journal of Personality and Social Psychology, 57,* 1069–1081.

Ryff, C. (1995). Psychological well-being in adult life. *Current Directions in Psychological Science, 4,* 99–104.

Ryff, C. D., & Singer, B. (1996). Psychological well-being: Meaning, measurement, and implications for psychotherapy research. *Psychotherapy and Psychosomatics, 65,* 14–23.

Ryff, C. D., & Singer, B. (1998). The contours of positive human health. *Psychological Inquiry, 9,* 1–28.

Sapolsky, R. M. (2004). *Why zebras don't get ulcers* (3rd ed.). New York: Henry Holt and Co., LLC.

Seeman, T., Glei, D., Goldman, N., Weinstein, M., Singer, B., & Lin, Y. (2004). Social relationships and allostatic load in Taiwanese elderly and near elderly. *Social Science and Medicine* [electronic version], *59,* 2245–2257.

Seeman, T., Lusignolo, T., Albert, M., & Berckman, L. (2001). Social relationships, social support, and patterns of cognitive aging in healthy, high-functioning older adults: MacArthur studies of successful aging. *Health Psychology* [electronic version], *20,* 243–255.

Seeman, T., Singer, B., Ryff, C., Love, G., & Levy-Storms, L. (2002). Social relationships, gender, and allostatic load across two age cohorts. *Psychosomatic Medicine* [electronic version], *64,* 395–406.

Seleen, D. (1982). The congruence between actual and desired use of time by older adults: A predictor of life satisfaction. *The Gerontologist, 22,* 95–99.

Shaw, R. (2003). The agent-environment interface: Simon's indirect or Gibson's direct coupling. *Ecological Psychology, 15,* 37–106.

Sheldon, K. M., & Niemiec, C. P. (2006). It's not just the amount that counts: Balanced need satisfaction also affects well-being. *Journal of Personality and Social Psychology, 91,* 331–344.

Skully, D., Kremer, J., Meade, M., Graham, R., & Dudgeon, K. (1998). Physical exercise and psychological well-being: A critical review. *British Journal of Sports Medicine* [electronic version], *32,* 111–120.

Sternberg, E. (1997). Emotions and disease: From balance of humors to balance of molecules. *Nature Medicine, 3,* 264–267.

Strong, L., & Fiebert, M. (1987). Using paired comparisons to assess Maslow's hierarchy of needs. *Perceptual & Motor Skills, 64,* 492–494.

Szuba, M., Yager, A., Guze, B., Allen, E., & Baxter, J. (1992). Disruption of social circadian rhythms in major depression: A preliminary report. *Psychiatry Research, 42,* 221–230.

Taylor, S., Repetti, R., & Seeman, T. (1997). Health psychology: What is an unhealthy environment and how does if get under the skin? *Annual Review of Psychology, 48,* 411–448.

Taylor, S., & Seeman, T. (1999). Psychosocial resources and the SES-health relationship. In N. Adler, M. Marmot, B. McEwen, & J. Stewart (Eds.), *Socioeconomic status*

and health in industrialized nations: Social, psychological, and biological pathways (pp. 210–225). New York: New York Academy of Sciences.

Thompson, M. G., & Heller, K. (1990). Facets of support related to well-being: Quantitative social isolation and perceived family support in a sample of elderly women. *Psychology and Aging, 5,* 535–544.

Uchino, B. N., Cacioppo, J. T., & Kiecolt-Glaser, J. K. (1996). The relationship between social support and physiological processes: A review with emphasis on underlying mechanisms and implications for health. *Psychological Bulletin, 119,* 483–531.

Verbrugge, L. M. (1983). Multiple roles and physical health of women and men. *Journal of Health & Social Behavior, 24,* 16–30.

Walker, S., Sechrist, K., & Pender, N. (1987). The health-promoting lifestyle profile: Development and psychometric characteristics. *Nursing Research, 36,* 76–81.

Wells, A. J. (2002). Gibson's affordances and Turing's theory of computation. *Ecological Psychology, 14,* 140–180.

Whiteford, G. (2000). Occupational deprivation: Global challenge in the new millennium. *British Journal of Occupational Therapy, 63,* 200–205. Reprinted in Chapter 26.

Whiteford, G. (2001). The occupational agenda of the future. *Journal of Occupational Science, 8,* 13–16.

Whiteford, G. (2004). When people cannot participate: Occupational deprivation. In C. Christiansen & E. Townsend (Eds.), *Introduction to occupation: The art and science of living* (pp. 221–242). Upper Saddle River, NJ: Prentice-Hall.

Wicker, F. W., Brown, G., Wiehe, J. A., Hagen, A. S., & Reed, J. L. (1993). On reconsidering Maslow: An examination of the deprivation/domination proposition. *Journal of Research in Personality, 27,* 118–133.

Wicker, F. W., & Wiehe, J. A. (1999). An experimental study of Maslow's deprivation-domination proposition. *Perceptual and Motor Skills, 88,* 1356–1358.

Wicker, F. W., Wiehe, J. A., Hagen, A. S., & Brown, G. (1994). From wishing to intending: Differences in salience of positive versus negative consequences. *Journal of Personality, 62,* 347–368.

Wilcock, A. A., Chelin, M., Hall, M., Hambley, N., Morrison, B., Scrivener, L., et al (1997). The relationship between occupational balance and health: A pilot study. *Occupational Therapy International, 4,* 17–30.

Wong, P. T. P. (2000). Meaning of life and meaning of death in successful aging. In A. Tomer (Ed.), *Death attitudes and the older adult: Theories, concepts, and applications* (pp. 23–37). Philadelphia: Brunner-Routledge.

Yalom, Y. D. (1980). *Existential psychotherapy.* New York: Basic Books.

Yerxa, E. (2002). Habits in context: A synthesis, with implications for research in occupational science. *Occupation, Participation and Health, 22,* 104S–110S.

Youngstedt, S., O'Connor, P., & Dishman, R. (1997). The effects of acute exercise on sleep: A quantitative synthesis. *Sleep: Journal of Sleep Research & Sleep Medicine, 20,* 203–214.

Zerubavel, E. (1981). *Hidden rhythms, schedules and calendars in social life.* Chicago: The University of Chicago Press.

Zika, S., & Chamberlain, K. (1992). On the relation between meaning in life and psychological well-being. *British Journal of Psychology, 83,* 133–145.

Zuzanek, J. (1998). Time use, time pressure, personal stress, mental health and life satisfaction from a life cycle perspective. *Journal of Occupational Science, 5,* 26–39.

Part III.B. Cultural Contexts

CHAPTER 22

Culture: A Factor Influencing the Outcomes of Occupational Therapy

RUTH LEVINE SCHEMM

Overview

People can accomplish seemingly impossible goals if invested in the outcome; on the other hand, few people are interested in activities that have no personal meaning. This paper will explore one of the factors that can make therapy more meaningful to our patients. The concept is a complex pattern of living, which is called *culture*. As therapists, we search for activities that will stimulate and interest our patients as well as promote functional abilities. This is no easy task because few of our patients come from the same culture group that we do. This paper will define culture, review the importance of culture in occupational therapy practice, and describe how cultural beliefs and values affect assessment and treatment in occupational therapy.

Let us begin with a treatment vignette that offers an introduction to the concept of culture.

Case Study

Mrs. W., a 57-year-old, attractive, upper-middle-class, urban housewife with Guillian–Barre syndrome, was hospitalized and transferred to a rehabilitation center and then to home care. Mrs. W. occupied a first-floor bedroom suite in the newly purchased home of one of her daughters. The family reasoned that Mrs. W. could interact with family members, walk short distances, and join the family for meals. The physical therapist felt that Mrs. W. was almost ready to return to her own home if it were adapted to accommodate her needs. Mrs. W. lived in a newly constructed three-story townhouse in center city. Although the OTR felt that referral

This chapter was previously published, under the name of Ruth Ellen Levine, jointly in *Sociocultural Implications in Treatment Planning in Occupational Therapy* (The Haworth Press, Inc., 1987) and in *Occupational Therapy in Health Care*, 4(1), 3–16. Copyright © 1987, Informa Healthcare. Reprinted with permission.

to occupational therapy was perhaps too late for best results, she decided to visit the patient anyway.

On the day of the scheduled evaluation visit, the OTR was admitted into the gracious house by the maid because the daughter was conferring with an interior decorator. The OTR was led to the first-floor bedroom where Mrs. W. was propped up in bed while a full-time attendant fussed over her sheets and cleared her breakfast dishes. Mrs. W. ignored the therapist and continued her conversation with the attendant. After a few minutes, Mrs. W. briefly acknowledged the OTR and spent the next 15 minutes describing her symptoms as if the OTR was an unwanted, inexperienced newcomer. Mrs. W. praised "her" physical therapist and attributed her progress to his guidance and skill. The occupational therapist tried to guide their conversation toward the patient's previous interests and activities and her present views on self-care and independence, but Mrs. W. switched the conversation back to the physical therapist.

The OTR decided to define her role and the type of equipment that might improve Mrs. W.'s functional abilities. This seemed to make Mrs. W. act more defensively. The OTR tried to ameliorate her discomfort by pointing out useful safety rails and tub seats in an equipment catalog. Mrs. W. grew even more negative and told the OTR that she did not need adaptive equipment. The OTR soon realized that something was wrong with the interview but could not fathom why it was going so poorly. Mrs. W. became more upset as the therapist tried to win her approval by switching the topic to the other services offered by an occupational therapist, including work simplification and analysis of architectural barriers. Unfortunately, this topic also proved difficult, and Mrs. W. interrupted the OTR and told her that the physical therapist said that she was making excellent progress. The OTR tried to explain that she was impressed with Mrs. W.'s efforts, but this praise did not impress Mrs. W.

The OTR decided there was nothing else to do so she concluded the evaluation by telling Mrs. W. that she would close the case because Mrs. W. had no interest in adaptive equipment. Mrs. W. said she hoped that she would never see the occupational therapist again and told the OTR that she planned to report her to the physical therapist.

Later, the physical therapist called the OTR to find out what had gone wrong with the evaluation. He reported that Mrs. W. was angry and upset and claimed that the OTR insisted that she would need "handicapped" equipment for the rest of her life. The OTR was both hurt and confused and wondered what she had done to infuriate Mrs. W. After all, she was doing exactly what she had been taught in her training for home health care.

The negative outcome of this evaluation visit affected all of the team members—patient, caretakers, physical therapist, nurse, and the occupational therapist. Each person was interpreting events from their own perspective. The meaning of the communication was, in part, determined by the person's values, interests, goals, roles, and habits. Each person's culture became a filter or screen that either passed information through or blocked it. The vignette demonstrates that even though the therapist's professional manner was similar to that prescribed during her professional training, the patient interpreted the visit as an attempt to jinx her hard-won progress. In retrospect, the OTR may have realized that two different opinions about the value of adaptive equipment started the tangled communication. Within a short time, the OTR could not extricate herself from the negative meaning that "handicapped" things had for Mrs. W. The therapist moved her treatment agenda too quickly without hearing what the patient was really saying. Mrs. W. was frightened by her diagnosis and did not want to see, touch, own, or talk about anything that implied that she might not regain her independence. In Mrs. W.'s culture outward appearances were of vital importance, people who used adaptive equipment were handicapped, and the thought that other people might regard her as disabled was more stressful than being dependent on an attendant.

Historical Overview

Occupational therapy founders first considered culture as an important aspect of treatment planning because of their belief in the interrelationship between mind and body. If an activity generated a patient's interests it could also promote functional independence. In the first occupations training course, Tracy identified activities that matched the patient's lifestyle,[1] and Dunton agreed and emphasized the need to stimulate the patient's interests by prescribing activities based on personal and cultural values.[2] Hall and Buck claimed that "brain workers should be given work that was largely physical and those who worked with their hands, must have simpler, more primitive tasks."[3] Although the consideration of culture was not fully developed, the Founders searched for different ways to elicit a patient's interest through the use of novel experiences. In 1925 a committee of the American Occupational Therapy Association defined *occupational therapy* and formulated 15 principles, one-third of which emphasized the importance of considering the patient's interests and needs.[4] Thus, the early literature of the profession is filled with examples of attempts to consider the patient's culture during treatment.

As medical care became more scientific in the 1930s and 1940s, therapists began to concentrate more on the patient's pathology than on residual strengths; thus, decreasing their initial commitment to linking the patient's goals, interests and values, habits, and roles with the activity process. At the same time, many therapists were arts-and-crafts teachers who were committed to a philosophy that tended to encourage patients to refine their craft skills and produce an attractive end-product. It was believed that the quality product would enhance self-confidence. Other therapists concentrated on the benefits that occurred during the *doing* part of the activity process. Thus, ideological differences grew between the therapists and the diversionists.[5] Another factor that compromised initial consideration of culture during the Depression years was the scarcity of funds. Therapists had to treat large numbers of patients and market and sell patient projects in order to replenish department supply budgets. The patients' interests were subordinated to the department needs because some projects were more cost efficient than others.

The emphasis on arts and crafts with little concentration on the therapeutic use of activities may have prompted Eleanor Clarke Slagle to tell the 1930 graduating class at Sheppard and Enoch Pratt Hospital that "handicrafts are not enough" because " . . . the patient is being more and more considered in relation to his domestic and community life."[6]

Culture was as important in early practice as it must be today, because occupational therapy deals with goal-directed activities which are part and parcel of everyday life. Recently, modern therapists are rediscovering the importance of early beliefs that emphasized the interaction of mind and body during treatment. Theorists Mosey,[7] Fidler and Fidler (see Chapter 9),[8] Llorens,[9] Reilly,[10] Kielhofner and Burke,[11,12] Barris,[13] Nuse-Clark,[14] and Yerxa[15] all address the influence of culture in treatment. Using basic concepts from our past, present-day theorists still emphasize the importance of the patient's motivation, interests, goals, interests, values, habits, time-orientation, roles, caretaker network, and use of the nonhuman environment. All of these concepts are part of a person's culture.

Defining Culture

Culture has been described as a "blueprint" for human behavior, influencing individual thoughts, actions, and collectively influencing a particular society.[16] Culture can be viewed as a multifaceted influence which is learned by direct and indirect daily experiences based on what people do (cultural behavior), say (speech messages), make, and use (cultural artifacts). In short, a child learns a life pattern of beliefs and values which shape the way that he or she believes, thinks, perceives, feels, and behaves.[17] Culture is a way of life that encompasses kinetic or overt behavior, psychological expressions, and the material products of labor or industry. The major cultural transmission agents are behavioral and material elements simply because psychological states are not transferable.[18]

Kinetic or overt behaviors, the first elements of culture, are evident in actions performed by an individual and include body motions, speech patterns, distance selected during communication with others, and use of products and tools. People use their bodies in unique ways to indicate agreement, acceptance, rejection, discomfort, and other reactions.

Speech patterns are also culturally determined; rate of speech, expression and emphasis, pronunciation, and choice of words are part of a person's culture. Even the distance preferred between people during different activities is also culturally determined.[19] Tool use, as part of one's behavior, is another factor indigenous to one's culture: some people use handtools exclusively, others rely on sophisticated gadgets and technology, some others prefer to use only their hands in doing tasks. In examining culture one must also consider how people employ objects and other artifacts. For example, consider a patient who uses the same hammer over and over and seems to derive pleasure from completing

a task by using this object which almost seems like a nonhuman friend. In contrast, another patient may be careless with tools and abuse them without giving it a second thought. Still another patient may regard the use of tools with disdain because handmade objects can be purchased and "time is money."

Psychological aspects, the second elements of one's culture, include knowledge, attitudes, and values that are shared by members of a given cultural group. These factors cannot be readily observed because they take place in a person's mind. Psychological factors are therefore more difficult for an observer to assess and observe. Although these factors are subjective they still deserve some of our attention because people exhibit different reactions to events in their daily lives. On the other hand, measurement of psychological factors is not precise and individual reactions may be inconsistent and variable even under the same circumstances. For example, if you introduce yourself to a patient using your first name only some people may feel right at home, welcome your informality, and respond with warmth and humor. On the other hand, another person may find it annoying but tolerable and respond stiffly to requests for additional information. We can speculate that the first patient equates the informality with a type of relationship where the therapist and he are equal partners. The second patient may feel that she has just met the therapist, and the use of first names indicates a forced familiarity that makes the patient feel guarded. Thus we see that the same event can take on different meaning for each participant depending on one's cultural background.

The last element associated with culture, the "material products of labor or industry," are the objects and artifacts that comprise *the non-human environment*. This category includes signs, symbols, objects, tasks, roles, and social organizations used to create products in the environment. Consider the work produced by a given group of people, the way that ideas are transformed into reality, and the type of organization that is needed to produce the goods and services. Members of a group teach their children how to participate in their culture through a complex system of rewards and punishments which are conveyed through thoughts, actions, social beliefs, attitudes, communication patterns, perceptions, time orientation, and ways of handling animals, plants, and objects. In effect, a child is exposed to a pattern of beliefs, attitudes, perceptions, meanings, and emotions based on personal experiences in a particular setting.[20]

Culture imposes a conditioning variable that is internalized in the human psyche and not easily forgotten.[21] Values, interests, goals, habits, roles, time orientation, communication patterns, the ways in which one uses symbols and artifacts, selects nonhuman objects—all are well ingrained as one grows, making change difficult. In fact, Likroeber compared culture to the great coral reefs built by polyps. The polyps die, but their secretions leave a permanent record of their former life.[22] Thus, culture establishes a filter through which individuals interpret daily events. At the same time, one's group establishes patterns that become "commonly defined meanings and sanctioned behaviors favored by the group."[23] Individuals are never free of the group influence—sometimes subtle and sometimes more specialized—to meet individual physical and psychological needs.[24]

The Relevance of Culture in Occupational Therapy

Culture is a central component of occupational therapy because people judge the quality of their therapy through a filter which is comprised, in part, of past learning and emotions and which is based on three levels of beliefs: (1) the patient's perception of illness and health, (2) the patient's perception of therapy, and (3) the patient's belief in the meaning of his own life and activities. These factors overlap and are not discrete.

Illness is not the same to all individuals. Sociologists have long identified significant differences in the ways that members of specific cultures decide to seek health care, care for themselves, use family caretaker networks, take medication and follow prescribed remedies, participate in a healthful daily regime, assist other ill family members, and endure pain and suffering.[25,26,27,28,29,30] Occupational therapists cannot assume that people all react to the stress of illness, traumatic events, or other life disruptions in the same way. "Illness behavior" refers to the ways in which symptoms may be differently perceived, evaluated, and acted (or not acted) upon by different kinds of persons.[31] The behavior varies with a person's socioeconomic class, education level, community cohesiveness, and ethnic origin. The higher the social status of a population, the better educated and informed they will be about signs and symptoms of illness.[32]

Being "ill" certainly is not the same to everyone. Some people are not ill until they are incapable of performing daily roles, others are ill as soon as they note a slight change in their body, still others are ill only if the illness is labeled by the medical establishment and therefore given "official" sanction. Therapists must consider the issue of illness behavior in rehabilitation because of diverse reactions such as a patient who does not want to participate in therapy because he is "ill" and therefore is not *capable* of participation. This type of behavior was described in a case study depicting the progress of an elderly Italian–American, with a left hemiparesis, who maintained that he could not dress or toilet himself until his arm "got well." This response is logical if you understand the culture of the first-generation Southern Italian.[33,34]

Another question to consider is how well patients understand their treatment programs. Occupational therapy can only be perceived as meaningful and deserving of the patient's interest and cooperation if it is relevant to patients and their caretakers. Treatment is valued only if patients believe that they have been helped by it. If not, services are judged as irrelevant and inconsequential. Chances are that therapists who are capable of attending to the patient's cultural values by selecting relevant treatment activities are also able to convince the patient that therapy is important. Yet, it is difficult to tap into the interests of patients who have experienced a traumatic illness, accident, or event which has drained their energies and made adaptation seem overwhelming and taxing. Sharrott maintained that occupational therapists "play a profound role in creation, affirmation and experience of meaning" because therapy provides opportunities for patients to redefine their previous experiences in light of their present abilities and needs.[35] Effective therapy alters the patient's perception of meaningful existence by offering concrete feedback on daily performance in activities that are important in a patient's life roles. Unlike other treatment, occupational therapy mirrors the painful limitations wrought by traumatic incident, aging, development, or deprivation. But therapy sessions can alter the patient's perception of life by providing immediate evidence on what the patient CAN do rather than what is lost.[36]

Another factor frequently overlooked when designing therapy programs is the patient's beliefs and values regarding the nonhuman environment. Barris discussed the importance of the treatment environment because it should provide "adequate but not overbearing stimulation."[37] Patients will express culturally determined values about their environment, and these ideas should be respected. For example, some patients prefer to do their therapy activities alone and refuse to participate in a group project, whereas other patients like to be involved in the social interactions that evolve during work on a collective project. Relevance, or the link between therapy and the patient's reality, should become part of initial treatment planning because the therapist is responsible for developing a strong link between the patient's interests and the goals of the occupational therapy program. This is not to say that it is easy to develop therapy that is compatible with the patient's goals, values, and interests. These three factors—the patient's perception of illness and health, the patient's perception of therapy, and the patient's belief in the meaning of life and activities—are all considered in a successful therapy program.

Factors to Consider During Evaluation and Treatment

This section will use information presented in the earlier case study to demonstrate how the OTR could have improved her assessment if cultural factors had been considered during the evaluation visit.

Conceptual Framework

One way to systematically include culture in one's daily treatment is to select a conceptual framework or model that includes culture. Although many occupational therapy theories and models mention culture, the Model of Human Occupation[38,39] includes a conceptual structure that integrates data about the patient's values, goals, interests, personal causation, habits, and roles into occupational therapy.

Background

The next step is to observe and investigate the lifestyle of cultural group members. Consider the largest number of ethnic group members in your patient load and find out where group members live. Try to do a small-scale, informal ethnographic study by exploring a local store, restaurant, recreational center, or religious sanctuary.[40] During your visit use your clinical skills to observe the human and non-human environment and the way that group members interact. Consider the values that are conveyed through all of these cues.

For instance, if the OTR had visited Mrs. W.'s neighborhood, she would have found a row of exclusive townhouses in a village within center city. The colonial-style, three-story, brick houses have narrow stairways and small rooms—in no way a barrier-free environment. Each house faced an attractive courtyard with a few trees and benches in the center. Garages were hidden underground and could only be accessed by an enclosed walkway. The houses were situated near a cluster of exclusive stores where one could buy things like gourmet take-out food, imported wine, custom made tiles, designer clothing, or hand-made lampshades.

This upper-middle-class neighborhood conveyed an air of cosmopolitan homogeneity. Although the OTR could not assume that Mrs. W. shared all of her neighbors' values, she could still learn something about her patient's lifestyle. It is not realistic to visit every patient's neighborhood; nonetheless, one can choose the largest group among one's patients and gather some background information about them. This data is as important as looking up medication side-effects and unfamiliar medical diagnoses.

Reading offers another source of information. Research on particular cultural groups appears in sociological, anthropological, and historical journals. Books also depict life in a particular culture. For instance, Chute's novel about the pain, humiliation, and rage of a poverty-stricken New England family[41] offers insight into rural deprivation. Factual accounts are also useful, such as the story told by Wideman, a Black-American Rhodes scholar and English professor, who searches for an answer to why his brother, who was raised by the same parents in the same environment as the author is presently serving a life sentence for murder.[42] Television and film documentaries that portray family and community life are helpful in understanding different lifestyles. In short, the OTR should gather as much information as possible about a patient's cultural group before the evaluation visit.

Using the case-study as an example, the OTR did not adequately prepare for the evaluation visit. The nurse and the physical therapist could have been used as informants so the OTR could be introduced to the patient's lifestyle. The OTR tried to control the interview by taking charge and asking questions. Mrs. W. valued competition and outward appearances; moreover, it was important for her to act like the family matriarch. Thus, the OTR became a rival. During the first 15 minutes of the interview, the OTR could have satisfied Mrs. W.'s need for attention by listening to her description of her progress and offering support for her efforts. At the same time, the OTR could have thoroughly observed the environment.

Evaluation

The initial evaluation is a crucial time to establish trust and gather cues from the human and the non-human environment. There are a number of evaluation tools that can be used to direct these observations. Use a guide to begin your search for an effective instrument. The Kielhofner text *The Model of Human Occupation*[43] includes an overview of assessment tools or Asher's *Annotated Index of Occupational Therapy Evaluation Tools*[44] which includes profiles on 87 occupational therapy instruments, as well as information on where to find the tool.

Because no instrument is perfect, consider elements of the patient's lifestyle by observing values concerning life, death, health, productivity, work, family relations, human nature, time, meaningful activities, and religion. Be alert to ethnic myths and taboos which will impede care if misunderstood by the therapist. Use data gathered from the evaluation tools you use to refine your ideas about treatment. For example, Mrs. W. may have responded better if the OTR had explored one of her interests and then used the activity to observe Mrs. W.'s functional abilities.

Specific tools which could have been used in conjunction with other ADL, cognitive, perceptual, or motor evaluations are the Occupational Role History,[45,46] a semi-structured interview on occupational choice, work experience, and leisure satisfaction, or The Occupational Questionnaire[47] which collects data on the patient's use of time in daily activities and how that relates to the patient's values, interests, and personal causation. Two other useful tools are The Role Checklist, which assesses productive adult life-roles by indicating the individual's perceptions of past, present, and future roles[48] and the Time Battery for gathering qualitative and quantitative data on temporal adaptation and use of time.[49] The OTR should have selected a tool which seemed to provide appropriate ideas for treatment planning.

Even if the OTR had used better interviewing skills, completed an ADL Evaluation, and administered an instrument such as the Occupational Questionnaire, she would still need to compare this data with cues from the environment. Thus, the OTR's observation skills are fundamental to evaluation and treatment planning because patients may not always mean what they say. Examine the "extent to which the patient's beliefs, values, and customs are congruent with a trifold set of standards: from the patient's culture or ethnic group, from the therapist's own culture, and from the setting in which the treatment takes place.[50] Consider the extent that the patient is "like all other humans, like some other humans, and like no other humans."[51] Take

time to identify and label similarities and differences between the patient's culture and the therapist's. This will help to separate personal bias and needs from those of the patient. For example, not all patients want to be independent in self-care. Some want to direct their energies toward other activities and view assistance as a trade-off. This was certainly true for Mrs. W.

A final consideration is the setting in which treatment takes place. Is the therapist a guest in the patient's home or is the patient a visitor in the hospital? The answer to those questions will determine roles and relationships. Treatment must be appropriate for the setting. For example, the institution is not always the best place to teach cooking and toileting skills because the information must be retaught once the patient returns home. On the other hand, the home setting is not suitable for constructing complex equipment and hand splints.

Summary

This paper has explored the importance of culture in occupational therapy. Occupational therapy founders emphasized the need to consider the patient's interests in treatment. Today, we again realize that treatment must be meaningful to patients. Thus, cultural factors must be considered in evaluation and treatment. This is no easy task because we are all entrenched in our own value systems. However, although there are many differences among cultural groups, there are also many similarities. Occupations can serve as a "common light among cultures."[52]

N.B. Throughout this paper the author has used the term "patient" to refer to the recipient of treatment. The term "client" was eschewed because it did not reflect people who were receiving medical services.

References

1. Tracy, SE: *Studies in invalid occupations.* Boston: Whitcomb and Barrows. 1912.

2. Dunton, WR: *Occupational Therapy: A manual for nurses. Philadelphia:* WB Saunders Co. 1918.

3. Hall, H and Buck, MMC: *Handicrafts for the Handicapped.* New York: Moffatt, Yard and Company. 1916, p. xii.

4. American Occupational Therapy Association Committee. An outline of lectures in Occupational Therapy to medical students and physicians. *Occupational Therapy and Rehabilitation.* 5, 1925, p. 278.

5. Doane, JC: Presidential address delivered at AOTA annual meeting. Toronto, Canada, September 28–30,

1931. Reprinted as *Occupational Therapy and Rehabilitation, 10,* 1931, p. 365.

6. Slagle, EC: Address to Graduates, Sheppard and Enoch Pratt Hospital, Towson, Maryland, June 28, 1930. *Occupational Therapy and Rehabilitation, 9* 1930, p. 275.

7. Mosey, AC: *Occupational Therapy: Configuration of a Profession.* New York: Raven Press. 1981, p. 78.

8. Fidler, GS and Fidler, JW: Doing and becoming: the Occupational Therapy experience. In Kielhofner, G, *Health through occupation.* Philadelphia: FA Davis Company. 1983, p. 267–280.

9. Llorens, LA: *Application of a developmental theory for health and rehabilitation.* American Occupational Therapy Association. 1976.

10. Reilly, M: The modernization of Occupational Therapy. *Amer J Occup Ther 25,* 1971, p. 243–246.

11. Keilhofner, G and Burke, JP: Components and determinants of human occupation. In Kielhofner, G (Editor): *A Model of Human Occupation: theory and application.* Baltimore, Maryland: Williams and Wilkins. 1985, p. 12–36.

12. Kielhofner, G and Burke, JP: A model of human occupation, Part I. Conceptual Framework and content. *Amer J Occup Ther 34,* 1980, pp. 572–581.

13. Barris, R: Environmental interactions: an extension of the model of occupation. *Amer J Occup Ther 36,* 1982, pp 637–644.

14. Nuse-Clark, P: Human development through occupation: A philosophy and conceptual model for practice, part 2. *Amer J Occup Ther 33,* 1979, pp. 577–585.

15. Yerxa, E: Audicious values: The energy source for occupational therapy practice. In Kielhofner, G. (Editor) *Health through occupation.* Philadelphia: FA Davis. 1983, pp. 149–162.

16. Leininger, M: *Transcultural nursing: concepts, theories, and practices.* New York: John Wiley and Sons. 1978, p. 80.

17. Spradley, JP, McDurdy, DW (Editors): *Conformity and conflict.* Boston: Little, Brown. 1980, p. 2.

18. Linton, R. *The cultural background of personality.* New York: AppletonCentury-Crofts, Inc. 1945, p. 38.

19. Hall, ET: *The hidden dimension.* Garden City, New York: Anchor Books. 1969.

20. Laudin, H: *Victims of culture.* Columbus, Ohio: Charles E. Merrill Pub. Co. 1973.

21. Opler, M: *Culture and social psychiatry.* New York: Atherton Press. 1967, p. 14.

22. Likroeber, Al: quoted in Laudin, op. cit. p. 4.

23. Ibid. p. 184.

24. Ibid. p. 189.

25. Mechanic, D: Response factors in illness: the study of illness behavior. In Jaco, EG. (Editor): *Patients, physicians and illness.* New York: The Free Press. 1972, pp. 128–141.

26. Leininger, op. cit.

27. Saunders, L: *Cultural difference and medical care.* New York: Russell Sage Foundation. 1954.

28. Scott, CS: Health and healing practices among five ethnic groups in Miami, Florida. *Public Health Reports. 89* 1974, pp. 524–32.

29. Suchman, EA: Social patterns of illness and medical care. *Journal of Health and Human Behavior. 6,* 1965, pp. 2–16.

30. Wolff, BB and Langley, S: Cultural factors and the response to pain. A review, In Weisenberg, M (Editor): *Pain: clinical and experimental perspectives.* Saint Louis: The CV Mosby Co. 1975, pp. 141–143.

31. Mechanic, D. Religion, religiosity, and illness behavior. *Human organization. 22,* 1963, p. 202.

32. Suchman, EA: Sociomedical variations among ethic groups. *American Journal of Sociology. 70* 1964–5, pp. 319–331.

33. Lopreato, J: *Italian Americans.* New York: Random House, 1970.

34. Levine, RE: The cultural aspects of home care delivery. *Amer J Occup Ther 38,* 1984, pp. 736–737.

35. Sharrott, G: Occupational therapy's role in the client's creation and affirmation of meaning. In Kielhofner, G: *Health through occupation.* Philadelphia: FA Davis. 1983, p. 215.

36. Rogers, JC: The spirit of independence: the evolution of a philosophy. *Amer J Occup Ther 36,* 1982 pp. 709–715.

37. Barris, op. cit.

38. Kielhofner and Burke, op. cit.

39. Kielhofner, G. op. cit.

40. Merrill, SC: Qualitative methods in occupational therapy research: an application. *The occupational therapy journal of research. 5* 1985, pp. 209–222.

41. Chute, C: *The Beans of Egypt, Maine.* New York: Ticknor & Fields, 1985.

42. Wideman, JE: *Brothers and keepers.* New York: Penguin Books. 1984.

43. Kielhofner, op. cit.

44. Asher, IE: *Annotated index of occupational therapy evaluation tools.* Thomas Jefferson University, Department of Occupational Therapy, 1985.

45. Moorehead, L: The occupational history. *Amer J Occup Ther 23,* 1969, pp. 329–334.

46. Florey, LL & Michelman, SM: Occupational role history: a screening tool for psychiatric occupational therapy. *Amer J Occup Ther 36,* 1982 pp. 301–308. http://dx.doi.org/20.5014/ajot.36.5.301

47. Riopel, N & Kielhofner, G: *Occupational questionnaire.* In Asher, op. cit. p. 57.

48. Oakley, F: *The Role Checklist.* In Asher. op. cit. p. 58.

49. Larrington, G: *Time Battery.* In Asher. op. cit. p. 59.

50. Tripp-Reimer, T., Brink, PJ, Saunders, JM: Cultural assessment: content and process. *Nursing Outlook. 32,* p. 81.

51. Kluckholn, C: quoted in Brill, NI: *Working with people: the helping process.* Philadelphia: JB Lippincott, 1976, p. 19.

52. Malinowski, B: *Argonauts of the western pacific.* New York: EP Dutton and Co., Inc., 1961. p. 25.

CHAPTER 23

Culture Emergent in Occupation

BETTE R. BONDER, LAURA MARTIN, AND ANDREW W. MIRACLE

Culture influences occupation as well as perceptions of health, illness, and disability. Therapists are aware of the need to address culture in interventions. However, definitions of culture can be unclear, providing little guidance to therapists about how to recognize its effects in therapeutic encounters. A pragmatic definition of culture as emergent in everyday interactions of individuals encourages reconsideration of the main elements of culture, that it is learned, shared, patterned, evaluative, and persistent but changeable. Understanding of culture as emergent in interaction, including therapeutic intervention, suggests three important characteristics that therapists can cultivate to enhance clinical encounters: careful attention, active curiosity, and self-reflection and evaluation.

Introduction

Occupational therapists have long acknowledged that culture is an important aspect of occupation and of perceptions of health, disability, and illness. The founders of the profession emphasized that therapeutic activities should be prescribed based on the individual's personal and cultural values (Dunton, 1918). This recognition has led to many calls for cultural competence in the clinic (Barney, 1991; Dillard et al., 1992; Mirkopoulos & Evert, 1994; Wittman & Velde, 2002), a call now incorporated into standards for education of new therapists (American Occupational Therapy Association [AOTA], 1999). It is fair to say that "few occupational therapists are unaware of the importance of considering culture in the provision of occupational therapy services" (Fitzgerald, Mullavey-O'Byrne, & Clemson, 1997, p. 1).

This chapter was previously published in the *American Journal of Occupational Therapy, 58,* 159–168. Copyright © 2004, American Occupational Therapy Association. Reprinted with permission. http://dx.doi.org/10.5014/ajot.58.2.159

Before cultural factors can be addressed in care, therapists must have a clear understanding of what culture is. Anthropologists, who have a primary focus on defining and describing culture, have throughout their history debated the definition of the term and still have not reached consensus (Kuper, 1999). It is therefore not surprising that therapists likewise are somewhat unclear about exactly what the construct means. Too often, race and ethnicity are used as representations of culture. For example, in their book on cultural competency, Wells and Black (2000) discuss what it is that "White American health practitioners" (p. 138) must be aware of in their practice, suggesting that White Americans constitute a single cultural group and that race is a central characteristic of cultural group identity. The equation of race or ethnicity with culture leaves therapists to puzzle about whether culture is something that applies only to those who look different from themselves or speak a different language (Pope-Davis, Prieto, Whitaker, & Pope-Davis, 1993). Because effective therapeutic interventions address cultural factors as a way to enhance quality of life and optimal performance (Barney, 1991; Dyck & Forwell, 1997), this confusion about what constitutes culture has a potentially damaging impact on client care.

Defining Culture

In the occupational therapy literature, an array of definitions of *culture* can be found. One definition is "a state of manners, taste, and intellectual development at a time or place. It is the ideas, customs, arts, etc. of a given people at a given time" (Baptiste, 1988, p. 180). At approximately the same time, Levine (1987; see Chapter 22) described culture as "a 'blueprint' for human behavior, influencing individual thoughts, actions and collectively influencing a particular society" (p. 7). Krefting and Krefting (1991) called it "a filter or veil through which people perceive life's experiences" (p. 108). Christiansen and Baum (1997) define culture as referring to the "values, beliefs, customs and behaviors that are passed on from one generation to the next" (p. 61). Still another definition labels culture "an abstract concept that refers to learned and shared patterns of perceiving and adapting to the world" (Fitzgerald et al., 1997, p. 1).

Anthropologists have also developed multiple definitions for culture. Since it was first created by Edward B. Tylor (1871) and other late 19th-century scholars, use of the term has evolved. Not surprisingly, changes in usage have reflected the changed understandings of what it means to be human that have been in vogue at various times.

By the mid-20th century, the burgeoning influence of individual psychology began to affect scholarly approaches to culture. Sapir (1924/1949) and Wallace (1961) noted that the foundations for cultural traits resided in the minds of specific individuals; that is, while patterns of thinking and behavior might be widely shared across a society, the locus of culture is within individuals. Wallace's theory of mazeway as the mechanism for cultural change was explicit in this regard. For Wallace, culture change begins when a single individual incorporates a new element (e.g., through invention or borrowing) or when someone synthesizes traditional elements in a new configuration. If such innovation is perceived as useful, then additional individuals in the cultural group may adopt it and thus widespread change may be underway.

Geertz (1973) describes *culture* as "webs of meaning" in which people live. Kuper (1999) indicates that "in its most general sense, culture is simply a way of talking about collective identities" (p. 3). Holland, Lachicotte, Skinner, and Cain (1998) suggest that culture can be conceived in several different ways: as defining and determining individual human needs; as a superficial labeling of deep-seated needs; or as a formation of motivation during development. There has been considerable debate in anthropological circles about whether culture refers to behavior, or to the artistic expression of emotion, that is, culture in the sense of the arts and literature (Kuper, 1999).

Today, anthropologists (e.g., Reyna, 2002) work to explain the relationship between the biological and the cultural. Noting the work of anthropologists such as D'Andrade (1999) and Dressler and Bindon (2000), Handwerker (2002) concludes that a "theory of culture as cognitive elements and structure now dominates

ethnographic research" (p. 119). Moreover, there is a growing recognition by psychologists (e.g., Hermans & Kempen, 1998; Pepitone, 2000) that the "discipline can no longer assume an acultural or unicultural stance" (Segall, Lonner, & Berry, 1998, p. 1101). And, sociologists (e.g., Cerulo, 2001) have begun to consider culture and cognition, especially in the context of race and ethnicity.

All of these conceptualizations carry some common themes related to individuals' actions, and their attributions of meaning and value to those actions. Two main strategies have typically been employed to create the necessary specificity in defining culture.

A Descriptive Approach

One strategy for elaborating on definitions of culture has been an approach characterized by a detailed description of particular groups through "the set of characteristics that an observer might record in studying the collective life of a human group" (Kuper, 1999, p. 24). This descriptive approach is exemplified in the thorough accounts by early ethnographers of New World indigenous groups, or by such works as Eliot's (1948) list of English cultural traits. Such descriptions involve a systematic identification of the particular characteristics and material goods of a given society. A full description of all the technological, economic, political, kinship, and religious characteristics of a people, together with the details of their socialization practices, rituals, and value systems, has been assumed to provide a description of the culture of that people. Providing a list of the major traits, patterns of behavior, and material objects the people produce or use is believed to offer a good approximation of a particular cultural group at a given moment in time. Examples of this kind of description are now widely available at Web sites focused on diversity, or on culture and health (for an example, see Cross-Cultural Health Care Program, www.xculture.org/resource/library/index/cfm).

Producing these descriptions is a demanding task. It is impossible to describe every relevant cultural fact about a given people. Even if the task itself were manageable, such a list can tell us nothing of the choices a single member of the group has made within the range of possibilities each culture provides. This approach assumes that by describing what seem (to the describer) to be the significant traits of a culture, outsiders can gain an appreciation of what life is like, at least superficially, for the people involved. Most of the time, though, descriptive approach products simply summarize cultures with just a few key values or characteristics. The ethnographies that abound in anthropology are excellent examples of the descriptive approach (cf., Hendrickson, 1995), but require constant updating as cultural circumstances change (Hendrickson, 1996).

Such summaries can be useful. They provide snapshots of particular groups at particular points in time, and a general sense of the important values and behaviors of the group. They provide for the observer, or the therapist, a starting point from which further exploration of the values of the specific individual within the culture can begin. But they are inevitably superficial. The potential exists to create stereotypes, or to replace one stereotype with another, rather than to reach a genuine understanding of the culture as represented by its individuals. This strategy also inevitably results in a limitation of scope. As an example, Hendrickson (1995) focused her attention specifically on weaving, providing much less information about other aspects of life in the Guatemala highlands, the lives of men, for instance, or the activities of women in villages where weaving was not typical.

A Rules Approach

Another strategy for enhancing cultural understanding focuses on the rules for belief and behavior. This approach assumes culture serves as a cognitive model of reality for each of the group's members. For example, Skinner (1989) provides a list of rules for the behavior of young girls in Naudada, a Hindu community in central Nepal. The list indicates what good daughters and good wives do. On the list is a rule indicating that good wives die before their husbands. Knowing this rule, that it is unseemly to outlive one's husband, helps the outsider understand why the term *Radi* (widow) is a pejorative term in that culture. Thus, understanding a culture means knowing how the people living in that culture view reality, how they make distinctions among categories of things, and how they generally make decisions about right courses of action (Schneider, 1976). Of course, in taking this approach it is necessary to know (and to describe for others) most of the things that exist in the world of those people. In this sense, the rules approach subsumes the descriptive one, but adds a list of the rules by which the culture determines meaning, molds behavior, and incorporates new information.

Taking the approach of listing rules can be quite helpful in providing a starting place for interaction. Many guides to cultural competence for health-care providers emphasize this strategy, indicating, for example, what the rules are for interaction between genders, how to address someone from a particular cultural group, or whether or not to make direct eye contact (Galanti, 1997; Wells & Black, 2000). Knowing the rules can provide the therapist with a starting point for asking appropriate questions about the preferences of the individual.

However, like descriptive accounts, rules studies are always incomplete because not everything can be included. Nor can it ever be known with certainty that the model provided by such an approach really describes reality as understood by all the people in a society or even by most of them. By imposing a static model of culture, this method also fails to accommodate the ranges of variability or the combinations of cultural influences experienced by most individuals, especially those living in culturally heterogenous communities.

In spite of the consistent association between action and meaning and the many examples of rules-based and description-based accounts, definitions of culture remain relatively vague from the occupational therapist's point of view. They fail to provide guidance regarding precisely how culture relates to occupation, and, therefore, how therapists might address culture in assessing clients and designing meaningful and relevant interventions. We believe that too often therapists fail to recognize that everyone in an encounter has culture (in fact, identifies with more than one culture, as will be discussed below), and that the cultural experiences of every participant in an encounter affect the nature of the interaction (cf., Bonder, Martin, & Miracle, 2002). It is equally easy to dismiss as "not really cultures" the regional differences (e.g., Appalachian) and other factors (e.g., sexual orientation, bicultural identities) that individual clients may self-describe as components of their cultural identities. For purposes of creating interventions, therapists need a pragmatic definition that can guide the kinds of questions they ask, their interpretation of responses, and their design of treatment.

The Model of Culture Emergent

A third approach to culture, the one we adopt here, is based on a pragmatic definition of *culture* as emergent in the everyday interactions of individuals (Bonder et al., 2002). It has been developed to elaborate on and reconceptualize factors found in traditional definitions of culture. This definition emphasizes both group patterns and individual variation to explain the multiple influences experienced by people who live and work in culturally diverse settings, and to allow for the inter-active effects of noncultural influences from biological and psychological aspects of the person. Rather than attempt to define and delineate specific cultural groups, this approach suggests that the way any individual be-haves is based on the array of influences, both those general to the group and those unique to her or his development. This idea is based on a conceptualization of culture as a *symbolic system that emerges through the interaction of individuals.*

Culture emergent suggests that the symbolic aspects of culture and cultural identity emerge in interaction and are displayed primarily through talk and through action. Both language and action are symbols (Hol-land et al., 1998; Kuper, 1999; Tedlock & Mannheim, 1995) that result from cultural learning and convey the values of the group. Talk and action are "processed through the filter of interpretation. Actions are arti-facts, signs that are intended to convey meaning" (Ku-per, p. 105). This symbolic language is public, thus, by extension the values of the culture are public (Ku-per), and talk and action are conditioned by transient circumstances as well as by traditional patterns of be-havior (Sherzer, 1987; Urban, 1991). Krefting (1991) notes that "although culture is a shared phenomenon, sharing is seen in the context of transmission and so-cialization. Moreover, individuals learn culture from a number of different people and places, so each per-son's contact with and interpretation of the culture is unique" (p. 5).

Not only is culture uniquely expressed by the indi-vidual; its expression also changes constantly, based on new experiences and the influence of those expe-riences on perceptions. In these ways, "Culture is con-tested, temporal, and emergent" (Clifford, 1986, p. 19). Tedlock and Mannheim (1995) suggest that cultures emerge and are revised continuously in the interaction among individuals within the group through both dia-log and action.

The theoretical framework of *culture emergent* takes into account the interactions of individuals and cul-tural development as well as the process of change in culture over time (Tedlock & Mannheim, 1995). Thus, the focus is away from cultural group–cultural mind-set and toward individuals making choices within cultur-ally supported boundaries. The idea of culture emer-gent assumes that cultural patterns are dynamic and collectively negotiated by individuals through multi-ple interactions. The culture emergent approach views culture itself as having evolved from application of the social, problem-solving, task orientation of human be-ings. We assume that some cultural belief structures and behavior patterns are laid down in early childhood through learning and experience within the family and community, but we also assume that those structures and patterns are continually reevaluated. One only has to reflect on the differences between the values and behaviors demonstrated by his or her parents, perhaps on the issue of cultural diversity itself, and those rep-resented by his or her peers and profession to see that even patterns learned very early in life are susceptible to modification over time and experience.

This approach also conceptualizes culture as a cogni-tive model of reality, a model that is based on the cumu-lative learning experiences of the individual. However, this model is not a unitary one shared by everyone in so-ciety, but a differentiated one located in individuals. And, because all individuals have had different experiences in life, personal models always vary at least slightly, even among individuals who live in similar environments and have shared many similar experiences. Inevitably, some elements of culture may be shared with one set of individuals, while other elements may be shared with other sets. Moreover, because individuals continue to have new experiences throughout life, the model reflects the fact that culture adapts and changes, sometimes dra-matically though often slowly, through the actions of individuals. Culture emergent presupposes the individ-ual—not the group—as the key cultural actor, and en-courages careful examination of both the group and the individual. Within this framework, we highlight five im-portant characteristics of culture, emphasizing the ways in which the concept of culture emergent affects tradi-tional conceptualizations of culture.

Culture Is Learned

Most definitions suggest that culture is learned. It is transmitted from one generation to another through the process of enculturation, the acquisition of cultural knowledge that allows one to function as a member of a particular group. The learned aspect of culture sets it apart from the biological (Kuper, 1999). It is not in-herited, but must be transmitted from individual to individual. Observation and discourse are the primary means of cultural transmission. One learns culture through interaction with others, listening, observing, and assessing those interactions.

Enculturation, the acquisition of culture, occurs both through purposeful instruction and through modeling and observation. One learns the culture of a profession like occupational therapy in part through direct teaching in the course of the professional education experience. Faculty teach not only the facts required to plan and provide intervention, but also the value system of the profession, through, for example, explication of the professional code of ethics, the mind-set that supports client-based care, or the importance of evidence-based practice. This initial learning may require organization around specific rules taught by others (Holland et al., 1998).

In addition to this purposefully taught information, specific individuals such as occupational therapy students acquire information from experience, interaction, and the evaluative responses of others. This kind of learning enables the learner to form a gestalt that directs action in new situations (Holland et al., 1998). Observing and modeling more experienced therapists during fieldwork and the early years of practice is a mechanism for learning about and practicing particular kinds of professional behavior. Both the intentional teaching and the less formal modeling serve to enculturate students to the professional culture.

Culture emergent suggests that because culture is learned, it must be presumed that the learning process is ongoing, and that new behaviors, beliefs, and values emerge as individuals acquire new information and experience. Further, because culture is learned, it also is shared with those from whom it is learned and those to whom it is taught. Each interaction with another individual provides an opportunity for learning culture and for reinforcing elements already acquired. This interactive sharing and mutual reinforcement has the effect of binding the individual to others and to the group. It is the mechanism by which group identities are formed.

Culture Is Localized

Culture is created and expressed through discrete interactions with specific individuals in particular locations. It is from such interactions that one draws meaningful elements that will be shared with some but not all individuals within society. Thus, culture is situated in personally meaningful locales. It is from such interactions, in the immediate surroundings, that individuals learn meaningful elements that will be shared with some, even most, of the other persons within the group. Rosaldo (1999) suggests that "all knowledge is local" (p. 31). Even in an era of mass electronic communication around the world, information is processed based on local values, mores, and norms (Abu-Lughod, 1999; Kuper, 1999).

Professional settings offer a kind of well-defined environment for the emergence of localized knowledge. For example, knowing how the occupational therapy clinic is set up, or how the supplies are classified, or how patient visits are prioritized is largely learned from experience or observation in a particular setting. The specifics of such knowledge need not be shared with others in different parts of the organization or with therapists in other clinics, although in general every occupational therapy practitioner will need to have similar information, regardless of work setting.

However, interactions in multiple social settings also provide multiple contexts for learning culture. Thus, the concept of culture emergent suggests that every individual embodies multiple cultural components, some based on ethnicity, race, or country of origin, and others based on life experience in other contexts such as professional, geographic, religious, social, or family settings. Everyone is a bundle of cultural threads, and social context influences individual choices about displaying one or another of them. In every interaction, only part of an individual's identity is being exhibited, making all understanding about that identity incomplete (cf., Holland et al., 1998).

This localization of culture is part of what makes it meaningful. Meaning is assigned to any particular cultural factor based in part on the perspective of the individual. Perspectives can be communicated and shared with others, and can be broadened through experience and training. Nevertheless, at any given moment, each individual is responding to a particular view of an interaction, a view that our model terms *vantage*. Like the position adopted by Bakhtin (1981) and drawing directly from Hill and MacLaurey (1995), this notion suggests that at another moment, a similar interaction may carry different interpretations because of a change of *vantage*. Vantage effects are clearly evident, for example, in the differing interpretations of a client's behavior from the perspective of a physician and a therapist. Similarly, asking someone "how are you" in a clinical setting carries a very different connotation than asking the same question in a social situation.

Culture Is Patterned

Patterning is essential for social behavior and for the development and maintenance of societies (Fitzgerald et al., 1997). It is essential that individuals develop patterns for behavior, because patterns help minimize ambiguity and relieve us from having to renegotiate each interaction from scratch (cf., Holland et al., 1998). Patterns emerge from the repetition of specific samples of behavior and talk. Repeated patterns establish the normal and customary expectations that structure interactions.

Culture is patterned in two senses. First, it is patterned in that the components of culture are integrated, reflecting generalizable patterns within which individual actions have meaning. Culture emergent theory suggests a second form of patterning, that is, culture is patterned in the repetitive behaviors of individuals, which become so ingrained that they seem like empirical reality. Through ritual, daily routine, and habitual behaviors, individuals express their cultural identities and affiliations, as well as their individual preferences and characteristics (cf., Holland et al., 1998). For example, a woman dressing in India will have a different routine for donning her sari than a woman donning her pantsuit in the United States. Such routinized behaviors serve not only to structure daily life, but also to help shape an evaluative system for assessing one's own and others' behaviors. Both women must also make somewhat less routinized decisions while dressing, including determinations about the level of formality in dress that is required by a particular situation and personal preferences about style and color. These decisions reflect a degree of individual self-expression, even though the ranges in both cases are bound by culturally governed matters of availability, convention, and values. In general, we assume that the process of repetition leads to ritualization (i.e., assignment of symbolic meaning). Ritualized and routinized behavior leads to a shaping of the individual's "reality." From there it is only a short step to being the "right thing."

Culture Is Evaluative

Values are embedded in culture and are reflected in individual behavioral decisions and choices (Kuper, 1999). Values reflect the underlying organization of shared structures that facilitate social interaction. Society would not be possible without a significant level of shared values. Socialization within families and communities is one means of acquiring values. Ideally, there is considerable consensus about values within a society or a group, because commonality of evaluative perception is one of the factors that helps hold individuals together in social institutions. It is doubtful, though, that there is ever total agreement on values, even in small groups. Different cultures, different groups within a society, or different individuals within a group may agree or disagree on how to evaluate items or ideas.

Perhaps the most salient example of this difference in evaluation is one that is mentioned repeatedly in the occupational therapy literature. Occupational therapy is based on a set of values that holds independence to be an essential goal for individual well-being (Kinébanian & Stomph, 1992). However, in a number of cultures, independence is much less highly valued, with interdependence, or, in situations of illness or disability, dependence, being both expected and accepted (cf., Jang, 1995). Kinébanian and Stomph (1992) give the example of a Hindu man with hemiplegia who, although able to accomplish many tasks for himself, declined to do so, indicating that he was waiting for God to improve his physical status.

The idea of culture emergent emphasizes that individuals are shaped by their culture. However, it also emphasizes that socialization is not the same for all members of a given group. Individuals are continuously evaluating the applicability and relative weight of values in terms of personal relevance. Sometimes, contradictory values may exist, and decisions about which one to acknowledge are contingent on context. Spencer, Krefting, and Mattingly (1993) report that when one of the researchers was introduced as an occupational therapist, patients with traumatic brain injury identified their problems as double vision, instability in walking, and difficulty swallowing. When the same researcher was introduced as an anthropologist, patients identified their problems as loneliness, financial difficulties, and unhappiness about being labeled as retarded. In this case, patients' expectations about the culture of the researcher, either in terms of what they thought was expected of them or in terms of what they thought the researcher could help them with, imposed a screen in terms of what they identified as problematic. Gender, age, innate skills, and social position are among the variables affecting an individual's socialization experiences (Holland et al., 1998). These factors in turn affect the acquisition of values.

One's values, the concepts of what is desirable or abhorrent, change over the life course. Children, adolescents, young adults, middle-aged individuals, and elderly individuals may have differing value orientations as a result not only of differing needs and personal experience, but also because of what their interaction with the cultures around them has taught them. This variation is reflected in, and reflects, another important characteristic of culture emergent. While elements of culture are persistent, culture is also constantly evolving.

Culture Has Continuity With Change

Generally, culture is more or less stable through time. This consistency is an important characteristic of culture, essential if it is indeed to provide the values and beliefs that guide or pattern behavior. However, cultures are far from static (Sewell, 1999). They are constantly evolving (Sahlins & Service, 1960), and would, in fact, disappear if they did not. This is not to suggest that cultural difference is disappearing. Even in the face of global communication, differences persist, perhaps even sharpening (Clifford, 1986). This ability of cultures to incorporate new ideas, to borrow from other cultures, to assimilate new information, is a strength that enables cultures to persist.

One source of cultural change is the introduction of new technologies. As part of our research on the meaning of occupation for weavers in the highlands of Guatemala (Bonder & Martin, 2001), we found that weavers in small villages in the Guatemala highlands have begun to use the Internet to market their textiles as a way to maintain a traditional art that might otherwise disappear. By opening new markets selling on the Internet, they increased the revenue generated by this age-old activity, thereby sustaining themselves as well as the tradition.

Similarly, the cultural knowledge of an individual changes over the life course as new objects, situations, and interactions are encountered (Tedlock & Mannheim, 1995). The theory of culture emergent is particularly focused on this element of culture. Individual experiences serve to shape a unique person. However, across a society, many individuals may experience forces for change almost simultaneously and respond in similar ways. The progress of digital technology in the United States and elsewhere offers us many examples of such forces for change and their relationships not only to life activities (e.g., job tasks) but to identity (e.g., technophobes versus technophiles) and values (e.g., role of Internet in discussions of plagiarism and reevaluations of intellectual property rights). Within larger cultural groups, smaller groups change at their own pace, often in response to trends elsewhere in the system. So, for example, demographic changes at a societal level produce organization change at an institutional level (cf., Martin & Bonder, 2003). The concept of emergence helps explain why this is so and helps manage it.

Usually, cultural groups are continuous over time. Except in cases of wholesale extermination through contact-induced disease or forcible conquest, cultural change seldom means replacement, especially for individuals. Though new cultural components are added to an individual's knowledge base, preexisting components are not excised. For example, old ideas about technology may be supplanted. They cease to exist only when they are no longer learned by a new generation. Occupational therapists rarely work with their clients on shoeing horses or making soap or using typewriters. However, these used to be common cultural skills, and are still viable among some groups.

Culture changes in two ways. First, at the societal level, the collective patterns may change when many individuals alter their behavior over a short period of time, as a result of changes in the external context. For example, when environmental circumstances change, or when one group comes in contact with another on a widespread basis, cultural change is nearly inevitable and often invisible (Kuper, 1999). Second, the cultural knowledge of an individual continues to change over the life course as the person encounters new elements in the personal environment and incorporates them into life and interactions.

Implications for Practice

The idea of culture emergent has consequences for therapeutic intervention in occupational therapy as well as in other health-care encounters. It suggests a particular view of culture that has the potential to guide therapists' interactions.

Culture and Occupation

Culture is an important influence on occupational patterns, and occupational choices reflect cultural beliefs. A client's choice of activity level, engagement in particular occupations, and perceptions about the value of particular occupational outcomes are all influenced by his or her cultural beliefs. Kluckhohn and Strodtbeck (1961) suggest that every culture has a conception of human activity that conveys values that may be expressed through orientations on "being," "being-in-becoming," or "doing." In Western culture, the "being" orientation is somewhat devalued (Rowles, 1991), while other cultures value that orientation more highly than the Western orientation toward "doing" (Jang, 1995). Some Far Eastern cultures emphasize harmony with nature, acceptance of fate, and personal reflection as being more central than active doing of occupations. If the therapist values the Western "doing" culture, there may be a conflict with a client who values a "being" perspective more highly.

Examples of cultural influences on occupation are ubiquitous. For instance, gender roles in some cultures are rigidly defined, such that women and men may have relatively restricted choice of productive (work) roles. In our observations in Maya communities in the highlands of Guatemala, women typically look after the home, weave using backstrap looms, and provide child care. Men work in the fields or take jobs in town. Women rarely run for public office or hold leadership positions in the church. However, individual personality and personal experience definitely influence these roles. Some women become influential in village politics through activities with women's weaving cooperatives, or through church activities linked to their husbands' roles in the church (Bonder, 2001). As educational opportunities, political activism, and social support for expanded women's roles increase, individual women will exercise new choices, and, over time, may alter the description of "typical" Maya women's work (Bonder & Martin, 2001).

Cultural constructions of occupation also influence the experience of disability. When disability interferes with accomplishment of occupations strongly linked to cultural values, life-satisfaction can be compromised. We spoke with a Maya woman who could no longer weave because of arthritis and who felt a great sense of personal loss. However, for her, modifying the activity was not acceptable because of the rigidity of her definition of its structure in her culture. The idea of sitting on a chair instead of the floor was not consistent with her view of how weaving occurred, even though in other villages nearby, weavers had all begun to sit on low stools. Alternatively, another Maya woman whose disability interfered with her weaving was able to substitute other activities that promoted a sense of self-worth for her (Bonder, 2001).

In clinical encounters, therapists must carefully explore the cultural construction of specific occupations and occupational patterns. Without such exploration, a process that characterizes the critical thinking that is vital to effective practice (Wittman & Velde, 2002), important aspects of occupation will be overlooked. In exploring culture, however, it is vital to recognize the emergent nature of culture in the individual. Knowledge of cultural facts is useful only as a means of generating preliminary hypotheses that must be tested for the specific client. It is also essential to recall that the therapist, too, has culture. The values and beliefs that accompany that culture also influence the interaction and must be given careful attention. It is not possible for the therapist to be an entirely objective observer of a situation (Bakhtin, cited in Willeman, 1994).

Framing Encounters

Sue (2000) suggests that effective intercultural clinical interaction has three primary characteristics. The first of these is *scientific-mindedness*. Sue refers here to the recognition that clinical encounters are based on forming hypotheses based on prior knowledge, with the expectation that these hypotheses must be tested in the specific encounter. Experience with individuals from a particular culture may well lead to a set of assumptions about all individuals from that culture. However, as Mattingly (1998) notes, therapists who carry those assumptions into intervention without examining their applicability to the specific client may well fail in their efforts. One must also cultivate what Sue has labeled *dynamic sizing skills*. The clinician must recognize when cultural generalizations apply to a particular situation and when individual factors predominate. In order to do so effectively, the clinician needs at least some *culture-specific expertise*, knowledge about the general characteristics of cultural groups.

Thus, therapeutic encounters become something of a dance between the individual and the cultural. The therapist must recognize the limitations of cultural generalities, but, at the same time, possess a fund of knowledge from which to begin. As an example, a therapist planning treatment for a Maya immigrant woman who has had a stroke will find it helpful to know that in Maya culture women do the cooking, and that typical meals include vegetables, beans, and tortillas. Tortillas are the staff of life for Mayans, carrying much ritual, mythological, and symbolic content. It is also helpful to know that the tortillas are made through a process involving soaking of the corn, grinding it into meal, mixing the dough, shaping it by clapping the dough between the hands, and cooking on a stone over a flame. However, if the Maya woman is a secondor third-generation resident of the United States, she may make her tortillas using purchased cornmeal, on a griddle over an electric burner, and may even shape the tortillas using a tortilla press. In fact, she might prefer to serve peanut butter and jelly sandwiches made with purchased white bread. Different movements and procedures are required for the different kinds of cooking, and treatment must be molded accordingly.

Intervention Strategies

Understanding of culture as emergent in intervention suggests three important characteristics that therapists can cultivate to enhance clinical encounters. The first of these is attending carefully to the interactional moment (Tedlock & Mannheim, 1995). Because culture emerges in interaction, each interaction is a new situation. Previous information about specific cultures, about the diagnosis of the client, and about other relevant factors must be understood in the context of the immediate situation. Therefore, attention to word choice, facial expression, body posture, voice tone, gestures, and other clues to the feelings and attitudes of the individual can be identified only through careful attention. The symbols that convey information about a culture are public and observable (Sewell, 1999), assuming one is attending carefully.

Active curiosity about the meaning of these clues is the second characteristic that therapists can bring to clinical encounters. It is impossible to know all there is to know about every labeled cultural group, Hispanics, for example, or Blacks. And as we have established, even knowing those facts would not provide adequate information in a particular encounter. Asking questions to help interpret observations can provide vital information to assist in understanding of the individual and framing of intervention.

Finally, therapists can engage in self-reflection and evaluation of interactions in order to improve subsequent encounters (Rosaldo, 1999). It is impossible always to notice the important clues, to ask the right questions, and to draw the right inferences. Nor are therapists neutral observers (Kuper, 1999). Reflection about choices made in one encounter can assist therapists to improve the next interaction. Their own culture, like that of their clients, is unavoidable (Greenfield, 2000), emergent in their clinical encounters, and, thus, subject to change. Self-reflection and evaluation can ensure that the change enhances future therapeutic interactions.

Conclusions

It is well-established that culture affects occupation and that occupational therapists must acknowledge its impact on daily life and on intervention strategies. Failure to do so can prevent establishment of rapport, decrease trust, and lead to communication difficulties, all of which can reduce effectiveness of intervention (Krefting, 1991). However, culture is difficult to define and even more difficult to quantify. Efforts to group people on the basis of a set of cultural facts, as is done in much diversity training practice, are unlikely to be effective because these efforts fail to recognize the subtle but profound interplay of personal, experiential, and cultural factors in individual lives. Further, this approach fails to take into account the constant change that is part of individual lives.

The task of cultural understanding "involves observing what occurs between people in the intersubjective realm. These exchanges take place in the clear light of public interactions, they do not entail the mysteries of empathy or require extraordinary capacities for going inside people's heads or, worse, their souls" (Rosaldo, 1999, p. 30). Rather, the therapist, like a good ethnographer, "constructs data in a dialogue with informants, who are themselves interpreters" (Kuper, 1999, p. 214). Incorporation of the concept of culture emergent, that is, a definition of culture as a part of identity that emerges in individual interactional moments in specific locales, has the potential to enable clinicians to enhance clinical care by acknowledging the profound impact of culture, the unique nature of each individual, and the strategies that can lead to enhanced understanding and therapeutic collaboration.

References

Abu-Lughod, L. (1999). The interpretation of culture(s) after television. In S. B. Ortner (Ed.), *The fate of "culture": Geertz and beyond* (pp. 110–135). Berkeley, CA: University of California Press.

American Occupational Therapy Association. (1999). *Standards for accreditation of an occupational therapy education program.* Rockville, MD: Author.

Bakhtin, M. M. (1981). *The dialogic imagination: Four essays by M. M. Bakhtin.* In M. E. Holquist (Ed.). (C. Emerson & M. Holquist, Trans.). Austin, TX: University of Texas Press.

Baptiste, S. (1988). Murial Driver Memorial Lecture: Chronic pain, activity, and culture. *Canadian Journal of Occupational Therapy, 55,* 179–184.

Barney, K. F. (1991). From Ellis Island to assisted living: Meeting the needs of older adults from diverse cultures. *American Journal of Occupational Therapy, 45,* 586–593. http://dx.doi.org/10.5014/ajot.45.7.586

Bonder, B. R. (2001). Culture and occupation: A comparison of weaving in two traditions. *Canadian Journal of Occupational Therapy, 68,* 310–319.

Bonder, B. R., & Martin, L. (2001, November). *The meaning of weaving for Maya women in the Guatemala Highlands.* Paper presented at the Midwest Association for Latin American Studies, Cleveland, OH.

Bonder, B. R., Martin, L., & Miracle, A. W. (2002). *Culture in clinical care.* Thorofare, NJ: Slack.

Cerulo, K. A. (Ed.). (2001). *Culture in mind: Toward a sociology of culture.* New York: Routledge.

Christiansen, C., & Baum, C. (1997). Person–environment occupational performance: A conceptual model for practice. In C. Christiansen & C. Baum (Eds.), *Occupational therapy: Enabling function and well-being* (2nd ed., pp. 47–70). Thorofare, NJ: Slack.

Clifford, J. (1986). Introduction. In J. Clifford & G. E. Marcus (Eds.), *Writing culture: The poetics and politics of ethnography* (pp. 1–21). Berkeley, CA: University of California Press.

Cross-Cultural Health Care Program. (1996). *CCHCP Library.* Retrieved June 5, 2002, from http://www.xculture.org/resources/library/index.cfm

D'Andrade, R. (1999). Comment. *Current Anthropology, 40*(Suppl.), S16–S17.

Dillard, M., Andonian, L., Flores, O., Lai, L., MacRae, A., & Shakir, M. (1992). Culturally competent occupational therapy in a diversely populated mental health setting. *American Journal of Occupational Therapy, 46,* 721–726. http://dx.doi.org/10.5014/ajot.46.8.721

Dressler, W. W., & Bindon, J. R. (2000). The health consequences of cultural consonance. *American Anthropologist, 102,* 244–260.

Dunton, W. R. (1918). *Occupational therapy: A manual for nurses.* Philadelphia: Saunders.

Dyck, I., & Forwell, S. (1997). Occupational therapy student's first year fieldwork experience: Discovering the complexity of culture. *Canadian Journal of Occupational Therapy, 64,* 185–196.

Eliot, T. S. (1948). *Notes toward the definition of culture.* London: Faber & Faber.

Fitzgerald, M. H., Mullavey-O'Byrne, C., & Clemson, L. (1997). Cultural issues from practice. *Australian Occupational Therapy Journal, 44,* 1–21.

Galanti, G. (1997). *Caring for patients from different cultures* (2nd ed.). Philadelphia: University of Pennsylvania Press.

Geertz, C. (1973). *The interpretation of cultures.* New York: Basic Books.

Greenfield, P. M. (2000). What psychology can do for anthropology, or why anthropology took postmodernism on the chin. *American Anthropologist, 102,* 564–576.

Handwerker, W. P. (2002). The construct validity of cultures: Cultural diversity, culture theory, and a method for ethnography. *American Anthropologist, 104,* 106–122.

Hendrickson, C. (1995). *Weaving identities: Construction of dress and self in a Highland Guatemala town.* Austin, TX: University of Texas Press.

Hendrickson, C. (1996). Women, weaving, and education in Maya revitalization. In E. F. Fischer & R. M. Brown (Eds.), *Maya cultural activism in Guatemala* (pp. 156–164). Austin, TX: University of Texas Press.

Hermans, H. J. M., & Kempen, H. J. G. (1998). Moving cultures: The perilous problems of cultural dichotomies in a globalizing society. *American Psychologist, 53,* 1111–1120.

Hill, J. H., & MacLaurey, R. E. (1995). The terror of Montezuma: Aztec history, vantage theory, and the category of "person." In J. R. Taylor & R. MacLaurey (Eds.), *Language and the cognitive construal of the world.* Trends in linguistics, studies, and monographs, 82 (pp. 277–329). Berlin, Germany: Mouton de Gruyter.

Holland, D., Lachicotte, W., Skinner, D., & Cain, C. (1998). *Identity and agency in cultural worlds.* Cambridge, MA: Harvard University Press.

Jang, Y. (1995). Chinese culture and occupational therapy. *British Journal of Occupational Therapy, 58,* 103–106.

Kinébanian, A., & Stomph, M. (1992). Cross-cultural occupational therapy: A critical reflection. *American Journal of Occupational Therapy, 46,* 751–757. http://dx.doi.org/10.5014/ajot.46.8.751

Kluckhohn, F. R., & Strodtbeck, F. L. (1961). *Variations in value orientations.* Evanston, IL: Row, Peterson, & Co.

Krefting, L. H. (1991). The culture concept in the everyday practice of occupational and physical therapy. *Occupational and Physical Therapy in Pediatrics, 11*(4), 1–16.

Krefting, L. H., & Krefting, D. V. (1991). Cultural influences on performance. In C. Christiansen & C. Baum (Eds.), *Occupational therapy: Overcoming human performance deficits* (pp. 102–122). Thorofare, NJ: Slack.

Kuper, A. (1999). *Culture: The anthropologists' account.* Cambridge, MA: Harvard University Press.

Levine, R. E. (1987). Culture: A factor influencing the outcomes of occupational therapy. *Occupational Therapy in Health Care, 4,* 3–15. Reprinted as Chapter 22.

Martin, L., & Bonder, B. (2003). Achieving organizational change within the context of cultural competence. *Journal of Social Work in Long-Term Care, 2*(1/2), 81–94.

Mattingly, C. (1998). *Healing dramas and clinical plots: The narrative structure of experience.* Cambridge, MA: Cambridge University Press.

Mirkopoulos, C., & Evert, M. M. (1994). Nationally Speaking: Cultural connections: A challenge unmet. *American Journal of Occupational Therapy, 48,* 583–585.

Pepitone, A. (2000). A social psychology perspective on the study of culture: An eye on the road to interdisciplinarianism. *Cross-Cultural Research, 34,* 233–249.

Pope-Davis, D. B., Prieto, L. R., Whitaker, C. M., & Pope-Davis, S. A. (1993). Exploring multicultural competencies of occupational therapists: Implications for education and training. *American Journal of Occupational Therapy, 47*, 838–844. http://dx.doi.org/10.5014/ajot.47.9.838

Reyna, S. (2002). *Connections: Mind, brain and culture in social anthropology.* New York: Routledge.

Rosaldo, R. I. (1999). A note on the cultural essayist. In S. B. Ortner (Ed.), *The fate of "culture": Geertz and beyond* (pp. 30–34). Berkeley, CA: University of California Press.

Rowles, G. D. (1991). Beyond performance: Being in place as a component of occupational therapy. *American Journal of Occupational Therapy, 45,* 265–271. http://dx.doi.org/10.5014/ajot.45.3.265

Sapir, E. (1924/1949). Culture, genuine and spurious. In D. Mandelbaum (Ed.), *Selected writings of Edward Sapir.* Berkeley, CA: University of California Press.

Sahlins, M., & Service, E. R. (Eds.). (1960). *Evolution and culture.* Ann Arbor, MI: University of Michigan Press.

Schneider, D. M. (1976). Notes toward a theory of culture. In K. Basso & H. Selby (Eds.), *Meaning in anthropology.* Albuquerque, NM: University of New Mexico Press.

Segall, M. H., Lonner, W. J., & Berry, J. W. (1998). Cross-cultural psychology as a scholarly discipline: On the flowering of culture in behavioral research. *American Psychologist, 53,* 1101–1110.

Sewell, W. H. (1999). Geertz, cultural systems, and history: From synchrony to transformation. In S. B. Ortner (Ed.), *The fate of "culture": Geertz and beyond* (pp. 35–55). Berkeley, CA: University of California Press.

Sherzer, J. A. (1987). Discourse-centered approach to language and culture. *American Anthropologist, 89,* 295–309.

Skinner, D. (1989). The socialization of gender identity: Observations from Nepal. In J. Valsiner (Ed.), *Child development in cultural context* (pp. 181–192). Toronto, Ontario, Canada: Hogrefe & Huber.

Spencer, J., Krefting, L., & Mattingly, C. (1993). Incorporation of ethnographic methods in occupational therapy assessment. *American Journal of Occupational Therapy, 47,* 303–309. http://dx.doi.org/10.5014/ajot.47.4.303

Sue, S. (2000, June). *The provision of effective mental health treatment by service providers.* National Institutes of Health Conference "Toward Higher Levels of Analysis: Progress and Promise in Research on Social and Cultural Dimensions of Health." Bethesda, MD.

Tedlock, D., & Mannheim, B. (1995). Introduction. In D. Tedlock & B. Mannheim (Eds.), *The dialogic emergence of culture* (pp. 1–32). Urbana, IL: University of Illinois Press.

Tylor, E. B. (1871). *Primitive society.* London: J. Murray.

Urban, G. A. (1991). *Discourse-centered approach to culture: Native South American myths and rituals.* Austin, TX: University of Texas Press.

Wallace, A. F. C. (1961). *Culture and personality.* New York: Random House.

Wells, S. A., & Black, R. M. (2000). *Cultural competency for health professionals.* Bethesda, MD: American Occupational Therapy Association.

Willeman, P. (1994). *Looks and frictions: Essays in cultural studies and film theory.* Bloomington, IN: University of Indiana Press.

Wittman, P., & Velde, B. P. (2002). The Issue Is: Attaining cultural competence, critical thinking, and intellectual development: A challenge for occupational therapists. *American Journal of Occupational Therapy, 56,* 454–456. http://dx.doi.org/10.5014/ajot.56.4.454

CHAPTER 24

The Kawa Model: The Power of Culturally Responsive Occupational Therapy

MICHAEL K. IWAMA, NICOLE A. THOMSON, AND RONA M. MACDONALD

Introduction

Most well known conceptual models of rehabilitation have been raised out of Western social and cultural contexts and, as such, reflect the characteristics and features germane to Western interpretations and views of health and well-being. Given this pervasive pattern of cultural influence on theory development in the rehabilitation professions, health professionals and service users alike may wonder how inclusive and responsive contemporary models of rehabilitation practice are in meeting the broad spectrum of rehabilitation requirements of a diverse clientele.

Given the dominance of Western influences on rehabilitation theory, there may be a need to better address the rehabilitation requirements of diverse clientele—many of whom represent shared experiences and contexts of daily living that diverge from the cultures of the Western world. Alternative models and theory originating from outside of the familiar boundaries of Western life may help to illuminate the cultural dimensions of rehabilitation theory and raise the cultural responsiveness of contemporary rehabilitation practice and service delivery. The Kawa (Japanese for 'River') Model [1] is one such model to emerge from rehabilitation practice outside of the West. This article describes the Kawa Model's origins, basic concepts, principles, underlying ideology and possibilities for informing a more culturally responsive rehabilitation practice. Consideration of such a novel model, raised from a different cultural context and construal of the self-environment interface, might also shed some light on the influence of culture on familiar contemporary models in rehabil-

itation, illuminating strengths and shortcomings that remained unremarkable until now.

Culture Embedded in Rehabilitation Theory

If culture can be redefined to transcend individual embodiments of race and ethnicity and be re-stated as; 'shared experiences and common spheres of meaning, and the (collective) social processes by which distinctions, meanings, categorisations of objects and phenomena are created and maintained' [1, p 8] then health professionals representing a spectrum of disciplines may see that they may each possess their own respective culturally and contextually bound ideology, structure, content and practice forms. Each can possess in their cultures, a shared specialised language, tacit rules of conduct in carrying out its activities, established social practices that follow a pattern that help to identify its members from other professionals and certain institutional conditions of knowledge production [2] that help to reify its discourse. Critical examination of contemporary rehabilitation theory will reveal that conceptual models are culturally situated and that their specificity can often, despite best intentions, exclude both clients and therapists who abide in differing cultural contexts that sit outside of a standard or universal set of norms.

Self in Relation to Environs: A Context for Health and Well-Being

Culture can be identified at the core of most contemporary conceptual models of rehabilitation, and is particularly observable in how the 'self' is socially constructed and situated in relation to the surrounding environment or context. The interpretations and meanings individuals derive through what they do in the world may vary according to how this dualism of self vis-à-vis the environment is regarded and understood (Figure 24.1). The self, in Western social depictions, is evident in current occupational therapy conceptual models such as the Model of Human Occupation (MOHO) [3] and the Canadian Model of Occupational Performance (CMOP) [4]. These models construe the self as being not only focally situated in the centre of all concerns, but also understood to be rationally separate and superior in power and status to the environment and nature. Well-being is constructed to be contingent on the extent to which the self can act on and demonstrate its ability to control one's perceived circumstances located in the environment. Failure or compromise in controlling the environment is construed with such terms as dysfunction and disability. These terms are often pejorative in a socio-cultural context in which the self is required to be competent, able and in control (of one's environment and circumstances). In these worldviews, dependency can often represent an undesirable state of disability.

Self in Relation to Time: Implications for Rehabilitation

An independent self-centrally situated and agent upon a separated and subordinated environment also appears to coincide with a particular sensation of time. When the self is centrally located in relation to the environment at large, one's sense of entitlement to doing in the present (here and now) can also extend temporally into one's future. The relation between intention, one's immediate action on the environment, and some specific (future) objective is often rationally connected. It is not uncommon for people situated in the Western world to believe that individuals carry primary responsibility for their own destinies. 'You make your bed and lie in it', and 'you get what you pay for' are familiar adages in many Western spheres of shared experience. It should come as little surprise, then, to see that independence, autonomy, equality and self-determinism, are celebrated ideals that point to a common world view and value pattern shared between mainstream rehabilitation ideology and the broader Western social contexts from which they emerged [5].

Lying in contrast to this worldview is the East Asian and Aboriginal worldview [6]. In the primitive cosmological myth (Ibid), the 'self' is not central nor unilaterally empowered but rather construed to be one of many parts of an inseparable whole [6,7]. In this view of reality, one does not need to occupy nor wrestle control of

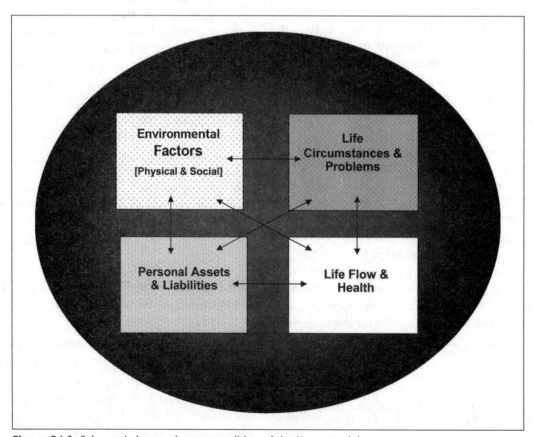

Figure 24.1. Schematic box and arrow rendition of the Kawa model.

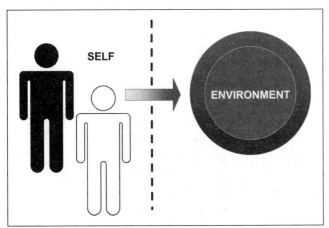

Figure 24.2. Diagrammatic representation of Western, rational, worldview in which the self and environs are regarded to be discrete, separate entities.

anything because in an integrated view of self and nature, one is already there amongst others (Figure 24.2). In this view of reality, health and disability states are also not imagined nor believed to be an individual-centred matter. Life circumstances are dependent on a broader whole, determined by a constellation of factors and elements located both within and outside of the physically defined body [8]. The self is decentralised and not accorded an exclusive privilege to exercise stewardship, nor unilateral control, over one's environment or circumstances. Hence, conceptual models of rehabilitation that are based on a tacit understanding of a central individual separate from a discrete environment are often incongruent with experiences of disability, health and rehabilitation for many who are situated outside of mainstream Western social norms.

Rehabilitation Professionals in Relation to Clients: Re-examining Power and Disability

The cultural features of Western-centric rehabilitation frameworks can also extend beyond the structure and content of a particular model, to its application forms. An examination of how concepts of a model are applied in practice can reveal how power and inequities are exercised. Embedded in universal frameworks, be it the *International Classification of Function (ICF)* [9] or other known rehabilitation models such as the MOHO [3] or the CMOP [4], is a tacit belief that a theory/model (assembled by well-meaning experts) should fit and benefit everyone. What appears to elude critical understanding is the top-down power dynamic whereby a limited set of (universal) concepts or categories of enquiry are established, through which

client narratives are translated and vetted. It is often assumed by the professionals using a model that the concepts are adequate to capture and explain the diverse client's health and disability issues and needs adequately. Problems become evident when clients and rehabilitation professionals who do not abide in the patterns, forms and meanings of everyday life experience embedded in a model are subjected to its use. Not all clients will necessarily regard autonomy, individualism and participation, for example, to represent their quintessential goals.

The universal concepts of a given model may not adequately and equitably represent clients' unique issues and views of normalcy. A practice that aims to be client centred should go beyond inquiring about client performance parameters and outcomes. It should ideally require critical acknowledgement of the client's unique experience of day-to-day life, in the context of their (cultural) realities, in their own concepts and in their own words.

One of the greatest challenges to providing culturally responsive disability services is the development of theoretical frameworks and procedures that privilege the unique narratives and needs of people experiencing disability. What are required are models that neutralise the familiar top-down applications of universal frameworks, and respond to the comprehensive needs of the whole person in appropriate context.

Recognising the multi-dimensional challenges that culture presents to the delivery of equitable disability services raises the important issue of the need for culturally responsive theory [10]. New conceptual and practice models may need to stray from any tendency to impose explanatory frameworks of health onto populations, out of cultural context. If rehabilitation is to achieve its aims of minimising the effects of disability and enabling people to resume better health states in safer cultural context, not only might the forms of practice need to undergo change but also the theoretical frameworks and knowledge systems that drive and inform them.

The Kawa Model

Origins of the Kawa Model

Faced with the challenges presented by existing rehabilitation and occupational therapy theory outlined in the previous section, a group of Japanese occupational therapists developed a new conceptual model of practice. Through a process of qualitative research, the therapists were led through an exercise of discussing their culturally situated views of what they felt was essential to their lives, including their explanations of wellness and their definitions and understanding of illness, health and disability. They were prompted to articulate and discuss what they and their clients lived for, and what they felt was essential to life and fulfilment. Through this exercise, they were encouraged to re-define occupation from East Asian cultural perspectives and re-align the purposes of occupational therapy to matters of essential importance to the Japanese person's life and world.

The research initially led to a cumbersome representation of their model along conventional, linear box and arrow structures (see Figure 24.1). At that early stage, it became readily apparent that there were fundamental differences in how self and environment were imagined and represented in established (Western) models and actually lived and experienced by the group participants. For a model to purposely explain self and context, the central placement of a distinctly defined self, adjacent to a separate but distinct environment commonly seen in conventional (Western) models, was non-existent (see Figure 24.2). Further consideration revealed comprehensions of self and environment-or context that were more diffuse and inseparably integrated by the Japanese than by their Western counterparts. Consistent with a worldview that imagined self and the world and all of its elements as integrated parts of an all-encompassing whole (see Figure 24.3), phenomena as complex as well-being and disability could not be adequately described and explained by linear diagrams that connect rationally defined categories through logical principles. These Eastern perspectives of wellness and disability states could not be readily contained in and explained by boxes/categories set in a logical sequence, familiarly observable in rational formulae or continua.

In this initial diagram, what was effectively captured was the interconnectedness of all elements and phenomena in the frame of life experience; that states of well being and disability are neither internally (in the body) nor externally (in the environment) isolated. The self and environment were inextricably connected in a manner in which a change in one or more components would effect a change in the greater whole.

In order to capture and better represent a conceptualisation of a diffuse self, unified, interdependent with and inseparable from other elements in the environment, the initial box and arrow diagram was aug-

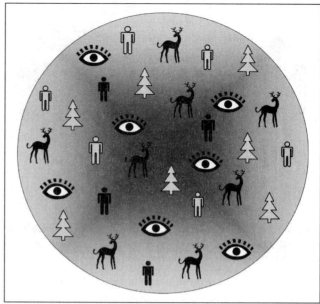

Figure 24.3. Diagrammatic representation of an alternate worldview in which the self, deities, and all parts of nature are inseparably inter-related; the individual human self is not situated solely at the centre 'of it all'.

mented by the addition of an alternate image. During a subsequent session, the research participants decided to employ a metaphor of nature (a river or Kawa in Japanese) to better explain the dynamic intricacies and fluid nature of the model. The use of such a metaphor contrasted dramatically to the familiar mechanical and 'system' metaphors frequently employed in the construction of Western conceptual models.

Structure and Components of the Kawa Model

The complex dynamic that characterises an Eastern perspective of harmony in life experience between self and context might be best explained through a familiar metaphor [11] of nature. In this metaphor, life is understood to be a complex, profound journey that flows through time and space, like a river (Figure 24.4). An optimal state of well-being in one's life or river, can be metaphorically portrayed by an image of strong, deep, unimpeded flow. Aspects of the environment and phenomenal circumstances, like certain structures found in a river, can influence and effect that flow. Rocks (life circumstances), walls and bottom (environment), driftwood (assets and liabilities), are all inseparable parts of a river that determine its boundaries, shape, flow-rate and overall quality (Figure 24.5). Occupational therapy's purpose, in concert with an interdisciplinary rehabilitation mandate, then, is to enable and enhance

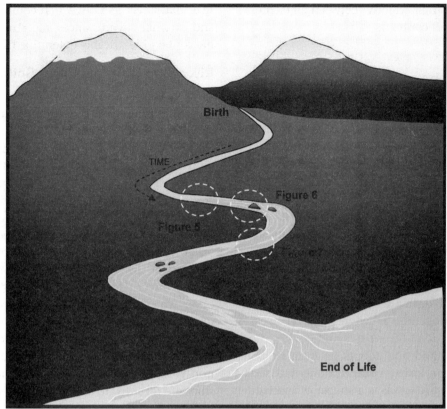

Figure 24.4. 'Life is like a river'; the river used metaphorically to represent the life journey.

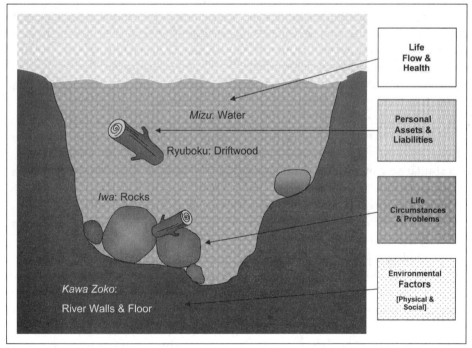

Figure 24.5. Four basic components of the Kawa (River) model; listed first in Japanese, followed by the English translation.

life flow by enhancing harmony (between all elements that form the overall context).

Water (Mizu)

Mizu—Japanese for 'Water' metaphorically represents the subject's life energy or life flow. Fluid, pure, spirit, filling, cleansing and renewing, are only some of the meanings and functions commonly associated with this natural element. Just as people's lives are bounded and shaped by their surroundings, people and circumstances, the water flowing as a river touches the rocks, sides and debris and all other elements that form its context. Water envelopes, defines and effects these other elements of the river in a similar way to which the same elements effect the water's volume, shape and flow rate.

When life energy or the water flow weakens, the client, whether individually or collectively defined can be described as unwell, or in a state of disharmony. When it stops flowing altogether, as when the river releases into a vast ocean, end of life is reached.

Just as water is fluid and adopts its form from its container, people in many collective-oriented societies often interpret the social as a shaper of individual self. Sharing a view of the cosmos that embeds the self, inextricably within the environment, collectively oriented people tend to place enormous value on the self embedded in relationships. There is greater value in 'belonging' and 'interdependence', than in unilateral agency and in individual determinism [12–14] celebrated in American life. In such experience, the interdependent self is deeply influenced and even determined by the surrounding social context, at a given time and place, in a similar way to which water in a river, at any given point, will vary in form, flow direction, rate, volume and clarity. The 'driving force' of one's life is interconnected with others sharing the same social frame or ba (Nakane), in a similar way in which water is seen to touch, connect and relate all elements of a river that have varying effect upon its form and flow.

With so much focussed on the independent and agent self, there may be a tendency to overlook or underestimate the importance that place and context plays in determining the form, functions and meanings of human occupation. From the vantage of the Kawa model, a subject's state of well-being coincides with life-flow. Occupational therapy's and rehabilitation's overall purpose in this context is to enhance life flow, regardless of whether it is interpreted at the level of the individual, institution, organisation, community or society. Just as there are constellations of inter-related factors/structures in a river that affect its flow, a rich combination of internal and external circumstances and structures in a client's life context inextricably determine his or her life flow.

River Side-Walls and River Bottom (Kawa Zoko)

The river's sides and bottom, referred to in the Japanese lexicon as Kawa Zoko, are the structures/concepts from the river metaphor that represent the client's environment. These are perhaps the most important determinants of a person's life flow in a collectivist social context because of the primacy accorded to the environmental context in determining the construction of self, experience of being and subsequent meanings of personal action. In the Kawa model, the river walls and sides represent the subject's social and physical contexts. The social contexts of the river walls represent mainly those who share a direct relationship with the subject. Depending upon which social frame is perceived as being most important in a given instance and place, the riversides and bottom can represent family members, workmates, friends in a recreational club, classmates, etc. In certain non-Western societies like those of Japan, social relationships are regarded to be the central [14] determinant, of individual and collective life flow.

The Kawa Zoko also represents the physical context of the client. This can include the home, work, built and natural environments. A foreboding set of stairs in the home or workplace; the lack of a ramp as an intermediate between road pavement and sidewalk, or even a heavy door separating where one is presently situated and where one would like to go, are rivers walls.

Aspects of the surrounding social and physical frame on the subject can affect the overall flow (volume and rate) of the Kawa. Harmonious relationships can enable and complement life flow. Increased flow can have an agent effect upon difficult circumstances and problems as the force of water displaces rocks in the channel and even create new courses through which to flow. Conversely, a decrease in flow volume can exert a compounding, negative effect on the other elements that take up space in the channel (Figure 24.6). If there are obstructions (rocks and driftwood) in the watercourse when the river walls and bottom are thick and constricting, the flow of the river is especially compromised. As can be readily imagined, the rocks in this river can directly butt up against the river walls and bottom, compounding and creating larger impediments to the river's usual flow. When applying the Kawa model in collectivist-oriented populations, these components and the perceptions of their importance are paramount.

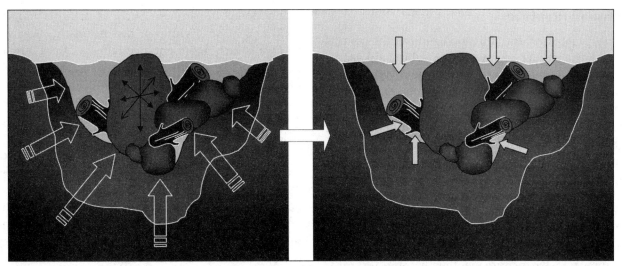

Figure 24.6. Specific problems have a tendency to combine with other aspects of the client's context of daily living and compound the overall impediment to life flow. Remaining channels of water flow are prime foci for rehabilitation intervention.

Like all other elements of the river, these concepts are always interpreted in relation to the whole, taking into consideration all other elements of the subject's context and their inter-relations/interdependencies.

Rocks (Iwa)

Iwa (Japanese for *large rocks*) represent discrete circumstances that are considered to be impediments to one's life-flow. They are life circumstances perceived by the client to be problematic and difficult to remove. Every rock, like every life circumstance, has a unique quality, varying in size, density, shape, colour and texture. Most rivers, like people's lives, have such rocks or impediments, of varying quality and number. Large rocks, by themselves or in combination with other rocks, jammed directly or indirectly against the river walls and sides (environment) can profoundly impede and obstruct flow. The client's rocks may have been there since the beginning, such as with congenital conditions. They may appear instantaneously, as in sudden illness or injury, and even be transient.

The impeding effect of rocks on the water flow can compound when situated against the river's sides and walls (environment). A person's bodily impairment becomes disabling when interfaced with the environment. For example, the functional difficulties associated with a neurological condition can change according to the environmental context. A (physically) barrier-free environment can decrease one's disability, as can social and/or political/organisational environments that are accepting of people with disabling conditions. Once

the client's perceived rocks are known (including their relative size and situation), the therapist can help to identify potential areas of intervention and strategies to enable better life-flow. The broader contextual definition of disabling circumstances necessarily brings into play the client's surrounding environment. Though often limited to narrow, medically oriented interventions in hospital institutions, occupational therapy intervention can therefore include treatment strategies that expand beyond the traditional patient, to his or her social network and even to policies and social structures of the surrounding institution or society that ultimately play a part in setting the disabling context.

The concepts and the contextual application of the Kawa model are by natural design flexible and adaptable. Each client's unique river takes its important concepts and configuration from the situation of the subject, in a given time and place. The definition of problems and circumstances are broad—as broad and diverse as the rehabilitation clients' worlds of meanings. In turn, this particular conceptualisation of people and their circumstances foreshadows the broad outlook and scope of occupational therapy interventions, when set in particular cultural contexts.

The subject, be it an individual or a collective, ideally determines specific rocks, their number, magnitude, quality and situation in the river. As with all other elements of the model, if the client is unable to express their own river, family members or a community of people connected with the issues may lend assistance and perspective.

Driftwood (*Ryuboku*)

Ryuboku is Japanese for 'driftwood', and in the context of the Kawa model represents the subject's personal attributes and resources, such as: values (for example, honesty, thrift), character (for example, optimism, stubbornness), personality (for example, reserved, outgoing), knowledge and experience (for example, advanced diploma, military service), special skill (for example, carpentry, public speaking) immaterial (for example, friends, siblings) and material assets (i.e. wealth, special equipment) that can positively or negatively affect the subject's circumstance and life flow.

Like driftwood in a river they are transient in nature and carry a certain quality of fate or serendipity. They can appear to be inconsequential in some instances and significantly obstructive in others—particularly when they settle in amongst rocks and the river-sides and walls. On the other hand, they can collide with the same structures, nudge obstructions out of the way, and even erode the constraining surfaces of river walls and rocks. A client's religious faith and sense of determination can be positive factors in persevering to erode or move rocks out of the way. For example, receiving a monetary gift or donation to acquire specialised assistive equipment can be the piece of driftwood that collides against existing flow impediments and opens a greater channel for one's life to flow more strongly. In another instance, a vocational counselor may assist in pushing away a large rock of unemployment.

Driftwood is a part of everyone's river and are often those intangible components possessed by each unique rehabilitation client. Effective therapists pay particular attention to these components of a client's or community's assets and circumstances, and consider their real or potential effect on the client's situation.

Spaces Between Obstructions (*Sukima*): The Promise of Occupational Therapy

In the Kawa model, spaces are the channels through which the client's life evidently flows. From an occupational therapy perspective, these spaces can represent a progressive way to define 'occupation'. When the metaphor of a river depicting the client's life flow becomes clearer, attention turns to the *sukima* (spaces between the rocks, driftwood and river walls and bottom). These spaces are as important to comprehend in the client's context as are the other elements of the river when determining how to apply and direct occupational therapy and rehabilitation. For example, a space between a functional impairment such as arthritis (an *Iwa/* rock) and a social group or person (in the river sides and walls) may represent a certain social role, such as parent, company worker, friend, etc. Such roles can be profoundly affected by impairment. Enabling the resumption of these roles when sudden impairment disrupts them may become an important rehabilitation objective.

Water naturally coursing through these spaces can work to erode the rocks and river walls and bottom and over time transform them into larger conduits for life flow (Figure 24.7). This effect reflects the latent healing potential that each subject naturally holds within their self and in the inseparable context. Thus, occupational therapy in this perspective retains its hallmark of purposeful activity and working with the client's abilities and assets. It also directs occupational therapy intervention toward all elements (in this case; a medically defined problem, various aspects and levels of environment) that comprise the context (see inner image, Figure 24.6).

Spaces, then, represent important foci for occupational therapy and the broader rehabilitation effort. They occur throughout the context of the self and environs; between the rocks, walls and bottom and driftwood. Spaces subsume the environment as part of the greater context of the problem and expands the scope of intervention to naturally integrate what, in the Western sense, would have been treated separately through the dualism of internal (pertaining to self and personal attributes) and external (environment constructed as separate and outside of the self). Spaces are potential channels for the client's flow, allowing client and rehabilitation professional to determine multiple points and levels of intervention (Figure 24.7). In this way, each problem or enabling opportunity is bounded by and appreciated in a broader context.

Rather than attempting to reduce a person's problems (i.e. focussing only on rocks) to discrete issues, isolated out of their particular contexts, similar to the rational processes in which client problems are identified and discretely named/diagnosed in conventional Western health practice, the Kawa model framework compels the occupational therapist and rehabilitation professional to view and treat issues within a holistic framework, seeking to appreciate the clients' identified issues within their integrated, inseparable contexts of daily life. Occupation is therefore regarded in wholes to include the meaning of the activity to self and community to which the individual inseparably belongs,

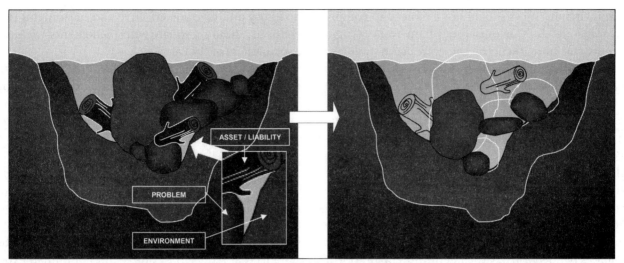

Figure 24.7. Each potential foci for intervention is multi-faceted, ideally requiring an inter-disciplinary, combined approach, resulting in decreasing impeding factors, and ultimately increasing life flow.

and not just in terms of biomechanical components, or embodied pathology and function.

Life circumstances rarely occur in isolation. By changing one aspect of the client's world, all other aspects of his or her river change. The river's spaces represent opportunities to problem solve and focus intervention on positive opportunities, which may have little direct relation to the person's medically defined condition.

By using this model, occupational therapists, in partnership with their clients are directed to stem further obstruction of life energy/flow and look for every opportunity in the broader context, to enhance it.

Harmony: The Essence of Human Occupation, and a Re-conceptualisation of Rehabilitation

What has been described so far is the underlying ontology of the Kawa framework. The Kawa model's central point of reference is not the individual but rather harmony—a state of individual or collective being in which the subject—be it self or community is in balance with the context that it is a part of. Here, the essence of such harmony is conceptualised as 'life-energy' or 'life flow'. Occupational therapy's purpose, in concert with the mandate of rehabilitation, is to help the client and community enhance and balance this flow. In this balance, there is co-existence, a synergy between elements that affirms interdependence. How can one come to terms with one's circumstances? How can harmony between the elements, of which one is merely one part, be realised? How and in what way can occupational therapists and their interdisciplinary partners assist this construction of well-being?

Using the Kawa Metaphor in Rehabilitation Practice

The Kawa model represents a novel addition to conventional rehabilitation conceptual model development in a number of ways. To begin with, the Kawa model is explicitly described as a culturally situated product, having originated outside of Western socio-cultural context. The model is also peculiar in regard to its structure, diverging from conventional scientific, rational form, taking the shape of a common metaphor of nature.

Similarities, as well as differences in interpretations of the river metaphor are bound to exist and will therefore be applicable in one form or another for some situations and inappropriate for others. Like people's experiences of wellness and disability, there is no one standard explanation or norm. In cases where the model cannot be adequately adapted to suit the client's construction of his or her state of well-being, or when the river metaphor holds less explanatory power in the client's context, the model should be placed aside for a more fitting alternative. Therefore, all universal assumptions and proprietary interpretations of the model and its applicability are dismissed, permitting and encouraging occupational therapists and rehabilitation professionals to alter and adapt the model in conceptual and structural ways to match the specific social and cultural contexts of their diverse clients.

A Client-Centred Perspective and Practice

To follow a client-centred approach and to respect diversity among people, the client's views of their realities and circumstances should not be forced to comply with someone else's manufactured framework of rigid concepts and principles. The therapist using the Kawa model can recognise the uniqueness of each subject's situation/context by using the river metaphor as a tool to draw out the client's narrative of day-to-day living experience. Rather than foisting a universal framework or model, with its predetermined concepts, principles, socio-cultural norms and rigid protocols on to each unique client, the client's emergent narrative—or 'river' is drawn out, centralised, and made to form the basis for the ensuing rehabilitation process.

Equipped with the Kawa framework, the occupational therapist or rehabilitation professional does not become dependent on a particular measurement tool or procedure to inform them of what their interventions ought to be. The structure and meanings of the river metaphor take shape according to the subject's views of their circumstances, bounded by a particular cultural context. Therefore, the Kawa metaphor is used to derive concepts that are meaningful and germane to the client's perspective of life and well-being. As the client's unique concepts and issues are determined, the therapist can proceed to select appropriate tools/instruments and methods that will explore the client's rehabilitation issues further and support a more comprehensive and culturally responsive treatment plan.

Discussion

The Kawa model is an example of how cultural views of reality and well being are tied to and expressed in theoretical material constructed in a particular socio-cultural context. The Kawa model shows a culturally specific way in which disability and health states are considered in a particular dynamic between people and the contexts in which they live. Such a different conceptual model not only portrays how certain non-Western people can view matters of well being and disability, but also may aid Western rehabilitation professionals to view the cultural features and biases within their own conceptual frameworks and classification systems.

A conceptual model based on a differing ontology supported with Eastern ways of knowing offers an alternate socio-cultural location from which to view and make sense of our conventional approaches founded and reified in explanations of Western spheres of shared experience. Ultimately, the models and theoretical frameworks employed by rehabilitation professionals to make sense of their clients' worlds of health and disability and to guide effective and meaningful interventions, should resonate with their clients' views and explanations of the same.

Rehabilitation clients participating in treatment are rarely regarded to be socially and culturally homogeneous. Each client brings a unique configuration of personal attributes coupled with a unique set of contextual conditions. Consequently, the formulae for wellness, as well as the structure and experience of disability, are just as unique and specific to each client's case. What is considered to be disabling in one context may be less or more so in another. Universally applicable theoretical precepts that carry social imperatives, such as autonomy and independence, or classification systems that reduce the complexities of human experience into rational categories have their own advantages and disadvantages. On the one hand, they may help rehabilitation professionals to standardise matters of wellness and disability and help to ensure a better level of care across a broad international spectrum. However, on the other hand, these classifications may also lead to disadvantaging those who fall toward the margins or even outside of a classification framework's normal categories.

As rehabilitation practice continues its foray into new cultural frontiers, the diversity of contexts in which people define what is important and of value in daily life in relation to their states of well being, will continue to broaden. Beyond race and ethnicity, conditions of poverty, limited access to technology, a global economy, diversity in health policy, continuation of population migration and deprivation of meaningful participation in society, to name but a few, represent some real-world contexts for the lives of millions of people. These increasingly familiar contexts will challenge the meaning and efficacy of occupational therapy and the meaning of rehabilitation in this era. These changing contexts will also push rehabilitation professionals to re-think their approaches to culturally responsive disability services. Rehabilitation models like the Kawa are offered to help comprehend the particular and culturally specific features of people's disability experiences- particularly for those clients whose life contexts fall outside of the explanatory powers of models raised from mainstream Western social contexts.

The non-Western occupational therapists who raised the Kawa model from their day-to-day practices seek to remind their international colleagues of the primacy and importance of nature as context, and how its laws need to be more fundamentally apparent in the epistemology, theory and practice in rehabilitation. The rhythms and cycles of nature continue to prevail and have yet to yield to mankind's attempts to transcend and subjugate them. In the Eastern perspective of humanity integrated in nature, occupational therapy may be appreciated less as an empowerment or enablement of the individual's dominion over nature and circumstance, but as an empowerment of bringing individuals' life force into harmony and better flow with nature and its circumstances. As long as there is a need for congruence between diverse selves and dynamic contexts of daily living, there is a need for culturally responsive occupational therapy and rehabilitation.

Readers may wonder why the field of rehabilitation needs newer and more models and frameworks like the Kawa model. Rehabilitation professionals have produced a number of substantial models like the *ICF* [9] and MOHO [3], which were developed by teams of experts, carrying the best intentions for recipients of rehabilitation care. As identified by the Kawa model's developers, however, all conceptual models are socio-culturally situated and privilege the norms of the contexts from which they had emerged. And unless these (universal) models are applied to a socially and culturally homogenous clientele who abide more or less in the same socio-cultural contexts of daily life, the practice forms that follow may exclude and even disadvantage the culturally diverse person with disability. Such clients may in many cases be compelled to adopt unfamiliar ideals, concepts and normative imperatives that resonate marginally with their own spheres of day-to-day experiences.

Along with the acknowledgement of the primacy of nature in human experience, the Kawa model also serves as a prototype for a new way of regarding and employing theoretical material in our rehabilitation professions. In this post-modern era of recognising cultural relativity, variations in world-views and interpretations of life, the notion of one rigid explanation of function and well-being for everyone will be increasingly difficult to tend. The same difficulty applies to occupational therapists and the meanings of their concept of occupation in a broader sense as it relates to meaningful activity in daily life. The notion of a universal explanation for occupation would potentially limit occupational therapy's cultural relevance and meaning to a narrower, exclusive scope of practice to societies and peoples who share similar views of life and experience with the social contexts that originally conceptualised the idea. The same may also apply to other rehabilitation professional groups and their respective ideas, views and concepts.

Occupational therapy and rehabilitation, in an ideal sense, should be as unique, flexible and diverse in approaches as its clientele changing its forms and approaches according to the clients' diverse circumstances and experiences of well-being. To move closer to that ideal, conceptual models and theory in rehabilitation should be better informed and drawn, at least in part, from diverse social landscapes and profound, complex contexts of the client-rehabilitation practice continuum. Perhaps, more culturally (rather than universally) responsive frameworks will emerge and offer alternative paths to overcoming the challenges of diversity in an increasingly global and challenging field of rehabilitation.

Declaration of interest: The authors report no conflicts of interest. The authors alone are responsible for the content and writing of the article.

References

1. Iwama M. *The Kawa model: culturally relevant occupational therapy.* Edinburgh: Churchill Livingstone-Elsevier Press; 2006.
2. Smith MJ. *Culture: reinventing the social sciences.* Buckingham: Open University Press; 2000.
3. Kielhofner GA. *Model of human occupation: theory and application,* 3rd ed. Baltimore: Williams and Wilkins; 2002.
4. Canadian Association of Occupational Therapists. *Enabling occupation: an occupational therapy perspective,* 2nd ed. Toronto: CAOT Publications; 2003.
5. Iwama M. *Situated meaning: an issue of culture, inclusion and occupational therapy.* In: Kronenberg F, Algado SA, Pollard N, editors. *Occupational therapy without borders—learning from the spirit of survivors.* Edinburgh:Churchill Livingstone; 2005.
6. Bellah R. *Beyond belief: essays on religion in a post traditional world.* New York: Harper & Row; 1991.
7. Gustafson JM. *Man and nature: a cross-cultural perspective.* Bangkok: Chulalongkorn University Press; 1993.
8. Shakespeare T. Cultural representation of disabled people: dustbins for disavowal? *Disabil Soc* 1994;9:283–299.
9. World Health Organization. *International classification of functioning, disability and health.* Geneva: WHO; 2001.
10. Iwama M. The issue is . . . toward culturally relevant epistemologies in occupational therapy. *Am J Occup Ther* 2003;57:582–588. http://dx.doi.org/10.5014/ajot.57.5.582

11. Lakoff G, Johnson M. *Metaphors we live by.* Chicago: University of Chicago Press; 1980.

12. Lebra S. *Japanese patterns of behavior.* Honolulu: University of Hawaii Press; 1976.

13. Doi T. *The anatomy of dependence.* Tokyo: Kodansha International; 1973.

14. Nakane C. *Tate shakai no ningen kankei* [Human relations in a vertical society]. Tokyo: Kodansha; 1970.

Part III.C. Sociopolitical Contexts

CHAPTER 25

Building Inclusive Community: A Challenge for Occupational Therapy

1994 ELEANOR CLARKE SLAGLE LECTURE

ANN P. GRADY

Preparation of the Eleanor Clarke Slagle Lecture promotes reflection on the values and philosophy of occupational therapy. I chose the topic *Building Inclusive Community: A Challenge for Occupational Therapy* because it provided me with an opportunity to explore my own values and the values of the profession regarding inclusion of all persons into the community they choose and into the world community at large. The topic particularly led me to review my own work in adaptation theory developed with Elnora Gilfoyle (Gilfoyle, Grady, & Moore, 1990) in light of changes occurring or being promoted in society regarding opportunities for inclusion of all persons in all aspects of living.

Ideas about inclusion; the meaning of community; the relationship between environment and community; the interaction between a person's past experience, present situation, and future hopes and dreams and its effect on the relationship that develops between an occupational therapist and a person seeking therapy services all became focal points for exploring our role in building inclusive community. The result has been some expansion of our understanding of the environment category of the spatiotemporal adaptation theory and exploration of the relationship between environment and community. In addition, exploring the concepts of the theory led to consideration of its relevance for enhancing our ability to plan with consumers of service who are creating or returning to their own community. Focal points for exploring the challenges related to building inclusive community include

- An understanding of the meaning of community building within a person's own environment and according to his or her choices.

- A review of current ideas about the nature of disability in relation to both philosophy and mandates for inclusion.
- An expansion of ideas about the role of environment in a person's adaptation to community living.
- A consideration of strategies for promoting choice and inclusion.

For as far back in time as we know, human beings have gathered together to share in daily living and use some form of symbols as means for communicating with each other, hence the building of community (Dance & Larson, 1972). To this day, we share meaning in our communities through symbols composed of pictures, words spoken in our own culturally determined language, and gestures or nonverbal expressions of our thoughts or feelings. Native Americans in the southwestern regions of our country choose to tell the stories of their community living and beliefs through petroglyphs, or rock art (Patterson-Rudolph, 1993). One expert in petroglyphs compared attempts at identifying subject matter and its significance to cloud watching in that no two people will interpret what they see in the same way. Petroglyphs were apparently not intended to represent words of a language as we know it, but instead were meant to convey more general concepts or global ideas about the society, such as ideas about religion, medicine, governance, art, war, and peace. An artist's rendition of petroglyphs titled "Circle of Friends" (see Figure 25.1) is chosen to represent ideas about community and inclusion that are central to the themes of this article. In rock art, spirals, concentric circles, and other geometric shapes are interpreted to be universal symbols used to convey conceptual ideas (Patterson, 1992). There are dozens of possible interpretations connected to each figure in the circle because rock art is interpreted not only according to the individual symbols present, but also by the figures that are

This chapter was previously published in the *American Journal of Occupational Therapy, 49*, 300–310. Copyright © 1995, American Occupational Therapy Association. Reprinted with permission. http://dx.doi.org/10.5014/ajot.49.4.300

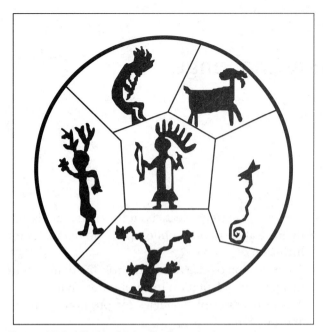

Figure 25.1. Circle of Friends petroglyph.

Note. Original metal sculpture by Kevin Smith, Golden, Colorado. Appears with permission of Kevin Smith.

combined in a panel, just like words in spoken language. For me, the Circle of Friends represents the encompassing nature of a community, whether it is the community that each of us constructs for ourselves or the larger environment in which we discover ourselves. The circle represents the wholeness of a community, and the figures relate to diversity that can exist within the community. Just as the circle is considered a symbol of inclusion and wholeness, the extension of the circle as a spiral is well known as a symbol of growth and continuity. Spirals frequently appear as symbols of continuity in Native American culture (Patterson, 1992). The spiral reflects evolution and renewal with growth emanating from continuous learning and new challenges. The spiral and its embedded circles will be used in this article to represent change and continuity.

Why is the idea of building inclusive community important to us as people and as occupational therapists? The idea is both profound and simple. Simply, we believe that people belong together regardless of real or perceived differences. All persons have the right to choose where they wish to live, work, learn, and play, and with whom they wish to spend time. On a deeper level, we believe that people belong together *because* of differences. There is a richness that characterizes a community constructed with appreciation for both differences and similarities among its members. The idea is not new, but as Winston Churchill said, "Men [and

women] stumble over the truth from time to time, but most pick themselves up and hurry off as if nothing had happened" (McWilliams, 1994, p. 413).

The Nature of Community and Choice

Community provides a context for actualizing individual potential and experiencing oneness with others (McLaughlin & Davidson, 1985). The human condition yearns for a greater sense of connectedness, expressed as a need to reach out, deeply touch others, and throw off the pain and loneliness of separation. The term *community* encompasses *communication* and *unity*. Yankelovitch said that the community evokes in the individual the feeling that "here is where I belong—these are my people, I care for them, they care for me, I am part of them, I know what they expect from me and I from them, they share my concerns. I know this place, I am on familiar ground, I am at home" (1981, p. 224).

There are established communities such as towns, neighborhoods, schools, and workplaces, and there are personal communities we create for ourselves, which include family, friends, acquaintances, how and where we spend our time formally or informally, and the relationships we build over time. Our personal communities do not necessarily depend on specific location or specific time, although they are often embedded in established communities. Building inclusive community refers to both the larger, more formal community context and the smaller, informal community that a person identifies as a personal community. Ideas about diversity and inclusion in community in this article apply to all people, but we as occupational therapists have particular concerns for assuring choice in community living for persons with disabilities and chronic health problems, as well as persons for whom disability and health issues can be prevented.

Personal community building begins at the center of the circle, where the person is embedded in family and close relationships (see Figure 25.2). Networks of informal support develop in the center of a personal community. Relationships grow because persons choose to be connected. The unique culture of personal community is created from family experience. Values are established: heritage, myths, and traditions are communicated. The foundation for building personal community is established within the family.

> We all come from families. Families are big, small, extended, nuclear, multigenerational,

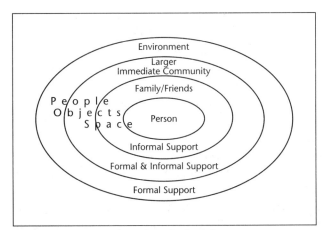

Figure 25.2. Personal community building.

with one parent, two parents, and grandparents. We live under one roof or many. A family can be as temporary as a few weeks, as permanent as forever. We become part of a family by birth, adoption, marriage, or from a desire for mutual support. Families are dynamic and are cultures unto themselves, with different values and unique ways of realizing dreams. Our families create neighborhoods, communities, states, and nations. (Shelton & Stepanek, 1994, p. 6)

For both children and adults, family provides a personal culture of embeddedness. Each person creates a community of family culture in the broadest sense of the concept of community. Like all cultures, each culture we create within our community is based on our values and may differ substantially from another's uniquely consummated community. However the family is constituted, whether we judge it adequate or not according to our value system, a person is embedded in his or her family and that is our starting place for inclusion. *A challenge for occupational therapy practitioners is understanding each person's unique community, including its culture and the context in which it was formed.*

The concept of community is broadened to include relations with acquaintances, coworkers, and schoolmates as well as locations like neighborhoods, workplace, and town. The community circle includes both formal and informal sources of support. The environment provides the context in which communities are formed. It is composed of persons, objects, and space—all of which can be combined for personal or formal community building. The environment generally provides formal support to persons in community. Community is not a static structure in the environment, but

an ongoing process of interaction among persons, objects, and space. Community provides familiarity with daily interactions that reduces the uncertainty experienced in new and challenging situations and creates a sense of belonging.

A sense of belonging in a community provides the comfort and security needed to explore and use one's gifts. According to Maslow's hierarchy, belonging is an important component in the development of self-esteem. Building blocks to self-esteem include a sense of safety in one's immediate community, a sense of self-acceptance, identity, affiliation with others and a sense of competence and mission. In some instances, we seem to expect children and adults with disabilities to demonstrate a sense of self-esteem before they can be included in a typical classroom or work or living environment, forgetting that belonging to a typical community is the means by which a person develops a sense of self (Kunc, 1994). *One of the challenges we often face is resolution of the conflict we have over the need for persons with disabilities to prove themselves capable before they are included in typical communities of their choice rather than creating opportunities for them to develop their capacities in their community with appropriate supports.*

Choice is a valued dimension of our community life. Choice means having alternatives from which to make a selection. As occupational therapists, we recognize the importance of choice in every person's pursuit of self-actualization, particularly as he or she fulfills occupational roles of daily living, work, school, and play and leisure. Choice in occupational therapy has traditionally meant that the person seeking services takes an active part in planning and carrying out a therapy program. Yerxa (1966) maintained that one of the most important roles an occupational therapist plays is providing choice in selection of therapeutic activities, interaction with the activities and, most important, establishment of objectives for a therapy program. Exercising choice in a therapeutic environment provides opportunities to explore capabilities and options for life outside the therapy setting. Making choices is another way of exploring personal values about daily living, relationships, roles, and the physical, psychological, social, and spiritual communities in which living needs to occur to pursue self-actualization. Making choices in therapy is only a prelude to the choices people need to make regarding their life in the community. How will I make a living? Where will I live? Where will my child go to school? What supports will I need to live fully in the community of my choice? *A challenge for occupa-*

tional therapy practitioners is fostering choice that reflects their consumer's priorities for living and accomplishing occupational tasks, even if there are differences between them regarding values or perceptions of expertise. Schön (1983) wrote that the interactive practitioner realizes that he or she is not the only one in the situation to have relevant and important knowledge. The consumer interacts by joining with a service provider to make sense of the situation and, by doing so, gains a sense of increased involvement and action—or choice.

Being part of a community provides opportunities for lifelong development. Persons with disabilities and their family members have a right to pursue and participate in all levels of their community, whether it is one they have known well or one they wish to build to accommodate new circumstances and fulfill new or old dreams. Each person creates a community of his or her own culture in the broadest sense of the concept. Like all cultures, each culture we create within our community is based in our values and may differ substantially from another's uniquely consummated community. Creating community opens doors to new cultural vistas with opportunities to cooperate with each other and participate in community activities. Inclusion in a community also means an end to loneliness and helplessness and the beginning of empowerment to fulfill dreams (McLaughlin & Davidson, 1985). Building inclusive communities with all persons provides opportunities for members of the community to experience different relationships. Each of us has the capacity for creating inclusive community through our work with individuals as well as our ability to influence society and its established institutions.

The Nature of Disability and Inclusion

A new sociopolitical environment is developing in which persons with disabilities are taking or creating social and political actions on their own behalf. Changing perceptions of disability and the histories of the civil rights movement in the 1960s and the women's rights movement in the 1970s resulted in substantial legislative action for disability rights. In his book *No Pity,* Shapiro (1993) chronicled the course of the disability rights movement in the United States. Shapiro stated that persons with disabilities insist simply on common respect and the opportunity to build bonds to their community as fully accepted participants in everyday life. In the past, disability was usually viewed as a medical problem with the expectation that, to be accepted,

persons with disabilities needed to be as much like persons without disabilities as possible without regard for their own uniqueness. Now, persons with disabilities are thinking differently about themselves. Many no longer think of their physical or mental differences as a source of shame or something to overcome in order to be like others or inspire others. In *Flying Without Wings,* Beisser, who contracted polio as an adult, said "When I stopped struggling, working to change, and found means of accepting what I had already become, I discovered that changed me. Rather than feeling disabled and inadequate, I felt whole again" (1989, p. 169). Beisser views disability as a difference among people. Considering disability as a difference is in itself neutral and changes the way persons with disabilities view themselves and are viewed by others. For example, in the village of Chilmark on Martha's Vineyard Island in Massachusetts, more than half the residents in the 1800s were genetically deaf (Groce, 1985). All the people in the village were fluent in sign language. It has been reported that spoken and sign language were used simultaneously or, if a person who was deaf joined a speaking group, group members immediately started to use sign as well as speech. Deafness was not a disability in Chilmark. Disability is a dimension of diversity not unlike ethnic background, color, religious, or gender differences (Shapiro, 1993). Differences do not necessarily equal limitations, but rather create opportunities for meaningful interaction (J. Snow, personal communication, 1994) as long as people are living together naturally.

Just as perceptions of disability are changing, so are the reasons that disability was so often seen as a limitation. The difference within the person is no longer viewed as the main problem; instead, the environment that cannot accommodate the person is considered responsible for society's failure to include persons with disabilities in the mainstream. Social considerations have led to a shift from the traditional medical view of disability to an interactional model that accounts for the relationship between person and environment. Gill (1987) summarized this shift in perspective as follows:

- According to the medical view, disability is considered a deficit or abnormality. In an interactional model, disability is a difference.
- In the medical view, being disabled is perceived as negative. In an interactional model, being disabled is in itself neutral.
- Medicine views disability as residing in the individual. In an interactional model, disability is derived

from problems encountered during interaction between the individual and their environment.

- In medicine, the remedy for disability-related problems is cure or normalization of the individual. In an interactional model, the remedy for disability-related problems is a change in the environmental interaction.
- Finally, the medical view identifies the agent of remedy as the professional. An interactional model has proposed that the agent of remedy may be the individual, an advocate, or anyone who affects the arrangements between the individual and society.

The last interactional category in Gill's summary can have a significant effect on the roles for occupational therapists. The shift from a medical perspective to an environmental framework is not difficult for us to understand. Occupational therapists have always recognized that disability was not an illness that could be cured by medicine. *The challenge for us is to promote the interactive model for practice regardless of the venue of our practice. A concurrent challenge is to increase support for more practice venues in the community where engagement in real occupation takes place.*

Change in perception of disability has fostered the disability rights movement and legislative action. The disability rights movement has focused on the rights of persons with disabilities to be included in society according to the choices they make for themselves and their families. The rights movement could also be called an *inclusion* movement. Inclusion in community means that all persons regardless of differences participate in natural environments for living, learning, playing, working, resting, and recreating. For persons with disabilities, participation may be with specific support from others or with adaptations to the environment. According to Gill (1987), inclusion means removal of barriers to power, which results in a greater number of alternatives or choices.

Shapiro (1993) identified the 1960s as the beginning of the disability independent living movement started by Ed Roberts and other students at the University of California–Berkeley. The movement spread to include action in Washington, DC, that initiated funding for independent living. Groups of parents of children with disabilities began to form around the country at about the same time, primarily to provide support to other parents in the same situations. The groups were often connected to existing organizations like United Cerebral Palsy or the Easter Seal Society. Later, parent organizations would emerge as independent, social change groups.

The 1970s saw adoption of Section 504 of the Rehabilitation Act (Public Law 93–112) prohibiting discrimination on the basis of disability. But Section 504 was not implemented for nearly 5 years after its adoption and was implemented only after a group led by Roberts and others staged a sit-in at the Department of Health, Education and Welfare office in San Francisco. Besides succeeding in obtaining regulations for Section 504, the event in San Francisco created an awareness that linked groups of adults around the country in a civil rights movement. Also in the 1970s, Public Law 94–142 was adopted as the Education for All Handicapped Children Act (1975), mandating public education in the least restrictive environment for children with disabilities who were 5 years of age and older.

In the 1980s, support was provided for that act through the establishment of statewide parent information and advocacy centers in every state. The legislation was expanded to include infants and toddlers with passage of the Education for All Handicapped Children Act Amendments of 1986 (Public Law 99–457). With this expanded legislation for education came the components of family-centered care, or respect for a family's central role as decision maker for a child, or support for an adult, which is now considered best practice across the life span. Public Law 94–142 and Public Law 99–457 were combined and expanded in reauthorization as the Individuals With Disabilities Education Act of 1990 (IDEA) (Public Law 101–476). Meanwhile, the Technology-Related Assistance for Individuals With Disabilities Act (Public Law 100–407) (1988) began the process of changing policy and availability of assistive technology for persons with disabilities in all states. The legislative decade of the 1980s culminated with the Americans With Disabilities Act of 1990 (ADA) (Public Law 101–336). ADA encompasses ideology from all previous legislation by ensuring that the barriers to inclusion be eliminated for persons with disabilities. Although far-reaching disability rights legislation was officially adopted in the 1980s, we are still struggling with implementation of all the laws in the 1990s.

The disability rights movement and legislation has focused primarily on removing physical and legal barriers to inclusion. Legislative mandates serve the purpose of forcing inclusion. The spirit of inclusion only comes with attitude change supported by community preparation and relationship building. In a midwestern city, 9-year-old Amy, who has cerebral palsy, visited Santa

Claus last year and had only one wish for Christmas—just one day in school when the kids did not tease her about her cerebral palsy. Clearly, Amy was present in school with her typical peers, and being there is a start. But she is not truly included since a community that accepts her for who she is has not been created. She needed a school community that gave her a sense of familiarity, caring, and belonging. She needed relationships that she could depend upon for support ("Disabled Girl Asks Santa," 1993). In another city, 14-year-old Kevin, who has Down's syndrome, has been with typical peers from the beginning of his school career. His inclusion has focused on preparation and relationship building that included Kevin along with the teachers and children in the building. When asked what it would be like if he was not included in typical school, he replied that he'd feel sad. "I like to be in school with my friends—I learn from them and they learn from me" (Kevin, personal communication, February 1993).

Inclusion is about relationships. Judith Snow, a consumer advocate in Canada, has said that the only real disability is having no relationships (personal communication, January 1994). Inclusion means participation. Inclusion in school is only the prelude to inclusion in life. Participation may require support not only in the traditional sense of personal assistance and adaptations, but also in terms of preparing the persons in the community to welcome differences into their community and help develop natural support systems. *A challenge for occupational therapy is development of programs that prepare persons and their families for life in the community while working to prepare the community and persons in it to welcome the gifts of diversity.* If we espouse the interactive model of disability, we can affect the arrangements between the individual and society and make unique contributions to the interactive model of change. We can assist with remediation of the person's physical or psychological problem to the extent that the manifestations of the problem can be changed. We can participate in modification of the person's environment so that it can accommodate the needs. We can assist with building community with the person or family in order to create a place for belonging that includes both the formal and informal sources of support. We can continue to promote inclusion as a value through our sociopolitical systems.

Building inclusive community sometimes requires change in value-based practices. The spiral (see Figure 25.3) serves as a model to illustrate that when we recognize differences in values, we may experience conflicts within ourselves or with others. If we cannot move be-

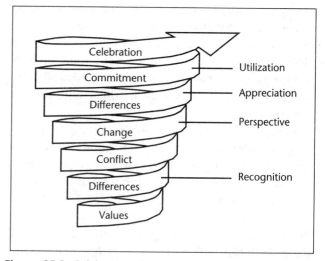

Figure 25.3. Celebrating diversity: Individual and society.

yond the downward spiral between values and differences, we will not be able to move beyond conflict. But if we move upward to change our perspective to one of appreciating differences, we can make a commitment to using differences in ways that productively build community. The spiral begins with a small, defined center focusing on personal values about differences. These values were established with past experience. As the spiral moves upward and widens, new experiences are included. The person uses past experience to respond to new situations. The response may be use of past behavior or of a new behavior that will modify old behaviors. For example, Bobbie wants to live alone in an apartment, but he cannot tie his shoes, button his shirt, prepare meals very well, or use the telephone to summon help. If your values about independence mean a person can only choose between doing everything alone or living in a segregated community, then Bobbie's proposal is different, causes conflict, and probably elicits a negative response. If you stay in a downward spiral of conflict between values and differences, you will continue to respond negatively to full inclusion for persons who cannot perform all tasks independently. But if you take an interactive view of disability, your perspective changes. You appreciate that Bobbie's disability resides in the community that cannot accommodate his differences. A change in perspective leads to modification of old behavior by new responses. A commitment to using rather than rejecting differences creates new possibilities for removing the barriers to inclusion. *The challenge for individual occupational therapists and the profession is making a commitment to inclusion in community for all persons with disabilities and chronic health problems.* The following values are proposed for occupational therapy:

- Every person has a right to be an integrated member of a community of choice.
- Every person has a right to active participation in decision making for self and family.
- Every person has a right to information and options as part of decision making.
- Every person has a right to choice of services delivered in natural environments in order to maximize success in occupational roles.

The Nature of Adaptation and Environment

To explore means for occupational therapists to meet the challenges of building inclusive community, I would like to turn to the spatiotemporal adaptation theory developed with my colleague Elnora Gilfoyle. The theory was developed when we were both involved in pediatric practice and education. During those years, pediatric occupational therapy and other disciplines focused knowledge development and research on typical child development as a means for designing programs for children who were not developing typically. Although the spatiotemporal adaptation theory articulated the importance of interaction between the child and the environment, it emphasized ways in which therapists could influence the child's development rather than ways in which the environment could be prepared to accommodate the child's function. In light of the shift from medical to interactive approach to disability, it seems appropriate to reexamine the categories of the theory, especially the environmental category of the model. The original categories in the theory included *movement, environment, adaptation, and spiraling continuum of development* (Gilfoyle et al., 1990).

In the theory, both development in children and ongoing functioning of adults is seen as a transactional process between a person and the environment; for example, movement provides a means for action and the environment presents a reason to act. The person influences and is influenced by the environment through a process of adaptation. According to Kegan, "adaptation is not just a process of coping or adjusting to events (of the environment) as they are, but an active process of increasingly organizing the relationship of self to the environment" (1982, p. 113). The relationship is transactional because persons organize themselves around events of the environment while simultaneously orga-

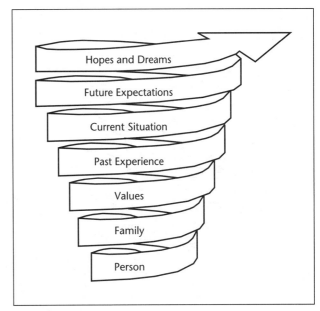

Figure 25.4. The person in life span.

nizing environmental events to meet their needs (Yerxa, 1992). Adaptation as a category of the theory is viewed as an ongoing process of change in behavior. The spiral again provides the model for the adaptation process (see Figure 25.4). Throughout the life span, a person uses past experience, including values established in early life, to adapt to current situations and prepare for future adaptations. Through adaptation, more complex behaviors evolve to respond to more extensive demands from the environment. If the demands of the current or future situations exceed the ability to adapt, the person may recall past behavior to respond until environmental events can be reorganized to elicit a higher level response. With adaptation as a process for organizing one's self and environment, interaction between person and environment sets up a system of relationships.

Environment as a category in the adaptation theory is all-inclusive. Environment represents the complete setting or surrounding in which a person lives, including self, other persons, objects, space, and relationships between all components in the environment (see Figure 25.2). According to Winnicott, a "good enough" (1965, p. 67) environment meets and challenges a person's need to grow and develop by adapting to stimulation from continually changing situations. Yerxa (1994; see Chapter 56) noted that persons need just the right challenge to make an adaptive response. Daloz said that

how readily we grow—indeed whether we grow at all—has a great deal to do with the nature of

337

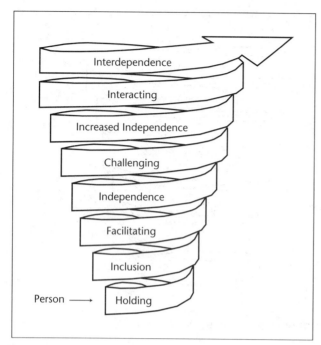

Figure 25.5. Environment–person relationships.

the world in which we transact our lives' business. To understand human development, we must understand the environment's part, how it confirms us, contradicts us and provides continuity. (1986, p. 68)

Environment–person relationships (see Figure 25.5) are conceptualized on a spiraling continuum from a *holding environment,* which promotes inclusion, to a *facilitating environment,* which promotes independence, to a *challenging environment,* which increases independence, to an *interactive environment,* which fosters interdependence. The holding environment begins in infancy and provides support through physical and psychological holding. Winnicott (1965) maintained that the holding environment is the context in which early development takes place. The infant experience can influence a lifetime. Kegan referred to holding as the "culture of embeddedness" (1982, p. 115), which means an environment that is for growth as well as for accumulating history and mythology. In the holding environment, the infant begins to acquire a culture based on values and traditions communicated during this phase. According to Kegan, there is no single holding environment in early life, but a succession of holding environments, a life history of embeddedness. Holding environments are psychosocial environments that hold us and let go of us. If the infant's experience

is satisfactory, it becomes a reference point whenever holding or support is needed later in life. The holding environment promotes a sense of inclusion or belonging, which usually precedes movement away from sources of support and is vital for all persons' development of independence.

The facilitating environment motivates a person to move beyond a familiar setting and on to new challenges and independence. It provides just enough support for moving, literally or figuratively, into new situations.

The challenging environment focuses on separating the person from embeddedness in order to develop and test potential. Just the right amount of challenge is needed if the person is to make an adaptive response to the situation. Increased independence evolves from successful adaptation to challenges.

Finally, the interactive environment promotes interplay between person and environment by combining a sense of self with an appreciation for relationships with others. Interactive environment supports interdependence. Winnicott stated that independence is never absolute. The healthy person does not become isolated, but relates to the environment in such a way that person and environment can be considered interdependent. The different functions of environment and the spiraling sequence of relating to environment can be useful for helping persons identify the environment they need to seek or create for their own health and well-being.

The role of the therapist is construction of Winnicott's "good enough" environment (1965), depending on the person's adaptation needs (Letts et al., 1994). A new parent of a child with significant health problems may need a supportive holding environment to learn the special care that will be given at home. A teenager with a spinal cord injury may seek a facilitating environment when he decides to go to college. He may begin assembling the sources for assistance and adaptations he will need to live independently as well as the advocacy skills he will need to act on his own behalf. A woman recovering from a head injury may have regained considerable function in a rehabilitation setting, but may be fearful of being back in her community. She will need challenge to regain her independence, but with enough support and facilitation to ensure progressively successful adaptation. She may want to reconstruct the life she led before the accident, or she may construct a new community and need resources for her new life. An infant may literally require a supportive environment to learn sensorimotor skills or speech or to focus on learning through play. For all of us, gaining and maintaining a balanced interaction between self and environment is a work in progress. We often need to challenge ourselves if we wish to move ahead. Or we seek facilitation for new situations, or support in difficult times. A challenge for occupational therapy practitioners is development of skill in analyzing environments and helping consumers to identify the type of environmental milieu that will facilitate their adaptation process.

Interactive Strategies for Choice and Inclusion

The promise of occupational therapy lies in our ability to continuously combine the mandates put forth in the early tenets of our discipline with our constantly changing practice environments. Occupational therapy emerged from both community and medical models of practice, although our philosophy is more related to what we know as the community-based model because occupations are practiced in community settings. For decades we tended to practice more in institutions or specialized settings, usually trying to simulate real-life settings to prepare persons to live in their community. Some of our more visionary colleagues set the course toward a future that focused on community consultation models of service delivery. The founders and leaders in our profession have fostered the importance of providing services in a person's own setting and according to the person's own choices and priorities for gaining or regaining specific skills for living. Our philosophy from the beginning of our profession has included the value of choice, relevance, and active participation through engagement in meaningful occupations. Occupation provides a context for organizing one's self and one's environment, thus promoting the transactional process of adaptation within a community setting (Engelhardt, 1977; Gilfoyle et al., 1990; Grady, 1992; Meyer, 1922; see Chapter 4; Schwartz, 1992; Yerxa, 1966). Therapy programs are designed to prevent or remediate the effects of disability or health issues and promote independent living in the community through occupations such as self-care and daily care of others, ability to play independently or with other children, ability to learn as a child and engage in lifelong learning as an adult, ability to be engaged in meaningful work to make a living or for one's own satisfaction or both, ability to balance work and recreation, and ability to blend all

occupational activity with rest. Although models for community service delivery have been promoted from within the profession, external mandates for change have also influenced expansion of our practice environments. The voices heard from our consumers, our colleagues, legislation at state and national levels, and rapidly changing payment systems direct us toward service delivery that focuses on consumers' priorities for goals and naturally occurring venues for activities. The new directions in practice allow us to combine our past experience and founders' mandates with the current realities of practice in ways that lead us to realize the future hopes and dreams of our consumers, ourselves as individuals, and the profession as a whole.

To build collaborative models of consumer-driven, community-based practice, we need to focus on a communication process that helps us understand other persons' unique culture and priorities for life occupations as well as meaning associated with past experiences, current situations, and hopes for the future. Recent developments in the field support a focus on communication that enhances a shift from medically focused to interactive models of practice in which the therapist serves as an agent of remedy to affect the arrangements between the individual and society. The use of narrative for storytelling has increased our understanding of a person's past and present experience. Reflective practice and clinical reasoning support our ability to gain insight into the interactive roles that can unfold between a therapist and a person seeking services. Ethnographic approaches to research have in general heightened our knowledge of persons living in their own environments (Clark, 1993; Mattingly & Fleming, 1994; Schön, 1983; Yerxa, 1994; see Chapter 56).

Therapist–consumer collaborative practice models mean that communication among the therapist, the person seeking services, the family members, and the close community members is critical. From the beginning, it is the relationships we build that are critical to our ability to collaborate effectively. Listening, talking, reflecting, informing, and demonstrating are all part of the ways we establish relationships. Human beings are uniquely constituted for giving and receiving information, making and sharing meaning. We have the capacity to use intrapersonal communication skills to explore the meaning of our own values and experiences, and interpersonal communication skills to link with another person's values and experiences. Intrapersonal communication refers to the creating, functioning, and evaluating of symbolic processes that operate within us. Such activities as thinking, reflecting, solving some problems, and talking with oneself are part of our unique intrapersonal communication system (Dance & Larson, 1972). Intrapersonal communication is active within us whenever meaning is attached to an internally or externally generated source of stimulation. Meaning associated with past events and current situations is deeply embedded in the intrapersonal system of both the persons seeking services and the service provider. Interpersonal communication serves to link us through verbal and nonverbal expression so that we can more explicitly share information and meaning. Through interpersonal communication, we can tell our stories; explore the meaning of relationships, events, and circumstances; reflect on similarities, differences, strengths, and challenges; and develop plans for working together toward future goals. Kegan said, "If you want to understand another person in some fundamental way, you must know where the person is in his or her evolution. You need to understand his or her underlying structure for making meaning" (1982, p. 113). The context in which we as therapists seek and receive the information shared by persons seeking services can enhance our communication and collaborative planning. A communication model of collaboration can be illustrated by the spiraling model of person in life span (see Figure 25.4). If we place spirals side by side and let one spiral represent the consultant therapist and the other represent a person seeking services, we can visualize the communication sequences that

occur. Communication moves from intrapersonal reflection to interpersonal linking through listening and speaking (see Figure 25.6). A closer look at the circle representing past experience provides details that can be shared about the meaning embedded in values and culture of childhood, family, and personal community (see Figure 25.7). We can discuss past experiences in terms of activities and relationships with family and close friends, with personal community, and with the larger environment. Exploring the past provides insight into the values that have directed past choices and the types of environments that the person has experienced. Discussing the current situation (see Figures 25.8 and 25.9) in the same context allows the therapist to understand the extent and meaning of the change that has occurred in the person's life as well as the priorities and types of environments that need to be foremost in planning together. The persons can glean considerable information about the therapist's perspective on the current situation on the basis of past experience. The interpersonal linking increases understanding and promotes collaborative goal setting between person and therapist. As much as we have moved toward collaboration in family-centered and person-centered planning, we are still sometimes heard to say that we are having difficulty with a person receiving services accepting the goals we have set for their therapy. Interactive strategies mean that persons receiving services set the goals and therapists collaborate to design programs with them that will help address the goals. Information shared and

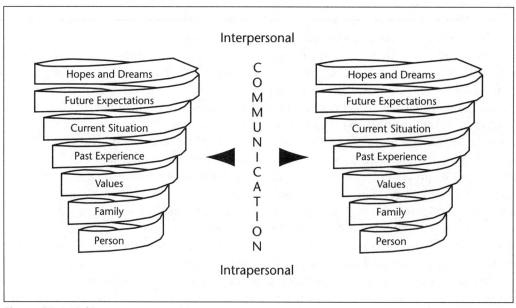

Figure 25.6. Linking past experiences.

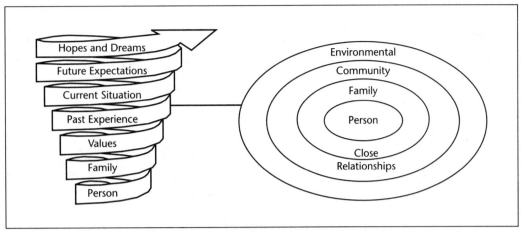

Figure 25.7. The link of past experience with personal community.

the meaning it holds for both consumer and therapist provide the basis for collaboratively planning the future (see Figures 25.10 and 25.11). According to Schön (1983), there is gratification and anxiety for the reflective, interactive practitioner in becoming an active participant in a process of shared inquiry. For a therapist or consumer who wishes to move from traditional to reflective communication, there is the task of reshaping expectations for the relationship. But if we are to be agents of remedy in the arrangements between a person and the environment, we need to be able to share with and receive comprehensive information from the persons who are seeking choices for inclusion in their community.

Summary

We have had an opportunity to focus on the challenges and opportunities for building inclusive community with the persons with whom we work in occupational therapy. We have gained understanding about the meaning of community and choice, reviewed current ideas about the nature of disability and mandates for inclusion, expanded ideas about environment and adaptation, considered strategies for promoting choice and inclusion, and related these concepts to the philosophy of occupational therapy. I had the extraordinary opportunity to explore my own values, past experience, current situation, and hopes for the future and I am forever changed by the ex-

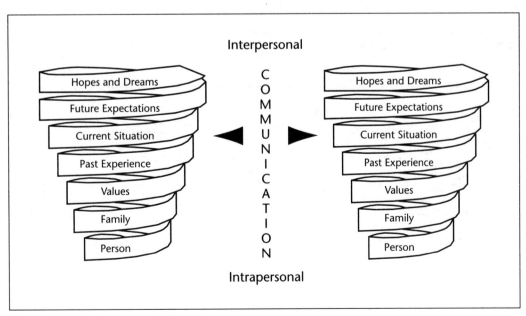

Figure 25.8. Linking current information.

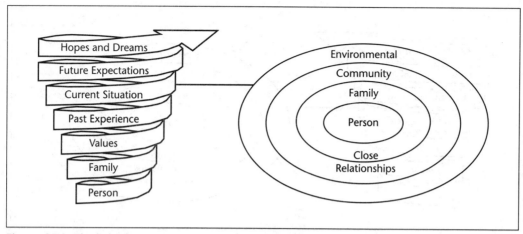

Figure 25.9. The link of current situation with personal community.

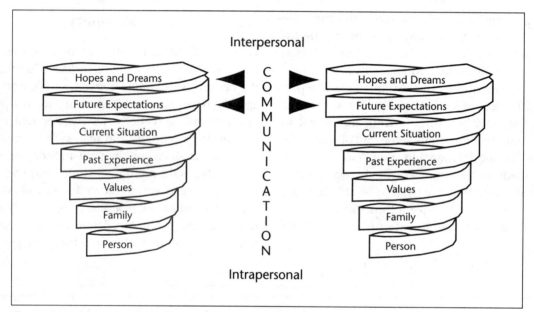

Figure 25.10. Exploring future possibilities.

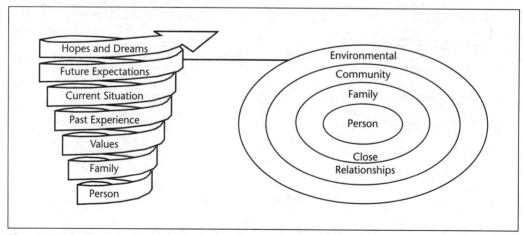

Figure 25.11. The link of hopes, dreams, and future expectations with personal community.

perience. As Emily Brontë reflected, "I've dreamt in my life—dreams that have stayed with me ever after, and changed my ideas: they've gone through and through me, like wine through water, and altered the color of my mind" (cited in *The Quotable Woman*, 1991, p. 185). Leading the development of inclusive community is right for occupational therapy and we all have it in us to do it. The challenges before us are as follows:

1. Understanding each person's unique community, including its culture and the context in which it was formed.
2. Resolving the conflict we have over the need for persons with disabilities to prove themselves capable before being included in typical communities of choice rather than creating opportunities for developing capabilities in the community with appropriate supports.
3. Fostering choice that reflects a person's priorities for living and accomplishing occupational tasks, even when there are differences regarding values or perceptions of expertise.
4. Promoting the interactive model for practice, regardless of the venue of practice.
5. Increasing support for more practice venues in the community where engagement in real occupation takes place.
6. Developing programs that prepare people and their families for life in the community while working to prepare the community to welcome the gifts of diversity.
7. Making a commitment to inclusion in community for all persons.
8. Developing skill in analyzing environments and helping people identify the type of environmental milieu that will facilitate their adaptation process.

Acknowledgments

I thank Ellie Gilfoyle for leading the Eleanor Clarke Slagle nomination process and for a lifetime of creative collaboration; my colleagues who supported the nomination and by doing so offered focus for the topic; Lou Shannon for ongoing support and inspiration; my colleagues at The Children's Hospital for their support; Anita Wagner, Jackie Brand, and all the other parents who enlightened me with their perspectives and changed the course of my family, who are in the center of my personal community. I also thank Carol Wassell from Instructional Services at Colorado State University for creating beautiful slides for the presentation and graphics for this article and Diane Brians for drawing the Circle of Friends.

This lectureship is dedicated to my parents, the late Marion and James Grady, with deep love and appreciation for the strong focus on family and community that they lived and instilled in their children.

References

Americans With Disabilities Act of 1990 (Public Law 101–336) 42 U.S.C. § 12101.

Beisser, A. (1989). *Flying without wings*. New York: Doubleday.

Brontë, E. (1991). Cited in *The quotable woman*. Philadelphia: Running Press.

Clark, F. (1993). Occupation embedded in a real life: Interweaving occupational science and occupational therapy. 1993 Eleanor Clarke Slagle Lecture. *American Journal of Occupational Therapy, 47*, 1067–1078.

Daloz, L. (1986). *Effective mentoring and teaching*. San Francisco: Jossey-Bass.

Dance, F., & Larson, C. (1972). *Speech communication: Concepts and behavior*. New York: Holt, Rinehart, & Winston.

Disabled girl asks Santa to end teasing. (1993, December 14). *The Denver Post*, p. 1.

Education for All Handicapped Children Act of 1975 (Public Law 94–142).

Education of the Handicapped Act Amendments of 1986 (Public Law 99–457).

Engelhardt, H. (1977). Defining occupational therapy: The meaning of therapy and the virtues of occupation. *American Journal of Occupational Therapy, 31*, 666–672.

Gilfoyle, E., Grady, A., & Moore, J. (1990). *Children adapt* (2nd ed.). Thorofare, NJ: Slack.

Gill, C. (1987). A new social perspective on disability and its implication for rehabilitation. *Occupational Therapy in Health Care, 7*, 1.

Grady, A. (1992). Nationally Speaking—Occupation as vision. *American Journal of Occupational Therapy, 46*, 1062–1065. http://dx.doi.org/10.5014/ajot.46.12.1062

Groce, N. (1985). *Everyone here spoke sign language: Hereditary deafness on Martha's Vineyard*. Cambridge, MA: Harvard University Press.

Individuals With Disabilities Education Act of 1990 (Public Law 101–476).

Kegan, R. (1982). *The evolving self*. Cambridge, MA: Harvard University Press.

Kunc, N. (1994). *The other side of therapy*. Port Alberni, BC: Axis Consultation and Training.

Letts, L., Law, M., Rigby, P., Cooper, B., Stewart, D., & Strong, S. (1994). Person–environment assessments in occupational therapy. *American Journal of Occupational Therapy, 48,* 608–618. http://dx.doi.org/10.5014/ajot.48.7.608

Mattingly, C., & Fleming, M. (1994). *Clinical reasoning: Forms of inquiry in a therapeutic practice.* Philadelphia: F. A. Davis.

Meyer, A. (1922). The philosophy of occupation therapy. *Archives of Occupational Therapy, 1,* 1. Reprinted as Chapter 4.

McLaughlin, C., & Davidson, G. (1985). *Builders of the dawn.* Summertown, TN: Book Publishing.

McWilliams, P. (1994). *Do it again!* Los Angeles: Prelude.

Patterson, A. (1992). *Rock art symbols of the greater Southwest.* Boulder, CO: Johnson.

Patterson-Rudolph, C. (1993). *Petroglyphs and Pueblo myths of the Rio Grande* (2nd ed.). Albuquerque, NM: Avanyu.

Rehabilitation Act of 1973 (Public Law 93–112), 29 U.S.C. § 794.

Schön, D. (1983). *The reflective practitioner.* New York: Basic.

Schwartz, K. (1992). Occupational therapy and education: A shared vision. *American Journal of Occupational Therapy, 46,* 12–18. http://dx.doi.org/10.5014/ajot.46.1.12

Shapiro, J. (1993). *No pity.* New York: Times.

Shelton, T., & Stepanek, J. (1994). *Family-centered care for children needing specialized health and developmental services.* Bethesda, MD: Association for the Care of Children's Health.

Technology-Related Assistance for Individuals With Disabilities Act (Public Law 100–407) (1988).

Winnicott, D. (1965). *The maturational processes and the facilitating environment.* New York: International Universities Press.

Yankelovitch, D. (1981). *New rules.* New York: Random House.

Yerxa, E. (1967). 1966 Eleanor Clarke Slagle Lecture—Authentic occupational therapy. *American Journal of Occupational Therapy, 21,* 1–9.

Yerxa, E. (1992). Some implications of occupational therapy's history for its epistemology, values, and relation to medicine. *American Journal of Occupational Therapy, 46,* 79–83. http://dx.doi.org/10.5014/ajot.46.1.79

Yerxa, E. (1994). Dreams, dilemmas, and decisions for occupational therapy practice in a new millennium: An American perspective. *American Journal of Occupational Therapy, 48,* 586–589. http://dx.doi.org/10.5014/ajot.48.7.586 Reprinted as Chapter 4.

CHAPTER 26

Occupational Deprivation: Global Challenge in the New Millennium

GAIL WHITEFORD

Occupational deprivation is, in essence, a state in which a person or group of people is unable to do what is necessary and meaningful in their lives due to external restrictions. It is a state in which the opportunity to perform those occupations that have social, cultural, and personal relevance is rendered difficult if not impossible. It is a reality for numerous people living around the globe today.

To highlight that occupational deprivation is a real and pressing phenomenon affecting the lives of many individuals, consider the situation of Trkulja Ljubica. She is a refugee living in Belgrade and reflects here on her former life:

> I remember my violets that remained blooming in the window of my kitchen. And all the flowers too. My violets flourished in various colors: blue, pink, white. I watched them there, one next to the other as if in conversation, not knowing that I would go from there and that my hand would not nourish them any more. Oh God, where is the end of this hell, when will I have violets and other flowers in my flat again? I always think how my violets dried up and died, dropping their gorgeous flowers. (Ljubica, 1996, p. 6)

Ljubica's story is part of a compelling collection of narrative accounts of the experience of refugeeism. This is the experience of being forcibly removed from home, family, and community, of being disenfranchised and of being unable to engage in the everyday occupations of life such as growing violets. In other words, it is preclusion from those everyday occupations that bring meaning and coherence to existence.

This is an experience that is difficult for many of us to imagine as we orchestrate the numerous occupations that compete for time on a daily basis. Most of us have the freedom and opportunity to make choices about what we will, or will not, do today based on personal preference and individual or social need. The lives of Bosnian women like Ljubica, as well as the numerous refugees around the world in Rwanda, Kosovo and, more recently, East Timor, stand in sharp contrast. Their lives speak of trauma, upheaval, dislocation, and occupational deprivation. While their situation is extreme, they are, however, not alone. Globally, groups of people that (arguably) include ethnic, cultural, and religious minority groups; prisoners; chronically unemployed people; political prisoners; child laborers; and women exist in the context of restricted occupational choice and diminished occupational opportunities.

In this article, definitions of occupational deprivation are presented and explored alongside the related phenomena of occupational disruption and dysfunction. Populations susceptible to the experience of occupational deprivation are identified, as are the impacts of occupational deprivation and the social, political, and economic contexts in which it occurs. Narrative accounts from individuals are included to highlight their realities. In conclusion, some ideas as to how occupational therapists can address occupational deprivation as part of their orientation toward social and occupational justice are posited for consideration.

Defining and Clarifying: What Is Occupational Deprivation?

Wilcock (1998) originally defined *occupational deprivation* as being characterized by "the influence of an external circumstance that keeps a person from acquiring, using, or enjoying something" (p. 145). Based on this original definition of Wilcock and on focused inquiry into the phenomenon, the author's definition of occupational deprivation is:

> A state of preclusion from engagement in occupations of necessity and/or meaning due to factors that stand outside the immediate control of the individual.

The intention of the latter is to highlight the occupational and meaning dimensions within the definition so as to bring to the foreground their importance and relevance both to occupational therapy (Christiansen et al., 1999) and to occupational science (Zemke and Clark, 1996).

The important concept tacit to both these definitions, however, is that *occupational deprivation* as a term implies that *someone or something external to the individual is doing the depriving.* This concept is of central importance in understanding occupational deprivation. The state of deprivation arises not as a result of limitations inherent within the individual, but due to forces outside his or her control. The forces and conditions that may cause such deprivation are complex and are discussed more fully below.

Occupational Disruption

There are two other occupational terms that, while sounding similar, describe quite different phenomena. These are occupational disruption and occupational dysfunction. Occupational disruption is a state that is usually temporary or transient rather than prolonged. Occupational disruption occurs when a person's normal pattern of occupational engagement is disrupted due to significant life events (such as having a baby), environmental changes (such as moving house or location), becoming ill, or sustaining an injury from which full recovery is expected. The most important thing to remember about occupational disruption is that it is a *temporary state and one that, given supportive conditions, resolves itself.* Occupational deprivation differs in that it usually occurs over time and in a context in which there is an absence of supporting conditions. More often, the forces that create a state of occupational deprivation, such as civil conflict leading to refugeeism or the economic constraints necessitating a redundancy, are experienced as hostile.

Occupational Dysfunction

Occupational dysfunction differs from occupational disruption in several key respects. Rather than con-

ceptualizing it as a discrete phenomenon, it can be viewed more usefully either as a byproduct of nonresolved occupational disruption, as a result of specific occupational performance deficits, or as arising from a prolonged state of occupational deprivation. It is a phenomenon that is "nested in a complex of factors all of which reflect and contribute to sustaining the performance, patterns of behavior, identities, choices and so on, that reflect a life in trouble" (Kielhofner, 1995, p. 156). Occupational dysfunction arising from a state of occupational deprivation may be characterized by atrophy of some of the innate human capacities for occupation (Wilcock, 1993; see Chapter 30).

Understanding and Identifying Occupational Deprivation

As may be evident, occupational deprivation is a relatively new term for a phenomenon that has arguably existed in human society for some time. The histories of human societies are characterized by groups of people subordinating others to themselves and depriving them of liberty (Toch, 1977) and, hence, occupational freedom. In today's world, occupational deprivation still results from such direct social and cultural exclusions, but may also exist as a byproduct of institutional policies, technological advancements, economic models, and political systems (Wilcock, 1998).

The Impact of Technology

If the impact of technology in particular is considered, it is evident that whole communities of people previously involved in both primary and manufacturing industries have been disenfranchised by mass unemployment due to new technologies in the workplace. As Tomlinson (1999) pointed out, technology never solves problems or creates better societies; rather, it serves to highlight social inequalities and political conflicts. That this is very much the case with the growing numbers of technology-driven redundancies is evident in the "ghosting" of the blue-collar worker (Toulmin, 1995). In an excellent analysis of the complex technological, economic, and market-driven forces that have an impact on unemployment, Jones (1998) suggested that the twin phenomena of high levels of unemployment and high levels of participation occur because:

> . . .males who were traditionally in work are now out of it and females who were traditionally out are now in. This phenomenon illus-

trates the development of a dual labor market and is broadly characteristic of most OECD countries. However, this is of no consolation to the unemployed, especially unskilled and semiskilled workers. (p. 129)

Maldistributed Labor

As indicated, economic conditions coupled with the new fiscal rationalism in many Western countries seem to be shaping occupational trends of concern. Of note is the paradoxical rise of chronic unemployment alongside overemployment; in other words, fewer people are doing more while lots of people are doing less. Bittman and Rice (1999) cited the Geneva-based International Labour Organization (ILO) which suggested that the new flexibility demanded of modern employees about when and for how long they worked resulted in a maldistribution of working hours. Such a maldistribution, they argued, generated still more unemployment as well as increasingly precarious employment, and had "the overall impact of reducing the bargaining capacity of organized labor" (p. 1).

Such an increasing trend toward maldistributed labor reflects an increasing polarization of working hours, creating a scenario of two distinct groups in society: those with too much to do and those with too little. Those in the latter category, that is, those deprived of opportunities to engage in the occupation of paid employment, have the time in which potentially to engage in other occupational pursuits but have little available financial resources with which to do so. This is problematic in a modern context because, as Lobo (1999) suggested, leisure has become commodified to the extent that it requires significant discretionary income. Increasingly, as he pointed out, you need money to be a leisure participant in Western society. This situation, that is, one in which people are already marginalized through lack of paid employment, lack of discretionary income and, subsequently, diminished opportunities to engage in leisure occupations, can over time evolve into a scenario of occupational deprivation.

Marginalization

Besides unemployed people, underemployed people and those living in poverty, Wilcock (1998) included prisoners of war, prison inmates, minority groups (particularly indigenous peoples), and women in her list of people who are most vulnerable to occupational deprivation. This list reflects a collection of those individuals

and groups who have traditionally had little or no legitimate "voice" in mainstream society. Voice and representation reflect levels of participation in mainstream forms of cultural production (Giroux, 1996). If you are occupationally deprived, such legitimate participation is difficult if not impossible. When this is the case, engagement in nonlegitimated occupations, such as vandalism and participation in occupational groups like gangs (Snyder et al., 1998), may become a seemingly attractive alternative.

Certainly, from an occupational perspective, such participation represents an understandable response. However, while there exist some perceived individual benefits in terms of identity construction and structured time use, engagement in such occupations is also potentially dangerous. Involvement has the potential for serious and negative consequences that represent a "downward spiraling trend" (Snyder et al., 1998, p. 134) at both personal and social levels. Antisocial activity, gang participation, and marginal group identity are modern and largely urban phenomena and certainly beyond the scope of full exploration in this article. However, if framed as essentially occupational phenomena, that is, as byproducts of sustained, socially constructed occupational deprivation, they warrant further inquiry as a matter of some urgency.

The Experience of Refugeeism

Refugees, as suggested above, are another group within society that are potentially at risk of becoming occupationally deprived. The experience of refugeeism is profound and life changing, leading to potentially serious and pervasive problems (Faderman, 1998). While the temporary accommodation (which in some instances becomes long term) of refugee camps may be experienced as a holding space affording few normative occupational opportunities, the country of resettlement can prove as hostile to full occupational participation. To highlight this point, it is worth considering a case illustration. Boua Xa Moua (1998) is an Hmong refugee who resettled in the USA. His story is compelling in that his dream of a new life in relative security sours as he finds himself isolated and occupationally restricted. He feels robbed of his previous legitimated social roles and describes his sense of being unable to "do" in the confusing and restricting world of contemporary urban USA:

> Life in America is very tough . . . I can't do anything, I would rather go back if I had the choice.

I have been here so long but I have not learned how to speak English or how to read and write . . . whenever you want to go anywhere, all the time, you have to wait for someone. I mean if they don't come you can't go where you want because you don't know how to go . . . Like I said, if I would have a choice, I would have remained in Laos, or if I could. I would like to go back now. It's much nicer and peaceful back home. Here everything feels too lonely. Everything is too much. I always find myself lost in this world. (Boua Xa Moua, 1998, p. 101)

This account suggests that resettlement in another country does not necessarily predicate a successful outcome for refugees. Societal structures, economic and language barriers, as well as cultural and religious differences, can prevent community integration and occupational participation (Wilcock, 1998). Even when financial status is secure through employment, the deprivation from occupations of meaning can have a devastating and long-term impact. As Boua Xa Moua (1998) reflected, there is little left but to wish for the place in which a meaningful occupational identity existed: home.

The Human Costs of Occupational Deprivation

A decade ago, Yerxa (1989) stated that "Occupation is not just something nice to do, rather, it is wired into the human" and that "Individuals are most true to their humanity when engaged in occupation" (p. 7). What happens, then, when people are deprived of this apparently innate feature of existence, of something so central to our humanity, as Yerxa put it? What are the consequences, both personal and social, of occupational deprivation?

There are few answers in the literature because, currently, there is a lack of existing research dealing with the negative consequences of occupational deprivation. This, in turn, is due to the fact that occupational deprivation (like numerous emergent occupational concepts) has been relatively recently framed as such within the occupational therapy profession. In order best to understand it, as well as other occupational phenomena and their respective relationships to health and well-being, focused inquiry using a range of methodological strategies is required in the near future (Law et al., 1998). In the absence of an in-depth

research base to draw upon, the following reflections on the impacts of occupational deprivation are based upon the author's experience of undertaking an occupational needs assessment of a special assessment unit in a high-security prison (Whiteford, 1995, 1997).

Lack of Meaningful Time Use

One of the most problematic dimensions associated with the direct experience of occupational deprivation is time use. Consistent with the study by Christiansen et al. (1999) pointing to the positive relationship between time spent engaging in meaningful occupation and perceived well-being, lack of time spent engaged in meaningful occupations in the prison setting appeared detrimental to health and well-being. The dynamic relationship among time use, sense of efficacy, and identity seemed, in the penal context, to be compromised by prolonged occupational deprivation.

Evidence of this came from the inmates' narratives. Many of those interviewed had experienced repeated psychotic breakdowns due to gross disturbances in orientation: they were unable to "locate" themselves in time. With few occupations (except eating) to provide structure and punctuate the day, and with little variation in time-use patterns between days of the week and months of the year, they reported feeling "adrift" in an undifferentiated sea of time. Many comments reflected a sense of hopelessness born of a deteriorating sense of efficacy because, where there is little or no perceived control over occupational choices, "there is no sense of efficacy" (Kielhofner, 1995, p. 45).

The prisoners' descriptions reflected these themes and varied from "Time is long and it passes slowly" to "The days go fast but time is slow" and "Time is nothingness." Additionally, they commented that increased occupational opportunities had the potential to "Keep my mind occupied and diverted from thoughts that make me crazy," "Give me an opportunity to bring a picture of something I have in my head to life," "Give me a chance to change my behavior," and "To let out anger and frustration" (Whiteford, 1997, p. 129).

Maladaptive Responses

Not surprisingly, sleep was reported by the inmates as a predominant response to their occupationally deprived state. Sleep, however, was not the only maladaptive response; the prison unit also had a high rate of suicide and suicide attempts. While acknowledging the multiplicity of factors that may have contributed to it, this disturbing feature of life in the unit was discerned by the author to be, at least in part, due to pervasive occupational deprivation. Clearly, this is an area requiring further investigation.

Barrier to Community Reintegration

The major concern with respect to these inmates is that, for them, the experience of occupational deprivation appeared to be a significant barrier to successful community reintegration. They had, to varying degrees, adapted to the occupationally barren environment, reflected in the inmate comment "I've spent most of my life in institutions so the bars don't bother me" (Whiteford, 1997). With severely restricted occupational role repertoires and diminished capacities for structuring and using time effectively, the inmates faced the challenge of living successful occupational lives in the communities to which they would ultimately return. Prolonged occupational deprivation very probably diminishes the likelihood of adaptive responses to new environments, a scenario that could be remediated through the conscious creation of "occupationally enriched" (Molineux & Whiteford, 1999) prison environments.

Wider Impact of Occupational Deprivation

While these observations have been drawn from interactions with a population of occupationally deprived prisoners, it can be argued that diminished opportunities to engage in occupations of meaning for any individual or group of people may potentially have similar results. After all, what we do in life is inextricable from the meaning we ascribe to it (Hasselkus, 1997). Atrophied occupational capacities (Wilcock, 1995), diminished self-efficacy beliefs, and truncated identity constructions may all be byproducts of this dehumanizing phenomenon. Understanding just what impact this has on individuals, families, communities, and societies is a central challenge in the new millennium and worthy of immediate attention.

Future Challenges

The cogent question, then, is how should occupational therapists address occupational deprivation? There are three dimensions to how this can be done.

Adopting an Occupational Perspective

First, it requires occupational therapists to make a conceptual shift to an occupational perspective: to view the world through occupational eyes, seeing phenomena that have previously been viewed from other perspectives (for example, medical, psychological, and social) as essentially occupational phenomena (Townsend, 1999). An occupational perspective is a requisite to considering the occupational needs of people as individuals and within society separately from consideration of how these can be met through the provision of therapeutic interventions. Such a perspective will serve to centralize the role of occupational therapists in being the key agents in the future to address challenging occupational phenomena. Although it has been suggested that there is a "renaissance" of occupation in occupational therapy (Whiteford et al., 2000), it still seems that a gap exists as to how occupation is incorporated into practice. This is an issue when, as Wood (1998) suggested, other professional groups are embracing occupation as pivotal to their interventions.

Acting at a Broader Social and Cultural Level

Second, occupational therapists need to think and act at a broader social and cultural level. Armed with an occupational perspective of society, there is a need to invest more energy into influencing social and institutional structures and policies, which preclude people from full occupational participation. In doing this, the profession comes closer to realizing occupational therapy's social vision (Townsend, 1993).

Embracing Occupational Justice

Third, occupational therapists need to embrace the concept of "occupational justice": to mobilize resources with the aim of creating occupationally "just" societies, societies based on people and their need, and indeed right, to do. Occupational justice is concerned with "economic, political and social force that create equitable opportunity and the means to choose, organize and perform occupations that people find useful or meaningful in their environment" (Townsend, 1999, p. 154). Dignity, as created through the opportunity to interact with the world in a meaningful way through living diverse occupational lives, not just those focused on material gain (Fromm, 1998), will be a central feature of an occupationally just future. Embracing the principles of equity, justice, diversity, and ecological sustainability will be central to the process of achieving this. In the excellent critique of a range of health promotion models presented by Wilcock (1998), that of "social justice" appears to provide the best blueprint for action in addressing occupational deprivation. The model is described as promoting:

. . . social and economic change to increase individual, community and political awareness, resources and equitable opportunities for health . . . participatory analysis of occupational disadvantage, underlying occupational determinants, and uncovering occupational injustice . . . social action for change of occupational policies toward occupational equity and justice [including] social and political lobbying. (p. 230)

Such action and activism represent a big, but necessary, brief for occupational therapy in the years ahead: the face of the new millennium is, to a greater or lesser extent, up to occupational therapists. This is because, as futurist Dator (paper given at the International Futures Conference, Auckland, 1992) suggested some time ago, we won't get the future we necessarily want, but we will get the future we deserve. It is a challenging prospect.

Summary

This article has explored occupational deprivation as a potentially challenging phenomenon in the new millennium. It has considered some definitions of the term and their origins and has explored some related occupational phenomena. The article has considered briefly the conditions that contribute to occupational deprivation and the individuals and groups most vulnerable to it. A consideration of the human and social cost of occupational deprivation preceded a call to arms for occupational therapists to address, through social and political action, this challenging problem now and in the future.

References

Bittman M, Rice J (1999) Are working hours becoming more unsociable? *Australian Social Policy Research Center Newsletter, 74,* 1–5.

Boua Xa Moua (1998) Boua Xa Moua's story. In: L Faderman, ed. *I begin my life all over: the Hmong and the American immigrant experience.* Boston: Beacon Press.

Christiansen C, Backman C, Little B, Nguyen A (1999) Occupations and well-being: a study of personal projects. *American Journal of Occupational Therapy, 53*(1), 91–99. http://dx.doi.org/10.5014/ajot.53.1.91

Faderman L (1998) *I begin my life all over: the Hmong and the American immigrant experience.* Boston: Beacon Press.

Fromm E (1998) *Between having and being.* New York: Continuum.

Giroux H (1996) *Living dangerously: multiculturalism and the politics of difference.* New York: Peter Lang.

Hasselkus B (1997) Meaning and occupation. In: C Christiansen, C Baum, eds. *Occupational therapy: enabling function and well-being.* Thorofare, NJ: Slack, 362–77.

Jones B (1998) Redefining work: setting directions for the future. *Journal of Occupational Science, 5*(3), 127–32.

Kielhofner G (1995) *A model of human occupation.* 2nd ed. Baltimore: Williams & Wilkins.

Law M, Steinwender S, Leclair L (1998) Occupation, health, and well-being. *Canadian Journal of Occupational Therapy, 65*(2), 81–91.

Lobo F (1999) The leisure and work of young people: a review. *Journal of Occupational Science, 6*(3), 27–33.

Ljubica T (1996) Violets. In: R Zarkovic, ed., *I remember: writings of Bosnian women.* San Francisco: Aunt Lute Books.

Moiineux M, Whiteford G (1999) Prisons: from occupational deprivation to occupational enrichment. *Journal of Occupational Science, 6*(3), 124–39.

Snyder C, Clark F, Masunaka-Noriega M, Young B (1998) Los Angeles street kids: new occupations for life programme. *Journal of Occupational Science, 5*(3), 133–39.

Toch H (1997) *Living in prison: the ecology of survival.* New York: MacMiilan.

Tomlinson J (1999) *Globalization and culture.* Cambridge: Polity.

Townsend E (1993) Occupational therapy's social vision. *Canadian Journal of Occupational Therapy, 60*(4), 167–83.

Townsend E (1999) Enabling occupation in the 21st century: making good intentions a reality. *Australian Occupational Therapy Journal, 46*(4), 147–59.

Toulmin S (1995) Occupation, employment, and human welfare. *Journal of Occupational Science: Australia, 2*(2), 48–58.

Whiteford G (1995) A concrete void: occupational deprivation and the special needs inmate, *Journal of Occupational Science: Australia, 2*(2), 80–81.

Whiteford G (1997) Occupational deprivation and incarceration. *Journal of Occupational Science: Australia, 4*(3), 126–30.

Whiteford G, Townsend E, Hocking C (2000) Reflections on a renaissance of occupation. *Canadian Journal of Occupational Therapy, 67*(1), 61–69.

Wilcock A (1993) A theory of the human need for occupation. *Journal of Occupational Science: Australia, 1*(1) 17–24. Reprinted as Chapter 30.

Wilcock A (1995) The occupational brain: a theory of human nature. *Journal of Occupational Science: Australia, 2*(2), 68–73.

Wilcock A (1998) *An occupational perspective of health.* Thorofare, NJ: Slack.

Wood W (1998) It is jump time for occupational therapy. *American Journal of Occupational Therapy, 52*(6), 403–11. http://dx.doi.org/10.5014/ajot.52.6.403

Yerxa E (1989) An introduction to occupational science: a foundation for occupational therapy in the 21st century. In: J Johnson, E Yerxa, eds. *Occupational science: the foundations for new models of practice.* New York: Haworth.

Zemke R, Clark F (1996) *Occupational science: the evolving discipline.* Philadelphia: FA Davis.

CHAPTER 27

Occupational Justice and Client-Centered Practice: A Dialogue in Progress

ELIZABETH TOWNSEND AND ANN A. WILCOCK

This paper reports our ongoing, international dialogue about the relationship among occupation, justice, and client-centered practice. We will discuss two foundations informing the dialogue, four exploratory cases of occupational injustice, implications for occupational therapy's client-centered practice, and concluding reflections. The question that frames our discussion is how do occupational therapists work for justice? Dialogue on this question seems timely as occupational therapists around the world articulate what distinguishes this numerically small, rather invisible profession and its contributions to individuals, populations, and societies.

Foundations of the Dialogue

When we first met in 1997 in South Australia, we discovered a strong synergy of ideas about justice, occupation, and the convergence of those interests in what we began to describe as occupational justice. In sharing our visions of an occupationally just world, we are raising questions about how individuals and populations could flourish as equal citizens in daily lives comprised of health-building occupations (Townsend & Wilcock, 2004; Wilcock & Townsend, 2000).

Occupational therapists already understand that participation in occupations is the means or medium of occupational therapy, and ideally is also the ends or outcomes (Gray, 1998; see Chapter 10; Rebeiro, 1998). History tells us that visions are what propel people to reach beyond what is. John Locke's (Locke, 1690) Essay Concerning Humane Understanding and Southwood Smith's social reforms in the British Industrial Era (Guy, 1996) remind us of the power inherent in articulating and critiquing beliefs, principles, and reasoning. With

awareness of the power of visions to spur action, we are pursuing a dialogue about what could be possible if societies utilize participation in the daily life occupations of a community, including but not limited to work, as both a means and a benchmark to advance occupational justice for individuals and populations.

With World War II as an early life marker, we both grew up in white, middle-class families of British culture. Wilcock moved as an occupational therapist from Britain to Australia to see the world and challenge her ideas in urban and rural communities. With her British cultural background, Townsend left Toronto to see the world and challenge her ideas by working in East Africa then in Prairie, Ontario, and Atlantic communities in rural and urban Canada. On the one hand, we express Western concerns for individual meaning, fulfillment, choice, identity, and autonomy, as well as for citizen participation, empowerment, and civil society. On the other hand, we recognize that daily life, including occupational therapy as a profession, is embedded in a complex environment of power relations. We value cultural differences and Eastern concerns for belonging in community, understanding that communities shape individuals and groups while individuals and groups shape their communities. While optimistically seeking to understand how occupation produces health, well-being, and justice, our critiques attempt to identify forces that produce alienation, deprivation, marginalization, and imbalance. Over the 5 years since 1997, we have been exploring justice from the perspective of two complementary knowledge foundations: occupation and client-centered practice (see Table 27.1).

Wilcock's research, using a history of ideas methodology (Wilcock, 1998, 2001), has generated historical, analytic knowledge about humans as occupational beings and an occupational perspective of health. She found that people in each historical era have implicitly or explicitly employed occupation as the mechanism to sur-

This chapter was previously published in the *Canadian Journal of Occupational Therapy, 71*, 75–87. Copyright © 2004, Canadian Association of Occupational Therapists. Reprinted with permission.

Table 27.1. Two Foundations to Explore Occupational Justice

Knowledge Foundations	Concerns for Justice	Example of Occupational Injustice
1. Occupation Humans are occupational beings. Their existence depends on enablement of diverse opportunities and resources for participation in culturally defined and health-building occupations (Wilcock, 1993, 1998).	Denial of universal access to opportunities and/or resources to participate in culturally defined, health-building occupations is unjust.	Occupational alienation Occupational deprivation Occupational imbalance
2. Client-centered practice Enabling of social inclusion is a justice-oriented, client-centered practice to create diverse opportunities and resources for people to participate in culturally defined, health-building occupations (Townsend, 1993, 1998).	Lack of enabling, client-centered practices restricts the opportunities and/or resources required for diverse people to participate in the occupations of a society.	Occupational deprivation Occupational marginalization Occupational imbalance

vive and promote health and well-being. Underlying occupational determinants, such as the type of economy, social structure, and belief system, shape health. Wilcock reasoned that because occupations are central to human existence, injustices occur when, for example, populations experience occupational alienation or deprivation.

Townsend's research, using an institutional ethnography methodology (Townsend, 1998; Townsend, Ripley, & Langille, 2003), has generated social, analytic knowledge about occupational therapy's social vision of client-centered approaches for enabling empowerment through occupations. She found that occupational therapists may enable some people to flourish, but professional dominance, standardized treatment and documentation, market-driven economies, insurance, laws, and political conditions can overrule our good intentions. Townsend reasoned that injustices occur when client-centred, empowerment approaches are overruled to the extent that populations are occupationally underdeveloped or marginalized.

Language of the Dialogue

Occupational therapy is not alone in its interest in justice, nor even in occupation. Many research and practice fields have an interest in everyday life, participation, occupation, and justice, expressed in diverse ways, examples being found in adult education, community development, community psychology, law, and social work. There are many theories about how social, political, legal, and economic practices determine possibilities and limits for promoting justice and civil society. Survivors of potentially disabling conditions, such as Galipeault, Gidden, Little, Moore, and Sherr Klein (Townsend, 2003a) all highlight their fundamental need to participate in various occupations as empowered citizens.

What, then, distinguishes this profession and its contributions to individuals, populations, and societies? We perceive that occupational therapists' best practices offer a unique synthesis and application of knowledge, skills, and attitudes about three interconnected pillars of knowledge: occupation, enabling, and justice. To distinguish occupational therapists' interests in justice, we use the language of *occupation* to describe participation in various aspects of daily life. We use the language of enabling to describe therapy that uses participatory, empowerment-oriented approaches, what occupational therapists have named client-centered practice. And we use the language of justice to talk about determinants and forms of occupational well-being and social inclusion that take differences in people and contexts into account.

Use of the term occupation to encompass all participation in daily life is as problematic in English as it is in other languages. Popular, research, and government references to occupation in English focus narrowly on work (Jarman, 2003), or aggressively on the military occupation of territory. As occupational scientists and therapists, we make strategic, political use of the term occupation to bring issues of participation in daily life to visible, public attention. We ally ourselves with those who use the term "enabling" to encompass culturally variable processes that invite active client participation in the decision-making and priorities of therapy as well as in daily life occupations—despite the tensions of going against the grain in hierarchically organized systems (Byrne, 1999; Deegan, 1997; Polatajko, 2001; Townsend et al., 2003). Whereas concerns for social justice have raised issues about equality, we want to bring to public awareness the injustices that persist when participation in occupations is barred, confined, restricted, segregated, prohibited, undeveloped, disrupted, alienated, marginalized, exploited, excluded, or otherwise restricted.

It seems that societies tolerate an occupational apartheid (Kronenberg & Simo Algado, 2003). Occupational apartheid may describe situations where occupations are classified, paid, valued, and enhance life for some, while in the same places and times occupations are taken for granted, exploited, and trivialized for others (Townsend, 2003b). It seems that occupational therapists innately know that everyday injustices are right in front of our eyes (H. Fujimoto, personal communication, July 2003). We assert that justice is an implicit, invisible foundation of occupational therapy's occupation-focused, client-centered practice (Townsend, 1993; Wilcock, 1993; see Chapter 30).

Methods

To draw others into our dialogue on occupational justice, our starting point was to review the literature and to organize workshops. We wanted to generate open discussion and critique, without confining participants to questions on a survey or other impersonal research tool.

Occupational Justice Workshops

Workshops and presentations on occupational justice in Australia, Britain, Canada, Portugal, Sweden, and the United States were the first initiatives to draw others into the dialogue. Participants to date have been occupational scientists and therapists, plus a few from sociology, urban and rural planning, social work, and nursing. Their words and phrases illustrate a range of responses to the questions What is occupation? What is justice? and What is occupational justice? (see Table 27.2) Typical comments to date have been:

- This concept feels like a good fit with occupational therapy.
- What is the difference from social justice? Do we need another concept?
- Occupational justice is interesting, but I can't see what I can do about it in my practice.
- There's already too much emphasis on theory [in occupational therapy] and new graduates have less and less skill to actually practice.
- Until the concepts are clearer, there is nothing new in this idea of occupational justice.
- I want to know more about this concept—it makes sense to my practice [as an occupational therapist].
- At last there is a name for something I have felt was behind my occupational therapy practice.

Literature Review

We will highlight references that we find particularly helpful in supporting or challenging our thinking on occupational justice. To understand the breadth of occupation and the relationships among occupation, health, and justice, we honor the contributions of Americans Mary Reilly (1962) (see Chapter 7) and Elizabeth Yerxa (1967, 1979, 1993) in particular who reminded us that occupation is our domain of interest as occupational therapists. Contemporary authors include Karen Rebeiro (2001) in Canada who is drawing in the voices of mental health consumers' experiences of marginalized participation in occupations. Borell and colleagues (2001) in Sweden are building a body of

Table 27.2. Word Associations: *Occupation, Justice,* and *Occupational Justice*[1]

Occupation	Justice	Occupational Justice
• Doing	• Equality	• Enablement of fairness and equal opportunity (possibly with different resources)
• Action	• Fairness	
• Being	• Opportunity	• No discrimination based on ability, age, or other factors
• Everyday life	• Resources	
• Work	• Shared power	• Social commitment to universal design and accessibility
• Leisure	• Empowerment for all	
• Parenting	• Rights	• Enabling everyone to flourish to their greatest potential individually or as members of communities
• Performance	• Responsibilities	
• Participation	• Social network	
• Meaningful doing	• Politics	
• Engagement	• Regulations	
• Meditation	• Doing the right thing	
• More than activity	• Ethics	
• Not a technique/task	• Moral principles	
• Vocation	• Civil society	
• Census classification	• Citizen participation	

[1]Words and phrases from workshop discussions between 1999 and 2002.

research that illuminates how older adults experience their occupations, becoming diminished in scope and highly controlled by caregivers. Forces that support and limit the occupational development of children with disabilities have been identified in Sweden and the United States (Hemmingsson & Borell, 2002; Royeen, Duncan, Crabree, Richards, & Clark, 2000).

In looking beyond individual experiences of occupation, from his professional and academic perspective that bridges Western (Canadian) and Eastern (Japanese) epistemologies, Iwama (1999, 2003) has asked if we are listening to understand the cultural context of occupations. Fujimoto (H. Fujimoto, personal communication, July 2003) echoes this call to cultural relevance in her formulation of occupational justice for children who are ventilator-dependent. Whiteford (2000; see Chapter 26) contributes a global, structural perspective on contexts that produce occupational deprivation as a form of injustice, using examples that range from refugee and aboriginal contexts, to the occupational contexts of prisoners, women, and those who are geographically isolated in the Australian outback.

Outside more than inside occupational therapy, the concept of enabling has been repeatedly emphasized. Dunst and his colleagues (Dunst, Trivette, & Deal, 1988) in social work and Noyes (2000) in nursing have described enabling as a participatory, empowerment-oriented process. Enabling is also a policy and legal concept used to describe how regulations undermine or enable social inclusion in community health, building, design, and legislation (Rosenau, 1994). In the Ottawa Charter for Health Promotion, the World Health Organization (1986) recommended enabling, advocating, and mediating as three necessary approaches for promoting health for all. McKnight (1989) articulated links among enabling, empowerment, and health. Labonte (1989) affirmed that enabling the empowerment of poor people in inner cities promotes health when they form new action communities, for instance to grow their own food.

The broad view of occupation that occupational scientists and therapists use expresses a critical, social perspective on occupations. We have drawn insights on occupations, enabling, and justice particularly from Elizabeth Casson, a physician and founder of occupational therapy in Britain (Wilcock, 2002), from Adolf Meyer (1922; see Chapter 4), a psychiatrist who contributed to the founding of occupational therapy in the United States, and from Goldwin Howland (Howland, 1944), a Canadian physician whose vision advanced

occupational therapy in this country following World War I. Dorothy Smith's (1987, 1990a, 1990b) sociology for women has been helpful in theorizing and tracing the interconnectedness of governance, from policies to media images, embedded in the everyday world. She described how power relations are formed and perpetuated invisibly and often unconsciously through a multiplicity of work processes, similar to our broad view of occupations.

To develop an understanding of justice, we have been guided by both general writings, as well as research on particular instances of injustice. Justice is an ethical, moral, and civic concept (Adelson, 1995; Bores, 2000; Rawls, 1975; Young, 1990) which is applied in various ways to particular circumstances. Underlying Western conceptions of justice may be beliefs about individual autonomy, or what constitutes scientific knowledge (Heitman, 2000). For instance, the notion of individual rights is based on the Enlightenment view of individual agency and moral capacity (Ignatieff, 2000). Whereas Irani (1995), Grammenos (2003), and Zanetti (2001) have emphasized that justice may be viewed outside Western thinking not as a matter of equal distribution of rights or goods, but as matters of trust and loyalty versus exploitation and betrayal. Because justice is culturally bound, ideas, beliefs, principles, and reasoning about civic governance and state regulation tend to establish justice within particular social and institutional frameworks (Armstrong, 2000; McKay, 2000; Metz, 2000).

In specific jurisdictions, such as correctional services, the North American concept of restorative justice has developed to consider debates about the long-term impact on crime rates of rehabilitation or punishment approaches with prisoners (Pogge, 2000). From a consumer perspective, justice related to mental illness is construed as a matter of empowerment (Deegan, 1997). In North American health services, the concept of distributive justice has been used to assess the equality of distribution of particular medical services across various populations (Cookson & Dolan, 2000; Daniels, Kennedy, & Kawachi, 1999; Emanuel, 2000). Principles of justice have been used to guide rationing and spending cuts in health services (Cookson & Dolan, 2000). These views of justice present health as a commodity that can be modified by rationing and distribution.

Two influential sources in developing our occupational perspective of justice have been Iris Morton Young (1990) and Vicki Schultz (2000), researchers in American law. Young challenges the distributive paradigm of justice based on sameness and individual rights by proposing that "issues of decision-making power and procedures, division of labor, and culture" (p. 15) require a paradigm based on enablement of opportunities that respond to differences across social groups. Only in examining power as a social relation rather than as a commodity for distribution, Young argues, can we understand how taken for granted injustices persist—injustices that oppress everyday life for women, persons with disabilities, persons of color, and immigrants. Writing in the Columbia Law Review, Schultz provides a feminist critique of work that has applicability for other populations who are denied fair opportunities or rewards for their work. She envisions a "social order in which work is consistent with egalitarian conceptions of citizenship and care" (p. 1886). To her, work can be structured negatively or positively: "if people's lives can be constrained in negative ways by their conception of their occupational roles, they can also be reshaped along more empowering lines by changing work or the way it is structured or understood" (p. 1891).

Exploratory Theory of Occupational Justice

A brief overview of an exploratory theory of occupational justice (Townsend & Wilcock, 2003) summarizes our own beliefs, principles, ideas, and reasoning to date, as highlighted in Table 27.3. We believe that people are occupational as well as social beings. We recognize that, individually or as members of particular communities, we have differing occupational needs, strengths, and potential which require differing forms of enablement to flourish. With an acknowledged Western view of individual autonomy exerted within an environment or context, we support the principle that occupations are the practical means through which humans exert citizen empowerment, choice, and control. It seems that various forms of participation—doing, being, or becoming through occupations—are essential in promoting health, well-being, and social inclusion in various cultural, economic, institutional, social, and political contexts. Occupational determinants, forms, and outcomes, such as unemployment and poverty, create or limit possibilities for occupational justice. Occupational justice appears to complement and extend understandings of social justice. An occupational perspective, we believe, sparks new perspectives and insights on injustices particularly related to participation in occupations.

Cases of Occupational Injustice

We propose four cases (see Table 27.4) which emerged when we discussed occupational justice together and with workshop participants. The four cases imply the possibility of extending concepts of social justice by defining occupational rights:

- To experience occupation as meaningful and enriching;
- To develop through participation in occupations for health and social inclusion;
- To exert individual or population autonomy through choice in occupations;
- To benefit from fair privileges for diverse participation in occupations socially excluded from full citizenship without participation in the typical range of occupations of a community.

Occupational Alienation

The case described as occupational alienation focuses on the right of populations as well as individuals to experience meaningful, enriching occupations, con-

Table 27.3. An Exploratory Theory of Occupational Justice[1]

Ideas about occupational justice	Reasoning about occupational determinants, forms, and outcomes
• People are occupational as well as social beings • Humans' occupational needs differ with each person • Differing forms of enablement address a variety of occupational needs, strengths, and potentials	• Occupational experiences and environments are determined by economic, policy, cultural, and other determinants • Media, parenting, education, and employment are examples of occupations that shape and are shaped by other occupations • Potential outcomes of occupational injustice are, for example, occupational alienation or occupational marginalization
Beliefs and principles about occupational justice	**Occupational justice versus social justice**
• Humans participate in occupations as autonomous yet interdependent agents in their societal context • Health depends on participation in health-building occupations • Empowerment depends on enabling choice and control in occupational participation	Emphasis in occupational justice on: • Participation in all daily occupations • Differences in occupational participation • Enablement of differences in occupational participation

[1]Townsend & Wilcock, 2003.

Table 27.4. Proposed Occupational Rights

Right to experience occupation as meaningful and enriching
Occupational injustice: occupational alienation

Right to develop through participation in occupations for health and social inclusion
Occupational injustice: occupational deprivation

Right to exert individual or population autonomy through choice in occupations
Occupational injustice: occupational marginalization

Right to benefit from fair privileges for diverse participation in occupations
Occupational injustice: occupational imbalance

*Injustices noted are examples only. They are not categorically limited consequences of restricted rights.

trasted against experiences of alienation. Whereas social justice might address freedom to choose where and how to live, from an occupational perspective, the underlying concern is whether choices are available for all populations to experience meaning and enrichment as they participate in occupations. Occupational alienation is named here as a social condition of injustice, not a psychological state.

With awareness of the complex and problematic notions of meaning and enrichment, we associate occupational alienation with prolonged experiences of disconnectedness, isolation, emptiness, lack of a sense of identity, a limited or confined expression of spirit, or a sense of meaninglessness. Such experiences may occur whether or not people are busy or wealthy. Occupational alienation may be a community or population experience of spiritual emptiness or lack of positive identity. Experiences of meaning and enrichment, enjoyment, health, identity, and quality of life within chosen places and routines appear to be derived from participation in one's occupations (Barnes, 2000; Blair, 2000; Christiansen, 1999 [see Chapter 34]; Hasselkus, 2002; Nygård & Borell, 1998; Primeau, 1996; Tindale, 1999; Vrkljan, 2001). Lack of opportunities or resources to enable occupational meaning and enrichment, then, is viewed as unjust.

Prime examples of occupational alienation occur when people are physically removed from their own cultural occupations through slavery, refugee confinement, or industrial policies that require them to work in demeaning jobs that pay them low wages, possibly great distances from their home or loved ones. Persons with physical or mental disabilities or persons who live in homes for seniors may experience occupational alienation if they are required to participate in occu-

pations that they find meaningless. If the only choices offer no meaningful or enriching occupational experiences for some, then these people may experience occupational alienation, even through others may find the same choices meaningful or enriching. Sheltered workshops for adults with disabilities, senior activity centers, and workfare programs for people without paid employment may carry a managerial and professional vision of meaningful occupation. Yet the actual experience for some may be demeaning, soulless, tiresome, coercive participation in occupations they find meaningless. The concept of occupational alienation may help us to understand the tragedies of aboriginal and other peoples who are denied opportunities and resources to experience meaningful cultural rituals and language. Occupational alienation may offer insights on the desperation of people who are displaced from their homes and communities through mass relocation or war. Consideration of occupational alienation might explain the apparently soulless behavior of people who are institutionalized for long periods without meaningful, enriching participation in occupations.

The right not to be occupationally alienated speaks to the importance of what Fearing and Clark (Fearing & Clark, 2000) have described as occupational dreams. With attention to the dreams of populations or communities as well as individuals, the case of occupational alienation makes visible and conscious the social conditions required for humans to develop through participation in the range of daily life occupations that are typical of a community.

Occupational Deprivation

Whiteford (2003) defines occupational deprivation as "a state of prolonged preclusion from engagement in occupations of necessity and/or meaning due to factors that stand outside the control of the individual" (p. 222). Whiteford's cases of occupational deprivation consider geographic isolation, unsatisfactory conditions of employment (underemployment, unemployment, and overemployment), incarceration, sex-role stereotyping, refugeeism, and disability (pp. 223–239). She distinguishes the prolonged nature of occupational deprivation from temporary occupational disruptions related to injuries, or moving to a new home.

In North America and other jurisdictions, the right to work may be a fundamental value and concept associated with social justice. Yet we know that life is more than work, and work does not necessarily promote health and social inclusion. As knowledge about the impact of daily life expands, it is becoming clear that humans need to do more than work. Humans need the right to develop through participation in occupations for health and social inclusion. Of particular concern in naming occupational deprivation as a form of injustice are those who are confined or otherwise limited from participating in work. Occupational deprivation may also arise when populations have limited choice in occupations because of their isolated location, their ability, or other circumstances.

One of Whiteford's (2003) examples of occupational deprivation is geographic isolation. She describes the daily lives of aboriginal women who live in remote Australian communities with too little companionship and opportunity to flourish. The concept of occupational deprivation might be useful for explaining the losses to children with a disability if they cannot participate in the natural school and play opportunities available around their home. Given the normative expectations of ability and competence, people who are old or living with a disability may also be socially excluded from participation in transportation, health care, recreation, shopping, farming, mining, fishing, industry, business, public service, or other occupations typical of their communities.

The case of occupational deprivation recognizes that the right to work is not sufficient to capture what people need and want to do to flourish from birth to death. One might say that being deprived of occupations is the ultimate punishment. Those who work or live in prisons, locked forensic mental health hospital wards, or refugee camps know the power of occupational deprivation—we call it isolation. When we want to control or punish others, we deprive them of something to do. The argument that occupational deprivation is a matter of justice is that participation in the range of occupations is the day-to-day means through which we exercise health, citizenship, and social inclusion. We are denied these opportunities when deprived of occupations.

Occupational Marginalization

Advocates for social justice have fought for the universal right to vote, a right that enables individuals to exert their macro decision-making power to determine political leadership and exercise citizenship. From an occupational perspective, marginalization may occur despite people having the macro-decision right to vote. Occupational marginalization speaks to the need for humans to exert micro, everyday choices and de-

cision-making power as we participate in occupations. Occupational marginalization may not be overt discrimination to bar certain groups, for instance, from paid occupations or recreation.

Rather, occupational marginalization operates invisibly, a major force of injustice being normative standardization of expectations about how, when, and where people "should" participate. Humans need to participate in and make choices about their occupations for physical, mental, and spiritual health (Frank & Engelke, 2001; Wilcock, 1998). People also need to exert self-determination and decision-making capacities in what they do (Sprague & Hayes, 2000). In its support for the *International Classification of Function (ICF)*, the World Health Organization (1980, 2001) has defined participation restrictions as a matter of citizenship and justice as well as health. Yet managerial systems persist in seeking efficiencies through standardization efficiencies that control time, places, policies, laws, and funding (Stein, 2001; Wells, 1990), potentially overruling the empowerment approaches of client-centered practice.

In their discussion of sociological and geographic perspectives on the environment, O'Brien, Dyck, Caron, and Mortenson (2002) remind us that "spaces may be socially constructed around ideas of normalcy and ablement and therefore create environments which are exclusionary for people with disabilities by restricting their physical access or social opportunities" (p. 231). To date, people who are chronically sick or disabled remain stigmatized and excluded from mainstream life (Dewolfe, 2002). Occupational marginalization may occur, for instance, when people with disabilities are excluded from employment opportunities and have few expectations that employment is even possible (Nagle, Cook, & Polatajko, 2002). A common image that the body is an absent presence, not a determinant of life, may result in social policy that overlooks physical differences (Twigg, 2002). In other words, regulatory policies, built environments, funding, and laws, more than bodily impairment, may undermine opportunities for client-centered practice (Campbell, 2002).

The case of occupational marginalization emerged with recognition that humans, individually and as populations, need to exert micro, everyday choices and decision-making power as we participate in occupations. Moreover, we need choices related to participation in a wide range of occupations. The argument is that choice and control in what we do to participate in occupations is the basis of our empowerment as humans, and empowerment is a determinant of health for individuals and populations.

Occupational Imbalance

Occupational imbalance is used as a population-based term to identify populations that do not share in the labor and benefits of economic production. The right to equal privileges and pay for equal work is a cornerstone of social justice principles. An occupational perspective, oriented to meaning, enrichment, health, social inclusion, choice, and everyday decision-making raises questions about the right to fair privileges as the just rewards for diverse participation in the occupations of a family, community, or nation.

Occupational imbalance can be described as a form of occupational apartheid if one recognizes three major occupational classes: unoccupied, underoccupied, and overoccupied. Underemployed people are at risk for ill health because they are less likely to experience sufficient mental, physical, and social exercise that provides meaning and enrichment in their lives. Overemployed people are also at risk for ill health because they are too busy to look after themselves, their families, or their communities. Therefore, unemployment is not only an economic status; it is a matter of injustice. People without paid employment may be unoccupied, if historical and present circumstances leave them in an environment where there is very little to do. Or unemployment may release people from paid occupations but leave them underoccupied, without opportunities to participate in occupations through which they can derive meaning and empowerment. It is important to recognize that unemployment may also result in overoccupation. Those who are unemployed may experience ill health because they become overoccupied with survival through multiple paid and unpaid occupations. While occupational imbalance may ring with concerns born of a Western work ethic, this case speaks to being occupied too much or too little to experience meaning and empowerment. Occupational imbalances relate to market rewards for work, as well as to the need for a range of occupations that promote health-giving routines and social inclusion.

Occupational segregation associated with gender, disability, race, or other forms of difference are actually forms of occupational imbalance, possibly also occupational alienation, occupational deprivation, occupational marginalization, or possibly occupational apartheid (Kronenberg & Simo Algado, 2003). To examine occupational imbalances in a community, we could identify conditions where occupations are classified, paid, valued, and enhance life for some, while in the same places and times occupations are taken for granted, exploited, and trivialized for others (Townsend, 2003b).

There are huge dilemmas in addressing occupational imbalances, because we are not only referring to having too little or too much to do, but also to the privileges and benefits associated with occupations. An imbalanced division of labor may be associated with imbalanced economic conditions. There may be economic and class gaps between those who are highly rewarded for their occupations, and those who receive few benefits for their participation in occupations. Therefore, an analysis of occupational imbalance needs to target the typical values and institutionalized practices of paying less for homemaking, child care, and physical labor than for intellectual or managerial occupations. The existence of welfare systems is an acceptance that some social groups are disadvantaged because they cannot survive without economic assistance in their participation in occupations. One is left asking, Would occupational justice be advanced by having a system of guaranteed wages, or a communal system of resource sharing, regardless of differences in daily life participation? What would an economy look like if societies calculated an economic value for the participation of children, persons with disabilities, seniors, and others whose occupations are not currently counted in economic calculations?

Implications for Occupational Therapy's Client-Centered Practice

Why is this discussion relevant to occupational therapy practice, beyond being a topic of interest? Our response is that occupational therapy exists as a profession to address occupational injustices. We believe this because occupational therapists' primary populations of concern are those who are vulnerable to injustices because their participation in occupations is restricted by injury, chronic illness, disability of various types, mental illness, incarceration, old age, or other circumstances. Moreover, occupational therapists' values, beliefs, and practical approaches advocate that we work as professionals in client-centered, just ways with persons who are active agents in therapy and their own lives. The most explicit link to occupational justice can be found in our goals and objectives to collaborate with clients to promote social inclusion, using various enabling methods that emphasize client decision-making about their participation in occupations (Townsend, 1993). The broad implication is that, in health, community services, employment support, housing, school, transportation, corrections, higher education, private business, and other systems worldwide, occupational therapists can choose to either advocate consciously with others for justice, or comply with occupational injustices through silence and inaction. Given occupational therapists' populations of concern, professional values, beliefs, and client-centered intentions, and focus on social inclusion, occupational justice is an implicit issue, whether or not we choose to make it explicit.

However, we know that occupational therapists' good intentions may be overruled by policies and funding priorities which are not yet organized to support client-centered practice (Sumsio & Smyth, 2000; Townsend, 1998; Wilkins, Pollock, Rochon, & Law, 2001). Occupational therapists' and others' enabling, client-centered approaches go against the grain of professionals' traditional, hierarchical decision-making about those who are dependent on their services (Cervaro & Wilson, 1999; Townsend, 2003a). Moreover, today's corporate efficiency models emphasize standardization over attention to justice (Stein, 2001).

In light of these difficulties, what actions can occupational therapists take? First, occupational therapy clinicians, educators, managers, policy makers, or researchers who want to make justice more explicit can extend the dialogue summarized here by developing a personal and professional self-critique and a social critique. The implication is to develop critical, reflexive rather than technical, prescriptive practice (Falardeau & José Durand, 2002; Stern, Restall, & Ripat, 2000). We advocate dialogues and research that combine critical analysis of

the everyday lives of our populations of concern, the systems in which we work, and our profession, with hope and visions of possible futures. Dialogues could consider how to use client-centered approaches more explicitly in order to counter professionals' traditional, structured dominance and authority (Campbell, Copeland, & Tate, 1998; Griffin, 2001). Dialogues could also brainstorm cases as a way of developing greater cultural competence to address clients' diversity in the areas, settings, and populations that we encounter (Whiteford & St. Clair, 2002).

Second, with critical reflection, occupational therapists can brainstorm possible actions, examples being the actions suggested in Table 27.5. As difficult as it sounds, those focused on working with individuals might collectively make time away, through professional development in-service sessions or retreats, from the pressing demands of individualized caseloads. The profession might develop strategies for change if we learn what limits us in the use of simulated and real occupations as therapy in health and other systems. Justice might be more consciously incorporated in occupational therapy curricula by educators. And justice could be made explicit in student projects in academic or fieldwork settings, encouraging students to learn to critically appraise the power relations that control clients' and occupational therapists' opportunities. Because management and research occupational therapists are positioned to gather and use data, these occupational therapists can develop critiques of policies on time use, service types, travel costs, and other issues to determine what supports and limits client-centered practice. Researchers might employ qualitative, critical, and/or quantitative methods to develop guidelines for

Table 27.5. Working for Occupational Justice Through Client-Centered Practice

Occupational therapy clinicians and practitioners with individual clients	• Consider client participation in occupations and what occupations are used in therapy • Examine policy support for client participation in all decision-making re: all aspects of services • Seek practice opportunities with groups, communities, and populations as well as with individuals
Occupational therapy educators	• Consider visibility of occupation, enabling approaches, and justice in curriculum • Incorporate student projects with occupational justice theme • Enable students to critically appraise power, economic, cultural, social, and political issues that impact equity and occupational justice
Occupational therapy managers	• Consider how policies on time use, service types, travel costs, and other data support and capture client-centered approaches targeting occupational justice rights
Occupational therapy researchers	• Employ qualitative methods with participants to explore experiences of occupational justice/injustice • Employ quantitative methods with participants to measure occupational participation, etc. • Employ critical theories/methods, e.g., critical ethnography, PAR (participatory, action research), liberation, and emancipatory approaches with participants to analyze and change social structures and policies

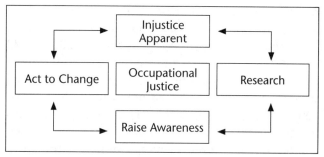

Figure 27.1. Client-centered activism for occupational justice.

evidence-based practice that would make occupation, enabling, and justice more explicit and known to others. Historical research could be taken to provide the facts and analysis about this profession's grounding in moral treatment and the therapeutic use of occupation with those who live with various restrictions in daily life (Friedland, 2001).

Third, the profession might engage with our communities. Taking a client-centered, action-research approach to matters of justice (Figure 27.1) could crystallize debate around apparent occupational injustices that occupational therapists confront every day. Looking beyond an individual's local family or work environment, as a profession we could record and talk publicly about social determinants of health (the economy, national priorities and policies, and societal values) and how these impact the individuals and groups with whom occupational therapists work. Occupational therapists can contribute to society by using our knowledge pillars (occupation, enabling, justice) to address health and social inclusion.

Examples of potential contributions would be to educate the public on the therapeutic power of occupation (Pierce, 2001; see Chapter 61). We could use a sociological and geographic analysis of the environment (O'Brien et al., 2002) as a basis for enabling changes in the social and physical environment while involving those who tend to be socially excluded as participants (Dunn, 2000; Fazio, 2001). Use of participatory evaluation tools, such as the Canadian Occupational Performance Measure, can remind us to attend closely to clients' goals and to involve clients in designing interventions (Wressle, Eeg-Olofsson, Marcusson, & Henriksson, 2002). Client-centered evaluation of community-based services would enable us to partner with clients to determine the relevance and impacts of our practice on people's lives (Hebert, Thibeault, Landry, Boisvenu, & Laporte, 2000). Explicit justice-oriented work would involve us in more alliances with consumers who are

advocating for greater empowerment in and beyond health services (Deegan, 1997; Sherr Klein, 1997). Qualitative inquiry (Hammell, 2002) would open up insights on clients' own perceptions of their involvement and decision-making in occupational therapy services. Evaluation studies that include client perceptions of occupational therapy services and outcomes would help to identify issues that may not be visible from a professional perspective (McKinnon, 2000). Action toward justice for and with persons with a disability should motivate and empower (them) to make appropriate, constructive responses. Actions consistent with occupational justice would develop community awareness through community groups, the Internet, and the media and provide role play or other opportunities for clients to practice the skills for becoming their own advocates. An international perspective would enable occupational therapists to take into account diverse Western and Eastern cultural constructions of occupation, enabling, and justice.

Reflections and Conclusions

This paper has highlighted an ongoing dialogue about occupational justice both to record it and to draw others into a widening circle of inquiry. We posed the question Do occupational therapists work for justice? Our answer is that occupational therapists may work for justice. We recognize that some occupational therapists are more interested in the methods and techniques of practice than in activism. Moreover, we cannot always see where injustices lie from our own position of power and privilege, even when that power is limited as it is for occupational therapists. Occupational therapists may be caught in our own experiences of occupational injustice as we struggle to keep up with workloads, let alone consider idealistic notions of justice. With acknowledgement of the struggle, we view the work of enabling occupational justice as congruent with worldwide activism. Dialogue about occupational justice seems timely as occupational therapists around the world articulate what distinguishes this numerically small, rather invisible profession and its contributions to individuals, populations, and societies.

References

Adelson, H. L. (1995). The origins of a concept of social justice. In K. D. Irani & M. Silver (Eds.), *Social justice in the ancient world* (pp. 25–38). Westport, CT: Greenwood Press.

Armstrong, H. (2000). Reflections on the difficulty of creating and sustaining equiable communicative forums. *Canadian Journal for Studies in Adult Education, 14,* 67–85.

Barnes, C. (2000). A working social model? Disability, work, and disability politics in the 21st century. *Critical Social Policy, 20,* 441–457.

Blair, S. E. (2000). The centrality of occupation during life transitions. *British Journal of Occupational Therapy, 63,* 231–237.

Borell, L., Lilja, M., Sviden, G. A., & Sadlo, G. (2001). Occupations and signs of reduced hope: An explorative study of older adults with functional impairments. *American Journal of Occupational Therapy, 55,* 311–316. http://dx.doi.org/10.5014/ajot.55.3.311

Bores, A. (2000). A comparison between the ethics of justice and the ethics of care. *Journal of Advanced Nursing, 32,* 1071–1075.

Byme, C. (1999). Facilitating empowerment groups: Dismantling professional boundaries. *Issues in Mental Health Nursing, 21,* 55–71.

Campbell, J. (2002). Valuing diversity: The disability agenda—We've only just begun. *Disability and Society, 17,* 471–478.

Campbell, M., Copeland, B., & Tate, B. (1998). Taking the standpoint of people with disabilities in research: Experiences with participation. *Canadian Journal of Rehabilitation, 12,* 95–304.

Cervaro, R. M., & Wilson, A. L. (1999). Beyond learner-centred practice: Adult education, power, and society. *Canadian Journal for the Study of Adult Education, 13,* 27–38.

Christiansen, C. (1999). Defining lives: Occupation as identity: An essay on competence, coherence, and the creation of meaning. *American Journal of Occupational Therapy, 53,* 547–558. Reprinted as Chapter 34.

Cookson, R., & Dolan, P. (2000). Principles of justice in healthcare rationing. *Journal of Medical Ethics, 26,* 323–379.

Daniels, N., Kennedy, B. P., & Kawachi, I. (1999). Why justice is good for our health: The social determinants of health inequalities. *Daedalus, 128,* 215–251.

Deegan, P. (1997). Recovery and empowerment for people with psychiatric disabilities. *Social Work in Health Care, 25,* 11–24.

DeWolfe, P. (2002). Private tragedy in social context? Reflections on disability, illness, and suffering. *Disability and Society, 17,* 255–267.

Dunn, W. (2000). *Best practice occupational therapy: In community service with children and families.* Thorofare, NJ: Slack.

Dunst, C., Trivette, C., & Deal, A. (1988). *Enabling and empowering families: Principles and guidelines for practice.* Cambridge, MA: Brookline Books.

Emanuel, E. J. (2000). Justice and managed care: Four principles for the just allocation of health care resources. *Hastings Center Report, 30,* 8–16.

Falardeau, M., & José Durand, M. (2002). Negotiation-centered versus client-centered: Which approach should be used? *Canadian Journal of Occupational Therapy, 69,* 135–142.

Fazio, L. (2001). *Developing occupation-centered programs for the community.* Upper Saddle River, NJ: Prentice-Hall.

Fearing, V., & Clark, J. (2000). *Individuals in context: A practical guide to client-centered practice.* Thorofare, NJ: Slack.

Frank, L., & Engelke, P. (2001). The built environment and human activity patterns: Exploring the impacts of urban form on public health. *Journal of Planning Literature, 16,* 202–218.

Friedland, J. (2001). Knowing from whence we came: Reflecting on return-to-work and interpersonal relationships. *Canadian Journal of Occupational Therapy, 68,* 266–271.

Grammenos, S. (2003). *Illness, disability, and social inclusion.* Brussels: Centre for European Social and Economic Policy.

Gray, J. M. (1998). Putting occupation into practice: Ocupation as ends, occupation as means. *American Journal of Occupational Therapy, 52,* 354–364. http://dx.doi.org/10.5014/ajot.52.5.354 Reprinted as Chapter 10.

Griffin, S. (2001). Occupational therapists and the concept of power: A review of the literature. *Australian Occupational Therapy Journal, 48,* 24–34.

Guy, J. R. (1996). *Comparison of the art of the possible: Dr. Southwood Smith as social reformer and public health pioneer.* Cambridgeshire: Octavia Hill Society.

Hammell, K. W. (2002). Informing, client-centered practice through qualitative inquiry: Evaluating the duality of qualitative research. *British Journal of Occupational Therapy, 65,* 175–194.

Hasselkus, B. R. (2002). *The meaning of everyday occupation.* Thorofare, NJ: Slack.

Hebert, M., Thibeault, R., Landry A., Boisvenu, M., & Laporte, D. (2000). Introducing an evaluation of community-based occupational therapy services: A client-centered practice. *Canadian Journal of Occupational Therapy, 67,* 146–154.

Heitman, E. (2000). Ethical values in the education of biomedical researchers. *The Hastings Center Report, 30,* S40–S44.

Hemmingsson, H., & Borell, L. (2002). Environmental barriers in mainstream schools. *Child Care, Health, and Development, 25,* 57–63.

Howland, G. W. (1944). Occupational therapy across Canada. *Canadian Geographical Journal, 28,* 32–40.

Ignatieff, M. (2000). *The rights revolution.* Toronto, ON: House of Anansi.

Irani, K. D. (1995). The idea of social justice in the ancient world. In K. D. Irani & M. Silver (Eds.), *Social justice in the ancient world* (pp. 3–8). Westport, CT: Greenwood Press.

Iwama, M. (1999). Are you listening? Cross-cultural perspectives on client-centered occupational therapy practice: A view from Japan. *Occupational Therapy Now, 1,* 4–6.

Iwama, M. (2003). Toward culturally relevant epistemologies in occupational therapy. *American Journal of Occupational Therapy, 57,* 582–588. http://dx.doi.org/10.5014/ajot.57.5.582

Jarman, J. (2003). What is occupation: Interdisciplinary perspectives on defining and classifying human activity. In E. Townsend (Ed.), *Introduction to occupation: The art and science of living* (pp. 47–62). Upper Saddle River, NJ: Prentice-Hall.

Kronenberg, E., & Simo Algado, S. (2003). *The political nature of occupational therapy.* University of Linkoping, Linkoping, SW.

Labonte, R. (1989). Community empowerment: The need for political analysis. *Canadian Journal of Public Health, 80,* 87–88.

Locke, J. (1690). *An essay concerning humane understanding.* London: T. Basset.

McKay, S. (2000). Gender justice and reconciliation. *Women's Studies International Forum, 23,* 561–570.

McKinnon, A. L. (2000). Client values and satisfaction with occupational therapy. *Scandinavian Journal of Occupational Therapy, 7,* 99–106.

McKnight, J. L. (1989). Health and empowerment. *Canadian Journal of Occupational Public Health, 76*(Suppl. 1), 37–38.

Metz, T. (2000). Arbitrariness, justice, and respect. *Social Theory and Practice, 26,* 24–45.

Meyer, A. (1922). The philosophy of occupation therapy. *Archives of Occupational Therapy, 1,* 1–10. Reprinted as Chapter 4.

Nagle, S., Cook, T. V., & Polatajko, H. (2002). I'm doing as much as I can: Occupational choices of persons with a severe and persistent mental illness. *Journal of Occupational Science, 9,* 71–82.

Noyes, J. (2000). Enabling young ventilator-dependent people to express their views and experiences of their care in hospital. *Journal of Advanced Nursing, 31,* 1206–1215.

Nygård, L., & Borell, L. (1998). A life-world of alternating meaning: Expressions of the illness experience of dementia in everyday life over three years. *Occupational Therapy Journal of Research, 18,* 109–136.

O'Brien, P., Dyck, I., Caron, S., & Mortenson, P. (2002). Environmental analysis: Insights from sociological and geographic perspectives. *Canadian Journal of Occupational Therapy, 69,* 229–238.

Pierce, D. (2001). Occupation by design: Dimensions, therapeutic power, and creative process. *American Journal of Occupational Therapy, 55,* 249–259. http://dx.doi.org/10.5014/ajot.55.3.249 Reprinted as Chapter 61.

Pogge, T. W. (2000). On the site of distributive justice: Reflections on Cohen and Murphy. *Philosophy and Public Affairs, 29,* 137–169.

Polatajko, H. (2001). The evolution of our occupational perspective: The journey from diversion through therapeutic use to enablement. *Canadian Journal of Occupational Therapy, 68,* 203–207.

Primeau, L. A. (1996). Running as an occupation: Multiple meanings and purposes. In R. Z. F. Clark (Ed.), *Occupational science: The evolving discipline* (pp. 275–286). Philadelphia: F. A. Davis.

Rawls, J. (1975). A Kantian conception of equality. *The Cambridge Review,* 94–99.

Rebeiro, K. (1998). Occupation-as-means to mental health: A review of the literature and a call for research. *Canadian Journal of Occupational Therapy, 65,* 12–19.

Rebeiro, K. (2001). Enabling occupation: The importance of an affirming environment. *Canadian Journal of Occupational Therapy, 68,* 80–89.

Reilly, M. (1962). Occupational therapy can be one of the great ideas of 20th century medicine. *American Journal of Occupational Therapy, 16,* 1–9. Reprinted as Chapter 7.

Rosenau, P. V. (1994). Health politics meet post-modernism: Its meaning and implications for community health organizing. *Journal of Health Politics, Policy and Law, 19,* 303–333.

Royeen, C., Duncan, M., Crabree, J., Richards, J., & Clark, G. F. (2000). Effects of billing Medicaid for occupational therapy services in the schools: A pilot study. *American Journal of Occupational Therapy, 54,* 429–433. http://dx.doi.org/10.5014/ajot.54.4.429

Schultz, V. (2000). Life's work. *Columbia Law Review, 100*(7), 1981–1964.

Sherr Klein, B. (1997). Foreword in *Enabling occupation: An occupational therapy perspective* (pp. vii–x). Ottawa, ON: CAOT Publications ACE.

Smith, D. (1987). *The everyday world as problematic: A feminist sociology.* Toronto, ON: University of Toronto Press.

Smith, D. (1990a). *The conceptual practices of power: A feminist sociology of knowledge.* Toronto, ON: University of Toronto Press.

Smith, D. (1990b). *Texts, facts, and femininity: Exploring the relations of ruling.* New York: Routledge.

Sprague, J., & Hayes, J. (2000). Self-determination and empowerment: A feminist standpoint analysis of talk about disability. *American Journal of Community Psychology, 28,* 671–695.

Stein, J. G. (2001). *The cult of efficiency.* Toronto, ON: House of Anansi.

Stern, M., Restall, G., & Ripat, J. (2000). The use of self-reflection to improve client-centered practice. In V. G. Fearing & J. Clark (Eds.), *Individuals in context* (pp. 145–158). Thorofare, NJ: Slack.

Sumsion, T., & Smyth, G. (2000). Barriers to client-centredness and their resolution. *Canadian Journal of Occupational Therapy, 67,* 15–21.

Tindale, J. (1999). Variance in the meaning of time by family cycle, period, social context, and ethnicity. In W. E. Pentland, A. S. Harvey, M. P. Lawton, & M. A. McColl (Eds.), *Time use research in the social sciences* (p. 155). New York: Kulwer Academic/Plenum Publishers.

Townsend, E. (1993). Muriel Driver Lecture: Occupational therapy's social vision. *Canadian Journal of Occupational Therapy, 60,* 174–184.

Townsend, E. (1998). *Good intentions overruled: A critique of empowerment in the routine organization of mental health services.* Toronto, ON: University of Toronto Press.

Townsend, E. (2003a). Power and justice in enabling occupation. *Canadian Journal of Occupational Therapy, 70,* 74–87.

Townsend, E. (2003b). *Occupational justice: Ethical, moral, and civic principles for an inclusive world.* Keynote presentation at the Annual Conference of the European Network of Occupational Therapy Educators, Czech Republic, Prague, October.

Townsend, E., Ripley, D., & Langille, L. (2003). Professional tensions in clientcentered practice. *American Journal of Occupational Therapy, 57,* 17–28. http://dx.doi.org/10.5014/ajot.57.1.17

Townsend, E., & Wilcock, A. A. (2004). Occupational justice. In C. Christiansen & E. Townsend (Eds.), *An introduction to occupation: The art and science of living* (pp. 243–273). Upper Saddle River, NJ: Prentice Hall.

Twigg, J. (2002). The body of social policy: Mapping a territory. *Journal of Social Policy, 31,* 421–439.

Vrkljan, B. (2001). Meaning of occupational engagement in life-threatening illness: A qualitative pilot project. *Canadian Journal of Occupational Therapy, 68,* 237–246.

Wells, L. (1990). Responsiveness and accountability in long-term care: Strategies for policy development and empowerment. *Canadian Journal of Public Health, 81,* 382–385.

Whiteford, G. (2000). Occupational deprivation: Global challenge in the new millennium. *British Journal of Occupational Therapy, 64,* 200–210. Reprinted as Chapter 26.

Whiteford, G. (2003). When people cannot participate: Occupational deprivation. In C. Christiansen & E. Townsend (Eds.), *An introduction to occupation: The art and science of living* (pp. 221–242). Upper Saddle River, NJ: Prentice Hall.

Whiteford, G., & St. Clair, V. W. (2002). Being prepared for diversity: In practice: Occupational therapy students' perceptions of valuable intercultural learning experiences. *British Journal of Occupational Therapy, 65,* 129–137.

Wilcock, A. A. (1993). A theory of the human need for occupation. *Journal of Occupational Science: Australia, 1,* 17–24. Reprinted as Chapter 30.

Wilcock, A. A. (1998). *An occupational perspective of health.* Thorofare, NJ: Slack.

Wilcock, A. A. (2001). *Occupation for health: A journey from self-health to prescription* (Vol. I). London: British Association and College of Occupational Therapists.

Wilcock, A. A. (2002). *A journey from prescription to self-health* (Vol. 2). London: British Association and College of Occupational Therapists.

Wilcock, A. A., & Townsend, E. (2000). Occupational justice: Occupational terminology interactive dialogue. *Journal of Occupational Science, 7,* 84–86.

Wilkins, S., Pollock, N., Rochon, S., & Law, M. (2001). Implementing client-centered practice: Why is it so difficult to do? *Canadian Journal of Occupational Therapy, 68,* 70–79.

World Health Organization. (1980). *International classification of impairments, disabilities and handicaps: A manual of classification relating to the consequences of disease.* Geneva: Author.

World Health Organization. (1986). *Ottawa charter for health promotion: An international conference on health promo-*

tion, retrieved March 2003 from the Health Canada web site: www.hc-sc.gc.ca/hppb/phdd/docs/charter.

World Health Organization. (2001). *International classification of functioning, disability and health (ICF).* Geneva: Author.

Wressle, E., Eeg-Olofsson, A., Marcusson, J., & Henriksson, C. (2002). Improved client participation in the rehabilitation process using a client-centered goal formation structure. *Journal of Rehabilitation Medicine, 34,* 5–11.

Yerxa, E. J. (1967). 1966 Eleanor Clarke Slagle Lecture: Authentic occupational therapy. *American Journal of Occupational Therapy, 21,* 1–9.

Yerxa, E. J. (1979). *The philosophical base of occupational therapy: 2000 AD.* Rockville, MD: American Occupational Therapy Association.

Yerxa, E. J. (1993). Occupational science: A new source of power for participants in occupational therapy. *Occupational Science: Australia, 1,* 3–10.

Young, I. M. (1990). *Justice and the politics of difference.* Princeton, NJ: Princeton University Press.

Zanetti, V. (2001). Global justice: Is interventionalism desirable? *Metaphilosophy, 32,* 196–211.

CHAPTER 28

Well-Being and Occupational Rights:
An Imperative for Critical Occupational Therapy

Karen R. Whalley Hammell and Michael K. Iwama

Introduction

Social analysts and policy-makers have recently focused their attention on the concept of wellbeing among people in the "Western" world (1) as well as among those living in poorer nations (2) and it has been argued that the global community has moved towards conceiving "development" as the "creation of conditions where all people in the world are able to achieve well-being" [(3), p 349–50, (4)].

Well-being has been of interest to Eastern and Western philosophers for many centuries, with some concluding that "human well-being is ultimately an issue of engagement in living" [(5), p 2]. This suggests that well-being is a concept with which occupational therapists should be concerned and, indeed, one of occupational therapy's core assumptions is that engagement in occupations influences well-being (6,7). Some occupational therapists have called for the profession's theories and practices to focus on well-being rather than exclusively on health (8–10), although it has also been observed that occupational therapy's current theories and practices appear preoccupied, not with well-being, but with dysfunction (9).

This paper is based on the premise that the ability and opportunity to engage in occupations that contribute to well-being is an issue that concerns occupational rights. The aims of this paper are to outline well-being and its centrality to human rights; to explore the relationships between well-being and occupation, and between well-being and occupational rights; and to highlight the consequent imperative to address issues of occupational rights through engagement in critical occupational therapy practices.

Critical Occupational Therapy

This paper takes a critical approach to occupational therapy, congruent with its concern with addressing occupational rights. Critical theories strive to link a concern with individuals' subjectivity with a focus on the structural, social, and political contexts of their lives (11). Thus, for example, critical race theories, critical disability theories, queer theories, and post-colonial theories probe the impact of social structures and constructions on the lives of individual people. Critical theories challenge conventional ideologies and assumptions, assert that theories are never objective or politically neutral, and expose imbalances of power such as those in professional/client, theorist/theorized, and researcher/researched relationships (12).

Congruent with these principles, practice that aspires to the name "critical" aims to confront injustices and inequalities, and strives towards a more just society (11,13). Thus, critical occupational therapy is a committed form of practice that recognizes the impact of inequities such as class, gender, race, ethnicity, economics, age, ability, and sexuality, acknowledges that well-being cannot be achieved by focusing solely on enhancing individuals' abilities, and thus endeavours to facilitate change at both individual and environmental levels (adapted from Mendes (14)).

Occupational Justice and Occupational Rights

Occupational therapy theorists have articulated and promoted the concept of occupational justice (15,16), a concept that derives from principles of human rights, equality, and a belief in the dignity of all human beings. Justice refers to the general principle that individuals should be treated fairly and equitably, and receive what they deserve (17), and includes dimensions of distributive, retributive, and corrective justice (18). Drawing from these fundamental principles, those who work, for example, towards "social" justice and "environmental" justice advocate for more equitable distribution of economic resources within and between societies and for redress of the inequitable distribution of environmental burdens (such as exposure to toxins).

Philosophers explain that although justice is fundamentally concerned with the distribution of resources, benefits and burdens in society, it does not address the causes of injustice or inequality in the distribution of those resources, benefits, and burdens (19). Moreover, they explain that, in contrast to notions of justice (with its predominant focus on distribution), the concept of rights "refer[s] to doing more than having" and to the conditions that enable or constrain action [(19), p 25]. Rights, therefore, are about the opportunity to act.

Because occupational therapy is clearly concerned with the conditions that enable or constrain actions, and particularly with doing, we contend that our profession should be focused on occupational rights. Although "the language of rights has its roots in European thought and history, concepts of human rights can be found in every religious and cultural tradition" [(20), p 68, (21)]. Therefore, while justice invokes metaphorical images of scales and balances, requires a judgement to be made about what constitutes fairness, and is a concept open to charges of moral relativism, rights state, unequivocally, what all people are entitled to expect (19,20) and thus offer a clearly definable mandate to occupational therapists.

Human Rights and Well-Being

Human rights are a set of universally endorsed principles that centre on two essential entitlements: freedom and well-being (22,23). Freedom is defined as the right of every human being to participate in shaping the decisions that affect his/her own life and that of his/her society (22). Clearly, this dimension of human rights supports occupational therapists' espoused client-centred approach to practice (9), with its philosophical ideal of enabling people to participate in shaping the decisions that inform their occupational therapy interventions, their occupations, and their lives.

Principles of human rights also assert that all people are entitled to well-being, which is defined by philosophers as the ability and conditions needed to achieve one's purposes by action (22). This focus on both abilities and conditions is important.

Because human well-being is impacted by the occupations in which we are able, or compelled, to engage, we contend that human rights are associated with occupational rights.

Occupational Rights

Occupational rights have been defined as "the right of all people to engage in meaningful occupations that contribute positively to their own well-being and the well-being of their communities" [(9), p 62]. Occupations are defined in this paper as being everything that people do during the course of their everyday lives (24). Instances of occupational deprivation, occupational alienation, occupational marginalization, occupational injustice, and occupational apartheid are unambiguously identifiable as violations of occupational rights. Clearly, for example, when civilians in Burma are "forced to serve as porters for the military, to build and maintain roads, to construct military camps, and to labour on infrastructure projects" (25), this constitutes a violation of their occupational rights. Less dramatic—but more common—examples of the violation of occupational rights are found in many residential institutions, where elderly and disabled people are routinely denied the opportunity to engage in those personally meaningful and fulfilling occupations that would contribute positively to their experience of well-being. When occupational therapists employ the language of rights, their mandate for enabling occupation becomes clear.

Well-Being

It is puzzling that occupational therapists have not expended much effort in asking present or potential clients how they define well-being, despite espousing the importance of well-being to occupational therapy and despite also claiming a client-centred approach to practice (26). Occupational therapists have explored people's experiences of well-being while engaged in daily occupations (27) and have sought to articulate a framework of "occupational well-being" that is based on the belief that well-being is enhanced when individuals' occupational needs are met (28). To date, however, little effort has been made by occupational therapists to determine how well-being is defined by a range of present or potential clients (although see Wilcock et al. (29)).

Synthesizing the work of multiple theorists [e.g. (1,6,27–31)] *well-being* is defined in this paper as a state of contentment—or harmony—with one's:

- physical/mental health (inseparable, not dualistic concepts);
- emotional/spiritual health (spiritual health is a concept defined, understood, and experienced by the person);
- personal and economic security;
- self-worth (sense of being capable, and of being valued by others);
- sense of belonging (which includes the ability to contribute to others and to maintain valued roles and relationships, and which may include a sense of belonging and of connectedness to the land and nature);
- opportunities for self-determination (defined as the ability to enact choices and counteract powerlessness);
- opportunities to engage in meaningful and purposeful occupations;
- sense of hope.

These concepts are not mutually exclusive but interrelated.

Relationships Between Well-Being and Occupation

Although our profession's theories of occupation assume a positive relationship between occupation and well-being, occupational therapy researchers have generated few data to support the premise that engagement in occupations contributes positively to human well-being (6,27). Hammell (26) suggested that this may be the inevitable consequence of focusing on three specific categories of occupation—self-care, productivity, and leisure—that were designated without reference to clients' experiences of occupation or to their perspectives or perceptions of well-being. A significant body of research evidence demonstrates that occupations that promote interdependence contribute positively to well-being (32; see Chapter 14), but current theories of occupation, with their individualistic focus on self-care, productivity, and leisure, provide little space for consideration of the importance to an individual's well-being of contributing to the well-being of others (32; see Chapter 14). Nor do these categorizations enable consideration of the collective occupations that contribute to community development and collective well-being (33).

Researchers in many other health and social science disciplines have generated a significant body of evidence to support the assumption that well-being is impacted by engagement in occupations. For example, research demonstrates that engagement in meaningful occupations is associated with positive physical/mental health and longevity (34–36). Moreover, engagement in valued occupations is found to contribute to self-worth and to self-determination through the ability and opportunity to enact choices and counteract powerlessness (37). Researchers in countries as diverse as Bangladesh, Canada, China, and Slovenia have found that engaging in occupations with and for others generates a sense of belonging, and that this is important to a sense of well-being (27,37–39). Moreover, research among people in seemingly hopeless medical circumstances shows that envisioning a future engaged in meaningful occupations contributes to a sense of hope, which is identified as integral to positive well-being (40,41).

Theories of occupation more rarely acknowledge that engagement in occupations may have a negative impact on well-being, yet "over employment, under employment and unhealthy jobs have . . . been identified as contributors to mental ill-health. Exclusion from meaningful work is recognised as a contributor to mental and psychological distress, and the workplace is both a potential contributor and threat to well-being" [(42), p 207]. Although occupational therapy theorists often extol the value of paid work (Yerxa, [(43), p 416; see Chapter 31] for example, asserted that "work is supportive of health even under poor conditions") it is apparent that work does not inevitably contribute positively to well-being (32).

Although occupational therapy theory has long identified the importance of the environment to occupational performance and engagement, there has been an apparent reluctance to formulate critical approaches to research and theory, such that attention to the structural, social, and political contexts of clients' lives informs efforts to confront those injustices and inequalities that constrain occupational opportunities (although there are notable exceptions, such as Letts (44), Strong & Rebeiro (45), Ripat et al. (46)). Moreover, there has been little attention to the occupational nature of communities, or to the relevance of existing models of occupation to occupational therapy practice in community development and community well-being (33).

Relationships Between Well-Being and Occupational Rights

Philosophers and economists note that if people's abilities are constrained by the available social, political, and economic opportunities, they will be unable to achieve well-being (19,47). And if ability is of little use without opportunity—as Napoleon Bonaparte asserted (48)—then conditions that constrain opportunity are of central relevance to occupational therapy.

Researchers have observed direct and indirect impacts of environmental factors on individuals' well-being. For example, traditional role assumptions may limit people's occupational choices; and structural factors may create social isolation for disabled people due to a lack of accessible transportation (Fook, cited in Mendes (14)). Moreover, racism, patriarchy, sexism, homophobia, violence, poverty, and social exclusion shape the anxiety and depression experienced by many individuals (42).

Some occupational therapy theories explicitly emphasize the importance of the environment (physical, social, cultural, institutional) to the ability and opportunity to engage in occupations that contribute positively to well-being (e.g. Townsend & Polatajko (49), Law et al. (50)). Regrettably, however, occupational therapy's practices often reveal a preoccupation with individuals' abilities (and more particularly, their inabilities) rather than a commitment to enhancing opportunities through addressing the conditions of people's lives. This preoccupation with changing individuals is reinforced by the proclamations of some of the profession's elite forerunners. For example, one of occupational therapy's most frequently cited beliefs is that "man, through the use of his hands as energized by mind and will, can influence the state of his own health" [(51), p 2; see Chapter 7]. Critical theorists would observe that this statement reflects both sexist and ableist ideals (32). Perhaps even more importantly, social commentators have noted that this sort of emphasis on individual will-power advances a specific, right-wing political ideology (52), observing that it is both erroneous and oppressive to promote the premise that powerless people could control their own lives and improve their well-being if they just decided to do so (2).

In reality, of course, many of the world's population have little or no choice, control, or opportunity to exercise their will to affect their lives (32). Many people, for example, lead lives blighted by poverty, disability, and disease, and their daily occupations—the uses of their hands—are associated with powerlessness, unremitting drudgery, high risks of injury, illness, and premature death (53). Opportunities for social participation and occupational engagement of many more people are constrained by inequities of class, caste, and education, and by patriarchy, sexism, homophobia and heterosexism, ableism, racism, and by factors such as political

oppression, geographical displacement, natural disasters, and wars (32).

Sherry [(21), p 69] observed that: "African culture does not promote the concept of individuals being in complete control of their own fate, and this is certainly not the lived experience of the majority, who live their lives vulnerable to disease, poverty, conflict, the elements and other factors way beyond their control". Clearly, the well-being of those who experience inequitable conditions that constrain their occupational opportunities and occupational rights cannot be enhanced solely by enhancing their individual abilities and skills, and this requires consideration of environment/occupation interfaces.

The Role of the Environment in Theories of Occupation

Although occupational therapists acknowledge that occupations are influenced by the environment (49,50), much of the occupational therapy theoretical literature focuses predominantly on individual issues such as volition, personal causation, habituation, mastery, and motor skills. Clearly, only the privileged can indulge in theory that minimizes oppressive economic, cultural, religious, social, political, legal, and policy constraints on people's lives (54)! It is important to acknowledge that because occupational therapy's dominant theories have all been developed in middle-class, urban areas of the English-speaking nations of the wealthy Western ("minority") world these theories inevitably reflect the specific perspectives of a privileged global minority (32 [see Chapter 14], 55–57). Therefore, it should not be surprising that oppressive conditions—such as poverty, discrimination, social inequality, marginalization, social exclusion, powerlessness, and exploitation—that constrain the lives of so many of the global population—have not been central theoretical concerns. However, these oppressive conditions are faced, to a greater or lesser degree, by people in every nation of the world.

It is especially important for occupational therapists to acknowledge that although their dominant theories have been devised by privileged, able-bodied, urban-dwelling residents of the minority world, 80% of disabled people live in the majority world, and 90% of these people live in rural areas (58). Moreover, because disabled people are among the poorest of the poor in every country, a profession ostensibly concerned with the well-being of disabled people ought to be centrally concerned with the negative consequences of poverty for well-being and for occupational rights, not solely, but especially, for disabled people. As Sherry [(59), p 37] observed: "It is not possible to talk about occupational therapy in Africa without addressing the realities of poverty" indeed "in situations of poverty, environmental factors may be more disabling than impairments themselves, and entire communities may be subject to occupational deprivation and injustice as a result of social, political, environmental and economic factors. The effects of poverty go far deeper than material deprivation" (p 40).

Reflecting specific Western understandings of people and their relationships to the world, the Model of Human Occupation (MOHO(60)), and the Canadian Model of Occupational Performance and Engagement (CMOP–E(49)) assert that individuals engage with their social and physical environment through occupation and that they are influenced by, and interact with, but are divisible from the environment. In contrast, the Kawa Model (55,61) proposes that humans do not engage with the environment through occupation because they are already inseparable from the environment. This model reflects African, Asian, Pacific, south-east European, Indigenous and Middle Eastern perceptions (i.e. those of the majority of the global population): of the interconnectedness of community and individual well-being; and of an understanding that people are interdependent within families and communities (21,31,62–67).

In several African languages (68) the term *ubuntu*—translated from Zulu as "I am human because I belong, I participate, I share" [(69), p 281]—is used to describe the pre-eminent cultural importance of belonging—of being enmeshed in reciprocal relationships with other people—and is rooted in a belief in the connectedness of all people and all things (21,68). Indeed, ubuntu is said to encapsulate the essence of what it means to be human, and highlights "the importance of human rights through the principles of reciprocity, inclusivity and a shared sense of destiny between peoples" [(69), p 282].

Many of the world's people also perceive an indivisibility, interconnectedness, and "oneness" of all life, understanding themselves to be interconnected with nature, the land and oceans (21,31,62–64,66,67). Within such modes of thinking, body, spirit, family, and land are understood to be essential aspects of identity, human health, and well-being (31). For example, in Aotearoa/New Zealand, Maori identity "is linked to the earth by a sense of belonging to the land, being part of the land and being bonded together with the land" [(31), p 1760]. Ecological scientists articulate a similar perspective, understanding all life to be interconnected, such that humans are inseparable from their physical environments (70). Ecologists observe, for example, that large rodents (agoutis), which scatter and hoard seeds, are crucial to the regeneration of the Brazil nut tree (71). Given that Brazil nut trees provide one of the most socioeconomically important non-timber forest products in Amazonia, and that Brazil nuts are collected exclusively from natural forests (71), it is apparent that the economically productive occupations of the Brazil nut harvesters and processors are dependent not solely upon their hands and wills, but on the relationship between a tree and a rodent. These insights have relevance for the study of human occupation.

Importantly, occupational theorists who acknowledge and respect holistic ideas concerning human/environment interconnections neither reject nor challenge the veracity of the concept of human occupation but, rather, seek both to expand the present construction of the idea, and to be more inclusive of the knowledge held by the majority world. In the nursing literature it is suggested that "Unity of person and environment is a concept that can be used to convey an assumption that humans and environment are interconnected and change simultaneously. Simultaneous change negates the idea of conforming or adjusting to a stimuli [sic]; rather, it implies incorporating change, becoming a different person, and increasing options and awareness of choice" [(72), p 129–30]. This could also be a useful concept for occupational therapy.

Occupational theorists' discrepant theoretical perspectives concerning the nature of the relationship between individual people and their physical, social, cultural, economic, political, and legal contexts are not solely an intellectual issue because theories inform the subsequent focus for interventions. If individuals are perceived to be divisible from the conditions of their lives, such that their well-being is contingent upon their own hands and will, then interventions directed solely at enhancing individual skill, will, and abilities appear wholly appropriate. If, however, the individual and the environment are understood to be inseparable, such that both abilities and conditions determine whether one can achieve one's purposes by action (22), then occupational therapy interventions that are focused solely on enhancing individuals' abilities appear not just inadequate but naive.

To date, theories of occupational therapy and occupational science have privileged an individualistic/egocentric view of human occupation, thus shaping and limiting occupational therapy's concerns to individualistic views of occupation. For example, there is little development or expansion of our understandings of occupational engagement as a shared experience, despite evidence of the importance of engagement in occupations with and for others (26); there has been little exploration of ways in which self/environs are experienced as integral and inseparable during occupational engagement, despite evidence of the importance of occupational engagement in specific natural or homely environments (73,74); and there has been little acknowledgement that, for many of the world's people, the self is of less importance than the family collective (65). Moreover, occupational therapists have rarely explored how the occupations of one group or collective effect the occupations of another.

In 2010, the multinational corporation, British Petroleum (BP), incurred a catastrophic accident in the Gulf of Mexico which clearly demonstrated how the occupations of one large corporation and its workers affected, and continue to affect, the occupations and day-to-day realities of entire communities spread across a vast coastline. What began as an industrial accident that claimed the lives of several oil-field workers evolved into an environmental disaster with enormous physical, economic, social, and occupational consequences. Concerns were immediately raised about the local shrimp-fishing industry and its related occupations. Subsequently, it was apparent that social and occupational devastation was not limited to one occupation but was far more extensive, with a ruined leisure and tourism industry, widespread unemployment, bankruptcies, home foreclosures, out-migration from affected shoreline communities, mental health problems, and disruptions within families, communities, and daily life patterns. This example demonstrates that the occupations of some people can have consequences for the occupations of others; that people and their occupations are both integral to, and inseparable from, their multidimensional environment; and that people's abilities are enabled or constrained by the conditions of their lives.

Obviously, the claim that people are inseparable from their environments does not deny the importance of occupation to human well-being, and it does not erase the importance of individuals' physical, cognitive, and emotional capabilities to their occupational engagement. But it does prompt consideration of the embedded nature of humans in their social, cultural, political, economic, and physical milieu, and of the consequences of this embedding for the ability and opportunity to engage in occupations that contribute positively to well-being.

Affirming the Relationship Between Human Rights and Occupations

The World Federation of Occupational Therapists (75) has issued a position statement declaring that all people have the right to participate in a range of occupations that enable them to flourish, fulfil their potential, and experience satisfaction in a way that is consistent with their culture and beliefs. This official statement asserted the human right to equitable access to participation in occupation. If occupational therapists are to take seriously their espoused commitment to enabling equitable access to participation in occupation, the inequitable conditions of people's lives have to be addressed.

Well-Being and Critical Occupational Therapy: The Practice Imperative

Recognizing the gap in well-being between privileged and marginalized people is an important step in understanding the social determinants of well-being (76). The arguments presented in this paper suggest that occupational therapists can—and should—enhance human well-being by addressing occupational rights; by focusing not solely on individuals' abilities, but also on the opportunities derived from the conditions of their lives.

Clearly, when occupational therapists strive to change dimensions of the physical, cultural, social, political, legal, or economic environment to counter discrimination and to equalize opportunities this is a political act. What is important to understand is that when occupational therapists view disability as embodied, or as something that people have (reflected in the euphemism "people with disabilities") and strive to change individuals' abilities so that they can better fit within discriminatory environments this is also a political act. "Acquiescing to the inequities of the status quo might be politically conservative, but it is political" [(12), p 143].

However, occupational therapists—as individual professionals and as a profession—have not consistently engaged in public discourses about issues such as poverty, yet we know that poverty constrains opportunities for engagement in occupations that contribute to well-being.

Nor has our profession advocated for literacy. Yet *il*-literacy significantly diminishes opportunities for engagement in occupations that contribute to well-being. The right to community participation and to a range of occupational opportunities is denied to those disabled people who are confined in institutions due to public policy (77), yet our profession has not consistently spoken out when disabled people are segregated in residential institutions in which we ourselves would never choose to live (12).

More than two decades ago, Jongbloed and Crichton (78) claimed that rehabilitation professionals had an inauspicious record in the struggle to change social policies that might benefit disabled people, tending to reserve advocacy in political and institutional arenas for issues pertaining to their own professional self-interests. More recently, Cottrell (77) noted that "occupational therapists have historically shown limited response to entrenched societal constraints and discriminatory policies" (p 566). Pollard, Kronenberg and Sakellariou (7) observed: "Occupational therapy is said to be based on the belief that there exists a universal and fundamental relationship between people's dignified and meaningful participation in daily life and their experience of health, well-being and quality of life. [This] requires occupational therapists to view enabling access to meaningful occupations as a right, not just 'treatment' but a political endeavour" (p 3).

Some might choose to argue that a professional commitment to the occupational rights of individuals and of populations is neither practical nor possible. Clearly, however, it is, because there are some committed occupational therapists, in both emerging and mainstream practice settings, who find spaces for advocacy and activism—for individuals and populations—despite heavy workloads, restricted resources, and constraining management practices. Moreover, inaction and inertia are also political acts, as has already been noted: "Acquiescing to the inequities of the status quo might be politically conservative, but it is political" [(12), p 143].

Recognizing that enabling access to meaningful occupations is a human right, there are some occupational therapists who embrace their political role in addressing the inequitable conditions of people's lives to enable occupations that contribute to well-being. For example, occupational therapists engaged in critical practice assert the equal right of disabled boys and girls to participate in schooling with their peers, and advocate for wheelchair access to turn this right into reality; they work to enhance the occupational opportunities of people with severe persistent mental illnesses by requiring governments to adhere to their espoused obligations; and they compel polling stations to enable equal access to all people entitled to participate in voting. Occupational therapists engaged in critical practice advocate for the right of refugees to participate in culturally valued occupations, and help develop their opportunities to do so; and they encourage non-governmental organizations to include disabled women and men in their community-based, income-generating programmes. A professional commitment to overcoming structural barriers and to achieving the occupational rights of individuals and of populations is clearly possible.

Client-Centred Theory: Contesting Imperialism

In Australia, National Guidelines have been established to ensure that all research concerning the health of Indigenous Australians includes consultation and collaboration with Indigenous groups and is designed to produce outcomes of direct benefit to Indigenous people (79). But what about the occupational therapy research that informs our theories and practices? Do our study participants and clients deserve any less respect? Critical occupational therapy requires consultation and collaboration with disabled people and members of other marginalized groups in all our practices, such that our research, theories, interventions, and practice norms are meaningful and relevant to those people with whom we engage in the occupation of occupational therapy.

Perhaps the most important element of a critical practice of occupational therapy may be the recognition that knowledge dissemination must flow in both directions (80), and a commitment to ensure that this occurs. Post-colonial theorists have called for healthcare providers to consider the power relationships between themselves and the people they serve; and to eschew the tradition of developing and perpetuating theories and models that privilege their own perspectives while overlooking, ignoring, or silencing the perspectives of others (12,55,81). Throughout history, imperial cultures, such as the European colonialists, have exercised power and reinforced domination by establishing the parameters of permissible thinking and by suppressing challenging ideas (82); imperialistic theorists do the same (54). Sadly, occupational therapy has also exhibited imperialistic tendencies: "Contemporary history has witnessed the North and the West being positioned or positioning themselves both as the source of inspiration and provider of guidance or assistance for the South and the East" [(80), p 65]. In an effort to counter the tendency to colonialism and imperialism, those occupational therapists who aspire to critical practice will actively seek out perspectives that have been discounted, suppressed, or unacknowledged. And in this spirit, the conceptualization and definition of "occupational rights", and the actions required to address occupational rights, cannot be dictated in a colonial manner by Western theorists and therapists but must be informed by a diversity of cultural perspectives, such that our profession's theories and practices are both inclusive and relevant (54).

Conclusion

One of occupational therapy's core assumptions is that engagement in occupations influences well-being. Because occupational engagement is integral to human well-being, and because well-being is integral to human rights, this paper has argued that the ability and opportunity to engage in occupations is an issue that concerns rights. Moreover, there is increasing recognition that improving health and well-being globally can only occur with improvements in human rights; and it has been proposed that "an ethical approach to understanding, measuring and improving outcomes in rehabilitation requires an explicit perspective on human rights" [(23), p 965]. The World Federation of Occupational Therapists (75) affirms that all people have the right to participate in a range of occupations that enable them to flourish, fulfil their potential, and experience satisfaction congruent with their culture and beliefs; and asserts the human right to equitable access to participation in occupation.

This paper has argued that a philosophical commitment to occupational rights and to human well-being requires a critical practice of occupational therapy: innovative practice that acts on the knowledge that human well-being cannot be achieved solely by enhancing individuals' abilities, and that consequently endeavours to address the inequitable conditions of people's lives.

Acknowledgements

A summary of this paper ("Well-being and occupational rights") was presented at the World Federation of Occupational Therapists' 15th Congress in Santiago, Chile on 4 May 2010.

Declaration of interest: The authors report no conflicts of interest. The authors alone are responsible for the content and writing of the paper.

References

1. Edwards C, Imrie R. Disability and the implications of the well-being agenda: Some reflections from the United Kingdom. *J Soc Policy* 2008;37:337–55.

2. Gough I, McGregor JA. *Well-being in developing countries: From theory to research.* Cambridge: Cambridge University Press; 2007.

3. McGregor JA. Researching well-being: From concepts to methodology. In: Gough I, McGregor JA, editors. *Well-being in developing countries: From theory to research.* Cambridge: Cambridge University Press; 2007. p 316–50.

4. Gough I, McGregor JA, Camfield L. Theorising well-being in international development. In: Gough I, McGregor JA, editors. *Well-being in developing countries: From theory to research.* Cambridge: Cambridge University Press; 2007. p 3–43.

5. Ryff CD, Singer B. The contours of positive human health. *Psychol Inquir.* 1998;9:1–28.

6. Law M, Steinwender S, Leclair L. Occupation, health and well-being. *Can J Occup Ther.* 1998;65:81–91.

7. Pollard N, Kronenberg F, Sakellariou D. A political practice of occupational therapy. In: Pollard N, Sakellariou D, Kronenberg F. editors. *A political practice of occupational therapy.* Edinburgh: Churchill Livingstone Elsevier; 2009. p 3–19.

8. Christiansen C. Defining lives: Occupation as identity: An essay on competence, coherence, and the creation of meaning. *Am J Occup Ther.* 1999;53:547–58. http://dx.doi.org/10.5014/ajot.53.6.547. Reprinted as Chapter 34.

9. Hammell KW. Reflections on . . . well-being and occupational rights. *Can J Occup Ther.* 2008;75:61–64.

10. Watson R. A population approach to transformation. In: Watson R, Swartz L, editors. *Transformation through occupation.* London: Whurr Publishers; 2004. p 51–65.

11. Briskman L, Pease B, Allan J. Introducing critical theories for social work in a neo-liberal context. In: Allan J, Briskman L, Pease B, editors. *Critical social work: Theories and practices for a socially just world.* 2nd ed. Crows Nest, NSW, Australia: Allen & Unwin; 2009. p 3–14.

12. Hammell KW. *Perspectives on disability and rehabilitation. Contesting assumptions; challenging practice.* Edinburgh: Churchill Livingstone Elsevier; 2006.

13. Kinchloe JL, McLaren PL. Rethinking critical theory and qualitative research. In: Denzin NK, Lincoln YS, editors. *Handbook of qualitative research.* Thousand Oaks, CA: Sage Publications; 1994. p 138–57.

14. Mendes P. Tracing the origins of critical social work practice. In: Allan J, Briskman L, Pease B, editors. *Critical social work. Theories and practices for a socially just world.* 2nd ed. Crows Nest, NSW, Australia: Allen & Unwin; 2009. p 17–29.

15. Wilcock AA, Townsend E. Occupational justice. Occupational therapy interactive dialogue. *J Occup Sci.* 2000;7: 84–86.

16. Townsend E, Wilcock AA. Occupational justice and client-centred practice: A dialogue in progress. *Can J Occup Ther.* 2004;71:75–87.

17. Jary D, Jary J. *The Harper Collins dictionary of sociology.* New York: Harper Collins; 1991.

18. Honderich T. *The Oxford companion to philosophy.* Oxford: Oxford University Press; 1995.

19. Young IM. *Justice and the politics of difference.* Princeton, NJ: Princeton University Press; 1990.

20. Nipperess S, Briskman L. Promoting a human rights perspective on critical social work. In: Allan J, Briskman L, Pease B, editors. *Critical social work: Theories and practices for a socially just world.* 2nd ed. Crows Nest, NSW, Australia: Allen & Unwin; 2009. p 58–69.

21. Sherry K. Culture and cultural competence for occupational therapists. In: Alers V, Crouch R. editors. *Occupational therapy: An African perspective.* Johannesburg, RSA: Sarah Shorten; 2010. p 60–77.

22. Kallen E. *Social inequality and social justice: A human rights perspective.* Basingstoke: Palgrave; 2004.

23. Siegert RJ, Ward T, Playford ED. Human rights and rehabilitation outcomes. *Disabil Rehabil.* 2010;32:965–71.

24. Law M, McColl MA. *Interventions, effects, and outcomes in occupational therapy.* Thorofare, NJ: Slack; 2010.

25. Tisdall S. UN steps up pressure on Burma over crimes against humanity. "Gross violation of human rights" is junta state policy, draft report says. *Guardian Weekly* 19 March 2010; 10:3.

26. Hammell KW. Self-care, productivity, and leisure, or dimensions of occupational experience? Rethinking occupational "categories". *Can J Occup Ther.* 2009;76: 107–14.

27. Piškur B, Kinebanian A, Josephsson S. Occupation and well-being: A study of some Slovenian people's experiences of engagement in occupation in relation to well-being. *Scand J Occup Ther.* 2002;9:63–70.

28. Doble SE, Caron Santha J. Occupational well-being: Rethinking occupational therapy outcomes. *Can J Occup Ther.* 2008;75:184–90.

29. Wilcock AA, van der Arend H, Darling K, Scholz J, Siddall R, Snigg C, Stephens J. An exploratory study of people's perceptions and experiences of wellbeing. *Br J Occup Ther.* 1998;61:75–82.

30. Hay D, Clague M, Goldberg M, Rutman D, Armitage A, Wharf B, Rioux M, Bach M, Muszynski L, Drover G, Kerans P. *Well-being: A conceptual framework and three literature reviews.* Vancouver, BC: Social Planning and Research Council of BC; 1993.

31. Mark GT, Lyons AC. Maori healers' views on wellbeing: The importance of mind, body, spirit, family and land. *Soc Sci Med.* 2010;70:1756–64.

32. Hammell KW. Sacred texts: A sceptical exploration of the assumptions underpinning theories of occupation. *Can J Occup Ther.* 2009;76:6–13.

33. Leclair LL. Re-examining concepts of occupation and occupation-based models: Occupational therapy and community development. *Can J Occup Ther.* 2010;77:15–21.

34. Krause JS. Survival following spinal cord injury: A fifteen-year prospective study. *Rehabil Psychol.* 1991;36:89–98.

35. Krause JS, Kjorsvig JM. Mortality after spinal cord injury: A four year prospective study. *Arch Phys Med Rehabil.* 1992;73:558–563.

36. Ville I, Ravaud J-F, Tetrafigap Group. Subjective well-being and severe motor impairments: The Tetrafigap survey on the long-term outcome of tetraplegic spinal cord injured persons. *Soc Sci Med.* 2001;52:369–84.

37. Hammell KW. Dimensions of meaning in the occupations of daily life. *Can J Occup Ther.* 2004;71:296–305.

38. Hampton NZ, Qin-Hilliard DB. Dimensions of quality of life for Chinese adults with spinal cord injury: A qualitative study. *Disabil Rehabil.* 2004;26:203–12.

39. Waldie E. *Triumph of the challenged: Conversations with especially able people.* Ilminster, Somerset: Purple Field Press; 2002.

40. Hammell KW. The experience of rehabilitation following spinal cord injury: A meta-synthesis of qualitative findings. *Spinal Cord* 2007;45:260–74.

41. Reynolds F, Prior S. "Sticking jewels in your life": Exploring women's strategies for negotiating an acceptable quality of life with multiple sclerosis. *Qualitat Health Res.* 2003;13:1225–51.

42. Macfarlane S. Opening spaces for alternative understandings in mental health practice. In: Allan J, Briskman L, Pease B, editors. *Critical social work: Theories and practices*

for a socially just world. 2nd ed. Crows Nest, NSW, Australia: Allen & Unwin; 2009. p 201–13.

43. Yerxa EJ. Health and the human spirit for occupation. *Am J Occup Ther.* 1998;52:412–18. http://dx.doi.org/10.5014/ajot.52.6.412 Reprinted as Chapter 31.

44. Letts L. Enabling citizen participation of older adults through social and political environments. In: Letts L, Rigby P, Stewart D. editors. *Using environments to enable occupational performance.* Thorofare, NJ: Slack; 2003. p 71–80.

45. Strong S, Rebeiro K. Creating supportive work environments for people with mental illness. In: Letts L, Rigby P, Stewart D. editors. *Using environments to enable occupational performance.* Thorofare, NJ: Slack; 2003. p 137–54.

46. Ripat JD, Redmond JD, Grabowecky BR. The Winter Walkability project: Occupational therapists' role in promoting citizen engagement. *Can J Occup Ther.* 2010;77:7–14.

47. Sen A. *Development as freedom.* Oxford: Oxford University Press; 2001.

48. Wehmeyer ML. Self-determination and individuals with significant disabilities: Examining meanings and misinterpretations. *JASH—J Assoc Pers Severe Handicaps* 1998:23:5–16.

49. Townsend EA, Polatajko H. Enabling occupation II: *Advancing an occupational therapy vision for health, well-being & justice through occupation.* Ottawa, ONT: CAOT Publications ACE; 2007.

50. Law M, Cooper B, Strong S, Stewart D, Rigby P, Letts L. The Person–Environment–Occupation Model: A transactive approach to occupational performance. *Can J Occup Ther.* 1996;63:9–23.

51. Reilly M. Occupational therapy can be one of the great ideas of 20th century medicine. *Am J Occup Ther.* 1962;26:1–9. Reprinted as Chapter 7.

52. Bunting M. You have less control than you may think. *Guardian Weekly* 28 September 2009:19.

53. Mocellin G. Occupational therapy: A critical overview, Part 1. *Br J Occup Ther.* 1995;58:502–6.

54. Hammell KW. Resisting theoretical imperialism in the disciplines of occupational science and occupational therapy. *Br J Occup Ther.* 2011;74:27–33.

55. Iwama MK. *The Kawa model: Culturally relevant occupational therapy,* Edinburgh: Churchill Livingstone Elsevier; 2006.

56. Iwama M. Culture and occupational therapy: Meeting the challenge of relevance in a global world. *Occup Ther Int.* 2007;14:183–7.

57. Nelson A. Learning from the past, looking to the future: Exploring our place with Indigenous Australians. *Aust Occup Ther J.* 2009;56:97–102.

58. Marks D. *Disability: Controversial debates and psychosocial perspectives.* London: Routledge; 1999.

59. Sherry K. Voices of occupational therapists in Africa. In: Alers V, Crouch R, editors. *Occupational therapy: An African perspective.* Johannesburg, RSA: Sarah Shorten; 2010. p 26–47.

60. Kielhofner G. *A Model of Human Occupation: Theory and application.* 4th ed. Baltimore, MD: Lippincott Williams & Wilkins; 2007.

61. Iwama MK. The Kawa (river) model: Nature, life flow, and the power of culturally relevant occupational therapy. In: Kronenberg F, Algado SS, Pollard N, editors. *Occupational therapy without borders.* Edinburgh: Churchill Livingstone Elsevier; 2005. p 213–27.

62. Bellah RN. Beyond belief: *Essays on religion in a post traditional world.* New York: Harper & Row; 1970.

63. Chuang T. *Basic writings.* New York: Columbia University Press; 1964.

64. Gustafson JM. *Man and nature: A cross-cultural perspective.* Bangkok: Chulalongkorn University Press; 1993.

65. Heigl F, Kinébanian A, Josephsson S. I think of my family, therefore I am: Perceptions of daily occupations of some Albanians in Switzerland. *Scand J Occup Ther.* 2011;18:36–48.

66. Kupperman JJ. *Classic Asian philosophy.* Oxford: Oxford University Press; 2001.

67. Paluch T, Allen R, McIntosh K, Oke L. Koori occupational therapy scheme: Contributing to First Australian health through professional reflection, advocacy and action. *Aust Occup Ther J.* 2011;58:50–3.

68. Wanless D. Ubuntu—we all belong to each other. *Int Congregational J.* 2007;7:117–19.

69. Murithi T. A local response to the global human rights standard: The ubuntu perspective on human dignity. *Globalisation Soc Educ.* 2007;5:277–86.

70. Suzuki D. *The sacred balance.* Vancouver, BC: Greystone; 2002.

71. Tuck Haugaasen JM, Haugaasen T, Peres CA, Gribel R, Wegge P. Seed dispersal of the Brazil nut tree (Bertholletia excelsa) by scatter-hoarding rodents in a central Amazonian forest. *J Tropical Ecol.* 2010;26:251–62.

72. Chinn PL, Kramer MK. *Theory and nursing: A systematic approach.* 4th ed. St Louis, MO: Mosby; 1995.

73. Rowles GD, Beyond performance: Being in place as a component of occupational therapy. *Am J Occup Ther.* 1991;45:265–71.

74. Unruh AM, Smith N, Scammell C. The occupation of gardening in life-threatening illness. *Can J Occup Ther.* 2000;67:70–7.

75. World Federation of Occupational Therapists. *Position Statement on Human Rights.* Available online at: http://www.wfot.org/office_files/Human%20Rights%20Position%20Statement%20Final.pdf 2006. Reprinted as Appendix III.A.

76. Fejo-King C, Briskman L. Reversing colonial practices with Indigenous peoples. In: Allan J, Briskman L, Pease B. editors. *Critical social work: Theories and practices for a socially just world.* 2nd ed. Crows Nest, NSW, Australia: Allen & Unwin; 2009. p 105–16.

77. Cottrell RPF. The Olmstead decision: Landmark opportunity or platform for rhetoric? Our collective responsibility for full community participation. *Am J Occup Ther.* 2005;59:561–8.

78. Jongbloed L, Crichton A. A new definition of disability: Implications for rehabilitation practice and social policy. *Can J Occup Ther.* 1990;57:32–8.

79. Nelson A, Allison H. Relationships: The key to effective occupational therapy practice with urban Australian Indigenous children. *Occup Ther Int.* 2007;14:57–70.

80. Galheigo SM. What needs to be done? Occupational therapy responsibilities and challenges regarding human rights. *Aust Occup Ther J.* 2011;58:60–6.

81. Ramsden I. *Kawa whakaruruhau—cultural safety in nursing education in Aotearoa: Report to the Ministry of Education.* Wellington: Ministry of Education; 1990.

82. Mohanty CT. Cartographies of struggle: Third world women and the politics of feminism. In: Mohanty CT, Russo A, Torres L, editors. *Third world women and the politics of feminism.* Bloomington, IN: Indiana University Press; 1991. p 1–47.

Part III.D. Personal Contexts

Eudaimonic Well-Being: Its Importance and Relevance to Occupational Therapy for Humanity

CLAIRE HAYWARD AND JACKIE TAYLOR

Introduction

Wilcock, the influential occupational therapist and scientist, described the currency of occupational therapy as Doing, Being, Becoming and Belonging (Wilcock, 2007). Wilcock's dimensions are the result of her in-depth critical appraisal of and vision for occupational therapy and occupational science. However, an occupational therapist's understanding of occupation differs from that of the general public (McAvoy, 1992; Chow and Chung, 1996; Creek, 2003). So which dimensions of occupational therapy are most apparent to the general public and other stakeholders?

Occupational therapists' most visible work and outcomes are often involved with "doing" (Creek, 2003; Perrin et al., 2008). However, if occupational therapists' prime concern is understood to be function *(doing)*, we risk losing focus on *being* (Rowles, 1991; Hammell, 2004, 2007; Perrin et al., 2008). This could contradict the complex and multidimensional nature of occupational therapy (Creek, 2003) and risk compromising the practice of authentic occupational therapy (Yerxa, 1966). This also creates a potential misunderstanding of the profession, for others to conclude as some occupational therapists do (Wilding and Whiteford, 2009) that the end of occupational therapy is what is performed rather than why it is performed or the experience of doing (Doble and Santha, 2008), in turn misconstruing occupational therapy as being simply task focused.

The way in which the relevance and utility of occupational therapy is understood and evaluated by the individuals and populations it is intended to benefit is also of critical importance (Royeen, 2002). A poorly rounded perception of occupational therapy places the

profession in jeopardy, especially in times of global economic pressure (Clouston and Whitcombe, 2008).

If being is a core construct of occupational therapy theory, then a positive experience of being, that is to say "well" being, must also be a key aim for occupational therapy practice. "Being" as it relates to occupation incorporates many elements and is indeed difficult to define (Wilcock, 2006), although in essence, in an occupational therapy context, it relates to the subjective experience of occupation (Doble and Santha, 2008). This is a view echoed by George Berkeley, the American philosopher who considered subjectivity the primary activist in being (Berkeley, 1713). Dige (2009) proposes an occupational therapy interpretation of well-being as "[that] which consists of the wholehearted and successful carrying out of valuable activities".

Doble and Santha (2008) also cite an imbalance between doing and being and suggest that the focus of occupational therapists on occupational performance detracts from concepts of occupational satisfaction and fulfilment. They argue that the subjective experience of occupation has been marginalized. Although the call to re-focus on the subjective experience of occupation is not new, it appears to have been overshadowed by the health and illness agenda (Hammell, 2007). This may be in part due to the modern medical focus on the measurable and finite (Wilcock, 2006). In may also be due to the impenetrability of our professional terminology. While the words "occupational satisfaction" for occupational therapists may clearly suggest the positive subjective experience of occupation, these words may have little if any meaning for those outside the culture of occupational therapy. In contrast, *well-being* is a term widely used and valued in contemporary society (Godfrey, 2000; Carlisle et al., 2009) and has resonance for many stakeholders of occupational therapy and those we serve. Evidence for this includes the recently unveiled plans by the British government to measure and collect data on national levels of well-being (Stratton, 2010), with other countries considering similar proposals to direct government policy as part of a global shift away from measures of wealth (Bok, 2010; Stratton, 2010).

But what is well-being? How does it map to occupational therapy philosophy and terminology? Occupational therapy theorists have developed models over time that aim to capture the belief system and skills of the profession (Duncan, 2005; Boniface et al., 2008). Despite the lack of priority accorded to "being" in occupational therapy practice as previously contended, occupational therapy theory, philosophy and models do consistently include the role that the concept of being plays in occupation and health using the language and constructs of the author(s). Indeed Imperatore Blanche and Henry-Kohler (2000) state that "The cosmovision of occupational therapy philosophy is that occupation is important to the health and well-being of the individual."

Occupational therapy has explored some of the constructs that comprise being: integrity, spirituality, identity, personal causation, motivation, volition, satisfaction and the subjective experience of occupation are some examples of these. However, the explicit use of the term "well-being" does not feature within the primary occupational therapy models.

The belief, widely accepted by occupational therapists (Ivarsson and Müllersdorf, 2009), that the relationship between occupation and well-being is strong and proven (Pentland and McColl, 2008; Perrin et al., 2008) has been challenged (Hammell, 2009a; see Chapter 14). Hammell asserts that occupational therapy must critically appraise its long-held assumptions and begin to develop models that reflect the diverse populations facing occupational challenges. As one illustration of this, Hammell gives the example of a man caring for his dying wife and asks the question: what occupational subset is this contributing to—self-care, leisure or productivity? Occupational therapy divided into these domains can be seen to be in direct opposition to the client-centered approach that occupational therapists espouse (Pierce, 2001 [see Chapter 61]; Hammell, 2009a [see Chapter 14], 2009b) This argument links back to the excessive focus of domains of occupation which are doing-centric (Hammell, 2003; Corr et al., 2005). The notion of well-being as a means of conceptualizing occupational therapy outcomes could be useful in this context and could offer a foil both to the arguments against task-focused domains and the "doing" focus.

Taylor (2008) surmised that "Subjective experience and the personal meaning of an occupation may defy the rigidity of commonly employed categories" (p. 18).

Occupational therapists' interpretations of well-being allow for many complex and competing factors and influences. Hocking notes that one occupation in itself may have both positive and negative outcomes for the individual but yet still be seen as enhancing well-being. In this way, an occupation may, at face value, be detrimental to well-being (for example, many hours of caring for an ill relative), but when seen in the context of the values of that person, it may actually engender a sense of well-being in spite of those superficial detractors (Hammell, 2009b; Poulin et al., 2010). The somewhat paradoxical effect of experiencing well-being despite what can be considered as barriers to health or wellness is noted by other disciplines and researchers (Albrecht and Devlieger, 1999; Seligman et al., 2004; Dolan et al., 2008).

Well-being has been described as having a spiritual dimension (Hammell, 2001; Egan and Swedersky, 2003; Kang, 2003; Morris, 2007). Spirituality in occupational therapy has long been seen as an important consideration in occupational theory and has been conceptualized as separate from religion (Kang, 2003). Hammell (2001) defines the notion of spirituality (which Hammell terms "intrinsicality") as "philosophy of meaning that informs life choices and life satisfaction".

Being can be seen to offer opportunities for client centredness. It has been noted that whilst the "doing" aspect of an occupation may be conducted in a remarkably similar way from one individual to another, the subjective experience of that doing (i.e. the "being") will always be unique. In this sense, it can be argued that a focus on being demands the therapist to recognize the individual experience of each client (Hammell, 2007).

Occupational Outcomes Re-considered

There is a significant risk that, without the adequate consideration for "being" in occupational therapy, important benefits to clients are overlooked and undervalued. Corr et al. (2005), in their study comparing definitions of occupational therapy and the reported experiences of consumers, confirmed that those who receive occupational therapy also define the outcome of that intervention as more than mere doing and identified results which encompass many dimensions of being.

"It is the definition of 'purposeful' and 'activity' that is crucial here: the meaning and action taken will be different for each individual and success may lie not in terms of measurable outcomes but in the client's perception that his or her quality of life has improved. There may be no physical signs that any measurable improvement has taken place, but the client, nevertheless, may feel that his or her journey has taken a more favourable path and that life has a meaning that cannot be expressed in purely logical terms." (Kelly and McFarlane, 2007).

This suggests that the subjective, well-being output of occupation should be both highlighted and evaluated. Reflecting this, Doble and Santha (2008) propose the use of well-being as the product of occupational therapy intervention, in part as a countermeasure to the use of the terms of participation and activity, given credence by the *International Classification of Functioning, Disability and Health* (WHO, 2001), which lacks the subjective experience of occupation (Borell et al., 2006; Polatajko et al., 2007; Doble and Santha, 2008).

The impact of a shift to well-being as an end product of occupational therapy could be significant and positive. If well-being was recognized as an outcome, occupational therapists would need to re-consider outcome measures and how interventions are evaluated.

Occupational Therapy and Eudaimonic Well-Being

Occupational therapy and occupational science draw from a range of related disciplines (Wilcock, 2006) including psychology (Creek and Hughes, 2008). Concluding a review of literature relating to the link between health and occupation, Creek and Hughes (2008) underlined the need for occupational therapists to use the evidence from these knowledge bases to underpin the profession. Hesse (2009) contends that occupational therapy should embrace the research base of psychology to better inform and professionalize its practice. The relevance of well-being to occupational therapy has been outlined; occupational therapists should therefore utilize the "body of internationally relevant theory and evidence" (Carlisle et al., 2009) from psychology which exists around the science of well-being to further explore this construct.

Psychology literature describes two main traditions in the study of well-being: hedonic and eudaimonic well-being (Deci and Ryan, 2008; Dolan et al., 2008). Hedonic well-being primarily relates to the experience of happiness through the attainment of pleasure and the avoidance of pain (Kahneman et al., 1999). This understanding of well-being has been critiqued by many academics, religious leaders and philosophers throughout the ages; indeed, Aristotle found hedonic well-being "to be a vulgar ideal, making humans slavish followers of desires. He posited, instead, that true happiness is found in the expression of virtue" (Ryan and Deci, 2001, p. 145).

Eudaimonic well-being occurs "when people's life activities are most congruent or meshing with deeply held values and are holistically or fully engaged" (Ryan and Deci, 2001) and is associated with a sense of an authentic existence, which may involve meeting challenges and feeling stretched in one's skills and abilities. Waterman et al. (2008) assert that eudaimonic well-being is fostered by "doing what is worth doing", which may or may not engender happiness. Eudaimonic experience is seen to be a dynamic process, aimed at achieving self actualization through engaging in activities. This poses the question for occupational therapists: if a person is doing what is not worth doing (i.e. not congruent with one's values and beliefs), then is this occupation?

Spirituality, a familiar and important area of inquiry and practice for occupational therapists, is seen as a dimension within eudaimonic well-being (van Direndonck and Mohan, 2006). This interpretation of spirituality as an inner resource, independent of religion or denomination, is comparable with the definitions proposed by occupational therapy researchers. Its inclusion within the landscape of eudaimonic well-being serves to underline the relevance of the concept for the occupational therapy professionals.

Eudaimonic well-being provides a framework of understanding for those activities that we may value and desire, which may even bring happiness but may not promote wellness. This can provide a useful construct to occupational therapists, considering the concept of occupations, such as producing illegal graffiti, that may produce apparently contradictory outcomes (e.g. producing graffiti may bring happiness for the individual but may have a negative impact on others in the community or may be considered a criminal offence). This duality also allows for those occupations, like caring for a sick relative as mentioned previously, that present both health-promoting and health-inhibiting consequences but are ultimately deemed as producing well-being. Ryff and Keyes (1995) and Ryff and Singer

(1996) contend that eudaimonic living creates psychological well-being and offers evidence to suggest that this creates physical health. Psychological well-being is seen as having the following dimensions: autonomy, personal growth, self-acceptance, life purpose, mastery and positive relatedness (Deci and Ryan, 2008). Bauer et al. (2006) explored eudaimonic well-being and its relationship to narrative identity; they concluded that people who are able to experience higher levels of eudaimonic well-being view challenging life experiences, which include significant pain and adversity, as transformational opportunities. Indeed experiences of hardship, trauma and grief are considered an integral part of living through eudaimonic lifespan, a view reflected by Joseph Campbell, the comparative mythologist who suggested that to find life's meaning we should be "participating joyfully in the sorrows of the world" (Campbell, 2008). This consolidatory approach which considers the challenges of life as integral to it brings the utility of the psychology theory base further into the realm of occupational therapy.

In discussing what promotes or engenders well-being, consideration of that which restricts it is also necessary. To the eye of an occupational therapist, barriers to well-being may also present barriers to occupation. However, this is a dangerous link to automatically make. Equating reduced occupational performance with reduced well-being of either tradition, hedonistic or eudaimonic, is a potential trap propagated by the mainstream occupational therapy focus on "doing". Research certainly suggests that people with restricted occupations in terms of function, doing and activity often report high levels of well-being (Albrecht and Devlieger, 1999). Hammell (2004) references a wealth of disability research which shows that physical disability and/or illness (and consequent disruption or reduction in "doing") can lead to a re-evaluation of the meanings subscribed to occupations and to experiencing higher levels of well-being than when previously "well" or non-disabled In a later paper, Hammell (2008) warned against occupational therapy's preoccupation with health, illness and impairment, a call echoed by many others, and proposed that occupational therapists move to consider the well-being of all. A focus on those who live in poverty and oppression, those who are migrants and those who are homeless has been some suggestions for areas of practice (Kronenberg et al., 2005). These groups again may be perceived, when the westernized viewpoint is continued, to be lacking in their ability to do, to perform activities and to func-tion. As such, the risk exists that we perpetuate in ascribing a potentially alien value base to these groups to assume that they are in "need" of occupational therapy based on their ability to participate in leisure, self-care and productivity. When the literature base of psychology is consulted, there are many examples of people living in poverty (for example) who report higher levels of well being than those in more affluent, western environments (Seligman et al., 2004; Waterman et al., 2008). A key challenge for occupational therapy, then, is not to replace the focus of the recent past on health and illness with other "causes".

Eudaimonic Well-Being for Humanity

The notion of eudaimonic well-being provides fresh impetus and direction towards a future state of occupational therapy which is owned by its recipients rather than tethered by its historical past. The inclusion of eudaimonic well-being provides a vision for occupational therapy which is for humanity, for all, allowing occupational therapy to be defined by those who may benefit from it, not its practitioners. Perhaps, the key question we should be asking this century is "Does this person experience optimum eudaimonic well-being through occupation?" It demands that we recognize that eudaimonic well-being may thrive in lives where disease or injury reside or where social, financial or political limitations exist. It challenges us to make the deeply personal and subjective experience of occupation our keystone. Such steps may feel counterintuitive; in times of international financial austerity, we may wish to court those who commission our services, focusing on the tangible, the traditional and the more easily demonstrable. Voices from mainstream medical groups have argued that, despite the frequent use, the term well-being, meeting the well-being needs of populations, should not be the central focus of health care (Fitzpatrick, 2010). Occupational therapy re-focused on eudaimonic well-being may turn away from those medical establishments and organizations that have for so long been both the hand that feeds us and the arm that holds us back.

Pentland and McColl (2008) introduced the notion of "occupational integrity"; this concept underlines the importance of the subjective experience of occupation and embodies the values-based concept of eudaimonic well-being:

"Occupational integrity expands the focus of therapy beyond 'doing' to interventions at the level of the person and identity, helping clients to identify their strengths, values and purpose, what is meaningful and satisfying for them, and then designing and living their lives in congruence with that" (p. 138).

Occupational integrity aligns the notion of occupation within the context of cultural, political, moral, social and spiritual influences and moves occupational therapy theory beyond occupational performance and therefore towards the pursuit of eudaimonic well-being. This is crucial if occupational therapists are to realize the profession's vision of a just and inclusive society (Kronenberg et al., 2005). Well-being in general terms has also been clearly linked to this new political and rights-based occupational therapy movement (Hammell, 2007) and has been shown to be sensitive to cultural influences (Piškur et al., 2002; Wilcock, 2006).

Eudaimonic well-being, it is contended, can be derived not simply from participation in occupation, or from occupational balance, but from the lived experience of occupational integrity. Occupational integrity asks the questions: *"What do I really value, and how do my occupational choices reflect those values? How can I put my life together in a way that honours my values?"* (Pentland and McColl, 2008, p. 137).

Carlisle et al. (2009) equate the negative elements of westernized culture to modernity and propose eudaimonic well-being as an antidote to modernity, defining modernity as the following:

"a worldview that tends towards objectification, reductionism and materialism: a view of the world as lacking in any inherent meaning, design or purpose; and a view of the person as fundamentally separate, unique and alone." (p. 1577).

They suggest, as do Ryan and Deci (2001) and Csikszentmihayli (1993), that eudaimonic well-being must be defined in a global context, considering the well-being of all humanity. This opportunity to recognize and renew connections to others, to values and to spiritual beliefs has been described as offering a renewed sense of connectivism (Arai and Pedlar, 2003; Carlisle et al., 2009).

The eudaimonic interpretation of well-being can be seen to reflect the post-modernist perspective which values local narratives (Mitchell, 1996), prioritizes subjectivity and temporality (Weinblatt and Avrecht-Bar, 2001) and rejects universality. Weinblatt and Avrecht-Bar (2001) state that the term "subjective meaning" is in itself a post-modern term and asserts the utility of a post-modern perspective in enabling an occupational therapist to provide functional interventions which are practical for the client.

One of the central criticisms of the current occupational therapy theory is that it represents a westernized perspective, where a universal and singular truth external to the self is predominant (Iwama, 2005, 2006; Hammell, 2009a [see Chapter 14]). In contrast, many other cultures value instead the interrelatedness of life and the success of the collective (Iwama et al., 2009 [see Chapter 24]). Iwama advocates that a position of cultural relativism (i.e. truth relative to each individual) is essential for the genuine cultural competence of the occupational therapy profession. The dimension of connectivism, also apparent in eudaimonic well-being, has been described as mythic (Kelly and McFarlane, 2007) and an antidote to the "cult" of westernized occupational therapy (Iwama, 2006; Kelly and McFarlane, 2007; Hammell, 2009b). The inherent respect for, and impact of, values and culture in eudaimonic well-being (Ryan and Deci, 2000; Dolan et al., 2008) therefore supports Iwama's (2005) recommendation of cultural relativism. This link between cultural sensitivity and the subjectivity of well-being has also been made in occupational therapy literature (Piškur et al., 2002; Watson, 2006; Wilcock, 2006).

As well as providing a mechanism for improved cultural relevance, moving away from hedonic notions of eudaimonic well-being has been proposed as a catalyst for change from social ills such as overly consumerist attitudes and the apparent decline in life satisfaction in the west (Carlisle et al., 2009).

However, there is also a critical tension here; in the eudaimonic tradition, the definition of well-being is subjective and unique to each person, achieved only when living a life representative of one's values and culture. However, the occupations that satisfy the eudaimonic well-being of one person or group may negatively affect that of another (Carlisle et al., 2009). These two notions of sustainable ecology and sustainable communities are brought together by Wilcock (2006) in the "Occupation-focused Ecosustainable Community Development Approach" (OESCD). Wilcock highlighted that occupational therapists have a key role to play in authentic moves to promote communal occupation-focused initiatives but recognized that "Occupational therapists . . . who chose to take an OESCD approach need, initially, to enable people to recognize the impact of what they do, be, and become in communal and environmental terms" (p. 220).

In other words, it is important to consider the macro level of well-being and to engage the "being" before the "doing". Therefore, occupational therapists have a significant potential role to play both in considering the occupations which engender eudaimonic well-being for individuals and communities and in considering the impact on wider communities.

Conclusion

The current climate of occupational therapy is one of lively discourse, change, threats and opportunities. Prominent occupational therapists have called for a re-conceptualization of occupational therapy that aims to benefit all. Hammell (2009a; see Chapter 14]) asserts that occupational therapy must critically appraise its long-held assumptions and begin to develop models that reflect the diverse populations facing occupational challenges (Imperatore Blanche and Henry-Kohler, 2000).

If we consider "being" in occupational therapy as the subjective experience of occupation, (eudaimonic) well-being can be seen as the expression of occupational integrity. In this way, occupation could be defined as "doing" which engenders eudaimonic well-being, reflective of culture and values. If we therefore reframe the goal of occupational therapy as achieving eudaimonic well-being, we may be able to mitigate the imperialist, westernized and ablest bias levelled at the occupational therapy profession by some (Kronenberg et al., 2005; Pentland and McColl, 2008; Hammell, 2009a [see Chapter 14], 2009b) and move wholeheartedly towards a professional theoretical base which is for all humanity. This shift in focus could continue the renaissance in occupation as a means (Pollock and McColl, 2003) but allow for a more critical appraisal of the utility of the term occupation (or occupational satisfaction or balance) as an end. Well-being, internationally recognized as vital to human experience (World Health Organization, 1946), more specifically eudaimonic well-being, offers a new way of conceptualizing the outcome of occupational therapy, which allows practitioners to be inclusive of our new politicized and rights-based practice agenda (Creek and Hughes, 2008), giving recognition to the importance of considering the sustainability of our social and natural environment.

The call for a renewed exploration of occupation and well-being in a contemporary world is not new (Rowles,

1991; Wilcock et al., 1998; Hammell 2004; Doble and Santha, 2008; Hammell, 2008; Taylor, 2008). However, this paper has made links between current thinking in psychology and modern occupational therapy theory and research. Eudaimonic well-being is proposed as a key concept for occupational therapy but one that is currently missing from the debate, literature and research of our profession. The opportunities offered by such a current (Bauer and McAdams, 2010), well-described and evidenced concept should be seized by occupational therapists. In considering who might benefit from the skills of occupational therapists in using occupation as a means, we should start by exploring those people or groups who experience a lack of self-defined eudaimonic well-being.

Well-being has been shown to transcend traditional boundaries of physical and mental health and societal and cultural norms and reflects the aspirations of international agencies such as the World Health Organization. This construct therefore has much to offer to an internationalized community of occupational therapists, going beyond the borders of the previously sacred domains of occupational therapy.

References

Albrecht G, Devlieger P (1999). The disability paradox: high quality of life against all odds. *Social Science & Medicine 48:* 977–988.

Arai S, Pedlar A (2003). Moving beyond individualism in leisure theory: a critical analysis of concepts of community and social engagement. *Leisure Studies 22:* 185–202.

Bauer J, McAdams D (2010). Eudaimonic growth: narrative growth goals predict increases in ego development and subjective well-being 3 years later. *Developmental Psychology 46*(4): 761–772.

Bauer J, McAdams D, Pals J (2006). Narrative identity and eudaimonic well-being. *Journal of Happiness Studies 9*(1): 81–104. http://dx.doi.org/10.1007/s10902-006-9021-6.

Berkeley G (1713). *Principles of Human Knowledge: Three Dialogues.* Oxford: Oxford University Press.

Bok D (2010). *The Politics of Happiness: What Government Can Learn from the New Research on Well-Being.* New Jersey: Princetown University Press.

Boniface G, Fedden T, Hurst H, Mason M, Phelps C, Reagon C, Waygood S (2008). Using theory to underpin an integrated occupational therapy service through the Canadian model of occupational performance. *British Journal of Occupational Therapy 71*(12): 531–539.

Borell L, Asaba E, Rosenberg L, Schult M-L, Townsend E (2006). Exploring perspectives of "participation" among individuals living with chronic pain. *Scandinavian Journal of Occupational Therapy* 13: 76–85.

Campbell J (2008). *The Hero with a Thousand Faces*. (4th ed) California: New World Library.

Carlisle S, Henderson G, Hanlon PW (2009). 'Well-being': a collateral casualty of modernity? *Social Science & Medicine* 69(10): 1556–1560. http://dx.doi.org/10.1016/j.socscimed.2009.08.029.

Chow S, Chung J (1996). The perception of occupational therapy by special school teachers. *Occupational Therapy International* 3(2): 94–104.

Clouston T, Whitcombe S (2008). The professionalisation of occupational therapy: a continuing challenge. *British Journal of Occupational Therapy* 71: 314–320.

Corr S, Neill G, Turner A (2005). Comparing an occupational therapy definition and consumers' experiences: a qualitative methodology study. *British Journal of Occupational Therapy* 68(8): 338–346.

Creek J, Hughes A (2008). Occupation and health: a review of selected literature. *British Journal of Occupational Therapy* 71(11): 456–468.

Creek J (2003). *Occupational Therapy Defined as a Complex Intervention*. London: College of Occupational Therapists.

Csikszentmihayli M (1993). Activity and happiness: Towards a science of occupation. *Journal of Occupational Science* 1(1): 38–42.

Deci EL, Ryan RM (2008). Hedonia, eudaimonia, and well-being: an introduction. *Journal of Happiness Studies* 9(1): 1–11. http://dx.doi.org/ 10.1007/s10902-006-9018-1.

Dige M (2009). Occupational therapy, professional development, and ethics. *Scandinavian Journal of Occupational Therapy* 16(2): 88–98.

Van Direndonck D, Mohan K (2006). Some thoughts on spirituality and eudaimonic well-being. *Mental Health, Religion and Culture* 9(3): 227–238.

Doble S, Santha J (2008). Occupational well-being: rethinking occupational therapy outcomes. *Canadian Journal of Occupational Therapy* 75(3): 184–190.

Dolan P, Peasgood T, White M (2008). Do we really know what makes us happy? A review of the economic literature on the factors associated with subjective well-being. *Journal of Economic Psychology* 29(1): 94–122. http://dx.doi.org/10.1016/j.joep.2007.09.001.

Duncan E (2005). *Foundations for Practice in Occupational Therapy*. Edinburgh: Churchill Livingstone.

Egan M, Swedersky J (2003). Spirituality as experienced by occupational therapists in practice. *American Journal of Occupational Therapy* 57: 525–533. http://dx.doi.org/10.5014/ajot.57.5.525

Fitzpatrick M (2010). Health and well-being? *The British Journal of General Practice* 60(570): 61.

Godfrey A (2000). Policy changes in the National Health Service: implications and opportunities for occupational therapists. *British Journal of Occupational Therapy* 63(5): 219–224.

Hammell KW (2001). Intrinsicality: reconsidering spirituality, meaning(s) and mandates. *Canadian Journal of Occupational Therapy* 68(3): 186–194.

Hammell KW (2003). Intrinsicality: Reflections on meanings and mandates. In M.A. McColl (Ed.), *Spirituality and occupational therapy* (pp. 67–82). Ottawa, ON: CAOT Publications ACE.

Hammell KW (2004). Dimensions of meaning in the occupations of daily life. *Canadian Journal of Occupational Therapy* 71(5): 296–305.

Hammell KW (2007). Reflections on. . . a disability methodology for the client-centred practice of occupational therapy research. *Canadian Journal of Occupational Therapy* 74: 365–369.

Hammell KW (2008). Reflections on. . . well-being and occupational rights. *Canadian Journal of Occupational Therapy* 75(1): 61–64.

Hammell KW (2009a). Sacred texts: a sceptical exploration of the assumptions underpinning theories of occupation. *Canadian Journal of Occupational Therapy* 76: 6–13. Reprinted as Chapter 14.

Hammell KW (2009b). Self-care, productivity, and leisure, or dimensions of occupational experience? Rethinking occupational "categories". *Canadian Journal of Occupational Therapy* 76(2): 107–114.

Hesse PW (2009). Psychology and occupational therapy—can we learn from each other? *Ergotherapie & Rehabilitation* 48(9): 19–24.

Hocking C (2003). Creating occupational practice: a multidisciplinary health focus. In Brown G, Esdaile SA, Ryan SE (eds). *Becoming an Advanced Healthcare Practitioner* (pp. 189–215). Edinburgh: Butterworth Heinemann.

Imperatore Blanche E, Henry-Kohler E (2000). Philosophy, science and ideology: a proposed relationship for occupational science and occupational therapy. *Occupational Therapy International* 7(2): 99–110.

Ivarsson A-B, Müllersdorf M (2009). Occupation as described by occupational therapy students in Sweden:

a follow-up study. *Scandinavian Journal of Occupational Therapy* 16(1): 57–64.

Iwama M, Thomson N, Macdonald R (2009). The Kawa model: the power of culturally responsive occupational therapy. *Disability and Rehabilitation* 31(14): 1125–1135. Reprinted as Chapter 24.

Iwama M (2006). *The Kawa Model: Culturally Relevant Occupational Therapy.* Edinburgh: Churchill Livingstone Elsevier.

Iwama M (2005). Occupation as a Cross-cultural Construct. In Whiteford G, Wright-St Clair V (eds). *Occupation and Practice in Context.* Sydney: Elsevier.

Kang C (2003). A psychosocial integration frame of reference for occupational therapy. Part 1: Conceptual foundations. *Australian Occupational Therapy Journal* 50: 92–103.

Kahneman D, Diener E, Schwarz N (eds). (1999). *Well-being: The Foundations of Hedonic Psychology.* New York: Russell Sage Found.

Kelly G, McFarlane H (2007). Culture or cult? The mythological nature of occupational therapy. *Occupational Therapy International* 14(4): 188–202. http://dx.doi.org/10.1002/oti.237.

Kronenberg F, Algado S, Pollard N (2005). Preface. In Kronenberg F, Algado S, Pollard N (eds). *Occupational Therapy Without Borders* (pp. xv–xvii). Edinburgh, UK: Churchill Livingstone Elsevier.

McAvoy E (1992). Occupational who? Never heard of them! An audit of patient awareness of occupational therapists. *British Journal of Occupational Therapy* 55(6): 229–232.

Mitchell D (1996). Postmodernism, health and illness. *Journal of Advanced Nursing* 23: 201–205.

Morris D (2007). Personal spiritual well-being, perceptions of the use of spirituality, and spiritual care in occupational therapy practice. Dissertation Abstracts International: Section B: *The Sciences and Engineering* 68(3-B): 1599.

Pentland M, McColl M (2008). Occupational integrity: another perspective on "life balance." *Canadian Journal of Occupational Therapy* 74(3): 135–138.

Perrin T, May H, Anderson E (2008). *Well-being in Dementia: An Occupational Approach for Therapists and Carers,* 2nd Ed., China: Churchill Livingstone Elsevier.

Pierce D. (2001). Occupation by design: Dimensions, therapeutic power, and creative process. *American Journal of Occupational Therapy* 55: 249–259. http://dx.doi.org/10.5014/ajot.55.3.249 Reprinted as Chapter 61.

Piškur B, Kinebanian A, Josephesson S (2002). Occupation and well-being: A study of some slovenian people's experiences of engagement in occupation in relation to well-being. *Scandanavian Journal of Occupational Therapy 9:* 63–70.

Polatajko HJ, Davis J, Stewart D, Cantin N, Amoroso B, Purdie L, Zimmerman D (2007). Specifying the domain of concern: Occupation as core. In Townsend EA, Polatajko HJ (eds). *Enabling Occupation II: Advancing an Occupational Therapy Vision of Health, Well-being and Justice Through Occupation* (pp. 13–26). Ottawa, ON: CAOT Publications ACE.

Pollock N, McColl MA (2003). How occupation changes. In: McColl MA, Law M, Stewart D, Doubt L, Pollock N, Krupta T (eds). *Theoretical Basis of Occupational Therapy* (pp. 63–80). Thorofare, NJ: Slack.

Poulin M, Brown S, Ubel P, Smith D, Janovic A, Langa K (2010). Does a helping hand mean a heavy heart? Helping behavior and well-being among spouse caregivers. *Psychology and Aging* 25(1): 108–117.

Rowles GD (1991). Beyond performance: being in place as a component of occupational therapy. *American Journal of Occupational Therapy* 45: 265–271.

Royeen C (2002). Occupation reconsidered. *Occupational Therapy International* 9(2): 111–120.

Ryan RM, Deci EL (2001). On happiness and human potentials: a review of research on hedonic and eudaimonic well-being. *Social Sciences* 52: 141–166.

Ryan RM, Deci EL (2000). Self-determination theory and the facilitation of intrinsic motivation, social development, and well-being. *American Psychologist 55:* 68–78.

Ryff CD, Keyes C (1995). The structure of psychological well-being revisited. *Journal of Personal Social Psychology* 69: 719–727.

Ryff CD, Singer B (1996). Psychological well-being: meaning, measurement, and implications for psychotherapy research. *Psychotherapy and Psychosomatics 65:* 14–23.

Seligman ME, Parks AC, Steen T (2004). A balanced psychology and a full life. *Philosophical Transactions of the Royal Society of London, Series B, Biological Sciences* 359(1449): 1379–1381. http://dx.doi.org/ 10.1098/rstb.2004.1513.

Stratton A (2010). Happiness index to gauge Britain's national mood. *The Guardian.* Retrieved 15th November 2010 from http://www.guardian.co.uk/lifeandstyle/2010/nov/14/happiness-index-britain-national-mood.

Taylor JA (2008). *The construction of identities through narratives of occupations.* (Doctoral thesis, University of Salford, unpublished).

Waterman AS, Schwartz SJ, Conti R (2008). The implications of two conceptions of happiness (hedonic enjoyment and eudaimonia) for the understanding of intrinsic motivation. *Journal of Happiness Studies 9:* 41–79. http://dx.doi.org/10.1007/s10902-006-9020-7.

Watson RM (2006). Being before doing: the cultural identity (essence) of occupational therapy. *Australian Occupational Therapy Journal 53:* 151–158.

Weinblatt N, Avrecht-Bar M (2001). Postmodernism and its application to the field of occupational therapy. Canadian *Journal of Occupational Therapy 68*(3): 164–170.

Wilding C, Whiteford G (2009). From practice to praxis: reconnecting moral vision with philosophical underpinnings. *British Journal of Occupational Therapy 72*(10): 434–414.

Wilcock A (2007). Occupation and health: are they one and the same? *Journal of Occupational Science 14*(1): 3–8.

Wilcock A (2006). *Occupation: Being Through Doing in an Occupational Perspective of Health.* 2nd Ed. United States: Slack.

Wilcock A, van Der Arund H, Darling K, Scholz J, Siddall R, Snigg C, Stephens J (1998). An exploratory study of people's perceptions and experiences of well-being. *British Journal of Occupational Therapy 61*(2): 75–82.

World Health Organization (1946). *Preamble to the Constitution of the World Health Organization* as adopted by the International Health Conference, New York, Official Records of the World Health Organization 2 p100.

World Health Organization (2001). *International classification of functioning, disability and health.* Geneva: WHO.

Yerxa E (1966). Eleanor Clarke Slagle lecture: authentic occupational therapy. *American Journal of Occupational Therapy 21*(1): 155–173.

CHAPTER 30

A Theory of the Human Need for Occupation

ANN WILCOCK

"It is the unique blend of biology and culture that makes the species 'Homo sapiens' a truly unique kind of animal. . . . Humans are different, not so much for what we do . . . but rather the fact that we can do more or less what we want."[1]

Occupation, that is, purposeful activity, is a central aspect of the human experience. In developing a theory of the human need for occupation, an exploration of occupational evolution as well as the biological and the sociocultural aspects of occupational behavior is necessary. This paper, which is based on a study of human occupational behavior throughout history, explores the proposition that, although in most instances the conception, expression, and execution of occupation is unique and motivated by sociocultural values and beliefs, the need to engage in purposeful occupation is innate and related to health and survival.

All animals appear to have some special characteristic which is paramount to their survival. This varies among and within species. For some it is speed, for others the ability to camouflage, and for yet others, highly developed visual or auditory capacities. Many animals possess qualities and characteristics once thought unique to humans, which is not surprising as all mammalian brains have neuronal circuitry and systems which enable then to receive, attend to, interpret, communicate with, and act upon information from the environment. In fact *"there is no strong evidence of unique brain–behavior relationships in any species within the class Mammalia."*[2] The difference among species is in the degree of capacities. Ethologist Konrad Lorenz contends that:

"Among humans . . . "perceptions of depth and direction, a central nervous representation of space, Gestalt perception and the capacity for abstraction, insight and learning, voluntary movement, curiosity and exploratory behavior" and "imitation" . . . are more strongly developed than any of them is among an animal species, even if they represent for those animals a fulfilment of the most vital life-furthering functions."[3]

The difference between humans and the other mammals is manifest in the size of the human brain. It is 6.3 times larger than expected for mammals of the same body size[4], with the difference mainly attributable to an increase in association areas of the cortex. These are responsible for the mediation of cognitive processes such as the capacities noted by Lorenz, and complex communication, language, thinking, forward planning, problem solving, analysis, judgement, and adaptation. It is these highly developed cognitive capacities, along with consciousness, which are the special survival characteristics of humans, enabling them to adapt to and meet the challenge of many different environments and dangers.

These differences in degree of cognitive capacity are central to the occupational nature of humans who go beyond survival needs in their pursuit of occupation because they free them from the functional constraints of most animals, enabling them to use their apparently strong drive to engage in daily, new, or adventurous occupations. People are able to undertake activities with individuality of purpose; to think about the effects, conceptualize, and plan beforehand; and to reflect and mentally alter future behavior as a result of outcomes. Children, through play, the predominant occupation of the young, learn practical skills to enable them to survive, to interact with others, to choose future roles, in fact to develop according to their environment and cultural values. Occupation provides the mechanism for social interaction, and societal development and growth, forming the foundation stone of communal, local, and national identity, because not only do individuals engage in separate pursuits, they are able to plan and execute group activity to the extent of national government or to achieve international goals, for individual, mutual, and community purposes. As Marx suggests *"History is nothing but the activity of man pursuing his aims."*[5] Individuals dream and communities plan what they will "do" in the future. Such dreams and plans often predict potential accolades for what will be achieved, reflecting how occupations are the outward expression of culturally desired intellectual, moral, and physical attributes. Occupation is the mechanism by which individuals demonstrate the use of their capacities by achievements of value and worth to their society and the world. It is only by their activities that people can demonstrate what they are or what they hope to be. Occupational achievement usually results in self development and growth experiences, which Hegel and Marx described as *"labour as man's act of self creation."*[6]

Marx founded much of his philosophy on the idea that labor is the collective creative activity of mankind, in fact, is *"man's species nature."*[7] As people engage in occupation to master their environment and improve human opportunities, well-being, and survival, the physical and social environment is altered. The more sophisticated the occupation, the greater the change to the environment, which in turn causes further change to and development of people, and *"by thus acting on the external world and changing it, he at the same time changes his own nature."*[8] In the same vein, Braverman proposes that people are the special product of purposeful action, arguing that occupation which *"transcends mere instinctual activity is the force which created human kind and the force by which humankind created the world as we know it."*[9]

The idea that occupation is not just the object of human function but is an integrated part of each person's being in relationship with the world suggests the need to explore the biological purpose of the human need to "do." This need is so much a part of our being that we have, to this time, paid scant attention to its purpose, other than, in post-industrial societies, as an objective of living. In considering people as occupational beings it is implied that humans need to engage in occupation in order to flourish, and that as Selye observes, purposeful use of time is a biological necessity because *"our brain slips into chaos and confusion unless we constantly use it for work that seems worthwhile to us."*[10] Further, Sigerist argues that work is essential in maintaining health *"because it determines the chief rhythm of life, balances it, and gives meaning and significance. An organ that does not work atrophies, and the mind that does not work becomes dumb."*[11]

Biological Need

Because basic biological needs are now obscured by millions of years of acquired values, present day awareness may not reflect human needs which were, and probably still are, fundamental to healthy survival. In fact, the study of biological needs has been neglected of late either because, as Allport remarked on fashion in scientific inquiry, *"we never seem to solve our problems or exhaust our concepts; we only grow tired of them,"*[12] or because of a false dichotomy between disciplines concerned with the study of biology and sociology which mirrors the Cartesian division of mind and body. In the long-running nature-versus-nurture debate, the need to consider both is poorly recognized except perhaps by disciplines such as ethology, sociobiology, and occupational therapy.

Biological mechanisms aimed at ensuring survival are basic to all animals, and the proposition put by Omstein and Sobel in "The Healing Brain"[13] that *"the major role of the brain is to mind the body and maintain health"* appears more logical than some of the lofty purposes attributed to it by those seeking to differentiate humans from their animal heritage. The brain, they argue, by making *"countless adjustments"* is able to maintain stability between *"social worlds, our mental and emotional lives, and our internal physiology."* It is contended here that biological "needs" have an integral role in this process.

It was in the early 1930s that the "concept of need" as a *"central motivating variable"* made its debut into academic psychology, eventually replacing the notion of instinct, although unlike instinct it does not have a *"repertoire of inherited, unlearned action patterns."*[14] Many needs theorists of the time were influenced by physiological discoveries such as those pertaining to homeostasis, and the notions propounded about "drives" as persistent motivations, organic in origin, which *"arouse, sustain, and regulate human and animal behavior."* These were seen as distinct from external determinants of behavior such as *"social goals, interests, values, attitude and personality traits."*[15] Dashiell in "Fundamentals of Objective Psychology,"[16] for example, argues that

"The primary drives to persistent forms of animal and human conduct are tissue conditions within the organism giving rise to stimulations existing the organism to overt activity. A man's interest and desires may became ever so elaborate, refined, socialized, sublimated, idealistic; but the raze basis from which they are developed is found in the phenomena of living matter."

Lorenz in examining *"the purposefulness of the anatomic characteristic as well the behavior patterns of every living creature"*[17] observes that humans do lack *"long, self-continued chains of innate behavior patterns"* but that they have more *"genuinely instinctive impulses than any other animal."*[18] It is such impulses which express biological needs. In the 1973 *Dictionary of Behavioral Science*, "Need" is described as:

"the condition of lacking, wanting or requiring something which if present would benefit the organism by facilitating behaviour or satisfying a tension."

and also as

"a construct representing a force in the brain which directs and organises the individual's perception, thinking and action, so as to change an existing, unsatisfying situation."[19]

The view held here accepts and extends this concept, arguing that "needs" relate not only to correction of disequilibrium but to facilitating what is required for living organisms—plants, animals, or humans to fulfil potential and flourish.[20,21] With this view, biological needs are seen as inborn health agents which recognize the organism as a "whole in interaction with the environment" as part of an open system. They do not differentiate among physical, mental, or social issues in the way of modern society, or as does medicine, psychology or sociology, but work as part of *"a flow of processes"* within the biological hierarchy relating structures and function,[22] and are integral to the collaboration between biological rhythms and homeostasis as described by Campbell.[23]

Using a cybernetic—that is, a transfer of information and feedback model to assist understanding of the processes, it is proposed that needs have a three-way role in maintaining the stability and health of the organism (Figure 30.1). They serve to warn after a problem occurs, to protect and prevent potential disorder, and to prompt and reward use of capacities so that the organism will flourish and reach potential. To warn and protect, needs are experienced as a form of discomfort which calls for some kind of action to satisfy or assuage the need. Examples of these experiences are pain, fatigue, hunger, cold, fear, boredom, tension, depression, anxiety, anger, or loneliness. To prevent disorder and prompt use of capacities, needs are experienced in a positive sense, such as a need to spend extra energy, walk, explore, understand or make sense of, utilize ideas, express thoughts, talk, listen or look, spend time alone or with others, and so on. The third category of needs considered here to be integral to the healthy survival of individuals are those that reward use of capacities, such as the need for purpose, satisfaction, fulfillment and pleasure. Pleasure and happiness have been recognized as powerful human needs by many, such as, Aristotle 2,300 years ago, and current writers such as Argyle[24] and Csikszentmihalyi.[25] These three categories of needs are structured physiologically to provide both motivation and feedback.

Founded on these notions about biological needs and following an exploration of human occupation from early in evolution, a theoretical framework attributing a place for purposeful occupation in maintaining and

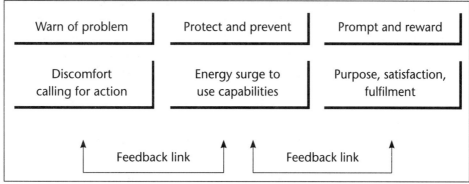

Figure 30.1. Needs: Three-way role in health.

Provide for immediate bodily needs of sustenance, self-care, shelter, and safety.	Develop skills, social structures, and technology aimed at superiority over predators and the environment.	❸ Exercise and develop personal capacities enabling the organism to be maintained and to flourish.

Figure 30.2. Occupation: Three major functions in species survival.

enabling the health of individuals and survival of the species is proposed. Three major functions of occupation are identified. They are:

- To provide for immediate bodily needs of sustenance, self-care, and shelter;
- To develop skills, social structures, and technology, aimed at safety and superiority over predators and the environment;
- And to exercise personal capacities to enable maintenance and development of the organism.

It is assumed that occupational behaviors of early humans of the hunter–gatherer period reflect basic phylogenic needs of humans more closely than those of the present day because they would be less affected by culturally acquired knowledge, values, and behavior. Within hunter–gatherer societies the direct provision of daily requirements formed the foundation of occupational behaviour. This simple occupational structure did not obscure innate physiological needs, but catered for them to the extent that the environment was able to furnish these needs, and people were able to adapt to changes of habitat. Virey, French physician–philosopher in "L'Hygiene Philosophique,"[26] asserted that humans in a state of nature are endowed with an instinct for health which permits biological adaptation and which civilized humans have lost, and it has been observed *"that people living a culturally primitive life (with less medical care) are generally more physically perfect than those from affluent societies."*[27] This view is supported by reports from explorers in their initial contacts with people of primitive cultures which suggest that they appeared both happy and healthy. For example, Captain James Cook recorded in his Journal, 1768–1771, that he found the natives of the Pacific Islands he visited happy, healthy, and full of vigor, and of the Australian aborigine he wrote *"they are far happier than we Europeans . . . they live in tranquility . . ."* and *"they think themselves provided with all the neces-*

sarys of Life, and that they have no Superfluities (sic)."[28] On the whole, health and well-being seem to have sat easily with the unequivocal lifestyle.

The occupational technology and social structures of this prolonged era aimed at safety and superiority over predators and the environment were in accord with the natural world and are generally considered not to have disturbed the environmental balance. The *"overexploitation of natural resources"* does not occur in the ecology of plants and animals, because human hunter–gatherer cultures *"influence their biotope in a way no different from that of animal populations."*[29] While some may argue this assertion, it is supported, on the whole, by observation of cultures such as that of the Australian aborigine which does not appear to have overexploited the environment, and *"in full tribal life . . . presented an excellent example of a society working in rhythm with its environment."*[30]

From such simple beginnings social structures and technology have become dominant and self-perpetuating forces, with most people seeming to accept whatever eventuates as an inevitable and useful progression, to the extent they are seldom considered as having grown from basic human needs. In fact, the needs of people pale into insignificance beside the drive to create more and more sophisticated technology, and more regulated societies which are no longer in step with ecology. The exercise of personal capacities to enable maintenance and development of the organism is perhaps the most primary and least appreciated function of human occupation. The organism, and all its parts, have to be active in order to remain healthy. Maslow observed that:

"capacities clamor to be used, and cease their clamor only when they are well used. That is, capacities are also needs. Not only is it fun to use our capacities, but it is also necessary for growth. The unused skill or capacity or organ can become a disease centre or else atrophy or disappear."[31]

In other words, capacities need exercise to maintain homeostasis and health, and the expanded human brain with its capacity to think, surmise, problem solve, anticipate, and plan for the future imposes upon the need for activity, the need for purpose. For millions of years, basic survival provided the purpose for required activity. With changes to occupation and purpose due to cultural evolution, particularly over the last 200 years, the balanced use of capacities is compromised, and ultimately long-term health and survival of the species may be under threat.

Sociocultural Factors

This may have come about because biological needs are not easy to distinguish from socioculturally acquired needs and wants, and neither are they omnipotent. They are subject to scrutiny of, and adaptation by, cognitive and intellectual capacities which are the most recent evolutionary processes of the human brain. These are primarily responsive to the sociocultural environment with a functional capacity to formulate acquired needs. Although acquired and biological needs work in partnership, acquired needs are able to override biological needs because of the hierarchical structure of the central nervous system. *In evolution, new structures of body and brain are often added on to existing ones,* but are involved in the same functions. *A tension can exist between the old and the new. Such tensions are especially pronounced in . . . humans [who are] equipped with a powerful cortex [which] can say 'no.'"*[32]

However, it can be argued that the biological mechanism of needs has focused human energies toward developing sociocultural structures to meet those needs. Humans' intellectual, cognitive, and cultural capacity has enabled them through engagement in occupation, to satisfy, in large measure, the three categories of needs identified earlier. Because of this, and despite diverse challenges, humans, unlike other mammals, have been successful survivors—to the point of overpopulation. In post-industrial countries, action to satisfy or assuage discomfort, such as food production, the regulation of temperature, and measures to reduce pain, have reached a level of sophistication far beyond the simple methods used by all other animals living in natural habitats. To prevent disorder, humans have developed ways of using their capacities in adaptive, inventive, and exploratory fashions to the extent that they provide purpose, reward, and the pursuit of happiness.

The human brain's capacity to adapt to and indeed construct social environs different from those in which humans evolved appears to alter the significance of biological needs, so that *"even phylogenetically evolved programs of . . . behavior are adjusted to the presence of a culture."*[33] This has led to *"culture itself"* creating *"norms of human behavior that, in a certain sense, can step in as substitutes for innate behavior programs."*[34]

Humans' ability for sociocultural adaptation enables infants at a very early age to assimilate and retain information from the environment, before a conscious appreciation of meaning or significance is possible. This early absorption of observed behaviors enables ontogenic development to be in step with sociocultural expectations. Attitudes, as well as behavior are absorbed and adopted, and it is those formed before intellectual capacities are sufficiently advanced to allow for adequate understanding or refuting, that have the strongest, because "unconscious," hold on individuals. While this mechanism was central to early humans' healthy survival because it allowed essential learning to occur from birth and stimulated cognitive capacities to develop, in latter-day cultures, despite these benefits, what is absorbed may have little to do with health. Sociocultural survival as observed by infants is, in post-industrial societies, concerned, in large part, with material things. In addition, infants are encouraged to hide many physiological actions, such as yawning or scratching, because they are counter to sociocultural rules. In this way biological needs are gradually suppressed to the point where, in order to meet social expectations, they are not adequately recognized. It is from views such as this that sociologists developed one of the fundamental postulates of the modern discipline, that human actions are limited or determined by past and present environments, and that humans are the products and the victims of their society.[35]

In a continuous but accelerating process, occupation has increased in complexity and division along with sociocultural change. In large part changes to the sociocultural world can be traced to occupational technology and the human need to exercise intellectual capacities to meet challenges imposed by social and ecological environments. Purposeful use of time is an issue of great complexity which has been poorly recognized because it forms the substance of everyday life and is taken for granted."[36] As Primeau, Clark, and Pierce[37] describe, each day, people weave together their own particular multiplicity of occupations within the context of contemporary society, with its many stresses, pressures, regulations, and changing values. The gradual evolution of complex occupational structures in response to cultural forces has led to the present situation in which it is difficult to tease out the survival and health maintaining behaviors which were once dominant in human occupation and, on the whole, health and well-being seem to sit uneasily amid the rush and stresses of present-day occupational structures.

This raises the question of whether occupational structures, the social environment and political agendas which support these structures, provide people with opportunities for health-enhancing, balanced and stimulating use of physical, mental, and social capacities and whether the passion to continue developing technology, which is known to be to the detriment of the ecology, is also to the detriment of basic human needs.

John Maynard Keynes, the economist, in 1931 observed *"the struggle for subsistence, always has been hitherto the primary, most pressing problem of the human race. . . .Thus we have been expressly evolved by nature."* If this need is removed:

> *"mankind will be deprived of its traditional purpose. . . . Thus for the first time since his creation man will be faced with his real, his permanent problem—how to use his freedom, . . . how to occupy the leisure, to live wisely and agreeably and well. . . . It is a fearful problem for the ordinary person, with no special talents, to occupy himself, especially if he no longer has roots in the soil or in the custom or in the beloved conventions of a traditional society."*[38]

This suggests that if the human need to use cognitive capacities continues in the present direction without consideration of how basic biological needs for occupation can be met, health, well-being, and survival may well suffer. The human use of capacities has changed as occupation has changed and as technology builds upon technology. Human creativity has effectively changed *"manual work into machine work: machine work into paper work: paper work into electronic simulation of work, divorced progressively from any organic functions or human purposes, except those that further the power system."*[39] This changed use of human energies and potentials via technology is primarily to meet production purposes rather than human needs. It is argued that the state of technology and the social structures which support it are not conducive to the maintenance of occupational balance for the ma-jority of people, the result being boredom or burnout. Ironically, in part, boredom or burnout is caused by the drive for human creativity and cognitive capacity. In part it is also caused by the arbitrary dividing of occupation resulting from cultural evolutionary forces which makes it difficult to consider occupation from a holistic perspective. This impedes the conscious awareness of the need to balance mental, physical, and social occupations as integral aspects of health; to balance energy expenditure and rest; and social activity and solitude. Additionally, although affluent societies appear to have an abundance of occupational choices offering opportunity for the exercise and development of physical, mental, and social skills, the structures and values placed upon different aspects of occupation may well affect how successfully individuals access these opportunities. People may be restricted in their choice by many factors such as lack of time or material resources. They may be disadvantaged in comparison with early humans because they are not socialized into selecting occupations conducive to health. They may lack opportunity to provide for their own basic needs because changing occupational structures and technologies:

- Restrict freedom of action by ever-increasing rules and regulations,
- Replace ongoing human endeavor with technological labor-saving devices,
- Reduce the availability of paid employment,
- Create an addictive way of life out of step with sustaining the ecology.

It is argued here that post-industrial societies have reached a stage in which the need to use human capacities is being overlooked. We are now creating a world in which what has been created by the capacities of humans appears more important than the balanced use of capacities. Use of capacities and needs are subjugated to external purpose which, for mankind in a natural state, was the motivation to use capacities. The purpose takes on a life form of its own and becomes a primary sociocultural need, such as the apparently overwhelming need at present for technology or money. The greater the need for the created rather than for the creating, the less health enhancing it becomes (Figure 30.3).

People need to make use of their capacities through engagement in individually motivating and ongoing occupations, and if they are able, or encouraged to pursue this need, they will, apart from supplying sustenance for survival and safety, enhance their health. As was possible prehistory, the total range of an individual's purposeful and fulfilling occupations can provide individuals

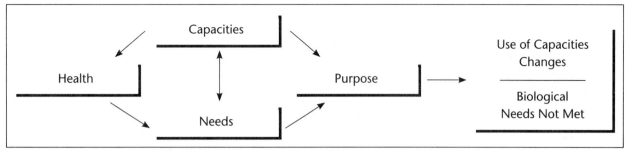

Figure 30.3. Capacities and needs are subjugated to external purpose.

with sufficient exercise to maintain homeostasis, to keep body parts and neuronal physiology and mental capacities functioning at peak efficiency, and enable maintenance and development of satisfying and stimulating social relationships. A range of occupations can provide balance among physical, mental, and social challenges and relaxation. This is part of the complex neural system aimed at maintenance of homeostasis, growth, and development because occupations act as a focus for integrating physical, mental, and social capacities.

Humans are occupational beings with a need to use time in a purposeful way. This need is innate and related to health and survival because it enables individuals to utilize their biological capacities and potential, and thereby flourish. Because of the adaptive capacity of the human brain the innate drive for purposeful occupation has been influenced over time by sociocultural forces and values which has added ever-increasing complexity to the relationship between biological needs and how people "spend their time."

This paper has proposed a theory of the primary functions of occupation and how they relate to health and survival, and it has proposed that sociocultural factors are deflecting occupation from its primary functions. It is desirable that following increased articulation and research into the possible consequences of the changes, political, social, and health policy can be influenced so that human rather than economic needs are central in future societies.

References

1. Leakey R, Lewin R. *People of the lake: man: his origins, nature, and future.* Penguin Books, 1978: 38–39.
2. Kolb B, Whishaw I Q. *Fundamentals of human neuropsychology.* 3rd ed. San Francisco: W H Freeman and Company, 1990: 106.
3. Lorenz K. *The waning of humaneness,* Munich: R Piper & Co Verlag, 1983. Translated USA: Little Brown and Company, 1987: 57–58.
4. Jerison H J. *Evolution of the brain and intelligence.* New York: Academic Press, 1973.
5. Marx K. The holy family. 1845: 125. In: Fischer E. *Marx in his own words.* London: Alien Lane The Penguin Press, 1970.
6. Marx K. Economic and philosophical manuscripts. 1843. In: Fischer E. *Marx in his own Words.* London: Alien Lane The Penguin Press, 1970: 31.
7. Marx K. Economic and philosophical Manuscripts. 1843. In: Fischer, E. *Marx in his own words.* London: Alien Lane The Penguin Press, 1970: 37.
8. Marx K. Capital 1.1867: 179–180. In Fischer E. *Marx in his own words.* London: Alien Lane The Penguin Press, 1970.
9. Braverman H. *Labor and monopoly capital: the deregulation of work in the twentieth century,* New York: Monthly Review Press, 1974.
10. Selye H, Monat A, Lazarus R S. *Stress and coping: an anthology.* 2nd ed. New York: Columbia University Press, 1985: 28.
11. Sigerist H E. *A history of medicine, Vol. 1,* primitive and archaic medicine. New York: Oxford University Press, 1955: 254–255.
12. Allport G W. The open system in personality theory. *Journal of abnormal and social psychology.* 1960, 61: 301–311.
13. Omstein R, Sobei D. *The healing brain: a radical new approach to health care.* London: MacMillan, 1988, p. 11–12.
14. Eysenck H S, Arnold W, Meili R. *Encyclopedia of psychology.* New York: Continuum Books The Seabury Press, 3979: 705–706.
15. Young P T. Drives. In: Sills D L, ed. *International encyclopedia of the social sciences.* The Macmillan Co & The Free Press. 1968: 275–276.
16. Dashiell J F. *Fundamentals of objective psychology.* Boston: Houghton Mifflin, 1928: 233–234.
17. Lorenz K. *The waning of humaneness,* Munich: R Piper & Co Verlag, 1983. Translated USA: Little Brown and Company, 1987: 21.

18. Lorenz K. *Civilized man's eight deadly sins,* translated by M. Latzke. London: Methuen & Co Ltd, 1974: 3–5.

19. Wolman B, ed. *Dictionary of behavioral science.* New York: Van Nostand Reinold Co, 1973: 250.

20. Anscombe G E M. Modern moral philosophy. *Philosophy.* 1958: 33.

21. Watts E D. Human needs. In Kuper A, Kuper J, eds. *The social science encyclopedia.* London: Routledge, 1985.

22. Bertalanffy L von. *General systems theory.* New York: George Baziller. 1968. 27.

23. Campbell J. *Winston Churchill's afternoon nap.* London: Paladin, 1988: 79

24. Argyle M. *The psychology of happiness.* London: Methucn and Co Ltd, 1987.

25. Csikszentmihalyi M. *Flow: the psychology of optimal experience.* New York: Harper and Row, 1990.

26. Virey. *L'hygiene philosophique.* Paris: Crochard, 1828.

27. Stephenson W. *The ecological development of man.* Sydney: Angus and Robertson, 1972: 217.

28. Wharton W J L, ed. *Captain Cook's journal during his first voyage around the world made in HM Bark Endeavour, 1768–1777.* London: Eliot Stock, 1893: 323.

29. Lorenz K. *Civilized man's eight deadly sins,* translated by M. Latzke. London: Methuen & Co Ltd, 1974: 12–13.

30. King-Boyes M J E. *Patterns of aboriginal culture then and now.* Sydney: McGraw-Hill Book Company, 1977.

31. Maslow A H. *Toward a psychology of being.* 2nd ed. New York: D Van Nostrand Company, 1968.

32. Campbell J. *Winston Churchill's afternoon nap.* London: Paladin, 1988: 14.

33. Lorenz K. *The waning of humaneness.* Munich: R Piper & Co Verlag, 1983. Translated USA: Little Brown and Company, 1987: 124.

34. Lorenz K. *The waning of humaneness.* Munich: R Piper & Co Verlag, 1983. Translated USA: Little Brown and Company, 1987: 124.

35. Shils E. Sociology. 799–810. In Kuyper A, Kuyper J, eds. *The social science encyclopedia.* London & New York: Routledge, 1985: 805.

36. Cynkin S, Robinson A M. Occupational therapy and activities health: toward health through activities. Boston: Little Brown and Company, 1990.

37. Primeau L A, Clarke F, Pierce D. Occupational therapy alone has looked upon occupation: future applications of occupational science to pediatric occupational therapy. *Occupational therapy in health care.* New York: Haworth Press, 1989: 6(4).

38. Keynes J M. Economic possibilities for our grandchildren. In *Essays in persuasion,* London: MacMillan, 1931.

39. Mufiiford L. *The condition of man.* London: Heinemann, 1944 and 1963.

CHAPTER 31

Health and the Human Spirit for Occupation

ELIZABETH J. YERXA

Reilly's (1962) fundamental hypothesis "that man, through the use of his hands as energized by mind and will, can influence the state of his own health" (p. 2) proposes a significant relationship between engagement in activity, as dictated by the human spirit for occupation, and healthfulness (see Chapter 7). I shall explore that connection by describing my views of occupation and health, sharing some assumptions, reviewing relevant ideas from an array of disciplines, and drawing implications for occupational science and its application in occupational therapy.

This article is based on my continuous search for ideas from other disciplines, a synthesis of which may contribute to the scholarly foundations of occupational therapy (occupational science) and should therefore be seen as a work in progress.

Views of Occupation and Health

The human spirit for activity is actualized, in a healthy way, through engagement in occupation: self-initiated, self-directed activity that is productive for the person (even if the product is fun) and contributes to others. Occupations are organized into patterns or the "elemental routines that occupy people" (Beisser, 1989, p. 166). These activities of daily living (ADL) are categorized by our culture as play, work, rest, leisure, creative pursuits, and other ADL that enable us to adapt to environmental demands. Dewey's (1910) criteria for a child's occupation were that it be of interest, be intrinsically worthwhile (relevant personally and socially), awaken curiosity, and lead to development. Engagement in occupation enables humans to learn competency.

I shall view health, not as the absence of organ pathology, but as an encompassing, positive, dynamic state of "well-beingness," reflecting adaptability, a good quality of life, and satisfaction in one's own activities. Notice that this perspective of health does not exclude persons with disabilities. They may have irremediable impairments but still possess the potential to be healthy, for example, by developing and using skills to achieve their vital goals (Pörn, 1993).

What is the connection between engagement in occupation and health? This question is crucial for humankind in the new millennium, for the 21st century will certainly usher in an unprecedented "era of chronicity" due to advances in medicine's ability to preserve life. What is thought about how people, including those with chronic impairments, achieve healthfulness through the use of their hands, minds, and will?

Assumptions

I always urge my graduate students to make their assumptions explicit, so I have to follow my own advice:

1. I shall view people as complex, multileveled (biological, psychological, social, spiritual), open systems who interact with their environments (Kagan, 1996) by using occupation to make an adaptive response to its demands. Consequently, human beings cannot be reduced to a single level, say that of the motor system, and retain their richness or identity. Similarly, water cannot be reduced to hydrogen and oxygen and still be wet and drinkable.

2. The occupational therapy profession is founded on an optimistic view of human nature (Reilly, 1962). Occupational therapists discover a person's resources and emphasize what that person can or might be able to do instead of the person's incapacities; what's right instead of what's wrong. We

are "search engines" for potential. Our profession is committed to improving life opportunities for all people, including those with so-called chronic impairments, a category that includes most of the persons we serve.

3. The postindustrial society is in danger of creating masses of throw-away people, a burgeoning underclass whose chronic impairments, homelessness, mental illness, and inadequate education and skills leave them outsiders in an increasingly technical, complex, and fast-paced society. In important respects, *most* of society, except for an elite superclass, may become an endangered species occupationally. As Beisser (1989) said when he lost the ability to work as a physician due to paralysis, "My place in the culture was gone" (p. 167). Similarly, for large segments of society, Rifkin (1995), an economist, predicted the "end of work." Work as we have known it may be replaced by a "technopoly" managed by an elite class who keeps the robots and computers operating, leaving millions without a job or a place in society. This endangerment to health and well-being is profound because our society lacks an agreed-upon, valued substitute for work. Because we often view work as an economic necessity rather than a biological, moral, and social imperative, we frequently fail to recognize the potential impact of unemployment and loss of occupational role on human health. The more than 70% of working-age persons with disabilities who are currently unemployed provides a window into the future (Bickenbach, 1993).

Relation of Engagement in Occupation to Health

Interests

Storr (1988), a British psychiatrist, proposed that our society has overvalued intimate relationships while paying too little attention to "work in solitude" as a source of health and happiness. Two opposing motives operate throughout life, one to bring us closer to people and another for autonomy. The second is as important as the first.

Creative persons classed among the world's great thinkers often lacked close personal ties. For example, Descartes, Newton, Kant, Nietzche, Kierkegaard, and Wittgenstein lived alone for most of their lives, finding their chief value in the "impersonal" (Storr, 1988). The

impersonal includes *interest* in doing almost anything from breeding carrier pigeons to designing aircraft. Such interest contributes to the economy of human happiness by fulfilling the need for autonomy, leading to both adaptation and creativity.

Storr (1988) criticized psychiatry and the social sciences for overlooking the importance of pursuing interests to meaning, happiness, discovery, creative contribution, and the human search for some pattern that makes sense out of life. Such pursuits can be a matter of life and death. Acting on interests may prevent mental collapse and subsequent death for persons in states of extreme deprivation. The capacity to be alone while pursuing one's unique interests is a valuable health resource, fulfilling the need for autonomy and achieving personal integration through activity one believes is worth doing. Interests energize occupation.

Satisfaction in Everyday Doing

When I become discouraged by the high-tech, business-oriented, specialist trajectory of our culture, I read Adolph Meyer (1931/1957). He never fails to revitalize my enthusiastic respect for the idea of occupation. Meyer (1922/1977 [see Chapter 4]) focused on the person's everyday doings and actual experiences as primary resources for health. Health was assessed by one's relative capacity for *satisfaction*, "doing and getting enough" in those cycles of activity and composure that mark the rhythms of life. Meyer's (1931/1957) formula for satisfaction included the components shown in Figure 31.1. His view of satisfaction and health suggests major concepts for investigation by occupational scientists. For example, *capacity* implies that people be viewed as individuals who have unique skills and resources; *opportunity* requires attention to environmental qualities such as novelty, affordances, attractors, and challenges that will stimulate activity; and *ambition* involves energizers of action such as interest, curiosity, will, desire, and personal perceptions of skills. In interaction, these contribute to satisfaction by influencing both performance (generating feedback) and mood (encompassing one's being).

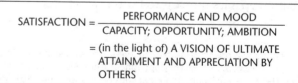

Figure 31.1. Formula for satisfaction (Meyer, 1931/1957, p. 81).

Meyer (1931/1957) placed this dynamic relationship within a cultural context, showing that both other people's appreciation of what we do and our own expectations of ourselves contribute to satisfaction. The formula suggests that health may be influenced by discovering or developing new capacities, changing the environment, nurturing ambition, improving performance, and modifying mood, all in ways appreciated by one's culture and acceptable to oneself. Meyer (1922/1977; see Chapter 4) proposed that occupational therapists provide opportunities rather than prescriptions in the spirit of this formula.

His formula applied to *all* people—physicians, psychiatric patients, and the public. Thus, health via satisfaction was possible for all, rather than requiring a special, separate track for those with psychopathology. Patients with mental illness were part of the mainstream of society, seeking the same satisfactions as anyone else, capable thereby of influencing their own health.

Meyer (1931/1957) saw potential everywhere; all people possessed assets and capacities: "A study and use of the assets, at the same time we attempt a direct correction of the ills, is the first important condition of a psychobiological therapy" (p. 157). But he was not blind to the challenge he posed: "To use the patient's assets is a more difficult problem than using something under our control" (p. 157). Capabilities discovered and nurtured could overcome psychiatric problems, which he viewed as problems of adaptation.

Meyer's (1931/1957) optimistic view of people emphasizing their resources, capabilities, habits, and skills that enable them to adapt to their environments with joy, satisfaction, and harmony places the spirit for occupation as central to human healthfulness. It is remarkable that his philosophy was applied in the early 1900s, long before the advent of psychotropic medications, because his patients must have exhibited severe symptoms rarely seen today. Yet he viewed even these persons as capable of healthy satisfaction through occupation.

Balance

Activity. Many theorists whose ideas are relevant to occupation and health propose the need for some sort of "healthy" balance. For example, Meyer (1922/1977; see Chapter 4) noted that people organize themselves in a kind of rhythm as they carry out their daily rounds of activity. To be healthy, people needed to be attuned to

the larger rhythms of night and day, of sleep and waking hours, of hunger and its gratifica-

tion and finally the big four—work and play and rest and sleep which our organism must be able to balance even under difficulty. (p. 641)

Meyer asserted that only by "actual doing" (p. 641) or performance could this balance be obtained. Consequently, all people needed to be provided with opportunities to work to achieve pleasure in their own achievement, and to learn a happy appreciation of time and the sacredness of the moment. This balance was learned through organizing one's own actions.

Pörn (1993), a contemporary philosopher, related health to people's ability to achieve their own goals through engagement in daily life activities and routines. He viewed people as acting subjects (not reacting objects). People, as actors, draw on three essentials: "a repertoire," an organized collection of abilities to act; an environment; and goals. Vital goals are personal objectives necessary for minimal happiness (p. 303). According to Pörn, health consists of achievement of a complex balance or equilibrium between people's environmental circumstances and the ability to realize their goals through a repertoire of abilities. Health is a kind of wholeness and general adaptedness that does not require freedom from pathology.

How could such healthfulness be assessed? We could look at the adequacy of one's repertoire (organized abilities to act), the appropriateness of one's environment (especially the opportunities it provides to exercise abilities), and the extent of realism in the person's goals in relation to both the environment and the repertoire.

How might health be fostered in a way that preserves and defends adaptation? This might be accomplished by addressing the repertoire (e.g., developing new skills for increased competence), the environment by its challenges, and the goals by helping the person alter his or her objectives. All three components need to be balanced for holistic care directed toward human agency.

Occupational therapists know this in their bones and hearts. In Sweden, they participated in research that validated Pörn's (1993) theory between persons with and without impairments. In this research, ability to achieve one's vital goals (via a repertoire of skills) was found to be more important to life satisfaction than degree of physical impairment among those with stroke (Bernspång, 1987).

Other theorists who have related balance to health include Csikszentmihalyi (1975), who posited the need for a balance between self-perceived skills and environmental demands, and Reilly (1962 [see Chapter 7], 1969, 1974), who related health to a balance between degree of environmental challenge and capacity for learning the skills, rules, and habits necessary to fulfill occupational role expectations. Offering a "just-right challenge" that enables an adaptive response promotes a crucial balance for health-promoting occupational therapy practice.

Information. Klapp (1986), a sociologist, proposed the need for another sort of balance concerning information and action. Today, health is threatened by the boredom that permeates postmodern life, creating a thick cloud over people's everyday experience. We feel trapped, satiated, habituated, and desensitized because we are bombarded by meaningless stimuli from the media, "noise" that requires no response. Listen to the monotonous, ever-urgent tones used by announcers and observe the sheer volume of noise created by the endless commercials and repetitive banality of the media. "Our ears are overwhelmed while we are denied a voice," Klapp observed (1986, p. 51). He defined information as "useful knowledge," contrasting it with "entropy" (p. 120), a tendency to randomness and confusion. When input does not arouse interest but continues relentlessly, people often escape into passivity or health-threatening "social placebos," such as alcohol, drugs, and other mood-altering addictions.

The desired balance that buffers boredom and contributes to health consists of "meaningful variety" that encourages learning and "meaningful redundancy," which is so familiar, reliable, and reassuring that it contributes to warm memories and a sense of community (Klapp, 1986, p. 118). (I think here of cultural rules and rituals.) People need to develop *skill* to respond to this overload of meaninglessness by learning to view their boredom as a signal for action. To be healthy, they need to be taught to create an individualized balance of meaningful variety and redundancy through discovering, developing, and acting on their own interests and by participating in the rules, habits, and rituals of their cultures.

Meyer's (1922/1977; see Chapter 4) vision of providing opportunities rather than prescriptions, contributing to performance and mood, offers occupation as an alternative to this health-threatening imbalance. Instead of escaping into unhealthy social placebos to alter their moods, people could learn to achieve their own balance of meaningful variety and meaningful ritual through engagement in activity worth doing.

Aristotle might have been right about the golden mean. Health as adaptation, satisfaction, and quality of life experience seems to require achievement of a desirable balance between environmental and personal attributes. Such a balance is highly individualized and is learned through opportunities to act on the environment as an agent. We need to learn much more about such healthy balances and how they might be fostered.

The Latent Consequences of Work

Recently a psychiatrist asked me, "Why is work so important to our patients? Why can't some other activity take its place?" Liebow's (1993) anthropological study of homeless women revealed their obsessive preoccupation with looking for and finding a job. Our own research with men who had spinal cord injuries found that they reserved the category of "work" almost exclusively for paid employment, even though they were engaged in many occupations that could have been called work (Yerxa & Baum, 1986). How is participation in the apparently significant occupation of work related to health as adaptation?

In technologically sophisticated societies, work is separated from other activities, such as leisure. Relationships that are largely based on work constitute a major source of societal structure and order (Argyle, 1987). Work appears to have a psychologically stabilizing effect on people. Leisure, to be satisfying in any important sense, needs to be viewed as the moral equivalent of work (Argyle, 1972) to fill its culturally significant role. People who are unemployed and have no organized leisure often become depressed, losing their sense of identify and purpose in life as well as their health.

Jahoda (1981) asked, why is work, as Marx observed, such a fundamental condition of human existence that people eat to work, not the other way around? She differentiated the "latent consequences" (p. 188) of work from its manifest outcome of earning a living. Latency meant the unintended but significant "by-products" of being employed (p. 188). Five latent consequences of employment seem relevant to health:

- Employment imposes a time structure on one's day.
- Employment implies regularly shared experiences and contacts with persons outside one's immediate family.
- Employment links persons to goals and purposes transcending their own.
- Employment defines important aspects of personal status and identity.
- Employment enforces activity, providing a predictable demand for action (Jahoda, 1981, p. 188).

Jahoda (1981) did not address the experience of "flow," that autotelic satisfaction in simply doing the work (Csikszentmihalyi, 1975), which is an important product for many people, nor did she discuss work's latent consequences for social units such as the family. However, her observations support the importance of work to health. Remove employment and you remove a person's strongest tie to reality (Freud, 1930), his or her place in the culture, threatening healthfulness. Work is supportive of health even under poor conditions. People may dislike their jobs, but they often dislike unemployment more (Argyle, 1987).

I still await the predicted utopia in which leisure becomes our major occupation. For leisure to be health promoting, it would have to convey the same latent consequences as work. Instead, the laboratory of unemployed persons with impairments and others who have lost their jobs due to corporate downsizing demonstrates the stubborn significance to health and quality of life of having work worth doing.

In many respects, the desire to engage in the occupation of work and its significance to human health and happiness are not fully appreciated until the opportunity to engage is taken away, whether by revolutionary social upheaval, as in today's postindustrial, increasingly automated society, or by the onset of impairment. Vash (1981), a woman who was severely paralyzed by polio as a teenager and later became a psychologist, put it this way: "The impact of disablement is largely contingent on the extent to which it interferes with what you are doing" (p. 15), not only the actual activities, but also the potential ones. Beisser (1989), who had been an ardent tennis player and medical student before he contracted polio, believed that "my place in the culture was gone" because he was no longer able to engage in the "elemental routines that occupy people" (pp. 166–167) and was disconnected from the familiar roles he had known in family, work, and sports. Yet the public, seeing Carolyn Vash and Arnold Beisser, would probably view inability to move as their most important characteristic, rendering them "disabled." Important though such impairment is, preoccupation with the loss of motor control blinds us to the significant loss of something important to do, the frustrated spirit for occupation, no longer served by their bodies, culture, or environment. Both of these articulate people believed that *this loss* was more important than their physical impairments. They echo Pörn's (1993) theory of health and Jahoda's (1981) latent consequences of work, revealing the connection between engagement in occupation and healthy adaptation.

Transcendence

The experiences of persons incarcerated under extreme conditions of deprivation and despair support the transcending effects of engagement in occupation that fosters survival and sanity (Storr, 1988). Frankl (1984), a psychiatrist who lived through Auschwitz, stated: "In the Nazi concentration camps, one could have witnessed that those who knew there was a task waiting for them to fulfill were most apt to survive" (p. 126). He reported that psychiatric investigations into Japanese, North Korean, and North Vietnamese prison camps reached the same conclusions.

The manuscript of Frankl's first book was confiscated when he was searched before incarceration. He felt this as a profound loss. His unfulfilled desire to rewrite the book not only helped him survive the rigors of camp life, but working on it, reconstructing the manuscript, and scribbling key words in shorthand on tiny scraps of paper, also enabled him to ward off attacks of delirium. Engagement in occupation, albeit mental, also enabled him to transcend his immediate disgust and despair. He visualized himself in a warm lecture room in front of an attractive audience. He was giving a lecture on the psychology of the concentration camp. By so doing, he rose above the suffering of the moment. Occupation enabled him to objectify and describe his oppressing situation from the "remote viewpoint of science" (Frankl, 1984, p. 95), transforming his emotions from despair into an interesting scientific study that he, himself, conducted.

Extreme environmental degradation reveals the potential transcending effects of occupation in stark clarity. People were more likely to survive such conditions when they had interests and tasks worth doing and were able to create transcending experiences that restored their sense of autonomy (Frankl, 1984).

Relevant Research on Occupation and Health

Hardy Personality

Kobasa (1982), an existentialist, believed that people construct a dynamic personality—"being in the world" (p. 6)— through their own actions. Because their life situations are always changing, they inevitably encounter stress. She asked, how do people confront unavoidable stresses and shape their lives successfully?

Her theory and research supported the idea of a "hardy personality" that resists stress and remains healthy. (In contrast to my definition, she defined health as lack of physical or psychiatric symptoms.) The three characteristics contributing to hardiness should interest occupational therapists:

- *Commitment*—"ability to believe in the value of who one is and what one is doing" (Kobasa, 1982, p. 6) involving oneself fully in life, including work, family, and social institutions. An overall sense of purpose, goals, and priorities acts as a buffer to stress.
- *Control*—"tendency to believe and act as *if* one can influence the course of events" (p. 7). Stress was viewed as a predictable consequence of one's own activity and subject to one's own direction.
- *Challenge*—a "belief that change rather than stability is the normative mode of life" (p. 7). Stress was viewed as an opportunity or incentive rather than as a threat. Hardy people search for new, interesting experiences and know where to turn for resources.

These three components contribute to "hardiness" or the ability to resist stress and maintain health. Kobasa hypothesized that when life is stressful, people with such hardiness would remain healthy. Her hypothesis was supported by research with male business executives, male general practice lawyers, and female medical outpatients in retrospective and prospective studies, using subjective and objective reports of illness indicators.

Kobasa's (1982) research connecting commitment, control, and challenge to hardiness in the face of stress supports the use of occupation as therapy to prepare people for engagement in the practical endeavors of everyday life. For if Meyer (1931/1957) was correct that people learn to achieve health in the doing, then such hardiness may be learned and developed through engagement in occupation. Gaining a sense of commitment in what one is doing, a sense of control over the course of events, and the seeking of challenges as a source of interest are products of one's adaptive responses to a "just-right" degree of challenge. In Kobasa's (1982) work, these products resisted the inevitable stressors of daily life and enabled people to maintain health. The most important piece missing from Kobasa's work is the *process* by which such characteristics are constructed by the person's actions in real life. I propose an important role for occupation.

Mortality

In today's world, engagement in some occupations is often trivialized, sometimes considered merely diver-

sion. This view may reflect our ignorance of the contribution of engagement in occupation not only to health, but also to actual survival.

In an 11-year study of the long-term survival of persons with spinal cord injuries, Krause and Crewe (1991) compared the characteristics of those still alive with those known to have died. The researchers hypothesized that the survivors would have superior medical and psychosocial adjustment. "Medical adjustment" measured by nonroutine medical appointments and hospitalizations, was expected to be the *most important* predictor of survival. But neither recent medical history nor emotional adjustment predicted survival. Instead, strong support was found for a relationship between *activity level* and survival. Those who were more active, vocationally and socially, in participating in a round of daily occupations were more likely to have survived. Activity level was more important than medical history or a mediating emotional state. The authors, both psychologists, concluded that "counseling must go beyond facilitating emotional adjustment" (p. 84). Rather, people need to be taught the skills to participate in life, skills that might influence *survival* itself.

In another study (Wright, 1983), 100 patients with severe disabilities underwent rehabilitation in a hospital that encouraged their maximum participation. Patients designed their own schedules and solved problems as they arose. If a wheelchair needed repair, the patients worked out how to get it done. One year after discharge, these more "occupationally autonomous" patients not only showed a greater degree of sustained improvement in activities of daily living, but also a *lower mortality* rate than did the control group.

Both theory and research demonstrate that an environment that provides opportunities for active engagement in life contributes to health, well-being, independence, and survival. We need to take another look at the trivialization of occupation. What could be less trivial than survival?

Conclusions

An increasing body of knowledge from an array of disciplines supports Reilly's (1962; see Chapter 7) great hypothesis. Humans can influence the state of their own health, provided that they are given the opportunity to develop the skills to do so. The human spirit for occupation, developed through eons of time in evolution, unfolding through development, and actualized through daily learning, needs to be nurtured to contribute to the health, quality of life, and survival of persons and society.

Occupational therapists and occupational scientists need to reaffirm that engagement in occupation, rather than being trivial, is an essential mediator of healthy adaptation and a vital source of joy and happiness in one's daily life. In the new millennium, the era of chronicity and the potential "end of work" as we have known it will pose particularly strenuous challenges: How can our profession help create an environment in which people have opportunities to engage in the "moral equivalent of work" and thus contribute to their own health? How can all people be provided with opportunities or "just-right challenges" to discover their interests and potential for something worth doing?

Occupational therapy could promote a new concept of health to replace the traditional view. Health, perceived as possession of a repertoire of skills enabling people to achieve their valued goals in their own environments, would then be possible for *all people,* including those with chronic impairments. A major objective would be to achieve "equality of capability" (Bickenbach, 1993). To do this, we need to learn much, much more about how human beings develop the adaptive skills, rules, and habits that enable competence as well as how occupational therapists might create a "just-right environmental challenge" to enable an adaptive response. Such "coaching" from occupational therapists could benefit all people who need to develop skills in order to survive, contribute, and achieve satisfaction in their daily life activities, whether or not they have impairments.

To serve humankind well requires that we discover much more knowledge about people as agents, in their own environments, engaged in daily occupations. We need to broaden our concept of ADL beyond self-care to include study of the daily routines that occupy people in real-life contexts. To learn what we need to know requires that we accept the challenge of becoming ardent students of life's daily activities, grappling courageously with the ambiguity and complexity of occupation, the occupational human, and the contexts in which occupation takes place. Only then will we fulfill our commitment to persons with chronic impairments and assure that our humanistic values are expressed in an occupational therapy practice that contributes to life opportunities and health for a new millennium.

Acknowledgments

A major portion of this article was presented as the Wilma West Lecture at the Ninth Occupational Science Symposium at the University of Southern California on April 12, 1996. It is respectfully dedicated to the memory of Wilma West, MA, OTR, FAOTA, who contributed so much of her spirit to occupational therapy.

References

Argyle, A. (1972). *The social psychology of work.* New York: Laplinger.

Argyle, M. (1987). *The psychology of happiness.* London: Methven.

Beisser, A. (1989). *Flying without wings: Personal reflections on being disabled.* New York: Doubleday.

Bernspång, B. (1987). *Consequences of stroke. Aspects of impairments disabilities and life satisfaction with special emphasis on perception and occupational therapy.* Unpublished medical dissertation, Umeå University, Umeå, Sweden.

Bickenbach, J. (1993). *Physical disability and social policy.* Toronto, Ontario: University of Toronto Press.

Csikszentmihalyi, M. (1975). *Beyond boredom and anxiety: The experience of play in work and games.* San Francisco: Jossey-Bass.

Dewey, J. (1910). *How we think.* Lexington, MA: Heath.

Frankl, V. (1984). *Man's search for meaning* (Rev. ed.). New York: Washington Square.

Freud, S. (1930). *Civilization and its discontents.* London: Hogarth.

Jahoda, M. (1981). Work, employment, and unemployment: Values, theories, and approaches in social research. *American Psychologist, 36,* 184–191.

Kagan, J. (1996, January 12). Point of view: The misleading abstractions of social scientists. *Chronicle of Higher Education, XLII,* p. A52.

Klapp, O. (1986). *Overload and boredom: Essays on the quality of life in the information society.* New York: Greenwood.

Kobasa, S. (1982). The hardy personality: Toward a social psychology of stress and health. In G. Sander & J. Sules (Eds.), *Social psychology of health and illness,* (pp. 3–32). Hillsdale, NJ: Erlbaum.

Krause, J. S., & Crewe, N. M. (1991). Prediction of long-term survival of persons with spinal cord injury: An 11-year prospective study. In M. Eisenberg & R. Glueckauf (Eds.), *Psychological aspects of disability* (pp. 76–84). New York: Springer.

Liebow, E. (1993). *Tell them who I am. The lives of homeless women.* New York: Penguin.

Meyer, A. (1957). *Psychobiology: A science of man.* Springfield, IL. Charles C. Thomas. Original work published 1931.

Meyer, A. (1977). The philosophy of occupation therapy. *American Journal of Occupational Therapy, 31,* 639–642. Original work published 1922. Reprinted as Chapter 4.

Pörn, I. (1993). Health and adaptedness. *Theoretical Medicine, 14,* 295–303.

Reilly, M. (1962). Occupational therapy can be one of the great ideas of 20th century medicine, 1961 Eleanor Clarke Slagle Lecture. *American Journal of Occupational Therapy, 16,* 1–9. Reprinted as Chapter 7.

Reilly, M. (1969). The educational process. *American Journal of Occupational Therapy, 23,* 299–307.

Reilly, M. (1974). *Play as exploratory learning.* Beverly Hills, CA: Sage.

Rifkin, J. (1995). *The end of work.* New York: Putnam.

Storr, A. (1988). *Solitude. A return to the self.* New York: Ballantine.

Vash, C. L. (1981). *The psychology of disability. Springer series on rehabilitation, 1.* New York: Springer.

Wright, B. (1983). *Physical disability: A psychosocial approach* (2nd ed.). New York: Harper & Row.

Yerxa, E. J., & Baum, S. (1986). Engagement in daily occupations and life satisfaction among people with spinal cord injuries. *Occupational Therapy Journal of Research, 6,* 271–283.

CHAPTER 32

Resilience and Human Adaptability: Who Rises Above Adversity?

1990 ELEANOR CLARKE SLAGLE LECTURE

SUSAN B. FINE

We work in a world of traumas and triumphs. Most of the persons we serve come to us out of necessity, struggling with the sequelae of disease and illness or the aftermath of natural or man-made disasters. We bring our expertise and compassion; they bring their bodies, minds, and compromised lives. Our worlds converge around a shared task: identifying and enhancing their capacities for daily living. We pursue problems of movement, perception, cognition, affect, and social capacity within the context of their roles and aspirations. Our contacts may be extensive, but often they are brief and only partially fulfilled. Our patients move on with varying degrees of functional ability—some with determination and buoyancy, other with little confidence that life is actually worth living. We remain, frequently knowing little about the factors that have influenced the outcome of our efforts, in spite of their compelling importance to our patients, our professional viability, and the health care system.

This Eleanor Clarke Slagle Lecture is a study of outcome—outcome that often defies the odds. It is a study of lives characterized by extraordinary hardships and remarkable abilities to move beyond them. It poses a core question: Who rises above adversity? It ventures beyond traditional concerns for pathology and vulnerability, beyond theoretical and statistical methods. In fact, its most valuable data come directly from the personal experiences of those confronted with chronic or terminal illness, physical and mental disabilities, abuse, impoverishment, the Holocaust, and other disasters. I have pursued many life narratives, not as a test of endurance in the face of human suffering (although it made for a more tearful year than most), not in search of heroes and heroines (although there were many),

but in an effort to more fully understand factors that influence resilient responses. The voices of the resilient send a powerful message: Personal perceptions and responses to stressful life events are crucial elements of survival, recovery, and rehabilitation, often transcending the reality of the situation or the interventions of others. The inner life (affective and cognitive processes and content) holds the potential for transforming traumas into varying degrees of triumph. Ironically, these same phenomena are often ignored in the clinical reasoning and practice of many health professions, including our own.

Consequently, this paper is intended to heighten the reader's appreciation of the powerful interaction among a person's inner psychological life, his or her relationship to the surrounding world, and his or her emerging functional capacities. It pursues these themes by first providing an overview of theoretical constructs about the human response to adversity. Second, it focuses on extreme life events and the personal and social meaning ascribed to them. Third, it addresses the phenomenon of resilience and the means by which persons in extreme situations have coped. Implications for occupational therapy practice are then considered.

Overcoming Adversity: A Human Condition

The experience of adversity and the drive to rise above it are themes that characterize the human condition. The inevitability of life's trials and tribulations and the struggles between good and evil are evident in religious traditions, myths, the arts, and everyday conversation. Although adversity is ultimately a personal experience, in the bigger scheme of things it is faceless and timeless. We have grown up with both the ascendance of Cinderella and the failure of Icarus. We share such maxims as "It's always something" (Radner, 1989) or "You

This chapter was previously published in the *American Journal of Occupational Therapy, 45*, 493–503. Copyright © 1991, American Occupational Therapy Association. Reprinted with permission. http://dx.doi.org/10.5014/ajot.45.6.493

have to take the bad with the good." These universal themes attempt to guide us in matters of social order and disorder.

The Law of Disruption and Reintegration

There is also a professional literature devoted to understanding the human response to disruptions, the search for order and balance, and the consequences of prolonged imbalance. Although taxonomies and belief systems vary, a central theme, linked to Cannon's (1939) work in biology and physics, identifies a recurring cycle of disruption and reintegration as a natural and necessary part of one's growing capacities to adapt to internal and external change (Flach, 1988). In today's lexicon we speak of risk, stress, coping, competency, crisis theory, and biopsychosocial models. The past has been marked by a more disparate array of assumptions.

The relationship of stress to disease has been the highest priority among clinicians since Hippocratic times. Attempts at developing broader, systematic constructs have emerged from a number of disciplines. Psychoanalysis has given us ego mechanisms of defense as a metaphor for mental processes that handle crisis and threats. Freudian views emphasize a hierarchy of defenses that transform conflict-ridden impulses into more acceptable thoughts and actions. Ego psychology promotes reality-oriented, purposeful, conflict-free capacities (i.e., attention, perception, and memory) that are future-oriented and that render one capable of transforming situations rather than being transformed by them. In this formulation, adaptive functioning is seen as the relative use of coping capacities over defense mechanisms (Anthony & Cohler, 1987). The growth and cumulative effects of coping resources and skills over the life span are reflected in Erikson's (1963) classic developmental theories.

A behaviorist tradition also emerged with an early emphasis on the consequences of concrete problem solving. Today, as cognitive behaviorism, it is concerned with the cognitive components of coping skills and the Eriksonian belief that "successful coping promotes a sense of self-efficacy, which in turn, inspires more efforts at mastering difficult situations" (Moos & Schaefer, 1984, p. 6).

Endocrinologist Hans Selye (1978) assumed importance in the disruption–reintegration debate. Half a decade of work on stress and its hormonal and neurochemical correlates has had a great impact on professional and popular views of prevention and disease management. Selye's original emphasis on the singular importance of the stressful event itself has been mediated by a growing belief that the physical or psychological impact of any demand will vary depending on how we interpret the situation and how able we are to do something about it (Lazarus & Folkman, 1984).

Moos and Billings (1982) elaborated by organizing coping skills into three areas: appraisal-focused coping (i.e., efforts to understand and find meaning in a crisis), problem-focused coping (i.e., attempts to deal with the reality and consequences of the crisis and create a better situation), and emotion-focused coping (i.e., handling the feelings provoked by the crisis).

The cognitive appraisal process (how we interpret personal experiences) is central to a great deal of contemporary thought on coping. Stress itself has been defined as a "relationship between person and environment that is appraised by the person as taxing or exceeding his or her resources and endangering his or her well being" (Lazarus & Folkman, 1984, p. 19). Although social psychology traditionally emphasizes the role of external stressors and cognitive strategies (i.e., logical analysis, mental preparation, cognitive redefinition, and avoidance or denial), internal phenomena must not be ignored. Personal theories of reality about oneself and one's world, developed over time and generally outside of awareness, serve as a filter through which we perceive, interpret, and respond to experiences (Janoff-Bulman & Timko, 1987). Disturbing thoughts and memories can also heavily influence the appraisal process (Houston, 1987).

The credibility of the cognitive appraisal paradigm is enhanced by the newly integrated discipline of psychoneuroimmunology, which is "the study of the intricate interaction of consciousness (psycho), brain and central nervous system (neuro) and the body's defense against external infection and aberrant cell division (immunology)" (Pelletier & Herzing, 1988, p. 29). The impact of personal mood and attitudes on the immune system has opened new doors for researchers and clinicians. Studies have found that one's immune system benefits from confronting traumatic memories, looking at life optimistically, and living at a mildly hectic pace (Goleman, 1989). This line of thought will no doubt continue to provide us with newer and different hypotheses about the laws of disruption and reintegration.

For now, contemporary biopsychosocial formulations represent a robust model. Capacities to meet challenging demands and stand up to disruptions depend on inborn and acquired skills, the material and interpersonal resources in the environment, and the psychosocial capacities to handle anxieties that arise when one is performing various life tasks. Successful adaptation is dependent on the degree of fit among these factors. Although mastery is both developed and sustained by manageable challenges, challenges that are too demanding or too dangerous defeat resources for coping and reintegration (White, 1976).

And dangers there are! The law of disruption and re-integration does not promise, or always deliver, a rose garden. Life events continually test the durability of the balance we try to maintain.

Ordeals Beyond Our Control

There are life events that are experienced as traumatic because they are severe ordeals beyond our control. Under circumstances of predictable, moderate stress, persons call on conventional patterns and solve problems with characteristic resources and adaptive styles. But extreme situations and the stress accompanying them are not conventional. By their nature they are beyond the range of the predictable; previous experiences have not prepared us for them. How does one prepare for a spinal tumor, a brain injury, a schizophrenic episode, or a devastating earthquake? How does one comprehend Auschwitz or Dachau, where

> Dreams used to come in the brutal nights,
> Dreams crowding and violent
> Dreamt with body and soul,
> Of going home, of eating, of telling our story.
> Until quickly and quietly, came
> The dawn reveille:
> *Wstawàch.*
> And the heart cracked in the breast. (Levi, 1965, p. xi)

Extreme experiences such as these are characterized by a lack of conventional social structure, a loss of anchor in reality, and a lack of ability to predict or anticipate outcomes (Torrance, 1965). Although we associate such phenomena with the high drama of hostage situations, prolonged combat, or concentration camps, they may also define the experience of persons whose lives are linked with ours on a daily basis, that is, our patients. Perhaps we ourselves have endured trauma or the sudden onset of a life-threatening illness.

> Being full of strength and vigor one moment and virtually helpless the next . . . with all one's powers and faculties one moment and

without them the next . . . such a change, such a suddenness, is difficult to comprehend and the mind casts about for explanations. (Sacks, 1984, p. 21)

There are those, like Lifton (1988), who view man "as a perpetual survivor . . . of 'holocausts' large and small, personal and collective, that define much of existence" (p. 12). Although the Holocaust was a horrifying reality, as a metaphor it illuminates many other ordeals, helping us to understand and negotiate them. The vivid words and images of those with illness and disability also reveal the deeper meaning of their experiences—meaning that defines the nature of their adaptive task and shapes the quality of their reintegration.

The Personal and Social Meaning of Trauma

There are many reasons to perceive extreme life events as threatening. The most stressful dimensions appear to be those that challenge personal assumptions about oneself and the structure of the world one lives in. Much of this is linked with the phenomenon of control: the ability (or the perceived ability) to change, predict, understand, or accept environmental transactions within a meaningful context (Potocki & Everly, 1989). The sense of being in control and the desire for such control are believed to be crucial aspects of personality affecting physical and mental health as well as recovery potential.

The perception of self, with its elements of body image, identity, and self-worth, were dominant themes in every narrative I encountered, whether the trauma occurred in Vietnam, Theresienstadt, a hospital in London, or a city in Arizona. The pervasive threat to, or loss of, identity was as potent a force as—and sometimes more significant than— any real threat to life and limb. The tattooed number on the arm of a concentration camp inmate had its counterpart in the history number on a hospital ID bracelet. As startling as this analogy may seem, in the eyes of the "number" it may well mean humiliation, a lack of personal validation, and varying degrees of dehumanization. Just as prisoners of war are stripped of rank, role, and place in their reference group, victims of fires suffer losses of important nonhuman anchors for personal identity (Rosenfeld, 1989). Stroke victims, made captive by their disease and an impersonal hospital environment, lose the ability and opportunity to act on their own behalf.

409

In losing one's identity, one must replace it with another. How one chooses the new altered self is no small task. "Feelings of fear, vulnerability . . . sadness over losses and weakness about not being able to control one's life or one's emotional reactions, contribute to feelings of defectiveness" (Marmar & Horowitz, 1988, p. 96). The impact of confinement, isolation, and perceptual distortions is described by neurologist Oliver Sacks following a near-death accident, serious leg injury, disturbing hospitalization, and role change from doctor to patient.

> I was physiologically, in imagination, and feeling . . . a pygmy, a prisoner, a patient . . . without the faintest awareness. How could one know one had shrunk, if one's frame of reference itself shrunk? (1984, p. 157)

Experiences that reflect a loss of self-control are often a central issue in psychiatric disorders as well. It is evident in schizophrenia, for example, when unpredictable symptoms turn "sparkles of light into demon eyes" (McGrath, 1984) or when a partially observing ego is "aware enough to recognize the dangers of not being able to control what I'm doing or thinking" (a patient, personal communication, October 1989).

Psychological stress, induced by threats of loss of self or failure, is also highly dependent on social values and the person's acceptance of the culture's definitions of what is valuable. Finding a new self or coming to terms with the only self one has ever known is reflected in the mirror others place before us. There is humiliation and pain generated

> by a gait to embarrass, to make children laugh, a clumsy countering locomotion . . . from only the most exacting, determined efforts to control. Inside my rolling head, behind my shocked, magnified eyeballs, my brain orders, with utmost precision, each awkward jerk of thigh, leg, foot. (Weaver, 1985, p. 43)

Jean Améry provides us with a powerful metaphor for thinking about a person's sense of his or her own body and place in the world when mastery and control of that body is violated through intentional political torture, abuse, or from the pain of illness and medical procedures.

> He who has suffered torture can no longer feel at ease in the world. Faith in humanity—

cracked by the first slap across the face, then demolished by torture, can never be recovered. (Améry, 1986, p. xiii)

There are, of course, many forms of torture. The torture that physical illness may bestow need not be limited to bodily discomfort or pain, but "visits upon [people] a disease of social relations no less real than the paralysis of the body" (Murphy, 1987, p. 4). Anthropologist John Murphy viewed his spinal tumor, growing paralysis, and confinement as an assault on his identity and a disruption of ties with others. In depicting his illness as an extended field visit to an unfamiliar culture, he identified a primal scene of sociology—the social confrontation of persons with significant flaws, where someone looks or acts differently and we are uncertain as to what to say or where to look. This robs the encounter of cultural guidelines, leaving those involved uncertain about what to expect and what to do. For Murphy, "it has the potential for social calamity" (p. 87).

This calamity is also experienced as being in limbo. Sacks (1984) viewed this as a by-product of his body agnosia and the empathic agnosia of his surgeon, who insisted that nothing was wrong. His disease and lack of a human foothold (i.e., adequate communication and validation) left Sacks with a sense of double nothingness. "Now doubly, I had no leg to stand on; unsupported, doubly" (p. 108). Kleinman (1988), in turn, characterized limbo, for those with chronic illness, as "the dangerous crossing of borders, the interminable waiting to exit and reenter normal everyday life . . . the perpetual uncertainty of whether one can return at all" (p. 181).

I heard this again and again: a common thread, a theme that plagued Holocaust survivors and Vietnam veterans as well as the physically and mentally disabled—the gulf between the self and others (family, friends, caregivers, society). Who will listen? Who will understand what we are experiencing? Who will believe where we have been and what we have endured? Who will validate us as we continue to deal with adversity and its imprints?

Resilience

For some, the imprints are so deeply etched that they succumb. Others endure under conditions that seem unsupportable to health. Redl's (1969) work with adolescents who have beat the odds inspired the concept of *ego resilience,* that is, the capacity to withstand pathogenic pressure, the ability to recover rapidly from a temporary collapse even without outside help, and the strength to bounce back to normal or even supernormal levels of functioning. Demos (1989) suggested that, in its most developed state, such buoyancy requires "an active stance, persistence, the application of a variety of skills and strategies over a wide range of situations and problems . . . [and] flexibility . . . to know when to use what" (p. 5).

The formal study of resilience emerged in epidemiological studies on susceptibility to heart disease over 25 years ago. It is only within the past 15 years, however, that more rigorous efforts have been made to extricate it from a disease model and focus instead on "good psychosocial capacities such as competence, coping, creativity, and confidence" (Anthony & Cohler, 1987, p. x). Although healthfulness remains a less-than-perfect body of knowledge, a variety of popular and scientific resources provide direction for the reader's ongoing investigation, including descriptions of personal experiences (Brown, 1990; Browne, Connors, & Stern, 1985; Cousins, 1979; Egendorf, 1986; Gill, 1988; Heller & Vogel, 1986; Miller, 1985; Minear, 1990; Nolan, 1987; Sheehan, 1982; Trillin, 1984), situational studies of combat (Elder & Clipp, 1988; Rahe & Genender, 1983), studies of disasters (Bolin & Trainer, 1978; Lifton & Olson, 1976) and illness (Cleveland, 1984; Cohen & Lazarus, 1973), studies of the invulnerable child (Anthony & Cohler, 1987; Dugan & Coles, 1989; Garmezy & Masten, 1986; Murphy & Moriarty, 1976), and longitudinal investigations of adaptation (Chess & Thomas, 1984; Vaillant, 1977; Werner & Smith, 1982).

Resilience has been chronicled in studies of famous men and women who were highly stressed and traumatized as children, among them, George Orwell, Charles Dickens, Anton Chekov, Kathe Kollowitz, Pablo Picasso, and Buster Keaton (Goertzel & Goertzel, 1962; Miller, 1990; Shengold, 1989). Resilience, however, is evident in all walks of life. What is less clear is how persons manage to marshal the necessary resources. What enabled young Ryan White, confronted with two life-threatening illnesses, humiliation, and rejection, to become so articulate a spokesman for AIDS? What contributed to the brutalized Central Park jogger's remarkable recovery and recent promotion in her highly competitive investment banking firm? These are questions whose answers have as many nuances as there are people and ordeals, for resilience is not all of one piece.

Resilience is made operational by cognitive and behavioral coping skills and the recruitment of social support. Lazarus and Folkman (1984) suggested that such skills do not come all at once. Rather, they are acquired through a developmental process—a process of selecting from available alternatives and having persons reinforce the skills that are necessary to make coping possible. Studies of vulnerability and competence in children and adolescents have provided valuable insight into some aspects of this multifaceted and shifting phenomenon. Theoretical models of stress resistance view the relationship between stress and personal attributes from several perspectives: as compensation (personal attributes help to improve adjustment when stress diminishes competence), as protection (personal traits interact with stress in predicting adjustment), or as a challenge (stressors enhance competence) (Garmezy, 1983). Dispositional attributes of the child, family cohesion and warmth, and the use of external support systems by parents and children are mechanisms that buffer stress and promote resilient responses. Temperament, sex, intellectual ability, humor, empathy, social problem-solving skills, social expressiveness, and an inner locus of control have been found to influence adaptation under adverse conditions (Garmezy, 1985). These phenomena, however, show variability over time and at different developmental periods (Werner & Smith, 1982) and are influenced by changing demands of the environment. Coping, for children and adults alike, reflects traitlike and situation-specific elements (Kahana, Kahana, Harel, & Rosner, 1988).

Resilience is often measured behaviorally on the basis of the person's competence and success in meeting society's expectations despite great obstacles. Internal indexes (thoughts and feelings) are often ignored, despite evidence that impressive social competence may well be heavily correlated with depression and anxiety (Miller, 1990; Peck, 1987). Clinicians and researchers are alerted to attend to the distinctions and interactions between adaptive behavior and emotional status. Resilience needs to be examined and understood from both perspectives.

Resilient Perspectives

Truly functional coping behavior has been characterized as not only lessening the immediate impact of stress, but also as maintaining a sense of self-worth and unity with the past and an anticipated future (Dimsdale, 1974). It involves two distinct tasks: a response to the requirements of the situation and a response to the feelings about the situation. Author Nancy Mairs (1986), struggling with multiple sclerosis, chronic depression, and agoraphobia, explained the process:

> Each gesture . . . carries a weight of uncertainty, demands significant attention: buttoning my shirt, changing a light bulb, walking down stairs. The minutiae of my life have had to assume dramatic proportions. If I could not . . . delight in them, they would likely drown me in rage and self-pity.

> Yet I am unwilling to forgo the adventurous life; the difficulty of it, even the pain, the . . . fear, and the sudden brief lift of spirit that graces . . . the pilgrimage. If I am to have it . . . I must change the terms by which it is lived. . . . I refine adventure, make it smaller and smaller . . . whether I am feeding fish flakes to my bettas . . . lying wide-eyed in the dark battling yet another bout of depression, cooking a chicken . . . [or] meeting a friend for lunch. . . . I am always having the adventures that are mine to have. (pp. 6–7)

Mairs accepted the challenge and altered her life-style in the face of unpredictable capacity while maintaining some semblance of control over her life through a commitment to scaled-down adventures. Even in the presence of many serious problems she demonstrated what Kobasa (1979) and colleagues have called *hardiness*. Hardiness is characterized by challenge, commitment, and control attributes. Challenge is expressed as a belief that change, rather than stability, is normal in life and is an incentive for growth rather than a threat to security. Control is expressed by feeling and acting as if one is influential rather then helpless. Influence is operationalized through the use of imagination, knowledge, skill, and choice. Commitment is a tendency to involve oneself rather then feel alienated from situations; it involves a generalized sense of purpose that allows one to find events, things, and people meaningful and to approach situations rather than avoid them.

In extraordinarily stressful situations (the ones that diminish social structure, connections with reality, and a sense of predictability), opportunities to operationalize commitment, control, and challenge orientations are greatly compromised. Nonetheless, cognitive and behavioral coping mechanisms and efforts to recruit so-cial support emerge and find expression in the most remarkable ways. The personal perspectives of the persons whose anecdotes follow are a tribute to the resourcefulness of the human mind and spirit. Their thoughts, feelings, and actions reflect the true character of resilience.

Hope and the Will to Overcome

Hope and the will to overcome are evident in the poignant poetry of children who found comfort and inspiration in the resilience of nature while confined in a Czechoslovakian camp in 1944:

> The sun has made a veil of gold
> So lovely that my body aches.
> Above, the heavens shriek with blue
> Convinced I've smiled by some mistake.
> The world's abloom and seems to smile.
> I want to fly but where, how high?
> If in barbed wire, things can bloom
> Why couldn't I? I will not die! (Anonymous, in *I Never Saw Another Butterfly*, 1978, p. 52)

Hope and the will to overcome emerge in others as a fierce, sometimes raging will to live, that is, "the burning desire to tell, to bear witness" (Gill, 1988, p. 59), "to testifying on behalf of all those whose shadows will be bound to mine forever" (Wiesel, 1990, p. 15), "to live not for oneself, but to lament those who died [in Hiroshima]" (Tamiki, 1990, p. 30).

Affiliation and the Recruitment of Social Support

Acquiring a sense of belonging to a social group or, for that matter, to all of life, is a powerful way to sustain oneself in the face of death or other extremes. It may manifest itself by turning one's attention inward to memories and images of loved ones, by participating in an organized underground movement, or by devising a tap code to communicate through cell walls to other Vietnam prisoners of war. It also emerges through the collaboration of a therapist and a severely mentally ill woman who is struggling against great odds to restore a semblance of autonomy and self-respect:

> You believed in me . . . were willing to take a chance on my being able to handle an apartment when my family felt it would be a waste of money. We had hopes; I didn't want to let you down . . . and I haven't. (a patient, personal communication, 1989)

Finding Meaning and Purpose

The identification of purpose, or finding meaning in an ordeal, was described by Viktor Frankl (1984) as "the last of human freedoms"—choosing one's attitude in any given set of circumstances, having at least the power and the control over how you interpret and explain what happens to you. Individuals find meaning and purpose in many different ways. Some find it in an increased commitment to religion, a political ideal, or a social cause. Others find it by using intellect and creativity to combat devastating fear. Many concentration camp victims and prisoners of war played chess and built houses, nail by nail, in their mind's eye; one man prepared a full German–English dictionary on scraps of paper during his incarceration and published it after his release. Others claimed that even forced labor was sustaining.

Interestingly, despite confining, constraining situations with extremely limited resources, many sought to find meaning and retain interests, values and skills through focused, self-regulating activity. "The prisoners who fared the best in the long run were those who . . . could retain their personality system largely intact . . . where previous interests, values and skills could to some extent be carried on" (Hamburg, Coelho, & Adams, 1974, p. 413). In situational studies of combat, illness, and the anticipated death of family members, Gal and Lazarus (1975) reported reductions in anxiety and feelings of helplessness even when activities did not provide actual control over the situation. In contrast, the vulnerable were described by Eitinger as those who "felt completely helpless and passive, and had lost their ability to retain some sort of self-activity" (Hamburg et al., 1974, p. 413). Our continuing efforts to understand the complex role of occupation in remediating illness and maintaining health may be greatly enhanced through studies of the spontaneous behavior of those in stressful situations.

The Capacity to Step Back

Frankl's (1984) disgust with his own trivial preoccupations with survival found him, in fantasy, lecturing on the psychology of concentration camps. Both he and his troubles became the object of a psychoscientific study undertaken by himself that later contributed to the development of a school of psychotherapy. Frankl demonstrated the capacity to step back and, in so doing, preserved a part of himself from extraordinary degradation, pain, and loss. Functioning somewhat like a solution to a figure–ground problem, this process provides one with the option of ignoring aspects of the situation that are out of one's control. It may appear as a differential focus on the good, or it may be marked by a heightened capacity for observation, that is, a period of exalted receptivity when details of events, faces, words, or sensations are retained (Levi, 1987). This is evident in the writings of Wiesel (1990), Cousins (1979), Heller and Vogel (1986), Brown (1990), and Nolan (1987). None perceived themselves to be victims or survivors, but rather, witnesses to their own experience.

There Is More to Oneself Than Current Circumstance Suggests

The discovery of the new or real self is artfully reflected in Frank's (1988) study of embodiment—the experience and meaning of disability in American culture. She described a young woman born with quadrilateral limb deficiencies who stressed her assets instead of her deficits—her womanly figure (like Venus de Milo's) and her ability to write better with her stumps than with her artificial arms. Interestingly, her rehabilitation team viewed her refusal to use prosthetics as poor adaptation.

Dugan and Coles (1989), in turn, described a 6-year-old Black girl who was initiating school desegregation in New Orleans in the face of mobs, violence, and threats to her life. She hoped she would "get through one day and then another," and if she did, "it will be because there is more to me than I ever realized" (p. xiv).

Novel Applications of Problem-Solving Strategies

Coping involves creative and reflective behavior (White, 1976). Resilience is manifest in the ability to turn a familiar way of solving problems into a novel application, one that may save a life. When Sacks (1984) sustained his injury while mountain climbing alone, he was at great risk for dying of exposure. He reported that there came to his aid a kinetic melody, rhythm, and motor music. "Now, so to speak, I was musicked along" (p. 30). Remembrances of the Volga Boatmen's Song gave him the strength and rhythm to "row" himself along the ground for many hours until he found help.

Transforming Dross Into Gold

Vaillant's (1977) longitudinal study of the life and coping strategies of a group of Harvard graduates documented the way in which the mature ego mechanisms

413

of altruism, humor, suppression, and sublimation function to transform disturbances into adaptive behavior, thus turning "dross into gold" (p. 16). This is, in part, the way the speechless, palsied Irish poet Christopher Nolan (1987) found his mellifluous voice:

> Fossilized for so long now, he was going to speak to anyone interested enough to listen. . . . Now he shared the same world as everyone else; he could choose how much to tell and craftily decide how much to hold back. His voice would be his written word. (p. 98)

The same mechanisms allowed comedian Buster Keaton to devote his life to making others laugh, while unable to laugh spontaneously himself (Miller, 1990). Long before Norman Cousins found health and fame in laughter and neuroscience linked it to our immune systems, humor was acknowledged to be one of the truly elegant defenses in the human repertoire (Lefcourt & Martin, 1986). "Like hope, humor permits one to bear and yet to focus upon what may be too terrible to be borne" (Vaillant, 1977, p. 386). This is precisely what ailing critic Anatole Broyard (1990) did when he quipped, "What a critically ill person needs above all is to be understood. Dying is a misunderstanding you have to get straightened out before you go" (p. 29).

Resilience is not a miraculous rescue. It can be a mere thread that wrestles itself to the surface of an otherwise despairing existence. It is reflected in the struggle of a 50-year-old chronically mentally ill woman who sustains her sense of altruism despite unrelenting suspiciousness, fear, and rigid thought processes. She is an ardent giver of small gifts, of greeting cards weeks before the actual event, and of postage stamps she hopes will acquire great value for the recipient's future grandchildren. The dignity and control she experiences in giving to others when she herself is in such great need allow her more comfort than she might otherwise have. It buffers her from the painful realization of how isolated and vulnerable she really is.

Hamburg et al. (1974) summarized the essence of survival under extreme duress by underscoring the importance of the maintenance of self-esteem, a sense of human dignity, a sense of group belonging, and a feeling of being useful to others.

How Durable Is Resilience?

Resilient responses to ordeals have phase-specific attributes. In the acute phase, energy is directed at minimizing the impact of the stress and stressor. In the reorganization phase, a new reality is faced and accepted in part or in whole. And then there is the rest of one's life. How durable is resilience? We know it is neither a single act nor a constant state. How and under what circumstances does it emerge, shift, or fail the person? Camus (as cited by Maquet, 1958) described its emergence: "In the depth of winter I finally learned that within me there lay an invincible summer." In contrast, Monette (1988) experienced its decline: "I used up all my optimism keeping my friend alive. Now that he's gone, the cup of my health is neither half full nor half empty. Just half" (p. 2).

The suicides of Primo Levi and Bruno Bettelheim prompt similar questions. Why did Levi, successful chemist and award-winning author who recorded his Holocaust experiences because there "were things that imperiously demanded to be told" (1987, p. 9), choose to die? Did cancer and the ill health of his mother chip away at the mission he had set for himself? Did a history of exemplary behavioral competence distract from the depression and anxiety that often accompany it? Did a major depression go untreated? What about Bettelheim? His essays bore witness to Nazi atrocities; his provocative style challenged a world he saw as too passive and naive. He enacted solutions to some of humanity's problems by developing therapeutic environments for severely disturbed children. Did retirement, physical ailments, or the loss of a familiar social network limit his ability to play out a meaningful life story? Did his resilience run out? Or was this last sorrowful act a measure of his need to be in control, exercising his own will, his way, while he could? He spoke prospectively of these issues in the introduction to *The Uses of Enchantment: The Meaning and Importance of Fairy Tales* (1977):

> If we hope to live not just from moment to moment, but in true consciousness of our existence, then our greatest need and most difficult achievement is to find meaning in our lives. . . . Many have lost the will to live, and have stopped trying, because such meaning has evaded them. An understanding of the meaning of one's life is not suddenly acquired at a particular age, not even when one has reached chronological maturity. (p. 3)

These anecdotes demonstrate the changing and highly personal nature of resilience, often attained at the cost of some degree of spontaneity and flexibility. This and the interplay among such factors as age, general health status, and changing roles and relationships may conspire to diminish the once raging will to live in some, while allowing others to continue to find meaning and commitment in changing life circumstances. Resilience appears to be less an enduring characteristic and more a process determined by the impact of particular life experiences on particular conceptions of one's own life history (Cohler, 1987), leading one, once again, to conclude that it is not so much what happens to people but how they interpret and explain it that makes a difference.

Integrating Personal Meaning, Behavior, and Reality: Implications for Practice

Who rises above adversity? Perhaps it is sufficient to say that human capacities can shrink, hibernate, and flourish under circumstances of extreme stress; the influence of personal perspective; and the people, places, and things in the environment. The lives I sampled in the course of this study heightened my appreciation for the richness of the coping process and the difficulties many face with the unrelenting demands of their illness and the ofttimes unresponsive health care system. Even a resilient outcome does not represent a simple linear trajectory. It often requires the empathic attention and skillful assistance of those, like us, who are empowered by training and, I hope, by inclination.

Ordeals Provide a Window of Opportunity

Physical and emotional disruptions, the circumstances that bring us and our consumers together, provide a window of opportunity. Timely and meaningful interventions can have a significant impact on the reintegration process. These interventions may involve us in multiple tasks, such as helping persons find meaning in their crises, helping them handle feelings provoked by their situation, helping them with the reality and consequences of their condition, and fostering the functional skills and behaviors that they will need to fulfill their potential. Unfortunately, individual needs and capacities do not necessarily run on the same time standard as that of third-party payers. Potential for resilience may be noted and nurtured, but not necessarily birthed in 6 inpatient days or 12 annual reimbursed outpatient visits. Illness, and certainly disability, is an ongoing process in which personal problems may constantly emerge to undermine technical

control, social order, and individual mastery (Kleinman, 1988). The conflicts that arise among individual needs, professional values, and the system's priorities pose real challenges to those who need access before the window of opportunity is shut. We must examine our own role in perpetuating this dilemma. We must reevaluate and, in some instances, reframe, short- and long-term practice models. Additionally, we must educate colleagues, administrators, and insurers to the personal and financial impact of psychosocial factors on recovery and rehabilitation outcome in all areas of specialization.

Many Factors Influence Individual Response to Ordeals

Many intervening variables affect patients' major life changes on the one hand and illness outcome on the other. The good news is that those who rise above adversity do not belong to an exclusive club. It is not a closed system. However, some people are their own best facilitators, while others need help. Neither group should face its ordeals at the hands of caregivers and environments that induce more stress by diminishing humanistic contacts and links with reality, by neglecting the person's need to predict or anticipate outcomes, or by ignoring the inner elements of coping and competency behaviors. It is troubling to note how well many of our treatment centers fulfill the criteria for extremely stressful, negative life events.

The variability of resilience may come as bad news for some, because it does not permit a simple recipe for treatment. Instead, we must commit ourselves to understanding the complexities of personality, coping capacities, and environmental influences and use them to identify goals, interventions, and environments that are meaningful to a given person under a given set of circumstances.

Transforming Adversity Into Possibilities

Murphy (1987) reminded us that "there is a need for order in all humans that impels us to search for systematic coherence in both nature and society, and when we can find none, to invent it" (p. 33). Thoughts, feelings, and actions, influenced by neurobiology and environment, are the means by which our patients attempt to invent coherence and order that is acceptable to themselves and the outside world (White, 1976). The experiences documented in the present paper are testimony to how innovative and powerful human thoughts, feelings, and actions can be.

These capacities are also our most elegant professional tools for transforming adversity into possibilities, when we take the time to conceive of them as such. As always, Sacks (1984) captured the essence of this phenomenon best:

> Rehabilitation involves action, acts . . . [and] must be centered on the character of acts—and how to call them forth, when they have come apart, disintegrated, been "lost"—or "forgotten." (p. 182)

Calling forth the character of acts involves the therapist's understanding and using the patient's thoughts and feelings, collaborating with him or her, establishing trust, and reaching for the personal context that is partner to external reality and individual potentials for functional behavior.

Professional Entreaties

How well do we call forth the character of acts? I believe that as a group we are far more effective at defining reality and assessing and promoting performance then we are at assessing and making use of patients' views of themselves and their situation. Although our clinical prowess has grown greatly, we are too often committed only to present manifest performance. These snapshot approaches to capacity fail to reflect the unique adaptive style and potential of each person. If we are to enhance outcome, we must integrate the patients' experience of their condition and their preexisting patterns of self-regulating activity with our concerns and strategies for functional mobilization.

Kleinman (1988) proposed the use of clinical miniethnographic methods for acquiring a better picture, much like an anthropologist does in assessing a different culture. The ethnographer draws on knowledge of the context to make sense of behavior, allowing herself to sample the subject's experience. Occupational therapists are ethnographers of sorts. We have unique access to information about activities of everyday living and what it is like to live with an illness or disability. We need only to acknowledge and actualize it. But do we? Do we draw out the patient's perception of his or her situation? Or do we focus only on those aspects of function we can see, palpate, or measure?

Practice has changed dramatically over the past 30 years, as much a product of our growth and development as it is a measure of new knowledge and shifts in the health care system. We certainly have not been idle.

It is therefore no surprise that we find ourselves pursuing the future with such vigor that we sometimes fail to look back to see if we have left something of value behind. I believe we are at great risk of leaving in our wake some of the most central and precious components of our practice—how people think and feel about themselves and the world in which they live. Evidence suggests that we may have already reframed the rehabilitation process to fit today's economy rather than to fit today's patients.

Our connections to the deeper personal experiences of our patients seem to be unduly mediated by professional objectivity, our personal reluctance to hear, and a narrow view of what belongs to a given area of specialization. Fleming (1989) identified the presence of practice dichotomies concerning the relative importance of the patient's personal phenomenological status and how best to relate to him or her. Although some therapists appear to use such information and their relationship in treatment, their ambivalence about acknowledging it relegates it to an underground practice and reflects troublesome conflicts in values. We must remind ourselves that psychosocial phenomena belong to everyone, irrespective of their diagnosis and health status. Practice that separates feelings from function and psychosocial from physical perpetuates disorder rather than fostering reintegration.

The profession's current efforts to examine the actuality of clinical reasoning show great promise for rescuing the person inside our patients and for allowing us to acknowledge the credibility of this element of clinical activity. Similarly, the study of resilient persons provides us with important opportunities to share their experience, rethink our beliefs about occupational therapy's domain of concern, and enrich the emerging science of occupation. Like the subjects of this paper, "each of us maintains a personal theory of reality, a coherent set of assumptions developed over time about ourselves and our world that organizes our experiences and understanding and directs our behavior" (Janoff-Bulman & Timko, 1987, p. 136). I believe that our responsiveness to the inner lives of others can add perspective to our professional assumptions and enhance our understanding of human performance capacity. In so doing, we will find ourselves far better able to help our patients refine their adventures, find meaning and purpose in their ordeals, discover there is more to themselves than current circumstance suggests, and transform the dross of their adversity into the gold of their accomplishments.

Epilogue

This is a work in progress. My purpose has been to examine the relevance of resilience to our practice. However, one person's efforts to orchestrate the chorus of resilient voices cannot do them justice. I urge the reader to explore this literature as well. It is likely to stimulate extraordinary personal and professional awakening. Moreover, it merits our collective thought and action, because the efforts of many are needed to give meaning to the hardships our patients endure and the difference occupational therapy can make.

Acknowledgments

I dedicate this lecture to three resilient women whose adaptive style and commitment to challenge have greatly enriched my personal and professional life: my mother, Elsie Babbitt; my mentor and friend, Gail Fidler; and my daughter, Deborah Fine. All three not only see the cup as half full, but strive to keep it overflowing for themselves and others.

References

Améry, J. (1986). *At the mind's limits: Contemplations by a survivor on Auschwitz and its realities.* New York: Schocken.

Anthony, E. J., & Cohler, B. J. (Eds.). (1987). *The invulnerable child.* New York: Guilford.

Bettelheim, B. (1977). *The uses of enchantment: The meaning and importance of fairy tales.* New York: Knopf.

Bolin, R., & Trainer, P. (1978). Modes of family recovery following disaster: A cross national study. In E. L. Quarantelli (Ed.), *Disaster theory and research* (pp. 233–247). London: Sage.

Brown, C. (1990). *Down all the days.* London: Mandarin.

Browne, S. E., Connors, D., & Stern, N. (1985). *With the power of each breath: A disabled women's anthology.* San Francisco: Cleis.

Broyard, A. (1990, April 1). Good books about being sick. *New York Times Book Review,* pp. 1, 28–30.

Cannon, W. (1939). *The wisdom of the body.* New York: Norton.

Chess, S., & Thomas, A. (1984). *Origins and evolution of behavior disorders: From infancy to early adult life.* New York: Brunner/Mazel.

Cleveland, M. (1984). Family adaptation to traumatic spinal cord injury: Response to crisis. In R. H. Moos (Ed.), *Coping with physical illness* (pp. 159–171). New York: Plenum.

Cohen, F., & Lazarus, R. S. (1973). Active coping processes, coping dispositions and recovery from surgery. *Psychosomatic Medicine, 35,* 375–389.

Cohler, B. J. (1987). Adversity, resilience and the study of lives. In E. J. Anthony & B. J. Cohler (Eds.), *The invulnerable child* (pp. 363–424). New York: Guilford.

Cousins, N. (1979). *Anatomy of an illness.* New York: Bantam.

Demos, E. V. (1989). Resiliency in infancy. In T. F. Dugan & R. Coles (Eds.), *The child in our times: Studies in the development of resiliency* (pp. 3–22). New York: Brunner/Mazel.

Dimsdale, J. E. (1974). The coping behavior of Nazi concentration camp survivors. *American Journal of Psychiatry, 131,* 792–797.

Dugan, T. F., & Coles, R. (1989). *The child in our times: Studies in the development of resiliency.* New York: Brunner/Mazel.

Egendorf, A. (1986). *Healing from the war: Trauma and transformation after Vietnam.* Boston: Shambhala.

Elder, G. H. Jr., & Clipp, E. C. (1988). Combat experience, comradeship and psychological health. In J. P. Wilson, Z. Harel, & B. Kahana (Eds.), *Human adaptation to extreme stress from the Holocaust to Vietnam* (pp. 131–154). New York: Plenum.

Erikson, E. (1963). *Childhood and society.* New York: Norton.

Flach, F. (1988). *Resilience: Discovering a new strength at times of stress.* New York: Fawcett Columbine.

Fleming, M. (1989). The therapist with the three-track mind. In *The AOTA Practice Symposium guide 1989* (pp. 70–73). Rockville, MD: American Occupational Therapy Association.

Frank, C. (1988). On embodiment: A case study of congenital limb deficiency in American culture. In M. Fine & A. Asch (Eds.), *Women with disabilities* (pp. 41–71). Philadelphia: Temple University Press.

Frankl, V. E. (1984). *Man's search for meaning.* New York: Washington Square Press.

Gal, R., & Lazarus, R. S. (1975, December). The role of activity in anticipating and confronting stressful situations. *Journal of Human Stress, 1,* 4–20.

Garmezy, N. (1983). Stressors of childhood. In N. Garmezy & M. Rutter (Eds.), *Stress, coping and development in children* (pp. 43–84). New York: McGraw-Hill.

Garmezy, N. (1985). Stress-resistant children: The search for protective factors. In J. E. Stevenson (Ed.), *Recent research in developmental psychopathology* (pp. 213–233). Elmsford, NY: Pergamon.

Garmezy, N., & Masten, A. S. (1986). Stress, competence and resilience: Common frontiers for therapist and psychopathologist. *Behavior Therapy, 17,* 500–521.

Gill, A. (1988). *The journey back from hell: An oral history—Conversations with concentration camp survivors.* New York: Morrow.

Goertzel, V., & Goertzel, M. G. (1962). *Cradles of eminence.* Boston: Little, Brown.

Goleman, D. (1989, April 20). Researchers find optimism helps body's defense system. *New York Times,* p. B15.

Hamburg, D. A., Coelho, G. V., & Adams, J. E. (1974). Coping and adaptation: Steps toward a synthesis of biological and social perspectives. In G. V. Coelho, D. A. Hamburg, & J. E. Adams (Eds.), *Coping and adaptation* (pp. 403–440). New York: Basic.

Heller, J., & Vogel, S. (1986). *No laughing matter.* New York: Avon.

Houston, B. K. (1987). Stress and coping. In C. R. Snyder & C. E. Ford (Eds.), *Coping with negative life events* (pp. 373–399). New York: Plenum.

I never saw another butterfly: Children's drawings and poems from Terezin Concentration Camp, 1942–1944. (1978). New York: Schocken Books.

Janoff-Bulman, R., & Timko, C. (1987). Coping with traumatic events: The role of denial in light of people's assumptive worlds. In C. R. Snyder & C. E. Ford (Eds.), *Coping with negative life events* (pp. 135–155). New York: Plenum.

Kahana, E., Kahana, B., Harel, Z., & Rosner, T. (1988). Coping with extreme trauma. In J. P. Wilson, Z. Harel, & B. Kahana (Eds.), *Human adaptation to extreme stress: From the Holocaust to Vietnam* (pp. 55–76). New York: Plenum.

Kleinman, A. (1988). *The illness narratives: Suffering, healing and the human condition.* New York: Basic.

Kobasa, S. C. (1979). Stressful life events, personality, and health: An inquiry into hardiness. *Journal of Personality and Social Psychology, 37,* 1–11.

Lazarus, R. S., & Folkman, S. (1984). *Stress, appraisal and coping.* New York: Springer.

Lefcourt, H. M., & Martin, R. A. (1986). *Humor and life stress: Antidote to adversity.* New York: Springer-Verlag.

Levi, P. (1965). *The reawakening.* New York: Collier.

Levi, P. (1987). *Moments of reprieve.* New York: Penguin.

Lifton, R. J. (1988). Understanding the traumatized self: Imagery, symbolization and transformation. In J. P. Wilson, Z. Harel, & B. Kahana (Eds.), *Human adaptation to extreme stress: From the Holocaust to Vietnam* (pp. 7–31), New York: Plenum.

Lifton, R. J., & Olson, E. (1976). The human meaning of total disaster. *Psychiatry, 39,* 1–17.

Mairs, N. (1986). *Plaintext: Deciphering a woman's life.* New York: Perennial Library.

Maquet, A. (1958). *Albert Camus: The invincible summer.* New York: Braziller.

Marmar, E. R., & Horowitz, M. J. (1988). Post traumatic stress disorder. In J. P. Wilson, Z. Harel, & D. Kahana (Eds.), *Human adaptation to extreme stress: From the Holocaust to Vietnam* (pp. 81–103). New York: Plenum.

McGrath, M. (1984). First person accounts: Where did I go? *Schizophrenia Bulletin, 10,* 638–640.

Miller, A. (1990). *The untouched key: Tracing childhood trauma in creativity and destructiveness.* New York: Doubleday.

Miller, V. (Ed.). (1985). *Despite this flesh: The disabled in stories and poems.* Austin, TX: University of Texas Press.

Minear, R. H. (Ed.). (1990). *Hiroshima: Three witnesses.* Princeton, NJ: Princeton University Press.

Monette, P. (1988). *Borrowed time: An AIDS memoir.* New York: Avon.

Moos, R., & Billings, A. (1982). Conceptualizing and measuring coping resources and processes. In L. Goldberger & S. Breznitz (Eds.), *Handbook of stress: Theoretical and clinical aspects* (pp. 212–220). New York: Macmillan.

Moos, R. H., & Schaefer, J. A. (1984). The crisis of physical illness: An overview and conceptual approach. In R. H. Moos (Ed.), *Coping with physical illness* (pp. 8–25). New York: Plenum.

Murphy, L. B., & Moriarty, A. (1976). *Vulnerability, coping and growth: From infancy to adolescence.* New Haven, CT: Yale University Press.

Murphy, R. F. (1987). *The body silent.* New York: Henry Holt.

Nolan, C. (1987). *Under the eye of the clock.* New York: Dell.

Peck, E. C. (1987). The traits of true invulnerability and posttraumatic stress in psychoanalyzed men of action. In E. J. Anthony & B. J. Cohler (Eds.), *The invulnerable child* (pp. 315–360). New York: Guilford.

Pelletier, K. R., & Herzing, D. L. (1988). Psychoneuroimmunology: Toward a mind–body model: A critical review. *Advances, 5,* 27–56.

Potocki, E. R., & Everly, G. S. Jr. (1989). Control and the human stress response. In G. S. Everly, Jr. (Ed.), *A clinical guide to the treatment of the human stress response* (pp. 119–136). New York: Plenum.

Radner, G. (1989). *It's always something.* New York: Simon & Schuster.

Rahe, R. H., & Genender, E. (1983). Adaptation to and recovery from captivity stress. *Military Medicine, 148,* 577–585.

Redl, F. (1969). Adolescents—Just how do they react? In G. Caplan & S. Lebovici (Eds.), *Adolescence: Psychosocial perspectives* (pp. 79–90). New York: Basic.

Rosenfeld, M. S. (1989). Occupational disruption and adaptation: A study of house fire victims. *American Journal of Occupational Therapy, 43,* 89–96.

Sacks, O. (1984). *A leg to stand on.* New York: Harper & Row.

Selye, H. (1978). *The stress of life* (2nd ed.). New York: McGraw-Hill.

Sheehan, S. (1982). *Is there no place on earth for me?* New York: Vintage.

Shengold, L. (1989). *The effects of childhood abuse and deprivation.* New Haven, CT: Yale University Press.

Tamiki, H. (1990). Summer flowers. In R. H. Minear (Ed.), *Hiroshima* (pp. 19–114). Princeton, NJ: Princeton University Press.

Torrance, E. P. (1965). *Constructive behavior: Stress, personality and mental health.* Belmont, CA: Wadsworth.

Trillin, A. S. (1984). Of dragons and garden peas: A cancer patient talks to doctors. In R. H. Moos (Ed.), *Coping with physical illness* (pp. 131–138). New York: Plenum.

Vaillant, G. E. (1977). *Adaptation to life.* Boston: Little, Brown.

Weaver, G. (1985). Finch the spastic speaks. In V. Miller (Ed.), *Despite this flesh: The disabled in stories and poems* (pp. 35–45). Austin, TX: University of Texas Press.

Werner, E. E., & Smith, R. S. (1982). *Vulnerable but invincible: A study of resilient children.* New York: McGraw-Hill.

White, R. W. (1976). Strategies of adaptation: An attempt at systematic description. In R. H. Moos (Ed.), *Human adaptation: Coping with life crises* (pp. 17–32). Lexington, MA: Heath.

Wiesel, E. (1990). *From the kingdom of memory: Reminiscences.* New York: Summit.

CHAPTER 33

Spirituality, Occupation and Occupational Therapy Revisited: Ongoing Consideration of the Issues for Occupational Therapists

LESLEY WILSON

Introduction

How can spirituality, something so universal and yet so individual, be explained in the pragmatic and practical world of occupational therapy? These are interesting times to reconsider spirituality because the general consciousness of people across the globe appears to be moving towards a more esoteric awareness. The materialism of the last few decades is increasingly rejected and lessons from popular explorations and positive psychology (for example, Frey and Stutzer 2001, Seligman 2002) suggest that people are not necessarily made happier by wealth or even health but by doing things that have meaning for them, such as spending time with friends, being creative, having a value system or simply having fun. A loss of such meaning in life's occupations may cause a person to become 'dispirited', which could eventually lead to illness and disease, both physical and psychological. It is for this reason that the nature of spirituality and its connection to wellbeing is worthy of ongoing consideration by occupational therapists.

The purpose of this opinion piece is to explore the spiritual dimensions of what we do and the place that occupation has in our spiritual lives from an occupational therapy perspective. The spiritual potential of occupation is considered alongside the capacity of an individual (occupational therapist or client) to engage with this dimension of occupation. Spirituality is a central tenet of several theoretical occupational therapy models and associated assessment tools (for example, Canadian Association of Occupational Therapists 1991, Iwama 2006, Kielhofner 2008). However, the inclusion of spirituality in the occupational therapy domain has not been without its detractors (Engquist et al 1997, Rose 1999, Unruh et al 2002) and

there are those who feel that occupational therapy should concentrate on strengthening its evidence base rather than ruminating on philosophical questions. Conversely, there is also a growing acceptance of spirituality and its integration into professional practice (Unruh et al 2004).

While the concept of spirituality seems embedded in the profession's philosophical underpinnings, it is still not so easy to see where or how it manifests in practice or even if it should. Recent occupational therapy practice research in this area has made some progress in addressing spirituality with specific client groups, for example those with physical disabilities (Schulz 2005, Feeney and Toth-Cohen 2008), within dementia care (Bursell and Mayers 2010) and in mental health (Bassett et al 2008), but the issues are still mostly being debated by academics rather than practitioners.

Definitions of Spirituality

Choosing a definition with which to work is a confusing business. Differentiating between religious and secular meaning adds to the complexity and stimulates further debate. According to Heriot (1992), *religion* refers to following a set of attitudes and beliefs in service to a God within a recognised framework, whereas *spirituality* is more concerned with personal interpretations of life and the use of inner resources. There is some evidence that people, particularly in later life, can in fact combine these two concepts without any discomfort (Langer and Ortiz 2002). Some would say that spirituality has several dimensions for them, irrespective or inclusive of their belief in a God; for example, viewing a beautiful sunset, listening to music, visiting a sacred site or walking in the mountains (Wilson 2007).

Greek philosophy and Hindu and Buddhist tradition view the spirit as the essence of the individual, which lives in the body (Pagels 1979, cited in Egan and De

Laat 1994). Christiansen (1997) regarded spirituality as a metaphysical phenomenon and other authors have stated that spirituality is an integral part of the person that permits us to be aware of the presence of spirit, which inspires us to connect with others attempting to make sense of our daily lives (Egan and De Laat 1997, McColl 2000, Urbanowski and Vargo 1994).

A recent American conference devoted to spirituality and palliative care, recognising the need for some consensus, put forward a definition that included the way in which human beings seek meaning and purpose as well as the experience of connectedness (Puchalski et al 2009). The *International Classification of Functioning, Disability and Health (ICF)* has a special category for defining religion and spirituality (d930), which emphasises engagement in activities and practices for finding meaning and establishing connection with a divine power (World Health Organisation 2001).

A working definition of *spirituality* proposed by Johnston and Mayers (2005) also incorporates the search for meaning and purpose in life and, in addition, relates this to the relationships experienced by an individual.

Although the benefits of engaging in meaningful occupation are well documented, the benefits of seeming to do nothing are less so. Wilcock (1998) explored some of these aspects, suggesting a distinction between doing, being and becoming and putting forward dimensions of reflection and contemplation within occupation that could arguably be connected to spirituality.

Thus, despite the attempts at uncovering the layers of defining attributes, the precise meaning of the term 'spirituality' is still poorly understood and succinct definitions remain elusive. The unique personal or transpersonal nature of the inner experience is perhaps too nebulous to set down clearly in words, although many have tried to do so (Jewell 2004). Smith (2008) agreed and proposed a more flexible approach, one not dependent on definitions.

Much has been written in the medical and nursing literature on the subject of spirituality in health care and some of this material has been synthesised in the last decade (for example, Aldridge 2000, MacKinlay 2001, 2008, Cox et al 2006, Coyte et al 2007, McSherry 2006 and White 2006). All are extremely useful contributions to the field and highlight the benefits and challenges of integrating spiritual care into multiprofessional practice. However, the complicated concept of *spirituality* is also highlighted as being a difficulty, which as has been seen is echoed in the occupational therapy literature.

A general lack of consensus persists, making any practical application in the traditional sense somewhat of a challenge. However, spirituality should not be assumed to be absent just because of an inability to articulate its presence. Neither should the inability to define it necessarily be seen as a negative factor, frustrating though it may be. It is inherent in the nature of spirituality.

Relevance to Occupational Therapy

Occupational therapists in particular are acutely aware of the subtle ways in which engagement in occupation can be used to communicate in a manner that words cannot. Spirituality manifests itself in the way of doing things as well as in the why and how. Thus, spirituality can be generally regarded as integral to the work of occupational therapists, although there are those who are still uncomfortable with the specifics of applying these ideas in practice and prefer not to engage at this level of awareness.

On a more direct practical level, the *ICF* focuses on the activities associated with religious and spiritual practice, such as attending places of worship or praying and chanting. These activities lend themselves to purposeful assessment and occupational therapists can assist clients to conduct the occupations associated with their spiritual needs (Bryant and Law 1990, Wilson 2005). However, the contemplative and intangible aspects of acknowledging a power beyond the human, which do not reveal themselves in obvious activity, remain more difficult to access.

Even for people who place faith in a God or have spirituality central to their everyday lives, it is often during a health crisis or at the end of life that spiritual needs emerge more strongly and a considerable body of literature relates to the older adult. Studies have shown that those older people with strong religious convictions have higher levels of life satisfaction, are less likely to be depressed and are more likely to be at ease with their personal past and the prospect of death (Ayele et al 1999, Coleman et al 2002). Schultz (2005) suggested that people with disabilities perceive and experience spirituality differently, depending on the age at which their disability had an impact on their lives.

Much of the literature has come from North America (for example, Egan and De Laat 1994, 1997, Christiansen 1997, Engquist et al 1997, Peloquin 1997, Farrar 2001, Rebeiro 2001, Unruh et al 2002). Both the *Canadian* and *American Journals of Occupational Therapy* have devoted special issues to the topic in 1994 and

1997, respectively. These and the relatively small number of United Kingdom studies highlight ambivalence and uncertainty amongst occupational therapists in incorporating spirituality in their work, despite broadly agreeing that it is important to do so (for example, Udell and Chandler 2000, Belcham 2004, Johnston and Mayers 2005, Hoyland and Mayers 2005, Bursell and Mayers 2010). It is this very dichotomy between thinking and doing that might be causing a rift. As a profession, it might be worth considering that there is room for both. After all, it is reflected in everyday life.

The difficult question is whether or not occupational therapists can encompass these diverse, strongly held opinions and also be tolerant of conflicting views. The guiding principle is, of course, to avoid subjecting clients to any interventions that might be inappropriately intrusive and practices that would be deemed unprofessional according to the accepted codes of professional conduct and ethical behaviour.

There are two pivotal points that an occupational therapist might explore when approaching the use of occupation with a spiritual perspective. These are the capacity of the client and his or her willingness or need to participate at a spiritual level and the capacity of the therapist to engage in a client-centred dialogue about spiritual matters—depending on the therapist's own experience and confidence, including the ability to recognise the appropriateness of explicitly using spiritual dimensions of occupation in the interaction and *when not to*.

Conclusion

Having briefly explored the place of spirituality in occupational therapy, it can be seen that it is not something that can easily be identified. Rather, it is part of a whole that cannot be separated from the whole. It is not something that can be taken out, examined, analysed and then put back again, for the very process of doing this changes it. Rather, it needs to be acknowledged as having holistic importance in people's lives and, if occupational therapists are fortunate enough to be in a position to facilitate this aspect of existence through engagement in life's occupations, then it should not simply be ignored.

Acknowledgement

Thanks to the anonymous *BJOT* article reviewers for their helpful comments.

References

Aldridge D (2000) *Spirituality, healing and medicine.* London: Jessica Kingsley.

Ayele H, Mulligan T, Gheorghiu S, Reyes-Ortiz C (1999) Religious activity improves life satisfaction for some physicians and older patients. *Journal of the American Geriatric Society, 47(4),* 453–55.

Bassett H, Lloyd C, Tse S (2008) Approaching in the right spirit: spirituality and hope in recovery from mental health problems. *International Journal of Therapy and Rehabilitation, 15(6),* 254–61.

Belcham C (2004) Spirituality in occupational therapy: theory in practice? *British Journal of Occupational Therapy, 67(1),* 39–46.

Bryant W, Law M (1990) A spiritual lift from a world of confusion. *Therapy Weekly,* 1 February.

Bursell J, Mayers CA (2010) Spirituality within dementia care: perceptions of health professionals. *British Journal of Occupational Therapy, 73(4),* 144–51.

Canadian Association of Occupational Therapists (1991) *Occupational therapy guidelines for client-centred practice.* Toronto, ON: CAOT Publications ACE.

Christiansen C (1997) Acknowledging a spiritual dimension in occupational therapy practice. *American Journal of Occupational Therapy, 51(3),* 169–80. http://dx.doi.org/10.5014/ajot.51.3.169

Christiansen C, Baum C, eds (1997) *Occupational therapy: enabling function and wellbeing.* Thorofare, NJ: Slack.

Coleman P, McKieran F, Mills M, Speck P (2002) Spiritual belief and quality of life: the experience of older bereaved spouses. *Quality and Ageing—Policy, Practice and Research, 3(1),* 20–26.

Cox J, Campbell AV, Fulford B, eds (2006) *Medicine of the person.* London: Jessica Kingsley.

Coyte ME, Gilbert P, Nicholls V, eds (2007) *Spirituality, values and mental health: jewels for the journey.* London: Jessica Kingsley.

Egan M, De Laat D (1994) Considering spirituality in occupational therapy practice. *Canadian Journal of Occupational Therapy, 61(2),* 95–101.

Egan M, De Laat D (1997) The implicit spirituality of occupational therapy practice. *Canadian Journal of Occupational Therapy, 64(1),* 115–21.

Engquist D, Short-DeGraff M, Gliner J, Oltjenbruns K (1997) Occupational therapists' beliefs and practices with regard to spirituality and therapy. *American Journal of Occupational Therapy, 51(3),* 173–80. http://dx.doi.org/10.5014/ajot.51.3.173

Farrar JE (2001) Addressing spirituality and religious life in occupational therapy practice. *Physical and Occupational Therapy in Geriatrics, 18(4)*, 65–85.

Feeney L, Toth-Cohen S (2008) Addressing spirituality for clients with physical disabilities. *OT Practice, 13(4)*, 16–18, 20.

Frey BS, Stutzer A (2001) *Happiness and economics*. Princeton, NJ: Princeton University Press.

Heriot CS (1992) Spirituality and aging. *Holistic Nursing Practice, 7(1)*, 22–31.

Hoyland M, Mayers C (2005) Is meeting spiritual need within the occupational therapy domain? *British Journal of Occupational Therapy, 68(4)*, 177–80.

Iwama M (2006) *The Kawa Model: culturally relevant occupational therapy*. Edinburgh: Elsevier Churchill Livingstone.

Jewell A, ed (2004) *Ageing, spirituality and well-being*. London: Jessica Kingsley.

Johnston D, Mayers C (2005) Spirituality: a review of how occupational therapists acknowledge, assess and meet spiritual needs. *British Journal of Occupational Therapy, 68(9)*, 386–92.

Kielhofner G (2008) *Model of Human Occupation: theory and application*. 4th ed. Philadelphia: Lippincott Williams and Wilkins.

Langer N, Ortiz LPA (2002) Assessment of spirituality and religion in later life: acknowledging clients' needs and personal resources. *Journal of Gerontological Social Work, 37(2)*, 5–21.

MacKinlay E (2001) *The spiritual dimension of ageing*. London: Jessica Kingsley.

MacKinlay E, ed (2008) *Ageing, disability and spirituality*. London: Jessica Kingsley.

McColl MA (2000) Spirit, occupation and disability. *Canadian Journal of Occupational Therapy, 67(4)*, 217–18.

McSherry W (2006) *Making sense of spirituality in nursing and health care practice*. 2nd ed. London: Jessica Kingsley.

Peloquin SM (1997) Nationally speaking: The spiritual depth of occupation: making worlds and making lives. *American Journal of Occupational Therapy, 51(3)*, 167–68. http://dx.doi.org/10.5014/ajot.51.3.167

Puchalski C, Ferrell B, Virani R, Otis-Green S, Baird P, Bull J, Chochinov H, Handzo G, Nelson-Becker H, Prince-Paul M, Pugliese K, Sulmasy D (2009) Improving the quality of spirituality as a dimension of palliative care: the Report of Consensus Conference. *Journal of Palliative Medicine, 12(10)*, 885–904.

Rebeiro KL (2001) Client-centred practice: body, mind and spirit resurrected. *Canadian Journal of Occupational Therapy, 68(2)*, 65–69.

Rose A (1999) Spirituality and palliative care: the attitudes of occupational therapists. *British Journal of Occupational Therapy, 62(7)*, 307–12.

Schulz E (2005) The meaning of spirituality for individuals with disabilities. *Disability and Rehabilitation, 27(21)*, 1283–95.

Seligman MEP (2002) *Authentic happiness*. New York: Free Press.

Smith S (2008) Towards a flexible framework for understanding spirituality. *Occupational Therapy in Health Care, 22(1)*, 39–54.

Udell L, Chandler C (2000) The role of the occupational therapist in addressing the spiritual needs of clients. *British Journal of Occupational Therapy, 63(10)*, 489–95.

Unruh AM, Versnel J, Kerr N (2002) Spirituality unplugged: a review of commonalities and contentions, and a resolution. *Canadian Journal of Occupational Therapy, 69(1)*, 5–19.

Unruh AM, Versnel J, Kerr N (2004) Spirituality in the context of occupation: a theory to practice application. In: M Molineux, ed. *Occupation for occupational therapists*. Oxford: Blackwell Publishing, ch. 3.

Urbanowski R, Vargo J (1994) Spirituality, daily practice, and the occupational performance model. *Canadian Journal of Occupational Therapy, 61(2)*, 88–94.

White G (2006) *Talking about spirituality in health care practice*. London: Jessica Kingsley.

Wilcock AA (1998) Reflections on doing, being and becoming. *Canadian Journal of Occupational Therapy, 65(5)*, 248–56.

Wilson L (2007) Spirituality and occupational therapy—the heart of what matters in occupation. *College of Occupational Therapists 31st Annual Conference Abstracts*. London: College of Occupational Therapists.

Wilson L (2005) Activity and participation, part 2. In: A McIntyre, A Atwal, eds. *Occupational therapy and older people*. Oxford: Blackwell Publishing, ch. 9.

World Health Organisation (2001) *International classification of functioning, disability and health*. Geneva: WHO.

CHAPTER 34

Defining Lives: Occupation as Identity: An Essay on Competence, Coherence, and the Creation of Meaning

1999 ELEANOR CLARKE SLAGLE LECTURE

CHARLES H. CHRISTIANSEN

The anthropologist Bateson (1996) has written that

> The capacity to do something useful for yourself or others is key to personhood, whether it involves the ability to earn a living, cook a meal, put on shoes in the morning, or whatever other skill needs to be mastered at the moment. (1986, p. 11)

In this article, I assert that occupations are key not just to being a person, but to being a *particular* person, and thus creating and maintaining an identity. Occupations come together within the contexts of our relationships with others to provide us with a sense of purpose and structure in our day-to-day activities, as well as over time. When we build our identities through occupations, we provide ourselves with the contexts necessary for creating meaningful lives, and life meaning helps us to be well.

In this article, an important distinction is made between being well and being healthy. The ultimate goal of occupational therapy services is well-being, not health. Health enables people to pursue the tasks of everyday living that provide them with the life meaning necessary for their well-being. As Englehardt said in describing the virtues of occupational therapy, *"people are healthy or diseased in terms of the activities open to them or denied them."* (1977, p. 672)

Overview

In addressing the complex topic of personal identity, I begin by reviewing key concepts from the literature,

noting particularly how our use of language gives us important insights into how we think about ourselves. I then discuss how identity is thought to be formed during the crucial developmental stages of our lives, and how it seems to be of immense importance to us as we make our way through the stages of life. After this, I consider how daily occupations serve the important purpose of enabling us to experience or realize our personal identities. I then address the implications of incomplete or blemished identities on personal well-being, and conclude with observations on the implications of identity-making for the practice of occupational therapy in the new millennium.

Propositions

My presentation is based on four propositions, all centered on the assertion that one of the most compelling needs that every human being has is to be able to express his or her unique identity in a manner that gives meaning to life. This assertion was influenced greatly by an ethnographic study of adaptive strategies reported in *The American Journal of Occupational Therapy* (McCuaig & Frank, 1991). That study described a middle-aged woman [Meghan] with severe athetoid cerebral palsy who had great difficulty with voluntary movement that profoundly affected her mobility and speech. Somehow, without much professional assistance, the woman was able to devise adaptive strategies so that she could use her limited voluntary movement and assistive technology to get along in daily life. Despite rather considerable postural deformities and difficulty with hearing, she was able to live in an apartment, requiring only modest assistance of friends and neighbors to live independently.

In considering the study, I found Meghan's motivations for choosing strategies, rather than the nature of

This chapter was previously published in the *American Journal of Occupational Therapy, 53,* 547–558. Copyright © 1999, American Occupational Therapy Association. Reprinted with permission. http://dx.doi.org/10.5014/ajot.53.6.547

her adaptations, of greatest interest. It seemed that one very important consideration underlying her choices—especially when they were to be viewed by others—was whether or not they would show her to be an intelligent, competent woman. In short, they were issues of identity.

I remember being surprised by this observation, thinking that someone as disabled as she was would be driven by the functional necessities of life, with little reserve time or energy to be consumed by thoughts of how she might be viewed in the eyes of others. But as I thought about it more deeply, I realized that life around me was teeming with indications[1] that people (with disabilities or without) are universally concerned about their social identity and acceptance by others. The ethnographic study also pointed squarely to the reality that daily occupation was the primary means through which the woman was able to communicate her identity as a competent person.

My further thinking and study about the relationships between daily occupations and selfhood led to four premises that may be useful to the process of considering identity issues in occupational therapy. Because there is yet much work to be done in establishing the validity of theories of how identity is constructed and maintained, each proposition must be viewed as tentative.

Proposition 1: Identity Is an Overarching Concept That Shapes and Is Shaped by Our Relationships With Others

Personal identity can be defined as the person we think we are. It is the self we know. Note that this is not the same as self-concept nor is it the same as self-esteem, although these important concepts are related to identity. Baumeister (1986, 1997), an often-cited authority on the study of identity, has noted that the most obvious things in daily life are sometimes the most difficult to define. We use the word *self* in our everyday language several times a day. When we say *self,* we include the direct feeling we have about our thoughts and feelings and sensations. This begins with the awareness of our body and is augmented by our sense of being able to make choices and initiate action. It also encompasses the abstract and complex ideas that embellish the self.

The term *self-concept* refers to the *inferences* we make about ourselves. It encompasses our understanding of

personality traits and characteristics, our social roles, and our relationships. We are motivated as adults to achieve some consistency in terms of how we view ourselves, and we want this view to be favorable. In general, we strive to maintain favorable views and to dispute or avoid feedback that is discrepant from our view of self (Swann, 1987; Swann & Hill, 1982). To the extent that we perceive discrepancies between our perceived and ideal selves, we are motivated to change.

A third concept is self-esteem. This refers to the evaluative aspect of the self-concept. Self-esteem is related to identity in the sense that our esteem is related to our ability to demonstrate efficacious action, which gains social approval and thus influences our overall concept of self (Baumeister, 1982; Franks & Marolla, 1976).

Finally, *identity* refers to the definitions that are created for and superimposed on the self. Identity is a composite definition of the self, and includes an interpersonal aspect (e.g., our roles and relationships, such as mothers, wives, occupational therapists), an aspect of possibility or potential (that is, who we *might* become), and a values aspect (that suggests importance and provides a stable basis for choices and decisions). Self-concept is entirely created in one's mind, whereas identity is often created by the larger society, even though it is often negotiated with others and refined by the individual as a result of those social negotiations (see Figure 34.1).

In summary, identity can be viewed as the superordinate view of ourselves that includes both self-esteem and the self-concept, but also importantly reflects, and is influenced by, the larger social world in which we find ourselves. This definition of identity leads logically to a second proposition:

Proposition 2: Identities Are Closely Tied to What We Do and Our Interpretations of Those Actions in the Context of Our Relationships With Others

It is interesting to note that in North America, after an exchange of names between strangers, the next part of a conversation often turns on the expression, "What do you do?" The resulting dialogue provides for shared meaning by situating each person in a context the other understands or attempts to understand through further dialogue.

This everyday exchange illustrates the close connection between doing and identity, and also points out the important role that language has in creating under-

---

[1]Consider the prevalence (and popularity) of monograms, tattoos, vanity license plates, titles, degrees, pierced body parts, autobiographies, and unique names (changed or not).

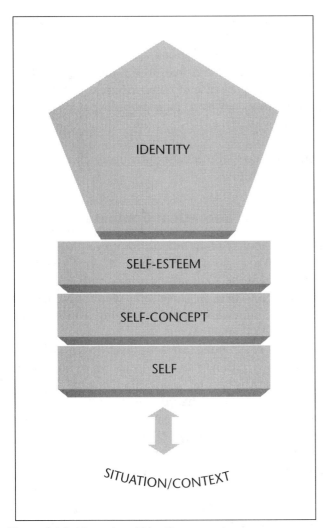

Figure 34.1. Hierarchy of identity concepts.

Piaget (1954) and others (Kagan, 1981) have shown that as infants and as toddlers, the experience of coming to know the world very much involves *doing.* As children, we learn that we can intentionally act on our environment and change it. It is this acting on the environment with observable consequence that gives us our sense of selfhood, that teaches us that we are active agents, separate from our environment.

As children explore cause-and-effect events, they learn that they can have an effect on inanimate objects, such as toys, and that they can also elicit reactions from animate objects, such as pets and other people. Mostly, a child's early experiences in this regard are positive because doting parents and grandparents tend to regard any behavior as cute and, as a consequence, are very forgiving of transgressions. Later, this tolerance becomes more selective, and parents can then also communicate disapproval when a child disobeys. Yet, already, children have become active agents in the world, exerting an effect on objects and on people. Using dolls or toy figures, they can even pretend that objects *are* people.

Thus, children learn that they can get the attention of others through their actions and that their actions can be approved or not. Studies have shown that *good* and *bad* are among the words most frequently spoken to young children (Kagan, 1981). Thus, very early on, a connection is made between behavior and social approval in a manner that influences our sense of self. The point to be made here is that already, at an early age, children know themselves as individuals capable of acting on the world, and they understand that their actions have a social meaning. They also begin to appreciate that their approval as individuals is often contingent on what they do (Keller, Ford, & Meacham, 1978).

This is to be the beginning of a lifetime of understanding the interdependence of self and the social groups to which we are connected. It is also the beginning of understanding ourselves as having an identity that is related to group membership. For example, as children we learn that we are members of a family, that we are male or female, and that we have other characteristics in common or in contrast with others.

Identity development continues to be influenced by social relationships as children mature. Beginning at preschool age, self-concept and identity are shaped by a person's competencies and capabilities in comparison to others and in relationship to social standards or expectations (Ruble, 1983). During adolescence, identity is shaped by more abstract concepts, such as interper-

standing and meaning. Were it not for our social existence, there would be no need for language and communication, and it is generally believed that thought itself is a product of language. That is, when we think, we carry on an internal dialogue with ourselves. Vygotsky (1981) maintained that language provides children with the tools to gain self-awareness and, consequently, voluntary control of their actions. Thus, our understanding of the world around us is shaped as much by language, a system of spoken and written symbols, as it is by direct experience.

For example, when we learn the word *stove* as toddlers, we are also apt to learn the words *hot* and *danger.* We may also discover that if we ignore our parents' admonitions and touch a hot stove, we may burn our fingers. At the same time, we may experience disapproval for not having behaved as our parents expected.

sonal traits, values, and preferences (Erikson, 1968). For adults, identity is oriented toward goals; often related to becoming a certain kind of person and not becoming another kind of person (Baumeister, 1986). Adolescent and adult identity development, although based more on abstractions, is nonetheless largely influenced by social phenomena.

Because symbolic communication involves behaviors as well as language, children learn also that a raised eyebrow or an awkward silence can be among many forms of communicating disapproval. As maturity develops, the task of understanding what constitutes social approval takes on even greater importance, and becomes even more challenging, because the feedback adults receive in social settings is much more ambiguous and indirect. At this point, it should be obvious that identity has no existence outside of interpersonal relationships. Our views of our goals, our behaviors, and ourselves are inextricably tied to our relationships with others.

Proposition 3: Identities Provide an Important Central Figure in a Self-Narrative or Life Story That Provides Coherence and Meaning for Everyday Events and Life Itself

When we interpret events, we evaluate them for personal meaning. If they are meaningful, they have significance to us, we respond emotionally to them, and they shape our behavior and perceptions of life. When people believe that they have no identity or that their identity has been spoiled, life becomes less meaningful and can become meaningless (Debats, Drost, & Hansen, 1995; Moore, 1997; van Selm & Dittmann-Kohli, 1998).

Our interpretation of life events and situations takes place within the framework of life stories or narratives. Other people are part of our life stories, and we are part of the life stories of others. Our lives are interwoven within the lives of others and, therefore, if our identities change, this influences our life as well as the lives of others. In this sense, identities are socially interconnected and distributed, yet understood in the context of ongoing life stories.

Proposition 4: Because Life Meaning Is Derived in the Context of Identity, It Is an Essential Element in Promoting Well-Being and Life-Satisfaction

Each of us hopes for a satisfactory outcome for the particular goals we are pursuing at the moment as well as

for the life we are leading, which we are aware will end at some point. To the extent that we can successfully weave together the various and multiple short stories that comprise our lives into a meaningful whole, we can derive a sense of coherence and meaning and purpose from our lives. I am proposing that our identities provide us with the context through which we interpret and derive meaning from the events we experience. Our identities also provide us with a view for future possibilities.

Theoretical Contexts

Having elaborated four propositions regarding identity, it is useful to create a context from which to view them and evaluate their implications for occupational therapy practice. There are three roots of selfhood that will serve as a framework for understanding. The first is the experience of reflexive consciousness, derived from the traditions of symbolic interactionism. This allows us to think about ourselves and the influence of our actions on others. The second is the interpersonal aspect of selfhood, the reality that identities are shaped within a social setting, where we receive acceptance, approval, and validation as worthwhile persons. The third is the agential aspect of identity, that aspect of demonstrating influence on the world around us that allows us to make meaning in our lives. When we create, when we control, when we exercise choice, we are expressing our selfhood and unique identities.

Reflexive Consciousness

The ability to think about ourselves and to have these thoughts modify our behavior is a distinctly human characteristic, and it depends on symbolic communication. Using symbols or language, we not only are able to categorize, think about, and act in socially influenced ways, but we also are able to reflect on ourselves from the perspective of others.

When we think about ourselves, we carry on the equivalent of an internal dialogue between two aspects of self, the experiencing self and the thought of self. These two aspects of the self can be labeled the *I* and the *me*. The I is the active creative agent doing the experiencing, thinking, and acting, and the me is the perspective or attitude toward oneself that one assumes when taking the roles of specific others or the generalized community. In this approach, the me's, or perspectives of the self, are the social selves—who we are in

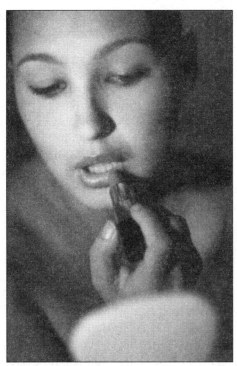

Figure 34.2. Reflexive self-consciousness—The dialogue between the *I* and the *me*.

Note. Image © 1999 PhotoDisc, Inc. Used with permission.

our own and others' eyes. Thought of in another way, when we consider the image of ourselves reflected in a mirror, the I is looking at and thinking about the me, all the while making grooming adjustments to improve it (see Figure 34.2).

The reflexive nature of the self is exemplified by everyday language that illustrates its duality. When we speak of self-discipline, we are talking about one aspect of the self keeping the other under control. Similarly, when we observe that Sue has "let herself go," we imply that she no longer has self-control or that she no longer cares about her public identity.

The Interpersonal Nature of Selfhood

The ideas of symbolic communication and the reflexive nature of the self are derived from a tradition of social psychology known as symbolic interactionism. This tradition goes back to the turn of the century and several prominent behavioral scientists of the time, beginning with William James (1892). Later, the famous sociologist Charles Horton Cooley (1902) made the observation that our views of ourselves are very much influenced by the reactions of others to what we do. He formulated what is known as the "looking glass

theory," which maintained that the reactions of others reflect their approval and disapproval and thus constitute a primary means of developing an awareness of ourselves.

The psychologist George Herbert Mead extended this thinking in the 1930s, advancing the theory even further. In *Mind, Self and Society,* Mead (1934) held that society is created, sustained, and changed through the process of symbolic communication. In other words, social reality is constructed and negotiated through interactions with others. In these interactions, people seek to present images of the self for others to see and evaluate. The primary purposes of these social selves are to gain approval from others and to be able to gain influence, which occurs through social status and power. Mead believed that by using the reflexive processes of communication, the dialogue between I and me, we are able to imagine how we appear to others or what reactions others will have to our behaviors.[2]

Because of the dependence on others for feedback about the self, Mead (1934) believed that there is a mutual interdependence of self and society. By seeking the approval of others, a person's behavior may be moderated, but this occurs only to the extent that people are capable of exercising the self-control necessary for them to gain social approval.

Many people are reluctant to accept a view of self that suggests that every action they take is calculated to gain the approval of others because it sounds manipulative or deceptive. However, in reality, people are not able to exercise conscious control over their behaviors in a manner that permits them to plan calculated actions at every moment in every social relationship. To a certain extent, however, the rules and conventions of social interaction are such that we preserve and enhance our identity through conformity and careful reflection about the anticipated results of our behaviors on others.

As expressions of identity, people often exhibit spontaneity and creativity that test the boundaries of conformity or risk social disapproval. Unconventional behavior is often risky. This is one of the things that makes the world such an interesting place. Occasionally, acts of spontaneity and creativity are embraced and

---

[2]It is worth noting that Mead's assertion that our identity is totally dependent on the feedback of others has been shown to be incomplete (Schrauger & Schoeneman, 1979), mainly because research has shown that people deceive themselves by perceiving that others evaluate them more favorably than is actually the case (Greenwald, 1980).

adopted by the larger group with the result that such innovations create change or progress in the culture. In this way, the reciprocal influence between self and society described by Mead (1934) is completed. That is, social expectations influence the individual, and the individual, through acts of creativity, sometimes influences the larger society. A proposal of symbolic interactionism views that the individual and society are interdependent. That is, they depend on each other for predictability and stability as well as for progress.

To summarize, the basic ideas underlying symbolic interactionism are that (a) we communicate symbolically much of the time and that the language of social life consists of both spoken and unspoken messages; (b) through our conversations with ourselves, we are able to modify our behaviors to gain social approval; and (c) the need for social approval encourages conformity, which promotes stability and predictability, but occasionally also yields individual creativity that, when adopted, serves to advance the social group.

Social Constructionism and Distributed Selves

In recent years, views of the social nature of self-identity have been extended with a school of thought called social constructionism. Theorists in this tradition propose that selves are distributed. That is, the person and their social context cannot be easily separated. Social constructionists argue that although we perceive a private and self-contained world inside our heads, it would be more accurate to describe this image as a snapshot from a constantly changing public panorama (Bruner, 1990; Gergen, 1991; Polkinghorne, 1988).

When we think of our multiple expressions of self, our children, our friendships, our marriages, our journals, and our daily interactions, we realize that our identities are indeed distributed throughout our social environments. These "pieces of self" are part of us. They define who we are, and yet they exist in other mediums, distributing identities well beyond the boundaries of a physical body. This distribution of the self only occurs through social interaction.

The social constructionist view suggests that people's identities not only are social, they also are multifaceted, yet they are perceived not so much as fragments, but as part of a comprehensive and understandable self (cf. Kondo, 1990). Ordinarily, we do not think of ourselves as fragmented, but as complex people with many dimensions of self. In short, we piece together our experiences to fashion an intelligible self, an identity that is comprehensible to both ourselves and others.

Life Stories

How is it that our identities can be complex and distributed while at the same time seem to be stable and predictable? The answer to this question lies in our understanding of our lives as evolving narratives or life stories. Through stories, we understand life events as systematically related. As Gergen and Gergen wrote: "One's present identity is thus not a sudden and mysterious event, but a sensible result of a life story" (1988, p. 55).

In a sense, our stories are unfolding and being rewritten as we live them. All narrative shares the similar characteristic of having a temporal order. That is, our life stories consist of events in progressive sequences. In order for our stories to have meaning, the events in our lives must be interpreted in ways that give them a relationship to each other. In this manner, they have coherence and unity. It helps that our everyday routines, our personality traits, and other factors, such as our genetic make-up, influence us in ways that provide a degree of consistency to our behavior. This makes it easier to interpret our life stories in an understandable way.

Making Sense of Experiences

The problem of how people make sense of their life experiences has been central to the work of McAdams (1997). He has analyzed life stories to derive insights into the processes people use to construct their identities within a coherent structure. His work suggests that one of the central purposes of the life story is to create unity and purpose in daily life. In constructing and interpreting life stories, people seek to fashion identities that make sense to themselves and others. Importantly, because people are not passive participants in their life stories, they can enact or create the events that express their identities in the manner they would like others to view them. This brings us to the third requirement of identity, that of human agency, or expressing the self through acting on the world around us.

Selfing: Shaping Identity Through Experience

It is the reflexive dialogue between the I and me that McAdams (1996, 1997) suggests ties human agency to identity. The I, he argues, is not a noun, but a process, which McAdams and others refer to as *selfing*. That is, by experiencing our actions and our lives as our own, we adopt them as part of ourselves, as belonging to the me. Selfing is responsible for human feelings of agency.

McAdams (1996) suggests that selfing is inherently a unifying, integrative, synthesizing process. Ego psychologists (e.g., Loevenger, 1976), building on Freud (as cited in Stachey, 1990), viewed the ego as the organizational medium of the mind that promotes healthy adaptation to life through learning, memory, perception, and synthesis (Kris, 1952). It permits the gaining of competence that White (1959) viewed as so important to successful adaptation. To quote McAdams: "The I puts experience together—synthesizes it, unifies it, makes it mine. The fact that it is mine—even when I see the sunset, I am seeing it; that when you hurt my feelings those were my feelings, not yours that were hurt—provides a unity to selfhood without which human life in society as we know it would simply not exist" (1997, p. 57). To *self* is to maintain the stance of the self in the world, it is the being and becoming that Fidler (Fidler & Fidler, 1978) has written about. In other words, selfing is the shaping of identity through daily occupations.

Occupations are more than movements strung together, more than simply doing something. They are opportunities to express the self, to create an identity.

Creating Life Meaning Through Selfing

When we create our life stories through doing, or selfing, as McAdams would say, we are living for a purpose, and deriving a sense of meaning in our lives in the process. Sommer and Baumeister (1998) have observed that people seek meaning in ordinary events along the same lines that they seek meaning in life generally. That is, they try to fulfill four basic needs. These needs are *purpose, efficacy, value,* and *self-worth*. By definition, our daily occupations, whether they pertain to work, leisure, or maintenance of self, are goal directed and, therefore, provide purpose in the moment. When we achieve success in reaching our goals, we derive a sense of efficacy and believe that we have some measure of control over our environments (Langer & Rodin, 1976).

Meaning is also derived from believing that we have done the right thing, that our actions are justifiable under the circumstances. Finally, and not least importantly, we derive meaning from our feelings of self-worth. We meet this need through the approval of others and by viewing our own traits and abilities favorably. We want to feel good about ourselves, and we want to believe that we are worthy of other people's attention and affection.[3]

This discussion should emphasize the important relationships between identity, occupations, competence, and meaning. There is clearly an important interplay between these concepts. We cannot gain the recognition of others without competent action, nor can we meet our needs for meaning without engaging in occupation in a way that receives social validation. Moreover, the things we do, even when validated by others as competent, must be understandable to ourselves within a meaningful life context.

Identity—Goals and Occupational Performance

It may be helpful here to elaborate on the important relationship between occupations and identity. To speak of occupation is to describe goal-directed activity in the context of living. Goals work as motivators precisely because we imagine how we will be affected directly or indirectly when the goal is met. Thus, goals serve as motivators because we view them in the context of self, whether we are dressing for the day or seeking a promotion. We put on the blue blazer because we imagine what we will look like and anticipate that it will be satisfactory or appropriate for the day's activities.

Similarly, when we work late, or when we willingly take on an added responsibility in volunteer activities, we imagine ourselves as being viewed as virtuous, hardworking, and worthwhile people. We may imagine getting praised, getting a promotion, or receiving a raise or recognition as a result of those efforts. These views of our identity in the future are imagined selves, and they are powerful motivators of goal-directed action. Markus and colleagues (Markus, 1977; Markus & Nurius, 1986) have called these motivating images *possible selves*. They have suggested that a goal can have an influence on behavior to the extent that an individual can personalize it

---

[3]The British psychologist and philosopher Rom Harré (1983) has used the term *identity projects* to refer to self-directed development and expression of self. Identity projects may take the form of pursuit of fame or status or recognition of some kind. Or they may be concerned with the more personal aspects of ourselves and the way we think about ourselves. This may involve developing our potentials to create and to relate to others, or enriching our experience and understanding. Harré (1998) has also written extensively about the importance of discourse in shaping agency. A complete treatment of his propositions is beyond the scope of this article, but highly recommended for readers interested in a more in-depth analysis of the psychology of selfhood.

by building a bridge of self-representations between the current state and the hoped-for state.

Possible selves can consist of both positive as well as negative images. They not only may represent what we would like to become, they also may represent what we are afraid of becoming. Either type of possible self can be a motivator. Thus, we may strive to become the wealthy self, the shapely self, or the well-respected and loved self; while we dread, and thus, try to avoid becoming the lonely, depressed, or incompetent self (Ogilvie, 1987).

Possible Selves as Images of Action

Markus and her colleagues have contended that possible selves give personal meaning and structure to a person's thoughts about the future. That is, when we think about actions we might take, we project images of ourselves into those thoughts, and we view ourselves taking the actions. In other words, possible selves provide a very useful and direct mechanism for translating thoughts into actions. Goals that individuals view as important, and to which they are committed, are effective because these goals are self-relevant and self-defining.

Goals differ between people because the nature of possible selves depends on the nature of one's core self or complex identity system. Goal-directed and motivated behavior and personal identity are thus reciprocally related. Studies (Pavot, Fujita, & Diener, 1997) have shown that as we perceive ourselves becoming more like the person we want to be, our life satisfaction increases. When we do not perceive ourselves as progressing toward our desired identities, we tend to exhibit signs of unhealthy adaptation (Heatherton & Baumeister, 1991).

Social Approval and Competent Performance

Social approval and competent performance are instrumental to our thoughts of actions that will help us avoid or realize possible selves. Research shows that people will go to great lengths to alter their behavior (and indeed, even their appearance) in order to gain social approval and avoid rejection (Crowne & Marlowe, 1964).

To a large extent, our ability to gain this approval depends on our ability to portray ourselves as competent people. Through implicit expectations associated with social standing and the performance of roles, social groups help define the levels of competence necessary for acceptance, approval, and recognition.

In other words, self-appraisal is highly dependent on the extent to which we believe that we will be accepted by others. Research has also shown that it is related to efficacious action or competent performance, meaning that we must demonstrate to others that we are competent people as part of the acceptance process (Franks & Marolla, 1976).

Competent Performance

To be competent suggests that we are effective in dealing with the challenges that come our way (White, 1971). If we experience success in the challenges we undertake, we enhance our view of ourselves as competent beings (Bandura, 1977; Gage & Polatajko, 1994). This encourages us to explore and to engage the world in ways that give us our sense of autonomy and selfhood.

As we experience successes, our views of ourselves as efficacious or competent become strengthened. Thus, completing a task successfully adds to our sense of being competent human beings and, in a sense, prepares us for new challenges by bolstering our self-confidence. The term *self-confidence* is an interesting expression because it establishes a clear link between our identity and our belief in the things that we can do. Rogers (1982) asserted that developing a sense of the self as a competent agent in the world requires the expression of choice and control. Through choice, we express autonomy and, through control, we express efficacy. Brewster Smith summed it up nicely in: "The crucial attitude toward the self is self-respect as a significant and efficacious person" (1974, p. 14).

Performance Deficits

If our identities are crafted by what we do and how we do it, then it follows that any threat to our ability to engage in occupations and present ourselves as competent people becomes a threat to our identity. On a daily basis, occupational therapists come into contact with persons whose identities are threatened by virtue of performance limitations. These identity crises may occur as the result of normal aging, which often deprives us of the sense of competence we once had, or result from congenital disorders, injuries, and diseases that leave lasting or progressive disability.

To the extent that disabilities interfere with the competent execution of tasks and roles, they threaten the establishment of an identity based on competence. In some cases, injury, disease and disability also result in bodily disfigurement, which further assaults the person's identity and increases the challenges associated with establishing an identity that receives social approval (Goffman, 1963). Facial scars or anomalies, involuntary movements related to motor planning deficits, balance disorders, and unwanted tics are among the many observable signs of disorders that gain unwanted public attention and increase the challenge of fashioning a social identity that is acceptable to self and others.

Stigma

Goffman (1959) suggested that a socially competent performance involves more than simply getting the job done. There are certain stylistic and procedural expectations that must be fulfilled in order for the person to be considered by others to have performed competently and credibly. When we convince others that we have performed credibly, we are engaging in what Goffman called *impression management.*[4]

It is widely acknowledged within the cultures of people with activity limitations that impression management is an important strategy to undertake. It is a practiced skill to develop such social proficiency that one's impairment is hardly noticed. Indeed, there is a word for this, *passing,* which means that one has hidden one's devalued characteristics from others successfully, so that one has been able to pass as "normal" or able-bodied.

The ability to manage the impressions of others is often so compelling that actual performance may be secondary to preserving identity by leaving a good impression. Studies of prosthetic and assistive technology devices show that their acceptance and use may be as dependent on appearance and perceived social acceptability as their functional benefits (Batavia & Hammer, 1990; Pippin & Fernie, 1997; Stein & Walley, 1983).

Of course, the easiest way to avoid rejection is to increase control and the possibility of rejection by avoiding social interaction altogether. In confronting the risk of social rejection, it is not unusual to find people with observable disability to retreat to the safety and emotional security of interactions limited to close friends and associates. These people, it is reasoned, know the person beyond the disfigurement. Avoidance strategies are more understandable when one considers that social disapproval is not simply an uncomfortable situation that evokes feelings of embarrassment or shame. It is, quite directly, an assault on one's identity.

Researchers have shown that while passing is a useful strategy for avoiding stigma, it can result in an unhealthy adaptation to disability if it results in denial. Successful adaptation to one's individual differences requires the ability to acknowledge one's differences and to integrate them into an identity that permits a confident expression of self (Weinberg & Sterritt, 1986). One of the challenges of acquired disability is reintegration into social patterns that promote acceptance of self and a more comfortable relationship with able-bodied persons. This comfort leads to more positive acceptance by those persons.

Disability and Identity Adaptations

A surprising number of studies have directly or indirectly studied the identity consequences of children and adults with chronic illnesses and disabling conditions. These have often shown that preserving and developing one's identity are often at the heart of adaptational strategies (Charmaz, 1994; Estroff, 1989; Monks, 1995; Ville, Ravaud, Marchal, Paicheler, & Fardeau, 1992; Weinberg & Sterrit, 1986).

For example, a study by Charmaz (1994) of men with chronic illnesses is relevant here. She found that when men did awaken to the changes in their bodies and accept the uncertainties of their futures, they engaged in reflection and reappraisals that often improved their awareness of self and personal priorities. It is noteworthy that reappraisals of productivity, achievement, and relationships were central to this process. As a result of these reappraisals, some men changed jobs, others retired or renegotiated their work assignments, and many followed health regimens, such as exercising, more devotedly.

One recurring theme in these and other studies of adaptation to illness and disability is the role of identity in creating a sense of coherence or continuity over time. When people experience loss and change, the continuity of their lives is disrupted. Identity is the great integrator of life experience. We interpret events that happen to us in terms of their meaning for our life stories. This gives life a sense of coherence.

[4]It is worth mentioning that stigma affects those with whom one shares identity. Consistent with the idea of distributed selves, spouses and family members may also endure the social cost of disfigurement, poor role performance, or deviance. For example, stigma accrues to families whose members have HIV or mental illness, or who have committed suicide.

Identity, Sense of Coherence, and Well-Being

People with a sense of coherence view their lives as understandable, meaningful, and manageable. The concept emanates from Aaron Antonovsky (1979), who proposed a model that would explain how some people are able to cope with stressors without experiencing the negative consequences to health experienced by others. Antonovsky proposed that a sense of coherence was central to this ability to cope with stress, suggesting that people who interpret their experiences within a meaningful and understandable framework, and who perceive that their challenges are manageable, are better equipped to deal with life's unexpected turns.

Research on the sense of coherence during the past 20 years has shown that people with this attribute, or way of viewing the world, are healthier and better adjusted than people without a strong sense of coherence. For example, significant relationships have been found between sense of coherence and blood pressure, emotional stability, global health, subjective well-being, and coping skills (Antonovsky, 1993). Sense of coherence is different from, but related to, another factor found in coping studies called hardiness (Kobasa, 1979).

Of importance to this discussion is the finding that sense of coherence seems to measure a human dimension that intersects with identity. Because it reflects one's efficacy or sense of agency, because it reflects meaning, and because it reflects a person's sense of how the events in their lives fit together, sense of coherence is related in important ways to the issue of identity (Baumeister & Tice, 1990; Korotkov, 1998). In fact, this relationship is borne out in studies of personal projects done by Little and others (Little, 1989; Christiansen, Backman, Little, & Nguyen, 1999). This research, using personal projects analysis (cf. Christiansen, Little, & Backman, 1998), seeks to connect occupations of everyday life with personality traits. Findings have shown a relationship between identity dimensions of personal projects and sense of coherence. This provides a small but important piece of evidence supporting the hypothesis that identity and sense of coherence are related, and possibly overlapping, concepts (see Figure 34.3).

Issues of coherence, personal identity, meaning, and well-being have been nicely tied together in research reported by Wong (1998). He has used an implicit theories approach to study how people define their lives as personally meaningful. Through analysis

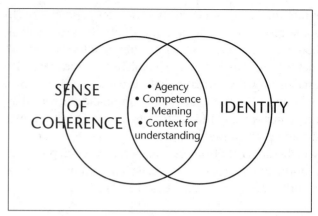

Figure 34.3. Concepts that link sense of coherence to identity.

of the responses of subjects in different age groups, he has identified nine factors that collectively provide a profile of an ideal meaningful life.[5] Four of these factors focus directly on the self. In these studies, Wong has found that when people have higher profiles on these factors, their subjective well-being increases.

We can summarize by noting that research has shown that people shape their identities through their daily occupations, which are performed in a social context that gives them symbolic meaning. Over time, our evolving identities and our actions are woven together to provide a coherent life story. The central place of occupations in shaping identity and creating life meaning is so powerful that one cannot help but marvel at their implications for occupational therapy practice.

Implications for Occupational Therapy Practice

Nearly 20 years ago, Bing (1981; see Chapter 2) provided a historical review of the people and ideas that have influenced occupational therapy since its inception. In his identification of themes that have provided particular relevance for the field, he included this principle: "The patient is the product of his or her own efforts, not the article made nor the activity accomplished" (p. 501). This principle suggests that the work of therapy involves identity building.

Therapy becomes identity building when therapists provide environments that help persons explore possible selves and achieve success in tasks that are instrumental to identities they strive to achieve, and when it

---

[5]The nine factors are achievement striving, religion, relationship, fulfillment, fairness–respect, self-confidence, self-integration, self-transcendence, and self-acceptance.

enables them to validate the identities that they have worked hard to achieve in the past.

Occupational Therapy as Identity Building

There is much opportunity for occupational therapy as a special and unique service that provides opportunities for people to establish, maintain, or reclaim their identities. Particularly in North America, the demographics of aging will bring the declines in function that are a threat to identity (Kunkel & Applebaum, 1992; Statistics Canada, 1993). It is no accident that late life depression is one of the most common mental health problems in adults 60 years of age and older. Although there are many causes of depression, late life depression can arise from a loss of self-esteem, a loss of meaningful roles, declining social contacts, and reduced functional status (Karp, 1994; Reker, 1997). Research on psychosocial theories of depression has shown that depression can be averted when people are given an opportunity to gain personal meaning from everyday activities, when their sense of optimism is renewed, and where they believe that there is choice and control in their lives (Baumeister, 1990; Brewer, 1993; Kapci, 1998; Rodin, 1986).

This was shown by investigators (Jackson, Carlson, Mandel, Zemke, & Clark, 1998) at the University of Southern California in their recent study of a program for well elderly persons. That successful program used lifestyle redesign to engage participants in occupations that provided both structure and meaning to the participants. The participants in the program showed less morbidity and higher morale than a control group, demonstrating clearly that occupations, through the mechanism of identity, provide the purpose, structure, and global meaning that is an essential need for all human beings. I suggest that the key link here is identity building.

Because issues of health and well-being are at stake, society needs services concerned with helping people establish and maintain their identities. The decline of abilities that comes with normal aging need not be interpreted or experienced as a decline in competence. The key to successful aging may very well be related to the acceptance of a changed body along with opportunities for demonstrating competence and control in mastering late life challenges that create the beginnings so necessary for satisfactory endings. Coming to terms with the end of life may be facilitated through occupations that lead to an enduring presence of self and the

sense that one can derive meaning from all that has happened during one's life.

Beyond the demographics of aging, there are other developments that call out for a profession that can help people find meaning in their lives. The recently released global burden of disease study contains some astonishing statistics. This study, completed at Harvard University but sponsored by the World Health Organization and the World Bank, is a careful epidemiological projection of the kinds of health-related problems the world will be dealing with in the year 2020 (Murray & Lopez, 1996).

The most interesting finding from the study is that unipolar major depression will become the second leading threat to life quality in the world. It is projected to increase significantly from 1990 levels in the developed countries. Besides dementia and osteoarthritis, other conditions showing major increases will be alcohol use and self-inflicted injuries. Although the projected pattern for the world in the year 2020 will show a general increase in overall health owing to the control of infectious diseases in the developing countries, many other health challenges will be of a nature that traditional medicine is currently unequipped to handle. Depression, self-inflicted injuries, and alcohol abuse have one thing in common—they are diseases of meaning; therefore, they can be linked to social conditions that permit people to lose their identity and sense of purpose and meaning in life.

Summary

In this article, I have made the claim that occupations constitute the mechanism that enables persons to develop and express their identities. I have asserted that identities are central features of understanding the world in an evolving self-narrative, and that the continuity provided by identity enables life to be comprehended in a manner that helps minimize the uncertainties and stresses of daily life. I have maintained that it is the imagined self that provides the context for motivation and purpose and that competence is interpreted as the capable expression of identity within a social world. And finally, and most importantly, I have argued that that identity is the pathway by which people, through daily occupations and relationships with others, are able to derive meaning from their lives.

As a profession concerned with enabling people to engage in meaningful daily occupations, occupational therapy is positioned uniquely to meet the challenges confronting people whose identity is threatened by impairments, limitations to activity, and restrictions on their participation as social beings. We have seen that, in the years ahead, our friends and colleagues will be challenged with assaults on their identities brought by age, health problems, and social conditions.

Englehardt (1986) once described occupational therapists as technologists and custodians of meaning. As an outsider, he saw the same opportunity and unfulfilled promise that Adolph Meyer (1922; see Chapter 4) described in the founding years of occupational therapy. Yet, a full and genuine appreciation of the power of occupation to enable health and well-being has not yet made its way across the landscape of the profession.

Just as individual persons create their unique identities and life meaning through occupations, so too do professions, which represent groups of people with shared purposes, values, and interests, realize their identities through collective action. Biomedicine will experience many great advances in the years ahead. But no genetic code, no chemical intervention, and no microsurgical technology will be invented to repair broken identities and the assault on meaning that accompanies them. Because of this, the new millennium will realize the health-enabling, restorative potential of occupation, and the promise of occupational therapy will be fulfilled.

Acknowledgments

This lecture is dedicated to my friend and mentor, Robert K. Bing, EdD, OTR, FAOTA; to my special colleague and friend, Carolyn Baum, PhD, OTR/L, FAOTA; to my parents; and especially to my wife, Pamela, a pediatric occupational therapist; and, not least of all, to my children, Carrie, Erik, and Kalle.

I thank Cindy Hammecker, Charles Hayden, and Natalie Sims for their invaluable assistance in the preparation of this paper. I am indebted to my colleagues Kenneth Ottenbacher, PhD, OTR, FAOTA, and Beatriz Abreu, PhD, OTR, FAOTA, for their expressions of confidence and support.

References

Antonovsky, A. (1979). *Health, stress and coping: New perspectives on mental health and physical well-being.* San Francisco: Jossey-Bass.

Antonovsky, A. (1993). The structure and properties of the Sense of Coherence Scale. *Social Science and Medicine, 36,* 725–733.

Bandura, A. (1977). Self-efficacy: Toward a unifying theory of behavioral change. *Psychological Review, 84,* 191–215.

Batavia, A. I., & Hammer, G. S. (1990). Toward the development of consumer based criteria for the evaluation of assistive devices. *Journal of Rehabilitation Research, 27,* 425–436.

Bateson, M. C. (1996). Enfolded activity and the concept of occupation. In R. Zemke & F. Clark (Eds.), *Occupational science: The evolving discipline* (pp. 5–12). Philadelphia: F. A. Davis.

Baumeister, R. F. (1982). Self-esteem, self-presentation and future interaction. A dilemma of reputation. *Journal of Personality, 50,* 29–45.

Baumeister, R. F. (1986). *Identity: Cultural change and the struggle for self.* New York: Oxford University Press.

Baumeister, R. F. (1990). Suicide as escape from self. *Psychological Review, 97*(1), 90–113.

Baumeister, R. F. (1997). Identity, self-concept and self-esteem. In R. Hogan, J. Johnson, & S. Briggs (Eds.), *Handbook of personality psychology* (pp. 681–711). San Diego, CA: Academic Press.

Baumeister, R. F., & Tice, D. M. (1990). Self-esteem and responses to success and failure. Subsequent performance and intrinsic motivation. *Journal of Personality, 53,* 450–467.

Bing, R. K. (1981). Occupational therapy revisited: A paraphrastic journey. 1981 Eleanor Clarke Slagle Lectures. *American Journal of Occupational Therapy, 35,* 499–518. Reprinted as Chapter 2.

Brewer, B. W. (1993). Self identity and specific vulnerability to depressed mood. *Journal of Personality, 61*(3), 343–364.

Bruner, J. S. (1990). *Acts of meaning.* Cambridge: Harvard University Press.

Charmaz, K. (1994). Identity dilemmas of chronically ill men. *Sociological Quarterly, 35*(2), 269–288.

Christiansen, C. H., Little, B. R., & Backman, C. (1998). Personal projects: A useful approach to the study of occupation. *American Journal of Occupational Therapy, 52,* 439–446. http://dx.doi.org/10.5014/ajot.52.6.439

Christiansen, C. H., Backman, C., Little, B. R., & Nguyen, A. (1999). Occupations and well-being: A study of personal projects. *American Journal of Occupational Therapy, 53,* 91–100. http://dx.doi.org/10.5014/ajot.53.1.91

Cooley, C. H. (1902). *Human nature and the social order.* New York: Scribner.

Crowne, D. P., & Marlowe, D. (1964). *The approval motive.* New York: Wiley.

Debats, D. L., Drost, J., & Hansen P. (1995). Experiences of meaning in life: A combined qualitative and quantitative approach. *British Journal of Psychology, 86*(3), 359–375.

Englehardt, T. (1977). Defining occupational therapy: The meaning of therapy and the virtues of occupation. *American Journal of Occupational Therapy, 31,* 666–672.

Englehardt, T. (1986). Occupational therapists as technologists and custodians of meaning. In G. Kielhofner (Ed.), *Health through occupation* (pp. 139–144). Philadelphia: F. A. Davis.

Erikson, E. H. (1968). *Identity, youth and crisis.* New York: W. W. Norton.

Estroff, S. E. (1989). Self, identity and subjective experiences of schizophrenia: In search of the subject. *Schizophrenia Bulletin, 15*(2), 189–196.

Fidler, G. S., & Fidler, J. W. (1978). Doing and becoming: Purposeful action and self actualization. *American Journal of Occupational Therapy, 32,* 305–310.

Franks, D. D., & Marolla, J. (1976). Efficacious action and social approval as interacting dimensions of self-esteem: A tentative formulation through construct validation. *Sociometry, 39*(4), 324–341.

Gage, M., & Polatajko, H. (1994). Enhancing occupational performance through an understanding of perceived self-efficacy. *American Journal of Occupational Therapy, 48,* 452–461. http://dx.doi.org/10.5014/ajot.48.5.452

Gergen, K. J. (1991). *The saturated self: Dilemmas of identity in modern life.* New York: Basic.

Gergen, K. J., & Gergen, M. M. (1988). Narrative and the self as relationship. In L. Berkowitz (Ed.), *Advances in experimental and social psychology* (pp. 17–55). San Diego, CA: Academic Press.

Goffman, E. (1959). *The presentation of self in everyday life.* Garden City, NY: Doubleday.

Goffman, E. (1963). *Stigma: Notes on the management of a spoiled identity.* Englewood Cliffs, NJ: Prentice-Hall.

Greenwald, A. G. (1980). The totalitarian ego: Fabrication and revision of personal history. *American Psychologist, 35,* 603–613.

Harré, R. (1983). *Personal being.* Oxford, U.K.: Blackwell.

Harré, R. (1998). *The singular self.* London: Sage.

Heatherton, T. F., & Baumeister, R. F. (1991). Binge eating as escape from self-awareness. *Psychological Bulletin, 110,* 86–108.

Jackson, J., Carlson, M., Mandel, D., Zemke, R., & Clark, F. (1998). Occupation in lifestyle redesign: The well elderly study occupational therapy program. *American Journal of Occupational Therapy, 52,* 326–336. http://dx.doi.org/10.5014/ajot.52.5.326

James, W. (1892). *Psychology: The briefer course.* New York: Henry Holt & Co.

Kagan, J. (1981). *The second year: The emergence of self-awareness.* Cambridge, MA: Harvard University Press.

Kapci, E. G. (1998). Test of the hopelessness theory of depression: Drawing negative inference from negative life events. *Psychological Reports, 82*(2), 355–363.

Karp, D. A. (1994). Living with depression: Illness and identity turning points. *Qualitative Health Research, 4*(1), 6–30.

Keller, A., Ford, L. H., & Meacham, J. A. (1978). Dimensions of self-concept in preschool children. *Developmental Psychology, 14,* 483–489.

Kobasa, S. C. (1979). Stressful life events, personality and health: An inquiry into hardiness. *Journal of Personality and Social Psychology, 37,* 1–11.

Kondo, D. (1990). *Crafting selves: Power, gender and discourses of identity in a Japanese workplace.* Chicago: University of Chicago Press.

Korotkov, D. L. (1998). The sense of coherence: Making sense out of chaos. In P. T. P. Wong & P. S. Fry (Eds.), *The human quest for meaning: A handbook of psychological research and clinical applications* (pp. 51–70). Mahwah, NJ: Erlbaum.

Kris, E. (1952). *Psychoanalytic explorations in art.* New York: International Universities Press.

Kunkel, S. R., & Applebaum, R. A. (1992). Estimating the prevalence of long-term disability for an aging society. *Journal of Gerontology: Social Sciences, 475,* S253–S260.

Langer, E. J., & Rodin, J. (1976). The effects of choice and enhanced personal responsibility for the aged: A field experiment in an institutional setting. *Journal of Personality and Social Psychology, 34*(2), 192–198.

Little, B. R. (1989). Personal projects analysis: Trivial pursuits, magnificent obsessions, and the search for coherence. In D. M. Buss & N. Cantor (Eds.), *Personality psychology: Recent trends and emerging directions* (pp. 15–31). New York: Springer-Verlag.

Loevenger, J. (1976). *Ego development.* San Francisco: Jossey-Bass.

Markus, H. (1977). Self-schemata and processing information about the self. *Journal of Personality and Social Psychology, 35,* 63–78.

Markus, H., & Nurius, P. S. (1986). Possible selves. *American Psychologist, 41,* 954–969.

McAdams, D. P. (1996). Personality, modernity, and the storied self: A contemporary framework for studying persons. *Psychological Inquiry, 7,* 295–321.

McAdams, D. P. (1997). Multiplicity of self versus unity of identity. In R. D. Ashmore & L. Jussim (Eds.), *Self and identity: Fundamental issues* (pp. 46–78). New York: Oxford University Press.

McCuaig, M., & Frank, G. (1991). The able self: Adaptive patterns and choices in independent living for a person with cerebral palsy. *American Journal of Occupational Therapy, 45,* 224–234.

Mead, G. H. (1934). *Mind, self and society.* Chicago: University of Chicago Press.

Meyer, A. (1922). The philosophy of occupation therapy. *Archives of Occupational Therapy, 1,* 1–10. Reprinted in Chapter 4.

Monks, J. (1995). Life stories and sickness experience: A performance perspective. *Culture, Medicine and Psychiatry, 19*(4), 453–478.

Moore, S. L. (1997). A phenomenological study of meaning in life in suicidal older adults. *Archives of Psychiatric Nursing, 11*(1), 29–36.

Murray, C.J.L., & Lopez, A. D. (1996). Alternative visions of the future: Projecting mortality and disability 1990–2020. In C.J.L. Murray & A. D. Lopez (Eds.), *The global burden of disease* (pp. 325–396). Geneva, Switzerland: World Health Organization.

Ogilvie, D. M. (1987). The undesired self: A neglected variable in personality research. *Journal of Personality and Social Psychology, 52,* 379–385.

Pavot, W., Fujita, F., & Diener, E. (1997). The relation between self-aspect congruence, personality and subjective well-being. *Personality and Individual Differences, 22*(2), 183–191.

Piaget, J. (1954). *The construction of reality in the child.* New York: Basic.

Pippin, K., & Fernie, G. R. (1997). Designing devices that are acceptable to the frail elderly: A new understanding based upon how older people perceive a walker. *Technology and Disability, 7*(1/2), 93–102.

Polkinghorne, D. (1988). *Narrative knowing and the human sciences.* Albany, NY: State University of New York Press.

Reker, G. T. (1997). Personal meaning, optimism, and choice. Existential predictors of depression in community and institutional elderly. *Gerontologist, 37*(6), 709–716.

Rodin, J. C. (1986). Aging and health: Effects of the sense of control. *Science, 233*(4770), 1271–1276.

Rogers, J. (1982). Order and disorder in medicine and occupational therapy. *American Journal of Occupational Therapy, 31,* 29–35.

Ruble, D. (1983). The development of social comparison processes and their role in achievement-related self-so-cialization. In E. T. Higgins, D. Ruble, & W. Hartup (Eds.), *Social cognition and social behavior: Developmental perspectives* (pp. 134–157). New York: Cambridge University Press.

Schrauger, J. S., & Schoeneman, T. J. (1979). Symbolic interactionist view of self-concept: Through the looking glass darkly. *Psychological Bulletin, 86,* 549–573.

Smith, M. B. (1974). Competence and adaptation: A perspective on therapeutic ends and means. *American Journal of Occupational Therapy, 28,* 11–15.

Sommer, K. L., & Baumeister, R. F. (1998). The construction of meaning from life events: Empirical studies of personal narratives. In P.T.P. Wong & P. S. Fry (Eds.), *The human quest for meaning: A handbook of psychological research and clinical applications* (pp. 143–161). Mahwah, NJ: Erlbaum.

Stachey, J. (Ed.). (1990). *The standard edition of the complete psychological works of Sigmund Freud.* New York: W. W. Norton.

Statistics Canada. (1993). *Population ageing and the elderly: Current demographic analysis.* Cat. No. 9I-533E. Ottawa, Canada: Government of Canada.

Stein, R. B., & Walley, M. (1983). Functional comparison of upper extremity amputees using myoelectric and conventional prostheses. *Archives of Physical Medicine and Rehabilitation, 73,* 1169–1173.

Swann, W. B. (1987). Identity negotiation: Where two roads meet. *Journal of Personality and Social Psychology, 53,* 1038–1051.

Swann, W. B., & Hill, C. A. (1982). When our identities are mistaken: Reaffirming self-conceptions through social interac- tion. *Journal of Personality and Social Psychology, 43,* 59–66.

van selm, M., & Dittmann-Kohli, F. (1998). Meaninglessness in the second half of life: The development of a construct. *International Journal of Aging and Human Development, 47*(2), 81–104.

Ville, I., Ravaud, J. F., Marchal, F., Paicheler, H., & Fardeau, M. (1992). Social identity and the international classification of handicaps: An evaluation of the consequences of facioscapulohumeral muscular dystrophy. *Disability and Rehabilitation, 14*(4), 168–175.

Vygotsky, L. S. (1981). The instrumental method in psychology. In J. V. Wertsch (Ed.), *The concept of activity in Soviet psychology* (pp. 134–143). Armonk, NY: M. E. Sharp.

Weinberg, N., & Sterritt, M. (1986). Disability and identity: A study of identity patterns in adolescents with hearing impairments. *Rehabilitation Psychology, 31*(2), 95–103.

White, R. W. (1959). Motivation reconsidered: The concept of competence. *Psychological Review, 66,* 297–333.

White, R. W. (1971). The urge toward competence. *American Journal of Occupational Therapy, 25,* 271–274.

Wong, P.T.P. (1998). Implicit theories of meaningful life and the development of the personal meaning profile. In P.T.P. Wong & P. S. Fry (Eds.), *The human quest for meaning: A handbook of psychological research and clinical applications* (pp. 111–140). Mahwah, NJ: Erlbaum.

Position Statement: Human Rights

Introduction

The WFOT fully endorses the UN Universal Declaration of Human Rights. The purpose of this Position Paper is to state the World Federation of Occupational Therapists (WFOT) position on human rights in relation to human occupation and participation.

Principles

- People have the right to participate in a range of occupations that enable them to flourish, fulfil their potential and experience satisfaction in a way consistent with their culture and beliefs.
- People have the right to be supported to participate in occupation and, through engaging in occupation, to be included and valued as members of their family, community and society.
- People have the right to choose for themselves: to be free of pressure, force, or coercion; in participating in occupations that may threaten safety, survival or health and those occupations that are dehumanising, degrading or illegal.
- The right to occupation encompasses civic, educative, productive, social, creative, spiritual and restorative occupations. The expression of the human right to occupation will take different forms in different places, because occupations are shaped by their cultural, societal and geographic context.
- At a societal level, the human right to occupation is underpinned by the valuing of each person's diverse contribution to the valued and meaningful occupations of the society, and is ensured by equitable access to participation in occupation, regardless of difference.
- Abuses of the right to occupation may take the form of economic, social or physical exclusion, through attitudinal or physical barriers, or through control of access to necessary knowledge, skills, resources, or venues where occupation takes place.
- Global conditions that threaten the right to occupation include poverty, disease, social discrimination, displacement, natural and man-made disasters and armed conflict. In addition, the right to occupation is subject to cultural beliefs and customs, local circumstances and institutional power and practices.

Strategies for Action

Occupational therapists have the knowledge and skills to support persons who experience limitations or barriers to participation in occupation. Occupational therapists also have a role and responsibility to develop and synthesize knowledge to support participation; to identify and raise issues of occupational barriers and injustices; and to work with groups, communities and societies to enhance participation in occupation for all persons. Achieving this is to achieve an occupationally just society. Challenges for Occupational Therapists and Occupational Therapy Associations lie in the following areas:

- Accepting professional responsibility to identify and address occupational injustices and limit the impact of such injustices experienced by individuals
- Raising collective awareness of the broader view of occupation and participation in society as a right.
- Learning to work collaboratively with individuals, organisations, communities and societies, to promote participation through meaningful occupation.
- Teaching and developing universal design, thereby promoting a society that is truly accessible to all.
- Responsibly addressing the issue of cultural sensitivity, and fostering cultural competency

Definition "Occupation"

In occupational therapy, *occupations* refer to the everyday activities that people do as individuals, in families and with communities to occupy time and bring meaning and purpose to life. Occupations include things people need to, want to and are expected to do.

Occupational Therapy's Commitment to Nondiscrimination and Inclusion

The occupational therapy profession affirms the right of every individual to access and fully participate in society. This paper states the profession's stance on nondiscrimination and inclusion.

Nondiscrimination exists when we accept and treat all people equally. In doing so, we avoid differentiating between people because of biases or prejudices. We value individuals and respect their culture, ethnicity, race, age, religion, gender, sexual orientation, and capacities, consistent with the principles defined and described in the *Occupational Therapy Code of Ethics and Ethics Standards* (American Occupational Therapy Association [AOTA], 2010). Nondiscrimination is a necessary prerequisite for inclusion. Inclusion requires that we ensure not only that everyone is treated fairly and equitably but also that all individuals have the same opportunities to participate in the naturally occurring activities of society, such as attending social events, having access to public transportation, and participating in professional organizations. We also believe that when we do not discriminate against others and when we include all members of society in our daily lives, we reap the benefits of being with individuals who have different perspectives, opinions, and talents from our own.

We support nondiscrimination and inclusion throughout our profession. Our concerns are twofold—for the persons who receive occupational therapy services and for our professional colleagues. In professional practice, our evaluations and interventions are designed to facilitate our clients' engagement in occupations to support their health and participation in the various contexts and environments of their lives. Contexts and environments include, but are not limited to, individuals' cultural, personal, temporal, virtual, physical, and social contexts as described in the *Occupational Therapy Practice Framework: Domain and Process* (AOTA, 2014). As occupational therapists and occupational therapy assistants, we assume a collaborative partnership with clients and their significant others to support the individual's right to self-direction.

We believe that inclusion is achieved through the combined efforts of clients, their families, and significant others; health, education, and social services professionals; legislators; community members; and others. We support all individuals and their significant others' rights to fully participate in making decisions that concern their daily occupations: activities of daily living, instrumental activities of daily living, rest and sleep, work, education, play, leisure, and social participation.

AOTA and its members recognize the legal mandates concerning nondiscriminatory practices. However, the concept of nondiscrimination is not limited to that which is dictated by law. This professional association, through its members, boards, commissions, committees, officers, and staff, supports the belief that all members of the occupational therapy professional community are entitled to maximum opportunities to develop and use their abilities. These individuals also have the right to achieve productive and satisfying professional and personal lives.

We are committed to nondiscrimination and inclusion as an affirmation of our belief that the interests of all members of the profession are best served when the inherent worth of every individual is recognized and valued. We maintain that society has an obligation to provide the reasonable accommodations necessary to allow individuals access to social, educational, recreational, and vocational opportunities. By embracing the concepts of nondiscrimination and inclusion, we will all benefit from the opportunities afforded in a diverse society.

References

American Occupational Therapy Association. (2010). Occupational therapy code of ethics and ethics standards (2010). *American Journal of Occupational Therapy, 64*(6, Suppl.), S17–S26. http://dx.doi.org/10.5014/ajot.2010.64S17

American Occupational Therapy Association. (2014). Occupational therapy practice framework: Domain and process (3rd ed.). *American Journal of Occupational Therapy, 68*(Suppl. 1), S1–S48. http://dx.doi.org/10.5014/ajot.2014.682006

Authors
Ruth H. Hansen, PhD, FAOTA
Jim Hinojosa, PhD, OT, FAOTA

for

The Commission on Practice
Mary Jane Youngstrom, MS, OTR, *Chairperson*

Adopted by the Representative Assembly 1999M4

Reference citations reviewed and updated by the Commission on Practice, February 2014
Debbie Amini, EdD, OTR/L, CHT, FAOTA, *Chairperson*

Adopted by the Representative Assembly Coordinating Council (RACC) for the Representative Assembly, 2014.

Note. This document replaces the 2009 document *Occupational Therapy's Commitment to Nondiscrimination and Inclusion,* previously published and copyrighted in 2009 by the American Occupational Therapy Association in the *American Journal of Occupational Therapy, 63,* 819–820. http://dx.doi.org/10.5014/ajot.63.6.819

To be published and copyrighted in 2014 by the American Occupational Therapy Association in the *American Journal of Occupational Therapy, 68*(Suppl. 3). Reprinted with permission.

AOTA's Societal Statement on Livable Communities

The demographic profile of the United States is rapidly changing, with an increasing number of older adults and persons with disabilities who desire to remain in their homes and communities as they grow older, a concept referred to as *aging-in-place*. According to the United Nations (2007), persons with disabilities have the same right as all other members of society to live in the community with opportunities to choose their place of residence and to have equal access to support services that promote full participation in all aspects of community living. To support these rights, society must create communities that enable all residents to live, work, play, and participate in locations of their choice (AARP, 2005; National Council on Disability, 2004). "A livable community is one that has affordable and appropriate housing, supportive community features and services, and adequate mobility options, which together facilitate personal independence and engagement of the residents in civic and social life" (AARP, 2005, p. 4).

The American Occupational Therapy Association's (AOTA's) *Core Values and Attitudes of Occupational Therapy Practice* (AOTA, 1993) and *Occupational Therapy Code of Ethics* (AOTA, 2005) support equality for all individuals, and are congruent with the goals of livable communities. Occupational therapy practitioners plan and implement strategies that promote their client's participation in community life by creating opportunities to establish, restore, or maintain the skills used in activities of daily living and other meaningful occupations and by supporting clients' who are advocating for their own and others' rights. Further, occupational therapy practitioners advocate for universal design and environmental modifications that remove barriers in homes and communities to ensure access to supportive community services, including transportation, personal care, health care, education, employment, and other services, and to facilitate engagement in social and civic activities. Occupational therapy promotes public health and civic engagement by advocating for and assisting in the creation of more livable communities through effective partnerships with individuals, private organizations, and government agencies. Supporting health and participation through active engagement in meaningful activities in the home and community contributes to health, wellness, and quality of life for all individuals (AOTA, 2006).

References

AARP Public Policy Institute. (2005). *Beyond 50.05—A report to the nation on livable communities: Creating environments for successful aging.* Washington, DC: Author.

American Occupational Therapy Association. (1993). Core values and attitudes of occupational therapy practice. *American Journal of Occupational Therapy, 47,* 1085–1086.

American Occupational Therapy Association. (2005). Occupational therapy code of ethics (2005). *American Journal of Occupational Therapy, 59,* 639–642.

American Occupational Therapy Association. (2006). *AOTA Board Task Force on Health and Wellness: Report to the Executive Board.* Retrieved February 4, 2008, from www.atoa.org/News/Centennial/AdHoc/2006/40407.aspx

National Council on Disability. (2004, December). *Livable communities for adults with disabilities: The 2004 report, executive summary.* Available online at http://www.ncd.gov/newsroom/publications/2004/pdf/livablecommunities.pdf

United Nations. (2007). *Rights and dignity of persons with disabilities, Article 19.* Retrieved May 11, 2008, from http://www.un.org/disabilities/documents/convention/convoptprot-e.pdf

Authors
Lisa Ann Fagan, MS, OTR/L
Cheri Cabrera, OTR

for

The Representative Assembly Coordinating Council (RACC):
Deborah Murphy-Fischer, MBA, OTR, BCP, IMT, *Chairperson*
Brent Braveman, PhD, OTR/L, FAOTA
René Padilla, PhD, OTR/L, FAOTA
Kathlyn Reed, PhD, OTR, FAOTA, MLIS
Janet V. DeLany, DEd, OTR/L, FAOTA
Pam Toto, MS, OTR/L, BCG, FAOTA
Barbara Schell, PhD, OTR/L, FAOTA
Carol H. Gwin, OT/L, *AOTA Staff Liaison*

Adopted by the Representative Assembly 2008CS85

Occupational Therapy's Perspective on the Use of Environments and Contexts to Support Health and Participation in Occupations

Purpose

This paper articulates the position of the American Occupational Therapy Association (AOTA) regarding how, across all areas of practice, occupational therapy practitioners[1] select, create, and use environments and contexts to support clients' health and participation in desired occupations.

Introduction

The value and purpose of occupational therapy is to support the health and participation of clients by engaging them in their desired occupations (AOTA, 2008). *Occupations* are activities that "reflect cultural values, provide structure to living and meaning to individuals; these activities meet human needs for self-care, enjoyment, and participation in society" (Crepeau, Cohn, & Schell, 2003, p. 1031). Where and how occupational therapy services are provided is based on the notion that clients' engagement in occupation is inextricably situated in environments and contexts. The *environment* refers to external physical and social aspects that surround clients while engaging in the occupation. *Contexts* are the cultural, personal, temporal, and virtual aspects of this engagement; some contexts are external to the client (e.g., virtual), some are internal to the client (e.g., personal), and some may have both external features and internalized beliefs and values (e.g., cultural) (AOTA, 2008). Occupational therapy practitioners view human performance as a transactive relationship among people, their occupations, and environments and contexts.

Using their expertise in analyzing these complex and reciprocal relationships, occupational therapy practitioners make recommendations to structure, modify, or adapt the environment and context to enhance and support performance. Both environment and context influence clients' success in desired occupations and therefore are critical aspects of any occupational therapy assessment, intervention, and outcome. This assumption is consistent with current educational and health care laws and policies that stipulate that assessment and intervention by providers take place in the natural and least restrictive environments that support the client's successful participation (Americans with Disabilities Act of 1990; Individuals with Disabilities Education Improvement Act Amendments of 2004; *Olmstead v. L.C. and E.W.*, 1999).

Occupational Therapy Process

Occupational therapy practitioners support people where life is lived. To support people to live meaningful lives in environments and contexts that best meet their needs and desires, practitioners interpret a wide range of laws, regulations, and standards as they seek to maintain the integrity and values of the profession to benefit clients. Table 1 reviews key legislation related to occupational therapy intervention and how these laws apply to practice.

---

[1]When the term *occupational therapy practitioner* is used in this document, it refers to both occupational therapists and occupational therapy assistants (AOTA, 2006). *Occupational therapists* are responsible for all aspects of occupational therapy service delivery and are accountable for the safety and effectiveness of the occupational therapy service delivery process. *Occupational therapy assistants* deliver occupational therapy services under the supervision of and in partnership with an occupational therapist (AOTA, 2010).

Table 1. Legislation and Court Cases Related to Occupational Therapy Practice

Federal Law/Court Case/Movement	Key Constructs	Application to OT Practice
Rehabilitation Act of 1973, Section 504	• Creates an obligation not to discriminate on the basis of special education needs for individuals with disabilities • Helps ensure students with disabilities receive the services, supports, and accommodations necessary to meet their needs • Specifically states "SEC. 504. No otherwise qualified handicapped individual in the United States, as defined in section 7(6), shall, solely by reason of his handicap, be excluded from the participation in, be denied the benefits of, or be subjected to discrimination under any program or activity receiving Federal financial assistance"	• Has implications for providing services to all individuals with disabilities in any program funded with federal funds • Addresses services for students with disabilities to ensure participation and access to the general education curriculum
No Child Left Behind Act (NCLB, 2001)	• Is the most recent re-authorization of ESEA (see below). • Expands accountability standards for public education • Includes children with disabilities in the accountability models developed to gauge student and school success	• Creates increased motivation for schools to use all existing resources to improve student achievement • Along with IDEA 2004, gives rise and momentum to models of schoolwide support such as response to intervention and positive behavioral supports • Creates broader opportunities for OT to benefit students with and without disabilities
Individuals with Disabilities Education Improvement Act (IDEA, 2004)	• Follows up on the Elementary and Secondary Education Act (ESEA) of 1965, which authorized grants to state institutions and state-operated schools devoted to the education of children with disabilities • Expands and renames the Education of All Handicapped Children Act of 1975 and the successor Individuals with Disabilities Education Act of 1997. • Reauthorizes and expands the discretionary programs, mandates transition services, defines assistive technology devices and services, and adds autism and traumatic brain injury to the list of categories of children and youth eligible for special education and related services • Requires that "removal of children with disabilities from the regular educational environment occurs only if the nature or severity of the disability is such that education in regular classes can not be achieved satisfactorily" [34 C.F.R. 300.114(a)(ii)].	• Clearly establishes OT as a primary service in early intervention and specifically identifies OT as a related service under Part B for school-age children • Changes how society views children with disabilities; opens doors for participation; and raises expectations of productivity, dignity, and independence

(continued)

Table 1. Legislation and Court Cases Related to Occupational Therapy Practice *(cont.)*

Federal Law/Court Case/Movement	Key Constructs	Application to OT Practice
Social Security Amendments of 1965 (Medicare)	• Establishes a national public health care program to meet the needs of older Americans and people with disabilities (Social Security Disability Insurance) who qualify for service on the basis of disability status and a sufficient work history • Under Part A, covers expenses associated with inpatient hospital stays, skilled nursing facilities, and some home health care • Under Part B, covers approved outpatient physician services, outpatient hospital services, certain home health services, and durable medical supplies and equipment	• Creates a system of health care financing and insurance for older Americans • Creates a steady funding stream for health care, including OT • Focuses mainly on specific health care issues and is not as involved in providing social supports and services as is Medicaid
Older Americans Act (OAA, 1965)	• Establishes a system and network for social, health, and community support for older Americans • Creates a network of local, regional, and state Area Agencies on Aging (AAAs) and provides broad federal grants to meet identified needs • Allows local AAAs to use funding to best meet the needs within their communities	• Provides flexible funding options that support OT services in community health and social services programs for seniors • Increases focus and desire for community-based living resources and aging in place
Omnibus Budget Reconciliation Act of 1987 (Federal Nursing Home Reform Act)	• Creates a set of national minimum standards of care and rights for people living in certified nursing facilities • Requires nursing homes to develop individualized care plans for residents that focus on maintaining or improving the ability to walk, bathe, and complete other ADLs absent of medical reasons • Requires nursing homes to develop individualized care plans for residents and training of paraprofessional staff • Protects residents' right be free of unnecessary and inappropriate physical and chemical restraints	• Creates opportunities for OT practitioners to facilitate balanced lifestyles and healthy routines in institutional care settings often in partnership with Nursing (Restorative Nursing Programs), Activities staff, and other departments • OT practitioners may advocate to support the needs of older adults and their families and caregivers by addressing environmental modifications and adaptations needed for maximum performance and safety, both in personal environments (e.g., wheelchairs, beds) as well as bedrooms, bathrooms, and common areas.
Americans with Disabilities Act (ADA) of 1990	• Extends previous civil rights legislation • Provides a clear mandate to end discrimination against people with disabilities in all areas of life • Includes five titles that address employment, state and local government services, transportation, public accommodations (i.e., public places and services), and telecommunications	• Supports initiatives and interventions that promote function and participation for people with disabilities across the life span • Supports independent living, accessibility, environmental modifications, and other reasonable accommodations

(continued)

Table 1. Legislation and Court Cases Related to Occupational Therapy Practice *(cont.)*

Federal Law/Court Case/Movement	Key Constructs	Application to OT Practice
Independent Living Movement (Batavia, 1999) 1972—First independent living center opens	• Is an important part of the broader movement for disability rights • Supports the premise that people with even the most severe disabilities should have the choice of living in the community • Supports an individual to use personal assistance services to manage his or her personal care, to keep a home, to have a job, to attend school, to worship, and to otherwise participate in the life of the community • Advocates for the removal of architectural and transportation barriers that prevent people with disabilities from sharing fully in all aspects of society	• Supports OT evaluation and intervention to be provided in natural environments where people live, work, and play and to adapt to and encounter the realities of the physical, social, attitudinal, and political contexts • Intervention includes consultation, program development, and advocacy with teachers in schools, supervisors in jobs, citizens' organizations, local governments, businesses, local media, and advocacy organizations
Olmstead v. L.C. and E. W. (1999)	• Affirms the right of individuals with disabilities to live in their community in 6–3 ruling by the U.S. Supreme Court against the State of Georgia • Requires states to place people with mental disabilities in community settings rather than in institutions • Dictates that the community placement must be appropriate; that the transfer from institutional care to a less restrictive setting is not opposed by the affected individual; and that the placement can be reasonably accommodated, taking into account the resources available to the state and the needs of others with mental disabilities	• Establishes precedent for an enforcement of a federal mandate for services to be provided in the least restrictive environment and in settings of choice for people with disabilities • Creates opportunities and obligations for OT practitioners to comply with the letter and spirit of the decision by designing intervention to support community living for people with disabilities and remove barriers such as attitudinal, physical, social, and policy related

Note. OT = occupational therapy; ADLs = activities of daily living.

Occupational therapy practitioners engage in a collaborative process with clients to identify clients' strengths and barriers to health and participation in society. As part of this process, practitioners consider a variety of personal, environmental, and contextual factors that guide the evaluation, intervention, and expected outcomes of occupational therapy services. Personal factors such as clients' age, time of intervention during the life course, service delivery environments, clients' or caregivers' goals, clients' occupational performance, and the services available can guide the decision-making process.

Occupational therapy practitioners "engineer" the environment as they consider the occupational needs of clients in their lived environments. They analyze performance in relation to how features of the envi-

Table 2. Case Studies: Environmental Considerations and Interventions for Specific Populations

Case Description	Environmental Considerations for OT Service Delivery	Selected Examples of OT Interventions Addressing Environments and Contexts	Research Evidence and Related Resources Guiding Practice
A **15-month-old boy** was born at 29 weeks' gestation. He has had difficulty sitting up, particularly during feeding, and achieving other developmental milestones. He is living at home with his family.	The focus of intervention is to support the entire family system to sustain their family life while addressing the developmental needs of the child. Intervention is provided in the home with recommendations as to how to adapt the natural environment to support the child's occupational performance and development.	• After discharge from the NICU, provide direct intervention in home to promote safety and establish child's developmental skills. • Collaborate with family to structure and modify the physical and social environments within the home to support occupational performance. • Educate caregiver in developmental principles, positioning, and activities to facilitate feeding and development. • Consult with family and other members of transdisciplinary team related to supporting family goals.	• Performing everyday activities in the natural setting provides reinforcement and support to achieve and enhance performance and competence (Dunst et al., 2001; Dunst, Trivette, Hamby, & Bruder, 2006). • Helping families accommodate to demands of daily life with a child with delays helps families develop appropriate and sustainable routines congruent with their values and child's developmental needs (Keogh, Bernheimer, Gallimore, & Weisner, 1998).
A **3-year-old boy** with social and emotional regulation challenges attends a center-based pre-school program.	The focus of intervention is to provide early childhood services in an inclusive classroom to enhance the child's opportunities for play with peers in naturally occurring situations that arise in the classroom. OT intervention is integrated into the classroom activities.	• Structure play group to promote peer social interaction skills. • Direct intervention with child and parents to promote self-regulation and establish routines to enable child's transitions throughout the day. • Consult with early childhood team to analyze demands of pre-school class and make recommendations for adaptations to support performance.	• Center-based early intervention services have a positive effect on children's social functioning (Blok, Fukkink, Gebhardt, & Leseman, 2005). • Preschoolers with disabilities perform as well, if not better, when placed in quality inclusive classroom settings and playgroups (Bailey, Aytch, Odom, Symons, & Wolery, 1999; Odom, 2000). • Parents of children with disabilities commonly report that they perceive inclusive classroom practices as contributing to their child's self-esteem, confidence, and happiness as well as reshaping their own expectations of their child's ability to develop and learn with others (Buysse, Skinner, & Grant, 2001).

(continued)

Table 2. Case Studies: Environmental Considerations and Interventions for Specific Populations *(cont.)*

Case Description	Environmental Considerations for OT Service Delivery	Selected Examples of OT Interventions Addressing Environments and Contexts	Research Evidence and Related Resources Guiding Practice
A **7-year-old student** with cognitive, motor, and speech delays participates in a special day class in a public school. He has difficulty processing sensory information, interacting with peers, focusing on academic tasks, using his hands for tasks, and maneuvering on equipment on the playground.	Guided by the child's needs, the IEP team, which includes the OT and the parents, determines that the child is having difficulty participating with typical peers and benefits from a special day class for students with behavioral challenges. Although such placements are viewed as more "restrictive," the regular classroom environment currently is overwhelming for the child. The goal of the tailored environment is to provide the structure necessary for the child to learn specific skills for participation in a less-restrictive environment in the future.	• Educate IEP team about the effect of the environment on sensory processing and the relationship to behavior in school setting. • Consult with IEP team and teachers to structure, adapt, and modify the classroom and playground environments so that the child has opportunities to meet sensory needs by participating in vestibular-, tactile-, and proprioceptive-based activities throughout school day. • Collaborate with student to help him establish strategies and routines for sensory regulation, emotional and behavioral de-escalation, and appropriate coping skills. • Develop a peer buddy system to promote appropriate social interactions with modeling and role play during social group. • Provide direct intervention to facilitate integration of sensory systems in an environment rich in sensory experiences and equipment.	• Student may attend to classroom instruction for longer periods of time when sensory needs are addressed (Schilling, Washington, Billingsley, & Deitz, 2003). • Teaching children self-regulation strategies (a cognitive approach to manage sensory needs) helps children manage their behavior (Barnes, Vogel, Beck, Schoenfeld, & Owen, 2008; Vaughn et al., 2003). • Supporting occupational performance and behavior in a school-age child improves participation at school (Schaaf & Nightlinger, 2007). • Suspended equipment and opportunities to carefully monitor various and safe sensory experiences is a hallmark of sensory integration intervention. These opportunities may be available only in a carefully designed environment (Parham et al., 2007).
A **28-year-old man** with schizoaffective disorder lives alone. He has difficulty organizing his daily routines to manage his medications. He was recently admitted to the hospital due to an acute exacerbation of his illness. He wants to be discharged home.	The intervention focuses on developing medication routines to help the client return to his apartment. If unable to manage his medications, he might need to move to a group home with more structured supervision. By analyzing the social and physical environment within the client's home and community, OT practitioners can identify external cues and resources to optimize client's occupational performance.	• Educate medical team and case manager about performance deficits that affect medication routines. • Request pharmacist/nurse to teach client how to read labels and practice filling medication box correctly. • Advocate for reminder calls for refills from pharmacy or others. • Teach client skills for medication management to establish habits and routines such as regular sleep/wake times; use of an alarm clock and calendar to track when to take and refill medication; or keeping of medication in a consistent location, such as on a nightstand.	Environmental supports are more likely to improve functional behavior for people with schizophrenia when the supports are customized for the person and situated in the person's home (Velligan, et al., 2000, 2006).

Table 2. Case Studies: Environmental Considerations and Interventions for Specific Populations

Case Description	Environmental Considerations for OT Service Delivery	Selected Examples of OT Interventions Addressing Environments and Contexts	Research Evidence and Related Resources Guiding Practice
		• Provide visual cues such as list of medications with pictures and purpose or reminder signs. • Establish connection with mental health support groups.	
Clients living in a shelter for homeless people desire to meet basic needs, remain safe, and reduce the potential for harm.	Using a consultative model, the intervention focuses on modifying the physical and social environment to promote safety and meet basic needs of the clients.	• Establish defined areas and organize schedules within the shelter to enable individuals to engage in self-care, education, work preparation, and play–leisure activities. • Design physically accessible spaces and equipment to enable individuals to complete basic activities of daily living. • Educate clients in life skills interventions to address the environment demands of homelessness. • Establish a self-governance and grievance committee to address safety within the shelter. • Post emergency procedures and community resources.	Life skills interventions have the potential to support the complex needs of individuals situated within the homeless context (Helfrich, Aviles, Badiani, Walens, & Sabol, 2006).
A **52-year-old successful businessman** had a right middle cerebral artery stroke with resulting left-sided weakness and decreased balance 1 year ago. He lives at home and has tried to return to his job as a financial consultant but struggled to maintain his productivity at work.	Because this client may not regain all performance skills, intervention focuses on designing environmental modifications in the home, work, and community settings that will support his heath and participation in occupations.	• Adapt activity demands for participation in necessary and desired occupations. • Modify home environment to optimize safety and reduce the impact of weakness and fatigue (Fange & Iwarsson, 2005; Stark, 2004; Stearns et al., 2000). • Consult with employer to modify the work environment by using assistive technology to change the task demands. • Set up an ergonomically advantageous setting by adjusting work routines and schedule to support work performance (Whiteneck, Gerhardt, & Cusick, 2004). • Consult with community agencies regarding access (e.g., transportation, public bathrooms, timing of crosswalk lights, safe railings).	• Specific strategies are effective to improve performance skills and participation in roles and routines after stroke (Ma & Trombly, 2002; Trombly & Ma, 2002). • OTs evaluate contextual factors of work environments (e.g., work tasks, routines, tools, equipment) and use this information to plan interventions that facilitate work performance (AOTA, 2005). • OT practitioners consult with community agencies, business owners, and building contractors, among others, to create environments that promote occupational performance for all (AOTA, 2000).

(continued)

Table 2. Case Studies: Environmental Considerations and Interventions for Specific Populations *(cont.)*

Case Description	Environmental Considerations for OT Service Delivery	Selected Examples of OT Interventions Addressing Environments and Contexts	Research Evidence and Related Resources Guiding Practice
Older adults living in an assisted-living facility are at high risk for balance and falls.	The focus of intervention is to maintain the clients' occupational engagement through a multifactorial approach such as strength and balance training; education; modifying activity demands; and creating a safe and supportive environment, including falls prevention.	Consult with facility administrators, architects, and facility staff to design environment that • Reflects a non-institutional character • Eliminates barriers to physical mobility • Provides lighting without glare • Clusters small activity areas together.	• The design of the social and physical environment influences the function and well being for older adults (Day, Carreron, & Stump, 2000). • OT practitioners advocate for and contribute to the creation of an environment where the demands do not exceed the capabilities of the client (Cooper & Day, 2003). • OT practitioners identify and modify environmental barriers (Davison, Bond, Dawson, Steen, & Kenny, 2005).
A **74-year-old woman** lives in an apartment in the inner city with her husband of 45 years. She has a moderate Alzheimer's disease. She has become lethargic and no longer initiates activities. Her husband now does all the shopping, cooking, and cleaning. He is overwhelmed with the demands of caregiving.	The intervention focuses on supporting the caregiver's and the care recipient's health and participation in desired occupations and activities and enabling them to remain in their home as they age.	• Educate caregiver about the disease process and the impact of the environment on the care recipient's occupational performance. • Recommend modifications to the home environment to manage daily care activities. • Provide emotional support as well as information on coping strategies and stress management to caregivers. • Facilitate use of community and family support. • Provide support and education for the uses of adaptive equipment in the home.	• Persons with dementia or Alzheimer's disease can live at home, remaining in their roles and contexts for a longer period of time, if given enough support from caregivers (Haley & Bailey, 1999). • An in-home skills training and environmental adaptation program (Gitlin et al., 2003) improves the quality of life for both the caregiver and the care recipient, with fewer declines in occupational performance of care recipients and less need for care giving (Gitlin, Hauck, Dennis, & Winter, 2005). Home-based OT is effective and cost efficient for community-dwelling elders and their caregivers (Graff et al., 2008). • Persons with Alzheimer's disease perform better at home than in unfamiliar environments; it is harder for them to adapt to new environments (Hoppes, Davis, & Thompson, 2003).

Note. OT = occupational therapy; NICU = neonatal intensive care unit; IEP = individualized education program.

ronment and context support learning and performance and generate practical solutions to solve problems. For example, practitioners recommend modifications to improve the physical accessibility of kitchens for clients who desire to engage in the occupation of cooking while using their wheelchairs. Practitioners also may add visual cues around the kitchen to structure cooking tasks to increase safety for people with cognitive limitations.

Occupational therapy practitioners recognize that the provision of service in environments and contexts are linked to the purpose of the intervention. Depending on the needs of clients, practitioners understand that environments and contexts will vary from natural to a modified environment that has a more planned structure. For example, a client with difficulty organizing his or her daily routine initially may function better in a structured social program. The intervention goal then is to diminish the need for structured programming to gain self-sufficiency in organizing and planning daily life.

The dilemma in decision-making about what type of environment and context best supports clients' participation in life along a continuum of natural to more structured directly relates to clients' occupational performance. With the value of participation and health, there is a drive toward customizing interventions to suit the person, population, or organization's desired abilities. For example, when someone needs to learn or relearn safety and emergency maintenance, it is optimal to teach him or her with the specific emergency alert system that he or she will actually use.

However, sometimes the natural environment and context initially may pose too many demands or not provide enough support. In such circumstances, it may be more advantageous for people to gain specific skills in occupational competence in a more structured environment and, with practice and feedback, incrementally learn to apply these skills and occupations to the natural environment. Occupational therapy practitioners are sensitive to how the structured or natural environments provide supports or barriers and continuously monitor and adjust these environments to support clients' occupational performance.

It is the intent that these structures be reduced as clients gain competence. For example, during inpatient rehabilitation, an adult with a spinal cord injury would practice community mobility and upon discharge to home would be able to use public transportation. In contrast, some individuals may be better able to participate in daily life occupations when they move from a natural to a more structured environment. For example, an adult with serious mental illness initially may experience enhanced occupational performance in a community group home rather than in a private home.

To narrowly define natural environment and structured environments may risk limiting clients' engagement or participation in meaningful occupations. Ultimately, interventions support clients where life is lived: in their homes, classrooms, playgrounds, work, and recreation or community centers, wherever their occupations take place. Providing intevention in these settings is consistent with the values and purpose of occupational therapy. Practitioners provide services in the natural enviroment and least restrictive environment whenever possible. They also realize that many factors such as limited financial, organizational, and personnel resources and the complexity of the client's condition may constrain this service delivery option. When this occurs, they make recommendations for continuing interventions beyond the immediate setting.

Providing opportunities for all members of society to engage in health-promoting occupations, flexibility in the analysis of the environment and context in which clients thrive is essential. Table 2 provides examples of how occupational therapy practitioners use and modify environments to support health and participation in occupations.

Summary

Occupational therapy practitioners work with a wide variety of clients across the life span. The goal of occupational therapy is to support health and participation in life through engagement in occupation (AOTA,

2008). Occupational therapists consider current educational and health care laws and policies as they make recommendations to modify, adapt, or change environments and contexts to support or improve occupational performance. On the basis of theory, evidence, knowledge, client preferences and values, and occupational performance, occupational therapists assess the intervention settings and environmental and contextual factors influencing clients' occupational performance. Interventions and recommendations focus on selecting and using environments and contexts that are congruent with clients' needs and maximize participation in daily life occupations. Practitioners' expertise is essential to support clients' health and participation in meaningful occupations.

Authors
Ellen S. Cohn, ScD, OTR/L, FAOTA
Cherylin Lew, OTD, OTR/L

With contributions from
Kate Hanauer, OTS
DeLana Honaker, PhD, OTR/L, BCP
Susanne Smith Roley, MS, OTR/L, FAOTA

for

The Commission on Education
Janet V. DeLany, DEd, OTR/L, FAOTA

Adopted by the Representative Assembly 2009CONov149

Citation. American Occupational Therapy Association. (2010). Occupational therapy's perspective on the use of environments and contexts to support health and participation in occupations. *American Journal of Occupational Therapy, 64*(Suppl.), S57–S69. http://dx.doi.org/10.5014/ajot.2010.64S57-64S69 Reprinted with permission.

References

American Occupational Therapy Association. (2000). Occupational therapy and the Americans With Disabilities Act (ADA). *American Journal of Occupational Therapy, 54,* 622–625.

American Occupational Therapy Association. (2005). Occupational therapy services in facilitating work performance. *American Journal of Occupational Therapy, 59,* 676–679.

American Occupational Therapy Association. (2006). Policy 1.44: Categories of occupational therapy personnel. In *Policy manual* (2007 ed., pp. 33–34). Bethesda, MD: Author.

American Occupational Therapy Association. (2008). Occupational therapy practice framework: Domain and process (2nd ed.). *American Journal of Occupational Therapy, 62,* 625–683.

American Occupational Therapy Association. (2010). Guidelines for supervision, roles, and responsibilities during the delivery of occupational therapy services. *American Journal of Occupational Therapy, 64.*

Americans with Disabilities Act of 1990, P.L. 101-336, 104 Stat. 327-378.

Bailey, D. B., Aytch, L. S., Odom, S. L., Symons, F., & Wolery, M. (1999). Early intervention as we know it. *Mental Retardation and Developmental Disabilities Research Reviews, 5,* 11–20.

Barnes, K. J., Vogel, K. A., Beck, A. J., Schoenfeld, H. B., & Owen, S. V. (2008). Self-regulation strategies of children with emotional disturbance. *Physical and Occupational Therapy in Pediatrics, 28,* 369–386.

Batavia, A. I. (1999). Independent living centers, medical rehabilitation centers, and managed care for people with disabilities. *Archives of Physical Medicine and Rehabilitation, 80,* 1357–1360.

Blok, H., Fukkink, R., Gebhardt, E., & Leseman, P. (2005). The relevance of delivery mode and other programme characteristics for the effectiveness of early childhood intervention. *International Journal of Behavioral Development, 29*(1), 35–47.

Buysse, V., Skinner, D., & Grant, S. (2001). Toward a definition of quality inclusion: Perspectives of parents and practitioners. *Topics in Early Childhood Special Education, 24*, 146–161.

Cooper, B. A., & Day, K. (2003). Therapeutic design of environments for people with dementia. In L. Letts, P. Rigby, & D. Stewart (Eds.), *Using environments to enable occupational performance* (pp. 253–268). Thorofare, NJ: Slack.

Crepeau, E. B., Cohn, E. S., & Schell, B. A. (Eds.). (2003). *Willard and Spackman's occupational therapy* (10th ed.). Philadelphia: Lippincott Williams & Wilkins.

Davison, J., Bond, J., Dawson, P., Steen, I. N., & Kenny, R. A. (2005). Patients with recurrent falls attending accident and emergency benefit from multifactorial intervention: A randomized controlled trial. *Age and Aging, 34*, 162–168.

Dunst, C., Bruder, M., Trivette, C., Hamby, D., Raab, M., & McLean, M. (2001). Characteristics and consequences of everyday natural learning opportunities. *Topics in Early Childhood Special Education, 21*(2), 68–92.

Dunst, C., Trivette, C., Hamby, D., & Bruder, M. (2006). Influences of contrasting natural learning environment experiences on child, parent, and family well-being. *Journal of Developmental and Physical Disabilities, 18*, 235–250.

Day, K., Carreon, D., & Stump, C. (2000). The therapeutic design of environments for people with dementia: A review of the empirical research. *Gerontologist, 40*, 397–421.

Education of All Handicapped Children Act of 1975, P. L. 94-142, 20 U.S.C., § 1400 et seq.

Elementary and Secondary Education Act of 1965, P. L. 89-10, 20 U.S.C.

Fange, A., & Iwarsson, S. (2005). Changes in ADL dependence and aspects of usability following housing adaptation: A longitudinal perspective. *American Journal of Occupational Therapy, 59*, 296–304.

Gitlin, L., Hauck, W., Dennis, M., & Winter, L. (2005). Maintenance of effects of the Home Environmental Skill-Building Program for family caregivers and individuals with Alzheimer's disease and related disorders. *Journals of Gerontology: Series A: Biological Sciences and Medical Sciences, 60*, 368–374.

Gitlin, L. N., Winter, L., Corcoran, M., Dennis, M. P., Schinfeld, S., & Hauck, W. W. (2003). Effects of the Home Environmental Skill-Building Program on the caregiver–care recipient dyad: 6-month outcomes from the Philadelphia REACH initiative. *Gerontologist, 43*, 532–546.

Graff, M., Adang, E., Vernooij-Dassen, M., Dekker, J., Jomsson, L., Thijssen, M., et al. (2008). Community occupational therapy for older patients with dementia and their care givers: Cost effectiveness study. *British Medical Journal, 336*, 134–138.

Haley, W., & Bailey, S. (1999). Research on family caregiving in Alzheimer's disease: Implications for practice and policy. In B. Vellas & J. Fitten (Eds.), *Research and practice in Alzheimer's disease* (Vol. 2, pp. 321–332). Paris: Serdi.

Helfrich, C., Aviles, A., Badiani, C., Walens, D., & Sabol, P. (2006). Life skills interventions with homeless youth, domestic violence victims, and adults with mental illness. In K. S. Miller, G. L. Herzberg, & S. A. Ray (Eds.), *Homeless in America* (pp. 189–207). New York: Haworth Press.

Hoppes, S., Davis, L. A., & Thompson, D. (2003). Environmental effects on the assessment of people with dementia. A pilot study. *American Journal of Occupational Therapy, 57,* 396–402.

Individuals with Disabilities Education Act Amendments of 1997, P. L. 105-17, 20 U.S.C. § 1400 et seq.

Individuals with Disabilities Education Improvement Act, P.L. 108-446, 20 USC Chapter 33 (2004).

Keogh, B. K., Bernheimer, L. P., Gallimore, R., & Weisner, T. S. (1998). Child and family outcomes over time: A longitudinal perspective on developmental delays. In M. Lewis & C. Feiring (Eds.), *Families, risk, and competence* (pp. 269–287). Mahwah, NJ: Lawrence Erlbaum.

Ma, H., & Trombly, C. A. (2002). Synthesis of the effects of occupational therapy for persons with stroke, part II: Remediation of impairments. *American Journal of Occupational Therapy, 56,* 260–274.

No Child Left Behind Act of 2001, P. L. 107-110, 20 U.S.C. § 6301.

Odom, A. L. (2000). Preschool inclusion: What we know and where we go from here. *Topics in Early Childhood Special Education, 20,* 20–27.

Older Americans Act of 1965, P. L. 89-73 42 U.S.C. 3056 et seq. (amended 2006, P. L. 109-365, 42 U.S.C. 3001).

Olmstead v. L.C. and E.W., U.S.C. 98–536 (1999).

Omnibus Budget Reconciliation Act of 1987 (Federal Nursing Home Reform Act), 42 U.S.C. 1396r, 42 U.S.C., 1395i-3, 42, CFR 483.

Parham, L. D., Cohn, E. S., Spitzer, S., Koomar, J. A., Miller, L. J., Burke, J. P., et al. (2007). Fidelity in sensory integration intervention research. *American Journal of Occupational Therapy, 61,* 216–227.

Rehabilitation Act of 1973, Section 504, P. L. 93-112, 29 USC § 794.

Schaaf, R. C., & Nightlinger, K. M. (2007). Occupational therapy using a sensory integrative approach: A case study of effectiveness. *American Journal of Occupational Therapy, 61,* 239–246.

Schilling, D. L., Washington, K., Billingsley, F. F., & Deitz, J. (2003). Classroom seating for children with attention deficit hyperactivity disorder: Therapy balls versus chairs. *American Journal of Occupational Therapy, 57,* 534–541.

Social Security Amendments of 1965, P. L. 89-97, § 332, 79 Stat. 403.

Stark, S. (2004). Removing environmental barriers in the homes of older adults with disabilities improves occupational performance. *Occupational Therapy Journal of Research: Occupation, Participation, and Health, 24*(1), 32–40.

Stearns, S. C., Bernard, S. L., Fasick, S. B., Schwartz, R., Konrad, R. T., Ory, M. G., et al. (2000). The economic implications of self-care: The effect of lifestyle, functional adaptations, and medical self-care among a national sample of Medicare beneficiaries. *American Journal of Public Health, 90,* 1608–1612.

Trombly, C. A., & Ma, H. (2002). A synthesis of the effects of occupational therapy for persons with stroke, part I: Restoration of roles, tasks, and activities. *American Journal of Occupational Therapy, 56,* 250–259.

Vaughn, S., Kim, A.-H., Sloan, C. V. M., Hughes, M. T., Elbaum, B., & Sridhar, D. (2003). Social skills interventions for young children with disabilities. *Remedial and Special Education, 24,* 2–15.

Velligan, D. I., Bow-Thomas, C. C., Huntzinger, C., Ritch, J., Ledbetter, N., Prihoda, T. J., et al. (2000). Randomized controlled trial of the use of compensatory strategies to enhance adaptive functioning in outpatients with schizophrenia. *American Journal of Psychiatry, 157*(8), 1317–1323.

Velligan, D. I., Mueller, J., Wang, M., Dicocco, M., Diamond, P. M., Maples, N.J., et al. (2006). Use of environmental supports among patients with schizophrenia. *Psychiatric Services, 57*(2), 219–224.

Whiteneck, G. G., Gerhardt, K. A., & Cusick, C. P. (2004). Identifying environmental factors that influence the outcomes of people with traumatic brain injury. *Journal of Head Trauma Rehabilitation, 19,* 191–204.

Part IV. The Conscious Use of Self: Joining With People to Enable Occupational Engagement

Behind all other of treatment tools and media is the basic tool, the occupational therapist.

—Le Vesconte (1948, p. 52)

The conscious and intentional use of one's self so that one becomes an effective tool in the occupational therapy process is one of the profession's most vital legitimate tools of practice (Baum, 1980; Mosey, 1996; Taylor, 2008). By its very nature, occupational engagement must be internally satisfying, individually determined, and self-directed; therefore, the person's participation in a collaborative relationship is essential (American Occupational Therapy Association [AOTA], 2014). The therapeutic relationship is embedded in occupational therapy's models of practice (Bruce & Borg, 2002; Kielhofner, 2009; Kramer & Hinojosa, 2010; Mosey, 1996), and its significance is supported by research (Darragh, Sample, & Krieger, 2001; Taylor, Lee, Kielhofner, & Ketkar, 2009). Due to the importance of this therapeutic tool, I have devoted Part IV of this text to exploring issues related to practitioners' ability to partner with the people they work with and enable person-directed, client-centered occupational engagement.

Interrelationships among the practitioner, the person, and occupation cannot be ignored. One cannot adequately understand the personal meaning of occupation without developing a positive therapeutic relationship. The practitioner may consider an occupation to be therapeutic and purposeful, but the person may chose not to engage in its related activity (Arnsten, 1990). As occupational therapy practitioners, we do not "do" an activity "on" or "to" a person; rather, we do activity *with* a person, thereby facilitating a therapeutic relationship (Gilfoyle, 1980). Partnership and a mutual cooperation develop (Yerxa, 1980), enabling the therapist to therapeutically use himself or herself (Sachs & Labovitz, 1994). This partnership has historically and traditionally been considered the art of occupational therapy practice (Gilfoyle, 1980; Mosey, 1996).

The vital importance of the conscious and intentional use of self to form therapeutic relationships that enable person-directed and client-centered occupational therapy is evident in all of the chapters in Part IV. However, many forces challenge our ability to practice this art. Shorter lengths of stay, greater productivity demands, increased emphasis on technology over people, and ongoing staff shortages are several trends that place pressure on occupational therapy practitioners to use mechanistic approaches and technological techniques instead of humanistic and holistic ones (Peloquin, 1994; Taylor, 2008; Yerxa, 1980).

Recognizing these challenges, the *Occupational Therapy Practice Framework: Domain and Process* (3rd ed.; *Framework;* AOTA, 2014) places a strong emphasis on the use of a client-centered approach that facilitates the person's engagement in occupation. However, an appreciation of this foundational tool of occupational therapy is insufficient. Practitioners must develop concrete skills for implementing this tool into practice (Fearing & Clark, 2000; Law, 1998; Sumsion & Smyth, 2000; Taylor, 2008). Several of this part's authors provide guidelines for developing the competencies needed to attain and sustain a client-centered approach. More strategies are provided in Part V to promote keeping this art of practice in occupational therapy.

The qualifications most desirable for the teacher of occupational therapy are: above all, infinite patience, the ability to teach and criticize without causing offense or discouragement, the power of inspiring confidence in others and last, but not least, an optimistic temperament and sense of humor.

—Moodie (1919, p. 314)

In Chapter 35, Devereux begins with a thoughtful analysis of the caring relationship, which she presents as the basis for our profession's philosophy and practice. She emphasizes that the development of a caring relationship between the person and the practitioner reinforces the holistic approach of our field, enabling us to make a unique societal contribution by being a caring profession. Devereux acknowledges that caring alone is insufficient for establishing an effective collaborative partnership with clients. However, her stance that caring is the foundation that enables the development of additional factors that are essential to the therapeutic relationship is one that any person who has had the misfortune to work with an uncaring practitioner can readily embrace. Devereux explores the characteristics of a therapeutic relationship and discusses how to develop a caring relationship with individuals to assist them in reconnecting to occupations that are meaningful. Equally important is her analysis of how the practitioner can care for himself or herself to be able to enter into and maintain caring therapeutic relationships. Devereux concludes with an exploration of how occupational therapy can maintain its caring focus in a complex and challenging health care system (see Active Reflection IV.1).

The benefits of forming therapeutic relationships on the basis of caring are clearly articulated by Devereaux. Her view that caring is an inherent part of the art of occupational therapy practice is strongly supported by the exploration of client-centered practice in Chapter 36. In this analysis, Law, Baptiste, and Mills define and discuss key concepts and issues related to the implementation of client-centered practice. They highlight the roots of the client-centeredness construct and describe its congruence with occupational therapy theoretical frameworks. Law and colleagues examine the client-centered concepts of *individual autonomy and choice, partnership, therapist and client responsibility, enablement, contextual congruence, accessibility,* and *respect for diversity* from a contemporary collaborative perspective and the traditional therapist-directed perspective. These concepts provide a basis for the authors' definition of *client-centered practice* and the formation of key assumptions about this approach.

> *There is no substitute for the exercise of reason and self-trust and the reward thereof is constant. Given the basic aim of wanting to help people help themselves, human beings tend to gravitate towards those ways of life which promise to transform their intangible aims into realities.*
>
> —Sokolov (1957, p. 15)

Law et al. realistically discuss implications for occupational therapy practice and challenges to the implementation of a client-centered approach. They provide two practice examples to illustrate client-centered concepts and assumptions and to raise consciousness about obstacles to the practice of client-centered occupational therapy. The authors end the chapter with a brief review of research about the efficacy of a client-centered approach in enhancing client satisfaction, increasing functional outcomes, and improving client participation in the occupational therapy process. Law et al. call for research on client-centered practices to increase the understanding of the effects of implementing approaches that promote the person's control of the occupational therapy process.

Since the publication of this seminal work, several studies have been published that examine client-centered practice and the therapeutic relationship (Brown & Bowen, 1998; Corring & Cook, 1999; Darragh et al., 2001; Mew & Fossey, 1996; Sumsion, 1999; Taylor et al., 2009; Tickle-Degnen, 2002). Given the number of occupational therapy practitioners who work with children, significant scholarship also has focused on family-centered practice (Brown, Humphry, & Taylor, 1997; Cohn, Miller, & Tickle-Degnen, 2000; Hinojosa, Sproat, Mankhetwit, & Anderson, 2002; Lawlor & Mattingly, 1998; Wilkins, Pollock, Rochon, & Law, 2001).

In Chapter 39, Kyler critically examines the historical roots of client-centered practice and the social and political precipitants to family-centered practice. In this work, Kyler identifies three theoretical models that provided the conceptual foundations for the emergence of client-centered approaches in occupational therapy. She critiques the approaches used in these models and analyzes the ethical ramifications of their use. Although there are philosophical similarities between client-centered care and family-centered care, Kyler articulates several key differences. She outlines core prin-

---

Active Reflection IV.1. Personal, Cultural, and Societal Influences on Caring

Think about the reasons you decided to become an occupational therapy practitioner.
- Did your personal values about caring influence your decision? Describe this influence.
- How does your culture view caring?
- How do your personal and cultural values influence your ability to formulate caring therapeutic relationships with others?
- Do you think the reality that occupational therapy is a predominantly female profession influences the profession's view of caring and society's view of the profession? Describe this influence.

Active Reflection IV.2. Impact of Practice Realities on Client-Centered Practice

Consider the complexities and constraints of today's practice environments.
- How can occupational therapy practitioners maintain focus on caring and ensure client-centered practice?
- What strategies and resources can practitioners use to create a humanizing environment in an often-dehumanizing system of care?
- How can you care for yourself when faced with the demands and stresses of practice?
- What personal attributes do you bring to the therapeutic relationship to enable client-centered practice?

---

ciples of family-centered care that can enable forming respectful partnerships between professionals and families. Kyler notes that information about client- and family-centered practice is pervasive in the field but contends that using this knowledge varies greatly. She supports her view by highlighting major occupational therapy documents and practice models that promote client-centered care and then critiquing the success of their application. Recognizing the barriers that limit the implementation of client- and family-centered care, Kyler proposes a more inclusive approach to engaging people in the therapeutic process.

According to Kyler, the relationship-centered approach recognizes the person as center to the therapeutic process; however, it does not consider health or illness to be solely determined by the individual's characteristics. Rather, social, political, economic, cultural, and environmental contexts are irrefutable determining factors of health and illness. Occupational therapy practitioners must consider the influence of these external determinants on the client, his or her family, and their communication and decision-making processes. Kyler views this shift in orientation as critical to contemporary relationship-centered practice. She advocates for occupational therapy practitioners to learn from the multidisciplinary literature on empowerment. Kyler believes integrating this knowledge with the best aspects of client-, family-, and relationship-centered care will enable occupational therapy practitioners to effectively partner with clients and their families (see Active Reflection IV.2).

A critical aspect of family-centered practice is the intentional inclusion of stakeholders beyond the client. To actively engage these individuals in the decision-making process about a client's care, the complexities of entering into familial relationships must be considered. Kyler explores the ethical conflicts that

may arise when the client's values and perspectives and his or her family or practitioner do not align. However, as she notes, realizing client-centered care and family-centered approaches can be difficult. Chapter 38 by Gitlin, Corcoran, and Leinmiller-Eckhardt presents a useful framework that can help practitioners bridge the gap between a philosophical commitment to client and family-centered care and its actual implementation in practice. They propose using an ethnographic approach when providing occupational therapy in the home. They argue that the practitioner's sensitivity to the inner life of a family enables caregivers to be active agents throughout the occupational therapy process. Gitlin et al.'s framework is founded on four key principles derived from ethnographic methodology: (1) identification of an informant, (2) use of an insider approach, (3) engagement in self-reflection, and (4) interpretation of information. They clearly describe the principles each term reflects. Gitlin et al. provide underlying strategies to use these principles to foster an understanding of the personal meaning of caregiving and its unique provision in a family. They realistically explore specific aspects of caregiving that can be viewed as problematic by family members (see Active Reflection IV.3).

An enhanced understanding of the family perspective allows occupational therapy practitioners to develop services that are congruent with, and respectful of, caregivers' values and belief systems and reflective of their unique needs. Gitlin et al. provide a series of excellent questions that are simple and straightforward and should always be asked of family caregivers who are recognized as lay practitioners. The answers to these questions can provide a wealth of information about each family's unique caregiving experience. This knowledge, combined with active reflection on the questions they pose to occupational therapy practitioners, can guide

---

Active Reflection IV.3. Application of the Ethnographic Approach

Review the case example provided in Chapter 38.
- Did the original plan of care proposed by the occupational therapist seem relevant and appropriate to you?
- What was your initial reaction when you read that the family caregivers rejected all of the therapist's recommendations?
- How did using the ethnographic approach influence the this case's outcomes?
- Can you think of a practice situation in which the ethnographic approach would have enabled client- and family-centered practice? Describe your application of this approach and its anticipated outcomes.

---

development and implementation of a family-centered plan. Gitlin et al. clearly and realistically illustrate the ethnographic framework and the application of their questions to a home-based caregiving situation.

Although this case example involves an older person, using these questions and the ethnographic framework is relevant to all caregiving experiences across the lifespan. Particularly relevant is this case's emphasis on the importance of using this framework to help identify and address potential ethical dilemmas. As the authors note, the caregiver (as the lay practitioner) has decision control when there is a conflict in beliefs or priorities. They advocate that occupational therapy practitioners actively use reflexivity to continually examine their personal and professional values and beliefs and analyze how these interact with the family's values and beliefs to shape occupational therapy service delivery.

The outcome of this openness to the personal perspectives and inner life of those we work with can lead to a new (and improved) view on the success of therapy. In her landmark study, Mattingly (1991; see Chapter 43) found that occupational therapy practitioners rarely measured success by goal attainment. Rather, they identified success as the self-confidence clients developed through their participation in therapeutic experiences that challenged them. Mattingly's participants reported that clients' ability to effectively meet challenges increased their confidence and engendered a commitment to take on new challenges. This perceived self-efficacy contributes to the person's motivation to act and implement his or her story. As a result, the ability to engage in the occupational therapy process can be highly influenced by one's judgment of his or her capabilities.

> *The treatment must not become too paternal; however, killing the patient's sense of responsibility for his own person. On the contrary, the patient's self-respect must be re-established by stimulating in all possible ways his pride in his appearance and achievements.*
>
> —Wilson (1929, p. 191)

Simply put, a person is less likely to engage in an activity that is viewed as beyond his or her capacities. Therefore, occupational therapy practitioners must consider the person's perceived self-efficacy when planning and implementing occupational therapy intervention. In Chapter 39, Gage and Polatajko explore the construct of perceived self-efficacy in depth. They consider the effects of perceived self-efficacy on activity selection, engagement, and performance. Perceived self-efficacy's origin, history, definition, parameters, and relationship to self-esteem, behavior, treatment outcome, and psychological well-being are discussed in a comprehensive manner. A literature review highlights relevant research, and clinical examples support the impact of perceived self-efficacy on performance.

Gage and Polatajko postulate that assessing and monitoring perceived self-efficacy and using real-life activities in the community (or those that closely approximate these) will result in better intervention outcomes and enhanced occupational performance. They question the use of reductionistic activities (e.g., pegboards) focused on mastery of component skills, because these have little relevance to attaining personal efficacy in the person's desired occupations. In contrast, the benefits of considering perceived self-efficacy in occupational therapy assessment, intervention planning, and intervention implementation are clear.

Gage and Polatajko challenge occupational therapy practitioners to identify and incorporate this construct into daily practice. Practitioners can consciously structure task experiences to be successful and intentionally provide a therapeutic relationship supportive of clients having a *real* voice about their treatment, thereby strengthening their perceived self-efficacy. This call for practitioners to empower clients so that they are in control of their therapeutic process, and to consciously establish relationships that are beyond those prescribed in the medical model, are supported by all of Part IV's authors.

In Chapter 40, Phelan provides a strong and targeted argument for the abandonment of outdated disempowering assumptions about disability. She maintains that traditional biomedical perspectives about disability, which have underpinned occupational therapy's philosophy, theories, and practice for decades, have resulted in a myopic view that ignores the social constructs of disability.

Phelan acknowledges that many contemporary occupational therapy models and tools of practice encourage adopting social constructivist perspectives; however, she contends that systemic power structures maintain the dominance of traditionalist views of disability (see Active Reflection IV.4). These prevailing viewpoints include conceptualizations of normal/nondisabled vs. abnormal/disabled, the disabled "hero" and overcoming disability, built environments, and social and attitudinal constructions of disability and identity. Phelan critically appraises these established constructs and the implicit and explicit

---

Active Reflection IV.4. Comparative Analysis of Social and Medical Models

---

Apply critical reflexivity to use a disability studies lens to review the theoretical and conceptual frameworks included in Part II of this text.
- Are components of the medical model and traditional views of disability evident in some of these frameworks?
- Which ones are congruent with a social model of disability?
- How would you use these models to guide occupation-based practice in a manner that is consistent with contemporary views of disability?

Active Reflection IV.5. Conscious Use of Self and the *Centennial Vision*

AOTA's (2007) *Centennial Vision* states, "We envision that occupational therapy is a powerful, widely recognized, science-driven, and evidence-based profession with a globally connected and diverse workforce meeting society's occupational needs" (p. 613).
- Are this statement and its identified strategic directions congruent with the art of occupational therapy as exemplified in client- and family-centered practice?
- How can practitioners' conscious and intentional use of self contribute to attaining the *Centennial Vision?*

---

assumptions that have dominated provision of services to persons with disabilities. She questions whether occupational therapy is an empowering profession if its philosophical base includes these disempowering views. Moreover, if the field's ultimate aim is the rehabilitation of persons with disabilities, with a primary focus on the remediation or compensation of impairments, we perpetuate damaging assumptions about disability.

In contrast, the conscious and intentional use of social constructionist views of disability allows occupational therapy practitioners to effectively challenge embedded practices. Phelan provides an excellent overview of contemporary perspectives of disability, as put forth in disabilities studies literature. She calls for occupational therapy practitioners to adopt a critical, reflexive lens informed by these perspectives and to include the social model of disability throughout the occupational therapy process. Phelan does not negate the importance of the individual's unique experience of impairment, but she advises this personal perspective must be integrated into the application of the social model of disability to ensure socially responsible occupational therapy.

Phelan's examination of the empowering potential of occupational therapy—if we move beyond a focus on the single person to consider institutional, social, cultural, and political contexts—is worthy of critical reflection. She challenges occupational therapy practitioners to rethink their preconceived beliefs about the people they work with and to actively use the tool of critical reflexivity, which, according to Phelan, enables the practitioner to move beyond reflection on actions to include the questioning of the underlying values, principles, constructs, and social conditions of knowledge production and its subsequent general acceptance. Most important, critical reflexivity requires the practitioner to actively challenge current practices that disempower people with disabilities.

Phelan's view that occupational therapy practitioners must adopt a disability studies lens is consistent with the perspectives of many of the authors of this part's chapters. Application of the social model of disability to occupational therapy is also supported by the *Framework*, which has moved away from the profession's historical allegiance to the medical model (with a primary focus on the attainment of independence) to emphasize social justice models that establish occupational justice as the desired outcome of occupational therapy (AOTA, 2014). This shift in the profession's guiding philosophies is also evident in AOTA's (2007) *Centennial Vision*, which identifies the field's overarching areas of practice as inclusive of disability and participation and health and wellness. Occupational therapy practitioners who embrace these significant changes in our profession's foci will be able to form effective partnerships with those they work with to enable client-centered and person-directed occupational engagement (see Active Reflection IV.5).

The reality that there are many obstacles to actualizing client-centered practice was a common theme in Part IV. Although awareness of barriers is first needed to find a solution, concrete actions are also needed to confront these challenges (Sumsion & Smyth, 2000). The next part of this text describes more tools of occupational therapy practice, several of which can be used to support client-centered practice. In particular, Chapter 44 provides a useful strategic framework on how to use clinical reasoning to enable client-centered practice.

Perhaps there is no profession which call for more ingenuity or more variety of training and experience.
—Shaw (1928, p. 200)

References

American Occupational Therapy Association. (2007). AOTA's *Centennial Vision* and executive summary.

American Journal of Occupational Therapy, 61, 613–614. http://dx.doi.org/10.5014/ajot.61.6.613

American Occupational Therapy Association. (2014). Occupational therapy practice framework: Domain and process (3rd ed.). *American Journal of Occupational Therapy, 68*(Suppl. 1), S1–S48. http://dx.doi.org/10.5014/ajot.2014.682006

Arnsten, S. M. (1990). Intrinsic motivation. *American Journal of Occupational Therapy, 44,* 462–463. http://dx.doi.org/10.5014/ajot.44.5.462

Baum, G. M. (1980). Occupational therapists put care in the health-care system. *American Journal of Occupational Therapy, 34,* 505–516. http://dx.doi.org/10.5014/ajot.34.8.505

Brown, C., & Bowen, R. (1998). Including the consumer in occupational therapy treatment planning. *Occupational Therapy Journal of Research, 18,* 44–62.

Brown, S. M., Humphry, R., & Taylor, E. (1997). A model of the nature of family–therapist relationships: Implications for education. *American Journal of Occupational Therapy, 51,* 597–603. http://dx.doi.org/10.5014/ajot.51.7.597

Bruce, M. A., & Borg, B. (2002). *Psychosocial frames of reference: Core for occupation-based practice* (3rd ed.). Thorofare, NJ: Slack.

Cohn, E., Miller, L. J., & Tickle-Degnen, L. (2000). Parental hopes for therapy outcomes: Children with sensory modulation disorder. *American Journal of Occupational Therapy 54,* 36–43. http://dx.doi.org/10.5014/ajot.54.1.36

Corring, D., & Cook, J. (1999). Client-centred care means that I am a valued human being. *Canadian Journal of Occupational Therapy, 66,* 71–82. http://dx.doi.org/10.1177/000841749906600203

Darragh, A. R., Sample, P. L., & Krieger, S. R. (2001). "Tears in my eyes 'cause somebody finally understood": Client perceptions of practitioners following brain injury. *American Journal of Occupational Therapy 55,* 191–199. http://dx.doi.org/10.5014/ajot.55.2.191

Fearing, V., & Clark, J. (2000). *Individuals in context: A practical guide to client-centered practice.* Thorofare, NJ: Slack.

Gilfoyle, E. M. (1980). Caring: A philosophy of practice. *American Journal of Occupational Therapy, 34,* 517–521. http://dx.doi.org/10.5014/ajot.34.8.517

Hinojosa, J., Sproat, C. T., Mankhetwit, S., & Anderson, J. (2002). Shifts in parent–therapist partnerships: Twelve years of change. *American Journal of Occupational Therapy, 56,* 556–563. http://dx.doi.org/10.5014/ajot.56.5.556

Kielhofner, G. (Ed.). (2009). *Conceptual foundations of occupational therapy* (4th ed.). Baltimore: Williams & Wilkins.

Kramer, P., & Hinojosa, J. (Eds.). (2010). *Frames of reference for pediatric occupational therapy* (3rd ed.). Baltimore: Lippincott Williams & Wilkins.

Law, M. (Ed.). (1998). *Client-centered occupational therapy.* Thorofare: Slack.

Lawlor, M. C., & Mattingly, C. F. (1998). The complexities embedded in family-centered care. *American Journal of Occupational Therapy, 52,* 259–267. http://dx.doi.org/10.5014/ajot.52.4.259

Le Vesconte, H. (1948). Our basic tools of treatment. *Canadian Journal of Occupational Therapy, 15,* 52–54. http://dx.doi.org/10.1177/000841744801500303

Mattingly, C. (1991). The narrative nature of clinical reasoning. *American Journal of Occupational Therapy, 45,* 998–1005.

Mew, M. M., & Fossey, E. (1996). Client-centered aspects of clinical reasoning during an initial assessment using the Canadian occupational performance measure. *Australian Occupational Therapy Journal, 43,* 155–166. http://dx.doi.org/10.1111/j.1440-1630.1996.tb01851.x

Moodie, C. (1919). The value of occupational therapy to the nursing profession. *Hospital Social Service Quarterly,* 313–315.

Mosey, A. C. (1996). *Psychosocial components of occupational therapy.* New York: Raven Press.

Peloquin, S. M. (1994). Occupational therapy as art and science: Should the older definition be reclaimed? *American Journal of Occupational Therapy, 48,* 1093–1096. http://dx.doi.org/10.5014/ajot.48.11.1093

Sachs, O., & Labovitz, O. R. (1994). The caring occupational therapist: Scope of professional roles and boundaries. *American Journal of Occupational Therapy, 48,* 997–1005. http://dx.doi.org/10.5014/ajot.48.11.997

Shaw, C. (1928). Occupation as an aid to recovery. *Occupational Therapy and Rehabilitation, 8*(3), 199–206.

Sokolov, J. (1957). 1956 Eleanor Clarke Slagle Lecture: Therapists into administrator: Ten inspiring years. *American Journal of Occupational Therapy, 11,* 13–19.

Sumsion, T. (1999). A study to determine a British occupational therapy definition of client-centered practice. *British Journal of Occupational Therapy, 62,* 52–58.

Sumsion, T., & Smyth, G. (2000). Barriers to client-centeredness and their resolution. *Canadian Journal of Occupational Therapy, 67,* 15–21. http://dx.doi.org/10.1177/000841740006700104

Taylor, R. (2008). *The intentional relationship: Occupational therapy and use of self.* Philadelphia: F. A. Davis.

Taylor, R. R., Lee, S. W., Kielhofner, G., & Ketkar, M. (2009). Therapeutic use of self: A nationwide survey of practitioners' attitudes and experiences. *American Journal of Occupational Therapy, 63,* 198–207. http://dx.doi.org/10.5014/ajot.63.2.198

Tickle-Degnen, L. (2002). Client-centered practice, Therapeutic relationship, and the use of research evidence. *American Journal of Occupational Therapy, 56,* 470–474. http://dx.doi.org/10.5014/ajot.56.4.470

Wilkins, S., Pollock, N., Rochon, S., & Law, M. (2001). Implementing client-centred practice: Why is it so difficult to do? *Canadian Journal of Occupational Therapy, 68,* 70–79. http://dx.doi.org/10.1177/000841740106800203

Wilson, S. (1929). Habit training for mental cases. Habit training for mental cases. *Occupational Therapy and Rehabilitation, 8*(3), 189–197.

Yerxa, E. J. (1980). Occupational therapy's role in creating a future climate of caring. *American Journal of Occupational Therapy, 34,* 529–534. http://dx.doi.org/10.5014/ajot.34.8.529

CHAPTER 35

Occupational Therapy's Challenge: The Caring Relationship

ELIZABETH B. DEVEREAUX

Caring exists only in relation to something; caring simply does not exist alone or in a vacuum. Before caring can exist or be relevant, it must be in relation to a living organism, a thing, or a thought. The relationship object may be tangible or intangible, the person may be self or other, and the living organism may be animal or human.

Occupational therapists are concerned about caring. We talk about this concern and act on it. In this paper my initial focus is on developing a caring relationship with the patient; this is followed by a discussion of the need to care for self as an integral part of developing any caring relationship with another and of the elements of therapeutic relationships. Finally, our functioning as caring professionals within the context and constraints of today's health-care environment is explored.

Relationship With the Patient

We are all attracted to a health-care profession because we are caring people. We value caring relationships, and the healthcare arena provides the structure within which our natural feelings and skills can find expression. Of even greater importance is the fact that we chose occupational therapy as the profession within the total health-care field. Occupational therapy does not do to, or for, the patient, but it instead does with. Through our treatment, we facilitate the patient's doing for him- or herself. When we treat a patient, it is with the awareness of the person, first, and the person who may have problems, second (1, p. 787). All health-care practitioners recognize the pathology when they look at a patient; however, occupational therapists not only see the pathology and deal with it as a part of the

treatment process, but we also recognize and focus on what is healthy about the individual. What is there to build on? What do we have to work with that can help this person learn, or relearn, the skills necessary to perform life tasks? We deal with the whole person, described by West (2) as "the mind–body–environment interrelationships activated through occupation" (p. 22). The concept of wholism is expressed eloquently in the report of the *Project to Identify the Philosophy of Occupational Therapy* (3).

> Embodiment or wholism is that perspective where mind and body are perceived as inextricably connected, integrated as one entity, in contrast to the dualistic perspective where mind and body are perceived as separate and hierarchically related entities (one entity superior to the other). . . . (p. 21)

To discuss a patient as "the kidney in room 319" or "the hand in the second treatment room" represents, to me, the height of dualism. Where and who are the people to whom these anatomic parts are vital? What right does anyone have to depersonalize them so? Ciardi (4) says, "If you don't really care, any reason is good enough" (p. 158). Menninger (5) and Thomas (6) advised that physicians and health-care providers should periodically become patients to experience, or reexperience, the patient role, to enhance sensitivity to what it's like to be a patient, and to see the effect of various provider behaviors on the patient's illness. Thomas said the following:

> One of the hard things to teach, is what it feels like to be a patient . . . (p. 222) being a patient is hard work . . . (p. 223). The nearest thing to a personal education in illness is the grippe. It is

almost all we have left in the way of on-the-job training. . . . (p. 221)

There is, of course, an emotional, or psychological, component to every physical illness. During the stress of illness, a person reverts to a dependent role, to the wish—the need—to be taken care of. The awareness of this wish sets up an inner struggle, a push–pull relationship, an ambivalence between dependence and independence. Not only do we want to be cared for, we also want to remain in control of (as much as possible) our lives and our relationships.

Patients sometimes resent both the need to be cared for and the people who fill the need. As caring professionals, it is our responsibility to know and understand the emotions of illness, to be sensitive to the many variations of these emotional manifestations in patient behavior, and to acknowledge this in empathic, yet therapeutic, responses as an integral part of our treatment. This is the essence of the holistic approach to treatment. Although we may know the complete history of the patient (e.g., employment, family, economic, interests, developmental, medical), if we do not in some way communicate to the patient our *understanding* of what his or her illness means to his or her life, our treatment reflects the dualistic mind–body dichotomy; thus, we are treating only "the kidney in room 319" or "the hand in the second treatment room." When patients know that we care enough to understand them as people, then we are contributing to their drive toward action (7), toward the reawakening of their drive for mastery of their environment. We then have helped patients to accept whatever level of dependency must be there for however long, and we have helped them reach for independence. This is an integral part of Reilly's (7) "nurturing of the spirit of man for action." (See Chapter 7.)

Several years ago a colleague and I were asked to consult with an occupational therapist working in a renal dialysis unit. This was the therapist's first job, and little about the role of occupational therapy treatment with renal dialysis patients had been published at that time. This pioneering therapist was questioning why she was there, her effectiveness, and whether she was actually "doing occupational therapy." She was particularly distressed about one patient, Charlotte (fictitious name), because Charlotte had been generally angry, hostile, and uncooperative, and was resistant to get involved in the discussion groups and other activities the therapist initiated. However, the therapist persisted in her attempts to engage Charlotte, and eventually Charlotte's behavior changed a great deal; Charlotte was involved and pleasant, and she even seemed to enjoy the activities and talked with the therapist and the other patients. The therapist was pleased but puzzled with this change in Charlotte's behavior. My colleague and I talked with the therapist about issues such as when is help helpful, patient resistance, and the concept of each patient having his or her own timing. We then went to talk with Charlotte. Charlotte told us about her husband at home who was even more seriously ill than she. She was concerned that her dialysis treatment 3 days each week took her away from caring for him. She told us about their two sons: one who had died from the same type of kidney disease Charlotte had and the other who was recently diagnosed as having this same disease. Charlotte talked of her anger, her despair, her feeling of hopelessness and helplessness, her inability even to drive a car, and her dependency on others for the trips to the dialysis unit. Charlotte said that each time she came for treatment, it reinforced the losses in her life caused by the illness. [Let me point out two important points here: (a) that being compliant by coming to treatment can have a negative and a positive component for the patient, that this action (of coming for treatment) prevents the denial of the illness, and (b) that the use of occupation during the treatment period helps the patient avoid getting caught in the emotional flooding of feeling the losses resulting from the illness and then connecting them to all the losses in his or her life.] She said that everything was out of control in her life but that she kept coming to dialysis because she could not function without it. She said the therapist accepted her in spite of her anger; one day, Charlotte reluctantly started working on a needlepoint project offered to her by the therapist, and an amazing thing happened. Charlotte said, "As I got involved, suddenly, I realized that this little piece of needlepoint was the only place I had any control in my life, but that I did have control here! Then I started looking around to see what other little things I could control. I knew I could not control my illness or that of my son or husband, and I couldn't drive, but I could control my behavior and I could become a more pleasant person and I could try to get and give more pleasure out of my time here. And that's what occupational therapy has meant to me so far, and I'm still looking for other places for me to control."

The story of Charlotte introduces another situation: some patients are simply not very lovable. We therapists dread the next treatment session of these patients, and we feel guilty that we do not like them. These patients are often noncompliant with treatment but are constantly demanding, and we frequently feel the impulse to grab them by both shoulders and say, "Hold still while I help you!" The therapist's anger and resentment may result in his or her becoming noncompliant also, if he or she becomes noncaring. As contradictory as it may seem, some manipulative patients learn to be powerful within the context of the dependent patient role; they have few behaviors that permit dependence and cooperation, while maintaining a sense of independence and coping within the patient role. As in Charlotte's case, a patient's resistance is often stirred by the mixture of emotions surrounding the disruptions in his or her life caused by the illness, the feelings of fear, anger, powerlessness, and the despair of having no hope for the future. In this type of situation, it is generally possible for the therapist to get under or around the resistance by empathetically understanding and acknowledging what the patient is experiencing.

Patients have their own timing for change, and we can facilitate this change, not by pushing, but by being supportive while they become sensitive to and in touch with that timing. We need to acknowledge that we cannot care for every patient. We need to accept that we cannot turn our caring feelings on and off at will. It is sometimes possible to refer a patient that we dislike to another therapist who can feel more positively for the patient, but at times this possibility is not an option. Whatever the situation, our responsibility is to deliver the best professional care. This "... in itself, is a kind of caring" (8, p. 235).

The same colleague who participated in the renal dialysis consultation (B. Bennett) recently commented (in a discussion, March 1984) that she wondered if the importance of what we do lies in our awareness. In her view, occupational therapy allows for and promotes "connectedness." Our patients are human beings who have had some aspect of human functioning taken away from them. They have been deprived of the mechanisms for connectedness in some part of their relationships. Occupational therapy may invent connectedness where perhaps none existed or create opportunities for reconnecting the patient to other human beings and the environment. We reawaken the patient's capacity to care. Often the patients are unattached to people and institutions. Daily life activities are often the connectors among people; that is, the mechanisms of caring. Occupational therapists care by

helping people disengage from despair and dysfunction and by helping them look forward, to see their loss as being able to be ameliorated through adaptation and occupation.

Occupational therapists are specialists in making caring happen. We know how to enrich all the transactions in the relationship with the patient. These become caring gestures. We augment the power of individuals to achieve their own objectives. In the same discussion mentioned earlier, Bennett continued that part of caring is knowing when to stop caring, to stop what she calls "emotional hemorrhaging"; walking the fine line between the two frequently becomes a balancing act. Finally, she added, when the structure of the treatment plan has been followed without the "spirit" of the plan, caring has been abandoned. (9) Caring implies quality of care and for us quality of life.

Occupational therapy is not the only caring profession. It demonstrates caring differently. To illustrate, a surgeon excised a malignant sarcoma from the hip joint of a middle-aged man and also removed about half the muscle tissue forming the buttocks on that side; the psychotherapist used family therapy to help the patient and his family deal with their fears of cancer, the changes in their lives, and the overwhelming feelings focused on his illness; the occupational therapist molded a special cushion allowing the patient to sit more comfortably while he drove a car and while he pursued his hobby of tinkering with cars. These "helpers" were all important to this patient, to his life, and to his quality of life. The occupational therapist's intervention was different in that it helped the patient reconnect to those occupations meaningful to him.

What is the market value of caring and who pays for it? Fromm (9) said, "... human energy and skill are without exchange value if there is no demand for them under existing market conditions" (9, pp. 70–71). In discussing employment settings for occupational therapists, Jantzen (10) said, "Caring for others and other altruistic motives seem to me rarely sufficient to generate dollars for salaries" (p. 72). The relationship between caring, *along with* the competence of the health-care professional, and patient treatment compliance and its effect on malpractice litigation is well documented. Menninger (5) stated the following:

> ... more often than not, the breakdown has been in the "caring" aspect the physician–patient relationship—not in the quality of technical care and treatment provided ...

Caring is an important aspect of health-care quality. (p. 837)

He further advocated including an assessment of caring within the professional standards review.

So far, caring has not been a part of the professional standards review. I do not believe that it ever will be, because the quality of caring is difficult to measure. However, every patient knows whether or not it is present. The ability of the health professional to develop a caring relationship with patients falls within the art rather than the science of health care. I am convinced that a profession that consistently provides treatment giving patients a clear sense of having both their physical and psychological needs well tended and contributed to will not only survive, but will also experience an increase in the demand for their services. Occupational therapy is such a profession.

Relationships With Self

The emphasis so far has been on the patient and on the development of the caring relationship as an integral part of the treatment. The focus now shifts to another relationship: that which we have with ourselves. Is it a caring relationship?

If I am not for myself, who will be?
If I am for myself alone, what am I?
If not now, when? (11, p. 237)

The meaning of these lines may be quite different for each person who hears them. Each individual's concept of self ". . . is composed of the thousands of perceptions varying in clarity, precision, and importance . . ." gathered since birth (12). Our own perceptions screen every experience in our world and interpret that experience uniquely for each of us, thus constantly shaping our self-concept. "The most important single factor affecting behavior is the self-concept" (8, p. 39). What we do at every moment in our lives is a product of how we see ourselves and the situations we are in. While situations may change, the beliefs, values, and purposes we have about ourselves are ever-present factors in determining our behavior. "Freud defined the ego (or the self) as that part of the mind which is aware of reality, stores up experiences (in the memory), avoids excessively strong stimuli (through flight), deals with moderate stimuli (through adaptation), and causes changes in the external world to its own advantage (through activity)" (12,

p. 86). The self is the star of every performance, the central figure in every act (8, p. 39). Therefore, we who are engaged in a helping profession need the broadest possible understanding of the nature, origins, and functions of the self-concept, not only for our own benefit but for that of our patients (8, pp. 6, 39).

The ability to develop caring relationships with others is in direct proportion to the ability to care for self. This caring for self is not an egocentric, narcissistic focus on self, but rather it is the sensitivity and knowledge of self that leads to personal growth. Just as Thomas (6) advocated a good case of the grippe to sensitize medical students to what it's like to be a patient (p. 222), I recommend that we occupational therapists perform an Activity Configuration on ourselves to gain a more objective view of how we use ourselves. How many "shoulds" have we grown up with that are no longer valid in our lives? Once when I was agonizing over whether or not to attend a meeting that I felt I "should" but did not really want to, a friend offered the perspective that "the world is not minimized by your lack of participation in it."

The process of helping others helps one's self: it is satisfying, therapeutic, and curative. There is an exhilaration in helping others that "is the result of something deeper than the power involved or the satisfaction of professional pride and a job well done." It is "the curative power of being human." The response of patients to genuine caring is enormous. It mobilizes "assets and self-curative resources on the part of a person being helped which too often he cannot tap on his own." Helping others increases our own self-esteem as we become aware of the strength and resources being mobilized for this effort and the power they activate in relationships (13, pp. 214–216).

Caring, for self and for others, ". . . orders other values around itself" (14, p. 51). A life that is ordered through caring has some telling features. It acquires a special kind of certainty, not a stewing need to feel certain and to seek guarantees. It is restful, yet dynamic, as opposed to static, giving security that retains vulnerability (14). "Such inclusive ordering requires giving up certain things and activities, and may thus be said to include an element of submission. But this submission, like the voluntary submission of the craftsman to his discipline and the requirements of his materials is basically liberating and affirming" (14, p. 53). Caring brings an order to our lives and relationships that frees our energy to be creative and productive, and provides parameters for our daily decisions. The energy thus freed, converted from negative to positive energy, has a direct effect on our productivity. Caring for self means choosing to attend to my needs first sometimes, not always second or third, because the less I give to me, the less I have to give to others.

We use relationships to define ourselves. As we look inward we see certain things about ourselves, but in the reflections from relationships we begin to see other facets of ourselves. Through relationships with our mothers, fathers, and others, we experience different levels of caring; our perceptions of that caring and how we use that information determine the kind of person we become. It is through this lifelong process that we learn to care for self and others. Our capacity to care and our ability to show we care are dependent on the kinds and quality of caring we receive. This is an ever-changing process for us, because once a word is spoken or an action has occurred, it becomes a part of our experience of the world. It is, in a psychic sense similar to the law of nature that for every action there is an equal and opposite reaction: we receive, we give; we give, we receive.

"One's actions are a part of one's existence" according to Pablo Casals (15). ". . . One feels it a duty to act, and whatever comes one does it—that's all—a very simple thing. I feel the capacity to care is the thing which gives life its deepest significance and meaning" (15, p. 156).

> If I am not for myself, who will be?
> If I am for myself alone, what am I?
> If not now, when? (11, p. 237)

The Elements of Therapeutic Relationships

It is self-evident that caring alone is not enough to establish an effective therapeutic relationship. Caring is the base; its presence enriches all other aspects of the relationship. The following are additional elements essential to the development of such a relationship:

1. *Competence.* We may be the most caring therapists in existence, but without the knowledge, skill, and ability to provide the needed treatment, we may develop only minimally therapeutic relationships. We have the responsibility to develop an ongoing continuing education program for ourselves. This personalized program should include studying the research being reported and translating treatment efficacy into treatment effectiveness. It should include studying the literature of related fields and studying our own. Developing and maintaining competence is also a part of caring . . . for ourselves and for our patients.

2. *Belief in the dignity and worth of the individual.* This element is conveyed in mostly subtle ways. It involves believing in the integrity of the individual, including his or her need for mastery and control, which we must not violate, but preserve as important.

3. *Belief that each individual has the potential for change and growth.* The individual already has the capacity to adapt and grow. The occupational therapist provides a road map in a sense and facilitates the journey of adaptation through "occupation to improve health and performance" (16).

4. *Communication.* True communication involves listening, hearing the words and the feelings behind the words, making sensitive observations, and sending clear messages.

5. *Values.* Values are reflected in our beliefs. They are our standards for living, and provide stability and meaning in our lives and parameters for our behavior. Values are the foundations of our selectivity, for saying, "This is good, this I believe; that is not good, that is not the way I will go."

6. *Touch.* Rather than elaborating on the use of this powerful therapeutic element here, I urge you to read again Huss's 1976 Slagle Lecture (17, pp. 11–18).

7. *Sense of humor.* A judicious use of humor can do much to bypass resistance or defuse a tense situation. It can introduce perspective for both patient and therapist. And it promotes health. In the introduction to Cousins' book, Bernard Lown, Harvard professor of cardiology, quoted the famous 17th-century physician Thomas Sydenham: "The arrival of a good clown exercises more beneficial influence upon the health of a town than twenty asses laden with drugs" (18, p. 24).

These are some of the elements necessary to therapeutic relationships. Individual therapists can expand this list by adding important elements from their experience. Taken individually, these elements are splinter skills; used collectively, they enable and enhance the use of self as a therapeutic tool. These elements become a part of us and a part of the treatment process; and, rather than requiring extra time to include, most often they save time, because we and our patients are in synchrony, and our actions and reactions are mutually supportive of our goals.

These same elements are eminently transferable to our relationships with co-workers, whether lateral, hierarchical, or interdisciplinary. Before staff members can relate to patients in a humanistic way, they have to be dealt with that way. How difficult it is for staff members to create a humanizing environment for patients within a setting where staff are being dealt with in a dehumanizing manner. I have observed that it is difficult to increase or even maintain productivity in situations like this.

Relationships Within Today's Health-Care Environment

No discussion of relationships in health care today is complete without some mention of how these relationships are affected by the complexity of the health-care system. The push for productivity makes it necessary for us to cut costs of providing services and maintain larger caseloads. At the same time, we are being asked to increase documentation. All of these demands make it difficult for us to retain our motivation to develop relationships with our patients that go beyond a superficial level.

Additionally, we are experiencing the initial impact of the prospective payment system. Patients are leaving health facilities before their complete rehabilitation needs have been addressed. We are participating in a health-care system that, for the first time, views our service as a cost as opposed to something directed toward supporting human function. Our educational programs face enrollment problems and decreased federal funding. These are definitely challenging times.

Along with the thrust for increased productivity and accountability in the health-care arena, a new round of regulation has emerged. "Health-care costs have been growing out of control and threaten to consume larger and larger shares of our national wealth. Even more perplexing is the fact that while we outspend other nations on health care we do not enjoy the best of health. We're clearly not getting our money's worth." (19, p. 6)

Not only is the federal government sending the message to the health-care system to do more, faster and better, with less, but also many states have enacted cost-containment legislation, and third-party payers are strictly following their criteria for reimbursement in the effort to control their risks. Now patients—the health-care consumers—are demanding more active participation in their own health care; that is, less dependence on and more accountability from their health-care providers. One of the fastest growing consumer groups is

the 35,000-member People's Medical Society, which has been in existence for just 1 year but adds 1,000 members each week. This past January, the organization asked all the physicians of West Palm Beach to sign a 10-point Code of Practice, which would include fees posting, complete and open discussion of proposed treatment, and the physician's particular competency to perform that treatment. Charles Inlander, the organization's executive director, said that the Code of Practice "simply affirms basic patient rights. We're only asking doctors the same questions they ask their Mercedes dealer's service department—up-front costs, prognosis, and 'You can't go ahead and do anything until I give you my full approval.' The only difference is we're not asking for the parts back" (20, p. D-2).

The shifting relationships in today's health-care environment are yet another phase of the action–reaction process that has its roots, at least in American medicine, in the beginning of this country. However, for our purposes, a few comments about the past decade will illustrate the pattern.

According to Starr (21), "Medicine, like many other American institutions, suffered a stunning loss of confidence in the 1970s!" (p. 379). Until then, the federal government had supported the beliefs that more medical services were needed and decisions regarding the delivery of these services should be made by the private medical sector. As costs continued to rise, but with no proportionate improvement in health care, government regulations and constraints increased as never before. This reaction was more than an economic one, because it included concern about the rights of patients, about the effectiveness of medical treatment, and about the moral values of medicine. Women, in particular, began to assume more responsibility for their own health, thereby diminishing the power, influence, and control of the medical profession (21, pp. 379, 380). It was no longer just a question of whether hospitalizations and surgery were necessary; rather, whether medical care made any difference in the health of the American people. "The nineteenth century doctrine of therapeutic nihilism—that existing drugs and therapies were useless—was revived in a new form. Now the net effectiveness of the medical system as a whole was [questioned]" (21, p. 408).

Starr's (21) comments indicate that the pendulum does swing—action, reaction—and that the "doctrine of therapeutic nihilism" (p. 408) appeared in both the 19th and 20th centuries, although in a different form the second time around. That pendulum will certainly swing again. While Starr's book focuses on the medical profession, we, as associates of that profession, must closely evaluate our capacity to address the effectiveness of our services and maintain the relationships that give us a position within the system itself. The turbulence within the health-care system today is but a reflection of the turbulence within society as it struggles to hold onto the old ways while also reaching to the new that are unknown. "One important characteristic to recognize is that if any one part of the system is changed, then all other parts within the system and any related system are changed as a result" (22, p. 800). Thus, the restructuring of society, from the changing profile of the labor force to the graying of America, affects the health-care system. Those of us who are in the health-care arena are scrambling to find our new place, to restore balance and security to our environment. In this competitive environment, it is important to do what we do well and maintain the relationships that will support our patients' needs, along with our own.

The greater the use of technology, the greater the depersonalization of the individual. Caring is the counterbalance: the "high touch" human response to the introduction of "high tech" (23, p. 39). From its beginning, occupational therapy treatment has been inextricably involved with high touch. We have helped our patients to do, participate, work, and enjoy, despite their dysfunction. Baum (24) has stated that, "As a profession, occupational therapy harnesses will and gives the individual control through activity. That is human, that is care" (p. 515).

Summary

The constraints in today's health-care environment make it extremely difficult to do the job we've been trained to do. With the possible exception of continuing competency, the elements of a therapeutic relationship described earlier do not increase the cost of health care, do not require additional time in the treatment process, and give the patient a clear sense of having both his or her physical and psychological needs well tended and contributed to. As occupational therapists, we have superb skills for developing and tending caring relationships. Let us continue to use them well.

Acknowledgments

The author thanks Carolyn Baum, MA, OTR, FAOTA; Binni Bennett, MSW; and Wanda Ellis-Webb for their invaluable support and assistance.

References

1. Devereaux E: Community home health care—in the rural setting. In *Willard and Spackman's Occupational Therapy*, 6th edition, Hopkins and H Smith, Editors. Philadelphia: Lippincott, 1983, p. 787.
2. West W: A reaffirmed philosophy and practice of occupational therapy for the 1980s. *Am J Occup Ther 38:22*, 1984.
3. *Project to Identify the Philosophy of Occupational Therapy.* Rockville, MD: AOTA, Jan 1983, p. 21.
4. Ciardi J: In *Choose Life*, B Mandelbaum, Editor. New York: Random House, 1968, p. 158.
5. Menninger W: "Caring" as part of health care quality. *JAMA 234:*836–837, 1975.
6. Thomas L: *The Youngest Science: Notes of a Medicine-Watcher.* New York: Viking, 1983, pp. 220–223.
7. Reilly M: Occupational therapy can be one of the great ideas of 20th century medicine. *Am J Occup Ther 16:*1–9, 1962. Reprinted as Chapter 7.
8. Combs A, Avila D, Purkey W: *Helping Relationships: Basic Concept for the Helping Professions.* Boston; Allyn & Bacon, 1971, pp. 6, 39.
9. Fromm E: *The Art of Loving.* New York: Bantam Books, 1956, pp. 70–71.
10. Jantzen A: The current profile of occupational therapy and the future professional or vocational? In *Occupational Therapy: 2001 AD*. Rockville, MD: AOTA, 1978, p. 72.
11. Ethics of the fathers (chapt 1, verse 14). In *Choose Life*, B Mandelbaum, Editor. New York: Random House, 1968, p. 237.
12. Appelton W: *Fathers and Daughters.* New York: Doubleday, 1981, p. 86.
13. Rubin T: *Through My Own Eyes.* New York: Macmillan, 1982, pp. 214–216.
14. Mayeroff M: *On Caring.* New York: Perennial Library, Harper & Row, 1971.
15. Casals P: In *Choose Life*, B Mandelbaum, Editor. New York: Random House, 1968, p. 156.
16. Representative Assembly: Occupation as the common core of occupational therapy. In *Policies of the AOTA, Inc.* Rockville, MD: AOTA, 1979, #1.12.
17. Huss J: Touch with care or a caring touch? *Am J Occup Ther 31:*11–18, 1977.
18. Cousin: Introduction. In *The Healing Heart, Antidotes to Panic and Helplessness.* New York: Norton, 1983, p. 24.
19. Schneiderman L: The "Molting" of America's welfare system. In *NASW News.* Silver Spring, MD: National Association of Social Workers, Sept 1983, p. 6.

20. Peirce N: Citizen's group going after more medical ac-countability. In *The Herald Dispatch*. Huntington, WV: Gannett Feb 19, 1984, p. D-2.

21. Starr P: *The Social Transformation of American Medicine*. New York: Basic Books, 1982, pp. 379–380, 408.

22. Baum C, Devereaux E: A systems perspective—Conceptualizing and implementing occupational therapy in a complex environment. In *Willard and Spackman's Occupational Therapy,* 6th edition, Hopkins and Smith, Editors. Philadelphia: Lippincott, 1983, p. 800.

23. Naisbitt J: *Megatrends*. New York: Warner Books, 1982, p. 39.

24. Baum C: Occupational therapists put care in the health system. *Am J Occup Ther 34:*515, 1980.

CHAPTER 36

Client-Centered Practice: What Does It Mean and Does It Make a Difference?

MARY LAW, SUE BAPTISTE, AND JENNIFER MILLS

Occupational therapists in Canada were one of the first health professional groups to describe and endorse a model of client-centered practice (Canadian Association of Occupational Therapists & Department of National Health and Welfare, 1983). Throughout the development of a clear framework for the unique contribution of the discipline of occupational therapy in Canada, the concept of client-centeredness has been constant (CAOT, 1991; Law et al., 1990; Townsend, Brintnell, & Staisey, 1990). The development of a client-centered approach reflects changes wanted by consumers who desire more control in defining health issues as well as changes in how health is viewed. According to the Ottawa Charter for Health Promotion (World Health Organization, 1986), health is viewed as a "resource for living." The implications of these changes have led to increased emphasis on consumer rights and public participation in health issues.

Although the Guidelines for the Client-Centred Practice of Occupational Therapy have been widely distributed and used in Canada (Blain & Townsend, 1993), there has been little discussion about the concepts and issues inherent in client-centered practice. In fact, in researching the literature for this paper, a definition of client-centered practice—along with a description of its concepts and assumptions, was not found. Because of the lack of discussion about the meaning of client-centered practice, it is difficult for therapists to understand and implement these ideas in their practice.

The purpose of this paper is to define and discuss concepts and issues fundamental to client-centered practice. Concepts such as individual autonomy and choice, partnership, therapist and client responsibility, enablement, contextual congruence, accessibility, and

respect for diversity will be examined. From these concepts, assumptions of client-centered practice emerge. The challenge of implementing the assumptions of client-centered practice on a day-to-day basis is illustrated through two occupational therapy practice examples. The paper concludes with a brief discussion of research evidence about the effectiveness of client-centered practice in enhancing client outcomes. The ideas raised in this paper should be of interest to occupational therapists in clinical practice, education, and research.

Client-Centeredness

The underpinnings of the construct of client-centeredness are found in original works of Carl Rogers just prior to World War II. Historically, the term *client-centered practice* first arose from Rogers in a book entitled *The Clinical Treatment of the Problem Child* (Rogers, 1939). Rogers recognized a number of key constructs of client-centeredness (1951). He emphasized the importance of cultural values, the dynamic nature of the therapist–client interaction, the need for a client to have an active role in approaching problems and concerns, and the need for openness and honesty within the clinical relationship (Rogers, 1951). The most important contributions of Rogers in articulating client-centered practice were the concept of listening and his discussion of the quality of therapist–client interactions. Growth of the client-centered movement continued into the mid-1960s with its main focus in utilization being within the discipline and practice of social work.

Though Rogers' interpretation of client-centered practice may be different from the occupational therapy interpretation, it is important to note from whence this term emerged. It was within the last two decades that the profession of occupational therapy in Canada articulated a congruence between the theoretical framework of occupational performance and the core value of client-centeredness (CAOT, 1991). In the development of these concepts for occupational therapy, the importance of the relationship between client and therapist reflects the contribution of Rogers' thinking. The initial version of the Guidelines for the Client-Centred Practice of Occupational Therapy (CAOT & DNHW, 1983) emphasized ideas about the worth of the individual and a holistic view of the individual. Ideas about client-centered practice have, however, evolved over time and now reflect the importance of client–therapist partnership, the rights of clients to make choices about occupations, the influence of a client's environment, and the need for intervention at a societal and policy level (Law, 1991; Polatajko, 1992; Townsend, 1993).

Concepts of Client-Centered Practice

There is increasing evidence that occupational therapists, as reflective practitioners, value a therapist–client relationship defined by trust, caring, and competence (Doble, 1988; Mattingly & Fleming, 1994; Peloquin, 1991). Client-centeredness is a philosophy of practice built on concepts that reflect changes in the attitudes and beliefs of clients and occupational therapists. There are a number of concepts which form the underpinnings of a client-centered approach.

Autonomy/Choice

It is recognized that each client is unique and brings that perspective to the occupational therapy experience (CAOT, 1991). Clients are experts about their occupational function. Only they can truly understand the experiences of their daily lives, express their needs, and make choices about their occupations. "The real experts on disability are the people who live with a disability" (Canadian Association of Independent Living Centers (CAILC), 1992, p. 58). Crabtree and Caron-Parker (1991) have suggested that Thomasma's freedoms—freedom from obstacles, to know one's options, to choose, to act, and to create new options—be the cornerstone of occupational therapy service.

Clients have the right to receive information to enable them to make decisions about occupational therapy services that will or will not effectively meet these needs. They expect that their opinions will be sought, their values will be respected, and that they will maintain their dignity and integrity throughout the therapy process (Polatajko, 1992). To enable this to occur, clients need to be provided with information in a format that is understandable and that will enable them to make decisions about their needs.

Partnership and Responsibility

Client-centered practice necessarily leads to a change in power so that clients have more say in defining the priorities of intervention and directing the intervention process (Kaplan, 1991; Sumsion, 1993). In client-centered practice, the goal of the client–therapist relationship is an interdependent partnership to enable the solution of occupational performance issues and the achievement of client goals. Assessment and intervention reflect the client's visions and values, taking into account the roles that they have and the environments in which they live. In such a therapist–client relationship, power is defined as a process by which the client and the therapist achieve together what neither could achieve alone (Crabtree & Caron-Parker, 1991; Law, 1991).

With partnership comes responsibility. The responsibilities of the therapist and client, in this practice model, change from responsibilities as viewed within a medical model. Traditionally, therapists have taken an active role in the assessment and definition of occupational performance issues and the delineation of methods to resolve those concerns. In a client-centered practice, the client has a more active role in defining both the goals of intervention and the desired outcomes of intervention. The role of the therapist shifts to one of facilitator in working with the client to find the means to achieve those goals (Kaplan, 1991). Client and therapist become partners in the intervention process. Therapists' responsibilities include providing information which will enable client choice and utilizing their expertise to facilitate a broad range of solutions to occupational performance issues (Matheis-Kraft et al., 1990; Sokoly & Dokecki, 1992). Clients have a responsibility to be active participants in the therapy process, both in defining issues for therapy intervention and in facilitating the intervention process. Such a partnership leads to the therapist and client working together, questioning issues, trusting, and learning from each other throughout the therapy process.

Clients may choose to define problems or seek intervention which puts them at risk to themselves or at risk for failure. Therapists recognize that such risks are often valuable learning experiences, provided that the client is competent to understand the consequences of risks and the therapist is not supporting actions which are unethical, could lead to harm, or could be considered as malpractice. In client-centered practice, it is important that therapists discuss openly with clients if they believe that the course of action the clients are undertaking puts them at risk. There may be situations when a therapist is uncomfortable with a client's choice, more because of a difference in values than the fact that the client is not competent to make that choice. Therapists must clearly outline when they cannot support clients in pursuing an action plan.

Enablement

Occupational therapy practice in the past has focused largely on remediation of functional difficulties by facilitating change in individual performance components. A client-centered approach in which clients define the central issues for occupational therapy intervention supports a shift from a deficit model of intervention to an enablement model (Polatajko 1992). Within such a model, therapists work with clients to enable them to achieve occupational goals that they have set for themselves. The occupational therapy process can focus on prevention, remediation, development, or maintenance of occupational performance (CAOT, 1991). Achievement of these goals is facilitated through a variety of means, including changes in individual skills, changes in environments, and changes in occupations. All intervention alternatives are explored. In the therapy encounter, the process of providing services is important. There is a need for increased emphasis on the use of listening and emphasis on the use of language that is understood by clients and provision of information to facilitate client decision-making (Baxendale, 1993). Peloquin (1993) found that clients desire more than simply technical competence from therapists. Clients value the caring which is shown by therapists who truly listen and learn from their experiences.

Contextual Congruence

The importance of clients' roles, interests, environments, and culture are central to the occupational therapy process within client-centered practice. Occupational therapy assessment and intervention using a client-centered approach places importance on the individualization of assessment and intervention (Dunn, 1993; Law, 1991; Law, Baptiste, et al., 1994). Consideration of the context in which a client lives demands a flexibility in the approach of the therapist in all intervention situations (Dunn et al., 1994). For example, the use of a set protocol of assessments and intervention for diagnostically defined types of clients is not supported within client-centered practice. Research about assessment has also indicated that results depend on

the environment in which the assessment occurs (Park, Fisher, & Velozo, 1993). In practice, there may be situations where therapists use different levels of client-centeredness, depending on the nature of the intervention and the needs of the client. One of the most challenging dimensions of client-centered practice is "how to adjust consultation style to the needs of the moment" (Moorhead & Winefield, 1991, p. 345). It is also important to note that a client of occupational therapy may not always be an individual. Clients can include other family members or can be communities, private companies, or organizations.

Accessibility and Flexibility

In client-centered practice, services are provided to clients in a timely and accessible manner. Services are constructed to meet the needs of the client, rather than the client fitting into a service model. A client-centered approach to practice is flexible and dynamic, with an emphasis on learning and problem solving. Therapists work to enable clients to access services with a minimum of bureaucratic red tape. The successful client-centered therapist exhibits an openness and honesty within the client–therapist relationship. This includes the provision of a welcoming service with attention paid to such details as parking, waiting lists, information brochures, and ongoing therapy procedures.

Respect for Diversity

Intervention based on clients' visions and values demonstrates a respect for the diversity of values that clients hold. It is important for therapists to recognize their own values and not impose these values on clients. What may seem to be an irrational choice by a client is often exactly what is right for that person at that time, based on all the information they have about their lives and values (Kaplan, 1991). The strengths and resources that a client brings to an occupational therapy encounter are recognized and used to facilitate the achievement of occupational performance goals. The client-centered approach recognizes that differences in values and opinions will occur, but supports a mediation approach to the resolution of these conflicts.

Definition and Assumptions of Client-Centered Practice in Occupational Therapy

One of the difficulties in discussing client-centered practice in occupational therapy has been the lack of a definition of client-centered practice. Using the concepts discussed in the previous section, a definition of client-centered practice in occupational therapy was developed. *Client-centered practice* **is an approach to providing occupational therapy, which embraces a philosophy of respect for, and partnership with, people receiving services. Client-centered practice recognizes the autonomy of individuals, the need for client choice in making decisions about occupational needs, the strengths clients bring to a therapy encounter, the benefits of client–therapist partnership, and the need to ensure that services are accessible and fit the context in which a client lives.** "The goal of the [client] centered philosophy is to create a caring, dignified and empowering environment in which clients truly direct the course of their care and call upon their inner resources to speed the healing process" (Matheis-Kraft, George, Olinger, & York, 1990, p. 128).

From the concepts and definition of client-centered practice, assumptions about practice can be developed. These assumptions can be used to guide the structure and process of occupational therapy practice as well as research directed at exploring the effects of a client-centered practice philosophy. They include:

- Occupational therapists using a client-centered approach recognize that clients and families are all different and unique and they know themselves best (King, Rosenbaum, Law, King, & Evans, 1994).
- Optimal client outcomes occur when clients and therapists work in partnership throughout the therapy process and focus on the resolution of client-defined occupational performance issues.
- Provision of information to clients about their occupational function will enable them to make choices about what services they need and the desired outcome.
- Optimal client outcomes occurs when occupational therapy services consider the environment and roles important to each client.

Implications for Occupational Therapy Practice

The concepts and assumptions of client-centered practice raise a number of client–therapist partnership issues that must be addressed. These include 1) defining the nature of the presenting occupational issues; 2) discussing and deciding on the need for intervention and the desired outcome; and 3) deciding the focus of occupational therapy intervention. In addressing these issues, it is important for therapists to determine who the client is, to respect the client's value system and culture, to facilitate the client in setting occupational goals, to provide education and information to facilitate personal choices and problem solving, and to use their skills to help the client achieve their occupational performance goals.

Because client-centered practice suggests a particular philosophical approach, it is difficult to list specific implications for practice. The challenges of basing intervention on priorities and client choice, increasing client participation in program planning, allowing clients to succeed but also to risk and to fail, changing therapist roles to enable facilitation, and broadening the focus of intervention are all critical challenges to be met and resolved. These ideas may not mean changing one's clinical practice entirely, as occupational therapists have always supported a holistic approach to practice. However, client-centered practice needs to be more clearly articulated in our day-to-day clinical activities and in how we approach interactions with clients.

Differences between a more traditional and a client-centered approach begin from the initial contact. In a recent survey, Neistadt (1995) found that the majority of occupational therapists use very informal methods to determine client priorities. In client-centered practice, considerable thought should go into how an occupational therapy encounter begins. For example, key questions (listed below) could be used by therapists to analyze the nature of this aspect of practice.

- How much power does the client have at initial contact?
- How much time is spent discussing the client's values and goals?
- How much of the occupational therapy assessment focuses on performance components compared to occupational performance issues?
- How much of the assessment process uses standardized assessment procedures as compared to procedures tailored to the needs of the client?
- Is the client aware of the system within which they are receiving service?
- Is the occupational therapy intervention plan addressing the roles and environments that are relevant to the client?
- Are educational materials tailored to the relevant needs of the client?

The following examples illustrate some of the key concepts and assumptions of client-centered practice as used within two occupational therapy clinical encounters.

Example 1

Mr. S. was a 76-year-old man who was admitted to an acute inpatient medical floor because of severe dehydration. Mr. S. was found at home, unable to get out of bed, incontinent, and unable to manage any aspect of personal care. His spouse had a history of moderately advanced dementia, and did not pursue medical attention until there was severe physical deterioration Occupational therapy was requested because of his dependence in basic activities of daily living. In therapy, Mr. S.'s main objective was to get well enough to return home. The occupational therapist worked with the client to facilitate a return to independence in self-care skills. Eventually, he was able to perform all aspects of personal care independently. After this stage of successful rehabilitation, the client had many options and choices to make regarding discharge from the hospital. Psychological assessment found Mr. S. to be competent to make his own decisions. The occupational therapist provided information regarding the risks and consequences of returning to his previous living arrangement. With this knowledge, Mr. S. made an informed decision to return to a home environment that was placing him at a fairly high safety risk, with minimal community supports accepted by his wife.

This case study highlights the concepts of autonomy/personal choice, client responsibility for goal setting, and respect for diversity of the client. It is an example of a situation that involved a client making an apparently irrational choice, but a decision that was accepted as right for him at that time. The degree of client-centeredness evolved throughout the therapy process. As Mr. S.'s acute medical crisis stabilized, he was able to assume more control for directing his therapy goals and interventions.

Example 2

Mrs. R. was a 39-year-old woman diagnosed with fibromyalgia. The home care occupational therapist was requested to assist with management of daily activities. Initial assessment found that, Mrs. R. had severe pain in the arms, neck, back, and legs; stiffness limiting range of motion; chronic fatigue; and problems sleep-

ing. In addition, other concerns included being a single mother of two young boys, geographic isolation, recent marriage separation, and financial difficulties.

To identify and prioritize problems and goals, the Canadian Occupational Performance Measure was administered (Law et al., 1994). The occupational performance problems identified were sleeping discomfort, preparing meals, use of toilet and bathing, playing with children, and pursuing meaningful roles outside the home. The process of setting occupational performance goals was challenging for Mrs. R., as she was quite focused on her individual physical problems. The use of the COPM, a client-centered assessment focusing on occupational performance areas, facilitated a shift in the therapy process from a deficit model to an enablement model of goal setting and intervention. The client-centered assessment process allowed subsequent intervention and education to be focussed on client priorities throughout the therapy process. This helped to ensure that these sessions were meaningful, and it allowed the client to assume responsibility for developing solutions which fit her lifestyle. Using the COPM also gave the client an indication of progress as the scores on the measure changed from 2.2 and 2.4 for performance and satisfaction to 5.2 and 4.9 after intervention.

Intervention involved providing education regarding the modification of her physical environment, implementing energy conservation and relaxation strategies, and counseling regarding a paced approach to resuming meaningful roles. By focusing on the potential functional outcomes, Mrs. R. was able to identify the need to implement changes in her lifestyle. For example, she decided that a scooter was acceptable because of the freedom it allowed for outings with her children. After this, the occupational therapist was able to provide her with practical methods of accessing a scooter for her regular use.

Central to this therapeutic process were the client-centered concepts of autonomy, personal control, partnership, responsibility, and enablement. The client–therapist relationship fostered skills in self-management for use by Mrs. R. in the present and for the future.

Challenges to Implementation

It must be recognized that working in a client-centered model of practice is challenging and complex. The therapist must be aware of obstacles that exist in the therapy process which may hinder the implementation of client-centered principles. Obstacles may arise from various sources, including the client, the therapist, and the organization.

Clients themselves may present barriers that alter the extent to which the therapy can be client-centered. For example, if a client does not have well-developed problem-solving skills, the therapist may have to be more directive than with other clients. As well, some clients may be reluctant to assume responsibility for their care. This creates an obvious challenge to the therapist, and challenges the therapist to act as a mediator to ensure that these issues are discussed and to work for potential solutions.

The therapist may also be the source of some obstacles toward client-centered practice. The process of giving more power/control to the client threatens the traditional view of the therapist as expert, and may elicit feelings of discomfort. In addition, separating personal and professional values from client values can be a challenge, especially when the client is making a decision that appears to entail unnecessary risk. One must be careful that the client-centered approach is not used to absolve therapists or the system of responsibility for providing excellent quality of service. If a client chooses not to adhere to recommendations, it is easy to assume that it is because the client is noncompliant. This may be the case, but it is important for the therapist to reflect back on the process and identify any barriers which may have prevented adherence. For example, did the client understand the rationale for such recommendations, any risks from nonadherence to them, and any other options which were available?

The third source of barriers may be at the organization or systems level. For example, in a program setting dominated by the medical model, it may be difficult to implement some concepts of client-centered practice such as autonomy, responsibility, and enablement. It may also be difficult to determine who is the primary client: the referred person, family, school, insurance company, hospital, or industry.

The obstacles will vary depending on the clinical setting, and the personal characteristics of the client and therapist involved. This discussion has highlighted only a few examples that may occur. It is important to be aware of the potential barriers to client-centered practice, so that they can be foreseen, identified, and solutions created.

Does Client-Centered Practice Make a Difference?

While occupational therapists may be comfortable with and support the philosophy of client-centered practice, it is important to determine whether the concepts and values inherent in client-centered practice make a difference, both in the service provision process and in client outcomes. A review of the occupational therapy literature yielded very few studies examining the effect of client-centered practice, so the review was expanded to examine studies in other disciplines as well.

Research findings indicate that providing respectful and supportive services, an aspect of client-centered practice, leads to improved client satisfaction and adherence to health service programs (Greenfield, Kaplan, & Ware, 1985; Hall, Roter, & Katz, 1988; Wasserman, Inui, Barriatua, Carter, & Lippincott, 1984). In a review of the service process, King, King, and Rosenbaum (1994) found that there is evidence that respectful and supportive treatment, information exchange, and practices enabling client professional partnerships are all significantly associated with increased client satisfaction.

Provision of information to clients to enable client decision-making has been shown to lead to both improved functional outcome and improved client satisfaction. In studies involving clients with diabetes or peptic ulcer disease, Greenfield, Kaplan, and Ware (1985) evaluated the effect of providing client education. Clients were randomized into two groups, an experimental group which received a 20-minute educational intervention about how to read their medical charts and ask for pertinent information, and another group receiving a standard education program. Clients receiving the experimental intervention were more satisfied with their services and had improved functional outcomes one month later. Moxley-Haegert and Serbin (1983), in a clinical trial comparing parent education about developmental issues to parent education about general parenting or a control group, found that parents who received developmental education were more able, after one year, to identify key issues related to their child's development and had increased adherence to service program suggestions. As well, children of parents who had received developmental education had improved developmental outcomes after one year.

Development of a client–therapist partnership has been demonstrated to lead to increased client participation, increased client self-efficacy, and improved satisfaction with service (Dunst, Trivette, Boyd, & Brookfield, 1994; Greenfield, Kaplan, & Ware, 1985). An individualized flexible approach to occupational therapy intervention, where the client defines goals which then become the focus of intervention, has been shown to lead to improved occupational performance outcome and improved satisfaction (Law, Polatjko, et al., 1994; Sanford, Law, Swanson, & Guyatt, 1994).

Conclusion

Client-centered practice is an approach to therapy that supports a respectful partnership between therapists and clients. It is the philosophical basis for the national occupational therapy guidelines published by the Canadian Association of Occupational Therapists (CAOT, 1991). Although client-centered practice is evident throughout the history of occupational therapy, its significance and implications for practice are only recently being explored in the occupational therapy literature and research. More research to understand the effect of promoting personal control and enablement through a client-centered approach is needed. It is important that the meaning and application of client-centered practice continues to be developed. The term client-centered is popular in many areas of health service, but using the term does not necessarily translate into a truly client-centered practice. As health care policy becomes influenced more by consumers, it is an opportune time for occupational therapists to integrate the concepts of client-centered practice into program planning and intervention.

References

Abramson, J. S. (1990). Enhancing patient participation: Clinical strategies in the discharge planning process. *Social Work in Health Care, 14,* 53–71.

Baxendale, B. (1993, June). *Being a patient . . . becoming a person.* Paper presented at the Canadian Association of Occupational Therapists Conference, Regina, SK.

Blain, J., & Townsend, E. (1933). Occupational therapy guidelines for client-centered practice: Impact study findings. *Canadian Journal of Occupational Therapy, 60,* 271–285.

Canadian Association of Independent Living Centres. (1992/ Fall–Winter). Research as an empowerment process for the Independent Living movement. *Abilities,* 58–59.

Canadian Association of Occupational Therapists. (1991). *Occupational therapy guidelines for client-centered practice.* Toronto, ON: CAOT Publications ACE.

Canadian Association of Occupational Therapists & Department of National Health and Welfare. (1983). *Guidelines for the client-centered practice of occupational therapy* (H39–33/1983E). Ottawa, ON: Department of National Health and Welfare.

Crabtree, J. L., & Caron-Parker, L. M. (1991). Long-term care of the aged: Ethical dilemmas and solutions. *American Journal of Occupational Therapy, 45,* 607–612.

Doble, S. (1988). Intrinsic motivation and clinical practice: The key to understanding the unmotivated client. *Canadian Journal of Occupational Therapy, 55,* 75–60.

Dunn, W., Brown, C., & McGuigan, A. (1934). The Ecology of Human Performance: A framework for considering the effect of context. *American Journal of Occupational Therapy, 48,* 595–607.

Dunst, C. J., Trivette, C. M., Boyd, K., & Brookfield, J. (1994). Help-giving practices and the self-efficacy appraisals of parents. In C. J. Dunst, C. M. Trivette, & A. G. Deal (Eds.), *Supporting and strengthening families (Vol. 1): Methods, strategies and practices.* Cambridge, MA: Brookline Books.

Greenfield, S., Kaplan, S. H., & Ware, J. E. (1985). Expanding patient involvement in care: Effects on patient outcomes. *Annals of Internal Medicine, 102,* 520–528.

Hall, J. A., Poter, D. L., & Katz, N. R. (1988). Meta-analysis of correlates of provider behavior in medical encounters. *Medical Care, 26,* 657–675.

Kaplan, R. M. (1991). Health-related quality of life in patient decision making. *Journal of Social Issues, 47,* 69–30.

King, G., Rosenbaum, P., Law, M., King, S., & Evans, J. (1994). *A framework for family-centered service.* Hamilton, ON: McMaster University, Neurodevelopmental Clinical Research Unit.

King, G., King, S., & Rosenbaum, P. (1994). *Interpersonal aspects of care-giving and client satisfaction, adherence, and stress: A review of the medical and rehabilitation literature.* Hamilton: McMaster University, ON, Neurodevelopmental Clinical Research Unit.

Law, M., Baptiste, S., McColl, M., Opzoomer, A., Polatajko, H., & Pollock, N. (1990). The Canadian Occupational Performance Measure: An outcome measurement protocol for occupational therapy. *Canadian Journal of Occupational Therapy, 57,* 82–87.

Law, M. (1991). The environment: A focus for occupational therapy. *Canadian Journal of Occupational Therapy, 58,* 171–179.

Law, M., Baptiste, S., Carswell, A., McColl, M. A., Polatajko, H., & Pollock, N. (1994). *Canadian Occupational Performance Measure Manual* (2nd edition). Toronto, ON: CAOT Publications: ACE.

Law, M., Polatajko, H., Pollock, N., Carswell, A., Baptiste, S., & McColl, M. (1994). The Canadian Occupational Performance Measure: Results of pilot testing. *Canadian Journal of Occupational Therapy, 61,* 191–197.

Matheis-Kraft, C., George, S., Olinger, M. J., & York, L. (1990). Patient-driven healthcare works. *Nursing Management, 21,* 124–128.

Mattingly, C., & Fleming, M. H. (1994). *Clinical reasoning: Forms of inquiry in a therapeutic process.* Philadelphia: F.A. Davis.

Moorhead. K., & Winefield, H. (1991). Teaching counseling skills to fourth-year medical students: A dilemma concerning goals. *Family Practice, 8,* 343–346.

Moxley-Haegert, L., & Serbin, L. A. (1983). Developmental education for parents of delayed infants: Effects on parental motivation and children's development. *Child Development, 54,* 1324–1331.

Neistadt, M. E. (1995). Methods of assessing clients' priorities: A survey of adult physical dysfunction settings. *American Journal of Occupational Therapy, 49,* 428–436. http://dx.doi.org/10.5014/ajot.49.5.428

Park, S., Fisher, A. C., & Velozo, C. A. (1993). Using the Assessment of Motor and Process Skills to compare performance between home and clinical settings. *American Journal of Occupational Therapy, 48,* 697–709. http://dx.doi.org/10.5014/ajot.48.8.697

Peloquin, S. M. (1991). Time as a commodity: Reflections and implications. *American Journal of Occupational Therapy, 45,* 147–154. http://dx.doi.org/10.5014/ajot.45.2.147

Polatajko, H. J. (1992). Naming and framing occupational therapy: A lecture dedicated to the life of Nancy B. *Canadian Journal of Occupational Therapy, 59,* 189–200.

Rogers, C. R. (1939). *The critical treatment of the problem child.* Boston: Houghton Mifflin.

Rogers, C. R. (1951). *Client-centered therapy.* Boston: Houghton Mifflin.

Sanford, J., Law, M., Swanson, L., & Guyatt. G. (1994). *Assessing clinically important change as an outcome of rehabilitation in older adults.* San Francisco: American Society on Aging Conference.

Sokoly, M. M., & Dokecki, P. R. (1992). Ethical perspectives on family-centered early intervention. *Infants and Young Children, 4,* 23–32.

Sumsion, T. (1999). Client-centered practice: The true impact. *Canadian Journal of Occupational Therapy, 60,* 6–8.

Townsend. E., Brintnell, S., & Staisey, N. (1990). Developing guidelines for client-centered occupational therapy practice. *Canadian Journal of Occupational Therapy, 57,* 69–76.

Wasserman, R. C., Inui, T. S., Barriatua, R. D., Carter, W. B., & Lippincott, P. (1984). Pediatric clinicians' support for parents makes a difference: An outcome-based analysis of clinician–parent interaction. *Pediatrics, 74,* 1047–1053.

World Health Organization. (1986). *Ottawa charter for health promotion.* Ottawa: Author.

CHAPTER 37

Client-Centered and Family-Centered Care: Refinement of the Concepts

PANELPHA (PENNY) L. KYLER

Introduction

Information on client-centered care is ubiquitous, generated by multiple sources and disseminated in a variety of forms. While people encounter information about client-centered care, the degree to which they use this information varies in accordance with a host of personal life events, circumstances and external forces. Based on a review of the literature, client-centered care has a variety of nuanced meanings; however, all include the importance of individual or family involvement. Similar to, yet different from, client-centered care is family-centered care. Family-centered care is the purposeful inclusion of multiple stakeholders in the decision-making process and is often fraught with concern and controversy. When to include and who to include in the decision-making process is not clear. Both terms have been used in occupational therapy and its literature. Revisiting these concepts in light of the historical roots of terms, the ethical implications and the application to today's clinical practice will lead to a refinement of the model of client-centered care as used in occupational therapy.

Client-centered care (Figure 37.1) is a concept that speaks to a universal standard of substantive inclusion of the primary individual as part of the decision-making health care process (Emanuel & Emanuel, 1992; Law, Baptiste, & Mills, 1995; Lawlor & Mattingly, 1998; Wilkins, Pollock, Rochhon, & Law, 2001). The terminology has come to education and health care from a variety of sources, but all share the motivational features of trying to establish a relationship that will provide a good outcome in keeping with the desires and values of the client. The client-centered approach focuses explicit attention on models designed to involve the person and empower him or her in contrast to previously prevalent expert-driven approaches (Bell, Kravitz, Thom, Krupat, & Azari, 2002; Charles, Gafni, & Whelan, 1999; Corring & Cook, 1999; Emanuel & Emanuel, 1992; Ende, Kazis, Ash, & Moskowitz, 1989; Guadagnoli & Ward, 1998; Law & Mills, 1998). Client-centered approaches emphasize professionals as agents of the person who intervenes in ways to help him/her act as autonomously as possible, protect that person's integrity, and strengthen family functioning.

Historical Roots of the Term

From a historical perspective, the term client-centered care has been part of a number of discipline specific foci. Before occupational therapy moved toward a client-centered approach, theoretical models of practice emphasized the integration of client-centered approaches to guide the therapeutic process (Emanuel & Emanuel, 1992; Law et al., 1995; Sumsin, 1999; Szasz & Hollender, 1956). In particular, the models identified by Rogers, (1951), Szasz and Hollender (1956) and Emanuel and Emanuel (1992) provide the historical context for today's occupational therapy practice. Prior

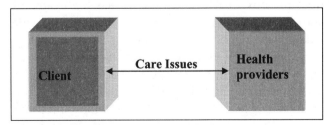

Figure 37.1. Client-centered care model.

Note. An inter-dependent partnership to enable solutions to occupational performance issues. Direct communication occurs between the client and provider regarding occupational performance issues.

This chapter was previously published in the *Occupational Therapy in Mental Health, 24,* 100–120. Copyright © 2008, Haworth Press. Reprinted with permission.

to Szasz and Hollender and Emanuel and Emanuel, Carl Rogers, a clinical psychologist, known for his contributions to counseling and psychotherapy provided the general overview of a client-centered theory. Rogers, in 1942, wrote *Counseling and Psychotherapy* and in 1945, was invited to set up a counseling center at the University of Chicago. While working at the University of Chicago, he published his major work, *Client-Centered Therapy* (Rogers, 1951), wherein he outlined his basic theory based upon years of clinical experiences. Rogers' therapeutic approach originally called non-directive, because he felt that the therapist should not lead the client, but rather be there for the client while the client directs the progress of the therapy, changed its name to client-centered. The Rogers therapeutic approach has three conditions: empathetic understanding, unconditional positive regard and therapeutic genuineness (Patterson, 1990). Rogers felt that the client was the one who should say for themselves what is wrong, find ways of improving, and determine the conclusion of therapy. Rogers' therapy was very "client-centered" even while he acknowledged the impact of the therapist (Boeree, 1998, p. 3). Today, though the terms non-directive and client-centered are still used, most people refer to Carl Rogers' approach as Rogerian therapy. One of the phrases Rogers used to describe his therapy is "supportive, not reconstructive" (Boeree, 1998, p. 6).

As psychiatrists, Szasz and Hollender in 1956 discuss the psychoanalytic, sociologic and philosophic considerations of physician–patient relationships clearly articulating three basic models of the physician–patient relationships. Szasz and Hollender (1956) proposed a "model of mutual participation" in which "essentially, the physician helps the client to help himself (p. 587)." They noted that this model was a far cry from the then dominant 1950s model of "activity–passivity" where the patient/client passively takes direction from the physician who actively directs the treatment and "guidance–cooperation" where physicians provide guided step-down choices and patients/clients cooperate in following those choices. The activity–passivity model was widely used in the management of chronic illnesses such as diabetes, arthritis and tuberculosis and was not only preferable, but essential, in controlling infectious chronic illnesses. The model embraced modes of interaction considered essential in medical relationships.

The three basic models each had positive and less than positive points. Model 1, or activity–passivity, is the oldest conceptual model. It is not an interaction, but an effect of one person upon another person; the physician is active and the patient is inanimate. This model is appropriate in emergency situations where the treatment takes place irrespective of the patient's contributions. Model 2, or guidance–cooperation, described the then prevalent model of medical practice where a patient seeks help and is ready and willing to cooperate. The physician placed in a position of power, also known as "transference reaction," directs the treatment and the patient willingly takes advice and, cooperates with treatment without indicating their treatment preference or individual concerns. Both parties are active and a certain degree of cooperation and collaboration exists similar to parent/physicians–child/patient mode. Model 3, or mutual participation, notes that there is some equality among the participants in the interaction. Szasz and Hollender indicate participants have some approximation of equal power, are mutually interdependent and engage in health care activities because the activity provides some satisfaction.

Nearly four decades later, Emanuel and Emanuel (1992) discuss four models of physician–patient interaction: (1) paternalistic, (2) informative, (3) interpretive and (4) deliberative. The paternalistic model, in which physicians use their skills to determine the patient's medical condition and stage in the disease process, identifies the test and treatment most likely to restore the patient's health, acknowledges the physician as a guardian figure who promotes the patient's well-being and objectively shares information. In the informative model, the physician is seen as a scientist. This second model, also called engineering or consumer model, outlines the physician's role as merely providing relevant information for the patient to select the intervention and implement the patient's selected intervention. The patient in this model has some degree of autonomy. In the third model, the interpretive model, the physician is seen as a counselor or advisor. The aim of the interaction is to clarify the patient's values and determine what the patient actually wants during the intervention. The physician provides information on the nature of conditions, risks and benefits of possible interventions. The patient values, while known, may not be fixed, thus the physician engages the patient in a joint process for understanding so the patient can come to know who he or she is and how the various medical options bear on his or her identity. The last model, the deliberative model, helps the patient choose the best health related values that can be realized in the clinical situation.

Concepts of Ethics With Client-Centered Care

Each patient-centered model has some ethical pluses and minuses, mainly focusing on concepts of patient autonomy and informed consent. Szasz and Hollender's model focus on paternalism in light of utilization ends where the health provider directs the care of the client who has little or no input into the treatment decisions. They use the prevalent medical model to provide a guidance–cooperation approach, yet do not address communication issues or difference of opinions between the physician and the client. Their stronger approach, based upon mutual participation, still indicates an imbalance in the nature of the communication and processes associated with client-centered care.

The Emanuels' informative model takes much of its position from business models that have been adopted in medicine, yet it has none of the true qualities essential for a physician–patient relationship such as caring about the values and beliefs of the patient. It further presupposes that the patient's values are known and fixed, yet people often come to medical encounters not knowing what they actually want, thus this model is seen as morally untenable. In the interpretive model, the physician may not have the skill to be attuned to what the patient wants and may unwittingly impose their own values under the guise of articulating the patient's values. Autonomy may exclude evaluative judgments. The deliberative model focuses on the physician's judgment of patient values, the nature of moral deliberation and whether patients actually see their physician as a person to engage in moral deliberations. Emanuel and Emanuel (1992) provide six points to justify their feeling that the best model is the deliberative model. The deliberative model (1) exemplifies the authors' ideal of autonomy; (2) personifies a physician that is caring and integrates the information and relevant values to make recommendations; (3) recognizes weak paternalism as the physician attempts to persuade the patient of the worthiness of certain things but does not impose; (4) recognizes that patient values are relevant and when disagreements over a course of action arise, the physician and patient discuss which values are more important and should be realized in medical care; (5) promotes health-related values and (6) stresses understanding rather than the provision of mere factual information.

Family-Centered Care

Families are social organizations which meet the normative development and situational needs of their members.

They are often the primary caregivers and advocates for their children. Through a variety of survey tools, including interviews and paper pencil instruments, the literature indicates that family-centered care (FCC) supports integration of the family into the process of promoting care (Blue-Banning, et al., 2004; Galvin et al., 2003; Macnab, 2000; Marino, 2000). FCC also has to have the necessary elements of rapport and clear communication (Espezel, 2003) including information shared with families, and facilitation of collaborative relationships (Hemmelgarn et al., 2001). Historically, the roots of family-centered care developed from the rights movement of the 1960s (Galvin, Boyers, Schwartz et al., 2000). In particular, women as care givers and medical decision-makers wanted more control over healthcare decisions. Also during that time and today, the federal laws P.L. 94–142 and Individuals with Disabilities Education Act (IDEA: P.L. 101–476) determined a focus that has changed from an emphasis that merely provided disabled children access to an education, to one that strengthens the role of parents in educational planning and decision making on behalf of their children (Galvin et al., 2000).

According to the Health Resources and Services Administration (HRSA), Maternal and Child Health Bureau (MCHB), in collaboration with the American Academy of Pediatrics (AAP), family-centered care assures the health and well-being of children and their families through a respectful family–professional partnership. It honors the strengths, cultures, traditions and expertise that everyone brings to the relationship. Family-centered care is the standard of practice, which results in high quality services.

The foundation of family-centered care is the partnership between families and professionals. Keys to these partnerships are:

1. Families and professionals work together in the best interest of the child and the family. As a child grows, he/she assumes a partnership role.
2. Everyone respects the skills and expertise brought to the relationship.
3. Trust is acknowledged as fundamental.
4. Communication and sharing are open and objective.
5. There is a willingness to negotiate.

Based on this partnership, family-centered care:

1. Acknowledges the family as the constant in a child's life.
2. Builds on family strengths.

3. Supports the child in learning about and participating in his/her care and decision making.
4. Honors cultural diversity and family traditions.
5. Recognizes the importance of community-based services.
6. Promotes an individual and developmental approach.
7. Encourages family-to-family and peer support.
8. Supports youth as they transition to adulthood.
9. Develops policies, practices, and systems that are family-friendly and family-centered in all settings.
10. Celebrates successes (Committee on Hospital Care, 2003; Ende et al., 1989).

The federal government has been investing in defining and implementing family-centered care for years. Concepts of family-centered care emerged as a moving force in the second half of the 20th century as part of the consumer movement and professional health and child development education. Additionally, Federal legislation of the late 1980s and 1990s, including Public Law 99–457, Education of the Handicapped Act Amendments 1986; Public Law 101–239 Omnibus Budget Reconciliation Act of 1989 and Public Law 101–476, Individuals with Disabilities Act and others lead the way in providing validation of the importance of family-centered care (Committee on Hospital Care, 2003).

Family-centered approaches are somewhat similar and yet markedly different from client-centered approaches. A family-centered approach engages the familial unit in the decision-making process. "The familial unit can be seen as a group of individuals with interrelated lives such that changes in one family member affect all other members" (Beisecker, 1990, p. 107). Embedded in the complex relationships of families and their obligations to persons about to make health care decisions are issues regarding social, financial, emotional and rehabilitative risks and burdens as they may affect the family unit. Family-centered care requires health care professionals to consider whether the family has enough information to make a decision, whether the family is properly motivated, and whether the treatment decisions are in accord with what the client would elect (Hyun, 2003).

Concepts of Ethics Within Family-Centered Care

Family-centered care may have some unintended consequences in that clients are especially vulnerable, in many cases have been placed in a healthcare facility,

and are not always in the position to defend their interests fairly. The client has a unique view and treatment decisions affect them in a very vivid and concrete way that does not affect the family members (Hardwig, 1990; Nelson, 1992). The imposition of family values on the uniquely personal perspective of the individual and their values and concepts of health is difficult and not always a tidy process. Issues of personal privacy and integrity filter throughout the family-centered care concept. Hardwig (1990) noted "A fundamental assumption of medical ethics: medical treatment ought to serve the interests of the client. This of course implies that the interests of family members should be irrelevant to medical treatment decisions or at least never ought to take precedence over the interest of the client" (p. 8).

Occupational Therapy Perspective on Client-Centered Care

Given the various perspectives on client-centered and family-centered care, the conundrum for occupational therapy has been to clearly define just what client-centered or family-centered care is and determine how to enfold or whether to enfold the philosophical underpinning of these concepts into clinical practice. The profession of occupational therapy between the years of 1980 and 1990 developed a series of guidelines regarding client-centered care (Figure 37.2).

Occupational therapy and particularly the Canadian occupational therapists, defined client-centered practice as a philosophy of practice that embraces autonomy, emphasizes the need for client choice in decision making, respects the individual, recognizes the need for partnership with the individual and understands the

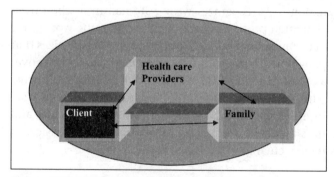

Figure 37.2. Family-centered care model.

Note. Family-centered care wherein communication is among the health provider, client and family. The family is seen as a partner in the decision-making processes.

need to ensure services are accessible and fit the context of people's lives (Law et al., 1995). Client-centered care, or family-centered care, may well be embedded philosophically in occupational therapy practice. It is embedded in the professional documents, and has recently been explicitly defined and incorporated in the American Occupational Therapy Association's *Practice Framework* which defines the profession and guides evaluation, intervention and outcomes (Johnson, Roter, Powe, & Cooper, 2004). This definition emphasizes therapists "... honoring the desires and priorities of clients" (AOTA, 2002, p. 660). The sharing of ongoing, unbiased and complete information during the course of occupational therapy sessions in an appropriate and supportive manner is essential for client buy-in. The recognition of the strengths of the individual and family and respect for different communication styles and different coping styles are essential parts of family-centered and client-centered care (Law, 1998).

Contextually, both the Szasz and Hollender and the Emanuel and Emanuel models are similar to concepts within occupational therapy's client-centered care. As noted in occupational therapy literature, The Occupational Performance Model (Canadian Association of Occupational Therapists [CAOT], 1997), Model of Human Occupations (Kielhofner, 2002), Occupational Adaptation Model (Shultz, 1992), and the Person–Environment–Occupational Performance Model (Christiansen, 1997), all indicate the client as an active participant, rendering constant collaboration between the client and therapist as essential to occupational therapy process and practice. These theoretical approaches note the importance of identifying client priorities and values to achieve successful outcomes. Additionally, the *Occupational Therapy Practice Framework* states "occupational therapists and occupational therapy assistants focus on assisting people to engage in daily life activities they find meaningful and purposeful" (Association, 2002, p. 4). The essence of client-centered care is to incorporate client-centered values into evaluation and intervention making the therapeutic process personally meaningful and purposeful.

Law (1998), reviewing the framework for client-centered care of six groups and her own writing, notes that certain concepts flow across a variety of client-centered care models. Each model indicates respect for clients, their families and the choices they make; have ultimate responsibility for decisions about daily occupations and occupational therapy services; emphasize person-centered communication; facilitates client participa-

tion in all aspects of occupational therapy services; is flexible and individualized; is enabling and focuses on the person-environment-occupation relationship.

Critique of Occupational Therapy's Concept of Client-Centered Care

Over the years that client-centered care has been part of occupational therapy, several authors have indicated how difficult this model is to attain in everyday practice (Clark, 1994; DeGrace, 2003; Falardeau, 2002; Hasselkus, 1988; Law et al., 1995; Rebeiro, 2000; Rosa & Hasselkus, 2005; Tickle-Degnen, 2002). The original model indicates a respect for clients yet it never clearly provides guidance regarding what is "respect"; hence the words are open to interpretation (Falardeau, 2002). The Canadian Guidelines for client-centered care also offered guidelines for a national model of practice that addressed areas or domains of concern and values. These guidelines note that occupational therapy should view the client as an active participant in the therapeutic process, develop a therapeutic relationship and respect the client's independence. This domain also indicates the client should have a therapist who understands internal locus of control and respects uniqueness of the individuals (McColl, 1994). However, Sumsin, in her study of 60 occupational therapists in the United Kingdom (Sumsin, 2000), indicated that there were several barriers to implementation of the guidelines for client-centered care. The most prevalent barriers to instituting client-centered care were the discordance of goals between the therapist and the client; the therapist's values and beliefs prevented them from accepting the client's goals and the therapist's lack of comfort with letting the clients choose for themselves. Another study of 19 therapists from Canada indicated that the underlying skills needed to implement the client-centered Canadian Occupational Performance Measure (COPM) were client insight, cognitive ability, emotional state and whether the client was English speaking (Toomey, 1995). The results of the Toomey study pointed out that the utility of the COPM depended upon the degree to which therapists incorporate the client-centered approach to their practice. Indeed the theoretical concept of client-centered care can be applied to all clients, yet occupational therapists seem to place artificial barriers for clients to meet. The barriers listed by occupational therapists in Toomey's study include whether an individual can speak or not speak English, and whether the client has the same beliefs or values as the therapists. These barriers automatically place the client and the therapist back at the activity–passivity model of interaction that is not in keeping with client-centered care. Given the studies by Sumsin, Toomey and others, occupational therapists have not been able to adequately integrate the philosophy of client-centered care into everyday practice. Several additional studies have suggested that client-centered practice has been associated with improved client satisfaction, increased compliance with medical programs, and better functional outcomes (Corring & Cook, 1999; Dunst, Trivette, & Deal, 1988; Eide, Quera, Graugaard, & Finset, 2004; Guadagnoli & Ward, 1998; Peloquin, 1990; Stewart, Belle Brown, Donner et al., 2000; Sumsin, 1993; Tamm, 1999), as well as increased family support.

What Is Missing? Models Revisited

The profession of occupational therapy has devoted a great deal of time defining and implementing client-centered care. Successive Canadian task forces (Townsend, 1990) issued three volumes outlining client-centered care with guidelines for implementation and outcome measures. The Task Force guidelines provided a national focus for clinical practice. The current model has come under review because three fundamental concepts—respect, power and partnership—have not been adequately defined (Falardeau, 2002) nor have they been adequately incorporated into occupational therapy services (Clark, 1994; Blain, 1993; DeGrace, 2003; Law, 1998). The failure to consistently define basic terms that are the roots of the philosophy of client-centered care unduly limits the ability of individuals to implement this philosophy. Occupational therapists believe in the philosophy of client-centeredness; however, some therapists feel an inability to actualize the philosophy because of the lack of support from their work organizations, the lack of understanding by the therapist of what client-centered really means and the inability to clearly define the nature of the power and partnerships between the participants in a client-centered practice. Therapists note that the level of the client, who the client really is, their cognition, family, language etc., limit their ability to truly implement a client-centered approach (Townsend, 1990; Wilkins, 2001; Peloquin, 1990; Law, 1998; Galvin, 2000).

A fundamental tenet espoused by both Canadians and American professional associations is to help clients achieve benefits from occupational therapy services and to recognize the importance of understanding clients in the context of his or her life experiences. As an example, the importance of occupational therapists understanding and embracing elements of family-centered care, and recognition that the family is the constant in a sick child's life while service providers may fluctuate cannot be understated.

Occupational therapists have to recognize that dialogues must take place in order for the clients and the families to gain benefit from the therapies even though there are still problems with the implementation of a specific client-centered care approach. Wilkins et al. (2001) note from three qualitative studies with three different populations (i.e., family-centered care for children and their families, community-based home care, facility-based care for older adults) that clients indicate the use of occupational therapy interventions did not meet their needs along with lack of trust of the therapists and a status differential between the client and the therapists as indicators for not having an effective client-centered approach.

Relationship-Centered Approach

To facilitate client involvement in the therapeutic process, meet their needs and increase their sense of trust, both the client and therapist should identify client strengths as well as community, environmental, and caregiver resources. With this information, the therapist and client can negotiate realistic targeted outcomes related to occupational performance (Sumsin, 1999). Another way to conceptually envision the involvement of multiple concerns for the client and therapist is a relationship-centered care approach (Figure 37.3) (Kyler, 2005). The phrase relationship-centered care captures the importance of the individual's limitations, societal participation, and function and interaction with their environment. Relationship-centered care is not a new term. The Pew Health Professions Commission, headed by Tresolini in 1994 discussed the concept, defined the term and provided guidance in creating the right environment for this philosophy to succeed. Relationship-centered care, the recognition of people as the foundation of any therapeutic or healing activity, moves away from a language of disease to language, which is neutral and covers a breadth of external influences that impact the person's ability to make healthcare decisions. Relationship-centered care is an iteration of the older Szasz approach that considers mutual participation merged with the newer Emanuel approach that considers the best healthrelated values in a particular clinical situation. Relationship-centered care

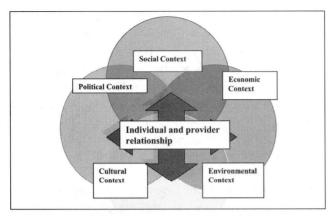

Figure 37.3. Relationship-centered care model.

Note. The relationship-centered approach includes consideration of the person, family, internal and external contextual influences in a fluid and changing manner. The bi-directional arrows between person and health care provider indicate a flow of external relationships. The central intersection of the circles represents relationship-centered care. The connecting arrows between the contextual issues represent the dynamic play of all contextual issues with one another, the person, family and the health care providers (Kyler 2005).

their sense of coherence (i.e., sense that life is comprehensible, manageable and meaningful) and ability to function in the face of changes in themselves and their relationships with their families and their environment (Law, 1998, p. 15). Clearly stated, occupational therapy needs to consider the relationship between external factors that are internalized and drive the decision-making processes.

In a relationship-centered approach, there are multiple layers of communication and external factors that impact the decision-making process. These layers are flexible and one adds or subtracts depending upon the individual and his or her needs and support system. A relationship-centered approach challenges occupational therapists to identify those factors inhibiting healing and to help clients and families strengthen and release their own healing power. Supportive family relationships are one of the factors promoting healing and the relationship between health professionals; the client and family assumes positive factors in promoting healing. Just as the relationship has the power to do well, it also has the potential for harm if, for example, the client or family feels misunderstood, demeaned or rejected (Law, 1998, p. 21). These multiple determinants are important deliberative components. Occupational therapists familiar with the *International Classification of Functioning, Disability and Health (ICF)* (Lollar & Simeonsson, 2005) (Figure 37.4) should be able to see similarities in this international model of classification which over the last several years has moved from a static model to an interactional model. Occupational therapists' interactions with clients and their families

indicates that the beliefs and values of health professionals have a fundamental impact on the health of the recipient of service (Tresolini, 1994). Determinants of health and illness lie not only within individuals, but also within social, economic, environmental, cultural and political contexts. These external contextual determinants are part of the client and/or family dynamics. These external determinants influence communication and decision-making processes. We are coming to understand health not as the absence of disease, but rather as the process by which individuals maintain

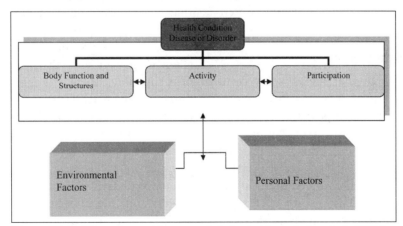

Figure 37.4. *ICF* conceptual framework (adapted from Lollar et al., 2005).

Note. The *ICF* framework is based on the ongoing influence of the environmental factors on body function is, activities and participation. This includes contextual issues such as age, education, socioeconomic status, family involvement etc. The arrows are purposefully bidirectional reflecting the fluidity of this framework.

are central to health care and for putting into action a paradigm that integrates respect, listening, caring, deliberation and decisions, hence an interactional focus that is built on the understanding of relationships that is client-centered. As noted, occupational therapists have indicated difficulty in using client-centered care because of external factors affecting those they serve. This paradigm supported by the *ICF* language encourages a focus on occupational therapists' ethical obligation to acknowledge the unique factors working within families and individuals as they go through any decision-making process. Those factors include biological, psychological, social, spiritual and economic dimensions. The perspective on health and illness is shaped by the relationships. These factors converge to indicate a more integrated approach to care (Tresolini, 1994).

Relationships are essential in the satisfaction of patient and occupational therapy practitioner. The relationship is how feelings and concerns are bought forth and how information is exchanged (Tresolini, 1994). In order to practice in a relationship-centered approach, occupational therapists must organize the information about the client and his/her family and the care provided. The occupational therapists must seek some sense of self-awareness and be open to hearing the perspective of the client, seek to preserve his/her dignity; listen and communicate openly. Relationship-centered care is based upon active collaboration with the patient and family in decision making and treatment. Relationship-centered care is about recognizing the person and the contributors to health; the client's perspective or realty, his/her illness and the lifelong process of growth and development within the biological, psychological, behavioral, social, economic spiritual and environmental contexts.

Lessons Learned From Others

Possible lessons for occupational therapy may come from studies of physicians' and nurses' interactions with clients and concepts of empowerment. Adopting a client-centered approach often requires the professionals to apply a shift in attitudes as they try to deliver good quality services. Many health professionals and other staff members assumed that they, as healthcare experts, know what is best for clients. An orientation to the client-centered, family-centered or relationship-centered approaches recognizes that clients' concerns and preferences are valid and important. The client comes to the decision-making process recognizing his or her preferences, values, goals and

expected outcomes. This approach also recognizes a contemporary vision of inclusion and dialogue among all parties that is a give and take and accepts the decision-making process as one where individuals make decisions based upon a dialogue and input by both the health providers and clients and families. While many have written about client-centered and family-centered care, the challenges of implementing client- and family-centered services are still prevalent for occupational therapy.

Some studies indicate lack of good communication skills between the provider and the client (Eide et al., 2004; Glass, 1996; Guadagnoli & Ward, 1998; Hasselkus, 1988). Lack of communication skills may not bode well for improved client satisfaction or for a client-centered, family-centered or relationship-centered approach. In client- [patient] centered literature, physicians are advised to ask questions to elicit from their clients those things that most concern them (Beisecker, 1990; Beisecker & Beisecker, 1993; Bell et al., 2002; Biley, 1992). In particular, in cancer the prospect of dealing with the client's fear may be anxiety provoking; however, in a study by Eide et al. (2004), no concerns were uttered by the clients after a direct inquiry from the physician. Sequence analysis associated with client's exhibiting cues showed that different behaviors by the clients and physicians were statistically significant. Clients seldom verbalize their concerns and emotions directly and spontaneously, but often exhibit indirect cues that something is problematic. Physicians and nurses who embrace client-centered and family-centered care recognize an informational asymmetry. A core skill for physicians that is translatable to occupational therapy is recognizing clients' emotions that are clinically relevant but not directly expressed. This skill of recognition of emotions is directly translatable to occupational therapy practice as are concepts of client empowerment. Also revisiting literature outside of occupational therapy, Emanuel and Emanuel (1992) discuss in their deliberative model concepts of enablement that are appropriate for occupational therapists to use in their clinical practice. As indicated, their model has six components including autonomy, lack of strong paternalism, integration of information and relevant values, resolution of disputes, promotion of health behaviors and true understanding of health information (p. 2226). The informed decision-making model views information sharing from physician to patient, but does not address the true processes of shared decision making. Information is enabling and empowering to clients and their families. The physician is outside the true decision-making process as their role is to just provide information. The shared decision-making approach proposes strong involvement of the participants, whether that is a single individual or an individual with their family. Shared decision making may change as family members and others enter into the process with the client and physician. This leads to different decision-making processes that the physician has to be flexible in addressing. Indeed in some cases clients wish to play a passive role if they are not motivated or they have learned that active engagement in the process is not welcomed by the physicians. The steps the parties take in working through an acceptable shared decision-making process includes: establishing a conducive atmosphere; eliciting the client's preference, values and lifestyle; transferring technical information including risks and benefits to the client; helping the client conceptualize the options and, physicians sharing treatment recommendations with clients or affirming the client's decision. This leads to recognition of the client's relationship to those external factors that influence their decision-making processes. Once again, models from medicine are congruent with occupational therapy values and beliefs as they echo client-centered family-centered and relationship-centered care at its best. Validation of participation, active listening, engagement, respect and trust are the benchmarks upon which the healthcare provider, whether occupational therapist or another discipline may provide the recipient of service with the best care.

Conclusion

Information on client-centered and family-centered care is ubiquitous and is embraced by many health care practitioners, including psychologists, primary care and pediatric practitioners, nurses, and occupational therapists. All incorporate some of the attributes of client-centered care, yet feel the ambiguity of language and pressed by time and financial constraints hinder fully implementing the philosophical concepts of client-centered care and family-centered care into clinical practice. Professional organizations and the United States government have, through policy papers and legislation, encouraged a client-centered or family-centered focus.

The occupational therapy literature provides a rich view of client-centered care, yet appears to not adequately define key terms important to the provision of client-centered care. Occupational therapy should address the clarity of language concerns and refocus on the external influences or relationships that impact the client's abil-

ity to successfully participate in life activities including healthcare decision making. One way posited to address the ambiguity of what client-centered or family-centered care really is, is to conceptually envision the multiple concerns of clients into a fluid relationship-centered approach with clearly defined terms. Building upon the work of the Canadian Occupational Therapy Task Force, utilization of the *ICF* language, the AAP family-centered standards of practice and statement of principles along with the visual schematic of the relationship-centered approach should move occupational therapy forward with a concise and cogent approach to relationship-centered care that is more in keeping with the current state of what many health professions indicate are acceptable standards of practice. As a vital and client-centered profession occupational therapy revisiting the topic may bring forth a cogent and workable approach that incorporates the best qualities of client-centered, family-centered and relationship-centered care. Using the salient qualities these three philosophical concepts offer may bring about a clinical focus that truly values information and concerns in context. Understanding and respecting what the client and family brings to making treatment decisions is critical and helps in the development of a dynamic occupational therapy treatment plan that will work for all involved.

References

American Academy of Pediatrics Committee on Hospital Care (2003). Family-centered care and the Pediatrician's role. *Pediatrics, 112*(3), 691–696.

American Occupational Therapy Association. (2002). Occupational therapy practice framework: Domain and process. *American Journal of Occupational Therapy, 56*, 609–639. http://dx.doi.org/10.5014/ajot.56.6.609

Beisecker, A. E. (1990). Patient power in doctor–patient communication: What do we know? *Health Communication, 2*(2), 105–122.

Beisecker, A. E., & Beisecker, T. D. (1993). Using metaphors to characterize doctor-patient relationships: Paternalism versus consumerism. *Health Communication, 5*(1), 41–58.

Bell, R. A., Kravitz, R. L., Thom, T., Krupat, E., & Azari, R. (2002). Unmet expectations for care and the patient-physician relationship. *Journal of General Internal Medicine, 17*, 817–824.

Biley, F. C. (1992). Some determinants that effect patient participation in decision-making about nursing care. *Journal of Advanced Nursing, 17*(4), 414–421.

Charles, C., Gafni, A., & Whelan, T. (1999). Decision-making in the physician–patient encounter: Revising the shared treatment decision-making model. *Social Science and Medicine, 49,* 651–661.

Committee on Hospital Care. (2003). Family centered care and the pediatrician's role. *Pediatrics, 112*(3), 691–696.

Corring, D. J., & Cook, J. V. (1999). Client-centred care means that I am a valued human being. *Canadian Journal of Occupational Therapy, 66*(2), 71–82.

Dunst, C. J., Trivette, C. M., & Deal, A. G. (1988). *Enabling and empowering families.* Cambridge, MA: Brookline Books, Inc.

Eide, H., Quera, V., Graugaard, P., & Finset, A. (2004). Physician-patient dialogue surrounding patients' expression of concern: Applying sequence analysis to RAIS. *Social Science and Medicine, 59,* 145–155.

Emanuel, E. J., & Emanuel, L. L. (1992). Four models of physician-patient relationship. *Journal of the American Medical Association, 267*(16), 221–227.

Ende, J., Kazis, L., Ash, A., & Moskowitz, M. A. (1989). Measuring patients' desire for autonomy: Decision making and information-seeking preferences among medical patients. *Journal of General Internal Medicine, 4*(1), 23–29.

Fearing, V. G., Clark, J., & Stanton, S. (1998). The client centred occupational therapy process. In M. Law (Ed.), *Client-centred occupational therapy* (pp. 67–87). Thorofare: Slack.

Galvin, E., Boyers, L., Schwartz, P. K., Jones, M. W., Mooney, P., Warwick, J., et al. (2000). Challenging the precepts of family-centered care: Testing a philosophy. *Pediatric Nursing, 26*(6), 625–633.

Glass, R. M. (1996). The patient–physician relationship. *Journal of the American Medical Association, 275*(2), 147–148.

Guadagnoli, E., & Ward, P. (1998). Patient participation in decision making. *Social Science Medical, 47*(3), 329–339.

Hardwig, J. (1990). What about the family? *Hastings Center Reports, 20*(2), 5–10.

Hasselkus, B. R. (1988). Meaning in family caregiving: Perspectives on caregiver/professional relationships. *The Gerontologist, 28*(5), 686–691.

Johnson, R., Roter, D., Powe, N., & Cooper, L. (2004). Patient race/ethnicity and quality of patient–physician communication during medical visits. *American Journal of Public Health, 94*(12), 2084–2091.

Kyler, P. (2005). The ethics of client-centered care models. In Purtilo, Royeen & Jensen. (Eds.), *Educating for moral action: A sourcebook in health and rehabilitation ethics* (pp. 159–168). Philadelphia: F. A. Davis.

Law, M. (1998). Does client-centred practice make a difference? In M. Law (Ed.), *Client-centred occupational therapy* (pp. 19–27). Thorofare: Slack.

Law, M., Baptiste, S., & Mills, J. (1995). Client-centred practice: What does it mean and does it make a difference? *Canadian Journal of Occupational Therapy, 62,* 250–257.

Law, M., & Mills, J. (1998). Client-centred occupational therapy. In M. Law (Ed.), *Client-centred occupational therapy* (chapter 1, pp. 1–18). Thorofare: Slack.

Lawlor, M. C., & Mattingly, C. F. (1998). The complexities embedded in family-centered care. *American Journal of Occupational Therapy, 52*(4), 259–267. http://dx.doi.org/10.5014/ajot./52.4.259

Lollar, D. J., & Simeonsson, R. J. (2005). Diagnosis to function: Classification for children and youth. *Developmental and Behavioral Pediatrics, 26*(4), 323–330.

Mew, M. M., & Fossey, E. (1996). Client-centred aspects of clinical reasoning during an initial assessment using the Canadian occupational performance measure. *Australian Occupational Therapy Journal, 43*(3/4), 155–166.

Nelson, J. L. (1992). Taking families seriously. *Hastings Center Reports, 22*(4), 6–12.

Peloquin, S. M. (1990). The patient–therapist relationship in occupational therapy: Understanding visions and images. *American Journal of Occupational Therapy, 44*(1), 13–21. http://dx.doi.org/10.5014/ajot.44.1.13

Stewart, M., Belle Brown, J., Donner, A., McWhinney, I. R., Oates, J., Weston, W. W., et al. (2000). The impact of patient-centered care on outcomes. *Journal of Family Practice, 49*(9), 796–804.

Sumsin, T. (1993). Reflections on. . . : Reflexions sur. . . : Client-centered practice: The true impact. *Canadian Journal of Occupational Therapy, 60*(1), 6–8.

Sumsin, T. (1999). A study to determine a British occupational therapy definition of client-centered practice. *British Journal of Occupational Therapy, 62*(2), 52–58.

Szasz, T. S., & Hollender, M. C. (1956). A contribution to the philosophy of medicine: The basic models of the doctor-patient relationship. *Archives on Internal Medicine, 97,* 585–592.

Tamm, M. (1999). Relatives as a help or hindrance- a grounded theory study seen from the perspective of the occupational therapist. *Scandinavian Journal of Occupational Therapy, 6,* 36–45.

Task Force on Guidelines for the Practice of Occupational Therapy. (1983). *Guidelines for the client-centred practice of occupational therapy; intervention guidelines for the client-centred practice of occupational therapy; toward out-*

come measures in occupational therapy: Ottawa Minister of National Health and Welfare 1983–87.

Tresolini, C. P., & Pew–Fetzer Task Force. (1994). *Health professions education and relationship-centered care.* San Francisco, CA: Pew Health Professions Commission.

Wilkins, S., Pollock, N., Rochhon, S., & Law, M. (2001). Implementing client-centred practice: Why is it so difficult to do? *Canadian Journal of Occupational Therapy, 68*(2), 70–79.

CHAPTER 38

Understanding the Family Perspective: An Ethnographic Framework for Providing Occupational Therapy in the Home

LAURA N. GITLIN, MARY CORCORAN, AND SUSAN LEINMILLER-ECKHARDT

It has been firmly established that families provide the majority of long-term care in the home to elderly persons with cognitive and physical impairments (Pepper Commission, 1990; Stone, Cafferata, & Sangi, 1987). To support family caregivers in these efforts, there has been an increased interest in developing and testing the effectiveness of a wide range of interventions (Knight, Lutzky, & Macofsky-Urban, 1993) and in identifying the particular contributions of occupational therapy (Clark, Corcoran, & Gitlin, in press; Corcoran & Gitlin, 1992; Hasselkus, 1989). However, the growing body of literature on caregiver interventions has suggested that family members tend to underuse formal health and human services (Knight et al., 1993), may indicate little need for assistance (Collins, 1992; Smyth & Harris, 1993), and sometimes express conflict with the goals that are established by health and human service professionals (Chiou & Burnett, 1985; Hasselkus, 1991; Kaufman, 1988). Furthermore, research on caregiver interventions such as home environmental modifications (Gitlin & Corcoran, 1993; Pynoos & Ohta, 1991), respite, psychoeducational counseling, and support groups has indicated that caregivers are selective in their use of prescribed strategies and do not uniformly benefit or demonstrate reduced stress from participation in these services (Knight et al., 1993).

Recent research in caregiving that has used naturalistic inquiry has demonstrated that caregiving in the home is a complex process that is imbued with meaning and purpose. The meaning of caregiving, or how a person makes sense of his or her experiences, influences how daily care is provided in the home and how caregivers define their needs (Albert, 1992; Gubrium & Sankar, 1990; Hasselkus, 1988, 1989). Other research has noted that caregivers vary in the way they adapt to their experiences and that they identify a range of factors as stressful and cope differently depending upon the particular stressor (Corcoran, 1992; Henderson & Gutierrez-Mayka, 1992; Williamson & Schulz, 1993). These findings underscore the highly individual and unique nature of each caregiving situation. The findings also suggest the existence of a "neglect of perspective" or the disregard by health-care professionals of the client's perspective on his or her own needs in developing services (Fine, 1993, p. 2).

Despite the evidence that caregivers define, approach, and react to their caregiving role in distinct ways, occupational therapists lack a framework for developing occupational therapy services that are based on the unique needs of the family members we seek to support. A framework from which to evaluate the specific and individualized needs of families and their elderly members with disabilities is increasingly important as we move toward a health care system that is community and home based.

Recently, there has been an increased interest in ethnography as an approach to research in gerontology (Gubrium & Sankar, 1994) and health services (DePoy & Gitlin, 1994), and as a basis for deriving clinical intervention strategies that overcome the potential conflict in perspectives between service provider and client (Hasselkus, 1990; Hill, Fortenberry, & Stein, 1990; Kleinman, 1988; Spencer, Krefting, & Mattingly, 1993). Ethnography is an approach to understanding culture or patterns of behavior and the meaning and interpretation by its participants. The purpose of ethnography is to understand another way of life as it is viewed and given meaning by participants. The ethnographer is interested in the values, meanings, and viewpoints of

This chapter was previously published in the *American Journal of Occupational Therapy, 49,* 802–809. Copyright © 1995, American Occupational Therapy Association. Reprinted with permission. http://dx.doi.org/10.5014/ajot.49.8.802

persons and how persons make sense of or perceive their own context.

It has been suggested that occupational therapists function in a fashion similar to ethnographers in that they strive to elicit the client's perspective and use this information to develop treatment protocols to fit the client's value and meaning structure. In her 1990 Eleanor Clarke Slagle lecture, Fine stated, "Occupational therapists are ethnographers of sorts. We have unique access to information about activities of everyday living and what it is like to live with an illness or disability. We need only to acknowledge and actualize it" (1991, pp. 500–501; see Chapter 32). A few occupational therapists have begun to identify how to actualize an ethnographic perspective. Hasselkus (1990) described the value of using ethnographic interviewing techniques as a tool in occupational therapy practice with family caregivers. Spencer et al. (1993) also suggested that constructs derived from ethnography are relevant and useful to occupational therapy and offer an important approach to practice.

Building on these works, we have developed a framework for evaluating the needs of family caregivers that uses concepts from ethnographs. This framework is intended to advance the efforts of occupational therapists to evaluate the caregiver's *inner life* as a basis from which to make treatment decisions and derive an individualized service approach in the home (Fine, 1993). It incorporates four key terms from ethnography (informant, emic, reflexivity, and interpretation) and the principles they reflect. The strategy is to use these principles and the actions they represent to derive an understanding of the perspective of the family member, the personal meaning of providing care, how care is provided in the home, and specific aspects that are perceived to be problematic. Specific occupational therapy strategies are then constructed that fit the fundamental values and belief system of the family unit or social–cultural context of the home.

This ethnographic framework has evolved through a number of funded research and training programs awarded to the first two authors. These programs have developed and evaluated the use of this framework under a number of conditions. Systematic case analyses involving family members caring for persons with disability suggest that occupational therapy intervention strategies are integrated into family routines and effectively used when occupational therapists use these principles to guide treatment. The outcomes of this research (Corcoran & Gitlin, 1992; Gitlin & Corcoran,

1993) as well as a description of a training approach based on some of these principles (Gitlin & Corcoran, 1991) have been reported elsewhere.

We examine the four key principles constituting the framework, their ethnographic foundations, and their clinical applications. A case example illustrates the framework in action in a home situation with family members caring for a person with dementia.

Four Key Principles of Ethnography

The four key principles of this framework, which are outlined in Table 38.1, are designed to enable an occupational therapist to modify traditional practice and evolve treatment strategies that target the values and meaning of the caregiver or family unit. These principles are not to be thought of as linear, step-by-step procedures for evaluation. Rather, they form a framework, or way of thinking about the caregiving situation, and can be used in combination with formal evaluations that are traditionally conducted in the home.

Principle One: Identify an Informant in the Home

As shown in Table 38.1, the first term in ethnography that is relevant to service delivery is that of identifying an informant or informants. In ethnographic methodology, an informant is a person with knowledge of the cultural system who informs the ethnographer of the values, beliefs, and activities of the group that is being studied. This person is a key source from whom the ethnographer learns about daily practices and behaviors and gains insight into the meaning of an activity or routine.

Table 38.1. Ethnographic Principles, Definitions, and Clinical Applications

Ethnographic Principle	Definition	Clinical Application
Informant	Individual with knowledge	Lay practitioner
Emic	Insider perspective	Uncovering personal meaning
Reflexivity	Self-reflection	Treatment planning
		Hypothesis development
		Hypothesis testing
		Self-questioning
Interpretation	Deriving an analytic framework	Treatment implementation: Putting it together

The clinical application of the term *informant* involves the principle of viewing the family member or primary caregiver as a lay practitioner. Hasselkus (1988) has used the term *lay practitioner* to refer to caregivers because of their primary role in managing, coordinating, and providing hands-on care to older adults with impairment. Through the act *of doing* and trial and error, family members develop a practice style, gain knowledge, and develop expertise or wisdom in providing care. Smith and Baltes have defined wisdom as "expert knowledge" about "fundamental life matters" (1990, p. 495). Applied to the case of caregiving, wisdom or expert knowledge of the pragmatics of providing daily care evolves over time as lay practitioners develop knowledge of how to perform caregiving tasks. This knowledge is situation specific and reflects a professional's *know how* as opposed to his or her formal or theory-based knowledge (Albert, 1992; Benner, 1984).

As an informant, the lay practitioner is an important source of information about caregiving routines and priorities of both the caregiver and the family member who is impaired. By viewing family members as practitioners, an occupational therapist recognizes their pivotal role and responsibility in the caregiving situation and their ultimate control over what therapeutic strategies evolve and are adapted. This principle encourages the occupational therapist to view his or her own role as that of an *enabler* as opposed to a prescriber.

Principle Two: Use an Emic Approach

The second principle is the use of an *emic* approach, that is, obtaining an insider perspective or the point of view of an informant as to how things are and why. In an ethnographic framework for service delivery, the occupational therapist interviews and observes the lay practitioner(s) to identify their perspective of the meaning that shapes their act of caregiving. This step is done in an effort to gain the family members' perspective and identify the unique meaning they have assigned to caregiving. Although a wide range of questions may be useful to gain an insider perspective, those included in Section I of the Appendix are straightforward and simple. They enable a caregiver to begin to tell the story of his or her caregiving experience. Other techniques to learn the inside view include observation of the physical environment, observation of a caregiving task, and active listening to how the lay practitioner constructs his or her story of the caregiving situation. Observation of the home environment in traditional occupational therapy evaluation typically focuses on accessibility

and safety. In an ethnographic approach, observation is expanded to include how caregivers set up objects for daily routines, the presence of photographs and other objects of meaning, and the extent to which caregivers have rearranged the home to accommodate the level of competence of the family member who is impaired.

Principle Three: Engage in Self-Reflection

The third principle is a dynamic activity in which the ethnographer engages in self-questioning in an attempt to understand the relationship of his or her own values and beliefs to those that exist in the cultural setting of the home. Through this constant comparison between the investigator's expectations and the way things are, insights are gained. Likewise, in working with a lay practitioner to identify and understand meaning, the occupational therapist remains reflexive or self-questioning and continually asks himself or herself four questions: (a) What do I see happening in this home? (b) Do I understand the perspective of the family members? (c) Is my vision of the family members' needs the same as those of the lay practitioner(s)? (d) In what ways are my values in this caregiving situation the same or different from those of the lay practitioner(s)?

Keeping notes as to one's own personal reactions to the caregiving situation, as well as one's discoveries, facilitates the reflexive discovery process. Through the act of self-reflection, the occupational therapist advances his or her own understanding of the family members' perspective and begins to formulate initial hunches or hypotheses about the meanings that underscore the actions of these lay practitioners. These initial hypotheses form the basis from which treatment planning emerges. As treatment progresses, the therapist continually tests these initial hypotheses by comparing observations of the family members' actions during treatment to his or her interpretive framework, discussed in Principle Four.

Principle Four: Develop a Framework for Interpreting Information

The fourth principle is based on the interpretive method used in ethnography. The interpretive process involves deriving an analytic framework from which to understand and explain behaviors and phenomena. Through interpretation, the ethnographer attempts to make sense of what is observed and uncover the underlying meanings and beliefs that guide behavior.

Likewise, the occupational therapist, on the basis of interview, observation, active listening, and reflexivity, derives an interpretation or analysis of the emic perspective, or how things work and what is important for the lay practitioner. Interpretation is a fluid, dynamic process by which the therapist continually refines his or her understanding of the family members' perspective on the basis of incoming information. The interpretative process is comparable to the clinical reasoning process by which a service provider attempts to fit the pieces together in the form of an effective treatment plan and its implementation (Fleming, 1991). In an ethnographic framework, the clinical reasoning involves skill in interpreting the meanings that underscore the family system and skill in adapting treatment strategies to fit the particular system meaning of the family unit. To refine an interpretive framework, the occupational therapist constantly observes the family members' behavior and returns to three fundamental questions: (a) What does the disability or impairment mean to the care receiver and the family member? (b) How do the family member and care receiver experience the caregiving activity? (c) On the basis of the underlying meaning that informs care, what is an appropriate treatment strategy to support the efforts of the family unit?

Refinement of the interpretive framework begins with the initiation of a home visit and does not end until the termination of treatment. As strategies are introduced, the occupational therapist evaluates how they are received and the extent to which they are incorporated into daily caregiving routines. Those strategies that are rejected by family members provide important information to the occupational therapist as to the beliefs and practices of the lay practitioner(s). Strategies that most closely match the beliefs and self-defined needs of family caregivers are those that will be embraced by family members and used effectively.

As displayed in Figure 38.1, this ethnographic framework for service delivery leads to the development of an individualized treatment approach. It uses a dynamic, iterative process, as in ethnography, in which treatments evolve and are continually refined in light of the observations and interpretations that are derived.

Case Example

A case example illustrates the four principles described previously as used in a five-visit occupational therapy intervention protocol with family members caring for an elderly person with dementia in the home. A detailed description of the intervention protocol has been published elsewhere (Corcoran & Gitlin, 1992; Gitlin & Corcoran, 1993).

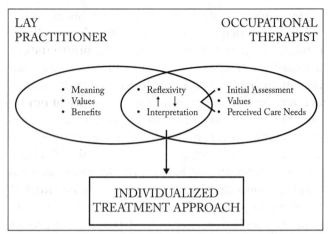

Figure 38.1. Ethnographic framework for service delivery.

In this case, there were two informants, or lay practitioners. Mrs. P, a frail, 90-year-old spouse, and her 85-year-old sister resided together in a two-story, twin home and cared for Mrs. P's 89-year-old husband. Mr. P suffered from moderate-to-severe dementia, aphasia, and physical decline including weight loss, rigidity, and movement problems. Mr. P needed constant supervision and assistance in bathing, eating, dressing, using the toilet, grooming, and ascending and descending stairs. Mrs. P and her sister reported that Mr. P was often "uncooperative," especially when descending stairs and during meals. Mrs. P and her sister appeared fatigued, stressed, and unsure how to accomplish the daily routines that they had established for Mr. P.

In an initial home visit, the occupational therapist was struck by the enormous difficulty imposed on the two elderly women in providing personal care to a resistive man twice their size and their use of caregiving techniques and routines that impeded the family members' functions and placed them at risk of injury.

The initial evaluation of the daily challenges faced by Mrs. P and her sister indicated four major areas of concern to the occupational therapist. These concerns included: (a) the risk of falling and injury to Mrs. P, her sister, and her husband, (b) the extremely poor nutritional state of Mr. P, (c) Mrs. P and her sister's struggle to maintain good hygiene for Mr. P, and (d) the overall level of stress and physical frailty of all three family members.

On the basis of these immediate concerns and an incomplete understanding of the meaning underlying the actions of the family members, the therapist initially offered recommendations to enhance safety and decrease caregiver stress. These initial recommendations included: (a) the use of formal home care services to assist in activities of daily living, (b) the implementation of major home adaptations such as installing a stair glide or moving Mr. P's bed downstairs to the dining room for safety, (c) medical intervention for Mr. P's poor nutritional status, (d) day care participation for Mr. P, and (e) preparation for the possibility of nursing home placement for Mr. P. These recommendations, which represent standard practice, were considered by the occupational therapist as critical for the well-being of both the care receiver and the caregivers. Each suggestion, however, was rejected by the lay practitioners (the caregivers).

Strategies to Understand the Caregivers' Perspective

The occupational therapist began to realize that Mrs. P and her sister rejected these suggestions because they presented a dramatic change to the daily routines and image of the household that they had constructed. In addition, these recommended interventions reflected only the formal provider perspective that focused on the medical and dysfunctional aspects of the situation. The occupational therapist recognized that she had an imprecise understanding of what was meaningful in this household and began to use several techniques to discover the beliefs and values that informed decision-making by the lay practitioners. She observed how objects were used in the home and the way caregiving tasks were performed, and she more closely listened to the language used by the lay practitioners to describe their daily routines. For example, the therapist noted that care objects in the home, such as a walker and commode, were kept out of sight until they were required. There were no signs or visual cues to encourage Mr. P's participation in basic self-care tasks, and the environment was not simplified to enhance his competence. As a consequence of the process of observing objects and behaviors, testing emerging hypotheses as to what was occurring in the home, and self-reflection over several home visits, the occupational therapist gained a better understanding of the emic perspective and a feasible, interpretive framework from which to develop specific, relevant solutions to fit this particular case.

Emic Perspective

The essential meaning of the caregiving activities for these two frail women was to maintain a sense of normalcy, or consistency, with the way things were before the onset of Mr. P's dementia. Their primary concern

in providing care was to preserve or maintain a sense of continuity in Mr. P's role in the home. From the perspective of Mrs. P and her sister, normalcy meant getting Mr. P through his daily routines of self-care, stair use, and eating as they had always done with minimal changes so as to preserve an image of what Mr. P used to do and how he used to be. The importance of maintaining normalcy and Mr. P's previous biographical roles were reflected in their stoic determination to enforce the basic routines that had always been followed in their adult lives, the language they used to describe their difficulties in the caregiving situation, and the types of caregiving concerns that they identified. For example, they preferred to label Mr. P's behavior as "uncooperative" in daily routines and rejected medical terms that suggested that Mr. P was *unable* to behave competently because of the underlying pathology. They were concerned about his poor eating habits primarily because these habits upset their meal routines. They also identified Mr. P's uncooperative behavior and stiffness when descending the stairs as a concern because it interfered with their expectation that he sit in the living room at a specific point in time during the day, as he used to do.

Mrs. P had rejected the occupational therapist's initial recommendations based on her wish to preserve her image and understanding of who Mr. P was and what he had liked to do. As she pointed out, Mr. P was never one to participate in groups and therefore he would not like a day care situation or nursing home. Whereas the occupational therapist had been concerned with the physical well-being of the caregivers and the medical status of the care receiver, the lay practitioners chose to preserve and be concerned with the biographical status of Mr. P. and to value the preservation of this status.

Interpretation

Through observation of daily tasks, open-ended interviewing, and reflexive self-questioning that occurred over all five home visits, the occupational therapist was able to derive an emic understanding and an interpretative framework of *normalization* for this particular family (Robinson, 1993). Individualized treatment strategies emerged from an iterative process that was based on continual evaluation of things observed and said, self-reflection of the therapist's own values and concerns, and refinement of the therapist's interpretive framework.

The therapist validated and tested her emerging interpretations of the caregivers' need to preserve Mr.

P's roles and a sense of normalcy by asking the caregivers validating questions, such as "Is this how you see it?" This technique invited the lay practitioners to comment on the accuracy of the therapist's hypotheses and understandings of what was meaningful and important to them. The therapist began to use the language of the lay practitioners to discuss what was happening in the caregiving situation and affirm their perspective. This communication required avoiding the use of medical or professional terminology and reframing problems with the vocabulary of the caregivers. An example was the use of the term "uncooperative" when describing Mr. P's actual inability to participate in life tasks.

On the basis of the meaning of caregiving in this home, the occupational therapist was able to offer a number of solutions to caregiving problems that were acceptable to the lay practitioners. The challenge to the occupational therapist was to uphold the biographical image of Mr. P while easing the lay practitioners' stresses and safety risks in performing caregiving tasks. In order to effectively communicate about caregiving strategies and routines, it was important for the therapist to link suggestions to the lay practitioners' goal of making Mr. P more "cooperative." Suggestions that fit this framework involved what may appear to be small changes in technique or routine (e.g., allowing Mr. P to initiate descending the stairs with the lay practitioners walking on either side, involving other family members to provide respite for the caregivers), minor home modifications for safety, and incorporation of techniques that enhanced Mr. P's role performance (e.g., use of visual cues, finger foods, and simplified instructions during eating). These modifications were accepted by the lay practitioners and easily incorporated in the routines that they had established long ago and sought to maintain. These solutions were acceptable because the occupational therapist framed them in terms of how well they maintained Mr. P's role as a family member and status as an independent person. In addition, these solutions did not change valued routines but modified lay practice to enhance safety and minimize the chance of injury.

In addition, on the final visit, the occupational therapist shared information about dementia and its progression with the lay practitioners and put together a packet of materials about other services that they could refer to in the future. This packet included information about day care, respite services, and nursing home placement. Although these services had not been acceptable to the lay practitioners, the information packet was welcomed. This approach to education enabled Mrs. P and her sister to control the information flow and the decision as to if and when additional assistance would be required.

Implications for Occupational Therapy

From an ethnographic point of view, informal caregiving represents a cultural activity in that it has meaning to its participants and reflects the caregiver's values and beliefs about the person and his or her disability. In an ethnographic framework for service delivery, a health-care professional suspends his or her own values and beliefs as to the appropriate course of treatment in an effort to discover what actually goes on in a family that is providing care and the value and meaning that underlie these activities. The four principles provide a framework to guide the clinical reasoning that needs to occur in working with lay practitioners. Mattingly and Fleming (1994) have asserted that a primary and challenging feature of clinical reasoning in occupational therapy is distinguishing the nature of *the good* for each particular client. The good refers to an image of what is beneficial and healthy for each client and is directed partially by the meanings assigned to the disability by the client. Occupational therapists are acutely aware of the need for knowledge about their clients' meaning structures (Fleming & Mattingly, 1994) and the difficulties associated with evaluating these perspectives accurately (Fine, 1993; Spencer, 1993). The ethnographic framework for evaluating the family members' perspective presented in this article can serve as a helpful structure for integrating the client's psychosocial, physical, and emotional dimensions in treatment planning. It can be used in combination with traditional formal assessment instruments of cognition, function, or health status, and can enable occupational therapists to gain insight into distinct caregiving practices and how these practices are embedded in the social and cultural context of the family unit.

An important implication of this framework for occupational therapy practice lies in its usefulness for identifying and addressing client-therapist ethical conflicts. Differences in priorities about the focus of treatment has been identified as a major form of ethical dispute between client and therapist (Corcoran, 1993; Gitlin, 1993; Hasselkus, 1991). For instance, Hasselkus (1991) noted that the principle of *autonomy* (listed first in the *Occupational Therapy Code of Ethics* [American Occupational Therapy Association, 1991]) may conflict with a client's cultural belief that one's elder is entitled to be dependent.

The case of Mrs. P illustrates our discomfort with these ethical dilemmas. For example, Mrs. P and her sister chose to uphold their biographical image of Mr. P as an independent, functioning husband who participated in daily routines, and they rejected the use of medical terms to describe the caregiving process. That is, they chose to continue practices such as his stair climbing at the risk of great personal injury. In this case, the occupational therapist needed to respect the lay practitioners' need to uphold these biographical notions even though the frailty of the caregiving situation remained disconcerting for her. Use of an ethnographic framework will not only help the therapist identify and validate the client's beliefs about disability, but also to continually explore the nuances of his or her own belief structure through the process of reflexivity.

An ethnographic framework for interviewing and service delivery is unlike a medical model approach and will therefore feel different to an occupational therapist in several ways (Levine & Gitlin, 1990). First, the family member as a lay practitioner is viewed as a partner in determining the most appropriate way of approaching the caregiving situation. This approach has the effect of empowering and reassuring family members while helping service providers to relinquish control. Second, intervention strategies are not dictated but evolve from interactions that reflect a blend of formal and practical knowledge. Third, decisional control to adapt new caregiving strategies or coping styles resides with the lay practitioner, whereas the service provider needs to remain flexible. Fourth, service providers must develop a different measure of success that includes the family members' acceptance and modification of suggestions to fit their situation.

Conclusion

The framework presented here is in direct contrast to the medical model approach in which standard treatment protocols emerge according to the condition, its pathology, considerations of dysfunction, and the assumption of the caregiving situation as a universal stressor. The intent of the framework presented here is to enable the occupational therapist to think beyond what *ought* to be done in a home-care situation to understand and respect what family members themselves emphasize as valued practice. It provides a systematic

way of thinking about occupational therapy practice with caregivers and shaping the clinical reasoning process in home-based occupational therapy.

The framework also has potential application to other practice areas in the profession of occupational therapy. For instance, therapists specializing in pediatrics may find that an ethnographic framework augments their efforts to collaborate with parents of children with disabilities. Likewise, occupational therapists practicing in the fast-paced arena of acute care may gain a useful way to establish the priorities of treatment and determine relevant discharge plans for their short-stay clients. Although this framework focuses on the caregiver, a similar process can be used to understand the perspective of the care receiver and how it may differ from that of the caregiver. In addition, the elements of this framework are appropriate for home-care situations in which the person who is impaired is the primary receiver of service.

As our health-care system undergoes dramatic revisions, the focus will be increasingly aimed at delivery of quality care in the community. Understanding individual perspectives and the unique meanings of the caregiving experience is critical to the development of services that are effective in assisting the family members in their ongoing caregiving efforts. Our experiences suggest that caregivers are receptive to the knowledge and skill of formal providers when this knowledge and skill is transmitted in a manner that is consistent with the beliefs and values of the family unit.

Appendix 38.A.
Examples of Useful Questions

I. To obtain meaning, ask lay practitioner:
   What is a typical day like for you?
   What most worries or concerns you?
   How is it now versus before?
   Tell me how you manage your day.
   What are your feelings about the future?
   What are some of your successes?
II. To verify meaning, ask lay practitioner:
   Is this how you see it?
   So you are saying that when _____ happens, you get frustrated.
   It sounds as though that really upset you.
III. To think reflexively, ask yourself:
   What do I see happening in this home?
   Do I understand the perspective of the family members?

Is my view the same as that of the lay practitioner(s)?

In what ways are my values in this care situation the same or different from those of the lay practitioner(s)?

IV. To derive an interpretive framework, ask yourself:

What does the disability or impairment mean to this person and the family member?

How does the family member experience the caregiving activity?

On the basis of an understanding of meaning, what is an appropriate treatment strategy to support the efforts of this family unit?

Acknowledgments

The framework presented in this article was developed on the basis of research supported by the National Institute on Aging (Grant No. AG10947). The first author's participation was also supported by a research grant awarded by the National Institute on Disability and Rehabilitation Research (Grant No. H133G00160). An earlier version of this article was presented at the Mental Health and Aging Symposium, Wills/Jefferson Hospital, Geropsychiatry, Philadelphia, Pennsylvania, October 29, 1993.

References

Albert, S. M. (1992). The autonomy of lay and professional knowledge in home health care. *Journal of Aging Studies, 6,* 227–241.

American Occupational Therapy Association. (1991). Essentials and guidelines for an accredited educational program for the occupational therapist. *American Journal of Occupational Therapy, 12,* 1077–1084.

Benner, P. (1984). *From novice to expert.* Menlo Park, CA: Addison-Wesley.

Chiou, I. L., & Burnett, C. N. (1985). A survey of stroke patients and their home therapists. *Physical Therapy, 65,* 901–906.

Clark, C., Corcoran, M. A., & Gitlin, L. N. (1995). An exploratory study of how occupational therapists develop therapeutic relationships. *American Journal of Occupational Therapy, 49,* 587–594. http://dx.doi.org/10.5014/ajot.49.587.

Collins, C. (1992). I don't need help! *Home Healthcare Nurse, 10(5),* 53–56.

Corcoran, M. A. (1992). Gender differences in dementia management plans of spousal caregivers: Implications for occupational therapy. *American Journal of Occupational Therapy, 46,* 1006–1012. http://dx.doi.org/10.5014/ajot.46.11.1006

Corcoran, M. (1993). Collaboration: An ethical approach to effective therapeutic relationships. *Topics in Geriatric Rehabilitation, 9(2),* 1–29.

Corcoran, M., & Gitlin, L. N. (1992). Dementia management: An occupational therapy home-based intervention for caregivers. *American Journal of Occupational Therapy, 46,* 801–808. http://dx.doi.org/10.5014/ajot.46.9.801

DePoy, E., & Gitlin, L. (1994). *An introduction to research: Multiple strategies for health and human services.* St. Louis: Mosby.

Fine, S. B. (1991). Resilience and human adaptability: Who rises above adversity? 1990 Eleanor Clarke Slagle Lecture. *American Journal of Occupational Therapy, 45,* 493–503. Reprinted as Chapter 32.

Fine, S. B. (1993, December). Psychosocial issues and adaptive capacities. *Mental Health Special Interest Section Newsletter, 16,* 1–7.

Fleming, M. H. (1991). Clinical reasoning in medicine compared with clinical reasoning in occupational therapy. *American Journal of Occupational Therapy, 45,* 988–996. http://dx.doi.org/10.5014/ajot.45.11.988

Fleming, M. A., & Mattingly C. (1994). Giving language to practice. In C. Mattingly & M. A. Fleming (Eds.), *Clinical reasoning: Forms of inquiry in therapeutic practice.* Philadelphia: F. A. Davis.

Gitlin, L. N. (1993). Therapeutic dilemmas in the care of the elderly in rehabilitation. *Topics in Geriatric Rehabilitation, 9,* 11–20.

Gitlin, L. N., & Corcoran, M. (1991). Training occupational therapists in the care of the elderly with dementia and their caregivers: Focus on collaboration. *Educational Gerontology, 17,* 591–605.

Gitlin, L. N., & Corcoran, M. (1993). Expanding caregiver ability to use environmental solutions for problems of bathing and incontinence in the elderly with dementia. *Technology and Disability, 2,* 12–21.

Gubrium, J. F., & Sankar, A. (Eds.). (1990). *The home care experience.* Newbury Park, CA: Sage.

Gubrium, J. F., & Sankar, A. (Eds.). (1994). *Qualitative methods in aging research.* Thousand Oaks, CA: Sage.

Hasselkus, B. R. (1988). Meaning in family caregiving: Perspectives on caregiver/professional relationships. *Gerontologist, 28,* 686–691.

Hasselkus, B. R. (1989). The meaning of daily activity in family caregiving for the elderly. *American Journal of Occupational Therapy, 43,* 649–656.

Hasselkus, B. R. (1990). Ethnographic interviewing: A tool for practice with family caregivers for the elderly. *Occupational Therapy Practice, 2,* 9–16.

Hasselkus, B. R. (1991). Ethical dilemmas: The organization of family caregiving for the elderly. *Journal of Aging Studies, 5,* 99–110.

Henderson, J. N., & Gutierrez-Mayka, M. (1992). Ethnocultural themes in caregiving to Alzheimer's disease patients in Hispanic families. *Clinical Gerontologist, 11,* 59–74.

Hill, R. F., Fortenberry, J. D., & Stein, H. F. (1990). Culture in clinical medicine. *Southern Medical Journal, 83,* 1071–1080.

Kaufman, S. R. (1988). Stroke rehabilitation and the negotiation of identity. In S. Reinharz & G. D. Rowles (Eds.), *Qualitative gerontology* (pp. 82–103). New York: Springer.

Kleinman, A. (1988). *The illness narratives.* New York: Basic.

Knight, B. G., Lutzky, S. M., & Macofsky-Urban, F. (1993). A meta-analytic review of interventions for caregiver distress: Recommendations for future research. *Gerontologist, 33,* 240–248.

Levine, R. E., & Gitlin, L. N. (1990). Home adaptations for persons with chronic disabilities: An educational model. *American Journal of Occupational Therapy, 44,* 923–929. http://dx.doi.org/10.5014/ajot.44.10.923

Mattingly, C., & Fleming, M. A. (1994). *Clinical reasoning: Forms of inquiry in therapeutic practice.* Philadelphia: F. A. Davis.

Pepper Commission. (1990). *A call for action. U.S. Bipartisan Commission on Comprehensive Health Care.* Washington, DC: U.S. Government Printing Office.

Pynoos, J., & Ohta, R. (1991). In-home interventions for persons with Alzheimer's disease and their caregivers. *Physical and Occupational Therapy in Geriatrics, 9*(3/4), 83–92.

Robinson, C. A. (1993). Managing life with a chronic condition: The story of normalization. *Qualitative Health Research, 3,* 6–28.

Smith, J., & Baltes, P. B. (1990). Wisdom-related knowledge: Age/cohort differences in response to life-planning problems. *Developmental Psychology, 26,* 494–505.

Smyth, K. A., & Harris, P. B. (1993). Using telecomputing to provide information and support to caregivers of persons with dementia. *Gerontologist, 33,* 123–127.

Spencer, J. C. (1993). The usefulness of qualitative methods in rehabilitation: Issues of meaning, of context, and of change. *Archives of Physical Medicine and Rehabilitation, 74,* 119–126.

Spencer, J., Krefting, L., & Mattingly, C. (1993). Incorporation of ethnographic methods in occupational therapy assessment. *American Journal of Occupational Therapy, 47,* 303–309. http://dx.doi.org/10.5014/ajot.47.4.303

Stone, R., Cafferata, G. L., & Sangl, J. (1987). Caregivers of the frail elderly: A national profile. *Gerontologist, 27,* 616–626.

Williamson, G. M., & Schulz, R. (1993). Coping with specific stressors in Alzheimer's disease caregiving. *Gerontologist, 33,* 747–754.

CHAPTER 39

Enhancing Occupational Performance Through an Understanding of Perceived Self-Efficacy

MARIE GAGE AND HELENE POLATAJKO

Occupational therapists enable clients to develop occupational performance skills with the expectation that these skills will be used outside the treatment setting and that the use of these skills will enhance their clients' occupational competence and their ability to cope with the life stresses associated with their deficits. Therefore, it is important for occupational therapists to understand the role of any factor that influences their clients' occupational performance, or their resultant ability to cope with their deficit in the community. Perceived self-efficacy is one such factor.

It is postulated that perceived self-efficacy explains part of the variance between a person's skill and the quality of that person's actual performance outside the protected clinical environment (Bandura, 1977, 1986; Shaffer, 1978). Furthermore, according to the Appraisal Model of Coping, the concept of perceived self-efficacy is one of 12 factors that influence a person's manner of coping with stressful person–environment interactions, such as those encountered by people with occupational performance deficits (Gage, 1992). Perceived self-efficacy has been found to be a significant behavioral determinant of actual performance and to influence psychological well-being (Allen, Becker, & Swank, 1990; Bandura, 1977, 1986; Bandura & Adams, 1977; Bandura & Wood, 1989; Ewart et al., 1986; Seydel, Taal, & Wiegman, 1990; Shunk, 1982; Toshima, Kaplan, & Ries, 1990; Wang & Richarde, 1987; Wassem, 1992). The most effective means of enhancing perceived self-efficacy is deemed to be through performance-based procedures (Bandura, 1977): the procedures upon which occupational therapy practice is traditionally based.

This article explores the construct of perceived self-efficacy, including origin, definition, relationship to self-esteem, parameters, history, relationship to behavior, outcome expectancy, psychological well-being, and the means of enhancing a client's perceived self-efficacy. The purpose of our review is to help occupational therapists recognize the goodness of fit between perceived self-efficacy and occupational therapy practice and thereby to identify the potential benefits of incorporating the attributes of perceived self-efficacy into day-to-day clinical practice.

Perceived Self-Efficacy

Origins of Perceived Self-Efficacy

Perceived self-efficacy is a concept originally developed as part of Social Cognitive Theory. Social cognitive theorists view human functioning as the result of triadic reciprocality: "behavior, cognitive and other personal factors, and environmental events all act as interacting determinants of each other" (Bandura, 1986, p. 18). The relative influence of each of these three factors varies from situation to situation, from person to person, and from environment to environment. Within the framework of Social Cognitive Theory, people are attributed with six basic capacities.

1. *Symbolizing capacity*—the ability to use symbols to transform experiences into models that guide future actions, which in turn are guided by thoughts; thoughts are sometimes inaccurate due to misinterpretation of the incoming information.
2. *Forethought capacity*—the ability to anticipate the potential outcome of future actions, set goals, and develop action plans.
3. *Vicarious capacity*—the ability to learn through observation of others and thereby abbreviate the learning period; this ability is vital to survival.

4. *Self-regulatory capacity*—the ability to make choices based on personal beliefs, rather than on the expectations of the external environment. Internalized standards are used to guide behavioral choices.

5. *Change capacity (plasticity)*—the ability to develop or change. The vast potential for human development is shaped by both direct and vicarious experiences into many forms, constrained only by biological limitations.

6. *Self-reflective capacity*—the ability to think about personal experiences and derive generic knowledge about one-self and the world in which one lives. One of the most powerful types of self-reflective thought is perceived self-efficacy (Bandura, 1986).

Each of these six capacities influences the degree of self-efficacy expressed for each task by any given person.

Definition of Perceived Self-Efficacy

The concept of perceived self-efficacy (or efficacy expectations) evolved primarily from the observation that traditional cognitive psychology models did not adequately explain the discrepancy between attained skills and the quality of performance output (Bandura, 1977). Traditional models attempted to explain the discrepancy between skills and performance as a function of the actor's expectation of outcomes or "action–outcome expectancy." Action–outcome expectancy theorists postulate that, given equivalent skills, performance differences are due to differences in the actor's belief that the response will lead to a desired goal. If this belief is strong, the actor will engage in the requisite behavior; if this belief is weak, the actor will not engage in the behavior even though he or she possesses the skill to do so.

Bandura (1977) suggested that a difference in outcome expectancy does not explain the total variance between skill and performance. He suggested that perceived self-efficacy is also a significant factor. Bandura (1986) defined *perceived self-efficacy* as:

> people's judgments of their capabilities to organize and execute courses of action required to attain designated types of performances. It is concerned not with the skills one has but with the judgments of what one can do with whatever skills one possesses. (p. 391)

Thus, Bandura (1977) asserted that one's belief in one's ability to use a specific skill partially explains why people of equivalent skill achieve at differing levels. This belief in one's ability to perform (i.e., perceived self-efficacy) develops as a result of the interaction of each of the six attributes of Social Cognitive Theory described earlier.

Relationship to Self-Esteem

Perceived self-efficacy should not be confused with the construct of self-esteem. *Self-esteem* is defined as "the dimension of self-concept that includes a negative and/or positive sense of self" (Daub, 1988, p. 57). Self-esteem is created by the person's analysis of his or her overall competency at factors that he or she considers to be socially relevant (Mayberry, 1990). Thus, a person may perceive himself or herself to be competent at many things but have low self-esteem due to a belief that these competencies are not socially relevant. Conversely, a person may express a low degree of perceived self-efficacy for one or more tasks yet have high self-esteem. Self-esteem and perceived self-efficacy should be highly correlated only when measuring perceived self-efficacy for a task that is highly socially relevant to the subject. A Nobel Prize winner may have high self-esteem in part due to the recognition of the value of his or her contribution to society. The same Nobel Prize winner may have low perceived self-efficacy for playing racquetball or gourmet cooking. However, his or her perceived self-efficacy for the activity that resulted in the Nobel Prize should be high and should correlate strongly with a measure of his or her self-esteem. Thus, perceived self-efficacy may contribute to a sense of self-esteem, but it is an independent construct.

Parameters of Self-Efficacy

Bandura (1977) identified three parameters of perceived self-efficacy: magnitude, strength, and generality. *Magnitude* refers to the relative level of difficulty of the task that is being rated. For example, Ewart and colleagues (1986) used different jogging distances to reflect differences in the magnitude of perceived self-efficacy for a group of subjects with postmyocardial infarction. Subjects who were completely confident that they could jog 1 mile were considered to have a greater magnitude of perceived self-efficacy than those who were completely confident that they could jog only a quarter of a mile and somewhat confident that they could jog 1 mile.

Strength of perceived self-efficacy refers to the degree to which people believe they can succeed at a given level of an activity; this degree can vary from total certainty to total uncertainty. The stronger the sense of efficacy, the more likely people are to persevere in the face of adversity and the less likely it is that failure will extinguish their efficacy expectations (Bandura, 1977).

Generality of perceived self-efficacy refers to the degree to which the person's perceived self-efficacy for one activity transfers to other similar or different activities. Successful performance of some tasks results in a strengthening of efficacy expectations for that task alone, whereas success at other tasks generalizes to tasks that are different from the original task (Bandura, 1977). Bandura does not identify the types of tasks that generalize or those that do not.

History of the Construct

Bandura postulated that, given the requisite skills and belief that the response will lead to a desired outcome, perceived self-efficacy would be an important determinant of successful performance. Bandura (1977; Bandura & Adams, 1977) tested the theory about perceived self-efficacy with an unspecified number of persons with snake phobias. Subjects were asked to state whether they were able to perform each of 18 tasks and to rate the strength of their expectations that they would succeed on a 100-point scale with 10-point intervals. The subjects were randomly assigned to one of three groups: vicarious experience, modeling (later called enactive experience), or no treatment. The subjects in the vicarious learning group observed an instructor handling snakes, while the enactive learning group first observed and then attempted the snake-handling techniques themselves. Of the subjects who achieved maximal performances during therapy (successfully achieved the snake-handling techniques), Bandura noted that not all expressed maximal efficacy expectations. Efficacy expectation and performance during the treatment sessions were examined as possible predictors of subsequent performance. Perceived self-efficacy was found to be the best predictor of subsequent performance. The higher the subjects' perceived self-efficacy at the completion of treatment, the better their performance when retested at a later date ($r = .75$, $p < .01$). This relationship existed regardless of whether the efficacy expectations were derived through vicarious or enactive experience. However, subjects who experienced enactive education produced higher, more generalized, and stronger efficacy expectations and increased performance attempts. Bandura (1977) stated that:

> on the one hand, the mechanisms by which human behavior is acquired and regulated are increasingly formulated in terms of cognitive processes. On the other hand, it is the performance based procedures that are proving to be most powerful for effecting psychological changes. As a consequence, successful performance is replacing symbolically based experiences as the principal vehicle of change. (p. 191)

Since his initial work, Bandura has examined the effect of perceived self-efficacy with a variety of subjects and found that perceived self-efficacy is a consistent predictor of performance (Bandura, 1982; Bandura, Cioffi, Taylor, & Brouillard, 1988; Bandura & Wood, 1989).

The construct of perceived self-efficacy has been applied in a variety of different clinical, educational, and organizational situations by many other authors. From January 1987 to December 1992, 933 articles referring to perceived self-efficacy have been printed in journals indexed by Psychlit alone. The following is a brief summary of the findings of a small sampling of these articles that were selected for their relevance to occupational therapy practice.

Clinical Examples

- Perceived self-efficacy for exercise was found to be correlated with an increase in exercise endurance in a sample of subjects ($n = 119$) with chronic obstructive lung disease (Toshima et al., 1990).
- Self-efficacy was found to explain 24 percent of the variance in adjustment to multiple sclerosis ($n = 62$) (Wassem, 1992).
- Self-efficacy for jogging proved superior to treadmill performance, depression, and type A personality in predicting adherence to exercise prescription in a sample ($n = 40$) of patients with coronary artery disease (Ewart et al., 1986).
- The results of a study of subjects ($n = 30$) diagnosed with arthritis indicated that a higher level of perceived self-efficacy for pain control after a cognitive behavioral education program was related to a lower level of perceived pain (O'Leary, Shoor, Lorig, & Holman, 1988).

Health Promotion Examples

- A scale, developed to measure perceived barriers to health-promotion activities, was found to be highly correlated (–.48) with perceived self-efficacy (Stuif-bergen, Becker, & Sands, 1990).
- In a sample (*n* = 600) of subjects participating in the Stanford Heart Disease Prevention Program, self-effi-cacy was found to be a better predictor of nutritional choices than demographic factors, social influences, and health knowledge (Slater, 1989). This study also found that cognitive control (the capacity to exer-cise control over one's own thinking and motiva-tion) predicted the level of perceived self-efficacy.
- Raising self-efficacy for health-promoting behaviors was found to be more effective than emphasizing the risk of not performing the health-promoting be-havior in two separate studies (Seydel et al., 1990).

Education Examples

- Attributional feedback from the researcher (feedback about who was responsible for past successes), as op-posed to feedback about future potential success or no feedback, was found to be related to faster math-ematical skill development and higher perceived self-efficacy in a sample (*n* = 40) of children ranging in ages from 7 to 10 years (Shunk, 1982).
- Subjects who were successful using strategies taught in a "learning to learn" program led to enhanced perceived self-efficacy and generalized to other ac-tivities requiring similar learning skills for a group of 4th graders (Wang & Richarde, 1987).

Perceived Self-Efficacy as a Behavioral Determinant

A strong sense of perceived self-efficacy for an activity is crucial to successful performance because "it deter-mines which activities people engage in, the amount of effort they expend before terminating the activity, and how long they will persevere in the face of adversity" (Bandura, 1981, p. 215). People are faced with frequent activity choices throughout their lives. The strength of their efficacy expectations for an activity affects whether they choose to engage in the activity or not. Strong ef-ficacy expectations result in engagement in an activity; whereas weak efficacy expectations result in avoidance (Bandura, 1986). This process of activity selection has a profound effect on human development, in that activity choices enlarge or restrict one's opportunities to develop new skills, or to enhance existing ones (Bandura, 1986).

Errors in judgment regarding one's performance, whether too optimistic or too pessimistic, may result in significant consequences (Bandura, 1986). In activities with a small margin of error (e.g., driving a car), overly optimistic efficacy expectations may prove disastrous. However, in activities with a greater margin of error, activities that are unlikely to result in harm to oneself or others, appraisals of performance that exceed actual ability are quite functional (Bandura, 1989).

For example, when a patient is attempting to learn to maneuver a wheelchair, a high expectation that he or she is capable of learning to propel the chair will result in more frequent attempts and learning will advance more quickly. On the other hand, if the patient be-lieves that he or she is unlikely to master propelling the wheelchair, he or she will avoid situations where this is a requirement and progress will be impeded. Bandura asserted (1989) that people must strive to exceed past performances, and that if efficacy expectations never exceeded past performance, the acquisition of new skills would not occur.

People with strong efficacy expectations will perse-vere in the face of adversity, due to a belief that they will ultimately succeed (Bandura, 1977). People with weaker efficacy expectations will quit when faced with obstacles, or refuse even to try. People who view them-selves as efficacious are more likely to expect things to go right (Bandura, 1989). They approach difficult tasks as challenges to master rather than threats to avoid. People who experience success react by raising their personal goals and being more committed to the activ-ity (Bandura & Wood, 1989). The stronger the sense of perceived self-efficacy, the higher the goals set and the stronger the commitment to attainment of the goals.

Although perceived self-efficacy is a crucial behav-ioral determinant, Bandura (1977) pointed out that perceived self-efficacy in the absence of skill, or a de-sire to perform, will not ensure successful performance. Attempts to enhance performance must be accompa-nied by an understanding of the influence of perceived self-efficacy on performance.

Outcome Expectations and Perceived Self-Efficacy

Perceived self-efficacy refers to a belief in one's ability to perform a certain task or behavior. It should not be con-fused with a belief that performance of a specified be-havior will result in a specific outcome (Bandura, 1977). Rogers (1983) referred to a belief that performance of a specified behavior will result in a specified outcome as response efficacy. Both perceived self-efficacy and response efficacy affect whether or not the person will elect to perform a certain task; however, they are distinct behavioral determinants (Bandura, 1977). That is, one must believe both that a specific action will lead to a desired goal and that one is capable of performing the specific action, or one will not act.

Bandura (1986) argued that theories that emphasize outcome expectations are based on animal research where measurement of perceived self-efficacy was impossible. He stated that "convictions that outcomes are determined by one's own actions can be either demoralizing or heartening, depending on the level of self-judged efficacy" (Bandura, 1986, p. 413). Therefore, an expectation that a certain behavior will result in a certain outcome is not sufficient to ensure successful performance unless one believes one has the skills to succeed at the required task.

Relationship to Psychological Well-Being

According to self-efficacy ideology, people can give up trying and become hopeless in two different ways: they may believe that their continued attempts will not bring positive results (response efficacy), or they may believe that they are unable to perform the tasks necessary to bring about the desired results (perceived self-efficacy) (Bandura, 1982). Different combinations of these two factors result in different self-assessments:

- If persons have a strong sense of perceived self-efficacy and a strong belief in the efficacy of the response, they will act in an assured manner and be dynamic.
- If persons have a strong sense of perceived self-efficacy but a weak sense of response efficacy, they will energize themselves to make changes in the system so that they can successfully attain their goal.
- If people have a weak sense of perceived self-efficacy and a weak sense of response efficacy, they will become resigned and apathetic.
- If people have a weak sense of perceived self-efficacy and a strong sense of response efficacy, they will become despondent and self-deprecating.

The relationship between perceived self-efficacy and psychological well-being was explored by Holahan, Holahan, and Belk (1984). Perceived self-efficacy was measured by asking a group of retired university faculty members how well they handled or could in the future handle each of the items on a list of daily hassles (self-efficacy/hassles scale) and a list of negative life events (self-efficacy/life events scale). The results indicated that higher levels of perceived self-efficacy were associated with lower levels of depression for both sexes. Additionally high levels of perceived self-efficacy were associated with lower levels of psychological distress for women and fewer psychosomatic complaints for men. Overall, the results indicate a significant association between perceived self-efficacy and psychological adjustment.

Perceived self-efficacy has also been shown to negatively correlate with depression. Davis-Berman (1990) administered the Physical Self-Efficacy Scale and the General Self-Efficacy Scale to a sample of 200 elderly residents of a retirement center. The Physical Self-Efficacy Scale consists of 22 items and includes questions about reflexes, muscle tone, and sports ability. The General Self-Efficacy Scale consists of two subscales, the General Scale and the Social Self-Efficacy Scale. The scale contains questions about one's general belief in one's ability to do things and one's ability to handle oneself in social situations. All three Self-Efficacy Scales were found to be inversely and significantly ($p > .01$) correlated to depression. (General Self-Efficacy $r = -.40$, Social Self-Efficacy $r = -.23$, and Physical Self-Efficacy $r = .50$). That is, persons with lower self-efficacy scores were more likely to be depressed.

Influencing the Strength of Perceived Self-Efficacy

Perceived self-efficacy is influenced through an ongoing evaluation of success and failure with each task people participate in over the course of their lives (Bandura, 1986). Bandura (1982) stated that perceived self-efficacy develops through successful experiences that create high efficacy expectations and failure experiences that lower efficacy expectations. Thus, the development of perceived self-efficacy is a dynamic process.

Perceived self-efficacy is constantly affected by four sources of information: personal performance accomplishments, vicarious experience (watching others of similar skill perform a task), verbal persuasion, and the person's physiological state (Bandura, 1977).

Personal Performance Accomplishments

Personal performance accomplishments, also called enactive experiences, are the most influential source of information about one's perceived self-efficacy (Bandura, 1986). Success, as perceived by the person, enhances perceived self-efficacy, and failure decreases it. Failure early in the development of a new skill is more likely to decrease perceived self-efficacy than failure after a firmly entrenched belief in the skill has been developed. When people believe they are efficacious, they attribute failure to the circumstances, poor effort on their part, or the use of poor strategies (Bandura, 1986).

Vicarious Experience

A great deal of human learning begins with observing others perform tasks (Bandura, 1986). Vicarious learning is developed more readily when the observer considers the person being observed to have similar skills to himself or herself. Children watch and then imitate their parents. In this process of observing activities, some learning occurs before the person is required to attempt any of the requisite behaviors. For example, children observe their parents driving cars for years before they begin. They observe how the wheel is turned, how to start the car, what the highway signs mean, and so on. This learning decreases the number of new skills that must be learned when the children reach an appropriate age and actually begin to drive the car. They already understand the component skills and now need to learn to execute them independently (Bandura, 1986). Vicarious learning is not as powerful a source of information as enactive learning, but it is still very important.

Persuasion

Persuasion is a frequently used means of convincing someone that his or her self-assessment is incorrect. However, it is the weakest form of information with respect to altering perceived self-efficacy (Bandura, 1986). Persuasion will be effective in altering beliefs only if the current belief is close to the belief that is being proposed. Subsequent performance quickly affirms or denies the new belief. Thus, accurate assessment of the other person's ability is required if persuasion is to succeed.

Physiological State

People read their level of somatic arousal as an indication of competency (Bandura, 1977). Thus, if your heart rate increases and you begin to sweat, you interpret these reactions as an indication that the activity you are approaching is in some way threatening. Strategies that decrease the level of arousal (relaxation techniques) have been found to enable people to feel more efficacious. This feeling of efficacy in turn leads to a willingness to attempt the behavior that had previously resulted in a state of physiological arousal, and to success experiences (Bandura, 1986).

Cognitive Appraisal

Personal performance accomplishments, vicarious experience, persuasion, and physiological arousal are the types of experiences that affect perceived self-efficacy. However, the degree to which these experiences influence perceived self-efficacy is determined by the person's cognitive appraisal and integration of these experiences (Bandura, 1982; Gist & Mitchell, 1992).

Gist and Mitchell (1992) developed a model to explain the effect of these experiences on perceived self-efficacy. They suggested that the cognitive appraisal and integration process has three components. The first component is the analysis of the requirements of the task. The more complex the task and the less previous experience one has with a task, the harder it is to accurately assess one's perceived self-efficacy for the task. The second component is the analysis of the degree to which success or failure is attributed to oneself rather than others or to chance. If one believes that one is successful due to a skill one possesses, then perceived self-efficacy for the task will be heightened. However, if one believes that one was successful because of chance, the actions of others, or the environment, perceived self-efficacy will not be affected. The third component is the analysis of personal and situational resources and constraints that affect the task at hand. This appraisal process involves the assessment of personal factors such as skill, motivation, anxiety, and desire, as well as situational factors, such as distractions, support of influential others, and competing demands.

The three cognitive appraisal processes will result in the subjects' determination of the degree of perceived self-efficacy for a task, which in turn affects the person's willingness to participate or persevere with the task in the future, and hence will affect actual future performance.

Generalizability

The development of perceived self-efficacy is largely situation specific, with a tendency to generalize to similar activities (Ewart, Taylor, Reese, & DeBusk, 1983). Ewart and his colleagues studied the relationship between perceived self-efficacy and activity for a group of patients with postmyocardial infarction. These patients participated in treadmill testing and filled in a perceived self-efficacy questionnaire before the treadmill test, after the treadmill test, and after a counseling session that followed the treadmill test. The perceived self-efficacy questions covered walking, running, climbing stairs, engaging in sexual intercourse, lifting objects, and an overall estimate of ability to tolerate physical activity. Perceived self-efficacy ratings for the activities that used the same physical skills as the treadmill (walking, running, and climbing stairs) showed the greatest increase. With the addition of counseling (a form of verbal persuasion), the efficacy ratings for the other activities increased. Assistance with interpretation of the treadmill experience was necessary before generalization could occur.

Control

The degree of control the person perceives that he or she has alters the influence of success or failure on the development of perceived self-efficacy. Bandura and Wood (1989) studied the influence of perceived control on perceived self-efficacy in a simulated manufacturing environment. The degree of perceived control and the amount of success the subjects experienced were regulated through the design of the experiment. Subjects were randomly assigned to one of four groups. Each group received instructions designed to alter their perception of two constructs, personal control and performance expectations. The four groups were low perceived control with high performance expectations, low perceived control with low performance expectations, high perceived control with high performance expectations, and high perceived control with low performance expectations. The groups that were given high performance standards experienced less success than those with low performance standards. Subjects who viewed the organization as controllable, regardless of whether they were in the high or low performance expectations group, had higher mean self-efficacy scores than those who thought that they had little control over the organization ($p < .02$). Subjects in the high control, high performance standards group showed increases in perceived self-efficacy over three trials, whereas subjects in the high control, low success groups showed decreases in perceived self-efficacy ($p < .05$). Subjects who were led to believe that the organization was difficult to control demonstrated low self-efficacy regardless of whether they were in the high or low performance expectation group; that is, their perceived self-efficacy was low regardless of whether or not they were experiencing success.

Discussion of the Literature

Adolph Meyer, a major contributor to the philosophical basis of occupational therapy practice, recognized the value of the feelings of satisfaction and achievement associated with successful completion of a project (1922; see Chapter 4). Thus, from the early days of occupational therapy practice, the value of successful experiences, that is, performance accomplishments, was recognized. Activity programs were structured to ensure success because success was believed to lead the patient to try another, more difficult task. Occupational therapists have often described this process as the enhancement of self-esteem (Christiansen, 1991; Meyer, 1922 [see Chapter 4]), yet the activities the occupational therapy client performs are not always socially relevant. Therefore, it is postulated that success with occupational therapy activities leads to an increase in perceived self-efficacy for these activities, which leads to a willingness to engage in and persist in future similar tasks. If the success experiences relate to socially relevant activities an elevation in self-esteem would also be predicted.

The occupational performance literature addresses the need to understand the effect of psychosocial factors on occupational performance (Christiansen, 1991; Pedretti & Pasquinelli-Estrada, 1985; Trombly, 1989). An underlying assumption appears to be that psychological factors affect only the acquisition of skill and that once the skill has been learned it will be used outside the protected clinical environment. However, just as Bandura (1977) noted that people do not always perform optimally even when they have the requisite skills, clinicians have stated that occupational therapy clients do not always perform at the level one might predict on the basis of clinical observation of skill (Gage, 1992).

The Model of Human Occupation, a model that guides occupational therapy practice, addresses the discrepancy between skill and performance through, among other things, a concept similar to perceived self-efficacy: personal causation (Oakley, Kielhofner, & Barris, 1985). *Personal causation* is defined as "the collective beliefs that an individual has efficacious skills, is personally in control, and will succeed in future endeavors" (Oakley et al., p. 148). This construct is equivalent to the construct of perceived self-efficacy.

When discussing the influence of inefficacy (a term that Kielhofner has used in the same view as perceived self-efficacy), Kielhofner stated that "occupational dysfunction is at the level of inefficacy when there is an interference with performing meaningful activity accompanied by dissatisfaction with performance" (1985, p. 69). He went on to state that "sources of inefficacy may be environmental constraints, disease processes, or imbalanced lifestyles" (p. 69).

The importance of the strength of the person's belief in his or her ability to perform the specific component parts of life roles is not articulated. One's perception of one's ability to perform is considered to be a major behavioral determinant (Allen et al., 1990; Bandura, 1977, 1986; Bandura & Adams, 1977; Bandura & Wood, 1989; Ewart et al., 1986; Seydel et al., 1990; Shunk, 1982; Toshima et al., 1990; Wang & Richarde, 1987; Wassem, 1992). Therefore, it is essential that the relationship of perceived self-efficacy to occupational performance be explored.

The terms *perceived self-efficacy* or *efficacy expectations* are beginning to appear in the occupational therapy literature. Crist and Stoffel (1992), when discussing the Americans With Disabilities Act as it applies to persons with mental impairments, discussed the value of perceived self-efficacy with respect to successful employment of persons with mental disabilities. Christiansen (1991) acknowledged that the "single characteristic of the individual that has the greatest influence on performance is one's sense of competence" (p. 20), yet this concept is given only four paragraphs in the occupational therapy textbook written by Christiansen and Baum.

There is a growing recognition that clients' perceptions of performance (perceived self-efficacy) are important. In the March 1993 issue of the *American Journal of Occupational Therapy,* professional leaders discussed the needs of the profession with respect to assessment. Authors cited the need to measure client perception of performance (Law, 1993), the need to identify the psychological factors that contribute to performance deficits and strengths (Bonder, 1993), and the need to develop means of remediating these psychological factors once identified (Bonder, 1993). Trombly stated that the overall goal of occupational therapy is to "enable the client to gain a sense of efficacy" (1993, p. 254). The Canadian Occupational Performance Measure (Law et al., 1991) uses client perception of performance as one outcome variable. However, there is a need to incorporate this belief into occupational therapy practices.

The influence of perceived self-efficacy on the person's ability to cope with the effects of disability has also been articulated by Gage (1992). She was interested in determining why patients of equal physical impairment and rehabilitation potential do not progress at the same pace, and why, given similar goals, these patients attain different levels of independent function. After

a review of the literature on coping, Gage formulated the Appraisal Model of Coping as a guide to assessment and intervention for occupational therapists. The Appraisal Model of Coping was based on the Cognitive Relational Theory of Coping and Emotion (Lazarus & Folkman, 1984) and Social Cognitive Theory (Bandura, 1977). *Coping* was defined by Lazarus and Folkman (1984) as the process through which people manage the demands and emotions generated by person–environment relationships.

The model presented by Gage identified 12 factors that influence the ability of persons to cope with their disability or any other life event that taxes personal resources. One of these 12 factors is perceived self-efficacy. In this model, perceived self-efficacy is considered by Gage to be particularly salient to the practice of occupational therapy because of its potential ability to explain the discrepancy between skill developed in therapy and occupational performance outside the protected clinical environment. However, the model is, as yet, conceptual and must be tested to determine the specific nature of the influence of perceived self-efficacy on coping with occupational performance deficits.

Enhancing Occupational Performance

A recognition that the client's level of perceived self-efficacy for a specific activity influences the likelihood of the client performing that activity outside the protected clinical environment has far-reaching implications for the practice of occupational therapy. This recognition brings with it an understanding that a client's ability to perform a specific skill in the clinical environment may not mean that the client will use the skill in his or her usual contextual environment. What good is treatment if it does not generalize to the use of the skill in the community?

Occupational therapists must learn how to evaluate their client's level of perceived self-efficacy and to develop techniques that not only improve clients' skills, but also enhance their self-efficacy for use of those skills in the community. As previously presented, empirical findings about the influence of perceived self-efficacy on clinical outcome are already available (Ewart et al., 1986; O'Leary et al., 1988; Toshima et al., 1990; Wassem, 1992). Although these studies do not specifically look at occupational performance activities or the influence of the occupational therapy process on perceived self-efficacy, they do provide information that is relevant to occupational therapy practice. Empirical studies have also investigated the relationship between perceived self-efficacy and the initiation or adherence to health-promoting behaviors (Seydel et al., 1990; Slater, 1989; Stuifbergen et al., 1990). The results of these studies are increasingly relevant to occupational therapists as more and more therapists become involved with primary and secondary prevention activities. In addition, the process of occupational therapy is often one of teaching new skills or teaching new ways to perform familiar activities. Thus, articles that present data about the relationship between perceived self-efficacy and learning are also relevant to occupational therapists (Shunk, 1982; Wang & Richarde, 1987).

It is important to remember that the articles cited in this paper are just a small sampling of the perceived self-efficacy literature available to occupational therapists. Occupational therapists working in various fields are encouraged to search the literature for articles that have valuable information about perceived self-efficacy within their area of practice. Occupational therapy research studies to add to this knowledge base are encouraged. There are many possible applications that arise from the attributes of perceived self-efficacy as presented in the section of this paper titled "History of the Construct." These themes can be categorized into three major categories: assessment, outcome, and therapeutic process.

Assessment and Outcome

Previous research has demonstrated a link between clinical outcomes and perceived self-efficacy (Allen et al., 1990; Bandura, 1977, 1986; Bandura, & Adams, 1977; Bandura & Wood, 1989; Ewart et al., 1986; Seydel, Taal, & Wiegman, 1990; Shunk, 1982; Toshima et al., 1990; Wang & Richarde, 1987; Wassem, 1992). Thus, it is important to derive ways to measure perceived self-efficacy for occupational performance activities that will enable the exploration of its relationship to outcome. For example, perceived self-efficacy is thought to explain the variance between development of skill and performance of that skill in the community. It is, therefore, important to explore the influence of increases or decreases in perceived self-efficacy for occupational performance activities on treatment outcomes. The level of perceived self-efficacy that is required before a client will use the skill independently in the community must be determined. The belief that the development of a skill is not sufficient to ensure successful occupational performance in the absence of an adequate level of perceived self-efficacy leads to a need to monitor a client's perceived self-efficacy during the treatment process. The ability to demonstrate occupational competence in the clinical environment should no longer indicate successful treatment outcome. Therapists must find ways to determine whether their clients are using these skills in the community. Because perceived self-efficacy is believed to be a good predictor of future performance, therapists need to establish the level of perceived self-efficacy that is likely to result in use of the skill in the community. This level may then be useful in the determination of when to discharge from therapy. However, individual variation will always necessitate individual follow-up to ensure that a given client has been successful.

Therapeutic Process

The section of this paper titled "Influencing the Strength of Perceived Self-Efficacy" provides occupational therapists with specific strategies for increasing perceived self-efficacy in the clinical environment. For example, perceived self-efficacy is enhanced through personal performance accomplishments; that is, by actually doing the activity or very similar activities. In fact, it is suggested that perceived self-efficacy for an activity performed in the occupational therapy department will only generalize to very similar activities. Thus, occupational therapists must use realistic activities that simulate the contextual environment of the client. This will be easy for therapists working in the community who provide services in the client's home; it will be more difficult for therapists working in institutional environments. The relevance of reductionistic activities such as peg boards and puzzles must be questioned. How does the mastery of these component skills relate to changes in perceived self-efficacy and actual performance for personally important life activities?

The role of vicarious learning with respect to the development of occupational competence must also be explored. If, in fact, a great deal of human learning begins with observing others perform tasks, it would be important for clients to observe the successful performance attempts of their peers. Bandura (1977) suggested that vicarious experience is most powerful when the participants consider themselves to have similar skills. Thus, modeling by the therapist may be ineffective, and consumer self-help groups might be encouraged.

Gist and Mitchell (1992) suggest that self-efficacy beliefs are most accurate when clients are rating familiar activities because they understand the relationship between the skills required to perform the task and the skills they possess. For occupational therapy clients the knowledge of the skills they possess has often been affected by the onset of a disabling condition. Although the clients are aware of the skills required for occupational performance activities, they may believe that their disability has robbed them of these skills. Thus, the occupational therapist must provide them with a safe environment within which to experiment with their altered level of performance and to develop a new understanding of their efficacy.

Therapists often try to convince clients that they are able to go home and live independently, or return to work, only to be confronted with a barrage of reasons why the client is not yet ready. These patients are labeled as fearful or, worse yet, as malingerers. Perhaps it is simply their perceived self-efficacy for home management or work activities that has not yet reached the level necessary to engage in the activity independently. If one accepts that persuasion is the least influential method of raising efficacy expectations, then the therapist must devise new intervention techniques. The treatment plan must incorporate vicarious learning and relevant personal performance accomplishments if success is to occur. The use of such simulations as Easy Street,[1] a stay in an activities of daily living (ADL) apartment located in the protected clinical environment, or a home visit with the therapist may be a better solution than attempts to persuade.

Perceived self-efficacy increases more when the client is in control. Thus, it is important for therapists to enable clients to articulate their needs and have a real voice in the therapeutic process. Tools such as the Canadian Occupational Performance Measure (Law et al., 1991) may create a feeling of control and enhance outcomes.

Summary

Perceived self-efficacy has great relevance to the practice of occupational therapy. It is consistent with the fundamental philosophical beliefs of the profession, may enhance and predict outcomes, and has a strong empirical basis that suggest specific changes to current occupational therapy treatment practice. Occupational therapists are challenged to develop, test, and publish these linkages.

Many of the attributes of perceived self-efficacy are relevant to occupational performance. By monitoring and working to enhance perceived self-efficacy, occupational therapists may be better able to explain the variance between development of skill and performance of that skill in the community, ensure successful occupational performance in the community, predict future performance, and enable occupational competence.

Acknowledgment

Funds for this study were obtained through a Health Services Research Grant awarded to the first author by Victoria Hospital, London, Ontario, Canada.

References

Allen, J. K., Becker, D. M., & Swank, R. T. (1990). Factors related to functional status after coronary artery bypass surgery. *Heart and Lung, 19,* 337–343.

Bandura, A. (1977). Toward a unifying theory of behavioral change. *Psychological Review, 84,* 101–215.

Bandura, A. (1981). Self-referent thought: A developmental analysis of self-efficacy. In J. H. Flavell & L. Ross (Eds.), *Social cognitive development: Frontiers and possible futures* (pp. 200–239). New York: Cambridge University Press.

Bandura, A. (1982). Self-efficacy mechanism in human agency. *American Psychologist, 37,* 122–147.

Bandura, A. (1986). *Social foundations of thought.* Englewood Cliffs, NJ: Prentice Hall.

Bandura, A. (1989). Regulation of cognitive processes through perceived self-efficacy. *Developmental Psychology, 25,* 729–735.

Bandura, A., & Adams, N. E. (1977). Analysis of self-efficacy theory of behavioral change. *Cognitive Therapy and Research, 1,* 287–310.

Bandura, A., Cioffi, D., Taylor, C. B., & Brouillard (1988). Perceived self-efficacy in coping with cognitive stressors and opioid activation. *Journal of Personality and Social Psychology, 55,* 497–488.

Bandura, A., & Wood, R. (1989). Effect of perceived controllability and performance standards on self-regulation of complex decision-making. *Journal of Personality and Social Psychology, 56,* 805–814.

Bonder, B. R. (1993). Issues in assessment of psychosocial components of function. *American Journal of Occupational Therapy, 47,* 211–216.

Christiansen, C. (1991). Occupational therapy: Intervention for life performance. In C. Christiansen & C. Baum (Eds.), *Occupational therapy: Overcoming human performance deficits* (pp. 3–43). Beckenham, Kent, England: Slack.

---

[1]Manufactured by Easy Street Environments, 6908 E. Thomas Road, Suite 201, Scottsdale, AZ 85251.

Crist, P. A. H., & Stoffel, V. C. (1992). The Americans With Disabilities Act of 1990 and employees with mental impairments: Personal efficacy and the environment. *American Journal of Occupational Therapy, 46,* 434–443. http://dx.doi.org/10.5014/ajot.46.5.419

Daub, M. (1988). Prenatal development through mid-adulthood. In H. L. Hopkins & H. D. Smith (Eds.), *Willard and Spackman's occupational therapy* (7th ed., pp. 50–75). Philadelphia: Lippincott.

Davis-Berman, J. (1990). Physical self-efficacy, perceived physical status, and depressive symptomatology in older adults. *Journal of Psychology, 124,* 207–215.

Ewart, C. K., Stewart, K. J., Gillilan, R. E., Kelemen, M. H., Valenti, S. A., Manley, J. D., & Kelemen, M. D. (1986). Usefulness of self-efficacy in predicting overexertion during programmed exercise in coronary artery disease. *American Journal of Cardiology, 57,* 557–561.

Ewart, C. K., Taylor, C. B., Reese, L. B., & DeBusk, R. F. (1983). Effects of early postmyocardial infarction exercise testing on self-perception and subsequent physical activity. *American Journal of Cardiology, 51,* 1076–1080.

Gage, M. (1992). The appraisal model of coping: An assessment and intervention model for occupational therapy. *American Journal of Occupational Therapy, 46,* 353–362. http://dx.doi.org/10.5014/ajot.46.4.353

Gist, M., & Mitchell, T. (1992). Self-efficacy: A theoretical analysis of its determinants and malleability. *Academy of Management Review, 17,* 183–211.

Holahan, C. K., Holahan, C. J., & Belk, S. S. (1984). Adjustment in aging: The roles of life stress, hassles, and self-efficacy. *Health Psychology, 3,* 315–328.

Kielhofner, G. (1985). Occupational function and dysfunction. In G. Kielhofner (Ed.), *A Model of Human Occupation* (pp. 63–75). Baltimore: Williams & Wilkins.

Law, M. (1993). Evaluating activities of daily living: Directions for the future. *American Journal of Occupational Therapy, 47,* 233–237. http://dx.doi.org/10.5014/ajot.47.3.233

Law, M., Baptiste, S., Carswell-Opzoomer, A., McCall, M. A., Polatajko, H., & Pollock, N. (1991). *Canadian Occupational Performance Measure.* Toronto: CAOT Publications ACE.

Lazarus, R. S., & Folkman, S. (1984). *Stress appraisal and coping.* New York: Springer.

Mayberry, W. (1990). Self-esteem in children: Considerations for measurement and intervention. *American Journal of Occupational Therapy, 44,* 729–734. http://dx.doi.org/10.5014/ajot.44.8.729

Meyer, A. (1922). The philosophy of occupation therapy. *American Journal of Occupational Therapy, 31,* 639–642. Reprinted as Chapter 4.

Oakley, F., Kielhofner, G., & Barris, R. (1985). An occupational therapy approach to assessing psychiatric patients' adaptive functioning. *American Journal of Occupational Therapy, 39,* 147–154.

O'Leary, A., Shoor, S., Lorig, K., & Holman, H. R. (1988). A cognitive–behavioral treatment for rheumatoid arthritis. *Health Psychology, 7,* 527–544.

Pedretti, L. W., & Pasquinelli-Estrada, S. (1985). Foundations for treatment of physical dysfunction. In L. Pedretti (Ed.), *Occupational therapy: Practice skills for physical dysfunction* (2nd ed., pp. 1–10). St. Louis: Mosby.

Rogers, R. W. (1983). Cognitive and physiological processes in fear appeals and attitude change: A revised theory of protection motivation. In J. T. Cacioppo, R. E. Petty, & D. Shapiro (Eds.), *Social psychophysiology* (pp. 153–176). New York: Guilford.

Seydel, E., Taal, E., & Wiegman, O. (1990). Risk-appraisal, outcome, and self-efficacy expectancies: Cognitive factors in preventive behavior related to cancer. *Psychology and Health, 4,* 99–109.

Shaffer, H. (1978). Psychological rehabilitation, skills-building, and self-efficacy. *American Psychologist, 33,* 394–396.

Shunk, D. (1982). Effects of effort attributional feedback on children's perceived self-efficacy and achievement. *Journal of Educational Psychology, 74,* 548–556.

Slater, M. (1989). Social influences and cognitive control as predictors of self-efficacy and eating behavior. *Cognitive Therapy and Research, 13,* 231–245.

Stuifbergen, A., Becker, H., & Sands, D. (May 1990). Barriers to health promotion for individuals with disabilities. *Family and Community Health,* 11–22.

Toshima, M., Kaplan, R., & Ries, A. (1990). Experimental evaluation of rehabilitation in chronic obstructive pulmonary disease: Short-term effects on exercise endurance and health status. *Health Psychology, 9,* 237–252.

Trombly, C. A. (1989). *Occupational therapy for physical dysfunction* (3rd ed.). Baltimore: Williams & Wilkins.

Trombly, C. (1993). The Issue Is—Anticipating the future: Assessment of occupational function. *American Journal of Occupational Therapy, 47,* 253–257. http://dx.doi.org/10.5014/ajot.41.3.253

Wang, A., & Richarde, R. S. (1987). Development of memory monitoring and self-efficacy in children. *Psychological Reports, 60,* 647–658.

Wassem, R. (1992). Self-efficacy as a predictor of adjustment to multiple sclerosis. *Journal of Neuroscience Nursing, 24,* 224–229.

CHAPTER 40

Constructions of Disability: A Call for Critical Reflexivity in Occupational Therapy

SHANON K. PHELAN

One of the primary goals of occupational therapy is to enable occupational engagement among people with disabilities. Within professional practice knowledge, there are many explicit and implicit assumptions about disability that underpin occupational therapy philosophy and define disability in a particular way. Disability is a foundational construct that lies beneath the surface of occupational therapy practices and tends not to be questioned by professionals in the discipline. Occupational therapy scholars such as Karen Whalley Hammell (2006) and Gary Kielhofner (2004) write about disability studies, asking occupational therapists to consider the critiques of rehabilitation in relation to occupational therapy practice. Applying this work to practice, I have embarked on a critically reflexive journey using a disability studies lens to begin to critique some of the implicit and explicit assumptions and pre-understandings in occupational therapy theory and practice. In my own practice as an occupational therapist in school health, I wrestled with tensions such as these, for example, with respect to handwriting and the expectations of normalcy (outlined by the funding agencies and the school systems). As I completed my progress notes at the end of my sessions, observing my own "abnormal" pencil grasp and my far from perfect penmanship, I felt a sense of unease, guilt, and almost inadequacy. Moments such as these initiated my critically reflexive journey and incited me to begin to rethink notions of disability within occupational therapy and within my own professional practice. Using critical reflexivity, this paper begins to question taken-for-granted notions of disability in order to consider how we may begin to rethink our assumptions about disability within occupational therapy theory and practice.

Critical Reflexivity

Reflexive action changes the form of the self: a reflexive practice never returns the self to the point of origin. (Sandywell, 1996, p. xiv)

Reflexivity invites one to "turn one's reflexive gaze on discourse—turning language back on itself to see the work it does in constituting the world" (Davies et al., 2004, p. 361). In this process, one begins to think critically about the world we take for granted. The process of reflection involves thinking about one's practice during (reflecting in action) or after (reflecting on action) an incident has occurred (Taylor & White, 2000). Reflexivity involves these aspects of reflection, in addition to the act of interrogating one's situatedness in society, history, culture, and how this may shape one's values, morals, and judgments at both individual and social levels. Kinsella and Whiteford (2009) suggest reflexivity surpasses reflection by introducing a critical dimension to question the conditions under which knowledge claims are accepted and constructed. Kinsella and Whiteford recently called for critical epistemological discussions within the discipline of occupational therapy in order to advance disciplinary knowledge, suggesting that it is more than a call. It is a responsibility. Epistemic reflexivity moves beyond the individual toward the social and begins to turn one's reflexive gaze on the social conditions under which knowledge is produced within the discipline (Bourdieu & Wacquant, 1992).

Critical perspectives have the potential to open new possibilities and new ways of seeing (Simon, 1992).

This chapter was previously published in the *Canadian Journal of Occupational Therapy, 78,* 164–172. Copyright © 2011, Canadian Association of Occupational Therapists. Reprinted with permission.

To be critical is to put current ideology up to question (common values and assumptions), to challenge conventional social structures, and to initiate social action (Crotty, 2007). A critical perspective allows us to gain awareness of power relationships within society and reveals the forces of hegemony and injustice (Crotty, 2007).

The term "critical reflexivity" will be used in this paper to further emphasize the necessity to examine discourse through a critical lens and to consider the possibility of praxis, as Freire (2007) defines it: reflection and action in order to transform the world around us. Critical reflexivity not only asks one to question current ideology, it also encourages one to enact change. Critical reflexivity invites new conversations with respect to conceptions of disability and begins to challenge current practices in occupational therapy. The objectives of this paper are (a) to critically examine how disability has been constructed in mainstream society by introducing perspectives from contemporary disability studies theories, and (b) to apply a critically reflexive lens to occupational therapy practice.

Emerging Perspectives on Disability

Much, but perhaps not all, of what can be socially constructed can be socially (and not just intellectually) deconstructed, given the means and the will. (Wendell, 1996, p. 45)

An emerging body of disability studies literature, critical theories of disability, and feminist disability literature discuss the notion of disability as socially constructed. This has been influential in the disability movement and on the development of new perspectives on disability (Marks, 1999). Social constructionist perspectives theorize disability as a social phenomenon, a product of societal constraints (Burr, 2003; Oliver, 1996; Shakespeare, 2006).

The social model of disability, made popular by the Union of Physically Impaired Against Segregation (UPIAS), distinguishes the notion of disability from impairment, such that people are "disabled" by social and attitudinal barriers while "impairment" is the biological limitation specific to the individual (Oliver, 1996; Shakespeare, 2006). The terms "disabled" and "impairment" and their corresponding definitions will be used in this paper to maintain the integrity of the scholarly work from which this paper draws. From this perspec-

tive, people are viewed as disabled only in settings and situations in which they are oppressed by societal structures and practices (Oliver, 1996; Shakespeare, 2006). This is contrary to the premise of the medical model, which has traditionally underpinned rehabilitation theory and practice (Hammell, 2006).

Traditionally, the medical model situates disability and impairment within the individual, using the biological impairment as the starting point for treatment (Williams, 2001). In rehabilitation professions, the focus of assessment and intervention has often been on the client's functional limitations, how these limitations affect activities of daily living, and how one might overcome his or her functional deficits in order to attain goals that allow one to function as close to normal as possible (Hammell, 2006, Williams). As an occupational therapist practicing in a pediatric setting, I often questioned why children with disabilities were receiving rehabilitation services to work towards a highly subjective "norm" that they had never known to exist, ignoring their unique life contexts. By reflecting on the differences between the biomedical model and the social model, I was able to understand this tension whereas previously it felt like a discomfort that I could not explain.

Although many occupational therapy theories, for example the Canadian Model of Occupational Performance and Engagement (Polatajko, Townsend, & Craik, 2007), encourage therapists to look beyond the individual and examine social, institutional, and environmental factors, in practice this may not always be the case when one is working within settings with limited resources and specific institutional policies and mandates. As a therapist, I often struggled with these tensions when receiving referrals focused on remediating impairment versus looking at the broader contextual issues that could also potentially contribute to inhibiting clients' participation in occupations. Despite shifts in occupational therapy philosophy toward a more holistic model of care, at times it feels that we, as therapists, are still overshadowed by dominant power structures strongly embedded in the systems we work within.

Merits of the social model notwithstanding, there are some critiques worth mentioning, particularly from feminist perspectives. Feminist scholars, such as Crow (1996), Morris (2001), and Wendell (1996), discuss disability as constructed by society; however, they argue that the individual experience of impairment must be acknowledged. They critique the social model as being narrow in its focus, not acknowledging the impairment experience and the realities of the struggles individuals may face at times, such as pain, illness, and suffering. Feminist perspectives advocate for social and cultural change to eliminate a large part of disability within society. However, they also recognize that there may be experiences of one's impairment that cannot be "fixed" and call for the implications of one's impairment to be recognized alongside disability (Crow, 1996; Wendell, 1996). This insight is important to consider in occupational therapy, creating a dialectic between the individual and the social, recognizing that the social model has a lot to offer the profession, yet realizing that it is always important to recognize individual experience.

In summary, these emerging perspectives on disability offer opportunities for occupational therapists to examine their current practices from new and relevant perspectives in order to continue to reinvent practice in a socially responsible way. Using these perspectives as a frame, constructions of disability will be discussed more deeply throughout the paper.

Constructions of Disability in Today's Mainstream Society

Drawing upon literature from several disability studies perspectives, a review of how disability has been constructed in dominant discourse will be discussed focusing on (a) constructions of "nondisabled" versus "disabled," (b) predominant metanarratives and representations of disability, (c) built environments and social structures, and (d) social and attitudinal constructions in light of disability and identity.

"Nondisabled" versus "Disabled"

Society and culture have constructed the notion of "nondisabled" versus "disabled," or "normal" versus "abnormal" as a means to make sense of our world and understand the disabled body (Davis, 1995, 2006; Linton, 1998; Marks, 1999). These categories are not fixed, as disability is culturally, socially, and historically situated. For example, Wendell (1996) discusses the pace of life as a factor that contributes to the social construction of disability. She suggests that as the pace and demands of society increase over time, there comes a time when more people are excluded from the "nondisabled" category as they can no longer meet expectations of normal performance (Wendell, 1996). Marks contends that social structures, practices, and symbols (such as the built environment, medical model, and popular media) reinforce, reproduce, and maintain these categories, mak-

ing it difficult to cross or break down barriers. He suggests that dichotomizing ability and disability creates a fear of becoming disabled, which further marginalizes and oppresses people with impairments.

Rather than accepting the nondisabled versus disabled dichotomy, some scholars take a more dynamic approach to ability and disability. From this perspective, people are viewed as only temporarily nondisabled, and at some point in a majority of people's lives, they may find themselves in a disability category (Davidson, 2006; Wendell, 1996). Wendell (2006) argues that if society accepted the notion that at some point everyone would become disabled to some degree, they would be more inclined to advocate for a society that provides the necessary resources for people of all abilities to contribute as full citizens.

Siebers (2006) writes that the prospect of becoming disabled creates fear within society, secondary to how disability has been constructed; the disabled body represents the image of Other. This is one reason that disability has become medicalized; something that medical science must treat and control (Siebers, 2006). People with disabilities and impairments are often portrayed as unhealthy even though many of them could be described as "without illness" (Wendell, 1996). Overall, the medicalization of impairments locates disability within the individual; taking responsibility away from society and placing it onto the person deemed "diseased" (Morris, 2001; Siebers, 2006; Wendell, 1996). Siebers draws attention to the merits of social constructionism, highlighting disability as the effect of an oppressive environment and advocating for advances in social justice rather than medicine and rehabilitation alone.

There is an expectation that people with disabilities must receive rehabilitation in order to reintegrate into society. Often times in rehabilitation services, including occupational therapy, people are given objects or devices such as wheelchairs, prostheses, or splints, which are seen as means to empower people. However, Siebers (2006) notes that this can occur without consideration of the reality of living with such devices. This is not to imply that assistive devices are not useful or that occupational therapists have gone wrong in any way, but that it is important to reflect on the meaning of such devices and the message they imply with respect to becoming closer to normal with respect to occupational patterns.

Looking back on my own practice experiences, I think about the many devices or adaptations that I prescribed to children in school and question what implicit messages might have been enacted for the child I was working with, his or her classmates and others within his or her social networks. One particular incident comes to mind; I was working with a teenager on handwriting. This client, very concerned, asked me, after we had completed a handwriting assessment requested on the referral, if he would be able to attend university or college if he did not have good handwriting. The client was proficient in keyboarding yet there was not enough funding within his private school to purchase a computer to make written communication easier for him. His handwriting was not "perfect," but looking at my own notes in front of me (which were barely legible in comparison) I found it hard to justify putting the client through such distress for something that seemed so trivial in the moment. Allowing him to see my handwriting and talking about my experience in postsecondary school, he was surprised and relieved that he still would be able to pursue his dreams despite what his handwriting looked like. This critical incident incited me to question norms set by society, specifically within education and occupational therapy contexts.

Finally, some scholars, for example Lennard Davis (1995, 2006), believe that there should be more emphasis on the construction of normalcy versus the construction of disability. Davis calls our attention to the fact that the concept of a "norm" implies that the majority of the population falls under the arch of a standard bell-shaped curve and those with disabilities are deviations to the norm. It is important to consider the context in which such norms have been constructed, as they are also situated in a particular historical and temporal period. I can recall an instance in practice when I conducted a gross-motor assessment with a child in kindergarten. The assessment suggested that the child was well below expectations of same-aged peers; however, the child's teacher reported that the child's performance was comparable to others in the class. After clinical observation of the child in class and at recess, I agreed with the teacher. There could be a variety of explanations for this, but, most important, I began to question whether such norms matched this specific context and, if perhaps, broader social factors were in play for this new generation.

The notion of normality has become, in Davis' view, hegemonic, such that the predominant view of the dominant group is seen as "natural" and universal for all, although it may actually be seen as a form of oppression for those outside of that dominant group. In addition, the notion of disability has also become, in Hammell's (2006) view, hegemonic as it "equates impairment with helplessness, dependency, loss, tragedy, incompetence, inadequacy and deviancy" (p. 76). Davis (2006) asserts that developing a consciousness of disability issues involves the task of reversing the hegemony of normality and taking on alternative ways of thinking about "the abnormal." This is a challenging task, but one that may be beneficial for occupational therapists to consider in theory and practice.

Metanarratives of Disability: Whose Voice Is Represented?

Although disability is frequently perceived as something to be feared and avoided, it is often represented differently, in a way that reinforces the need to become as close to "normal" as possible. Disability is often portrayed in popular media as appearing a particular way and is constructed by "nondisabled" individuals. Most often disability is represented by the image of "a young man in a wheelchair who is fit, never ill, and whose needs concern a physically accessible environment" (Morris, 2001, p. 9). Hutchinson and Kleiber (2000) view this image as one of heroic masculinity, implying that with "aggressive action and stoic perseverance in the face of overwhelming challenge" (p. 43), one can regain identity lost through the disability experience. These "disabled heroes" are readily accepted by nondisabled society because they speak to the possibility of overcoming the impairment, giving the false impression that one can defeat disability (Wendell, 2006) and also reinforcing negative connotations of disability.

Morris (2001) articulates the tensions between avoiding and embracing the experience of impairment as is, asserting that it is "dangerous because to articulate any negative feelings about our experience of our bodies may be to play into the hands of those who feel that our lives are not worth living" (p. 9). She goes on to say, "We are forced into situations of denying the experience of our bodies, of trying to conform to the outside world's view of what it is to be a full human being" (Morris, 2001, p. 10). Morris raises concerns that "if we don't express the experience of our bodies, others will do it for us. If we don't confront what we need as a result of illness, pain, and chronic conditions that inhibit our lives, then health services and support services will continue to be run in ways that disempower us" (p. 11). Wendell (1996, 2006) argues that allowing the nondisabled world to decide how disability is represented and who can be identified as "disabled" creates unequal power relations and excludes the voices of people with disabilities, which in turn may negatively affect their lives socially, economically, and psychologically.

This raises questions for occupational therapy practitioners, for example: How often do professional opinions (implicitly or explicitly) supersede the opinions of clients in clinical decision making? Do contemporary occupational therapy theory and practice privilege professional voices by design? Does the profession of occupational therapy inadvertently encourage "overcoming" disability or "disability heroism," which may unknowingly reinforce negative connotations of disability? These questions are difficult to consider as a therapist. Initially, for me, thinking about such questions invoked feelings of hostility and resistance, as they go against everything I feel I stand for as an occupational therapist. Yet, after deeper critical reflection, I began to realize that these questions are important to reflect on. Although we practice within client-centred models, we may be constrained by institutional structures and policies to act in the most client-centred way. We have been socialized in a society that has historically privileged the opinions of "professionals," which could potentially influence how decisions are made in practice and how disability is constructed. Notions of "overcoming" disability are inherently present within rehabilitation practices, which is problematic when thinking about perpetuation of negative connotations of disability. As hard as it is to question the foundations of our profession, it is with these questions and answers that we can begin to work towards becoming more socially responsible practitioners.

Built Environment and Social Structures

The built environment inevitably shapes the notion of disability as its structures inherently able or disable participation. Designers and architects are often nondisabled males who fail to consider accessibility of bodies that are different from the paradigmatic norm (young, male, fit/ideally shaped, and nondisabled) (Wendell, 1996). Aesthetics are are given priority over accessibility, and it is frequently assumed that bodies will conform to structures instead of structures conforming to bodies (Marks, 1999; Wendell, 1996). On the other hand, when accessible environments are designed they often lack aesthetic appeal, instead drawing attention to difference both by visual and auditory make-up (for example, alarms sound when lifts take people up and down stairs in public places). In these cases, "they reinforce associations of disability as something which can-

not be harmoniously included into the 'able' world" (Marks, 1999, p. 85). Creating "accessible" environments is seen as an accommodation rather than an act that facilitates the rights of others. In practice, as an occupational therapist in school health, I was called upon as a consultant when the school board was planning to make accessible rooms and washrooms. In these instances I worked with architects and school board representatives to suggest different options and adaptations to the environment. In the majority of these cases, the end result would be deemed "accessible" on paper; however, in reality it was not truly accessible. In the end, many of the subtle nuances (for example, sensor-activated lights, taps, dryers, etc.) were neglected, likely on the basis of cost and convenience. These "accommodations" did not make life for the children I worked with any more accessible. They continued to need assistance to use the toilet in the "accessible" washroom at school even though with the right design they would not be disabled in such an environment. More important, the children or others with disabilities were not always consulted with respect to their needs. These environments were considered accessible from a nondisabled perspective.

It has been suggested that restructuring our built world and implementing the concepts endorsed by universal design will assist in deconstructing the notion of disability (Marks, 1999; Wendell, 1996). Universal design involves architecture to provide access to the built environment for people of all abilities (Davidson, 2006). Although universal design promises access to all, it is important to consider that some designs will permit access for some users but act as barriers to others (Marks, 1999). In this sense, we cannot construct a perfect world, but we can do our best to design environments to deconstruct disability for the greatest number of people with diverse characteristics. In addition, Wendell (1996) recognizes that "disability cannot be deconstructed by consulting a few token disabled representatives" (p. 46.), as the experience of disability varies across impairments and the notion of normality is highly embedded in our culture, making it difficult to discern what the "problem" is—the person or society. Taking a more critical look at for whom our environment is built reveals embedded assumptions of who our culture and society deems as citizens (Marks, 1999). It is also equally important to look critically at social attitudes in deconstructing disability as the built environment is only one component of the complex creation of disability.

Disability and Identity: Social and Attitudinal Constructions

It has been suggested that the notion of disability, and acceptance of disability, affects a person's perception of self and identity (Wendell, 1996). Perceptions of self can be both positive (identifying with others with disabilities to contribute to understanding one's own experience) and negative (being labeled as disabled in society is often stigmatizing and oppressive) (Wendell, 1996). For many people with disabilities, their identities are constructed within a society in which they have often been excluded because they have been seen as deviants from the "norm" (Swain & Cameron, 1999). For this reason, many people avoid a social identity of being disabled or having a disability, and this can translate into a form of self-oppression (Swain & Cameron, 1999). Goffman (1968), an American sociologist, writes about both "inborn stigma" (for those born with disabilities) and "acquired stigma" (for those who acquire disabilities later in life). Goffman explains that those who are born with disabilities are either taught what to expect from society early on or are protected from society's notions of normality and normal identity. Those who acquire disability later in life must re-negotiate their identities. In both cases identities can be "spoiled" by stigmatization, and people with visible or nonvisible disabilities attempt to manage their spoiled identities through different strategies when encountering social interactions. For example, those with visible disabilities may focus on recovering their identities as "normal" and those with nonvisible disabilities may focus on whether or not they choose to disclose the extent of their disabilities (Goffman, 1968).

Even though many people would rather avoid the social stigma that is attached to having a disability, in many cases without such diagnosis or identity one may not receive many of the services needed (Wendell, 1996). Without such services, people with disabilities may not be able to participate in and contribute to society as they rightfully should be able to. I witnessed this tension often in practice as parents wrestled with the pros and cons of receiving a diagnosis for their child. The pressure to obtain a diagnosis was great because without one the opportunity for services diminished. In addition, parents wrestled with decisions of whether or not to reveal the diagnosis to his or her child in fear of "labeling" them and separating them from their peers. Reflecting on my experience as a therapist, tensions arise when a child does not understand why he

or she needs to see an occupational therapist at school and their classmates do not. This can result in confusion and frustration and, in some cases, resistance. This contributes to the complexity of constructing identities for persons living with disabilities.

Finally, children with disabilities may have different experiences forming identities. Literature has shown that children tend to focus on "sameness" with other children, which may be attributed to the avoidance of the negative experiences of being excluded by their peers and broader society (Connors & Stalker, 2007). Connors and Stalker assert "impairment effects, barriers to doing, and barriers to being" (p. 31) play a role in constructing a disabled childhood and identity, which may affect self-confidence and self-worth for the future. A dominant societal discourse illustrates childhood disability as personal tragedy and a place of extreme vulnerability, charity, and lack of agency. These images may be reproduced with each social encounter that a child with a disability engages in (Priestly, 1999). Priestly suggests that children's experiences of dominant images of disability contribute to a child's identity development and to the construction of disability as a social concept.

In summary, discussing notions of "nondisabled" versus "disabled," predominant metanarratives and representations of disability, built environments and social structures, and social and attitudinal constructions in light of disability and identity are just the tip of the iceberg when attempting to examine mainstream constructions of disability in relation to occupational therapy. Applying some of these ideas to current theories and practices will create opportunities for dialogue as a profession with respect to the foundations of our discipline.

Discussion

Voices bespeak conditions of embodiment that most of us would rather forget our own vulnerability to. Listening is hard, but it is also a fundamental moral act; to realize the best potential in postmodern times requires an ethics of listening. (Frank, 1995, p. 25)

In light of what has been discussed thus far, it is evident that critical reflexivity offers generative insights with respect to the examination of conceptions of disability within the occupational therapy profession. This discussion raises issues for the profession to consider with respect to constructions of disability and normalcy, both of which are embedded within the notion of rehabilitation.

Rehabilitation tends to focus strongly on impairments and remediating or "accommodating" for such impairments. Kielhofner (2004) draws our attention to three significant tensions between rehabilitation and disability studies perspectives that occupational therapists are encouraged to consider: (1) "Rehabilitation practices reinforce the idea that the disability is the disabled person's problem"; (2) "The rehabilitation professional is cast as the expert on the disabled person's condition, the implication being that the essence or meaning of disability is to be located in the objective descriptions of disability produced in professional classificatory and explanatory systems"; and (3) "Rehabilitation efforts enforce a version of normalcy that pressures disabled persons to fit in by appearing and functioning as much like nondisabled persons as possible" (p. 241). In addition, the notion of normalcy and standardized/nonstandardized norms is an issue to consider in occupational therapy. Hammell (2006) raises strong concerns regarding the constructions of norms within rehabilitation practices. Hammell asks us to begin to think more critically about how we define norms such as "normal" posture, gait, and handwriting, to name a few, and how such norms reinforce professional power and further dichotomize the nondisabled and disabled. Evidence-based practice asks therapists to rely on normed assessment to evaluate client needs; however, we must consider the risks and dangers associated with planning interventions with the sole purpose of helping clients approximate norms and ask ourselves what ideologies are we perpetuating? Is this truly our intention?

Although occupational therapists consider the person, occupation, and environment in context and are open to making adaptations in all realms, therapists are often asked to focus on the person and his or her impairment, secondary to the demands of health care settings that prioritize the biomedical model. When occupational therapists direct their intervention strategies towards environmental factors (physical, social, and institutional), they still tend to focus at an individual level. A critical disability studies perspective calls for interventions directed at socio-cultural and socio-political levels. Therapists' participation at this level would require renaming the role of occupational therapists and becoming a profession that focuses on social justice (Galheigo, 2005; Townsend & Whiteford,

2005). A broader understanding of disability, one that is explicitly focused on social justice and socio-cultural and socio-political issues may help occupational therapists carve out and articulate their niche amongst other health care professionals and align with the aims of therapists to be truly client-centred, "that is, practice where day-by-day actions are driven by a vision of changing systems to serve better those who experience occupational injustices" (Townsend & Whiteford, 2005, p. 112). This would call for advocacy by the professional body for a fundamental change in what are considered to be "traditional rehabilitation settings" in occupational therapy.

Client-centred practice is another concept that may require reconceptualization in light of a critically reflexive examination of disability. At first glance it would appear that client-centred practice would be the answer to the existing tensions between biomedical/rehabilitation perspectives and critical disabilities studies perspectives; yet, to an extent this may be misleading (Hubbard, 2004). Client-centred practice, as defined in our current system, locates the disability within the individual and places the individual at the centre of the model. A disability studies perspective, on the other hand, calls for accountability at a societal level and locates disability within society. It is important for the profession to reflect on and acknowledge the ways in which an unreflective adoption of the ideal of client-centred practice may unintentionally reinforce power structures and potentially contribute to forms of oppression (Hammell, 2006). As a profession, perhaps it is time to rethink and elaborate our understandings of client-centred practice in a way that expands beyond a focus on the individual and that considers broader social structures. In addition, it is important to critically reflect, both at individual and epistemic levels, on notions of power as professionals. In a recent study conducted by Mortenson and Dyck (2006), power relations in practice were evident at both interpersonal and institutional levels; however, institutional structures seemed to be more influential with respect to how occupational therapists enacted their practice. It is important to recognize, as Mortenson and Dyck suggest, that the health care system may be organized in a manner that denies true client-centred practice, a practice that seeks to share power between therapists and clients. Mortenson and Dyck call for more critical reflection on how client-centred practice has been constructed within institutional organizations. Such reflection could potentially allow therapists to become more aware of the implications of power relations in the context of client-centred practice from a perspective that acknowledges the ways in which disability may be socially constructed, perhaps even (unintentionally) by therapists themselves. This may lead therapists in a direction of advocacy for institutional and educational change, which may appear to be daunting at first glance. However, in order to see change we must begin to make change, even if the change begins at the micro-level and progresses to macro-level endeavors.

As a profession, we must also consider the language we adopt in our theories, models, and practice. The use of person first language has become routine, and it is likely unquestioned by most therapists, who are under the assumption that this is what people with disabilities want. Many disability scholars argue that such language further oppresses the individual, taking the onus off of society and placing it back onto to the person. Morris (2001) asserts that people with disabilities are "disabled" (i.e., by society), and the use of language in this way "describes the denial of our human rights, locates our experience of inequality as a civil rights issue, and, at the same time, creates a space to articulate our experience of our bodies" (p. 2). This is not to say one way is better than the other, but to begin to think about what political stance we want to take as a profession and how that can be represented not only in our actions but also in our language.

Wendell (1996) calls for notions of independence in rehabilitation practices to be challenged. Rehabilitation's focus on independence inadvertently depicts dependence in a negative light, further reinforcing dichotomies between ability and disability. Some scholars draw attention to notions of interdependence, recognizing the relational aspects of care and the reality that no one person is truly independent (Wendell, 1996). Whiteford and Wilcock (2000) suggest that occupational therapy may benefit by adopting notions of interdependence both theoretically and pragmatically, taking into account the uniqueness of each client and his or her family. Hammell (2006) asserts that by not contesting disciplinary preoccupations on independence, we are inadvertently reinforcing ideologies of physical independence as opposed to interdependence and reciprocity, which may potentially be offensive to people with disabilities.

Other scholars, such as Fine and Glendinning (2005), have explored notions of dependence, independence, interdependence, care, and dependency. Although they acknowledge that the notion of interdependence

deserves merit, they suggest rethinking the meanings that underpin the terms "care" and "dependency," recognizing the issues of power that permeate both constructs as these terms inevitably will still be used in policy making and research initiatives. Both positions warrant further exploration within occupational therapy theory and practice in order to begin to challenge the predominance of independence within our practices as therapists.

Perhaps the reason why many assumptions about disability appear not to be questioned in occupational therapy stems from a lack of exposure to different perspectives outside of our profession and from the predominance of the biomedical discourse. Hammell (2006) observed that health care professionals have been socialized in a culture in which their ideas and beliefs "appear not only to be natural and self-evident but benevolent and beneficial" (p. 31). This is what makes the dominant ideology so dangerous. Without engaging in critical and epistemic reflexivity such ideas and beliefs remain pristine, unquestioned, and maintained. Reading about critical disability studies and feminist critical disability studies is an eye-opening experience. For me, it shook the foundations of my professional identity, and it also became an "ah-ha" moment in which I began to understand some of the tensions that I felt as a therapist but could not name. Exposure to such literature and ideas during occupational therapy education may help to prepare future therapists for tensions they may encounter in practice in addition to helping them to become more aware and reflexive practitioners with respect to the disability experience and their roles as advocates (Franits, 2005; Kielhofner, 2005). As Hubbard (2004) suggests, "Our future clinicians cannot see through a lens they do not know exists" (p. 188).

Beginning to rethink notions of disability must begin with the voices of individuals living with disability, disability activist groups, and centers of independent living. One way of initiating this discussion may be to introduce disability studies literature into the occupational therapy curriculum (Block et al., 2005; Hubbard, 2004). In this sense, students will begin to hear from disabled persons/groups and listen to their narratives in order to understand disability from diverse perspectives. This may potentially invoke critical reflexivity at a personal level and create dialogue that can begin to deconstruct preconceived notions of disability, which have been deeply ingrained up until this point. Hubbard points out that curricula within the health professions has been developed "from the perspectives of clinician, teacher, and practitioner and casts people with disabilities into the role of patient, client, or student" (p. 187). This not only creates a dichotomy between persons with and without disabilities (Hubbard, 2004), but also reinforces and embeds notions of power, which casts those with disabilities as being "powerless." From an educational perspective, occupational therapy curriculum and fieldwork requirements may require more flexibility and modifications to ensure that people with disabilities can enroll in and successfully complete occupational therapy training with all of the same opportunities as their peers. This may help to break down dichotomies such as those between persons with and persons without disabilities, service providers and the "othering" of service recipients, and professional knowledge and the lived experience of disability.

Linton (1998) critiques the applied fields of rehabilitation for their lack of attention to disabled peoples' voices in their curricula. Linton asserts that "if rehabilitation professionals believe in self-determination for disabled people, they should practice what they teach by adhering to an active affirmative action program in their own departments; by adopting the books and essays of disabled people into their curricula; and by demanding that disabled people have an active voice in conference planning and on the platform at conferences" (p. 141).

To summarize, applying a critically reflexive lens informed by the perspectives of contemporary disability studies has offered opportunities to critically examine notions of rehabilitation, client-centred practice, disciplinary language, independence, and education within occupational therapy. Further examination of these issues may offer generative understandings of core constructs that inform our practice as occupational therapists.

Conclusion

Those who authentically commit themselves to the people must re-examine themselves constantly. (Freire, 2007, p. 60)

Reflexivity, critical or epistemic, creates uncertainty, which is one reason why many object to its practice (Taylor & White, 2000). Taylor and White (2000) assert that denying uncertainty does not eliminate it; they call for professionals to confront uncertainty in practice in order to move forward. In this paper, questions and issues are raised that may create discomfort for some and

comfort for those already wrestling with these tensions. This paper was intended to do exactly that, to disturb some of the foundational notions of disability implicit and explicit in occupational therapy, and ultimately to invite occupational therapists to engage in discussions about these tensions for the advancement of our practices. A critically reflexive examination of notions of disability reveals how powerful discourse is in naming reality and how such discourses may be oppressive. Bringing a disability studies lens to occupational therapy literature may challenge current practices and merits further investigation. Naming disability in a manner that is sensitive to humanity and the experience of persons with disability has the potential to inform models of theory and practice, which may enhance occupational therapy's mandate as a socially responsible discipline. It is acknowledged that this will not be an easy task as current practices are embedded within powerful institutions and discourses. This critically reflexive examination has revealed the ways in which occupational therapy and society at large are embedded in discourses that may reinforce negative connotations of disability. With this in mind, new understandings may pose a challenge to occupational therapists and other health professionals as well as to people with disabilities who have also accepted the dominant view. However, it is worth "making the familiar strange" to open the possibilities of making the strange familiar.

Key Messages

- Critical reflexivity invites conversation with respect to conceptions of disability within occupational therapy theory, practice, and education.
- Defining disability in a manner that is sensitive to the experience of persons with disability has the potential to inform theory and practice, enhancing occupational therapy's mandate as a socially responsible discipline.
- Bringing a disability studies lens to occupational therapy literature may challenge current practices and merits further investigation.

Acknowledgements

The author would like to extend thanks and appreciation to Dr. E. Anne Kinsella, Dr. Sandra DeLuca, Dr. Lilian Magalhães, and the manuscript reviewers for their generosity, support, and guidance during the researching and writing of this manuscript.

References

Block, P., Ricafrente-Biazon, M., Russo, A., Chu, K. Y., Sud, S., Koerner, L., . . . Olowu, T. (2005). Introducing disability studies to occupational therapy students. *American Journal of Occupational Therapy, 59*, 554–560. http://dx.doi.org/10.5014/ajot.59.5.554

Bourdieu, P., & Wacquant, L. (1992). *An invitation to reflexive sociology.* Chicago: The University of Chicago Press.

Burr, V. (2003). *Social constructionism* (2nd ed.). New York: Routledge Taylor & Francis Group.

Connors, C., & Stalker, K. (2007). Children's experiences of disability: Pointers to a social model of childhood disability. *Disability & Society, 22*, 19–33. http://dx.doi.org/10.1080/09687590601056162

Crotty, M. (2007). *The foundations of social research: Meaning and perspective in the research process.* Thousand Oaks, CA: SAGE Publications.

Crow, L. (1996). Including all of our lives: Renewing the social model of disability. In J. Morris (Ed.), *Encounters with strangers: Feminism and disability* (pp. 206–226). London: The Women's Press.

Davidson, M. (2006). Universal design: The work of disability in an age of globalization. In L. J. Davis (Ed.), *The disability studies reader* (2nd ed., pp. 117–128). New York: Routledge Taylor & Francis Group.

Davies, B., Browne, J., Gannon, S., Honan, E., Laws, C., Mueller-Rockstroh, B., & Petersen, E. B. (2004). The ambivalent practices of reflexivity. *Qualitative Inquiry, 10*, 360–389. http://dx.doi.org/10.1177/1077800403257638

Davis, L. J. (1995). *Enforcing normalcy: Disability, deafness, and the body.* New York: Verso.

Davis, L. J. (2006). Constructing normalcy: The bell curve, the novel, the invention of the disabled body in the nineteenth century. In L. J. Davis (Ed.), *The disability studies reader* (2nd ed., pp. 3–16). New York: Routledge Taylor & Francis Group.

Fine, M., & Glendinning, C. (2005). Dependence, independence or inter-dependence? Revisiting the concepts of "care" and "dependency". *Ageing & Society, 25*, 601–621.

Frank, A. W. (1995). *The wounded storyteller. Body, illness and ethics.* Chicago, IL: The University of Chicago Press.

Franits, L. E. (2005). Nothing about us is without us: Searching for the narrative of disability. *American Journal of Occupational Therapy, 59*, 577–579. http://dx.doi.org/10.5014/ajot.59.5.577

Freire, P. (2007). *Pedagogy of the oppressed. 30th anniversary edition.* New York: Continuum.

Galheigo, S. M. (2005). Occupational therapy and the social field: Clarifying concepts and ideas. In F. Kronenberg, S. S. Algado, & N. Pollard (Eds.), *Occupational therapy without borders. Learning from the spirit of survivors* (pp. 87–98). New York: Elsevier Churchill Livingstone.

Goffman, E. (1968). *Stigma: Notes in the management of spoiled identity.* Harmondsworth, UK: Penguin.

Hammell, K. W. (2006). *Perspectives on disability and rehabilitation: Contesting assumptions; challenging practice.* New York: Churchill Livingstone Elsevier.

Hubbard, S. (2004). Disability studies and health care curriculum: The great divide. *Journal of Allied Health, 33*, 184–188.

Hutchinson, S. L., & Kleiber, D. A. (2000). Heroic masculinity following spinal cord injury: Implications for therapeutic recreation practice and research. *Therapeutic Recreation Journal, 34*, 42–54.

Kielhofner, G. (2004). *Conceptual foundations of occupational therapy* (3rd ed.). Philadelphia: F. A. Davis Company.

Kielhofner, G. (2005). Rethinking disability and what to do about it: Disability studies and its implications for occupational therapy. *American Journal of Occupational Therapy, 59*, 487-496. http://dx.doi.org/10.5014/ajot.59.5.487

Kinsella, E. A., & Whiteford, G. (2009). Knowledge generation and utilisation in occupational therapy: Towards epistemic reflexivity. *Australian Occupational Therapy Journal, 56*, 249–258. http://dx.doi.org/10.1111/j.1440-1630.2007.00726.x

Linton, S. (1998). *Claiming disability: Knowledge and identity.* New York: New York University Press.

Marks, D. (1999). *Disability: Controversial debates and psychosocial perspectives.* New York: Routledge Taylor & Francis Group.

Morris, J. (2001). Impairment and disability: Constructing an ethics of care that promotes human rights. *Hypatia, 16*(14), 1–16. http://dx.doi.org/10.1353/hyp.2001.0059

Mortenson, W. B., & Dyck, I. (2006). Power and client-centred practice: An insider exploration of occupational therapists' experiences. *Canadian Journal of Occupational Therapy, 73*, 261–271. http://dx.doi.org/10.2182/cjot.06.008

Oliver, M. (1996). *Understanding disability: From theory to practice.* London: MacMillan Press Ltd.

Polatajko, H. J., Townsend, E. A., & Craik, J. (2007). Canadian model of occupational performance and engagement (CMOP-E). In E. A. Townsend & H. J. Polatajko (Eds.), *Enabling occupation II: Advancing an occupational therapy vision for health, well-being, and justice through occupation* (p. 23). Ottawa, ON: CAOT Publications ACE.

Priestly, M. (1999). Discourse and identity: Disabled children in mainstream high schools. In M. Corker & S.

French (Eds.), *Disability discourse* (pp. 92–102). Philadelphia: Open University Press.

Sandywell, B. (1996). *Reflexivity and the crisis of western reason: Logical investigations* (Vol. 1). London: Routledge.

Shakespeare, T. (2006). The social model of disability. In L. J. Davis (Ed.), *The disability studies reader* (2nd ed., pp. 197–204). New York: Routledge Taylor & Francis Group.

Siebers, T. (2006). Disability in theory: From social constructionism to the new realism of the body. In L. J. Davis (Ed.), *The disability studies reader* (2nd ed., pp. 173–183). New York: Routledge Taylor & Francis Group.

Simon, R. I. (1992). Pedagogy as political practice. In R. I. Simon (Ed.), *Teaching against the grain: Texts for a pedagogy of possibility* (pp. 55–75). Toronto, ON: OISE Press.

Swain, J., & Cameron, C. (1999). Unless otherwise stated: Discourses of labeling and identity in coming out. In M. Corker & S. French (Eds.), *Disability discourse* (pp. 68-78). Philadelphia: Open University Press.

Taylor, C., & White, S. (2000). *Practising reflexivity in health and welfare: Making knowledge.* Buckingham, UK: Open University Press.

Townsend, E., & Whiteford, G. (2005). A participatory occupational justice framework: Population-based processes of practice. In F. Kronenberg, S. S. Algado, & N. Pollard (Eds.), *Occupational therapy without borders: Learning from the spirit of survivors* (pp. 110–126). New York: Elsevier Churchill Livingstone.

Wendell, S. (1996). *The rejected body: Feminist philosophical reflections on disability.* New York: Routledge Taylor & Francis Group.

Wendell, S. (2006). Towards a feminist theory of disability. In L. J. Davis (Ed.), *The disability studies reader* (2nd ed., pp. 243–256). New York: Routledge Taylor & Francis Group.

Whiteford, G. E., & Wilcock, A. A. (2000). Cultural relativism: Occupation and independence reconsidered. *Canadian Journal of Occupational Therapy, 67*, 324–336.

Williams, G. (2001). Theorizing disability. In G. L Albrecht, K. D. Seelman, & M. Bury (Eds.), *Handbook of disability studies* (pp. 123–144). Thousand Oaks, CA: SAGE Publications.

Part V. Tools of Practice That Enable Occupational Engagement

Occupational therapy provides a mean of conserving and bringing into play whatever remains to the sick and injured of capacity for health functioning. The patient is aided in mobilizing his physical, mental and spiritual resources for overcoming his disability. The tedium and consequent depression occasioned by the enforced idleness of illness are relieved, suffering is diminished, the care and management of the patient presents fewer difficulties, convalescence is hasted, and the danger of relapse, invalidism and dependency is reduced.

—Kidner (1932, p. 239)

As evident in the above statement by Kidner (1932), occupational therapy has a strong legacy in using multiple resources to help a person engage in occupation and attain well-being. Moreover, as supported by this text's previous part, best practice in occupational therapy is consciously designed by the occupational therapy practitioner to be person directed and client centered. The entire occupational therapy process must be founded on a collaborative therapeutic relationship that is respectful of the person's unique identity, values, beliefs, and priorities (American Occupational Therapy Association [AOTA], 2014). It is important to recognize that occupational therapy practitioners' own personal identity, values, and beliefs also shape care (see Chapter 14).

Practitioners also bring their clinical reasoning skills and knowledge about the relationships between engagement in occupation and well-being to the occupational therapy process (AOTA, 2014). The *Occupational Therapy Practice Framework: Domain and Process* (3rd ed.; *Framework;* AOTA, 2014) describes *clinical reasoning* as a continuous process that "enables practitioners to identify the multiple demands, required skills, and potential meanings of the activities and occupations and gain a deeper understanding of the interrelationships between aspects of the domain that affect performance and those that will support client-centered interventions and outcomes" (p. S11). This text part provides foundational readings related to clinical reasoning and other tools of practice that comprise our professional expertise.

Rogers begins this examination in Chapter 41 with a discussion on the ethics, science, and art of clinical reasoning and a strong call for the individuation of the occupational therapy process. She poses three fundamental questions that occupational therapy practitioners should ask to ensure that interventions are congruent with the person's needs, values, goals, and lifestyle. Each question is explored in terms of the knowledge needed to answer it and the processes used to obtain this essential information, providing readers with clear guidelines and concrete suggestions for improving clinical reasoning skills.

Due to the need to individualize all decision making throughout the occupational therapy process, there is no cookbook of clinical solutions. Therefore, Rogers advocates using the art of clinical reasoning to consider the uniqueness of each person and address the complexities of clinical problems. She comprehensively explores the scientific, ethical, and artistic dimensions of clinical reasoning. Rogers substantiates these issues with several practice examples that highlight the benefits of becoming an inquisitive practitioner, enabling the transition from novice to expert practitioner.

The patient's attention must be engaged. Things which are done in a mechanical manner are not beneficial.

—Dunton (1913, p. 388)

In Chapter 42, Fleming expands on Rogers's exploration of the clinical reasoning process by reporting results of the AOTA/American Occupational Therapy Foundation's (AOTF's) Clinical Reasoning Study (Gillette & Mattingly, 1987). This landmark research project analyzed the reasoning processes used by therapists in solving problems in their day-to-day practice. After extensive study, four types of reasoning—procedural, interactive, conditional, and narrative—were identified.[1] The first three are discussed extensively in this chapter, and the last is explored in depth in the following chapter (Chapter 43). Fleming defines each type of reasoning and discusses their major characteristics, purposes, methods, values, and benefits. She provides case examples to substantiate implementing these principles into clinical practice and add humanness to the discussion (see Active Reflection V.1).

This chapter supports the notion that practitioners can "walk and chew gum at the same time" by holistically working with a person using a multi-track mind. The ability to use diverse perspectives in a health care system that devalues holism and supports concrete reductionist procedures is a critical skill needed throughout the occupational therapy process. In this study, experienced occupational therapy practitioners appeared to move smoothly and sometimes rapidly among the different types of reasoning or simultaneously use multiple types of reasoning as they analyzed, interpreted, and resolved different types of clinical problems throughout the occupational therapy process.

Fundamental to the thinking of occupational therapy practitioners is the use of a narrative model of reasoning. In Chapter 43, Mattingly argues that traditional scientific modes of reasoning are incongruent with the occupational therapy process because practitioners think with stories. This narrative thought process became evident during the aforementioned AOTA/AOTF clinical reasoning study, which found that occupational therapy practitioners actively listen to the stories told to them by their clients and relate stories about the people they work with to others. Mattingly presents a compelling argument for the value of this storytelling process. Storytelling helps practitioners understand an individual's uniquely personal experience of illness or disability. It also enables both practitioners and clients to make sense of this experience.

In addition to storytelling, Mattingly found that occupational therapy practitioners create stories that allow the person to remake the story of his or her life once it has been altered by an illness or disability experience. When occupational therapy practitioners create a prospective treatment story, they imagine the potentialities of the person's future. Mattingly terms this

---

> **Active Reflection V.1. Clinical Reasoning**
>
> Think about a particularly challenging individual with whom you worked or observed in a practice setting. Analyze this person's situation using all modes of clinical reasoning.
> - How could the insights that you gained from this analysis be used to guide the occupational therapy process?
> - What prospective story can you imagine for this person?

process *therapeutic emplotment*, because this envisioned future guides the occupational therapy process. The power of narrative reasoning in helping practitioners make sense of the uniquely human experience of living with illness and disability, and its effectiveness in helping us uncover different motivational possibilities to move people to act, is strongly supported by a case example. Mattingly's story of the development of the "NY Gang" is a stellar example of the power of client-centered practice based on narrative reasoning.

Given that there are organizational, social, political, and economic realities that can affect the provision of client-centered occupational therapy, practitioners need to know how to effectively integrate these pragmatics into their clinical reasoning process (Schell & Cervero, 1993). In Chapter 44, Restall, Ripat, and Stern present a useful tool to overcome barriers to the provision of client-centered services. The Client-centred Strategic Framework (CSF) was developed by these authors in response to their observation that implementing client-centered occupational therapy was often stymied by the many challenges presented by clinicians, clients, client–clinician relationships, practice contexts, and setting environments (see Active Reflection V.2). The CSF builds upon the previously published Client-centered Process Evaluation (Stern, Restall, & Ripat, 2000), which was designed to obtain client input, evaluate occupational therapy services, analyze practice contexts, and facilitate improvements in practice. It is comprised of five categories (i.e., personal reflection, client-centered processes, practice settings, community organizing, coalition advocacy and political action) that recognize the multidimensional and complex nature of client-centered practice.

[S]he has the pleasure of doing creative work in the form of handicrafts, and she will in the future feel a deeper interest in the patient's endeavor to overcome physical and mental obstacles through the work of his hands.

—Spainhower (1925, p. 380)

---

[1]Alternative perspectives on the types of clinical reasoning (including scientific, narrative, pragmatic, and ethical reasoning) were put forth by Schell and Cervero (1993) and Schell (1998).

Restall et al. elaborate on each CSF category and its unique relationship to the provision of client-centered occupational therapy. They challenge readers to consciously (and honestly) reflect on their personal views of, and experiences with, each dimension of client-centered practice. Because even the best of client-centered services can be thwarted by systemic barriers, their expanded view of client-centered occupational therapy to include setting, community, and social–political dimensions are particularly illuminating.

Restall et al. provide a clear outline of the complete CSF in a table that has concrete recommendations for specific actions practitioners can take to actualize client-centered principles within the realities of diverse practice settings. They describe a common challenge to the provision of client-centered practice and use this case to illustrate the conscious use of the strategies provided for each CSF category. This integrated case example provides a realistic exemplar on the use of the CSF to effectively problem solve the best way to provide client-centered occupational therapy. Most important, it demonstrates how the CSF can be used to help students and novice and experienced practitioners move out of their established comfort zones and implement innovations that can enhance existing client-centered practices and expand systemic supports for client-centered services through coalition building and political action. Those who add this strategic framework to their occupational therapy "toolbox" and consistently apply the strategies recommended by Restall et al. will find that they can capably and proactively address the challenges they face to client-centered practice.

In addition to struggling with barriers to client-centered practice, many occupational therapy students and novice practitioners frequently struggle with the basic question of what to actually say to a person about the planned occupational therapy intervention. Chapter 45 provides clear guidelines to help address this fundamental concern. In this chapter, Peloquin presents an outstanding discussion on linking purpose to procedures during each therapeutic interaction we have with our clients. She explores the effectiveness of a collaborative approach that involves people in the intervention process and examines the increased efficacy of intervention when individuals know the purpose of each given treatment session. Peloquin presents a clear rationale for discussing the relevance and purpose of any and all procedures with clients. Her stance that every intervention session provides the practitioner with an opportunity to link goals with a structured activity that is relevant to the individual is strong.

If the work is made a joke or a kindergarten exercise, then bedside occupations will do more harm than good. Equally fated will be too technical or matter of fact approach.

—Hall (1919, p. 12)

Peloquin provides concrete examples and realistic suggestions for developing this collaborative approach. Providing the purpose of each activity can increase a person's knowledge about the reasons for the intervention, thereby increasing the level of active participation in the session. Peloquin contends that the need to consistently integrate goal statements with occupational therapy intervention is critically important because of three realities: (1) current health care trends, (2) traditional occupational therapy assumptions supportive of the collaborative process, and (3) the often ambiguous nature of occupational therapy's primary modality of activity. The health care system's emphasis on informed consent, treatment accountability, and patient rights provide strong justification for incorporating a collaborative approach into each occupational therapy session.

One foundational tool of practice that can help occupational therapy practitioners effectively use the primary modality of activity and explain the purpose of occupational therapy intervention to clients is activity analysis. To achieve therapeutic goals there must be a match between a person who has been holistically assessed and an activity that has been thoroughly analyzed and synthesized (AOTA, 2014; McGarry, 1990; Mosey, 1996; Wilson & Landry, 2014). Activity analysis and synthesis have been major tools of occupational therapy practice from the profession's inception, and they have maintained their relevance and importance throughout the years. The need to analyze activities to determine how the demands of the activity relate to the person's skills and to successful performance is emphasized in the *Framework* (AOTA, 2014). Although the *Framework* provides an integrated view of activity analysis that includes the consideration of the activity's social, cultural, and physical environmental requirements (AOTA, 2014), traditionally, this process often focused on an activity's physical and kinetic demands (Licht, 1947; Murphy, 1943) or psychodynamic properties (Llorens & Rubin, 1962; Weston, 1961).

In Chapter 46, Creighton explores this reductionist view of activity analysis and traces the evolution of this process to its more recent holistic conceptualization. The origin of activity analysis in the early 1900s with the initial development of structural activity analysis on the basis of motion studies is discussed. The first systematic application of activity analysis in an occupational therapy clinic is presented. These early analyses emphasized the study of movement required by each activity and the subsequent adaptations of the activities to improve physical function or compensate for a movement deficit.

Creighton describes the evolution of activity analysis between World War I and World War II and the expansion of activity analysis to include activities' psychosocial characteristics. However, she states, these analyses continued to perpetuate a physical and psychosocial split reflective of the dichotomy between psychiatric and physical disabilities practices. Creighton examines the refinement of activity analysis into an integrated, holistic approach in the 1970s and 1980s as frames of reference were further developed. The current view of activity analysis as a multifaceted process that also considers environmental contexts according to a frame of reference is emphasized.

An insight may be gained as to why an occupation with qualities that hold attention and stimulate

may be good for one type of patient while another needs a craft with more sedative qualities.
—Spainhower (1925, p. 377)

Activity analysis is just one of the tools of occupational therapy practice that has evolved over the course of the profession's history. In Chapter 47, Reed critically examines many factors that determine whether the profession adopts, maintains, or discards a tool of practice. Occupational therapy practitioners have used many media and methods for intervention over the years (Bissell & Mailloux, 1981; Carmer, 1933; Freidland, 1988; Friedman, 1953; Llorens & Rubin, 1962; Morse, 1936; Murphy, 1943; Taylor & Manguno, 1991; Thompson & Blair, 1998), but the reasons for embracing or abandoning numerous media or methods are often unclear. In her Eleanor Clarke Slagle Lecture, Reed postulates that the lack of a rationale for using medium or method may lead to limited understanding of its therapeutic value for both the practitioner and the client.

This lack of awareness can compromise the therapeutic potential of the selected tool of practice. Reed suggests that eight factors—cultural, social, economic, political, technological, theoretical, historical, and research—influence the selection or abandonment of tools of practice in occupational therapy. Reed explores the nature of these influences, providing clear and relevant examples to highlight her points. She summarizes the effects of these eight factors by proposing 14 assumptions and providing three relevant, yet diverse, examples to illustrate how these factors and assumptions operate to affect the use of specific tools in occupational therapy practice. Reed emphasizes that the media, methods, and objectives of an activity must be consistent with each other for the activity to be purposeful and meaningful. She asserts that careful consideration of cultural, social, individual, and professional interests and values will ensure that the tools used in occupational therapy practice will have therapeutic value and be meaningful and purposeful to the individual (see Figure V.1 and Active Reflections V.3–V.5).

Daily we are impressed with the revival of interest in religion, the revanescence of handicrafts. . . . All about us are signs of the swing of the pendulum from crass materialism to a renewed acknowledgement of man's need for human kindness and compassion, for individual creative effort. What could be more assuring to people engaged in the practice of healing through doing?
—Sokolov (1956, p. 16)

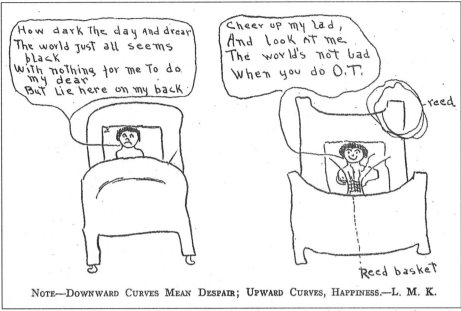

Figure V.1. Insights on the therapeutic value of occupational therapy tools of practice from 1922.

Source. From "Teaching Occupational Therapy to Student Nurses," by B. Spainhower, 1925, *American Journal of Nursing,* Vol. 25, p. 378.

Reed's call for practitioners to increase their awareness of the *why* of practice to ensure their interventions are consistent with occupational therapy philosophy is a timely one. Since the publication of Reed's address, tools of practice used by occupational therapists have expanded greatly, and this growth is likely to be exponential in the future (Hinojosa, 2007). Although it is not within this text's scope to review all tools of occupational therapy practice, I have included AOTA official documents concerning three tools that have had (or will have) important implications for the field in this part's appendices. For example, the use of physical agent modalities (PAMs) has become commonplace in physical rehabilitation practice settings (see Appendix V.A). However, the introduction of PAMs to occupational therapy practice was not universally heralded as advancement for the field. Some viewed these modalities as incongruent with the profession's focus on therapeutic occupation (Fidler, 1992; West & Wiemer, 1991).

Do we keep in mind the query, 'why do I do this? Is it effective and why'? A troublesome but stimulating and thought-provoking question.

—Morse (1936, p. 297)

Active Reflection V.4. Tools of Practice in Occupational Therapy

Reflect on the tools of occupational therapy practice presented in Appendixes V.A.–V.C.
- How have the influential factors identified by Reed affected the development and use of PAMs, CAM, and telerehabilitation in occupational therapy?
- Do you think adopting these contemporary tools of practice will contribute to the loss of occupational therapy's heritage, or are they appropriate tools that can enrich current and future practice?
- How can practitioners use these tools in a manner that is consistent with the occupational therapy's philosophical foundations?

Active Reflection V.5. Clinical Application of Practice Tools

Review the case provided in Exhibit V.1. Identify the tools of practice and principles of intervention that were used and those that were not used in the described session.
- How would you have increased the relevance of occupational therapy to Helen and engaged her and in the occupational therapy process? Describe your approach.
- Identify an evaluation method and an intervention approach that could potentially be used to facilitate Helen's engagement. Describe how you would have explained the purposes of your evaluation and intervention to Helen to facilitate her active participation in the occupational therapy process.

In 1966, West observed that in physical therapy "physical agent agents as [sic] heat, light, water, electricity, and ultrasound, among others, are used to aid the restoration of physical function . . . these media by their very nature are *applied to the patient and controlled by the therapist,* whereas the media and activities common to occupational therapy are primarily those in which *the patient himself actively engages or participates*" (West, 1966, p. 1709, italics added). To differentiate the use of PAMs by occupational therapy practitioners from their use by physical therapy practitioners, AOTA has published several position papers over the years that clarify that PAMs are preparatory or adjunctive methods to the therapeutic use of occupation (AOTA, 1997, 2003, 2008). In the most recent AOTA position paper on PAMS (AOTA, 2012; see Appendix V.A), it is clearly stated that "the exclusive use of PAMs as a therapeutic intervention without direct application to occupational performance is *not* considered occupational therapy" (p. S78, italics added).

Consistent with this view, Ahlschwede (1992) describes an approach to treatment that is realistic and congruent with occupational therapy's philosophical base. She states that the time "during which a patient's hand is sandwiched between hot packs is spent discussing occupational performance or daily living components, collaborative goal setting, and patient education, or addressing psychosocial concerns or issues that the patient may have" (p. 650). This interactive holistic approach is a strong contrast to the one presented in Exhibit V.1 (see also Active Reflection V.6).

> ### Active Reflection V.6. Ethical Decision Making
>
> Reflect on the case provided in Exhibit V.1 and its relationship to ethical practice.
> - Which principles of AOTA's (2010) *Occupational Therapy Code of Ethics and Ethics Standards (2010)* did this occupational therapy practitioner not consider?
> - What were the likely external factors that may have contributed to this practitioner's use of a meaningless activity in a manner that ignored the individual?
> - How could the structured approach to ethical decision making as described in Howowitz's chapter be used to ensure that future sessions with Helen are congruent with the occupational therapy profession's ethical standards and core values?

Similar to the use of PAMs, complementary and alternative medicine (CAM) has been proposed as appropriate for occupational therapy practitioners to use as "preparatory methods or purposeful activities to facilitate the ability of clients to engage in their daily life occupations" (AOTA, 2011, p. S27). Use of CAM has been identified as reflective of "the core of what occupational therapy is as a healing profession" (Haltiwanger & Stein, 2009, p. 2). The global recognition of CAM as a holistic, client-centered approach to be used and researched by occupational therapy practitioners is expanding (Haltiwanger & Stein, 2009). In the United States, AOTA (2011) has published an official statement on CAM (see Appendix V.B). This document examines the practice of CAM in the United States and describes how CAM can be appropriately, competently, and ethically used by occupational therapy practitioners. It proposes that including CAM into occu-

Exhibit V.1. Helen and the Disappearing Pegs

Helen was an elderly woman with multiple physical disabilities, including diabetes, bilateral lower-extremity amputations, expressive aphasia, upper-extremity (UE) weakness, and decreased UE range of motion. She had a feeding tube and was dependent in all ADLs. She was also perceived by many to have a major cognitive deficit, because her interactions with her environment were limited to moans and attempts to remove her feeding tube and slide out of her wheelchair.

One day, while waiting with my brother in the occupational therapy clinic, we observed a therapist place numerous pegs on the right side of Helen's lapboard and a basket on the floor to the left of her wheelchair. The therapist told Helen her activity for the day was to pick up each peg and drop it into the basket. She demonstrated the desired movement and then asked Helen to begin the activity. Helen dutifully picked up a peg, crossed her midline, and dropped the peg into the basket. The therapist praised Helen and told her to continue this activity until all of the pegs were placed in the basket. She then walked away to set up another patient with a "treatment activity."

Helen watched her walk away, and as the therapist began to talk to another client, Helen placed her forearm on her lapboard, and by moving her forearm across the surface, she placed all of the pegs in the basket in one fell swoop. A gasp of breath and then laughter came from both my brother and I as we witnessed her cleverness in completing her assigned task. Helen instantly turned her gaze at us. Giving us a stern look and placing her index finger to her lips, she nonverbally commanded us to "shh." We complied, and Helen serenely waited for the therapist to return.

After about 20 minutes, the therapist returned to shower Helen with profuse praise for doing the activity so well. A transporter was then summoned to take Helen back to her room. As she was wheeled past us, Helen gave us a profound wink and a smile. Thereafter, each time Helen saw my brother and I, she would wink and put her finger to her lips. This supposedly cognitively disabled woman turned out to be one sharp lady with a great sense of humor. It was tragic that so few ever got to know her and that the potential of occupational therapy was never realized for her.

Note. ADLs = activities of daily living.

pational therapy's scope of practice can enhance the comprehensiveness of the approaches used by occupational therapy practitioners to enable occupational engagement, promote health, and facilitate participation at the personal, organizational, and population level (AOTA, 2011).

Additional practice innovations that hold great promise for enabling participation in life and the attainment of occupational well-being include the use of assistive technology (Polger, 2006; Verdonck & Ryan, 2008), including service animals (Winkle, Crowe, & Hendrix, 2012); virtual reality (Bondoc, Powers, Herz, & Hermann, 2010), including Wii health and rehabilitation (Bacon, Farnworth, & Boyd, 2012; Brosnan, 2009); the Internet (Chiu & Henderson, 2005); and the emerging service delivery system of telehealth (Cason, 2012). The telehealth delivery model uses "information and communication technologies to deliver evaluative, consultative, preventative, and therapeutic services to clients who in a different location than the practitioner" (Cason, 2012, p. CE1).

Recognizing the potential that telehealth has for the provision of occupational therapy services without geographic constraints, AOTA (2013) published a comprehensive official document on its use (see Appendix V.C). In this document, the use of telehealth as a service delivery model that enables provision of occupational therapy in places where people live work, learn, and play is described. Practitioners' ability to improve access to occupational therapy in isolated and underserved communities by using telehealth technologies to provide teleevaluation, telerehabilitation, teleintervention, teleconsultation, and telemonitoring are clearly explained. Case examples and supporting research are provided. The need to use clinical reasoning to guide appropriate and competent use of telehealth technologies for occupational therapy service delivery is emphasized. Practitioner qualifications and supervisory guidelines for telehealth practice are highlighted. The ethical dimensions of telehealth and strategies for ethical practice using telehealth technologies are outlined.

The importance of using ethics to guide practice is explored in depth in this part's last chapter. In Chapter 48, Horowitz thoughtfully examines the impact that emerging areas of practice, changing health care environments, and increased demands on practitioners have on the ethical practice of occupational therapy. The reality that current practice requires occupational therapy practitioners to pay increased attention to cost-effectiveness and functional outcomes in an envi-

ronment that often challenges ethical practice is well supported by clinical examples. Horowitz reflects on how personal values and ethics influence one's ability to recognize ethical issues, challenges, and dilemmas. She explores the role of a profession's code of ethics and the societal expectation that a profession provide ethical practice in a morally responsible manner. Horowitz reviews Purtilo's Six-Step Approach to ethical decision making, which provides strategies that can effectively structure the problem-solving process needed when an occupational therapy practitioner is confronted with an ethical challenge, problem, or dilemma.

Horowitz advises that using this organized approach to ethical decision making can reduce practitioners' distress and thereby decrease the risk of burnout. A case study is provided to demonstrate the efficacy of using a structured approach to solving an ethical problem. The reality that additional resources and strategies are needed to ethically respond to the complexities of everyday occupational therapy practice is well-supported by this example and Horowitz's discussion. The need for occupational therapy practitioners to actively and continuously reflect on our profession's core values and ethics and our professional legal and social responsibilities to ensure that our actual practices remain ethically and morally congruent is strongly validated by Horowitz's analysis. Those who forget the vital importance of this reflective process and argue that systemic constraints force them to use reductionist interventions in an isolated manner will likely continue to scurry from treatment session to treatment session with little to no meaningful interaction with their clients, perpetuating stagnation and burnout. In contrast, those who continuously and actively reflect on their practice and maintain a holistic approach grounded in the profession's core beliefs (in spite of system limitations) will enjoy rich and empowering collaborations with their clients, sustaining growth and fulfillment.

I intend for the chapters in this part and throughout the text to provide readers with helpful information and practical resources that will enable them to readily choose the latter course of action. By using traditional and contemporary occupational therapy tools of practice that are purposeful and meaningful to the person in a collaborative and ethical manner, the art and science of occupational therapy can be actualized.

In this basket there must be variety. The man who colors reeds will not touch moccasins; the one who loves to print photographs sees no special attraction in rugs. There is always something interesting for each person.

—Tracy (1921, p. 398)

References

Ahlschwede, K. (1992). The Issue Is—Views on physical agent modalities and specialization within occupational therapy: A rebuttal. *American Journal of Occupational Therapy, 46*, 650–652. http:dx.doi.org/10.5014/ajot.46.7.650

American Occupational Therapy Association. (1997). Physical agent modalities position paper. *American Journal of Occupational Therapy 51*, 870–871. http://dx.doi.org/10.5014/ajot.51.10.870

American Occupational Therapy Association. (2003). Physical agent modalities. *American Journal of Occupational Therapy, 57*, 650–651. http://dx.doi.org/10.5014/ajot.62.6.691

American Occupational Therapy Association. (2008). Physical agent modalities: A position paper. *American Journal of Occupational Therapy, 62*, 691–693. http://dx.doi.org/10.5014/ajot.62.6.691

American Occupational Therapy Association. (2010). Occupational therapy code of ethics and ethics standards (2010). *American Journal of Occupational Therapy, 64*(Suppl.), S17–S26. http://dx.doi.org/10.5014/ajot.2010.64S17

American Occupational Therapy Association. (2011). Complementary and alternative medicine. *American Journal of Occupational Therapy, 65*(Suppl.), S26–S31. http://dx.doi.org/10.5014/ajot.2011.65S26

American Occupational Therapy Association. (2012). Physical agent modalities. *American Journal of Occupational Therapy, 66*(Suppl.), S78–S80 http://dx.doi.org/10.5014/ajot.2012.66S78

American Occupational Therapy Association. (2013). Telehealth. *American Journal of Occupational Therapy, 67*(Suppl.), S92–S102. http://dx.doi.org/10.5014/ajot.2013.67S69 Reprinted as Appendix V.C.

American Occupational Therapy Association. (2014). Occupational therapy practice framework: Domain and process (3rd ed.). *American Journal of Occupational Therapy, 68*(Suppl. 1), S1–S48. http://dx.doi.org/10.5014/ajot.2014.682006

Bacon, N., Farnworth, L., & Boyd, R. (2012). The use of Wii Fit in forensic mental health: Exercise for people at risk of obesity. *British Journal of Occupational Therapy, 75*, 61–67. http://dx.doi.org/10.4276/030802212X13286281650992

Bissell, J., & Mailloux, Z. (1981). The use of crafts in occupational therapy for the physically disabled. *American Journal of Occupational Therapy, 35*, 369–374. http://dx.doi.org/10.5014/ajot.35.6.369

Bondoc, S., Powers, C., Herz, N., & Hermann, V. (2010). Virtual reality-based rehabilitation. *OT Practice, 15*(11), CE1–CE4.

Brosnan, S. (2009). The potential of Wii-rehabilitation for persons recovering from acute stroke. *Physical Disabilities Special Interest Section Quarterly, 32*(1), 1–3.

Carmer, D. R. (1933). Handicrafts for threescore years and ten. *Occupational Therapy & Rehabilitation, 12*, 107–111.

Cason, J. (2012). An introduction to telehealth as a service delivery model within occupational therapy. *OT Practice, 17*(7), CE1–CE4.

Chiu, T., & Henderson, J. (2005). Developing Internet-based occupational therapy services. *American Journal of Occupational Therapy, 59*, 626–630. http://dx.doi.org/10.5014/ajot.59.6.626

Dunton, W. R. (1913, March 1). Occupation as a therapeutic measure. *Medical Record*, pp. 388–389.

Fidler, G. (1992). Against use of physical agent modalities. *American Journal of Occupational Therapy, 46*, 567. http://dx.doi.org/10.5014/ajot.46.6.567a

Freidland, J. (1988). Diversional activity: Does it deserve its bad name? *American Journal of Occupational Therapy, 42*, 603–608. http://dx.doi.org/10.5014/ajot.42.9.603

Friedman, I. (1953). Art in therapy: An outline of suggested procedures. *American Journal of Occupational Therapy, 8*, 169–170.

Gillette, N. P., & Mattingly, C. (1987). The Foundation: Clinical reasoning in occupational therapy. *American Journal of Occupational Therapy, 41*, 399–400. http://dx.doi.org/10.5014/ajot.41.6.399

Hall, H. J. (1919). *Bedside and wheelchair occupations*. New York: Red Cross Institute for Crippled and Disabled Men.

Haltiwanger, E., & Stein, F. (2009). Editorial: Occupational therapy and complementary and alternative medicine. *Occupational Therapy International, 16*(1), 1–5.

Hinojosa, J. (2007). Becoming innovators in an era of hyperchange [Eleanor Clarke Slagle Lecture]. *American Journal of Occupational Therapy, 61*, 629–637. http://dx/doi.org/10.5014/ajot.61.6.629

Kidner, T. B. (1932). Occupational therapy: Its aims and developments. *Occupational Therapy and Rehabilitation, 11*(4), 233–240.

Licht, S. (1947). Kinetic analysis of craft and occupations. *Occupational Therapy and Rehabilitation, 26*, 75–78.

Llorens, L., & Rubin, E. (1962). A directed activity program for disturbed children. *American Journal of Occupational Therapy, 16*, 287–290

McGarry, J. (1990). National perspective: Our special skill—Is it lost? *Canadian Journal of Occupational Therapy, 57,* 258–259.

Morse, H. (1936). Crafts in a general hospital. *Occupational Therapy and Rehabilitation, 15,* 295–299. http://dx.doi. org/10.1097/00002060-193610000-00003

Mosey, A. C. (1996). *Psychosocial components of occupational therapy.* New York: Raven Press.

Murphy, J. S. (1943). Crafts that interest men. *Occupational Therapy and Rehabilitation, 22,* 146–150.

Polger, J. M. (2006). Muriel Driver Lecture 2006: Assistive technology as an enabler to occupation: What's old is new again. *Canadian Journal of Occupational Therapy, 73,*199–205.

Schell, B., & Cervero, R. (1993). Clinical reasoning in occupational therapy: An integrative review. *American Journal of Occupational Therapy, 47,* 605–610. http:// dx.doi.org/10.5014/ajot.47.7.605

Schell, B. (1998). Clinical reasoning: The basis of practice. In M. Neistadt & E. Crepeau (Eds.), *Willard and Spackman's occupational therapy* (9th ed., pp. 90–100). Philadelphia: Lippincott Williams & Wilkins.

Sokolov, J. (1956). Therapist into administrator: Ten inspiring years [Eleanor Clark Slagle Lecture]. *American Journal of Occupational Therapy, 11,* 13–19.

Spainhower, G. (1925). Teaching occupational therapy to student nurses. *American Journal of Nursing, 25,* 376–381.

Stern, M., Restall, G., & Ripat, J. (2000). The use of self-reflection to improve client-centered processes. In V. Fearing & J. Clark (Eds.), *Individuals in context: A practical guide to client-centered practice* (pp. 145–158). Thorofare, NJ: Slack.

Taylor, E., & Manguno, J. (1991). Use of treatment activities in occupational therapy. *American Journal of Occupational Therapy, 45,* 317–322. http://dx/doi. org/10.5014/ajot.45.4.317

Thompson, M., & Blair, S. (1998). Creative arts in occupational therapy: Ancient history or contemporary practice. *Occupational Therapy International, 5*(1), 48–64. http://dx.doi.org/10.1002/oti.67

Tracy, S. E. (1921). Getting started in occupational therapy. *The Trained Nurse and Hospital Review, LXVII*(5), 397–399.

Verdonck, M., & Ryan, S. (2008). Mainstream technology as an occupational therapy tool: Technophobe or technogeek? *British Journal of Occupational Therapy, 71,* 253–256.

West, W. (1966). Occupational therapy philosophy and perspective. *American Journal of Nursing, 68,* 1708–1711. http://dx.doi.org/10.2307/3420981

West, N. L., & Wiemer, R. B. (1991). The Issue Is—Should the Representative Assembly have voted as it did, when it did, on occupational therapists' use of physical agent modalities? *American Journal of Occupational Therapy, 45,* 1143–1147. http://dx.doi.org/10.5014/ajot.45.12.1143

Weston, D. (1961). The dimensions of crafts. *American Journal of Occupational Therapy, 15,* 1–5.

Wilson, S., & Landry, G. (2014). *Task analysis: An individual, group, and population approach* (3rd ed.). Bethesda, MD: AOTA Press.

Winkle, M., Crowe, T., & Hendrix, I. (2012). Service dogs and people with physical disabilities partnerships: A systemic review. *Occupational Therapy International, 19,* 54–66. http://dx.doi.org/10.1002/oti.323

CHAPTER 41

Clinical Reasoning:
The Ethics, Science, and Art

JOAN C. ROGERS

A therapist, employed at a regional rehabilitation center, extracts cues from the records of acute hospitals, to judge the rehabilitation potential of patients referred for admission. Another therapist, working with persons with mental retardation, selects a treatment approach based on task analysis to teach self-care skills. A third therapist, serving on a geriatric assessment team, uses scores on a mental status examination and performance ratings in daily living activities to estimate patients' ability to continue living alone in their homes. A fourth therapist reviews patients' progress in manual dexterity to formulate a recommendation for or against hand surgery. These four therapists are using their clinical reasoning skills to collect and transform data about patients into decisions that have critical implications for the quality of life of their patients.

If we questioned the therapists about their decisions, each would probably comment on their potential fallibility. Some patients, denied occupational therapy because of a perceived lack of potential for rehabilitation, would make substantial gains in functional skills if intervention were initiated. Some patients with mental retardation will not benefit from the task breakdown approach to self-care training. Some geriatric patients admitted for institutional living could have been supported adequately in the community. Some patients undergoing hand surgery will lose functional abilities. The possibility of error in our clinical judgments and the potential ensuing negative consequences urge us to develop ways of improving our assessment and treatment decisions.

Despite the obvious importance of clinical judgment in the occupational therapy process, little attention has been given to explicating the thinking that guides practice. My research, albeit with a small number of occupational therapists, suggests that our cognitive processes are regarded as intuitive and ineffable. For example, when therapists were asked how they arrived at their treatment decisions, they commonly responded by saying, "I have never really thought about it" or "I don't know how I reached that conclusion. I just know." Cognitive activity constitutes the heart of the clinical enterprise. Our failure to study the process of knowing and understanding that underlies practice precludes an adequate description of clinical reasoning. This in turn prevents the development of a methodology for systematically improving it and for teaching it.

I intend to explore here the reasoning process through which we learn about patients so that we may help them through engagement in occupation. I will construct an intellectual device for viewing clinical reasoning from the perspective of the basic questions the therapist seeks to answer through clinical inquiry. The scientific, ethical, and artistic dimensions of clinical reasoning will be elucidated as these questions are explored. The device will be useful for directing and appraising our thoughts about treating patients and for developing a clinical science of occupational therapy. In developing my thoughts, I have relied on the basic scheme of clinical judgment presented by Pellegrino (1) for medicine and have adapted it to the occupational therapy process.

The Goal of Clinical Reasoning

The goal of the clinical reasoning process has an impact on each of the steps taken to achieve the goal. Hence, an appreciation of this goal provides insight on the whole process.

Patients come to occupational therapy when they, their physicians, family members, or caregivers perceive that they are not adequately performing their daily activities. Performance in self-care, work, and leisure occupations has been compromised because of the consequences of disease, trauma, abnormal development, age-related changes, or environmental restrictions. The disruptions in occupational functions are characteristically severe and enduring as opposed to transitory. To regain a former level of performance, maintain the current level, or achieve a more optimal one, the patient enlists the aid of the therapist. The therapist's task, therefore, is to select a right therapeutic action for the patient (1). In other words, the goal of clinical reasoning is a treatment recommendation issued in the interests of a particular patient. Decision-making is highly individualized.

The occupational therapy treatment plan details what a particular patient should do to enhance occupational role performance. The therapeutic action must be the right action for this individual. This implies that it must be as congruent as possible with the patient's concept of the "good life." Treatment should be in concert with the patient's needs, goals, lifestyle, and personal and cultural values. A therapeutic program that is right for one patient is not necessarily right for another. The ultimate question we, as clinicians, are challenged to answer is: What, among the many things that could be done for this patient, ought to be done? This is an ethical question. It involves a judgment to which facts contribute but that must be decided by weighing values. A salient criterion of an ethical action is its agreement with the patient's valued goals. The clinical reasoning process terminates in an ethical decision, rather than in a scientific one, and the ethical nature of the goal of clinical reasoning projects itself over the entire sequence.

Ethical decisions regarding treatment are not made in isolation from scientific knowledge. The patient comes to the therapist for expert advice regarding adaptation to chronic dysfunction. The factual basis for decision-making is provided by the therapist. When therapists set out to solve clinical problems, they are confronted with an unknown—the patient. Scientific methodologies are used to learn about the patient. Once the patient's condition is adequately understood, scientific and empirical knowledge is applied in the efforts to enhance occupational status. Although ethical considerations can override scientific ones, they do not displace the need to secure a scientific opinion.

Clinical Questions

To ascertain the right action for each patient, clinical inquiry focuses on three questions: What is the patient's current status in occupational role performance? What could be done to enhance the patient's performance? And what ought to be done to enhance occupational competence? These are the fundamental questions that I previously alluded to as guiding the clinical process. Each question will be considered first in terms of the knowledge needed to answer it, and, subsequently, in terms of the cognitive processes used to obtain the knowledge.

What Is the Patient's Status?

Assessment

The first question to be considered is the assessment question: What is the patient's occupational status? The occupational therapy assessment is a concise and accurate summary of a patient's occupational role performance that arises from an investigation of the patient. The occupational therapy assessment tells us what we need to know about the patient to plan a sound intervention or prevention program. To serve this function, the assessment includes several features: it indicates what is wrong with the patient, it indicates the patient's strengths, and it indicates the patient's motivation for occupation.

The word *assessment* is preferable to the terms *diagnosis* or *problem definition* for the evaluation of occupational status because it has a much broader meaning. Diagnosis and problem definition connote the identification of pathological, abnormal, dysfunctional, or problematic processes or states. To assess means to rate the value of property for the purpose of taxation. The word *assessment,* then, with its emphasis on the evaluation of the worth of something, is an appropriate term to apply to the process of collecting information to resolve clinical problems and to the statement that summarizes the results of that process. Occupational therapy is concerned with helping disabled persons to adapt to chronic disability more effectively. This may be accomplished by enhancing abilities as well as by remediating or reducing dysfunction. The occupational therapy assessment serves as the end point of evaluation and the starting point for treatment planning. To serve this pivotal function, the assessment must specify both assets and liabilities. Thus, diagnosis, or the determination of what is wrong with the patient, is only a part of the assessment.

Knowledge

The assessment process usually begins with diagnosis, because knowledge of dysfunction tells us what is wrong and requires correction or amelioration. The therapist seeks to ascertain the specific problems the patient is having in performing self-care, work, and leisure occupations. Disruptions in occupational role are commonly of two major types: an inability to perform socially defined age-appropriate tasks and an inability to coordinate these tasks effectively in daily life. To the extent that a person has disruptions in occupational role, or impairments that we can predict will result in such disruptions, that person is an appropriate candidate for occupational therapy. The occupational therapy diagnosis clearly articulates the disruption in occupational role that is of concern for treatment. For example, we might state that Tom Smith is totally dependent in hygiene and dressing and requires physical assistance with feeding. This diagnosis indicates that these are the major problems at this time.

The occupational therapy diagnosis has a temporal quality. Participation in daily living tasks may change over the course of an illness or other disorder. For example, as Tom Smith gains competence in self-care, the diagnosis may switch to dysfunctions in home management. Similarly, as an individual matures and needs and interests change, the occupational therapy diagnosis changes, and intervention is refocused. Thus, the range of problems that comprise the occupational therapy diagnosis is broad and variable, and the diagnosis may change over time.

Often, the occupational therapy diagnosis indicates not only the disruption in occupational role, but also the suspected cause or causes for this disruption. This is the etiological component of the diagnostic statement and it offers an explanation of why the individual behaves or fails to behave in some way.

The most prevalent perspective for defining the etiology of occupational role dysfunctions is based on the biopsychosocial model. This enables us to pinpoint the causes of performance dysfunctions in terms of biological, psychological, and social variables. For example, we might state that Ida Cox cannot dress herself because she has contractures in her upper extremities, thus attributing the cause to a biological variable. Or we might suggest that she cannot dress herself because of a memory problem, thus attributing the cause to a psychological variable. Or. we might conclude that the reason she is unable to dress herself is because she cannot reach her clothes from a wheelchair. In this case, the dressing dysfunction is attributed to the interaction of a biological variable, motor impairment, and a social variable, the man-made environment. Such attributions allow us to plan appropri-

ate treatment. We can plan to remediate the contracture or memory deficit or to circumvent their effects on performance. We can remove the architectural barriers.

An occupational therapy diagnosis stemming from the biopsychosocial model is so specific that it is applicable to only one patient. For instance, an occupational therapy diagnosis might state: Homemaking disability secondary to a lack of endurance for shopping to procure groceries, and postural instability in negotiating the stairs to the laundry facilities in the basement; ability is complicated by blurred vision in both eyes as a consequence of cataracts. Such a diagnosis is unlikely to be appropriate for more than one patient. Although the diagnostic statement is highly descriptive, it is also highly prescriptive. For example, the above diagnosis suggests such interventions as: employing homemaker services, scheduling and performing activities in such a way as to control fatigue, using good light with no glare, and using mobility aids or environmental supports.

In addition to a description of what the patient cannot do and why, the occupational therapy assessment includes a description of what the patient can do and how well it can be done. Although the problem is diagnosed, it is the person who is assessed. The need to acknowledge positive factors was well expressed by the little boy who reacted to the scolding he received about his report card by saying, "Daddy, I think your eyes need fixing. You only saw the D and not the four As." Knowing a person's problems or deficits tells us little about his or her strengths. The image of the patient drawn from problem behaviors is distorted. It needs to be supplemented with snapshots of the patient's occupational competencies and strengths to enable the therapist to construct a fair and valid impression of the patient.

The assessment of occupational competence requires a wide-angled lens. Occupational performance emerges from a complex network of transactions between the internal characteristics of the individual and the external properties of the surrounding environment. Just as features of a particular situation may account for a limitation of ability, so they may also allow the expression of ability. The qualities of the environment are important enablers of human performance. You cannot swim without water or play tennis without a partner. Both the physical and the social environments influence the patient's ability to occupy time productively. To assess occupational competence, the therapist evaluates the people, places, and objects associated with the patient's occupational endeavors to determine the extent to which they support occupation.

The final requirement of the occupational therapy assessment is to summarize the patient's motivation to engage in occupation. Who among us has never pondered over the patients with excellent potential who fail to achieve and those with intractable conditions who surpass all expectations? We cannot understand the patient without an appreciation of the way in which the urge toward competence has been habitually satisfied. The ontogenetic aspects of occupation have critical implications for recovery and growth. The patient's history of occupation informs us whether the present dysfunction is extenuated by a pattern of adaptive behavior or augmented by a career of maladaptive behavior. The patient's mastery of the environment is documented in occupational achievement, while exploration of the environment is recorded in the use of time. Because time is occupied by doing things of value, the patient's use of time provides insight into the varieties of occupations that are meaningful to him or her. The patient's past is reviewed to shed light on how occupational behavior is organized and to lend perspective to activities that are important and incidental to the life plan.

Historical assessment is directed toward a deeper understanding of the patient's occupational nature. The normative sequence of occupational endeavors begins in childhood play and self-care. Participation in arts and crafts, games, academics, chores, and part-time work are added to the repertoire through young adulthood. Productive occupation in the form of employment predominates in adulthood. This often changes to leisure pursuits during later maturity. The therapist thus captures the development and balance of self-care, work, and leisure occupations in studying the sequence of preschool, school age, worker, and retiree roles.

The yield of the occupational therapy assessment is a model of the patient that describes and explains his or her unique functioning in occupation. The model superimposes current functional abilities on disabilities, and relates these to environmental demands and to past performance. It is from this comprehensive model of the patient that future capacity is predicted and treatment goals are recommended.

Process

Having described the requirements of the occupational therapy assessment, I will now turn to the cognitive processes used to formulate it. What is involved in clinical inquiry? How do we go about the task of constructing a model of the patient? The approach used here for looking at the cognitive processes that undergird practice reflects an information-processing view of cognition. The human mind is thus conceptualized as a computer that has certain information-processing capabilities. It can do some things better than others and uses certain labor-saving strategies to overcome its limitations. A primary limitation of the human mind is its small capacity for short-term or working memory. Because of this limitation, data must be selected judiciously, processed serially, and managed through simplifying strategies (2). In assessment, the clinician has as intake to the information-processing system cues gathered from the patient or about the patient. The output is the conclusions summarized in the occupational therapy assessment. The conversion of intake data to output conclusions is a critical feature of clinical reasoning.

The therapist begins the assessment by choosing a plan for studying the patient. We say to ourselves, "Of all things that I could consider about this patient, what am I going to think about?" We typically respond to this question by constructing an image of the patient from the preassessment data and use this image to direct our plan. Our preassessment image tells us what to include and what to exclude as we observe the patient. Thus, the first labor-saving device the therapist uses is to limit the parameters within which the patient will be studied.

The preassessment image of the patient is derived from the conceptual frame of reference or postulate system of the therapist. A conceptual frame of reference represents a therapist's unique view of occupational therapy. It consists of facts derived from research studies, empirical generalizations drawn from experience, theories and models accepted by the therapist, and principles of practice obtained from instructors and colleagues. My frame of reference represents what I believe about occupational therapy practice. A frame of reference operates largely as an unconscious ideology in forming the preassessment image. The therapist links his or her frame of reference with the preassessment data to construct an image of the patient that furnishes the outline for the clinical investigation.

Two salient preassessment factors are the medical diagnosis and age. By knowing even these elementary facts. we can predict certain things about a patient. For example, if we know that a patient's dominant arm has been amputated, we can anticipate problems in manual dexterity and bilateral coordination. If, in addition, we know that the patient is 6 years old, rather than 76, we can expect to direct treatment toward habilitation of hand skills as opposed to rehabilitation.

The preassessment image of the patient is used to generate a series of testable working hypotheses. The therapist reasons that, if a particular hypothesis is valid, then it should follow that such and such will be found in further study of the case. For example, a therapist learns from the occupational therapy referral that the patient is a 40-year-old woman with depression. The therapist reasons that, if this patient is depressed, she is likely to be disheveled, to have a low level of involvement in activities, and to concentrate on events associated with negative affect. In other words, by knowing that the patient is depressed, the therapist is able to view the patient as a representative of the class of depressed patients, and, thus, hypothesizes that she will exhibit characteristics of depression. The therapist then sets out to perform the procedures needed to substantiate the hypothesis.

Up to this point, the reasoning process is essentially deductive in nature. The therapist recalls some general postulates from memory and applies them to a specific patient. The open-ended question of what is wrong with the patient has now been refined to a set of better-defined problems for exploration and resolution.

The working hypotheses provide a plan for acquiring cues from the patient to test the hypotheses. A cue is any bit of information that guides or directs the assessment (3). Cues arise from the observational process that employs three general types of data-gathering methodologies: testing or measurement; questioning, including history taking and interviewing; and observation. Accurate clinical decisions are dependent on the collection of good cues. Two tests of the goodness of cues are reliability and validity.

Cues can be used to test the working hypotheses developed from deductive reasoning. By comparing each cue to the working hypotheses, sense may be made of the data. The therapist reasons, "This is what I expect to find, now what do I find?" A cue may be interpreted as confirming a hypothesis, disconfirming a hypothesis, or noncontributary to a hypothesis. Thus, as information is collected about the patient, the therapist decides repeatedly whether or not a finding is related to the patient's problems. Confidence in each hypothesis increases or decreases, based on the interpretation of additional data. Extensive case data are reduced by eliminating, or holding in reserve, data that do not appear significant. Hypothesis testing is thus another of the mind's strategies for simplifying data management.

Hypotheses direct the collection of data and determine how they are organized and filed in memory. This organization prevents the mind from becoming overloaded with irrelevant facts and assists the therapist in retrieving information from memory.

Cues may also be combined to formulate new hypotheses. As cues are collected to test the validity of the deduced hypotheses, some cues may not fit well. Some of the performance problems we had expected to find will not be found, and others that we had not anticipated will become manifest. Our thinking begins to move from the classical, textbook picture of the disorder, to the disorder as it is uniquely manifested in this patient. The reasoning process now becomes inductive, with problem definition induced from empirical study of the patient, rather than deduced from the therapist's frame of reference. Additional cues may then be collected to test the inductively derived hypotheses. Clinical reasoning proceeds by developing hypotheses that pull together several inferences into a broader pattern or model of the patient.

After gleaning a clear perception of the patient's problems, the therapist then begins to search for cues indicative of the health of the patient as avidly as the search was conducted to identify dysfunction. Inductive reasoning and hypothesis testing are the basic processes through which the clinician assesses the patient's competencies, motivation for occupational achievement, and the environments in which the patient operates or will operate. These kinds of data are highly personal and hence are less likely to be deduced from knowledge of disease or disorder.

Data collection cannot continue indefinitely, and at some point the therapist decides that adequate information has been collected. How much data constitutes adequate data is dependent on the ethical consequences of an error in judgment (2,4). A recommendation to institutionalize a patient because he or she is unable to look after his or her self-care needs would require more evidence than that required for the prescription of a rocker knife. Regardless of how many data are collected, however, the database remains incomplete. The database represents only a sampling of the patient's behavior. The therapist's task is to use this incomplete information to make a judicious decision. Decision-making takes place under conditions of uncertainty.

Throughout the process of data collection, the therapist's preassessment image of the patient has been revised and elaborated, based on the accumulated cues. Once cue collection is stopped and no new information is being generated, hypothesis testing also ceases. The clinical reasoning of the therapist now resembles the dialectical process in which the therapist argues or defends the interpretation of the data in much the same way as a lawyer pleads a case in court. Does the patient have a dressing problem that is of concern? Is the cause of the patient's performance difficulties visual–perceptual problems? Is the mental status of the patient adequate for self-care? The evidence supporting or opposing each alternative is weighed with the objective of rendering one explanation more cogent than another. Inferences that are compatible are retained and others are rejected or modified as contradictions appear. Through the dialectical process the model of the individual patient is polished and repolished. In this way, the therapist arrives at a cohesive conception of the patient, and, having grasped the whole, reinterprets the parts in light of this understanding. Once a holistic picture of the patient has been devised, the function of the assessment moves from model building to decision-making.

What Are the Available Options?

The second of the three general questions guiding clinical inquiry is the therapeutic question: What can be done for this patient? Having proposed a model of the patient's occupational status, we then begin to explore the actions that could be taken to enhance occupational role performance. The intent is to generate a list of the treatment options available for the problems and assets presented by this patient. For example, suppose a patient's problems in self-care were attributed to hemiplegia subsequent to a cerebral vascular accident. To treat this problem, we might consider a neurological approach aimed at regaining controlled action in the involved arm, or a rehabilitative approach aimed at training the uninvolved arm to perform skilled activities, or a combination of these approaches. The aim, at this stage of clinical reasoning, is to foster an awareness of the range and kind of treatment possibilities. In effect, the therapist uses the model of the patient to construct a theory of practice for the patient.

Knowledge

The therapist's consideration of what could be done includes a review of the relative effectiveness of each treatment approach. If a particular treatment option is initiated, what results can be expected, and how long will it take to achieve them? Any hazards associated with the various treatments, or with no treatment, are evaluated in light of the potential benefits.

Decision-making concerning the appropriate action can approach certitude if the deleterious effects of a disorder without treatment are known, and if there is substantial evidence of how these effects can be altered by a particular treatment. We know, for instance, that if joints are not moved, contractures develop and the joints become immobile. Thus, movement becomes the scientifically acceptable treatment for preventing contractures.

For most occupational therapy approaches or procedures, however, the scientific evidence is not definitive. Rarely are the outcomes of research so specific that they allow us to know with 100 percent accuracy what will happen. Scientific findings generally emerge as probabilities rather than as certainties. They may, for example, tell us that 95 percent of the patients with right hemiplegia receiving self-care training will become independent in self-care. But when we apply this finding to Edith Jones, we do so with the recognition that her chances of becoming independent remain 50–50. The response of a patient to treatment cannot be predicted with certitude. Scientific knowledge can improve our chances of making accurate technical decisions but it cannot assure this. When the scientific evidence is inconclusive, the therapist has considerable leeway in devising treatment recommendations.

In the absence of scientific knowledge about the effectiveness of treatment options, clinicians rely on knowledge gleaned from their own clinical experience or from the experiences of others. Knowledge derived from practice rather than research indicates what works but may not indicate what works best.

Process

To draw up a list of the patient's treatment options, the therapist searches memory for relevant scientific and practice knowledge. Clinical experiences are stored and classified in memory and retrieved as needed for application to new patients. Each time a therapist treats a patient, a clinical experiment is performed in which the objective is to replicate a successful outcome of a past experiment (5). As a first step in reproducing the experiment, the therapist mentally reviews previous patients whose occupational status resembled the patient at hand. Although no two patients are exactly alike, the therapist assembles a subgroup of patients who are most similar to the patient under study (6). Treatment is selected for the new patient by analyzing and comparing the therapeutic actions and outcomes of the patients in the reference group. If there is a high degree of similarity between the patient being treated and previous patients, the therapist will select a treatment that is highly replicative. If the similarity is low, or if previous treatment was not very effective, the therapist will propose a treatment that is more inventive.

The cognitive process involved in the selection of treatment is again that of dialectical reasoning. The therapist argues one treatment option against another without recourse to new clinical data. The process of enumerating the patient's treatment alternatives relies heavily on the content of long-term memory. The more clinical experience therapists have, the more empirical data are available to guide decision-making. It is impossible for therapists to consider a treatment with which they have no familiarity. Similarly, clinicians cannot debate the scientific merits of one procedure over another, unless the procedure has been scientifically investigated and the research has been assimilated.

What Ought to Be Done?

The third and final question to be considered is the ethical question: What ought to be done to enhance occupational competence? Simply because a goal appears technically feasible for the patient does not mean that it should be set as a goal. And, simply because a treatment approach can be initiated does not imply that it should be instituted. We must avoid confusing action that can be taken with action that ought to be taken. From an ethical standpoint, decisive action must take the patient's valued goals into account. It must conform to the patient's definition of health, accomplishment, and the "good life."

Knowledge

Ethical principles arise from reflection on the nature of humanity and human dignity. Respect for individuals requires that each individual be regarded as autonomous. Each individual has a definite pattern and characteristic style for mastering the environment in the pursuit of occupational competence. The life plan is guided by personal and cultural values. Values give meaning and direction to one's life by inciting future goals and sustaining involvement in activity.

The concept of respect for the individual implies that the occupational therapy treatment plan should not interfere with the patient's intentions for recovery. To develop an appropriate plan, the patient's values are dis-tilled from the thematic continuity of the assessment of occupational status and taken into account in the review of technically feasible treatment options. When there is a range of possibilities for treatment goals and substantial lack of certitude concerning the technical merits of treatment alternatives, the therapist has considerable latitude in shaping recommendations. Expert advice is based more on opinion than fact. Ethical decision-making requires the therapist to search for an understanding of the patient's life rather than to make an evaluation of it. This understanding facilitates the selection of options to be discussed with the patient.

The goal of the clinical encounter is to devise a therapeutic plan that preserves the patient's values and represents a mutual understanding between the therapist and patient. Occupational therapy involves habit training and often requires major restructuring of the way in which personal values are to be satisfied. If habits are to be developed, patients must choose the objects and processes that they want to master in occupational therapy. Worthwhile achievement is the end product of personally deliberated decision-making. Occupational achievement begins with the choice to develop one's capabilities. It is the patient who restores, maintains, and enhances occupational performance. The patient, not the therapist, is the agent of change. The patient's active participation is required not only in determining and prioritizing the goals of treatment, but also in deciding on the methods to be used to achieve the goals. As a result of assuming personal responsibility for treatment decisions, the patient emerges from the assessment with an increased sense of self-determination and control, and a sense of commitment to accomplishing planned goals. In the capacity of expert advisor, the therapist guides patients through the decision-making process, and helps them fuse the intellectual and emotional aspects of decision-making into choices that are right for them.

It cannot be assumed that the goals selected by a patient for himself or herself will match those the therapist would select. Each may have a different view of the "good life." Because most persons with quadriplegia secondary to a spinal cord lesion at the level of the 6th and 7th cervical vertebrae can relearn dressing skills, the therapist may reason that Tim Robbins should work toward this goal. However, Tim may conclude that he would prefer to spend his limited energy relearning how to manage his home computer.

When the therapist and patient have different goals, the potential for conflict is high, and the resolution of conflict can easily be tipped in favor of the therapist's view. Two factors contribute significantly, to the therapist holding the balance of power (1). First, the therapist has the knowledge and skills to alleviate the problems facing the patient. The patient is thus dependent on the therapist for help. Second, the patient's position of dependency is compounded by the patient's vulnerability. As a result of disease or other disorders, patients sustain insults to functions regarded as integral to human life and living. The very fact that they need help may diminish their sense of autonomy. Adaptive functioning in basic life tasks, such as eating and dressing, may be impeded. Patients may even be unable to express their own values or make rational choices. Such impairments place a patient's moral agency at risk, and often make it easy to take advantage of the patient's right to control his or her life.

Process

The methods used to answer ethical questions differ from those used in science. While scientific questions are answered by accumulating data and testing hypotheses, ethical questions are resolved by coming to grips with values and making value judgments (7). To empower the patient to act as his or her own moral agent, the therapist provides the patient with the knowledge needed to participate effectively in decision-making. The patient's choice must not only be autonomous, it must also be informed. Patients are not adequately informed to make choices, unless they can anticipate the results of their choices. The ethical and scientific dimensions of clinical reasoning are closely intermingled. The therapist presents the possible options for treatment, projects the outcomes of each option, explains how the outcomes are achieved, and outlines a time sequence for goal attainment. Together the therapist and patient consider each recommendation and evaluate the consequences of each alternative in terms of the patient's occupational potential and goals. If necessary, the therapist tempers unrealistic expectations, corrects inaccurate information, and points out any inconsistencies in rationalization. In effect, the therapist assists the patient in imagining what might occur, if treatment is to be undertaken or rejected. The strength of arguments for one action over another is assessed by dialectic. Greater weight is assigned a position according to the importance it holds for the patient. The selection of treatment becomes more difficult as the merits of one action over other actions become more ambiguous. The therapist makes known his or her preferences for the patient's treatment as well as the rationale for this decision. The patient ends the deliberation by making a choice.

Once the patient has determined the course of action, the therapist supports or confirms the decision. The therapist captures the persuasive elements of the dialectical argument, and uses them to instill in the patient a belief that treatment X is the best course of action and should be undertaken. At the same time, the therapist strives to bolster the patient's belief that he or she can carry out the treatment and achieve the goals. The reasoning process ends, therefore, in persuasive rhetoric, which we call "motivating the patient." In situations where therapists judge that they cannot lend support to the patient's choice, responsibility for providing occupational therapy services is terminated.

The therapist is privileged to help the patient select from the available opportunities those that are to be brought to fruition. As the patient executes and fulfills his or her choice, the therapist learns about the healing power of occupation. Occupational choice rekindles the will to live, and mobilizes the mind to discipline the body, in enacting the creative processes associated with reversing disability. The subtle wisdom of participation in self-initiated and self-directed occupation becomes apparent as confidence is rebuilt and hope is restored. Choices are not confined to the outset of treatment. Assessment and planning are ongoing processes and there are repeated occasions to consider if treatment should be continued, terminated, modified, or supplemented.

This discussion of the ethical dimension of clinical reasoning has been based on three cogent assumptions: 1. that patients can serve as their own moral agents; 2. that the patient's choice is the ultimate one; and 3. that the therapist acts independently. None of these conditions may be met in a particular situation, which introduces further complications into the already complex process of ethical decision-making. Surrogates may substitute for patients in the planning process because patients are too young, too impaired mentally, or too emotionally disturbed to participate in decision-making. The rights of family members and the values and resources of society may limit the choices patients can make. The conjoint decision of therapist and patient may be modified or set aside by the health care team. These are vital issues that cannot be avoided in clinical decisions.

In summary, the data collected in clinical inquiry play three roles in clinical reasoning. First, clinical data are used to describe the patient's occupational status.

This description includes an indication of the patient's adaptive skills, performance dysfunctions and their presumed causes, and competency motivation. Second, clinical data are used to conjure up a group of patients who have an occupational status and history comparable to the patient under consideration. These patients serve as a reference group for the identification of treatment options and prediction of treatment outcomes. Third, clinical data are used to identify therapeutic options appropriate to the specific needs of the patient, and to recommend a course of action consistent with the patient's values. As the clinical reasoning process moves from an assessment of occupational status, to a review of treatment options, to a selection of the right action, the scientific mode of reasoning gives way to nonscientific intellectual processes. Choosing a course of action involves many value considerations. The closer we come to making a clinical judgment, the less use is made of facts and hypothesis testing, and the more reliance is placed on the dialectical process, opinion, and persuasion.

Perfecting Clinical Inquiry

Now that what is involved in clinical study has been considered, it seem appropriate to ponder how our habits of inquiry can be improved. My suggestions are intended to be directional rather than comprehensive.

Model of the Patient

The therapist's understanding of the patient is highly dependent on the development of a model of the patient. It is pertinent to point out that studies conducted with counseling professionals have consistently supported the value of inductive theory building for practice, as opposed to the application of deductive theory. McArthur (8), for example, found that psychologists who applied existing theories in a doctrinary fashion turned out to be the poorest appraisers of personality. The critical element in devising a model of the patient is meticulous attention to the cues obtained from the patient. The ability to use assessment-related data to develop hypotheses is a vital professional skill.

Although hypotheses have adaptive value for organizing and managing data, they represent strong conceptual biases. In collecting and interpreting data, we have a tendency to overlook evidence that does not support our hypotheses. This is accompanied by an inclination to overemphasize positive evidence. In other words, we are psychologically prone to affirm our ideas,

and feel less compelled to refute them (4, 9). Agnew and Pyke (10) drew a salient comparison between the blindness imposed by hypotheses and that generated by love. They commented: "The rejection of a theory once accepted is like the rejection of a girlfriend or boyfriend once loved—it takes more than a bit of negative evidence. In fact, the rest of the community can shake their collective heads in amazement at your blindness, your utter failure to recognize the glaring array of differences between your picture of the girl or boy, and the data." (p. 128) The rigid application of a conceptual bias emerged as a major concern in my study of occupational therapists' thinking (11). The medical diagnosis was used to formulate the preassessment image of the patient and that image remained stable, even in the face of cues portending a revision.

Once cognizant of the pitfalls involved in hypothesis use, the therapist can initiate steps to avoid them. Obtaining a second opinion through consultation is one method commonly used to check the validity of one's interpretation. Consultants should perform their own assessments without reference to the patient's database. Objectivity will be destroyed if consultants read reports or participate in discussions about the patient before conducting their own evaluations. The consultant's final opinion, however, should be based on the total available data (5).

A fixed data collection schedule is another mechanism used to prevent premature closure of hypothesis generation. The Occupational Therapy Uniform Evaluation Checklist (12) is an example of a fixed data collection schedule. It specifies the boundaries of occupational therapy practice and lists the variables to be reviewed for assessment. The Checklist forces the therapist to examine occupational performance from a panoramic view rather than microscopically. In so doing, it fosters the search for information that might suggest hypotheses the therapist might not otherwise have entertained. Adherence to a fixed routine assures the therapist that observations will be conducted that afford a fair and adequate opportunity to disprove as well as to confirm favorite hypotheses (13).

Research on the assessment process suggests that practitioners' "favorite" hypotheses concentrate on the dysfunctional aspects of patient performance (14, 15). We seem to be more interested in exploring why Alice Thompson falls so often than in ascertaining why she maintains her balance for so long. This preoccupation with problematic behaviors probably stems from the fact that they are the reason for the patient's referral to occupational therapy and constitute the focus of interventive efforts. Our first response to the question concerning the patient's occupational status is that it is dysfunctional. Our image of the patient changes as we collect additional cues and make adjustments in the initial picture. However, once our thoughts are anchored in dysfunction, it becomes difficult to switch our focus and too few modifications may be made in the image (16). Wright and Fletcher (14) point out that the perception of strengths and weaknesses as a unit, that is, as belonging to one person, requires the therapist to integrate two dissimilar qualities and that such synthesis is difficult. The same rationale may also be used to explain why practitioners are prone to see more pathology in their patients than the patients themselves perceive. Patients live with disability and adapt to it. Professionals regard disability as something to be eliminated. From this vantage point it is hard for professionals to see how disability can have any positive implications. Unfortunately, an emphasis on negative perceptions results in a skewed image of the patient. Dysfunctions are overestimated and abilities are underestimated (14).

Research also indicates that practitioners are more likely to hypothesize that a patient's problems are caused by factors within the patient as opposed to factors in the patient's physical and social milieu (14, 15). For instance, we are more apt to attribute a patient's distress to an inability to deal with authority figures than to an unreasonable supervisor. One reason for this tendency is that we generally have a clearer picture of patients than we do of the situations in which they live, work, and play. We generally see patients in health-care settings and rarely sample their behaviors in natural settings. Thus, the patient's environment has a quality of vagueness about it compared to the patient, who appears more real. Another explanation for our neglect of the environment is that it is often impossible or very difficult to change the environment. Even if the patient's supervisor is irrational, the patient still has to learn to manage the situation or to find another job. Nevertheless, it should be recognized that our "clinic-bound" view of the patient may lead us to ignore or underestimate impediments to occupational performance residing in the environment. Furthermore, because patients often attribute their difficulties to situations rather than to themselves, there is a potential conflict between the therapist's and patient's perceptions of causation. The validity of the patient's causal attribution should not be dismissed lightly by the therapist because patients are attuned to situational exigencies by their struggle for occupational competence.

Recognizing the distortion that may occur because of the exploration of hypotheses oriented toward dysfunction rather than function, and emphasis on the person as opposed to the environment, the therapist can take steps to countermand these biases. The data collection schedule can be arranged to include both assets and liabilities for every aspect of occupational performance evaluated. Because a patient's self-perceptions of competence are as important for participation in activity as is competence itself, the checklist should also highlight the patient's subjective impressions of occupational status. The schedule can also be extended to include the physical and social environments. These additions will serve to remind us of the significance of these variables for occupation and to foster the habit of routinely evaluating them.

Integration of Data

The challenge presented to the mind by the occupational therapy assessment is intensified by the need to integrate the wide variety of information gathered about the patient. Although we may isolate aspects of human functioning for the purposes of data management, humans function as unities or wholes. Competence requires the individual to function as an integrated organism, with the physical, mental, emotional, and social dimensions of occupational behavior interacting with the surrounding human and nonhuman environment. The selection of treatment proceeds from a holistic conception of the patient. If the therapist is to manage the array of complex clinical data required to understand occupational behavior, a simplifying strategy is needed to ward off chaos in the information-processing capabilities of the human mind. Clinical judgments are not made on the basis of one or two test scores. And, although the statistical integration of clinical data may be possible in some situations, it is impractical in most. We need a labor-saving device to assist the mind in integrating data. General systems theory provides such assistance.

According to the systems metaphor, data are framed in terms of relationships among systems and systems are ordered hierarchically based on increasing levels of complexity. In the assessment of a patient with a traumatic spinal cord injury, for example, we would look at the effects of disorder on other biological systems, such as the musculoskeletal and integumentary. At the same time, the rules of systems hierarchy would direct our attention to factors in the psychological system, such as competency motivation, which will strongly influence the recovery of the biological system as well as the social reintegration of the patient. Although the assessment checklist is useful for reminding us of the spectrum of occupational performance, general systems theory provides rules for organizing the list so that the assessment data can be meaningfully related and stored in memory.

Occupational Therapy Assessment

Once an occupational therapy assessment has been made, viable therapeutic approaches are selected. The selection of treatment rests on a comparison between the patient under consideration and similar patients previously treated. Thus, the effective application of treatment requires that patients be accurately identified and grouped together according to characteristics that are salient for occupation. If the results of a clinical experiment are to be replicated, we must begin with a patient who closely resembles those used in the original experiment.

At the present time, occupational therapy has no meaningful way of systematically describing occupational role performance and of differentiating homogeneous subgroups based on occupational characteristics. The medical diagnosis is inadequate for delineating the diverse levels of occupational performance that occur in patients with the same diagnosis. It also lacks utility for identifying the similar levels of occupational performance that occur in patients with different medical diagnoses. Occupational therapy lacks a standardized way of classifying the functional disabilities that result from disease and other disorders. In the absence of an agreed-upon system for thinking about, remembering, and expressing our clinical observations, each therapist develops his or her own idiosyncratic system for describing occupational performance. To the extent that these informal descriptions facilitate a comparison of patients, based on salient occupational characteristics, the inferences resulting from the comparison will be valid. However, until a systematic scheme for describing and organizing clinical data is developed, we will not be able to communicate meaningfully with each other, either in informal exchanges in the clinic, or in more scientific dialogue in our journals.

Selection of Treatment

We have seen that a treatment recommendation is largely based on the therapist's recall of similar cases.

Some memories are more easily recalled than others (6). We are more likely to think of patients treated recently than those treated in the past. It is easier to remember patients who are seen frequently than those treated less often. Exceptional cases, either of success or failure, make strong impressions. Inferences gleaned from patients who happen to come to mind are likely to be less accurate than those derived from systematic analysis. Although we can all recount our brilliant successes, how many of us know what our batting average is? How good are we as judges of occupational potential? By keeping a score of the accuracy of our clinical predictions, our judgmental abilities can be improved. Checking our initial predictions against discharge data is something that can be readily incorporated into the clinic routine. Did the patient accomplish what I predicted he or she would? If not, why not? Because the ultimate test of treatment is what happens after discharge, mechanisms should also be sought for testing the accuracy of our discharge predictions with follow-up data.

A common error made by therapists in arriving at a clinical judgment is to assume that the patient is like oneself (17). This assumption enables us to know the patient through ourselves. In using the self as a referent, one rationalizes, "I will treat the patient as I would wish to be treated if I were in this situation." This kind of reasoning risks denying the validity of the patient's values. The therapist ascribes meaning to the patient's situation according to his or her own criteria. The patient is presented with a decision, rather than a list of options, and the choice of occupation is denied. Respect for the individual implies giving the patient the same opportunity to express and achieve what the patient sees as worthwhile as one would desire for oneself. We must be sensitive to the human spirit and curb the offering of pseudo choices of activity that have little meaning for the patient.

Instrumentation

The validity of clinical reasoning is grounded in the collection of good cues. This is a critical point to consider as we concentrate our energies on developing assessment instruments for practice. The nature of the phenomena we are interested in evaluating dictates the appropriate kind of instrumentation. As clinicians, our primary interest lies in evaluating performance in self-care, work, and leisure occupations. Our concern is with the ability to do and that doing is observable. You do not need to infer that I can dress from my grip strength, or mental acuity. You can observe my ability. Performance is not an abstract construct as is intelligence, anxiety, or sensory integration. We can see performance. Furthermore, we know that performance in occupation depends on the environment or situation as much as it does on the patient. Recognizing the interplay between the patient and the environment leaves us with two fundamental ways of evaluating occupational performance. First, we can go into the environments where our patients live, work, and play and observe their performance. Second, we can simulate the occupational environments of our patients by providing test stimuli, such as beds, chairs, games, arts and crafts, and work and collect a series of behavior samples in our clinics. In this case, the validity of our evaluation depends on how well we approximate the places where function is to occur.

There is inherently little uniformity in the occupational environments of our patients and, if we try to establish that uniformity, we will obscure the validity of our evaluation. The strength of occupational therapy assessment lies not in placing patients in contrived and standardized situations and recording their responses, but rather, in observing them in real-life settings and evaluating their adaptive competence. Thus, development of occupational therapy instrumentation depends on a conceptualization of the task environment, because this constitutes the test stimulus that evokes behavior. Our description of occupational behavior will be incomplete until we can mesh it with a description of the task environment.

The Art

Our exploration of the intellectual technology of clinical reasoning has focused on the scientific and ethical aspects. We have not considered the art except by implication and innuendo. In the peroration, I return to the therapist who says, "I don't know how I know, I just know that I know." While the scientific dimension of clinical reasoning is directed toward specifying the correct treatment from a technical standpoint, and the ethical dimension is geared toward selecting the treatment that meets the patient's criteria of right occupational role performance, the artistic dimension pursues excellence in achieving a right action—and it does this in the face of individuality, indeterminacy, and complexity (6). Artistry involves the orchestration of broad strategies for grappling effectively with the uncertainties inherent in clinical practice.

Skill in Thinking

Artistry is knowing as it is revealed in our actions (6). It is exhibited in knowing what to do and how to do it, rather than in knowing about something. In the early stages of acquiring a skill, such as dressing or piano playing, our actions are slow and clumsy. We have to think a lot about what we are doing and we make a lot of errors. But as skill develops, our actions become smooth, flexible, and spontaneous, and our thinking becomes automatic. We get a feel for the skill and that feeling allows us to repeat our performance. You know how to touch the piano keys to play a Mozart piano concerto, and your artistry is apparent in your music. If you were to describe your "knowing how to" play the piano, you would find this difficult, if not impossible, just as someone else would find it difficult to acquire the skill of piano playing by following your instructions.

Clinical reasoning may be viewed as a skill akin to piano playing. The skill consists of reducing the ambiguities inherent in clinical practice to manageable risks, and by so doing, enabling the formulation of prudent decisions (6). In each clinical transaction, the therapist is challenged to apply the theories and techniques of occupational therapy to a particular patient. Our textbooks inform us of the implications of blindness, hemiplegia, and age-related changes, but the hiatus between theory and practice becomes readily apparent when 90-year-old John Green, accompanied by his loving wife and devoted daughter, stands before us with hemiplegia, blindness, and the beginning signs of brain failure. Who among us has not experienced the gap between what we learned in school and what we need to know in the clinic?

Clinical problems are not neat. They are messy and complex. Everything that could be known about the patient is not known and much of the data collected are flawed and imperfect. Clinical problems deal with the uniqueness of patients rather than with their similarities. And, as Gordon Allport (18) reminds us, uniqueness is not equivalent to the sum of the ways in which a person deviates from the hypothetical average human. Unlike the simple cause-and-effect problems associated with basic science, clinical problems involve a complex interplay of multiple variables, the effects of which are largely unpredictable. The outcomes of occupational therapy treatment cannot be guaranteed. Clinical problems change as patient's progress and regress and as the occupational opportunities provided by the environment fluctuate.

No one can provide "cookbook" recipes for dealing with situations in which uniqueness, uncertainty, complexity, and instability are the chief characteristics. There are no formulas or algorithms that tell us how to use the interneuronal processes associated with perception, memory, reasoning, and argument. In the clinical situation, the therapist is under pressure to act and to act now. One cannot interrupt an assessment to go to the library and read up on a critical point. In handling the uncertainties contained in clinical practice, therapists rely on their accumulated experience, conceptual and judgmental heuristics, intuition, and insight to "apply their knowledge" and make clinical judgments. In spite of defective data and incomplete information, artistic inquiry enables the therapist to make prudent decisions and to know why a treatment will work for a particular patient.

The artistry of clinical reasoning is exhibited in the craftsmanship with which the therapist executes the series of steps that culminates in a clinical decision. It is expressed in the interpersonal skills through which the therapist invites involvement in decision-making, builds trust, explains treatment alternatives, and offers encouragement. Artistry manifests itself in the adeptness with which the therapist gathers cues: by selecting questions, probing for information not volunteered, clarifying discrepancies, administering tests, and observing performance. The degree of perfection with which the data to be processed are obtained influences the reliability and validity of the data, and hence sets limits on the quality of the final judgment. The art extends to grouping cues effectively, recognizing patterns, and depositing in memory organized reference images. The knowing derived from perceptual acuity, such as that needed to discern spasticity and achievement motivation, is also contained in the art of clinical reasoning. Linking the model of the patient with the appropriate memory structures to build a theory of practice for the patient requires considerable acumen. Artistic insight reaches its peak in combining evidence and opinion to support arguments convincingly, thus bringing closure to the decision-making process. Although each of these processes is difficult to master in and of itself, getting them coordinated and "on line" so that one can think "on one's feet" is an even vaster task.

Experts and Novices

The automation of clinical reasoning is not merely a matter of thinking faster. Experts think differently from novices. Because of the limited capacity of short-term memory, the human mind can only consider five to nine units of information at a time (16). This is why we find it difficult to remember telephone numbers. If I asked you to remember 9 1 9 9 6 6 2 4 5 1, chances are you would have forgotten the number long before you arrived at a telephone to dial it. However, if you knew that the area code for Chapel Hill is 919, and that all university numbers begin with the prefix 966, it is likely that you would have remembered the number 919-966-2451 correctly. Memory is aided by organizing and chunking information into larger units. By chunking telephone digits into familiar patterns, the number of units to be remembered is reduced and falls within the capacity of working memory.

Evidence is accumulating that expert and novice problem solvers differ in their use of problem-solving strategies, such as chunking (19). The expert sees and stores cues in patterns and configurations, whereas the novice records individual cues. Experts chunk data into larger information units than novices do. The expert creates memory structures by classifying data according to how they are to be applied in practice. The novice's memory structures, on the other hand, arise from features more peripheral to functional usage. The novice relies on conceptual principles to get things out of memory. The expert retrieves knowledge on the basis of situational cues as well as on conceptual stimuli. As the reasoning process unfolds, experts monitor their own thinking and understanding, which enables them to curtail errors and omissions. The ability to think faster is thus a result of thinking more efficiently, more functionally, and more critically.

Simply because our knowledge is in our action does not mean that we cannot think about it. When skill breaks down, and we strike a discordant note, drop a stitch, or fall off a bicycle, we step back, slow down our pace, and reflect on our actions. In clinical reasoning, skill breakdown occurs when clinical data are incongruous with our expectations and experience. Artistic inquiry is spurred by perplexity. As long as we are assessing patients whom we perceive as highly similar to those we have treated in the past, the clinical encounter presents no challenges, our intuitive understanding of the situation remains tacit. However, when we are no longer able to see things as we previously saw them, or do things as we previously did them, our curiosity is engaged, our anxiety is aroused, and we become inquisitive practitioners.

Expert clinicians are those who are competent in action and, simultaneously, reflect on this action to learn from it (6). They create opportunities for introspection by critically examining their reasoning to disclose bias and inconsistency. Artistic inquiry is also initiated through reframing, that is, by looking at the clinical situation from a new perspective. For example, a therapist might reason, "What would happen if this patient with low back pain were treated by diverting attention from back pain to pleasurable activity, instead of with exercises to improve body mechanics?"

As thinking becomes less automatic and more conscious, through self-criticism and reframing, it also becomes more accessible to explanation. Although our explanations and descriptions of clinical reasoning may never be complete, they can become progressively more adequate through reflection, and the artistic dimension can be better understood. The conversion of our practice into theory revolves around a cycle of concrete experience, reflective thinking, conceptual integration, and active experimentation.

In conclusion, the clinician functions as a scientist, ethicist, and artist. The scientific, ethical, and artistic dimensions of clinical reasoning are inextricably intertwined, and each strand is needed to strengthen the line of thought leading to understanding. Without science, clinical inquiry is not systematic; without ethics, it is not responsible; without art, it is not convincing. The intentions and potentials of chronically disabled patients are difficult to discern, but a therapist of understanding will elicit them, and use them to help patients discover health within themselves.

Acknowledgments

Sincere appreciation is expressed to the following individuals for their critical review of the ideas presented in this paper: Anne Blakeney, David Hollingsworth, Teena Snow, and Joyce Sparling.

References

1. Pellegrino ED, Thomasma DC: *A Philosophical Basis of Medical Practice*, New York: Oxford University Press, 1981.
2. Scriven M: Clinical judgment. In *Clinical Judgment: A Critical Appraisal*, HT Engelhardt, SF Spicker, B Towers, Editors. Dordrecht, Holland: D. Reidel Publishing Co., 1979, pp. 3–16.
3. Cutler P: *Problem Solving in Clinical Medicine: From Data to Diagnosis*, New York: Basic Books, Inc., 1979.
4. Sober E: The art of science of clinical judgment: An informational approach. In *Clinical Judgment: A Critical Appraisal*, HT Engelhardt, SF Spicker, B Towers, Editors. Dordrecht, Holland: D. Reidel Publishing Co., 1979, pp. 29–44.
5. Feinstein AR: Scientific methodology in clinical medicine, III. The evaluation of therapeutic response. *Am Intern Med 61:* 944–966, 1964.
6. Schön DA: *The Reflective Practitioner: How Professionals Think in Action,* New York: Basic Books, Inc., 1983.
7. Brody H: *Ethical Decisions in Medicine,* Boston: Little, Brown, and Co., 1981.
8. McArthur C: Analyzing the clinical process. *J Counseling Psychol 1:* 203–208, 1954.
9. Koester GA: A study of diagnostic reasoning. *Educ Psychol Measurement 14:* 473–486, 1954.
10. Agnew NM, Pyke SW: *The Science Game,* Englewood Cliffs, NJ: Prentice Hall, 1969.
11. Rogers JC, Masagatani G: Clinical reasoning of occupational therapists during the initial assessment of physically disabled patients. *Occup Ther Res 21:* 95–219, 1982.
12. Shriver D, Mitcham M, Schwartzberg S, Ranucci M: Uniform occupational therapy evaluation checklist. In *Reference Manual of the Official Documents of The American Occupational Therapy Assocation,* 1983.
13. Elstein AS, Shulman LS, Sprafka SA: *Problem Solving: An Analysis of Clinical Reasoning,* Cambridge, MA: Harvard University Press, 1978.
14. Wright BA, Fletcher BL: Uncovering hidden resources; A challenge in assessment. *Prof Psychol 13:* 229–235, 1982.
15. Bateson CD, O'Quin K, Pych V: An attribution theory analysis of trained helpers' inferences about clients' needs. In *Basic Processes in Helping Relationships,* TA Wills, Editor. New York: Academic Press, 1982, pp. 59–80.
16. Matlin M: *Cognition,* New York: Holt, Rinehart, and Winston, 1983.
17. Sarbin TR, Taft R, Bailey DE: *Clinical Inference and Cognitive Theory,* New York: Holt, Rinehart, and Winston, 1960.
18. Allport GW: *Pattern and Growth in Personality,* New York: Holt, Rinehart, and Winston, 1961.
19. Feltovich PJ: Expertise: reorganizing and refining knowledge for use. *Professional Education Researcher Notes,* December 1982/January 1983, pp. 5–9.

CHAPTER 42

The Therapist With the Three-Track Mind

MAUREEN HAYES FLEMING

The primary purpose of the American Occupational Therapy Association/American Occupational Therapy Foundation Clinical Reasoning Study was to identify the reasoning strategy that occupational therapists used to guide their practice. The designers of this study assumed that there was one reasoning style that is typical of clinical reasoning in occupational therapy. They decided that ethnography was the research method (Gillette & Mattingly, 1987) most likely to enable them to identify this typical or best reasoning style. However, as investigators, Mattingly and I soon realized that the occupational therapists in the study employed a variety of reasoning strategies.

During the early stages of the research project, when we were still searching for a single reasoning style, the apparent use of several forms of reasoning led us to believe that the therapists' thinking was inconsistent or scattered. Further analysis of the videotapes of treatment sessions, interviews, and group discussions with the therapist–subjects gave us deeper insight into their reasoning processes. They employed different modes of thinking for different purposes or in response to particular features of the clinical problem. The occupational therapists in the study seemed to use at least four different types of reasoning: narrative reasoning (Mattingly, 1989, 1991), procedural reasoning, interactive reasoning, and conditional reasoning (Fleming, 1989). These last three types of reasoning are discussed in the present chapter.

Another insight was that each type of reasoning seemed to be employed to address different aspects of the whole problem. Eventually, we realized that the therapist–subjects attended to the patient at three levels: (a) the physical ailment, (b) the patient as a person, and (c) the person as a social being in the context of family, environment, and culture. We then saw that each type of reasoning was employed to address a particular level of concern. The procedural reasoning strategy was used when the therapist thought about the person's physical ailments and what procedures were appropriate to alleviate them. Interactive reasoning was used to help the therapist interact with and understand the person better. Conditional reasoning, a complex form of social reasoning, was used to help the patient in the difficult process of reconstructing a life now permanently changed by injury or disease.

These three reasoning strategies appeared to be distinctly different, yet the therapist–subjects seemed to shift rapidly from one form of reasoning to another. They changed reasoning styles as their attention was drawn from the original concern to treat the physical ailment to other features of the problem, such as the particular person's response to the present activity. Using procedural reasoning, the therapist–subjects readily moved back to the physical problem that they had been pursuing earlier. They analyzed different aspects of the problem simultaneously. They used different thinking styles without losing track of some aspects of the problem while they temporarily shifted attention to another feature of the problem. We began to think about these styles of reasoning as different operations that interacted with each other in the therapist's mind. We referred to these operations as different *tracks* for guiding thinking. Thus, we developed the notion of the occupational therapist as a therapist with a three-track mind. The track analogy helped us envision how a therapist thought about the multiple and diverse issues that pertained to the patient's problems and the therapist's ability to influence them.

This chapter was previously published in the *American Journal of Occupational Therapy, 45,* 1007–1014. Copyright © 1991, American Occupational Therapy Association. Reprinted with permission. http://dx.doi.org/10.5014/ajot.45.11.1007

Procedural Reasoning

The therapist–subjects used what we called *procedural reasoning* when they were thinking about the disease or disability and deciding on which treatment activities (procedures) they might employ to remediate the person's functional performance problems. In this mode, the therapists' dual search was for problem definition and treatment selection. In situations where problem identification and treatment selection were seen as the central task, the therapists' thinking strategies demonstrated many parallels to the patterns identified by other researchers interested in problem solving in general and clinical problem solving in particular (Coughlin & Patel, 1987; Elstein, Shulman, & Sprafka, 1978; Newell & Simon, 1972; Rogers & Masagatani, 1982). The problem-solving sequence of diagnosis, prognosis, and prescription, which is typical of physicians' reasoning, was commonly used. However, the words the therapists used to describe this sequence were *problem identification, goal setting,* and *treatment planning.*

Experienced therapists in the study used forms of reasoning similar to the problem-solving strategies identified by many investigators who study physicians. For example, therapists used all three problem-solving methods described by Newell and Simon (1972)—recognition, generation and testing, and heuristic search. They also displayed characteristics identified by Elstein et al. (1978), such as cue identification, hypothesis generation, cue interpretation, and hypothesis evaluation. They interpreted patterns of cues, much like the ones that Coughlin and Patel (1987) identified among physicians and medical students. The structural features of the hypotheses generated by the therapists were similar to those of medical students in a study by Allal (as cited by Elstein et al., 1978), that is, hierarchical organization, competing formulations, multiple subspaces, and functional relationships.

One characteristic of reasoning common to all of the physicians and medical students in the studies by Elstein et al. (1978) was generation and evaluation of competing hypotheses. Physicians always looked for more than one potential cause of the problem presented. They devoted a considerable portion of their reasoning efforts to seeking additional cues and rearranging hypotheses in their minds in order to either support or negate more than one possible cause of the presenting ailment. Competing hypothesis generation was also a strategy commonly used by the occupational therapists. The experienced therapists in this study typically generated two to four possible hypotheses regarding the cause and nature of aspects of the person's problem. They generated several hypotheses about potential treatment activities as well. However, there was a tendency among the newer therapists to seek the right answer rather than to generate hypotheses about possibilities. When they generated hypotheses, they tended to consider only one or two of them.

Elstein et al. (1978) noticed a phenomenon that they referred to as *early hypothesis generation,* which they interpreted as being an attempt on the part of the physician to define, or mentally enter, the appropriate problem space, as theorized by Newell and Simon (1972). Newell and Simon hypothesized that abstract thinkers categorized problems or phenomena in different spaces or areas of the possible source of the problem or avenue of inquiry. A similar notion was advanced by Feinstein (1973), who suggested that physicians' thinking would be improved if they systematically searched for sources of the problem using a reverse hierarchical method. Using this method, physicians would think of what area of the body was involved, then what system, then what organ, then what process, until the problem space was sufficiently defined and specific problems could be identified. Experienced therapists seemed to quickly identify and search within the appropriate problem spaces. Novice therapists had more difficulty with this task.

It makes sense that occupational therapists who work in a medical center, as did the subjects in the Clinical Reasoning Study, and for whom part of their education contained long hours of medical lectures, would use a thinking style similar to that used in medical decision-making. That therapists frequently used these logical reasoning styles was expected. However, it was surprising that therapists often did not use these styles. This phenomenon led us to search for other modes of thought that the therapist–subjects might be using.

In discussions with the therapists, a few persistent themes emerged. At first, these themes did not seem to be explicitly linked to clinical reasoning. Some seemed to be distractions from discussing reasoning. Later, we found that these seeming distractions were important to the therapists' thinking about clinical problems. Our misunderstanding of these possible distractions was a result of our initial failure to recognize that therapists viewed clinical problems from more than one perspective. After examining these perspectives, we achieved a greater understanding of how therapists think in general and how they think differently about different aspects of the patient's situation.

We were able to identify these perspectives by analyzing several of the persistent themes that flowed through the therapists' conversations. One such theme was that the therapist–subjects often questioned what aspects of the person and the disability were appropriate for them to treat. In one group discussion, we were analyzing a videotape in which a therapist was attempting to encourage an outpatient to solve a problem. The personal care attendants he hired all quit after only a few weeks of working with him. The therapist was unable to convince the patient that this was a problem. He engaged in a wide range of what therapists referred to as avoidance tactics. Clearly the therapist and the patient had differing points of view on this issue. As the problem was discussed, many therapists in the group interpreted it as a value conflict between the patient and the therapist. There were at least two value conflicts here. One was the that the therapist thought it was unsafe for the patient to live alone without someone to assist him in accessing the bed, the tub, the toilet, or his wheelchair. The patient had fallen many times while attempting these moves by himself, and his solution was to call the fire department in his small town and have someone come to his house and pick him up. The patient viewed this as a simple solution, whereas the therapist viewed it as poor judgment and irresponsibility. Another conflict was that the therapist believed that the patient should keep himself and his home cleaner. The patient did not agree with this. The group of therapists focused on whether the therapist should have pursued the discussion. The concern was whether or not the therapist, who specialized in treating physical disabilities, should have been discussing personal issues with the patient. Some group members believed that discussions of personal issues were under the aegis of psychiatric therapists only. A therapist who worked in a psychiatric setting then said that in her hospital, occupational therapists were not supposed to discuss personal issues; only psychiatrists were to discuss personal issues. In her setting, therapists could only discuss observable behaviors and relate them back to possible implications for such concerns as how one behaves at work. The discussion became more intense regarding the role of the different types of occupational therapists and what they could and could not do or discuss with their patients. It was clear that the group members had different opinions regarding the appropriate depth and range of their interaction with patients. This difference was not divided along specialty lines. One therapist said, "Well, I work in physical disabilities and I talk about all sorts of things with my patients."

Others confirmed her position. The therapists were not in agreement regarding their role in discussing the more personal issues and what they considered to be intimate or embarrassing aspects of the person's thoughts, feelings, bodily functions, or history. Some believed that therapists should treat the whole person. However, others believed that their role was to treat only the physical aspects of the person's disability or functional limitation. Still other therapists were undecided about their stance on these issues.

A related issue came up weeks later in a discussion group with experienced therapists. Their concern was to identify exactly what constitutes treatment. They wanted to define which of the therapist's actions were part of the therapeutic process and which were not. These therapists were generally comfortable with the notion of treating the whole patient, but they were not sure whether their conversations with patients were part of the treatment. Because the therapists in this particular hospital tended to see patients on a fairly long-term basis, they knew the patients as individuals quite well. There seemed to be confusion regarding whether the therapist's understanding of the individual person and his or her concerns was part of therapy or simply an artifact of the therapist's personality. Some therapists felt strongly that the relationship with the patient was an essential element of the therapy. Others saw it as an adjunct to therapy. Still others saw it as not a part of therapy. Some believed that personal discussions were inappropriate.

It seemed that these two related issues of what aspects of the person an occupational therapist treats and what actions of the occupational therapist constitute the therapeutic process were sources of conflict for the therapists. There were two types of conflict. The opinion held by some therapists that occupational therapists should treat the whole person conflicted with the opinion that therapists should treat only the physical problems. Another conflict was that some therapists were uncertain about which of these two points of view or perspectives was the right one. This conflict seemed to be created, at least in part, by a perceived conflict between the medical model perspective and the humanistic perspective.

Therapists who had strong beliefs that their relationship with patients was an effective part of therapy thought that those beliefs were in conflict with the perspective of the medical setting. Issues such as what constitutes therapy, the role of the therapist, turf boundaries, and the necessity for scientific evidence as a validation of practice all served to deny or devalue the importance of therapists' concerns for the patient as a person. This feeling was so pervasive that some therapists had difficulty appreciating the depth and complexity of their practice. They seemed confused and wondered whether they should accept their own interpretations of their practice or the interpretations of individuals and groups around them. The discussions were full of comments like the following:

> Well, I know I was supposed to be teaching the lady bathing techniques. After all, that's my job—that's what I get paid for. But she really wanted to talk to me about her grandchild. So I did and she felt better and we understood each other better. Besides, what was I going to say? "Don't talk to me while you take a bath"? She has been much better at learning the bathing since that session, by the way. Of course, I put on the chart, "bathing training," but I sort of felt guilty even though I know I did the right thing. I know I wasn't wasting time chatting, but it could have looked that way.

The therapists believed that the physicians, administrators, and especially the insurance companies did not value their interactions with patients. They further believed that these various authorities would criticize them for interacting with patients and taking time away from what the authorities considered the real treatment. It soon became clear that those therapists who valued their relationship with the patient persisted in interacting with them as people regardless of the requirements of the hospital and reimbursement agencies. Therapists talked to, listened to, understood, and were respected by their patients. Therapists and patients valued these interactions. Most therapists valued interacting with patients but did not report talking with patients.

This process of conducting essentially two types of practice, one focused on the procedural treatment of the person's physical body and the other focused on the phenomenological person as an individual, is discussed by Mattingly (1991). The point here is that while two practices were conducted, only one was reported—the procedural practice. The interactive practice, which was the unreported practice, we called the underground practice. Later, we saw that although often underground, this sort of practice was important both to patients and therapists. It also had a logic or

reasoning strategy of its own and a particular way of guiding therapists' thoughts and actions. We called this *interactive reasoning*.

Interactive Reasoning

Interactive reasoning took place during face-to-face encounters between the therapist and the patient. It was the form of reasoning that therapists employed when they wanted to understand the patient as an individual. There were many reasons why a therapist might want to know the person better. The therapist might want to know how the person felt about the treatment at the moment or what the patient was like as a person, either out of sheer interest or in order to more finely tailor the treatment to his or her specific needs or preferences. Further, the therapist might be interested in this patient in order to better understand the experience of the disability from the person's own point of view. This is what Kleinman (1980) called the *illness perspective*, as contrasted with the *disease perspective*. The therapists wanted to know what the illness experience was like for a person. They wanted to understand the patients from their own point of view. Interactive reasoning occurred when therapists took the phenomenological perspective (Kestenbaum, 1982), although the therapists did not typically use that term to explain a shift to the humanistic point of view.

Several people have been interested in the clinical reasoning study and have analyzed various videotapes made during the data-gathering stage. Some have examined different aspects of interactive reasoning. The depth of these analyses is impressive, as is the complexity of the interactive reasoning strategies discovered. A compilation of those analyses shows us that therapists appeared to employ interactive reasoning for at least eight reasons or purposes, as follows:

1. To engage the person in the treatment session (Mattingly, 1989, identified six such strategies).
2. To know the person as a person (Cohn, 1989).
3. To understand a disability from the patient's point of view (Mattingly, 1989).
4. To finely match the treatment goals and strategies to this patient with this disability and this experience. Therapists call this process *individualizing treatment* (Fleming, 1989).
5. To communicate a sense of acceptance, trust, or hope to the patient (Langthaler, 1990).
6. To use humor to relieve tension (Siegler, 1987).

7. To construct a shared language of actions and meanings (Crepeau, 1991).
8. To determine if the treatment session is going well (Fleming, 1990).

It seems that although the therapists did not initially recognize interaction and interactive reasoning as central to their practice, they used it at least as an adjunct to practice on many occasions for various reasons. Perhaps particular interactive strategies were used for particular therapeutic reasons. Some of the reasoning styles or strategies identified and the hypothesized reasons for their use are similar to new concepts about reasoning that have been proposed by various psychologists and philosophers. Gardner (1985), for example, proposed that there are many useful ways to think and that hypothetical deductive reasoning is not necessarily the only, or even the best, way to think. Many forms of reasoning have been suggested by investigators who study how persons think about themselves and their experience within the cultural context (Berger & Luckman, 1967; Bruner, 1986, 1990). Many are concerned with how such elusive processes as values, norms (Perry, 1979), and symbolic meanings (Koestler, 1948) are used to guide, gauge, frame, and formulate thought and action (Bernstein, 1971; Dreyfus & Dreyfus, 1986; Geertz, 1983; Schön, 1983). Others examine properties of problems and relate them to particular problem-solving strategies. Some propose that features of the problem will influence individuals and, in effect, direct them to select a particular problem-solving method. Such features may include salient characteristics of a task or problem (Hammond, 1988), the context (Greeno, 1989), individual interests and talents (Gardner, 1985), or experience (Dewey, 1915).

The notion that characteristics of the presumed problem will prompt a particular thinking process seemed to be borne out in our observations of the therapists in the clinical reasoning study. The therapists shifted from one form of thinking to another. They often noted subtle cues and responded to them rapidly, then returned to another task and thinking mode without "skipping a beat," as one observer commented.

If such numerous reasoning strategies exist, and if the therapists had different purposes in mind for using interaction as a therapeutic medium, then it also seems likely that the purpose of the interaction would prompt the use of a particular reasoning strategy. For example, in trying to understand the person as a person, therapists' reasoning resembled what Belenky, Clinchy,

Goldberger, and Tarule (1986) described as *connected knowing,* which they linked to empathy. In trying to understand the disability from the patient's point of view, therapists used a phenomenological approach similar to that advocated by Paget (1988). Therapists' interactions with patients created an understanding of the person as an individual within a culturally constructed point of view, or what Schutz (1975) called a *reciprocity of motives.*

When individualizing treatment, therapists appeared to be functioning intuitively rather than analytically. Hammond (1988) proposed, however, that intuitive reasoning is as effective and complex as analytical reasoning. Intuitive reasoning is employed in response to problems that are not well defined. Tasks in which there are many cues from several sources and that require perceptual rather than instrumental measurement, Hammond argued, induce the person to use intuitive methods of problem solving. He further asserted that in these situations, analytical reasoning would be less effective than intuitive reasoning.

The interactive reasoning strategies that Mattingly (1989) identified indicate that therapists use several ways to engage the patient in treatment. To be effective, some of these strategies require complex interpretations of subtle interactive cues. The 23 interactive strategies that one therapist used in treatment, which were identified by Langthaler (1990), seem to suggest that the therapist was partially influenced by psychoanalytic theorists such as Rogers (1961) and occupational therapy theorists such as Fidler and Fidler (1963) and Mosey (1970). This finding is not surprising, because occupational therapy students are required to read the works of these theorists. The complexity, subtlety, and facility with which some therapists used numerous interaction forms, however, suggest processes far more complex than could be accounted for by professional education alone.

We also had a strong sense that the therapists' reasoning about and interaction with patients was directly related to their values. Their sense of the importance of patients as individuals leads one to draw parallels to beliefs about ethical and moral decision-making, such as those expressed by Gilligan (1982), Kegan (1982), and Perry (1979). The task of monitoring the patient's feelings about the treatment and yet managing that treatment, which is often difficult and sometimes painful or distasteful, seems to require a considerable amount of what Gardner (1985) referred to as *interpersonal intelligence.* Gardner postulated two kinds of interpersonal intelligence: "The capacity to access one's own feeling life" and the "ability to notice and make distinctions among other individuals in particular among their moods, temperaments, motivations and intentions" (p. 239). Interactive reasoning requires active judgment (Buchler, 1955) on several levels simultaneously. This requires that the therapist analyze cues from the patient, transmit his or her interpretation of the patient, and interpret the patient's interpretations of the therapist's interpretations quickly and accurately. This reciprocal process is one that Erikson (1968) considered essential to identity formation and future social interaction capabilities. Possibly, the therapist's ability to interact successfully and therapeutically is strongly linked to his or her personal and professional identify. Gardner hypothesized that interpersonal intelligence is based on a well-developed sense of self. Certainly it is linked to professional self-confidence. Novice therapists reported that in their first year of practice they did not have the confidence, nor did they believe they had the right, to interact with patients as individuals. They reported that they "stuck to the procedural" until they were confident in their use of those skills. We observed therapists even in the second year of practice going back and forth between the procedural and interactive modes of treating their patients. In the experienced senior therapists, procedural and interactive forms seemed to flow together, each enhancing the other.

We therefore found that interaction, which at first seemed like a distraction from treatment or, at best, an adjunct to it, was a necessary and legitimate form of therapy. Interactive reasoning was used effectively by most therapists to guide this aspect of their treatment. It appears that procedural reasoning guides treatment and interactive reasoning guides therapy. Although interactive reasoning is far more difficult to map than procedural reasoning, we will continue to make observations and develop theory in this area.

Conditional Reasoning

The concept of conditional reasoning is perhaps the most elusive notion in our proposed theory of a three-track mind. Yet we are firmly, if intuitively, convinced that there is a third form of reasoning that many therapists used. This reasoning style moves beyond specific concerns about the person and the physical problems placed on them to broader social and temporal contexts. The term *conditional* was used in three different ways. First, the therapist thought about the whole con-

dition, which involved the person, the illness, and the meanings the illness had for the person, the family, and the social and physical contexts in which the person lived. Second, the therapist needed to imagine how the condition could change. The imagined new state was a conditional (i.e., temporary) state that might or might not be achieved. Third, the success or failure of treatment was contingent on the patient's participation. The patient must participate not only in the therapeutic activities themselves, but also in the construction of the image of the possible outcome, that is, the revised condition.

Conditional reasoning seems to be a multidimensional process involving complicated, but not strictly logical, forms of thinking. In using conditional reasoning, the therapist appears to reflect on the success or failure of the clinical encounter from both the procedural and interactive standpoints and attempts to integrate the two. Thinking then moves beyond those immediate concerns to a deeper level of interpretation of the whole problem. The therapist interprets the meaning of therapy in the context of a possible future for the person. The therapist imagines what that future would be like. This imagined future is a guide to bringing about a revised condition through therapy. This thinking process is essentially imagination tempered by clinical experience and expertise.

The therapists tried to imagine what the person was like before the injury. Similarly, they tried to estimate or imagine what the possibilities were for the person's future life. By imagining, therapists mentally placed the person in contexts of current, past, and future social worlds. The therapists used imagination in order to best match the treatment selections to the specific interests, capacities, and goals of the person. Thus, the therapists were able to make their current treatment relevant to the individual patient. The present treatment, therefore, was not simply a link to future performance, but also was imagined within the context of a life in process.

Perhaps this form of reasoning is best described by example. Cathy, a pediatric therapist, was the most articulate about using this form of reasoning. Cathy usually treated very young children who lived in the community and had come to an outpatient early intervention program. The child's mother or guardian was usually present, and Cathy invariably included the mother in the session. The mother might be enlisted to hold the baby in an advantageous position or to help sustain the child's interest. Cathy would often talk to the mother while simultaneously working with the child. She often asked questions like, "Does he do this at home?" "Does he usually cry in this sort of situation?" "What does he like to do?" "Does he usually have difficulty calming himself down?" These were not diagnostic history-taking questions in the medical procedural sense. Cathy said she asked these questions to construct an image of what the child was really like on a day-to-day basis. She told us that she used this image to structure her treatment and imagine possible goals for the child. As she said:

> I see this little child and his movement patterns and his difficulties, and then I imagine what he will be like in 2 years and then when he is 5 (years old) and maybe going to school. I think of what I can do to help him develop the skills that he will need to function in school and in the community and what he will be like and how his family will be with him.

Here Cathy describes a process of imagining and integrating images of the past, present, and future for this child given the variables of the child himself, his developmental delays and disabilities, his family situation, the social and educational opportunities available to him, what he might be able to do in the future, and how she might enable that future condition to come about.

Clearly, it takes professional experience to be able to project the possible developmental pattern and potential rate of success in attaining a future developmental level. It also requires a mind that is imaginative, curious, and interested in future possibilities. Conditional reasoning involves a way of thinking that may include a systems perspective and that extends to the future (Mattingly, 1989), yet it moves beyond this perspective to an analysis of present interactions (Kielhofner, 1978; Mattingly, 1989), so that one can envision how these interactions might help create a better life for the child.

Having constructed these images, which changed slightly over time and throughout the course of treatment, the therapists used images as a way of interpreting the importance of the patient's treatment. Therapists would mentally compare the patient's abilities today and the relative success of today's treatment session against images of what the person was like before. They also compared where the patient was today to where they wanted the patient to be in the future. Each therapist would envision the patient today and estimate how close that was to where he or she thought the pa-

tient should be at this point in the course of treatment. They would mentally check to see how far the patient had come toward attaining the future the therapist had in mind. The evaluation of today's treatment was made in the context of past and future possibilities. Therefore, the particular state of things today would serve as a mental mile marker for indicating progress toward a distant, and perhaps only dimly perceived, future.

One reason that we called this conditional reasoning was because a change in the present condition was conditional on the therapist's and the patient's participation in effective therapy. This condition was dependent not only on the therapist's ability to engage the patient in treatment in the sense discussed in the interactive section, but also on building a shared image of the person's future self. This image building was often accomplished through stories or narrative, as described by Mattingly (1991). However, in many aspects of therapeutic interaction, the images that the therapists helped to build were often based in action. Pediatric therapists often included the mother in creating a mental image of the child in the future. This image was projected into the distant future, such as when a therapist wondered what an infant she was treating would be like in school several years later. Therapists projected images into the near future as well. They also used images as a way of extending therapy into the home setting. Cathy said to the child's mother, "Would he do this at home? Could he just sit quietly and look at something and have this nice position? Could the kids maybe hold him like I am doing while they watch TV?" Here she created a visual image, based on action in the present, of the child in a near-future situation. This was done not only to enhance the therapy, but also to build an image of the child as a participant in the family, rather than just as a disabled baby.

One technique for conveying these images that therapists often used was to tell patients that they were getting better and to produce evidence of this by saying such things as, "Remember when you could not do this? Now you can." Sometimes the therapists would also use this technique for themselves. Therapists commented that when they were discouraged with a patient's progress, they found it helpful to remind themselves of how far the patient had come. This technique helped both the patient and the therapist focus on the importance of their joint participation in this enterprise of treatment. It helped them through difficult, frustrating, and boring times and allowed them to place the moment in a more positive, though abstract and distant, context. Most importantly, it seemed to remind them that the condition was changing. Such changes were often quantitative, such as increased range of motion, and would be noted in the person's chart. But qualitative changes and their meanings were equally important to therapists and patients. Although these changes were not reported in the patient's chart, they did indicate progress toward that shared future image that the therapist and patient jointly constructed and worked toward. Meaningful progress was best measured through the therapist's and patient's collective memory. Therapists were not simply saying, "This is progress. Remember how bad things were before?" Instead, they were saying, "If you have come this far, maybe we will get to where you imagined you would be, even though you are discouraged today."

Putting It All Together: Treating the Whole Person

The therapists in the Clinical Reasoning Study often used two phrases to describe their treatment—*putting it all together* and *treating the whole person*. Treating the whole person did not mean that the therapists were in charge of the patient's whole medical and psychological treatment. In fact, in the traditional medical sense of the word *treatment,* occupational therapists are peripheral to the patient's treatment. The phrase was intended to convey the belief that therapists concern themselves with the patient as a person, that is, as an individual with many facets, interests, and concerns. By saying that they treat the whole person, therapists mean that they treat the person as a whole, not as the sum of ill and healthy parts.

The phrase *putting it all together* seemed to mean that although the therapists often had to think only about the disability or only of the individual patient at a given moment, they were concerned that they eventually thought and did something about the patient as a whole person, that is, person, illness, and condition. Although they used several types of reasoning and addressed several different types of concerns, therapists always wanted their reasoning to track back to making a better life for the patient as a person. Their ultimate goal was to use as many strategies as necessary to improve the individual functional performance of the person. Because functional performance requires intentionality, physical action, and social meaning, it is not surprising that persons who concern themselves with enabling function would have to address problems of the person's sense of self and future, the physical body, and meanings and social and cultural contexts—contexts in which actions are taken and meanings are made. Because these areas of inquiry are typically guided by different types of thinking, it seems necessary that therapists become facile in thinking about different aspects of human beings using various styles of reasoning. Perhaps these multiple ways of thinking guide the therapists in accomplishing and evaluating the mysterious process of "putting it all together" for the person. This process, which enables the whole person to function as a new self in the future, seemed to be guided by a complex yet unidentified form of reasoning that was both directed and conditional.

Conclusion

The Clinical Reasoning Study showed that therapists use several different types of reasoning to solve problems and to design and conduct therapeutic processes. Further, the particular reasoning processes are selected to guide inquiry into different aspects of the person's problem or of the therapist's intervention. As part of this research process, we developed a theory about these reasoning processes and constructed concepts to which we added terminology in order to discuss these concepts among ourselves and with the therapists. Thus, we referred to the type of reasoning that was used to guide those aspects of practice that are concerned with the treatment of the patient's physical ailment as *procedural reasoning. Interactive reasoning,* we propose, is a type of reasoning that therapists used to guide their interactions with the person. *Conditional reasoning* is both an imaginative and an integrative form of reasoning that the more proficient therapists used to think about the patient and his or her future, given the constraints of the physical condition within the patient's personal and social context. The therapists who were part of this study confirmed our assumptions that they use different forms of reasoning for different parts of the problem and found these concepts and terms useful in understanding and explaining their reasoning and practice.

References

Belenky, M. F., Clinchy, B. M., Goldberger, N. R., & Tarule, J. M. (1986). *Women's ways of knowing.* New York: Basic.

Berger, P., & Luckman, T. (1967). *The social construction of reality.* Garden City, NJ: Anchor.

Bernstein, R. J. (1971). *Praxis and action.* Philadelphia: University of Pennsylvania Press.

Bruner, J. (1986). *Actual minds, possible worlds.* Cambridge, MA: Harvard University Press.

Bruner, J. (1990). *Acts of meaning.* Cambridge, MA: Harvard University Press.

Buchler, J. (1955). *Nature and judgement.* New York: Columbia University Press.

Cohn, E. S. (1989). Fieldwork education: Shaping a foundation for clinical reasoning. *American Journal of Occupational Therapy, 43,* 240–244.

Coughlin, L. D., & Patel, V. L. (1987). Processing of critical information by physicians and medical students. *Journal of Medical Education 62,* 818–828.

Creapeau, E. B. (1991). Achieving intersubjective understanding: Examples from an occupational therapy treatment session. *American Journal of Occupational Therapy, 45,* 1016–1025.

Dewey, J. (1915). The logic of judgments of practice. *Journal of Philosophy, 12,* 505.

Dreyfus, H. L., & Dreyfus, S. E. (1986). *Mind over machine.* New York: Macmillan.

Elstein, A., Shulman, L., & Sprafka, A. (1978). *Medical problem solving. An analysis of clinical reasoning.* Boston: Harvard University Press.

Erikson, E. H. (1968). *Identity, youth, and crisis.* New York: Norton.

Feinstein, A. R. (1973). An analysis of diagnostic reasoning, Parts I & II. *Yale Journal of Biology and Medicine, 46,* 212–232, 264–283.

Fidler, G., & Fidler, J. (1963). *Occupational therapy: A communication process in psychiatry.* New York: Macmillan.

Fleming, M. H. (1989). The therapist with the three-track mind. In *The AOTA Practice Symposium program guide* (pp. 70–75). Bethesda, MD: American Occupational Therapy Association.

Fleming, M. (Ed.). (1990). *Proceedings of the Clinical Reasoning Institute for occupational therapy educators.* Medford, MA: Tufts University.

Gardner, H. (1985). *Frames of mind: The theory of multiple intelligences.* New York: Basic.

Geertz, C. (1983). *Local knowledge: Further essays in interpretive anthropology.* New York: Basic.

Gillette, N. P., & Mattingly, C. (1987). The Foundation—Clinical reasoning in occupational therapy. *American Journal of Occupational Therapy, 41,* 399–400.

Gilligan, C. (1982). *In a different voice: Psychological theory and women's development.* Cambridge, MA: Harvard University Press.

Greeno, J. (1989). A perspective on thinking. *American Psychologist, 44,* 134–141.

Hammond, K. H. (1988). Judgment and decision-making in dynamic tasks. *Information and Decision Technologies, 14,* 3–14.

Kegan, R. (1982). *The evolving self: Problems and process in human development.* Cambridge, MA: Harvard University Press.

Kestenbaum, V. (1982). *The humanity of the ill: Phenomenological perspectives.* Knoxville, TN: University of Tennessee Press.

Kielhofner, G. (1978). General systems theory: Implications for theory and action in occupational therapy. *American Journal of Occupational Therapy, 32,* 637–645.

Kleinman, A. (1980). *Patients and healers in the context of culture.* Los Angeles: University of California Press.

Koestler, A. (1948). *Insight and outlook: An inquiry into the common foundations of science, art, and social ethics.* Lincoln, NE: University of Nebraska Press.

Langthaler, M. (1990). *The components of therapeutic relationship in occupational therapy.* Unpublished master's thesis. Tufts University, Medford, MA.

Mattingly, C. (1989), *Thinking with stories: Story and experience in a clinical practice.* Unpublished doctoral dissertation, Massachusetts Institute of Technology, Cambridge, MA.

Mattingly, C. (1991). What is clinical reasoning? *American Journal of Occupational Therapy, 45,* 979–986.

Mosey, A. C. (1970). *Three frames of reference for mental health.* Thorofare, NJ: Slack.

Newell, A., & Simon, H. (1972). *Human problem solving.* Englewood Cliffs, NJ: Prentice Hall.

Paget, M. (1988). *The unity of mistakes.* Philadelphia: Temple University Press.

Perry, W. (1979). *Forms of intellectual and ethical development in the college years.* New York: Holt, Rinehart & Winston.

Rogers, C. (1961). *On becoming a person.* Boston: Houghton Mifflin.

Rogers, J. C., & Masagatani, G. (1982). Clinical reasoning of occupational therapists during the initial assessment of physically disabled patients. *Occupational Therapy Journal of Research, 2,* 195–219.

Schön, D. (1983). *The reflective practitioner: How professionals think in action.* New York: Basic.

Schutz, A. (1975). *On phenomenology and social relations.* Chicago: University of Chicago Press.

Siegler, C. C. (1987). *Functions of humor in occupational therapy.* Unpublished master's thesis, Tufts University, Medford, MA.

CHAPTER 43

The Narrative Nature of Clinical Reasoning

CHERYL MATTINGLY

Many professions identify good thinking with a process that resembles the scientific method—an application in practice of empirically tested abstract knowledge (theories) and generalizable factual knowledge. Here reasoning involves the recognition of particular instances of behavior in terms of general laws that regulate the relationship between the cause and a caused state of affairs (see Mattingly, 1991, for a related discussion of this point). There are many debates within the philosophy of science about whether this model of objective knowledge characterizes even the hard sciences, such as physics (Kuhn, 1962; Putnam,1979; Rorty, 1979). Also debated is whether the scientific method provides an appropriate model with which to characterize professional reasoning (Dreyfus & Dreyfus, 1986; Schön, 1983, 1987). I enter these debates in arguing that a narrative model of reasoning, as opposed to scientific reasoning in the traditional sense, is fundamental to the thinking of occupational therapists.

Therapists think with stories in two distinct, but equally important, ways—through storytelling and story creation. Storytelling constitutes an extremely important and underrated mode of discourse in occupational therapy. Recently, there has been a surge of interest in the health professions in eliciting stories from patients (Coles, 1989; Kleinman, 1988). It became clear in the course of the American Occupational Therapy Association/American Occupational Therapy Foundation Clinical Reasoning Study that therapists not only listen to the stories that their patients tell them, but also tell stories about their patients. Furthermore, an important part of this storytelling involves the therapist's understanding of the patient's way of dealing with disability and with puzzling about how to approach a problematic patient. The creation of clinical stories in clinical time is the second way in which occupational therapists use narrative in their reasoning process. I call such creation *therapeutic emplotment*.

Narrative Reasoning and Storytelling: Making Sense of the Illness Experience

What does it mean to say that occupational therapists think about their patients through the telling of stories and that this constitutes a primary form of thinking in their therapeutic practice? Jerome Bruner (1986, 1990), a psychologist noted for his studies of cognitive development, argued that humans think in two fundamentally different ways. He labeled the first type of thinking paradigmatic, that is, thinking through propositional argument, and the second, narrative, that is, thinking through storytelling. The difference between these two kinds of thinking involves how we make sense of and explain what we see. When we look at something and try to understand it through propositional argument, we are trying to take a particular and see it in general terms, as an instance of a general type. For example, when we see a patient with a set of symptoms, we may note that we are seeing a severe case of Parkinson's disease. According to Bruner, in linking the particular symptoms to a general disease category, we are thinking propositionally.

Conversely, when we are thinking narratively, we are trying to understand the particular case. Specifically, we are trying to understand a particular person's experience. Narrative thinking is our primary way of making sense of human experience. We do this primarily through an investigation of human motives (Burke,

This chapter was previously published in the *American Journal of Occupational Therapy, 45,* 998–1005. Copyright © 1991, American Occupational Therapy Association. Reprinted with permission. http://dx.doi.org/10.5014/ajot.45.11.998

1945; Gardner, 1982). We think narratively when we want to explain not whether someone has Parkinson's disease, but rather, why this patient's wife is so unwilling to have her husband be discharged home. The difference between these two modes of thinking in occupational therapy is illustrated by the way in which therapists use storytelling to talk about their cases over lunch or to present cases to colleagues in weekly departmental staff meetings.

At University Hospital in Boston, where the Clinical Reasoning Study took place, the therapists drew on two modes of talking to discuss patients. Case presentations consisted of two distinct parts: "chart talk" and storytelling. The first, chart talk, involved a familiar biomedical presentation. When speaking chart talk, therapists focused on the pathology in general. The items ordinarily addressed were (a) key symptoms; (b) major typical physical impairments and primary needs, especially activities of daily living needs; (c) assessment goals and other ways of rating a patient's extent of impairment; and (d) typical treatment modalities and strategies.

The second form of case presentation was through storytelling. Here the therapists shifted their focus from a discussion based on pathology to one based on the specific patients they had worked with and their experiences of disability. One example of such storytelling comes from a staff meeting in which an affiliating student was doing a presentation of a patient with Parkinson's disease. After discussing Parkinson's disease as a pathology, she turned to describe her problems with a specific patient with Parkinson's disease whom she was treating and how his wife was responding to her husband's disability. As part of her description of treating the patient, she recounted her interchanges with his wife. Here is part of the student's story:

He [the patient] said that something would have to be changed because his bedroom was downstairs in the basement. His wife wanted to keep him downstairs but finally agreed that he could have a bedroom in the living room. He progressed rapidly, and after a week and a half he was smiling, becoming more social. His wife told me, "He does nothing at home." I don't know if she could hear what we were telling her. We said, "He is not just sitting around. Many times he simply can't do anything because of the disease." When the wife heard that he would be on medication and that this would improve his functioning, she said to

him, "Good. There's a lot of chores around the house you can do." I don't know how much she heard of what we were telling her.

This story triggered a storytelling exchange in which others around the table offered their own experiences in treating patients with Parkinson's disease, emphasizing how the disease was experienced by the patient, the family, or themselves rather than its general medical features. Nearly all of the speakers told stories that elaborated on themes raised by the initial story. What does this storytelling have to do with clinical reasoning? When the student told her story about the wife of the patient with Parkinson's disease, she identified a critical problem for clinical reasoning: What is she supposed to do with the patient's wife? How should she best treat this patient, given his wife's feelings? How does the wife really feel? What are this wife's denial and anger about? Or is the wife displaying something that is being mistaken for denial or anger? These are all narrative questions whose answers require a kind of clinical reasoning that is fundamentally narrative in form. To return to Bruner's (1986, 1990) distinction, when we think in propositional arguments, we try to transcend particulars and strive for abstraction (i.e., for truths that transcend any particular historical situation). But narrative is rooted in the particular. Whereas propositional arguments are concerned with understanding phenomena in terms of general causes, narratives are concerned with the likely connections among particular events. Bruner gave a simple example to illustrate the difference. The statement "if x, then y" belongs to propositional argument. An occupational therapist is relying on propositional reasoning when she says, "If you see these symptoms, then you probably have a case of Parkinson's disease." Such if–then statements are aimed at providing an abstract description of a causal relationship that holds up generally or, ideally, universally across concrete individual cases.

This genre of descriptive and explanatory statements can be contrasted with a very different mode of explanation. Bruner (1986) gave the following illustration, borrowed from E. M. Forster (1927). The statement, "The king died, and then the queen died" (pp. 11–12) is a narrative statement that not only concerns the particular, that is, some specific king and queen, but also, suggests causes that lead one to wonder about intentions. Did the queen die of grief? Was the queen murdered? We investigate the meaning of a narrative statement by trying out different motivational possibilities; we search for what guided the action that the statement reports. And human action, unlike a pathological process, is motivated. Narratives make sense of reality by linking the outward world of actions and events to the inner world of human intention and motivation. To ask in a narrative sense why something happened is to ask what motivated the actors to do what they did. In the philosophy of history, this mode of narrative explanation has been called "explanation by reason" (Dray, 1971, 1980). In a story, a person's actions are accounted for—or explained—by their placement in some specific historical context that shows how and why they were begun, what other actions unfolded as a result, and how they evolved over time. So when we hear about a particular patient with Parkinson's disease whose wife complains that he does not do enough housework and we want to explain what is going on, we start asking the narrative questions enumerated earlier.

In moving between chart talk and storytelling, therapists present the clinical problem in different ways. The shift in presentation from an abstract discussion of Parkinson's disease to a story of a patient with Parkinson's disease who has an uncooperative wife involves much more than a move from the general to the concrete or from the objective to the subjective.

In chart talk, the focus is on a disease. The disease is the main character. But in storytelling, it is the patient's situation or experience with the disease that is the central clinical problem. The therapist might ask, What is the best way to treat the patient with Parkinson's disease who is going home to this particular wife? The severity and nature of the patient's dysfunctions are still important, but they are only one part of the picture that the therapist has to put together with the unique features of one patient's situation.

Therapists often speak of expert practice as involving the ability to "put it all together" for a particular patient. I suggest that what they mean by this involves a thinking that is essentially narrative. The therapist takes what he or she knows in general of a disease process, appropriate theoretical frames of reference, and relevant experience with similar patients and applies all of this generalized and abstract knowledge to a particular case, such as that of the patient whose wife thinks he should be able to do household chores and resists having his bed moved up to the first floor where he will have access to the bathroom.

Medical anthropologists have made an extremely useful distinction in looking at health care by separating disease from illness experience (Good, 1977; Good & Delvecchio-Good, 1980, 1985; Kleinman, 1988; Kleinman, Eisenberg, & Good, 1978). Although traditionally medicine has focused on the diagnosis and treatment of disease, anthropologists argue that much more attention needs to be given to treatment of the illness experience, which involves the way in which the disease affects the person's life. Physiologically, the same disease can result in a very different illness experience, depending on the patient's particular life history and life possibilities. The patient with Parkinson's disease whose wife learns all she can about the disease and welcomes her husband home is likely to have quite a different illness experience than the patient whose wife wants to relegate him to the basement.

What anthropologists have argued to the medical community during the last decade or two, occupational therapists have known for a long time: To effectively treat persons with long-term disabilities, one must treat the whole patient, which involves looking beyond the disease to how that disease is experienced by that particular patient. Treatment of a patient's illness experience is integral to good occupational therapy and it is where the heart of clinical reasoning lies; it is also where the thorniest reasoning puzzles present themselves. Reasoning about how to treat the illness experience is often the most difficult thing to teach the affiliating student or new therapist. How does a supervisor help a novice therapist to examine what is going on with this patient's wife and what therapeutic approach would best help this patient make the transition back home to this wife? Notably, when one addresses the illness experience, as opposed to the disease alone, it is often hard to establish who has the disease. Although a disease obviously belongs to one person—the patient—the illness experience, especially in the case of serious life-changing illnesses, is likely to be shared by the whole family.

Puzzling over how to treat a patient with Parkinson's disease, given how his wife is responding to the illness, involves narrative reasoning, because it involves consideration of the disease from the patient's and family's points of view. The therapist must try to imagine how it feels to the patient and to various family members to have this disease, how they are experiencing it, and how it enters and changes the life story of a patient and his or her family.

Narrative Reasoning and Story Making: Creating Clinical Stories

Therapists create as well as tell stories. The narrative nature of clinical reasoning manifests itself not only in the work therapists do to understand the effect of a disability in the life story of a particular patient, but also in the therapist's need to structure therapy in a narrative way, as an unfolding story. This is perhaps the most interesting and subtle use of narrative reasoning in occupational therapy practice. Therapy can be seen as a kind of short story within the patient's longer life story. The therapist enters and exits the patient's life, playing a part for only a short time. Often, this part occurs at a critical juncture in the patient's life, a turning point triggered by the onset or downturn of an illness. Sometimes it occurs at a critical juncture in an entire family's life, as is often true in pediatric therapy when a family is learning to adjust to a newborn with a disability or when a child with a disability begins school. If disability is considered in narrative terms as something that interrupts and irreversibly changes a person's life story, then work with a patient can be seen as one chapter in that life story.

Although this narrative language is not a familiar way for therapists to describe their own practice, it serves to highlight how intensely therapists want to make therapy itself an occasion for patients to remake life stories that can no longer continue as they once did when a disability was absent or less serious. The therapist enters the life story of a patient and has the task of negotiating with the patient what role therapy is going to play within the unfolding illness and rehabilitation story that the patient is living through. To be meaningful, occupational therapy must serve as a coherent short story within a larger narrative whole.

In each new clinical situation, then, the therapist must answer the question, What story am I in? To answer this question, the therapist must make some initial sense of the situation and then act on it. The process of treatment encourages, perhaps even compels, therapists to reason in a narrative mode. They must reason about how to guide their therapy with particular patients by imagining where the patient is now and where this patient might be at some future point after discharge. It is not enough for therapists to know how to do a set of tasks that have an abstract order based on a general or typical treatment plan; therapists must be able to picture a larger temporal whole, one that captures what they can see in a particular patient in the present and what they can imagine seeing sometime in the future. This picturing process gives them a basis for organizing tasks.

In her study of clinical reasoning among nurses, Benner (1984) noticed this narrative mode of reasoning in her subjects, although she did not focus on its narrative nature per se. The need for a narrative framework was suggested by a nurse quoted in Benner's study who worked in an intensive care nursery. She described what she considered to be the most essential kind of thinking she wanted her newly graduated students to evince at the end of their 3-month affiliation with her:

> To my mind, moving the child from Point A to Point B is what nursing is all about. You have to perform tasks along the way to make that happen, but performing the task isn't nursing. . . . I wanted to see a light going on—that OK, here's this baby, this is where this baby is at, and here's where I want this baby to be in six weeks. What can I do today to make this baby go along the road to end up being better? It's that kind of thing that's just happening now. They're [the student nurses] just starting to see the whole thing as a picture and not as a list of tasks to do. (p. 28)

This example emphasizes both the imagistic character of what the clinician needs to know, in contrast with the knowledge of tasks, and the context-specific nature of those images. Therapists in the Clinical Reasoning Study spoke similarly about picturing the patient and especially about having future images of who the patient could be. They believed that what they often held most vividly in mind when treating patients was not plans or objectives, but rather, pictures of the potential patient, that is, the future patient. For example, one of the pediatric therapists said, "You know, when I treat that 18-month-old child, I see the child at 3, then I see the child at 6, learning to hold a pencil. I have all these pictures in my head." The therapists described their difficulty when the patients or their families held different images of the future and their dilemma about the extent to which they should give patients or families their therapeutically based pictures, which were often more pessimistic. The therapists were frequently in the difficult position of trying to give hope to a patient while also having to let the patient know of his or her dark prognosis. The patients and their families could be extremely depressed about conditions that were even worse than they had imagined. The therapists spoke of these images as necessary but dangerous: necessary because the therapist and patient needed some guiding pictures, but dangerous because these pictures could blind the therapist or patient to what was realistically possible.

The therapists in the Clinical Reasoning Study were, like Benner's (1984) nurses, also conscious of the need to create specific images appropriate to a particular patient. General treatment goals devised from general knowledge of functional deficits and developmental possibilities were insufficient guides to practice, in the therapists' view. Instead, they worked with much more concrete guides, images, and stories, which were the "wholes" that allowed them to selectively choose what aspects of their knowledge base were appropriate to the situation. These images were organized temporally and teleologically, thus giving the therapists a sense of an ending for which they could strive.

Although these images of the future were often not formulated in words, unless there was some need to explicitly communicate them, they were part of what I call a prospective treatment story. In this prospective story, the therapists envisioned a possible and desirable future for the patient and imagined how they might guide treatment to bring such a future about.

The treatment approaches and treatment paths that the therapists tried to follow were often guided by such stories. These stories, derived from particular experiences and stereotypical (collectivized) scenarios, were projected onto new clinical situations in order to help therapists make sense of what story they were in and where they might go with particular patients. The therapists then attempted to enact their projected stories in the new clinical situations, working improvisationally to narratively pull in and build on whatever happened in a clinical session so as to add to the story's plot line. The therapists saw a possible story, which they recognized as clinically meaningful, and they tried to make that story come true by taking the individual episodes of their clinical encounters and treating them as parts of a larger, narratively unfolding whole. Prospective treatment stories were based on what therapists observed and inferred about the patient's larger life history, which involved both the patient's past and future. The therapeutic stories that the therapists imagined took their power and plausibility as part of a larger historical context that included a past that began before therapy started and a future that would extend after therapy had ended.

Notably, the prospective story cannot be equated with treatment goals and plans, although these will be incorporated into the story. Therapists try to create significant therapeutic experiences and not simply reach a set of objectives in the most efficient way possible. They are concerned that the whole process of therapy unfold in such a way that patients will have powerful experiences of successfully met challenges; such challenges will motivate them to believe in therapy and work hard at it. In listening to therapy success stories, I found it rare for the success of therapy to have been measured by the reaching of the final goal. Rather, most of the therapists counted success as the generation of therapeutic experiences along the way, in which patients developed increasing confidence and commitment to take on challenges. The whole treatment story mattered.

Therapists in the Clinical Reasoning Study also worked to create significant experiences for their patients, ones worth telling stories about, because if therapy was to be effective, then the therapists had to find a way to make the therapeutic process matter to the patient. Each therapist faced the problem of constructing therapeutic activities that were meaningful enough to elicit the patient's active cooperation. The patients had to see something at stake in therapy. Otherwise, why should they bother to try? If the patient did not try, therapy did not work. This was partly because the therapists required the patients to do things in therapy that the patients did not necessarily feel ready to do or believe to be worth the effort. But more important, the patients had to become committed because they had to take up the therapeutic activities. Therapists were often with patients only a short time—just a few weeks or less. They might teach a few skills or improve the patient's strength a bit, but generally their effectiveness depended on the use of therapy as a catalyst to help patients begin to see how they might do for themselves even when the therapist was no longer present.

For example, a therapist is working with a spinal cord–injured patient, teaching him to move checkers pieces with a mouth stick. It is not enough for this patient to learn to move these checkers pieces for the therapy to be successful; he must also take up a point of view that comes with being committed to the tremendous concentration needed to perform this previously trivial task. He must absorb a vision about why he should work so hard at something that was once so easy. This is just as critical as the skills he acquires. The therapeutic time together itself must provide a kind of existential picture of how he might live his life in the future with his disability. Therapy will not ultimately work, not in any catalytic way that patients will take home when they leave the hospital, if they are not strongly committed to the process. Without experiencing treatment activities from a committed stance, they will not see any future in them. They will not see the point.

If the patient is to become committed to the therapeutic process, then both the patient and the therapist must share a view about why engaging in any particular set of treatment activities makes sense. Coming to share such a view requires that both the therapist and the patient see how these treatment activities are going to move the patient toward some future that he or she can care about. Such a view is not reducible to a general prognosis or even to a shared understanding of a treatment plan. The therapist and patient must come to share a story about the therapeutic process; they must come to see themselves as in the same story. This is a kind of future story, a story of what has not yet happened, or has only partly happened—an as yet unfinished story.

How is such a story constructed? Generally it is not constructed through any explicit storytelling, but rather, through the sharing of powerful therapeutic experiences that point to a prospective story—a path that therapy will take. Clinical reasoning requires that the therapist (a) see possibilities for creating important experiences in which the patient will be staked, (b) make moves to act on those possibilities, (c) respond to the moves the patient makes in return, and (d) build on the experience by showing the patient a future in which this therapeutic experience becomes one building block. In the language of narrative, the experience becomes one episode in a much longer story. The therapist tells the story not in words but in actions that create an experience the patient can care about.

I follow the work of the philosophers Ricoeur (1984) and White (1987) in describing this therapeutic work as "emplotment." The clinician's narrative task is to take the episodes of action within the clinical encounter and structure them into a coherent plot. A plot is what gives unity to an otherwise meaningless succession of events. Quite simply, "emplotment is the operation that draws a configuration out of a simple succession" (Ricoeur, 1984, p. 65). What we call a story is precisely this rendering and ordering of a succession of events (e.g., a series of treatment activities) into parts belonging to a larger narrative whole. When a therapeutic process has been successfully emplotted, it is driven and shaped by a sense of an ending (Kermode, 1966). To have a single story is to have made a whole out of a succession of actions. These actions then take their meaning by belonging and contributing to the story as a whole. A story, Ricoeur wrote, "must be more than just an enumeration of events in serial order: it must organize them into an intelligible whole, of a sort such

that we can always ask what is the 'thought' of this story" (p. 65).

Narratives give meaningful structure to life through time. The told narrative builds, to borrow from Ricoeur's (1984) argument, on action understood as an as yet untold story. Or, in Ricoeur's provocative phrase, "action is in quest of narrative" (p. 74). Therapists are in a quest to transform their actions and the actions of their patients into as yet untold stories.

This can be translated into more familiar clinical language through a narrative reading of treatment goals. When an occupational therapist makes an assessment of the patient, the outcome is a set of treatment goals. Goals, according to Ricoeur (1984), are not predictions of what will happen; rather, they express the actor's intentions and preferences. These goals express a therapeutic commitment. They capture what the therapist intends to accomplish over the course of therapy. Treatment goals are an expression of what the therapist has committed himself or herself to care about with a particular patient.

As occupational therapists have argued (Rogers, 1983 [see Chapter 41]; Rogers & Kielhofner, 1985), a primary task of clinical reasoning is the individualization of treatment goals. Narratively, individualization involves the construction of a particular story of the treatment process rather than reliance on a generic line of action that strings together standard goals and activities.

Therapeutic Emplotment: A Case Example

A wonderful illustration of this process of narratively structured treatment is given by O'Reilly (1990), who, as part of the Clinical Reasoning Study, described her work with a head injury group. O'Reilly recounted a situation in which she was asked to take over a failing head injury group that was poorly attended. The first thing that bothered her was its name—the Upper Extremity Group. She described her first visit to the group, "I enter the large OT/PT treatment area where I see several residents scattered about at tables and exercise equipment. . . . At one table, a resident diligently puts small pegs into a pegboard. . . . What is most memorable is the silence. Except for the clang of the pulley weights, a dropped peg or the therapist's quiet voice, there is not a sound in this room" (p. 2).

O'Reilly noticed that several of the group members were not present, and when she went to inquire, they told her, "That [expletive deleted] group is a waste of time." She tried several strategies to entice members back, but nothing worked. She puzzled:

> I wonder, "What's wrong with this group?"
> I make mental lists:
>
> 1. The name—I'll talk to the residents about that.
> 2. The activities—no meaning, no purpose, no life-related goals, no goals that belong to the patients.
> 3. No interaction among members with the therapist.
> 4. Nobody is having fun—the residents are bored and the therapist is bored (and boring?).
> 5. Is there any progress that the residents experience?
> 6. What are the reasons for attending or not attending? and there is no direction—no theme.
> (O'Reilly, 1990, p. 2)

Although O'Reilly did not use the language of story to describe the problems she noticed, this list could easily be restated in narrative terms. Her statement that the group has no direction and no theme could be recast to say that there is no plot to this group; there is no story for which the group members are a part. The group is not going anywhere, narratively speaking. Any particular group activity is not an episode in an unfolding story that members share. The activities of the group are focused on broken body parts, as the group name (Upper Extremity Group) implies. Although the exercises may help improve body functioning, they carry no intrinsic meaning to the group members, because group activities are in no sense a short story in the larger life story of the patients.

The therapist pondered what to do by beginning to think about individual group members. Her mode of puzzling represents a shift from a biomechanical framing of the members' disability to seeing their disability as having personal meaning in their lives. She described her reasoning in this way: "I think about the people. What do they want? What do they need? They are all so young; so far from home. They want to get out. They want to go home. HOME! They're all from New York. That's it! NEW YORK! I have a theme with which to begin" (O'Reilly, 1990, p. 2).

O'Reilly was reasoning in narrative terms. She was not telling a story, but she was beginning to envision a prospective story that all the group members could be a part of. She wrote:

> I have a theme with which to begin, but I don't know a thing about New York. The Program

Director is from New York . . . I dash to her office. "New York," I blurt. "The Upper Extremity Group, they're all from N.Y. Tell me something about N.Y., anything, everything." She lists: "Empire State Building, Statue of Liberty, Long Island Ferry, the subway." Laughingly, "You could have a New York Subway Group." I reply, "We could be on the subway. They can take me to New York. What does it look like—is there graffiti? We can do graffiti. I need a new room, away from the big treatment room. Can we use the small meeting room?" Program Director replies "yes" and adds that she has a map of the N.Y. subway and will bring it in. "I'll be the conductor . . . I have a blue blazer." She says, "I think I have a funny little hat that will pass for a conductor's hat." We laugh through all the possibilities of this activity. This is going to be FUN! (O'Reilly, 1990, p. 3)

In deciding to create a therapy group around a New York theme, O'Reilly could not only locate therapy in the relevant past of these patients, but also locate it within the future that they desire. This study dealt with young people in a chronic long-term care facility in Massachusetts, one that residents rarely ever leave. These patients wanted to go home.

O'Reilly invented the ingenious idea of turning a therapy room into a New York subway station. She also devised a way of generating some interest in the group:

> I go straight to Mike's room and ask him to make sure everyone comes to group today. "I have a different type of activity planned, and I'd really like to talk to everyone so that we can make some plans together." Mike states that he hates the [expletive deleted] group. I tell him that I understand that and that perhaps he could gather everyone for me, and come for awhile. "Then, if you are really unhappy with the activity, you can leave." He agrees. I hand him a small bag containing poker chips and ask him to give one to each group member on the attached list and have them bring the chips to group. "Okay, but what the [expletive deleted] are these for?" "It's a surprise. See you at 1:30." (O'Reilly, 1990, p. 3)

Notably, in announcing the group, she introduced a key narrative element critical to any dramatic story—the element of suspense. In any good story, the reader will want to know what will happen next. To prepare for the meeting of the group, the therapist lined three walls of the therapy room with white paper. She labeled spots with street names and subway stops and hung a subway map on the fourth wall.

Just as the group was scheduled to begin, O'Reilly stood outside the door in a subway conductor's uniform (trying not to feel too foolish in front of other surprised hospital colleagues) and waited for group members to arrive. She, herself, also felt unsure about what would happen:

> I put out materials, don my conductor's uniform and stand outside the door, on which a sign reads: NEW YORK THIS WAY. As I await the passengers, my stomach churns with anxiety and excitement, and I wonder where this subway ride will take us. (O'Reilly, 1990, p. 3)

She described the following scene:

> As the members arrive, escorted by Mike, I take their tokens, explaining that it's commuter fare for a ride on the New York Subway. Nancy grins, Eileen looks puzzled. Bobby shrugs. Mike says, with a great laugh, "You are crazy!" As these travelers enter the room, I hear snickers and queries like, "What the [expletive deleted] is she doing?" and comments like, "It's better than the other room." Then snickers, laughter, recognition. They go from stop to stop, reading, commenting, all smiling! [As they turn to her, she explains] "You folks are all from N.Y. Right? This is a N.Y. subway station. You've all ridden on the subway, right? M. tells me that there's graffiti, words and pictures on the walls, in the subway. We're going to do graffiti. You do remember graffiti, don't you?" "Yeah," laughs Mike, "but nothing I could write HERE!" With that, I close the door, and say, "You can draw or write anything you want in this room. The only rule is that you use the tools that I give you." These tools have been chosen with particular concern for the motor deficits of individual patients: "Large colored pencils and wrist weights for Mike who has a tremor, but brush and paint for Bobby who's working on gross motor skills, crayons for Nancy who needs to strengthen wrist and fingers, mark-

ers for Eileen who can't tolerate resistance." (O'Reilly, 1990, p. 4)

O'Reilly described the reaction of her "travelers" to this new activity:

> Eileen asks, "Where are we supposed to be?" "Anywhere you'd like to be, and when you finish working at one place, you can move to another. It's up to you." Nancy starts: "This is neat . . . just like when I was a kid." We're off!

From this point on, drawing, writing, conversation, and laughter are continuous. So much activity fills this room that it is difficult to remember details. Words, pictures, memories, and feelings cover the walls:

> "This place sucks." "My ass is stuck in Mass." "Home sweet Home." And on and on. . . . I go from one participant to another, asking about their work or just watching. After 35 minutes, I ask the group to finish up their artwork so that we can talk a bit and plan for our next group session. Stickball wins unanimously. Since, I admit, I know nothing about stickball, I ask the group to write out rules and equipment we'll need and get it to me on Tuesday. They agree, and, in fact, begin to work immediately. As I leave to see my next client, I tell the group,"You guys can hang out here for awhile. Just be sure to take your words and pictures with you when you leave." Thinking . . . clean up can wait. (O'Reilly, 1990. p. 4)

The end result of this therapeutic intervention was the beginning of the "New York Gang," as they came to call themselves. They met not only twice a week but also informally on the weekends, at which time they planned a series of events and activities. Their ventures included "making giant pretzels and cooking hot dogs to sell from a makeshift pushcart; taking a trip to a simulated Central Park; and filling a photo album with pictures of the group, home, drawings, postcards, and *New York Times* clippings" (O'Reilly, 1990, p. 4). The therapist had begun a story that spawned additional episodes. She set a therapeutic story in motion. The first group session that O'Reilly described in her case not only had a coherent plot, that is, a beginning, middle, and end (making graffiti), but also, because of her success, that session became just one episode in an unfolding therapeutic story in which patients became a cast of characters in the New York Gang. Even the name of the group came from the group members themselves. Specific biomechanical interventions were integrated in a meaningful way as activities allowed group members to act their part in this drama, and the task of writing things on the wall allowed each person to express an individual voice as well.

When O'Reilly initially devised the idea of doing something with a New York theme, the prospective story that she had begun to envision (and that she had concretely begun when she fixed up a room and donned a conductor's uniform) was much more than a set of treatment goals. Specific goals were incorporated in the narrative plot that she started. The success of this therapeutic intervention was ensured when the patients themselves took the story up and began to create new episodes that the therapist could not have imagined.

Narratively speaking, the shift of names from the Upper Extremity Group to the New York Gang represents a shift from a series of interactions in which therapeutic time is treated as a mere succession of activities, that is, as a procedural movement not grounded in context or in a picture of the patient, to narrative shaping of the therapeutic interaction in which therapeutic time has been emplotted by the clinician's picture of how to create an important therapeutic experience for the patients. The therapeutic efficacy of this intervention is about much more than meeting specific treatment goals. It is about creating an experience that gives the participants a vision of themselves as actors in the world, that is, as more than just patients.

Conclusion

Narrative thinking is central in providing therapists with a way to consider disability in the phenomenological terms of injured lives. Narrative thinking especially guides therapists when they treat the phenomenological body; that is, when they are concerned with their patients' illness experience and how the disability is affecting their lives.

In this article, I examined two kinds of narrative thinking. One is narrative as a mode of talk that therapists rely on to consider certain kinds of clinical puzzles. Because narratives are predominantly about human actions, they provide a particular vantage point from which one can view the nature of clinical practice and pose clinical problems. The stories that the therapists

told portrayed disability from an actor-centered point of view. They were personal, even individualistic, built on the structure of actors acting. Disability itself shifted from a physiological event to a personally meaningful one, that is, to an illness experience. General physiological conditions were shadowed as background context. What was brought to center stage were the ways that particular actors, with their own motivations and commitments, had done things for which they could be praised or blamed.

The second form of narrative thinking, which occurs in occupational therapy in a more subtle way, is story making, which involves the creation rather than the telling of stories. The telling of stories is always retrospective—a way of considering past events—whereas story making is largely prospective, playing out images that therapists have of what they would like to happen in therapy. Story making as therapeutic emplotment concerns the way in which therapists work to structure therapy narratively, thus creating dramatic therapeutic events that connect therapy to a patient's life. Often, the search for a meaningful therapeutic story appears to be triggered by resistance or alienation of the patient to the initial therapeutic activities offered, as in the case of the members of the Upper Extremity Group. Whatever the impetus, therapists try to create clinical experiences in which there is a significant occurrence or event for the patient in therapy, one in which the therapy itself is a meaningful short story in the larger life story of the patient.

References

Benner, P. (1984). *From novice to expert. Excellence and power in clinical nursing practice.* Reading, MA: Addison-Wesley.

Bruner, J. (1986). *Actual minds, possible worlds.* Cambridge, MA: Harvard University Press.

Bruner, J. (1990). *Acts of meaning.* Cambridge, MA: Harvard University Press.

Burke, K. (1945). *A grammar of motives.* Berkeley, CA: University of California.

Coles, R. (1989). *The call of stories.* Cambridge, MA: Harvard University Press.

Dray, H. (1971). On the nature and role of narrative in historiography. *History and Theory, 10,* 153–171.

Dray, W. (1980). *Perspectives on history.* London: Routledge & Keegan Paul.

Dreyfus, H., & Dreyfus, S. (1986). *Mind over machine: The power of human intuition and expertise in the era of the computer.* New York: Free Press.

Forster, E. M. (1927). *Aspects of the novel.* Harcourt Brace Jovanovich.

Gardner, H. (1982, March). The making of a storyteller. *Psychology Today,* pp. 49–63.

Good, B. (1977). The heart of what's the matter: The semantics of illness in Iran. *Culture, Medicine, and Psychiatry, 1,* 25–28.

Good, B., & Delvecchio-Good, M.J. (1980). The meaning of symptoms: A cultural hermeneutic model for clinical practice. In I. Eisenberg and A. Kleinman (Eds.), *The relevance of social science for medicine* (pp. 165–196). Norwell, MA: D. Reidel.

Good, B., & Delvecchio-Good, M. J. (1985). *The cultural context of diagnosis and therapy.* Unpublished manuscript.

Kermode, F. (1966). *The sense of an ending: Studies in the theory of fiction.* London: Oxford University Press.

Kleinman, A. (1988). *The illness narratives. Suffering, healing, and the human condition.* New York: Basic.

Kleinman, A., Eisenberg, L., & Good, B. (1978). Culture, illness, and care: Clinical lessons from anthropologic and cross-cultural research. *Annals of Internal Medicine, 88,* 251–258.

Kuhn, T. (1962). *The structures of scientific revolutions.* Chicago: University of Chicago Press.

Mattingly, C. (1991). What is clinical reasoning? *American Journal of Occupational Therapy, 45,* 979–986.

O'Reilly, M. (1990). *The New York subway.* Unpublished data, Tufts University Clinical Reasoning Institute, Boston.

Putnam, H. (1979). *The meaning and the moral sciences.* Boston: Routledge & Keegan Paul.

Ricoeur, P. (1984). *Time and narrative* (Vol. 1). Chicago: University of Chicago Press.

Rogers, J. (1983). Clinical reasoning: The ethics, science and art. *American Journal of Occupational Therapy, 37,* 601–616. Reprinted as Chapter 41.

Rogers J. C., & Kielhofner, G. (1985). Treatment planning. In G. Kielhofner (Ed.), *A model of human occupation* (pp. 136–155). Baltimore: Williams & Wilkins.

Rorty, R. (1979). *Philosophy and the mirror of nature.* Princeton, NJ: Princeton University Press.

Schön, D. (1983). *The reflective practitioner. How professionals think in action.* New York: Basic.

Schön, D. (1987). *Educating the reflective practitioner.* San Francisco: Jossey-Bass.

White, H. (1987). *The content of the form: Narrative discourse and historical representation.* Baltimore: Johns Hopkins University Press.

CHAPTER 44

A Framework of Strategies for Client-Centred Practice

GAYLE RESTALL, JACQUIE RIPAT, AND MARLENE STERN

Client-centred practice is a commonly used term in occupational therapy and other health professions. Although there is intellectual acceptance of its approach within occupational therapy daily practice, practical barriers to implementation continue to exist. To help therapists overcome these we have developed the Client-centred Strategies Framework (CSF). It consists of five categories of strategies: personal reflection, client-centred processes, practice settings, community organizing and, coalition advocacy and political action. The strategies identified within the CSF are intended to challenge clinicians to expand their thinking about the possible approaches they might use to be more client-centred. Some of the strategies will seem comfortable and congruent with clinicians' current levels of knowledge, skills, attitudes and experiences. Others will encourage exploration beyond current comfort zones and challenge clinicians to move in new and exciting directions for personal and professional growth. Each category will be described and its application illustrated through a case study developed from our collective experiences on how an occupational therapist could use the CSF.

Barriers to Client-Centred Practice

Client-centred practice is a complex construct that is contextually framed by the clinician, the client and the environments in which they interact (Canadian Association of Occupational Therapists [CAOT], 1997). Core concepts of client-centred practice that have emerged from the literature include developing partnerships with people receiving services, providing clients with informed choices about their health care, facilitating client decision making and ensuring that services are accessible and fit into the context of client's lives (CAOT, 1997; Fearing & Clark, 2000; Law, 1998; Law, Baptiste & Mills, 1995; Sumsion, 1999). Evidence is mounting that using a client-centred approach has a positive effect on the occupational therapy process (Law et al., 1995; Rebeiro & Cook, 1999). This evidence has given increased credibility to using this approach. Despite a belief in and an increasing understanding of what client-centred practice is, some occupational therapists continue to have difficulty implementing this approach (Brown & Bowen, 1998; Law et al., 1995; Law & Mills, 1998; Neistadt, 1995; Stern & Restall, 1993; Sumsion & Smyth, 2000). Occupational therapists face the challenge of applying the client-centred approach in a variety of health care environments, some of which are solidly supportive of this model and many that are not.

Many barriers to client-centred practice have been identified and can be grouped into clinician barriers, client barriers, client–clinician relationship barriers and contextual or environmental barriers. Clinician barriers may relate to perception of client safety, clinician confidence and clinician values (Sumsion, 1999). Client barriers can consist of issues related to social environment, family, level of education, culture or problem-solving skills. Client–clinician relationship barriers often relate to expectations placed on the relationship by either partner and by past experiences. Environmental barriers can relate to time pressures that clinicians may experience, the approaches used by other team members, and the philosophy of the program (Wilkins, Pollock, Rochon & Law, 2001).

Some authors have provided insight as to how these barriers may be resolved (Baum, 1998; Sumsion, 1999; Wilkins et al., 2001). Client-centred practice and the

This chapter was previously published in the *Canadian Journal of Occupational Therapy, 70*, 103–112. Copyright © 2003, Canadian Association of Occupational Therapists. Reprinted with permission.

strategies that enhance this practice will evolve as clinicians, health care environments, and the capacities and expectations of clients change. Using a framework for selecting strategies provides clinicians with a tool that can inform the choice and modification of strategies. This can occur over time and within a variety of contexts.

Development of the Framework

The Client-centred Strategies Framework was developed as both a companion to the Client-centred Process Evaluation (CCPE) (Restall, Stern, & Ripat, 2000) and as a tool to be used independently. The CCPE is described in *Individuals in Context, A Practical Guide to Client-Centred Practice* (Stern, Restall, & Ripat, 2000) as a tool to facilitate therapists to evaluate their practice, obtain feedback from their clients, analyze their practice environments and consider alternative strategies for improving practice. This process is accomplished through the use of clinician and client questionnaires (Part 1—Therapeutic Process and Relationship, Part 2—Environmental Scan), a reflection summary form, client-centred strategies, and an action plan form. Conversations with practising clinicians using the CCPE during its development led to the conclusion that while the strategies section of the CCPE was useful, clinicians desired more information on the strategies and support for their use. The CSF was developed to address this need. The CSF builds on the Client-centred Process Evaluation (Restall et al., 2000) and draws on current knowledge of the concepts of client-centred practice (CAOT, 1997; Fearing & Clark, 2000; Law, 1998; Sumsion, 1999) and the therapeutic process described in the Occupational Performance Process Model (Fearing, Law & Clark, 1997).

The CSF may be beneficial to students, novice clinicians and experienced clinicians. For example, it could assist clinicians who are struggling with a challenging clinical issue by identifying strategies and actions that could be used to resolve it. Others may use the CSF to further develop their professional knowledge, skills, and attitudes about client-centred practice. The framework has the potential to push the client-centred comfort zone of clinicians and challenge them to actualise strategies beyond those routinely chosen. Some of the strategy categories are intended to encourage clinicians to move beyond the traditional domains of addressing client performance issues for occupational therapists (i.e., working directly with an individual client) to less traditional domains that involve a systems perspective (i.e., community organizing or political and coalition advocacy). Finally, the CSF may be used to facilitate discussion of client-centred issues between clinicians and clients, family members, colleagues and communities.

The Client-Centred Strategies Framework

The CSF encourages conscious and purposeful use of strategies with consideration of the context, and clinicians' professional and personal development needs. It presupposes that clinicians have the ability to make changes that will enable client-centred practice. Covey's (1989) concept of a circle of influence suggests that each person can take action on the matters over which they have control. Using the CSF can help clinicians be proactive in creating a context for client-centred practice. The circles of influence that the individual clinician may influence include intrapersonal behaviours and actions, issues that are external to the person and require negotiation, co-operation or action by other people and processes that occur within political, social or organizational systems. Choosing whether to exert that influence at an intrapersonal, interpersonal or systemic level is the first step in using the CSF. The client-centred strategies chosen will then correspond to where the clinician chooses to act on that circle of influence.

The ideas that are presented within the five strategy categories are not new. We have simply arranged actions into a framework that encourages addressing client-centred issues from a variety of perspectives. Clinicians can selectively choose strategies from the categories or create their own.

Each of the five categories will be described with examples of strategies. A case example will be used to illustrate application of the strategies. Figure 44.1 provides additional suggestions for actions within each category.

Personal Reflection

Personal reflection is the process of cognitively and affectively exploring clinical experience to gain greater insight into client-centred practice. Through this category of strategies clinicians improve client-centred processes by making changes within themselves. Self-reflection is the exploration of the clinician's own knowledge, values and beliefs about a whole range of personal and professional experiences and tasks. It facilitates a better understanding of how personal values and beliefs shape one's practice. Through self-reflection, clinicians explore and resolve the differences between

Personal Reflection	Client-centred Processes	Practice Settings	Community Organizing	Coalition Advocacy and Political Action
Embark on a journey of reflection by: • utilizing structured reflective mini workbooks and tools • keeping a professional journal and reflecting on your practice **Enhance communication skills by:** • developing assertiveness skills • becoming a more effective negotiator **Learn more about yourself by:** • reflecting on and clarifying your values and beliefs • identifying your strengths as a clinician • exploring your potential role as a leader in client-centred practice **Learn more about client-centred practice by:** • reading client-centred practice literature • going to a conference with a focus on client-centred practice • finding a mentor who embodies client-centred practice principles • organizing a study group that uses case examples of applying client-centred approaches • observing other therapists practice and identifying opportunities for client-centred practice • asking others to observe your practice and identifying opportunities for client-centred practice	**Evaluate the use of client-centred processes by:** • using structured evaluation tools that measure client-centred processes • conducting studies that investigate cost effectiveness, efficiency or client satisfaction with client-centred practice • reviewing documentation to determine congruence with client-centred principles **Facilitate receipt of client-centred care by:** • educating clients about client-centred approaches • encouraging clients to discuss their values • teaching clients advocacy skills • coaching and encouraging clients to question health care providers **Model client-centred behaviours by:** • providing clinical services in an environment that is meaningful to the client • using assessment tools and processes that are based on client-centred frames of reference	**Advocate for a client-centred workplace by:** • revising mission statements, job descriptions, performance appraisal tools and policies to reflect client-centred care • incorporating client perspectives into program planning and evaluation • organizing support networks with colleagues around client-centred issues with the goal of improving service quality • learning from strategies used by other client-centred organizations • conducting environmental audits to determine the extent to which the environment is welcoming to people with varying abilities, cultures, and lifestyles **Communicate to treatment teams about client-centred practice by:** • reporting on use of client-centred approaches with individual clients and the outcomes of the approaches • talking with colleagues about client-centred practice and its impact within practice settings	**Inform communities about client-centred health services by:** • writing media releases, editorials, and letters to the editor • drafting and circulating position statements that support client-centred practice • serving as resource to self help groups • advocating for clients to assume leadership positions on health related boards **Engage in community development by:** • partnering with persons who are working to build healthier communities • assisting in the formation of client and resident advisory committees • providing support and expertise to community members attempting to overcome barriers to client-centred health services • facilitating the leadership skills of community members **Engage in community planning by:** • conducting needs and capacities assessments in communities • advocating for clients to have meaningful participation in community planning • illustrating how broad system structures, policies, and resource allocation can support or impede full participation of all people in communities	**Demonstrate a position on client-centred practice by:** • collaborating with other groups, organizations, professional associations and government bodies that support client-centred principles • advocating for funding models that give clients more control over how services are purchased and used • supporting community and self help groups who are advocating for legislation and policies that are congruent with client-centred principles • advocating for policy planning that crosses government departments **Influence persons of influence by:** • meeting with and writing politicians about the status and benefits of client-centred practice • speaking publicly about client-centred issues

Figure 44.1. Client-centred Strategies Framework.

577

what one would like to do and what one does (Schon, 1987). A solid foundation of knowledge of client-centred practice is helpful as a basis for enhancing personal reflection. A clinician's values, beliefs and skills all contribute to assumptions and the resultant behaviour toward the client (Kinsella, 2001).

The process of clarifying values can be a powerful tool in understanding the comfort or discomfort one feels when pursuing a certain course of action. Sometimes a clinician will have difficulty accepting a client's choices because the choices may be different than the clinician's deeply ingrained value system. Clarifying values assists the clinician to understand their reaction to, and resistance of behaviours when the client's values are different than their own. The clinician then makes decisions about what he or she can morally support with a client. When a situation arises where values seem to be in conflict, clarifying and articulating values helps illuminate an appropriate course of action that allows the clinician to remain true to his or her own values while supporting the client in the enablement of chosen occupations.

Clinicians' behaviours in therapeutic situations are shaped by ingrained beliefs about the world and people. These beliefs have been called mental models, a term that is often used to understand why people behave the way they do (Senge, Roberts, Ross, Smith, & Kleiner, 1994). Reflecting on mental models can help clinicians to better understand the assumptions and biases that they hold when interacting with clients. If this awareness is combined with vigilance in reflecting on the impact clinicians' verbal and non-verbal behaviours have in particular situations, clinicians will be better able to make difficult choices within therapy interactions that promote client-centred processes.

Clinicians enter into interactions with clients with a set of personal skills in addition to personal values and beliefs. Identifying those skills that are assets to enhancing client-centred practice can lead to clinicians choosing to improve skills that will facilitate their use of client-centred approaches. For example, embarking on a path of personal development can give clinicians the self-confidence and skills to negotiate goals with clients, assertively advocate on their behalf and trust their own ability to develop and sustain client-centred relationships within environments that may appear disempowering.

The process of self-reflection can be both daunting and exhilarating. It takes a certain level of personal confidence to challenge one's beliefs and values and to commit to developing personal skills. Beliefs or values that are uncomfortable to admit to, and that confront current levels of understanding of self and perceptions of a situation may be uncovered. At these times, time and mental energy is needed to re-explore the mental models held about a situation and create new or modified models that are consistent with newly discovered perceptions.

Journeys of personal reflection would not be complete without evaluating one's own application of client-centred approaches. Using a structured means to analyse, particularly from clients' perspectives, whether the approach is being used, can provide clinicians with greater insight into the need for change. The client questionnaire from the Client-centred Process Evaluation (Restall et al., 2000) can be used as one such tool. Other means include discussion with the client, the use of client satisfaction surveys, and the use of tools like the Measure of Process of Care (King, Rosenbaum, & King, 1995).

Here is the story of Dana. This story illustrates an approach to using the CSF. It begins by describing how Dana began to work through a client-centred practice issue using Personal Reflection.

Dana is a sole charge occupational therapist in a small town in western Canada where she has lived for 8 years. She works at the town hospital which has an attached personal care home. The population in the town and surrounding area is aging, and rooms in the personal care home are scarce. Dana received a referral for a 73-year old man named Maurice. The referral indicated that Maurice lives alone, recently lost his wife and has shown a gradual decrease in his ability to maintain his personal care and his home. Depression was being considered as a differential diagnosis. On speaking to the physician, Dr. Ryan, Dana learned that the physician and Maurice's son, Robert, felt it would be best for Maurice to move into the personal care facility. She also learned that Maurice wanted to remain at home.

Dana considered her potential involvement with Maurice, his son and the physician and found herself challenged to be client-centred, as she considered who the real client was. She consulted the Client-centred Strategies Framework to identify some methods that she might use to assist her. She felt that the Personal Reflection category would be a good place to start.

Dana hoped that Internet access would help her reconnect with other occupational therapists and grow professionally as she explored client-centred practice. She learned of a number of occupational therapy on-line discussion groups. Through the group discussion, she obtained the ideas of others on the issue of identifying who is the client. Through a personal values clarification exercise, she identified that she also valued independence and the right to make one's own decision, consistent with those of her client but somewhat contrary to those of his son and the physician. She realized that although Robert and Dr. Ryan had a right to be concerned, Maurice was capable of making his own decisions. Dana wanted to help facilitate Maurice's choices for independence. She thought that by initiating a discussion between Maurice, Robert and the physician, and encouraging Maurice to advocate for himself, she could ensure that Maurice's concerns were heard.

Facilitating Client-Centred Processes

This category of strategies involves the clinician's active and conscious facilitation of client-centred interactions with the client. Clinicians who have a solid knowledge base for client-centred practice can create opportunities to hone their skills in the use of these processes.

Client-centred practice is multi-dimensional and may manifest itself differently with different clients and in different contexts. The way clinicians relate to clients and the non-verbal space that is created by the interaction is fundamental to many concepts of client-centred practice. Specific strategies to facilitate the client-centred processes when working with clients with cognitive impairments (Hobson, 1999), physical impairments (Gage, 1999), in mental health settings (Kusznir & Scott, 1999) and with the older adult (Hobson, 1999) have been explored. These strategies illustrate the need for clinicians to be sensitive and knowledgeable of the common client-centred practice issues that groups with different abilities experience.

Clinicians who interact with clients in ways that give them their full attention and give clients the opportunity to talk about things that are important to them, (Corring & Cook, 1999) create a space for client-centred practice. Fearing (2000) discussed how therapists can "co-create healthy and enabling environments with clients through our presence, our communication and

our presentation" (p. 15) and described the value of mental, physical, spiritual and emotional presence on the client-therapist relationship.

However, despite the best intentions to interact with clients using these approaches, time pressures, personal and work priorities and stresses, and individual clinician values will get in the way. To help overcome these realities clinicians can use assessment processes and outcome measures that engage the client and focus on issues that are central to their lives, such as Goal Attainment Scales (Kiresuk & Sherman, 1968) and the Canadian Occupational Performance Measure (COPM) (Law et al., 1998). These structured tools and others individualized to the client (Donnelly & Carswell, 2002) facilitate the engagement of the clinician and the client in understanding what is relevant and important to the client's life.

We return to the case study to illustrate Dana's use of these strategies.

Dana completed a functional assessment with Maurice. She found that he was physically able to manage his self-care and home management tasks other than heavy housework and lifting. Although he could make himself a simple meal, he acknowledged he was not eating well; his wife, Margaret, had been the primary cook and he did not enjoy the task.

Dana again consulted the CSF and thought that the client-centred processes category would help. Using this as a guide, she decided to review and use the Occupational Performance Process Model (Fearing et al., 1997) to structure her involvement and the COPM to identify issues that were of concern to Maurice.

She spent time listening to Maurice tell his story, how he grew up on a farm near the town, took over the farm from his father and met and married Margaret. With pride, he spoke of how they raised Robert who had gone on to university in the city to become a teacher. Maurice talked about how difficult it had become five years ago when he could no longer keep up the work at the farm due to his arthritis and he needed to sell it and buy a small bungalow in town. At that time, he felt "lost" and "useless". He cried as he spoke of the loneliness since the sudden death of his wife a year ago. He talked of his lack of desire to take care of himself and his home, his poor appetite and sleeplessness.

Using the COPM she discovered that, more than anything, Maurice wanted to be independent. He wanted to have privacy and manage as much of his own self-care as possible. He told her he would like to become more involved in the community. He had never been involved in any structured leisure activities but did indicate an interest in horticulture and gardening. He missed Margaret's company and wanted to be able to make new friends.

Practice Settings

This group of strategies involves creating practice environments that facilitate client-centred practice. Practice settings include systems and physical environments within the organizations where occupational therapy services are provided.

Many clinicians prefer to operate in the clinical domain and leave the system's administrative tasks such as mission statements, job descriptions, performance appraisal tools and program evaluations to administrators. However, clinicians who participate in these tasks can influence client-centred documentation and processes within facility operations. An environmental scan can be conducted to determine the supports and barriers to client-centred practice within their environment (Stern et al., 2000) and be used to report and discuss findings with colleagues and managers. Offering to initiate or participate in task groups to develop or revise documents that support client-centred practice will ensure documentation that guides practice is consistent with the client-centred approach. Client-centred practice settings require partnerships between clinicians and those who have ultimate responsibility for the systems that support service delivery. Clinicians have suggested that they would have greater ease and comfort with using a client-centred approach if they had management and peer support for its use (Sumsion & Smyth, 2000). Clinicians can take responsibility to ensure their managers are familiar with the concepts and applications of client-centred approaches.

As uncomfortable as it may initially feel, stating clients' desired outcomes using their words at team meetings and in documentation is a way of modeling client-centred approaches to peers. Goals can be established and outcomes reported using client-centred outcome measures such as the COPM. On an individual or team basis, using structured tools such as The Measure of Processes of Care (King et al., 1995) or the CCPE (Restall et al., 2000) and unstructured tools such as focus groups can solicit client feedback on their perspective of how client-centred they found services. This information may be used to guide changes to individual and team service delivery.

Colleagues can mentor and coach each other to increase confidence in practice. Asking to observe a colleague who models client-centred approaches can assist clinicians to develop a further understanding of the verbal and nonverbal behaviours that demonstrate respect, care, genuine concern and a connection with a client. These strategies were highly ranked in Sumsion and Smyth's (2000) study as methods to resolve barriers to being client-centred.

While the hospital room or therapy department may be the most convenient and expedient places for therapy, they may not be the most comfortable places for meaningful exchanges for some clients and clinicians. Enabling choices for location of therapy sessions, such as home, school or workplace, demonstrates care and respect for clients while also modeling client-centred approaches. Although health policies and systems are encouraging more client-driven care, most recipients of health care services do not feel empowered to direct their care. When service providers model client-centred approaches, clients feel more comfortable in directing their health care.

The environments in which the interaction and chosen occupations occur also have a significant impact on the client's desire and comfort with addressing occupational performance issues. Rebeiro (2001) explored the importance of the environment in enabling occupational performance and found that an affirming social environment, which is the creation of a just-right environment based upon client-driven needs, is likely to have an impact on the person's confidence to participate in therapy.

This is how Dana worked to influence her practice setting.

In preparation for a meeting with Dana, Maurice, Robert and Dr. Ryan, Dana assisted Maurice to articulate his goals and desires. Maurice was concerned that he would not be fully understood and was concerned if the meeting was held in Dr. Ryan's office. Dana and Maurice requested that the meeting take place in Maurice's home and all eventually agreed. The meeting was held and everyone stated his or her concerns. Through the discussion, Dana identified that perhaps the real problem was that the town did not have a range of housing options for seniors. Supportive housing could provide many of the things that Maurice wanted—a meal program and opportunity for socialization. It could also provide Robert with the security of knowing that his father was not alone. All agreed that this might be a solution. With the aging population of the town, perhaps this was something that other town residents would also be interested in having. While this idea was being explored, increased home care supports would be put in place for Maurice.

Community Organizing

This group of strategies involves organizing people around issues that promote empowerment and enable communities to address client-centred practice issues. Community organizing (Labonte, 1992; Registered Nurses Association of British Columbia [RNABC], 1992) can be either professionally driven or grassroots driven. In either case occupational therapists can provide leadership, support and encouragement to community groups who are attempting to organize around issues related to client-centred practice.

Community organizing strategies use community building practice as a way of engaging and empowering communities. This group of strategies maximizes the collective effort of people and organizations to take action toward change. Although individual clinicians may not feel that they have the power or ability to make the types of changes that are necessary to change systems, individual energies aimed at supporting communities to influence change may be well within their power and ability.

Communities can be defined in many different ways including a locality such as a group of people living in the same neighbourhood or a group of people who may have something else in common such as people receiving the same type of health services. Community building informs how strategies in this category can influence broad systems and issues. Walter (1999) conceptualizes community building practice as incorporating several dimensions, including community development, and community planning.

Community development is the process of developing relationships that involve mutual respect, equity, inclusiveness and co-ordinated effort. Inherent in community development is shared leadership and power.

Occupational therapists who engage in community development are considered as equal partners to others in the community. Even if they take a leadership role in forming a community organization such as an advisory group (professionally driven organization), the goal is for the group to increase its leadership capacity and for leadership and power to be shared among participants. The values and principles inherent in client-centred practice (Law & Mills, 1998) are similar to those inherent in community development practice (Minkler, 1999). As a method to enhance client-centred practice, community development strategies empower individuals to organize and make changes that will improve their quality of life.

Community planning is another dimension of community building practice that can be implemented as community organizing strategies. Community planning assumes that there are relationships between people and organizations and that the groups created from these relationships have the resources and capacity to plan, organize, implement and evaluate projects.

As a strategy to enhance client-centred processes, occupational therapists can participate in community planning activities that assess the needs and capacities of communities. Community needs and capacity assessments can be done to inform an already identified issue or to identify issues that are named and framed by the community. A potential drawback of this process is that when issues are defined by a community, the concerns of a less powerful minority such as people with disabilities, may be ignored in preference of the issues of the more powerful majority (Lysack & Kaufert, 1999). Keeping this limitation in mind, occupational therapists can initiate, support, and provide expertise to community needs and capacity assessments that will allow community members to voice their priorities and concerns. Clinicians can assist individuals to identify their needs and capacities so that these individuals can give voice to needs and desires and offer their capacities in service of the community. Therapists can also use the results of community health assessments to inform their own program planning and evaluation activities.

Community planning includes other processes such as resource allocation and policy development, the implementation of project structures and the measurement of outcomes. To improve client-centred processes clinicians can use community planning to articulate how resource utilization, policies, and structures can support or impede client-centred practice. More importantly, therapists can advocate for clients to have meaningful participation in planning health services though participation on groups such as advisory bodies, implementation committees and boards of directors. Occupational therapists using this set of strategies enable clients to participate fully and to assume leadership within these planning groups.

Dana's value for community organizing assisted Maurice to achieve his goals.

> Dana felt that establishing supportive housing in the town would be a big project. She required the assistance of others in advocating for such a facility. Reviewing the CSF, she decided to set up a town hall meeting to find if there was interest in such a project. She asked Maurice to join her in presenting the idea to the town residents. Over 300 residents attended the town hall meeting and support for the idea was unanimous. Several residents suggested that a working group to get this project going was needed, which Maurice and Dana then organized. At the meeting, an advisory board for the new housing project was established.

Coalition Advocacy and Political Action

Client-centred practice occurs in a context larger than the client-therapist relationship; it is influenced by attitudes, established systems, and political, economic and social trends. Changes that will enable the delivery and receipt of client-centred services will not evolve by individual action only. Coalitions comprised of professional and lay groups can collectively influence change.

Coalition and political advocacy are strategies that work to bring together diverse individuals and groups to advocate for system changes through policy change, resource development, and ecological change (McElroy, Bibeau, Steckler, & Glanz, 1988). Political action is an extension of coalition advocacy; it refers to advocacy that is targeted at elected politicians.

Coalition advocacy activities are organized around one specific issue or a variety of issues targeted at creating significant change. Advocacy efforts can be directed locally (e.g., health care professionals joining together to change hospital policies around clinic hours) or nationally (e.g., AIDS Vaccine Advocacy Coalition advocating for changes to government policy and legislation). Joining or creating coalitions to advocate for policies, resources and environments that support

client-centred practice can be a powerful means of influencing change.

Occupational therapists use their advocacy skills when promoting the needs and wishes of individual clients to their treatment teams. They also use advocacy skills when involved in professional organizations whose mandates may include making presentations to, or responding to, government initiatives on issues of importance to their clients and the profession. Increasingly professional groups have realized greater effectiveness in reaching their target audiences by partnering with other professional organizations and lobbying together around common issues. Advocacy and coalition building can be strong forces in creating environments that are conducive to client-centred processes.

Therapists can tap into existing local coalitions and support client-centred practice or work towards putting client-centred initiatives services on the agenda. Coalitions can include Family or Client Advisory Committees and health care lobby groups. Groups may choose to partner with others and create a larger coalition to exert greater influence on decision makers.

Occupational therapists can also provide leadership and support to the establishment of new coalitions. Therapists who choose such endeavours should keep in mind that coalition advocacy is a very time intensive process that has no guarantee of success. It requires commitment, resources and patience to maintain relationships and sustain momentum. Coalition activities need to be well-timed (Johnson, Grossman, & Cassidy, 1996) and consider the environmental context related to political, economic and social trends.

Coalitions can conserve resources by avoiding duplication and maximizing the power of the individuals and groups through collective action. They also have more credibility than an individual (Aspen Reference Group, 1997). Several success factors for coalition advocacy efforts are factors congruent with client-centred practice, including: openness, inclusiveness and diversity, building upon strengths, and empowering stakeholders (Wolff & Kaye, 1995).

Improved accessibility for persons with disabilities, smoking laws and stronger penalties for impaired drivers resulted from the efforts of individuals and coalition advocacy groups targeting elected politicians. Getting the message to the politicians requires deliberate planning. Clinicians can learn from groups who have ventured down this road, by consulting members of successful coalitions on effective and ineffective strategies, targeting individuals with previous experience to join existing advocacy groups, and finding out if members of existing coalitions want to join in client-centred advocacy efforts.

Dana used advocacy strategies to gain support for the housing initiative in the following way.

> Government support through funding for the new supportive housing project remained an issue. The working group developed a draft proposal and Dana took it upon herself to telephone her local government representative to arrange a time to present the project. Other members of the group also requested their government representatives be present. At the presentation, the government representatives expressed full support for the idea and commended the group on how well they had worked together to develop the project idea and proposal. Two years later, the supportive housing project was completed and Maurice moved in. Today, he remains an active member on the advisory board and leads the other residents in caring for a co-op garden.

Conclusion

The value and belief in a client-centred approach to practice has been evident in the profession of occupational therapy since its establishment at the beginning of the twentieth century. Despite immense changes over the past century, client-centred concepts remain fundamental to the practice of occupational therapy. The development of theory and research that supports the client-centred approach is well on its way to becoming an established body of knowledge in occupational therapy. As theory will drive practice, from that theory will naturally come application. To apply the theory of client-centred practice, the Client-centred Strategies Framework has been proposed and its application illustrated through Dana, a story that identifyed, explored and developed strategies to operationalize client-centred practice theory. The challenge for clinicians is to continue to remain true to the client-centred practice approach, and to explore strategies that may be beyond their current comfort zone to overcome barriers. If occupational therapists want to continue to provide leadership in the area of client-centred practice, this is a challenge that the authours hope they will address and accept. It is hoped that the Client-centred Strategies Framework will assist in this journey.

Acknowledgements

We wish to acknowledge the clients and clinicians that we have each known who have inspired us to seek as many ways as possible to promote the concepts of client-centred practice. The University of Manitoba, School of Medical Rehabilitation Endowment Fund is acknowledged for its financial support. Virginia Fearing and Laurel Rose provided helpful suggestions for an earlier draft of this paper. Parts of this paper were presented at the 2002 annual meeting of the Canadian Association of Occupational Therapists in Saint John, New Brunswick.

References

Aspen Reference Group (1997). *Community health: Education and promotion.* Gaithersburg, MA: Aspen.

Baum, C. (1998). Client-centred practice in a changing health care system. In M. Law (Ed.), *Client-centred occupational therapy* (pp. 29–47). Thorofare, NJ: Slack.

Brown, C., & Bowen, R. (1998). Including the consumer in occupational therapy treatment planning. *Occupational Therapy Journal of Research, 18*, 44–62.

Canadian Association of Occupational Therapists (CAOT). (1997). *Enabling occupation: An occupational therapy perspective.* Ottawa, ON: CAOT Publications ACE.

Corring, D., & Cook, J. (1999). Client-centred care means that I am a valued human being. *Canadian Journal of Occupational Therapy, 66*, 71–82.

Covey, S. (1989). *The 7 habits of highly effective people: Powerful lessons in personal change.* Toronto, ON: Simon & Schuster.

Donnelly, C., & Carswell, A. (2002). Individualized outcome measures: A review of the literature. *Canadian Journal of Occupational Therapists, 69*, 84–94.

Fearing, V. (2000). Environments that enable therapist and client occupations. In V. Fearing., & J. Clark. (Eds.), *Individuals in context: A practical guide to client-centred practice* (pp. 15–24). Thorofare, NJ: Slack.

Fearing, V., & Clark, J. (Eds.). (2000). *Individuals in context: A practical guide to client-centred practice.* Thorofare, NJ: Slack.

Fearing, V., Law, M., & Clark, L. (1997). An occupational performance process model: Fostering client and therapist alliances.n *Canadian Journal of Occupational Therapy, 64*, 7–15.

Gage, M. (1999). Physical disabilities: meeting the challenges of client-centred practice. In T. Sumsion (Ed.), Implementation issues. *Client-centred practice in occupational therapy: A guide to implementation* (pp. 89–102). London: Churchill Livingstone.

Hobson, S. J. G. (1999). Using a client-centred approach with persons with cognitive impairment. In T. Sumsion (Ed.), Implementation issues. *Client-centred practice in occupational therapy: A guide to implementation* (pp. 51–60). London: Churchill Livingstone.

Hobson, S. J. G. (1999). Using a client-centred approach with elderly people. In T. Sumsion (Ed.), Implementation issues. *Client-centred practice in occupational therapy: A guide to implementation* (pp. 61–74). London: Churchill Livingstone.

Johnson, K., Grossman, W., & Cassidy, A. (Eds.) (1996). *Collaborating to improve community health: Workbook and guide to best practices in creating healthier communities and populations.* San Francisco, CA: Jossey-Bass.

King, S., Rosenbaum, P., & King, G. (1995). *The measure of processes of care* (MPOC). Unpublished manuscript, McMaster University, Hamilton, ON.

Kinsella, E.A. (2001). Reflections on reflective practice. *Canadian Journal of Occupational Therapy, 68*, 195–198.

Kiresuk, T., & Sherman, R. (1968). Goal attainment scaling: A general method for evaluating comprehensive community mental health programs. *Community Mental Health Journal, 4*, 443–453.

Kusznir, A., & Scott, E. (1999). The challenges of client-centred practice in mental health settings. *Client-centred practice in occupational therapy: A guide to implementation* (pp. 75–88). London: Churchill Livingstone.

Labonte, R. (1992). Heart health inequities in Canada: Models, theory and planning. *Health Promotion International, 7*, 119–128.

Law, M. (1998). *Client-centered occupational therapy.* Thorofare, NJ: Slack.

Law, M., Baptiste, S., & Mills. (1995). Client-centred practice: What does it mean and does it make a difference. *Canadian Journal of Occupational Therapy, 62*, 250–257.

Law, M., Baptiste, S., Carswell, A., McColl, M.A., Polatajko, H., & Pollock, N. (1998). *Canadian occupational performance measure (3rd ed.).* Ottawa, ON: CAOT Publications ACE.

Law, M., & Mills, J. (1998). Client-centred occupational therapy. In M. Law (Ed.), *Client-centred occupational therapy* (pp. 2–18). Thorofare, NJ: Slack.

Lysack, C., & Kaufert, J. (1999). Disabled consumer leaders' perspectives on provision of community rehabilitation services. *Canadian Journal of Rehabilitation, 12*, 157–166.

McElroy, K., Bibeau, D., Steckler, A., & Glanz, K. (1988) An ecological perspective on health promotion programs. *Health Education Quarterly, 15*, 351–377.

Minkler, M. (Ed.) (1999), *Community organizing and community building for health.* New Brunswick, NJ: Rutgers University Press.

Neistadt, M. (1995). Methods of assessing clients' priorities: A survey of adult physical dysfunction settings. *American Journal of Occupational Therapy, 49*, 428–436.

Rebeiro, K. (2001). Enabling occupational: The importance of an affirming environment. *Canadian Journal of Occupational Therapy, 68*, 80–89.

Rebeiro, K., & Cook, J. (1999). Opportunity not prescription: An exploratory study of the experience of occupational engagement. *Canadian Journal of Occupational Therapy, 66*, 176–187.

Registered Nurses Association of British Columbia (RNABC) (1992). *Determinants of health: Empowering strategies for nursing practice.* Vancouver, BC: Author.

Restall, G., Stern, M., & Ripat, J. (2000). Client-centred process evaluation. In V. Fearing., & J. Clark. (Eds.), *Individuals in context: A practical guide to client-centred practice* (pp. 165–177). Thorofare, NJ: Slack.

Schön, D. (1987). *Educating the reflective practitioner.* San Francisco, CA: Jossey-Bass.

Senge, P.M, Roberts, C, Rosser, B., Smith, B.J., & Kleiner, A. (1994). *The fifth discipline fieldbook.* New York: Doubleday.

Stern, M., & Restall, G. (1993, June). *Client-centred practice and the medical model.* Paper presented at the annual meeting of the Canadian Association of Occupational Therapists, Regina, Saskatchewan.

Stern, M., Restall, G. & Ripat, J. (2000). The use of self-reflection to improve client-centred processes. In V. Fearing., & J. Clark. (Eds.), *Individuals in context: A practical guide to client-centred practice* (pp. 145–158). Thorofare, NJ: Slack.

Sumsion, T. (1999). *Client-centred practice in occupational therapy. A guide to implementation.* London: Churchill Livingstone.

Sumsion, T., & Smyth, G. (2000). Barriers to client-centredness and their resolution. *Canadian Journal of Occupational Therapy, 67*, 15–21.

Walter. C. (1999). Community building practice: A conceptual framework. In M. Minkler (Ed.), *Community organizing and community building for health* (pp.68–83). New Brunswick, NJ: Rutgers University Press.

Wilkins, S., Pollock, N., Rochon, S., & Law, M. (2001). Implementing client-centred practice: Why is it so difficult to do? *Canadian Journal of Occupational Therapy, 68*, 70–79.

Wolff, T., & Kaye, G. (Eds.) (1995). *From the ground up: A workbook on coalition building and community development.* Amherst, Mass: AHEC/Community Partners.

CHAPTER 45

Linking Purpose to Procedure During Interactions With Patients

SUZANNE M. PELOQUIN

This article describes a rationale and some methods for incorporating statements of purpose, or goal statements, into the daily practice of occupational therapy. Given the clinical pressures generated by brief lengths of stays in care facilities, occupational therapists need to recommit themselves to meaningful relationships with their patients. The need for this renewed commitment sharpens when one considers three realities basic to practice: current trends in health care, traditional occupational therapy assumptions, and the often ambiguous nature of activity, occupational therapy's primary modality. Each of these realities provides a context within which the process of discussing goal statements with patients will be explored.

Rosen (1974, p. 292) used the term *therapy set* to refer to statements or directives that inform patients about a therapeutic procedure, motivate them to cooperate, and heighten their expectations of the benefits to be derived from treatment. When this treatment approach is used, patients (a) understand what they are doing and why they are doing it and (b) feel encouraged to engage in the process.

As applied to occupational therapy, a communication in psychiatric practice that encourages informed patient involvement might be the following:

> We'd like to have you join us in the 9 am craft group today. You will probably experience this as a pleasant hour since you enjoy working with your hands. Our main interest in having you attend this group, however, is that your participation will give you an opportunity to

use several skills, such as your ability to concentrate, to solve problems, and to organize your thoughts.

Effectiveness of the Collaborative Approach

Although the purpose of this article is not to investigate the effectiveness of enlightening patients about and involving them in their therapy, but to explore a rationale for the use of such a collaborative approach in occupational therapy practice, some brief discussion of the effectiveness of the approach seems indicated. Rosen (1974) cited several studies involving subjects receiving desensitization therapy procedures accompanied by different forms of "therapy set." He indicated that two primary approaches dominated the research on the effectiveness of informing and involving the patient. The first group of studies investigated the extent to which varied instructions might alter subjects' expectations for a therapeutic outcome. The second group of studies explored the effects of changing subjects' knowledge of the procedure through instructions. In the first approach, control groups were given a general therapeutic orientation, whereas experimental groups were given instructions that might influence their expectations of the treatment outcome positively. Small between-group differences that failed to achieve statistical significance were reported in these studies (Lomont & Brock, 1971; McGlynn, 1971; McGlynn & Mapp, 1970; McGlynn, Mealiea, & Nawas, 1969; McGlynn, Reynolds, & Linder, 1971; McGlynn & Williams, 1970; Woy & Efran, 1972). In the second approach, groups given therapeutic orientation were compared with groups who believed they were being studied for physiological reactions only. In this approach, subjects' knowledge of the purpose of the procedure was being manipulated. Most studies of this type demonstrated significant effects attributable to the type of instruction given (Borkovec, 1972; Leitenberg, Agras, Barlow, & Oliveau, 1969; Miller, 1972; Oliveau, Agras, Leitenberg, Moore, & Wright, 1969; Rappaport, 1972). Subjects who knew that the purpose of the treatment was therapeutic had better therapeutic outcomes.

In his own study, Rosen (1974) concluded that subjects aware of the purpose of procedures designed to make them less afraid of snakes demonstrated significantly higher mean behavioral changes, that is, became more desensitized to the offending stimulus, than subjects unaware of the purpose. Those informed that test procedures were therapeutic demonstrated more confident behavior in approaching snakes than those told that the procedures were simply experimental.

The collaborative approach's focus on patients' expectations resembles a construct called "expectancy of therapeutic gain." Historically, this construct emerged from research on the placebo effect described in the medical literature (Wilkins, 1973). Cartwright and Cartwright (1958) explained that in the 1950s the concepts of anticipation, belief, confidence, and conviction emerged in psychotherapy, giving rise to the concept of the placebo effect. Frank (1959) said that a patient's expectancy of benefit from treatment may in itself have enduring and profound effects on his or her physical and mental health. Krause, in 1967, wrote that the client's beliefs about treatment determine his or her valuation of the process, and that this valuation determines his or her motivation to participate. Kielhofner (1985) echoed this conviction in his conceptualization of volition as the human subsystem that provides the energy and desire for choosing an action, that energy being generated by what a person believes to be interesting and valuable.

Wilkins (1973) proposed that an individual's expectancy of therapeutic gain may be treated as either (a) an attitude that the individual brings to a situation concerning how much benefit he or she will receive or (b) a state that can be induced by instructions delivered about the effectiveness of procedures to which he or she will be exposed. The idea of the collaborative approach is predicated on the assumptions that instructions can induce an expectancy of therapeutic gain and that creating a state of expectancy potentiates the therapeutic procedure.

There is justification for the use of the collaborative approach in occupational therapy when one considers its efficacy; there is additional justification for its use when one reflects on current demands in health-care practice.

Current Demands in Health Care

In light of the current emphasis on bioethical issues such as informed consent and patients' rights, there is sound reasoning for incorporating a collaborative approach into each occupational therapy procedure. Engelhardt (1986) described the patient's status as that of a stranger in a strange land:

> Patients, when they come to see a health care professional, are in unfamiliar territory. They enter a terrain of issues that has been carefully defined through the long history of the health care professions. A patient is unlikely to present for care with as well-analyzed and considered judgments as those possessed by health care professionals. . . . The patient in this context is a stranger, an individual in unfamiliar territory who does not fully know what to expect or how to control the environment. . . . Things no longer happen as usual; they no longer take place in their taken for granted ways. As an outsider in a strange culture, the patient always runs the risk of being a marginal person. (pp. 256–257)

The caregiver must explain this new and strange land to the patient, thereby reducing the patient's sense of being a marginal person. The caregiver must augment the patient's sense of belonging by providing him or her with access to information and by giving him or her control in the form of consent over the treatment process (Engelhardt, 1986).

Current emphasis on patients' rights reminds those in positions of power that the ultimate power is changing hands. Patients have the right to know the precise relevance and nature of their treatment and to choose it or reject it on the basis of their understanding of its value to them (Bloomer, 1978). This patient/consumer right gives the practitioner a powerful incentive for explaining procedures and for collaborating with patients throughout treatment.

Clinicians face a demand from agencies, both accrediting and reimbursing, to be accountable for the treatment they provide. They face requests from patients and their families to prove the utility of their service and to clarify the expected outcome of their treatments. Current trends to exact statements of purpose from therapists can be perceived as the public's validation of a professional and ethical response that is their due.

Traditional Occupational Therapy Thinking

Even before the emergence of current trends, traditional occupational therapy assumptions supportive of the collaborative approach were well represented in the literature. The assumptions can be summarized as follows: The patient is rational. The patient is a collaborator with the therapist. The patient is free to choose or reject therapeutic services. The therapist, in turn, is a teacher and a motivator in the therapy process.

Excerpts from *Willard and Spackman's Occupational Therapy* highlight these assumptions. McNary (1947) wrote: "An activity entered into without a purpose is not occupational therapy" (p. 10). If the patient is the one entering into the activity, it is he or she who must understand the purpose. It then becomes the therapist's responsibility to share that information. Edgerton (1947) said that "the ability to relate an activity to the need of the individual is one of the characteristics that distinguishes the occupational therapist from the . . . crafts instructor" (p. 42). Here is a clear endorsement of any procedure that communicates the relevance of a therapeutic activity. If occupational therapists resent having their role minimized by others, they must take measures to ensure that they are not sabotaging themselves by failing to define their work so that others will recognize it unmistakably as therapy.

Wade (1947) said that "if the patient is unable to participate actively in the plan, its existence should be kept in his consciousness as a justification for the task" (p. 90). When meaningful collaboration with the patient is not possible, the therapist still retains responsibility for explaining the plan on some level. When the patient is elderly, psychotic, young, or cognitively impaired, it may seem easier to abandon explanations in favor of expediting the procedure. Therapists are encouraged to do otherwise. At whatever level of comprehension is possible, caregivers need to inform. The information may be brief, simple, and even reductionistic. The information is nonetheless "placed in the patient's consciousness." When in doubt about the potential for awareness, one communicates.

An anecdotal contribution to *Reader's Digest* ("Speedy Recovery," 1987) illustrates a response that even patients assumed to be minimally aware can furnish. A nurse's aide described her patient as a 96-year-old woman immobilized after a stroke. The aide's task was to get the patient out of bed. She communicated her plan to her assistant as follows: "I'll take an arm and a leg on this side, you take an arm and a leg on that side and then. . . ." The explanation was interrupted by the patient's saying in a weary voice: "Oh, God, she's not even going to make a wish!" (p. 53).

This anecdote clearly reminds therapists that the presence of a significant disability does not justify excluding the patient from an active understanding of any procedure. Exclusion constitutes treatment of the patient as a marginal person. The publication of this anecdote as a humorous short in a popular magazine reflects perhaps the universality of the situation. The treatment is all too familiar. The poignancy of the story lies in the fact that the patient's best defense was that of taking the offensive by being more humane and personable than the caregiver.

Current literature supports these examples taken from the past. Reed and Sanderson (1983) described several attitudes and assumptions about the occupational therapy process consistent with those underlying the idea of the collaborative approach. They emphasized salient points made more subtly 40 years ago by encouraging therapists to regard the client as a *valuable, worthwhile person,* even if the client does not respond readily to the program" (p. 153). Here stands a declaration of the patient's right to challenge services offered on the basis of his or her understanding of them. A consequent responsibility for the therapist is to maintain the patient in high regard and to respond to the challenge with information. "The client has a right to be informed, but also the information should be in a manner that is comprehensive and at a rate that can be absorbed by the client" (p. 154).

Reed and Sanderson (1983) drew up a list of patient's rights that included the following:

1. A person has the right to decide whether to seek and accept health care services within legal limitations.
2. A person has the right to determine the state of health and level of wellness that person will seek to attain and maintain, as long as the decision does not threaten or endanger the health and wellness of other persons.
3. A person has the right to be consulted regarding the objectives, goals, and methods to be used in individual health care plans. (p. 71)

These three rights merit observance during daily sessions when specific treatments are being proposed. The patient's right to be consulted and to decide needs to be reinforced daily. Providing the patient with the necessary information at each session can operationally reaffirm his or her rights.

Motivating the patient becomes an inevitable therapist responsibility if one endorses the patient's right to choose. Reed and Sanderson (1983) identified the last step of the occupational therapy process as being "to facilitate and influence client participation and investment" (p. 81). This step constitutes a directive to communicate the rationale, the importance, and the relevance of the therapy process in such a manner as to facilitate the patient's investment in a successful outcome.

Traditional occupational therapy has been a process of teaching, motivating, and collaborating with the patient during therapeutic activity. More recently, proponents of a psychoeducational approach to occupational therapy have contrasted it with traditional occupational therapy. Fine and Schwimmer (1987) described the psychoeducational approach to occupational therapy as a derivation from social learning theory:

> The life skills curriculum (LSC) is further differentiated from its traditional counterpart by structuring the educational format and techniques, emphasizing the patient's active participation in setting and evaluating treatment goals, identifying learning needs and influencing the teaching-learning process, planning the integration and continuity of problem-solving and communication skills among all groups, providing multiple opportunities to practice skills through graded repetition and homework assignments, and matching treatment tasks to patient's problems and priorities. (p. 3)

Excerpts from traditional and more current literature, cited earlier, support the premise that traditional occupational therapy (a) has incorporated the tenets of social learning theory to a considerable extent and (b) has promoted active involvement in goal formulation all along.

The Public's Knowledge of Occupational Therapy

The rationale for using the collaborative approach sharpens considerably when we reflect on the profession's unclear image. "Occupational therapy is not understood well by the average client because it is not a common profession, such as medicine, nursing, engineering, law, teaching or the ministry" (Reed & Sanderson, 1983, p. 161). Practitioners often find themselves explaining the word *occupational,* differentiating occupational therapy functions from those of other therapies, and otherwise clarifying their professional roles. If the public expects physicians, nurses, and engineers, whose professions are better understood, to clarify their procedures, the expectation increases for those representing less well understood professions.

Occupational therapy is often not understood; it can, in fact, often be misunderstood. A particularly noteworthy example of that misunderstanding appears in Joyce Rebeta-Burditt's novel *The Cracker Factory* (1977). In the story a young female patient, a self-described alcoholic, writes from the psychiatric hospital to a friend:

> I should write to you every day. I could not only unravel the Gordian knot in my psyche, but appear to be busy and involved when Brunhilde, the misplaced Viking lady, comes tapping on my door every afternoon in an effort to intimidate me into going to Occupational Therapy. She marches around the seventh floor telling all the patients that their doctor has "ordered" Occupational Therapy and they must come IMMEDIATELY. She herds them out in the hall where they mill around until she lines them up in two columns and goose steps them out the door. . . .
>
> Patients are forever trying to hide by taking a shower or even [having] a fit, but she doesn't care. Wet or screaming, it makes no difference. She drags them along anyway. . . .
>
> I go sometimes and hate myself for it. I sit and dab grout on a metal shell and try to decide what color ashtray I'm going to mess up that day. I listen to the conversations around me, and the tape recorder in my head jots down snatches and fragments and I smile and pretend that I am not listening in. (pp. 114–115)

Fiction will often exaggerate or satirize those aspects of our functioning that create interesting reading material, such as the domineering qualities of Brunhilde and the perceived irrelevance of occupational therapy. Fiction also mirrors reality. In this case the reality is that occupational therapy is sometimes misunderstood.

The consequence of this misunderstanding can be significant. Patients uninformed of the purpose of occupational therapy are free to infer its meaning based on their observations. The result may well be compliance with the procedure. It might as easily be noncompliance accompanied by hostility. One probability is that patients who are uninformed or misinformed will be less able to generalize to their life situations those concepts the therapist had hoped might be learned in therapy.

The Ambiguous Nature of Activity

Because occupational therapists use activity as a primary modality, they increase the risk of being misunderstood. Any single activity can have many therapeutic possibilities. Proficiency in activity analysis enables clinicians to recognize the multiple goals that can be attached to any one activity. Therapists need to apply that theoretical concept clinically and consider its practical consequences. Therapeutic methods can easily confuse patients. A patient can be given leather stamping as a task to achieve a wide range of goals, including (a) the enhancement of grip strength, (b) the redirection of nervous energy through gross-motor release, or (c) the use of organizational and problem-solving skills in the planning of a balanced design. If the only focus patients have is the one they can infer while doing the task, the relationship between the leather-stamping activity and the treatment plan may elude them. Because they do not clearly understand the therapeutic concepts supporting the activity, they may be less apt to apply them to their personal life situations.

A pleasant staff development exercise that illustrates the multifaceted aspect of any activity is the following: Divide the total group into five working subgroups. Provide each small group with a bowl of sliced oranges. The primary activity will be to eat the oranges. From the list given in the appendix to this paper, provide each group with a different set of written directions. Allow each group to complete the activity as directed. Following the group activity, ask a representative from each group to share both the directions given and the results of their activity. Reports from the representatives will reflect the different end points that one task with different directions can have. The exercise can stimulate reflection on the importance of clarifying the specific focus of a planned activity.

Methods of Providing a Collaborative

Approach

A collaborative approach can be used creatively. Therapists can provide feedback formally or informally, use the printed or the spoken word, and communicate the purpose of occupational therapy procedures at various phases in the treatment process. Any method used that communicates the purpose of or the expectations for the treatment can qualify.

In an earlier article (Peloquin, 1983), I endorsed integrating information about the expectations and relevance of the occupational therapy program into the structure of an initial interview format in an acute-care psychiatric setting. The three-part interview stresses the continuous provision of feedback to the patient. My conviction remains that, if nothing else, we give patients methods of self-help when we provide them with informative goal statements that they can readily apply to their personal environments after discharge.

One way to enlighten patients is to give them printed materials. A general description of the occupational therapy program might be a suitable accompaniment to the initial contact between a patient and a therapist. The descriptive introduction might include a statement of the various purposes of the occupational therapy program. Next, a brief, goal-oriented paragraph at the top of an occupational therapy schedule might serve as a motivational reinforcement. Posters listing typical occupational therapy goals for various groups can be displayed in both residential and treatment areas. In more financially comfortable settings, pamphlets or video messages discussing the programmatic goals of occupational therapy might be used as part of a general hospital orientation.

Feedback can be provided in formal groups and individual orientations. On a daily basis, a brief discussion can either precede or follow each activity group. More articulate patients can be asked to help clarify the purposes and expectations of various groups for new patients. Less organized patients can be reminded informally on the way to and from groups about the specific purpose of each group. Brief personal contacts reminding patients about individualized goals can occur during large parallel groups.

It might be helpful to include here a few illustrations of how the collaborative approach can be incorporated into occupational therapy. Each illustration includes vocabulary that can be adjusted upward or downward to match the intellectual level of the patient population being addressed. Any verbal delivery of the feedback needs to reflect, in its tone, rate, and inflection, the therapist's perception of the patient as intelligent. A singsong or overly didactic delivery, suggesting condescension, could vitiate or at least compromise the purpose of the feedback. A respectful intent requires respectful delivery.

An introductory explanation of a psychiatric occupational therapy program might read, in part, as follows:

Occupational therapy adds to your total treatment by encouraging you to use activities and occupy your time in a therapeutic way. Purposeful activity has an organizing and beneficial effect on an individual. Because it involves the total person, activity meets several mental health needs.

Occupational therapy offerings here include crafts, exercise, greenhouse, relaxation, communication, and life skills groups. By participating in these activities you help ready yourself to return to your community. During group and individual sessions, you can set goals and practice skills essential to your coping more effectively outside of the hospital.

You will have daily opportunities to plan and organize tasks, to solve problems, to improve your physical condition, to interact effectively with others, to make decisions, to boost your self-confidence, to learn new ways of relaxing and coping with different life situations. Activity becomes therapy because of the adaptive skills you practice when you are active.

A poster mounted in the clinical area to provide information about a typical occupational therapy craft group might list some of the following goal statements:

Why Crafts?

To improve your concentration
To organize your thoughts
To have you solve problems
To help you make decisions
To exercise your work skills
To boost your self-confidence
To increase your independence
To help you interact with others
To increase your sense of control
To keep you alert and involved.

A poster describing the purposes of a communication group might read as follows:

Why Communication Group?

To improve your listening skills
To help you share and interact
To increase your self-awareness
To help you identify your feelings
To help you express yourself

To help you better deal with anger
To increase your assertiveness
To help you clarify your thoughts
To help you make or keep friends.

A discussion at the end of a particular group might follow a basic outline such as the following, addressing a different goal from day to day. The following format has been used with groups of adults having cognitive problems:

1. *Explain the purpose of the group:* "One of the goals for this particular group is to have you use your cognitive or thinking skills. During the course of this hour each of you has had some opportunity to use a number of thinking skills, such as concentrating, problem solving, decision making, comprehending instructions, or organizing your activity."

2. *Set the stage for a discussion:* "Take a minute to think about the thinking skills you used while working on your project. I'll be asking a few of you to share with the rest of us how you used your skills during the past hour."

3. *Facilitate a brief discussion of skills used, making sure to clearly link for patients the various task steps they completed with the cognitive skills they used:* Examples of therapist responses might be
   a. "That's right, Jim. You had to follow several complex verbal instructions today. I also noticed that you were doing a lot of planning and organizing for the design you want to put on your belt tomorrow."
   b. "Lorene, you're feeling that you didn't use your thinking skills today, but I noticed that you had to make several color choices when you were painting. That's decision making. You also had to pay attention to the shapes you were painting. That required you to concentrate on what you were doing. You really were using thinking skills for the better part of the hour."

4. *Summarize what was accomplished and encourage patients to return to the next session.*

Formulating and providing a set of goals in collaboration with the patient can be a creative process evolving from the basic premise that patients have rights, capabilities, and a vested interest in knowing the relevance of therapy. Using the collaborative approach can potentiate our therapeutic activities by communicating their value to patients in the real world outside the treatment setting. An old proverb says, "Give a man a fish and you have fed him for a day; teach a man to fish and you have fed him for a lifetime." Sharing goal statements with patients can give them an understanding of a process that can provide a link to improved functioning.

Summary

There is a rationale for a collaborative approach with patients in the daily practice of occupational therapy. Effective collaborative procedure (a) provides patients with knowledge about what they are doing and why they are doing it and (b) encourages patients to engage in the process.

The effectiveness of this approach has not been established conclusively, but studies suggest that subjects exposed to the therapeutic purpose of desensitization procedures tend to have better therapeutic outcomes than those unaware of the purpose. Current emphasis on the patient's right to be informed and on the therapist's responsibility to inform reflects the public's growing insistence that practitioners explain the utility of the treatments they provide to the patient.

Excerpts from past and present literature indicate that assumptions underlying the practice of traditional occupational therapy reflect similar assumptions underpinning the use of a collaborative approach. These assumptions describe the patient as rational, as having rights, and as a collaborator in therapy. The therapist is assumed to be a teacher and a motivator in the therapeutic process, the person who articulates the relevance of therapy and encourages the patient's participation.

The general public often lacks understanding of the occupational therapy process. Additionally, the versatility and multiple possibilities associated with any activity can confuse the patient about its purpose. The uninformed patient might be less inclined to participate in therapy and less able to generalize helpful concepts from the experience.

Feedback to patients can be provided in a number of creative ways throughout treatment. Providing such feedback need not require a major time investment, but can represent the therapist's renewed commitment to the therapeutic alliance and to the goal directedness of occupational therapy practice.

Acknowledgments

I thank Lillian Hoyle Parent, MA, OTR, FAOTA, for her support and encouragement in the preparation of this paper.

The topic of this paper featured in a workshop entitled "Goal Formulation: Clinical Leverage in Challenging Times," which I co-presented with Debora Davidson, MS, OTR. The workshop was sponsored by the Department of Occupational Therapy at the University of Texas Medical Branch Hospitals, L. Randy Strickland, EdD, OTR, FAOTA, Director.

Appendix 45.A

1. You have been given orange sections as a help in your discussion. The tangible and sensual experience of the orange will enable you to complete your task. As you are eating the sections, discuss as a group the various memories you have that are associated with eating oranges. Appoint a spokesperson who will later present a 30–60 second summary of your discussion.

2. You have been given orange sections as a help in your discussion. The actual taste of the orange will help you to better focus on your task. As you are eating the sections, discuss as a group as many dishes or recipes as you can think of that use oranges. Appoint a spokesperson who will later present a 30–60 second summary of your discussion.

3. You have been given orange sections as a help in your discussion. The visual and tactile experience of the orange will help you in your task. As you are eating the sections, discuss as a group as many functions as you can think of that an orange might have aside from its function as a food item. Appoint a spokesperson who will later present a 30–60 second summary of your discussion.

4. You have been given orange sections as a help in your discussion. The sight of the orange will help you in your task. As you are eating the sections, discuss as a group as many other natural items as you can think of that share a similar color. Appoint a spokesperson who will later present a 30–60 second summary of your discussion.

5. You have been given orange sections as a help in your discussion. The smell of the orange will help you in your task. As you are eating the sections, discuss as a group as many other items as you can think of that share a similar odor, or that have the orange scent. Appoint a spokesperson who will later present a 30–60 second summary of your discussion.

References

Bloomer, J. S. (1978). The consumer of therapy in mental health. *American Journal of Occupational Therapy, 32,* 621–627.

Borkovec, T. D. (1972). Effects of expectancy on the outcome of systematic desensitization and implosive treatments for analogue anxiety. *Behavior Therapy, 3,* 29–40.

Cartwright, D. S., & Cartwright, R. D. (1958). Faith and improvement in psychotherapy. *Journal of Counseling Psychology, 5,* 174–177.

Edgerton, W. B. (1947). Activities in occupational therapy. In H. Willard & C. Spackman (Eds.), *Occupational therapy* (pp. 40–59). Philadelphia: Lippincott.

Engelhardt, H. T., Jr. (1986). *The foundations of bioethics.* New York: Oxford University Press.

Fine, S. B., & Schwimmer, P. (1986, December). The effects of occupational therapy on independent living skills. *Mental Health Special Interest Section Newsletter,* pp. 2–3.

Frank, J. D. (1959). The dynamics of the psychotherapeutic relationship. *Psychiatry, 22,* 17–39.

Kielhofner, G. (1985). The human being as an open system. In G. Kielhofner (Ed.), *A Model of Human Occupation: Theory and application* (pp. 2–11). Baltimore: Williams & Wilkins.

Krause, M. S. (1967). Clients' expectations of the value of treatment. *Mental Hygiene, 51,* 359–365.

Leitenbheerg, H., Agras, W. S., Barlow, D. H., & Oliveau, D.C. (1969). Contributions of selective positive reinforcement and therapeutic instructions to systematic desensitization therapy. *Journal of Abnormal Psychology, 74,* 113–118.

Lomont, J. F., & Brock, L. (1971). Cognitive factors in systematic desensitization. *Behavior Research and Therapy, 9,* 187–195.

McGlynn, F. D. (1971). Experimental desensitization following three types of instructions. *Behavior Research and Therapy, 9,* 367–369.

McGlynn, F. D., & Mapp, R. H. (1970). Systematic desensitization of snake-avoidance following three types of suggestion. *Behavior Research and Therapy, 8,* 197–201.

McGlynn, F. D., Mealiea, E. L., & Nawas, M. M. (1969). Systematic desensitization of snake avoidance under two conditions of suggestion. *Psychological Reports, 25,* 220–222.

McGlynn, F. D., Reynolds, E. J., & Linder, L. H. (1971). Systematic desensitization with pre-treatment and intra-treatment therapeutic instructions. *Behavior Research and Therapy, 9,* 57–63.

McGlynn, F. D., & Williams, C. W. (1970). Systematic desensitization of snake-avoidance under three conditions of suggestion. *Journal of Behavior Therapy and Experimental Psychiatry, 1,* 97–101.

McNary, H. (1947). The scope of occupational therapy. In H. Willard & C. Spackman (Eds.), *Occupational therapy* (pp. 10–22). Philadelphia: Lippincott.

Miller, S. B. (1972). The contribution of therapeutic instructions to systematic desensitization. *Behavior Research and Therapy,* 159–169.

Oliveau, D. C. (1969). Systematic desensitization in an experimental setting: A follow–up study. *Behavior Research and Therapy, 7,* 377–380.

Oliveau, D. C., Agras, W. S., Leitenberg, H., Moore, R. C., & Wright, D. E. (1969). Systematic desensitization, therapeutically oriented instructions and selective positive reinforcement. *Behavior Research and Therapy, 7,* 27–33.

Peloquin, S. M. (1983). The development of an occupational therapy interview/therapy set procedure. *American Journal of Occupational Therapy, 37,* 457–461.

Rappaport, H. (1972). Modification of avoidance behavior: Expectancy, autonomic reactivity, and verbal report. *Journal of Consulting and Clinical Psychology, 39,* 404–414.

Rebeta-Burditt, J. (1977). *The cracker factory.* New York: Macmillan.

Reed, K. L., & Sanderson, S. R. (1983). *Concepts of occupational therapy.* Baltimore: Williams & Wilkins.

Rosen, G. M. (1974). Therapy set: its effects on subjects' involvement in systematic desensitization and treatment outcome. *Journal of Abnormal Psychology, 83,* 291–300.

Speedy recovery. (1987, July). *Reader's Digest,* p. 53.

Wade, B. D. (1947). Occupational therapy for patients with mental disease. In H. Willard & C. Spackman (Eds.), *Occupational therapy* (pp. 81–117). Philadelphia: Lippincott.

Woy, J. R., & Efran, J. S. (1972). Systematic desensitization and expectancy in the treatment of speaking anxiety. *Behavior Research and Therapy, 10,* 33–49.

Wilkins, W. (1973). Expectancy of therapeutic gain: An empirical and conceptual critique. *Journal of Consulting and Clinical Psychology, 40,* 69–77.

CHAPTER 46

The Origin and Evolution of Activity Analysis

CYNTHIA CREIGHTON

In 1911, industrialization had resulted in unprecedented economic growth for the United States. The average employee worked a 9- to 12-hour shift, 6 days per week, for a wage of approximately $2 a day. The automobile assembly line had not yet been invented.

Two books that would revolutionize industry were published that year: The Principles of Scientific Management (Taylor, 1911) and Motion Study (Gilbreth, 1911). Taylor, past president of the American Society of Mechanical Engineers, proposed in his text that management in business and industry be approached as a true science with clearly defined rules and principles. An important element of Taylor's new system of management was the study and standardization of jobs to increase productivity. Soon, efficiency experts were observing and timing workers in shops and factories nationwide. As a laborer shoveled ore or cut metal, the consultant identified the fundamental operations, the most efficient tools, and the optimum speed for the task.

Gilbreth (1911), 10 years younger than Taylor and also an engineer, was the first to use the term *analysis* when discussing the systematic study of jobs. He believed that the worker's movements should be the focus of such studies. Gilbreth outlined the steps in analyzing a task as follows: "1. Reduce . . . practice to writing. 2. Enumerate motions used. 3. Enumerate variables which affect each motion" (p. 5). Three categories of variables were considered in a motion study: characteristics of the worker (e.g., physical build, experience, temperament), characteristics of the surroundings (e.g., lighting, tools), and characteristics of the motion (e.g.,

direction, length, speed). Gilbreth documented these in chart form and in photographs. The purpose of analyzing a job was to identify and teach the "definite best" (most productive and least fatiguing) method of performance (p. 93).

Gilbreth (1911) also discussed adapting activity to make it more efficient:

> A careful study of the worker will enable one to adapt his work, surroundings, equipment and tools to him. "This will decrease the number of motions he must make, and make the necessary motions shorter and less fatiguing." (p. 10)

In his own bricklaying business, he made adaptations such as reversing the position of materials for left-handed workers and placing stock on a scaffold so the bricklayer no longer had to stoop when picking it up. In 1913, he began founding small museums of devices designed to simplify work and prevent fatigue (Gilbreth & Gilbreth, 1920).

Gilbreth and his wife, Lillian,[1] became well known both at home and abroad as consultants to the business community (Yost, 1949). In 1914 and 1915, Gilbreth visited hospitals in Europe to analyze surgeons' work. World War I had begun, and he met disabled veterans and learned about the groundbreaking research of Jules Amar.

Amar (1918) was a French physiologist appointed by his government to investigate scientific management and apply its principles to the training and re-employing of wounded soldiers. At that time, France led the world

This chapter was previously published in the *American Journal of Occupational Therapy, 46,* 45–48. Copyright © 1992, American Occupational Therapy Association. Reprinted with permission. http://dx.doi.org/10.5014/ajot.46.1.45

[1]Lillian Gilbreth also applied motion study methodology to organizing the Gilbreth's home and raising 12 children while earning her doctorate at Brown University. The American public came to know the family through the books and films *Cheaper by the Dozen* and *Belles on Their Toes,* written by two of the children.

in the study of human physiology and the development of instruments to measure physiological functions; Amar began analyzing jobs in terms of their physiological requirements. He described the planes of motion in which work was performed and measured movements with simple goniometers. To document strength requirements, Amar attached spring dynamometers to tools such as a file, a plane, and a spade. He measured energy expenditure during work, using oxygen consumption, pulse rate and blood pressure, and urine and blood by-products as indicators. The results of the analyses were applied in a three-part program to re-educate soldiers (many of them with amputations). At the beginning of the convalescent period, exercise and crafts were used to strengthen stump muscles and build endurance. The patient was then fitted with a prosthesis or splint and taught to use it in vocational tasks.

Occupational Therapy and Motion Study

When Gilbreth returned from his travels, he and his wife presented papers to several professional groups about the application of motion study to "re-education of the crippled soldier" (Gilbreth & Gilbreth, 1920). The theme of the papers was as follows:

> In considering any type of activity to which it is proposed to introduce the cripple, we first analyze this activity from the motion study standpoint, in order to find exactly what way these motions may be adapted to the available, or motions are required to perform the activity and in what remaining, capable members of the cripple's working anatomy or eliminated by altering the device or machine itself. (pp. 45–46)

One in this series of papers was presented in March 1917 at the founding conference of the National Society for the Promotion of Occupational Therapy (NSPOT) at Consolation House in Clifton Springs, New York (NSPOT, 1918). Titled "The Conservation of the World's Teeth," it recommended that disabled veterans be retrained as dental assistants (Gilbreth & Gilbreth, 1920). During the meeting, Frank Gilbreth and Jules Amar were elected honorary members of the Society (NSPOT, 1918).

The Gilbreths clearly believed that engineers were best qualified to analyze and adapt jobs for people with disabilities (Gilbreth & Gilbreth, 1920). Still, in their presentations after the Consolation House conference,

they began acknowledging the contributions of George Barton and William Rush Dunton, Jr. (first and second presidents of the National Society). Barton and Dunton, in turn, began incorporating motion study into their work and their writings. A paper about Barton's practice with convalescents at Consolation House stated that he:

> considers what motions are possible or impossible, desirable or undesirable; then he finds some occupation which involves those possible and desired motions. . . . Failing to find such an occupation in his own knowledge, the "Director" turns to his "materia medica"—a huge fifteen-hundred page catalog of tools and machines—from which, by a visualization of each tool, how it is used and what motions are necessary for its use, he "compounds" his "prescription." (Newton, 1919, pp. 4–5)

Dunton (1919) discussed the work of both Amar and the Gilbreths in his second occupational therapy textbook and provided a bibliography of the Gilbreths' publications on motion study.

When the United States entered World War I, activity analysis was included in the new occupational therapy programs and in training courses that were developed to serve returning American soldiers. In early 1918, Elizabeth Upham wrote a curriculum plan for a proposed government course to train teachers of occupational therapy.[2] The plan, presented to the U.S. Senate and the Federal Board for Vocational Education, stated that students should study "1. Analysis of industrial, commercial and agricultural occupations in terms of therapeutic values. 2. Modification of processes, special devices and tools for special needs and fatigue prevention" (Dunton, 1918, p. 89). Upham's required reading list included selections from Amar's research.[3] Later that year, Upham became director of the first university-based occupational therapy school, at Milwaukee Downer College, Milwaukee (Reed & Sanderson, 1980).

The first systematic application of activity analysis in an occupational therapy clinic may also have been in 1918, at Walter Reed General Hospital in Washington, DC. Bird Baldwin (1919a), director of the new occupa-

---

[2]The term *occupational therapist* was not yet in use. Practitioners in the new discipline were called *teachers of occupation* or *reconstruction aides*.

[3]An English translation of Amar's most recent text had been published in 1918, making his ideas more accessible to American students.

tional therapy department, described the selection of therapeutic activities for patients as follows:

> First, the work must be one which involves as an essential part the movements required by the prescription, or in which these movements recur from time to time as the work is performed by the normal individual. In order to discover the activities in which certain specific movements were thus involved, a survey was made of all the shop and ward activities, and insofar as it was possible by observation and practice, each activity was analyzed into its constituent movements. (p. 449)

Baldwin's activity analyses were detailed but addressed primarily joint position and action. For example, his analysis of engraving described the position of each body part: Fingers flexed at all joints, thumb extended at the interphalangeal and metacarpophalangeal joints to guide the tool, shoulders rigid and slightly abducted. Other important requirements, such as muscle strength and vision, were not delineated, although they were clearly considered when patients' programs were planned (Baldwin, 1919b). Activities were also adapted by changing the tools or methods used when this was indicated to improve the patient's physical function or compensate for deficits.

Between the Wars

In the 1920s, after the NSPOT had become the American Occupational Therapy Association (AOTA), a standing committee of the organization began publishing a series of papers designed to help therapists establish new departments in curative workshops and state psychiatric hospitals (AOTA, 1924). Dunton and Association president Thomas Kidner were among the influential members of the committee. Their reports included guidelines for analyzing crafts[4] in terms of joint motion and muscle strength (AOTA, 1928). Crafts requiring active motion with strength were listed for each body joint, and actions of the two sides of the body were differentiated. No attempt was made to quantify the requirements (e.g., in degrees of range or grades of strength). These craft analyses remained a standard ref-

erence for occupational therapists working with physically disabled patients for many years.

In psychiatric occupational therapy, activity analysis took the form of classification of crafts according to their characteristics or applications. Louis Haas, another member of AOTA's standing committee, developed an early system of classification that was widely accepted (Haas, 1922). He analyzed and rated activities in terms of the types of tools and materials used, the noise involved, the potential for modifying methods, the appeal to various ages and sexes, and the simplicity or complexity of processes. As was typical in psychiatry, he was most interested in the characteristics of activities that would address patients' emotional and social needs (e.g., channel aggression, promote self-esteem).

World War II stimulated renewed interest in motion study, now sometimes called *work simplification*. Frank Gilbreth had died, but Lillian Gilbreth published a paper in an occupational therapy journal recommending that engineers and rehabilitation professionals work closely together to help handicapped soldiers (Gilbreth, 1943). The army's War Department (1944) printed a technical manual on occupational therapy that contained the most detailed activity analyses to date. In addition to the traditional breakdown of joint motions, this manual listed activities for strengthening individual upper-extremity and lower-extremity muscles. Charts rating the intensity of motion at each joint during the performance of various tasks were also included.

Activity Analysis Comes of Age

In 1947, Sidney Licht, a physician who had been chief of physical medicine in an army hospital during the war, wrote a paper calling for more precise analysis of activities used in occupational therapy for physical dysfunction. He suggested the name *kinetic analysis* for the study of specific motions required in an occupation. Licht stated that a kinetic analysis should be based on actual observation of an experienced worker using proper body mechanics. It should describe the starting position and cycle of motion for the activity. The type of muscle contraction and degrees of joint range should be specified, as should the size and shape of tools used. Although Licht's terminology was not generally adopted, the elements of such an analysis are addressed today.

Through the 1960s, occupational therapists continued to analyze activities either in terms of physical re-

---

[4]During this period, the term *crafts* was used more broadly than it is today. Early craft analyses included work-related and recreational activities such as tennis, typing, gardening, and bookbinding.

quirements or in terms of emotional and social properties. In the 1970s and 1980s, however, a new way of thinking about the theory base of the profession led to major changes in activity analysis. Theorists began to delineate frames of reference within which occupational therapy intervention occurred (e.g., developmental, biomechanical, behavioral). Because each frame of reference included a unique perspective on the selection and uses of activity, each required a different type of activity analysis. Llorens' (1973) analysis of activities for treatment of cognitive–perceptual–motor dysfunction focused on the sensory systems stimulated and the motor responses produced. Trombly and Scott (1977) differentiated biomechanical analysis (emphasizing range of motion and strength) from neurodevelopmental analysis (emphasizing postures and patterns of movement). Cubie (1985) discussed volitional, habituation, and performance analysis within the Model of Human Occupation. The cognitive requirements of tasks were Allen's focus (1985).

Conclusion

Today, activity analysis is viewed as a multifaceted process (Cynkin & Robinson, 1990; Hopkins & Smith, 1988; Lamport, Coffey, & Hersch, 1989; Mosey, 1986). A comprehensive analysis first places the activity within a cultural and environmental context. Then both its generic properties (e.g., steps, tools used, cost, safety considerations) and its characteristics related to a specific frame of reference are described. The activity is discussed as it is normally performed and as modified for remedial or compensatory applications with patients.

Okoye (1988) provided an example of activity analysis as it is currently applied in occupational therapy. She discussed the importance of the computer as a medium for skill development, education, and prevocational training in our computer age. She presents a form for analyzing a computer-based treatment activity in which the therapist lists the hardware and software needed and answers a series of questions about the characteristics of the activity. The form delineates the neuromotor requirements for accessing the computer (posture, alignment, coordination) and the basic cognitive and sensory integrative functions necessary (visual discrimination, attention, problem solving), because the persons most likely to have difficulty are those with severe physical or multiple handicaps. For each requirement identified, the therapist lists alternative positioning, equipment, or methods for access (e.g., breakaway

keyboard, audio reinforcement, software with slower speed options).

Although the original link with industrial engineering and other fields doing time and motion studies in the pursuit of productivity has been severed, occupational therapists continue to use activity analysis essentially as the founders did: to improve the functioning and quality of the lives of persons with disabilities.

Acknowledgment

This work was supported in part by Grant #H133G00139 from the National Institute on Disability and Rehabilitation Research.

References

Allen, C. K. (1985). *Occupational therapy for psychiatric diseases.* Boston: Little, Brown.

Amar, J. (1918). *The physiology of industrial organization and the re-employment of the disabled.* London: Library Press Limited.

American Occupational Therapy Association. (1924). Report of Committee on Installations and Advice. *Archives of Occupational Therapy, 3,* 299–318.

American Occupational Therapy Association. (1928). Report of Committee on Installations and Advice. *Occupational Therapy and Rehabilitation, 7,* 29–43, 131–136, 211–216, 417–421.

Baldwin, B. T. (1919a). Occupational therapy. American *Journal of Care for Cripples, 8,* 447–451.

Baldwin, B. T. (1919b). *Occupational therapy applied to restoration of function of disabled joints.* Washington, DC: Walter Reed General Hospital.

Cubie, S. H. (1985). Occupational analysis. In G. Kielhofner (Ed.), *A Model of Human Occupation: Theory and application.* Baltimore: Williams & Wilkins.

Cynkin, S., & Robinson, A. M. (1990). *Occupational therapy and activities health: Toward health through activities.* Boston: Little, Brown.

Dunton, W. R. (1918). Rehabilitation of crippled soldiers and sailors: A review. *Maryland Psychiatric Quarterly, 7,* 85–101.

Dunton, W. R. (1919). *Reconstruction therapy.* Philadelphia: Saunders.

Gilbreth, F. B. (1911). *Motion study.* New York: Van Nostrand.

Gilbreth, F. B., & Gilbreth, L. M. (1920). *Motion study for the handicapped.* London: Routledge.

Gilbreth, L. M. (1943). The place of motion study in rehabilitation work. *Occupational Therapy and Rehabilitation, 22,* 61–64.

Haas, L. J. (1922). Crafts adaptable to occupational needs: Their relative importance. *Archives of Occupational Therapy, 1,* 443–445.

Hopkins, H. L., & Smith, H. D. (Eds.). (1988). *Willard and Spackman's occupational therapy* (7th ed.). Philadelphia: Lippincott.

Lamport, N. K., Coffey, M. S., & Hersch, G. I. (1989). *Activity analysis handbook.* Thorofare, NJ: Slack.

Licht, S. (1947). Kinetic analysis of crafts and occupations. *Occupational Therapy and Rehabilitation, 26,* 75–78.

Llorens, L. A. (1973). Activity analysis for cognitive-perceptual-motor dysfunction. *American Journal of Occupational Therapy, 27,* 453–456.

Mosey, A. C. (1986). *Psychosocial components of occupational therapy.* New York: Rover.

National Society for the Promotion of Occupational Therapy. (1918). *Proceedings of the first annual meeting of the National Society for the Promotion of Occupational Therapy.* Towson, MD: Author.

Newton, I. G. (1919). *Consolation House.* Clifton Springs, NY: Consolation House.

Okoye, R. L. (1988). Computer technology in occupational therapy. In H. L. Hopkins & H. D. Smith (Eds.), *Willard and Spackman's occupational therapy* (pp. 340–345). Philadelphia: Lippincott.

Reed, K. L., & Sanderson, S. R. (1980). *Concepts of occupational therapy.* Baltimore: Williams & Wilkins.

Taylor, F. W. (1911). *The principles of scientific management.* New York: Harper & Brothers.

Trombly, C. A., & Scott, A. D. (1977). *Occupational therapy for physical dysfunction.* Baltimore: Williams & Wilkins.

War Department. (1944). *Occupational therapy.* Washington, DC: U.S. Government Printing Office.

Yost, E. (1949). *Frank and Lillian Gilbreth.* New Brunswick, NJ: Rutgers University Press.

CHAPTER 47

Tools of Practice: Heritage or Baggage?

1986 ELEANOR CLARKE SLAGLE LECTURE

KATHLYN L. REED

Over the years, occupational therapists have adopted or adapted numerous media and methods. The list is so long it staggers the imagination. Yet explanations for the changing practice scene are rare. Few therapists seem to know *why* media come and go or even *when* or *how* various media or methods became part of the occupational therapy tool kit. Why do occupational therapists drop some media or methods like so much excess baggage? Is occupational therapy losing its heritage or keeping up with the times?

The question of heritage first occurred to me during Mary Fiorentino's Slagle Lecture (Fiorentino, 1975). She said she used no arts and crafts in her clinic, implying that such media were no longer useful in the treatment tool kit of occupational therapists. Many people applauded her pronouncement as if occupational therapy finally had shed its 19th-century image and joined the 20th century. Her denunciation of arts and crafts set me thinking. Why did arts and crafts become a medium of occupational therapy in the first place? What about other media and methods, such as sanding blocks or work-related programs? Discussions with colleagues produced few answers except that arts and crafts had always been taught since the days of the founders. Therefore, I decided to investigate the literature, historical documents, and old photographs to find some answers.

The objective of this article is to suggest reasons why certain media and methods have evolved as the treatment of choice in occupational therapy in a particular period of time. Likewise, a discussion of why certain media and methods fall into disfavor is relevant.

Definition of Media and Methods

A *medium* is an intervening mechanism through which a force acts or an effect is produced (Morris, 1981). In therapy the medium is the means by which the therapeutic effect is transmitted. A sanding block, a weaving loom, a vestibular board, and a large plastic ball are all media or means by which the therapeutic effect of occupational therapy is activated. Of course, the same objects can be used for other purposes not related to the therapeutic effect of occupational therapy.

Methods are the manner of performing an act or operation: a procedure or technique (*Dorland's*, 1985). In therapy the methods constitute the steps, sequence, or approach used to activate the therapeutic effect of a medium. Examples include one-handed techniques, joint protection, work simplification, and activity configuration. Thus, media and methods are two sides of the same coin. Media provide the means, and methods provide the manner through which the therapeutic effect of occupational therapy is achieved.

Definitions describe but do not determine what will become a therapeutic medium or method. To discover how an object or approach becomes identified as having therapeutic potential, one must look outside a dictionary. Analysis of media and methods over several years has suggested to me that there are eight primary factors that account for which media and methods are selected or discarded from the occupational therapy tool kit. These factors are cultural, social, economic, political, technological, theoretical, historical, and research (Christiansen, 1981; Cynkin, 1979; Di Sante, 1978; English, 1975; Jantzen, 1964; Johnson, 1983; Kielhofner, 1985; Kielhofner & Burke, 1983).

Factors in Selecting and Discarding Media and Methods

Culture is the most pervasive but hidden factor in the selection of media and methods in occupational ther-

This chapter was previously published in the *American Journal of Occupational Therapy, 40*, 597–605. Copyright © 1986, American Occupational Therapy Association. Reprinted with permission. http://dx.doi.org/10.5014/ajot.40.9.597

apy practice (Cynkin, 1979; Kielhofner, 1985). Occupational therapy was organized around the concept of improving people's abilities to deal with their daily lives. Therefore, it is logical that activities, occupations, or daily living tasks would be selected and used as media and methods. The activities, occupations, and daily living tasks are determined by the culture in which a person lives. A simple example is eating utensils. In Western culture the knife, fork, and spoon are used, but in Eastern culture chopsticks are used to get food from the serving vessel to the mouth. Thus, an occupational therapy clinic in America likely will contain eating utensils that resemble knives, forks, and spoons, but an occupational therapy clinic in Japan likely will contain chopsticks or adaptations of chopsticks.

The social factor is more conspicuous than the cultural (Cynkin, 1979; Kielhofner, 1985). Media and methods are subject to social acceptance or nonacceptance, which often is influenced by marketing and advertising strategies and changing values. The marketing strategies and changing values in turn create fads or trends that influence purchasing decisions. An example is the ongoing issue of whether handmade or machine-made products are superior in quality and value. Is there a difference in the warmth provided by a sweater made of the same yarn when one is handmade and the other made by machine? Probably not. Why then would a person pay more for one than the other? Because social factors, such as perceived value, enter the picture.

The economic factor affects the selection or discarding of media because some media cost more to use and may or may not be reimbursable by third-party insurance. Building a 16-foot boat could be a very therapeutic occupational activity, but the cost is a little high for many therapists' budgets and probably not reimbursable through most health insurance plans.

The impact of political factors on media and methods has been well documented. Diversional methods of occupational therapy have been ruled out of reimbursable services for many years. More recently there have been disputes over the use of occupational therapy for people with hip replacements or sensory integrative dysfunction.

Technological factors can have a dramatic impact on the media and methods of occupational therapy. Perhaps the best example is the change that has occurred in splinting with the advent of plastics. Originally splints were made from plaster reinforced with wire. The process was tedious, and the product subject to frequent breakdown. Then came plastics, but they had to be heated at high temperatures and tended to become brittle with age. The advent of low-temperature plastics allowed a splint to be made in a few minutes in a small frying pan. Splints from this material last for many months without noticeable change in molecular structure.

Some media and methods develop directly from a given theoretical model. An example is the use of vestibular boards, which is a direct application of the sensory integration model. When a medium or method is associated only with one theoretical model, it is easy to determine the origin. However, some media and methods can be used within a variety of theoretical models, and thus identification becomes more difficult. Cooking, for example, can be viewed as essential to nutrition, a pleasurable reward, a social activity, a paid vocation, a leisure skill, or an educational task. How many theoretical models encompass cooking as a medium and method?

The historical factor influences media and methods because some media and methods have been associated with occupational therapy from the earliest records and their origin is now obscure. For example, the use of the bicycle jigsaw can be traced back to occupational therapy clinics in 1918, but the trail is difficult to follow beyond that point. Who built the first bicycle jigsaw, and what was the original therapeutic objective?

Finally, research influences the selection and discarding of media and methods. For example, the research on building muscle strength led to the concept of progressive resistive exercise, which in turn led to the development or adaptation of media that can be modified to provide increased resistance. Many floor looms were modified in the 1950s and 1960s to provide increased resistance to shoulder, arm, hand, and leg muscles.

Table 47.1. Factors in the Selection and Use of Media and Methods

1. Cultural factor
    Dominant culture
    Subdominant culture
	5. Technological factor
	    New invention
	    Modification of
	        known invention

2. Social factor
    Upper-, middle-, or
      lower-class custom
    Fad or tradition
	6. Theoretical factor
	    Organismic philosophy
	    Mechanistic philosophy

3. Political factor
    Family or extended
      family politics
    Local community politics
    State or national politics
	7. Historical factor
	    Significant
	    Incidental

4. Economic factor
    Budget of department
      or hospital
    Reimbursement policies
	8. Research factor
	    Supports statements
	    Refutes statements

These factors can be explained further in a set of assumptions about their effect on the selection and discarding of media and methods in occupational therapy. The 14 assumptions can be stated as follows:

1. Media and methods become tools of occupational therapy through one or more of the eight factors.

2. Media and methods disappear from the tool kit of occupational therapy because of one or more of the eight factors.

3. The factors may operate to change the selection or discarding of media and methods singly or, more often, in combination.

4. Occupational therapists should understand the effects of the eight factors on the media and methods used in occupational therapy practice. (See Table 47.1 for a list of subfactors.)

5. Media and methods are selected from the dominant existing culture.

6. The sociocultural meaning of a medium and its methods may change over time and be used for a different reason or be discarded.

7. When the sociocultural rationale for a medium or method is lost or changed, the medium may be used in therapy in ways that make little sense to patients or other health professionals.

8. Economic considerations affect the selection and discarding of media and methods and thus restrict their use if the price is too high or if the cost is not reimbursable.

9. Changes in political issues may restrict or facilitate both the selection and use of various media and methods in occupational therapy based on decisions to cover them under or to exclude them from health-care programs.

10. Technology introduces new possibilities or modifies existing ones, allowing new media or methods to emerge.

11. Media and methods may be selected because they operationalize an existing theoretical model recognized by the profession.

12. A medium or method may be used in more than one model. Therefore, the therapist must know why a medium or method is being used and change the explanation when a new model is adopted.

13. Historical precedent is the least desirable justification for the existence and continued use of a medium or method but the easiest to explain.

14. Selection and use of media and methods based on research and study is the most professionally re-sponsible approach to justifying the use of a medium or method but the most difficult to obtain.

To illustrate how the eight factors and 14 assumptions operate, I have selected three media and their methods from among the many possible choices. The three are arts and crafts, sanding blocks, and work-related programs. Arts and crafts will illustrate the cultural, social, technological, and historical factors; the sanding blocks will illustrate the theoretical and research factors; and work-related programs will illustrate the political and economic factors.

Arts and Crafts

The use of arts and crafts as media and methods in occupational therapy is directly attributable to the arts-and-crafts movement that was in full swing during the formative years of occupational therapy early in this century (Levine, in press-a, in press-b). The movement was designed as a cure for the social ills of a society struggling to deal with the impact of the Industrial Revolution. During the 1800s, Western civilization changed from an agrarian to a manufacturing economy; from a cottage industry to a mass-production society; from a consumer-driven marketplace to a producer-driven marketplace; from a patronage system to an industrial-wealth system; from pride in workmanship to concern for profit; and from an ordered society of similar cultural backgrounds to a disordered society of many cultures and customs. These factors all played a role in the demise of moral treatment. The arts-and-crafts movement provided a means of revitalizing the ideas of moral treatment in a new rationale, which the founders and early leaders of occupational therapy were quick to understand. Thus, the arts-and-crafts movement is the missing link between moral treatment, which dominated the practice of medicine in the 1800s, and the treatment models to follow.

The arts-and-crafts movement began in England. The original philosophy was based on the "conviction that industrialization had brought with it the total destruction of 'purpose, sense and life'" (Naylor, 1971). Mechanical progress had been gained at the expense of human misery and the destruction of fundamental human values. Thus, the arts-and-crafts movement "was inspired by a crisis of conscience" (Naylor, 1971). Its motivations were social and moral, and its aesthetic values derived from the conviction that a society produces the art and architecture it deserves (Naylor, 1971). To that idea could be added the thought that society produces the lifestyle it deserves.

Many people contributed ideas and thoughts to the arts-and-crafts movement, and not all agreed as to their importance. Therefore, a summary of concepts must be general. The arts-and-crafts movement did the following:

- Advocated the simplification of life and ordering of daily activity as opposed to the overcomplicated or idle life (Borris, 1986; Kornwolf, 1972; Lears, 1981; Shi, 1985; Wagner, 1904);
- Valued the "craftsman" ideal, in which occupation was pursued at its own pace and not on a production schedule (Borris, 1986; Kornwolf, 1972; Lears, 1981);
- Valued the standard of craftsmanship that gave an honest day's work for an honest day's pay, rather than exploitation of the worker or cheating by the employee (Borris, 1986; Kornwolf, 1972; Naylor, 1971);
- Favored returning to the land and the home as a means of escaping the crowded, unhealthy, unnatural conditions of the city and factory (Lears, 1981; Shi, 1985);
- Ennobled the power of handwork as useful, important, a joy, and a pleasure, as opposed to mindless, repetitive activity on an assembly line, which was viewed as drudgery (Borris, 1986; Lears, 1981);
- Promoted an appreciation of performing the process and the inherent satisfaction or pride in doing or making a product, as opposed to concern only for sale and profit (Naylor, 1971);
- Encouraged respect for the inherent properties of materials and opposed any deception designed to make a material look like something it was not (Kornwolf, 1972);
- Considered functionalism and fitness of purpose the best guide to decoration, as opposed to ornamentation that served no purpose (Borris, 1986; Kornwolf, 1972);
- Believed that manual training of children would increase knowledge of moral aesthetics and improve work skills, as opposed to intellectual learning only (Borris, 1986; Lears, 1981);
- Valued the creative spirit in the artist and abhorred the mindless copying of designs (Borris, 1986);
- Attempted to improve the standards of taste and aesthetics, as opposed to allowing moral decay (Borris, 1986; Shi, 1985); and
- Viewed people as more than mere machines; human beings as having morals, values, and a sense of purpose (Kornwolf, 1972; Shi, 1985).

One early influence of the arts-and-crafts movement on occupational therapy came from Jane Addams. In 1900 she started the Hull House Labor Museum, because she wanted young people to see that the complicated machinery of the factory had evolved from the simple tools that their parents had used in the old country before immigrating to America. She wanted to interest young people in the older forms of industry so they would see "a dramatic representation of the inherited resources of their daily occupation" (Addams, 1945). The Labor Museum not only showed how spinning, weaving, pottery, and many other crafts were done, but also provided classes to teach people how to do the crafts. Addams admonished educators, saying that "educators have failed to adjust themselves to the fact that cities have become great centers of production and manufacture, and manual labor has been left without historic interpretation or imaginative uplift" (Addams, 1900, p. 236). Thus, when the training courses for attendants were started in 1907, in conjunction with the Chicago School of Civics and Philanthropy, there was an emphasis on the idea that occupation should be used as a means of education and that education was to substitute for custodial care of the mentally ill (*20th Biennial Report*, 1909).

In 1914, Eleanor Clarke Slagle started the Community Workshop under the auspices of the Illinois Society of Mental Hygiene. Its purpose was to serve as a clearinghouse for cases of doubtful insanity whom the courts considered as showing promise of a return to usefulness if given a proper environment and trade (Favill, 1917). The environment was the Hull House Labor Museum. In 1917 the Community Workshop became the Henry B. Favill School of Occupations. The following year, the first course in curative occupations and recreation was offered (*Special Courses*, 1917). Again the Labor Museum at Hull House served as the laboratory until the school was moved to the headquarters of the Illinois Society of Mental Hygiene in late 1919.

Another person to incorporate the ideas of the arts-and-crafts movement into treatment was Herbert J. Hall. In 1904 Hall began his studies of alternate treatments to the "rest cure" for neurasthenia. He was assisted by Jessie Luther, OTR, the first curator of the Hull House Labor Museum (Luther, 1902). Hall states that the "modern Arts and Crafts idea appealed very strongly, because of the growing interest in the movement and because of the clean, wholesome atmosphere which surrounds such work, and because of the many-sided appeal which such a work as the making of pottery, for instance, has to most educated minds" (Hall, 1905). Hall believed that faulty living was the cause of neurasthenia and that what was needed was a change in occupation and habits. Manual work based on the life of the artisan (craftsman ideal) was recommended itself because it was simple. The "simple life," he felt, was best for neurasthenics because it offered the least food for the nourishment of neurasthenia and provided a structure of normality. Today the person with neurasthenia would be classified as suffering from stress or burnout. The "simple life" would be called stress reduction, and the "craftsman ideal" would be called time management.

In 1906 Hall received a grant from the Procter Fund of Harvard University for $1,000 to "assist in the study of the treatment of neurasthenia by progressive and graded manual occupation." His study at Marblehead, Massachusetts, probably was the first grant-funded research project on the use of occupation as a means of treating patients. He reported that 59 of 100 patients improved, 27 were much improved, and 14 received no relief (Hall, 1910).

The arts-and-crafts philosophy was summarized in the "Philosophy of Occupation Therapy" by Adolf Meyer (1922 [see Chapter 4]). He said, "Our industrialism has created the false idea of success in *production* to the point of overproduction, bringing with it a kind of nausea to the worker and a delirium of the trader. . ."—in other words, loss of the craftsman ideal. Meyer said, "The man of today has lost the capacity and pride of workmanship and has substituted for it a measure in terms of money." In other words, there was a loss of respect for hand work. And he said that there is "a real pleasure in the use and activity of one's hands and muscles." In other words, one can find pride and satisfaction in performing and doing. Furthermore, "Our body is not merely so many pounds of flesh and bone figuring as a machine."

A final example of the influence of the arts-and-crafts movement on occupational therapy is the regional location of the arts-and-crafts societies that developed to organize the work of the arts and crafts movement. The three major areas of the country that responded to the arts-and-crafts movement were New England, Chicago and the Midwest, and the Pacific area (Clark, 1972). There is a strong correspondence between these three areas and the areas where there are large numbers of occupational therapists today.

The specific location of the societies also influenced occupational therapy. Thirteen states had at least one known arts-and-crafts society in 1904 (West, 1904). Of the 13, nine (69 percent) developed early programs in occupational therapy before 1920. All 13 states have occupational therapy programs today (West, 1904).

Considering its influence, what happened to the arts-and-crafts movement? It was overtaken by World War I. The rules of the game changed for many people. The war effort provided its own sense of purpose. Some industries did hire craftsmen to improve designs, and machine-made products did improve in quality. City life improved as sanitation efforts made inroads against the piles of garbage. The expanding population meant that machine manufacture was the only means of providing products for everyone. Hand production was just too slow and too expensive.

How did the changes influence occupational therapy? What factors were changing the role of arts and crafts in practice? The cultural scene had shifted: Society was no longer struggling to adapt to city life, and the factory system had been integrated in the fabric of American life. The number of people living on the land would continue to decrease over the coming years. People had become used to the technological changes the factory had produced. Machine-made goods were acceptable and could be made in quantities unknown under the handmade system. Young therapists did not remember the arts-and-crafts movement and did not know what it represented. They only knew that arts and crafts always had been a part of occupational therapy's tool kit. Finally, a new philosophy was overtaking the profession. The humanistic ideas of the founding years were being challenged as unscientific and unmeasurable. The profession was being reformulated in such a manner that the arts-and-crafts philosophy made little sense. Not until the 1960s would the founding ideas resurface. Figure 47.1 illustrates the changing theory and philosophy of the arts-and-crafts ideology.

Sanding Blocks

Sanding blocks, or sandblocks, are a common sight in many occupational therapy clinics. Nearly all occupational therapists become acquainted with them during their education, and many have made sanding blocks. Yet, few can describe the origin and original purpose of the sanding block or trace the changes in thinking about their use over the years.

Woodworking and sanding can be traced to the beginning of occupational therapy history. The initial use of sanding blocks, however, is unclear. The first mention of them appears in 1934 in an article by Henrietta McNary. In the same article, the first description of an adapted

	1880	1890	1900	1910	1920	1930	1940	1950	1960	1970	1980	1990
Organismic	End of Moral Treatment	Rise of the Arts-and-Crafts Movement					Rise of the Developmental Model		Rise of Systems Model Return of Humanism			
Mechanistic				Flexner Report	Rise of the Orthopedics Model		Rise of the Biomedical Model	Dominance of the Psycho-analytic Model		Dominance of the Behaviorism Model		
				Medical Schools Increase Science Study								

Figure 47.1. Relative influence of organismic and mechanistic models on occupational therapy practice.

sanding block also appears. Its purpose was to improve opposition. The last article in our literature on a sanding block, a reciprocal sanding device, appears in 1965 (Mathews, 1965). In all, 14 different types of sanding blocks are presented. These are listed in Table 47.2.

The dates of the articles on sanding blocks coincide with the rise and fall of the orthopedic and kinesthetic treatment models of occupational therapy. The ortho-

pedic model followed the arts-and-crafts model. It was concerned with muscle strengthening and range of motion. Stretching contractures, exercise, and physical tolerance also were included. These concepts form the basis of the objectives for which the sanding block was used. A summary of these purposes or objectives is found in Table 47.3.

The use of sanding blocks has not disappeared, but the theories underpinning their development and use have been superseded by the sensorimotor and sensory integration models. As a result, some unusual uses of sanding blocks have surfaced. For example, one therapist was observed giving a patient a sanding block with no sandpaper and an incline plane made of formica. Because the patient did not want to make anything, the therapist explained that the purpose of the activ-

Table 47.2. Types of Sanding Blocks

1. Proximal sanding blocks
   (Abbott, 1957; *Photographs*, 1947)
2. Proximal interphalangeal sanding block
   (Abbott, 1957; *Photographs*, 1947)
3. Metacarpal phalangeal sanding blocks
   (Abbott, 1957; *Photographs*, 1947)
4. Distal sanding block
   (Abbott, 1957)
5. Opponens sanding block
   (Abbott, 1957)
6. Shoulder abduction sanding block
   ("Adapted," 1957; Bennett & Driver, 1957)
7. Spring squeeze sanding block
   (Gurney, 1959)
8. Grip sanding block
   (Hightower et al., 1963)
9. Reciprocal sanding device
   (Mathews, 1965)
10. Weighted sander or progressive resistive exercise sander
    (Svensson & Brennan, 1954)
11. Bilateral sander, horizontal or vertical handles
    (*Photographs*, 1947)
12. Wrist exercise sander (Blodgett, 1947)
13. Hemiplegia sander (Forbes, 1951)
14. Graduated sanding blocks—graduated straight
    handles or graduated round knob handles
    (*Photographs*, 1947)

Table 47.3. Purposes or Objectives of Sanding Blocks

Sanding blocks were adapted to provide the following:
1. Different hand grip position for active or passive stretching:
   a. Handles were added and enlarged.
   b. Holes or grooves were drilled or carved for finger and thumb placement.
   c. Straps were added to hold the hand in place.
   d. Gloves were used to position the hand.
   e. Construction was altered to provide a different grip than that normally used.
2. Dynamic exercise of wrist, elbow, or shoulder—usually range of motion
3. Increased grip strength of hand and fingers
4. Bilateral activity of the upper extremities
5. Reciprocal activity of the upper extremities
6. Improved trunk stability
7. Standing and physical tolerance

ity was bilateral exercise. In this example, the fundamental concepts of occupational therapy, performance through doing and the use of occupation toward some purpose, were overlooked or separated from the application. The medium of sanding blocks and the methods of setting up the activity to obtain selected objectives had been separated from the original concepts so the meaning and purpose of the activity were lost. The *motion* of sanding is a necessary but not sufficient part of the *activity* of sanding. The media, the methods, and the objective of an occupation must be consistent with each other. Three out of three—medium, method, and objective—must be the rule, not the exception.

Sanding blocks illustrate the factors of theory and research. The many adaptations of the sanding block are based on the theoretical concepts of the orthopedic and kinesthetic treatment models, which stress positioning the body part in the desired pattern of motion and then encouraging that motion to stretch, strengthen, or increase the motion of a particular body part or parts. Research supported the concept that increased amounts of resistance applied to a given muscle group would strengthen the muscle group involved. This concept became known as progressive resistive exercise.

Work-Related Programs

Work-related programs were a part of the early ideology of occupational therapy. The term *work-related programs* is used to represent all efforts to enable people to engage in productive occupations through occupational therapy, whether the effort is aimed at vocational education, vocational guidance, prevocational evaluation and training, vocational training or retraining, vocational readiness, work hardening, work adjustment, or career education.

Hall was very interested in helping patients find an alternate occupation that would be less stressful and more suitable to the person's needs. The "work cure" was based on the assumption that by substituting or bringing about "by a gradual process the conditions of a normal life, a life of pleasant and progressive occupations, as different as possible from the previous life, a person could overcome the mental and nervous problems in his life" (Hall, 1905).

George E. Barton said he was going to "try to prove that the hours of idleness in convalescence could be filled with pastimes which would be useful not only to pass the time, but to prepare the person for remunerative labor later on to get a job, a better job, or to do a job better than it was before" (Barton, 1914). Consolation House was created to serve the needs of people who were learning to put their lives back together and who needed assistance to find an occupation suitable to their abilities but not limited by their disabilities.

Slagle had experience in assessing people's fitness for a job at the Community Workshop at Hull House. At the founding conference of occupational therapy in Clifton Springs, New York, she spoke of a family of five who had been supported by charities for many years. After 1 year at the Community Workshop, the family was self-sufficient (Dunton, 1917).

Thomas B. Kidner, Vocational Secretary to the Military Hospitals Commission in Ottawa, Canada, was well acquainted with the vocational side of occupational therapy. In June 1918, he was loaned by the Canadian government to the United States as a special adviser on rehabilitation to the Federal Board for Vocational Education (FBVE). The FBVE had been created the previous year to establish a federal-state program in vocational education. In 1918 it had been given the authority and responsibility for the vocational rehabilitation of veterans ("Editorial," 1922). Elizabeth G. Upham (later Davis), who had been instrumental in starting the occupational therapy course at Milwaukee Downer College, also joined the FBVE in 1918. She wrote two documents illustrating the role of occupational therapy with the disabled veteran (Upham, 1918a, 1918b) and recommended that the FBVE be given control of military patients as soon as possible in order to prepare them for adjustment to normal life (Davis, no date). Had her recommendation been accepted, occupational therapy's role in vocational preparation would have been larger than it has been. Both Kidner and Upham left the FBVE in 1919.

The medical department of the army also had a plan for the rehabilitation of disabled soldiers. It had created a system of orthopedic reconstruction hospitals that included vocational workshops and employment bureaus (Gritzer & Arluke, 1985). The dispute over who would do what came to the floor of the U.S. Senate in July 1918. The medical department of the army was granted the exclusive right to all aspects of functional restoration and medical control over curative work. This action bound occupational therapy to medicine's domain. The FBVE, on the other hand, was given responsibility for vocational rehabilitation. The separation became more divided in 1920 when the Industrial Rehabilitation Act was passed without any coverage for medical services. Bulletin #57 of the FBVE makes it quite clear than any occupational work not related to the vocation for which the injured person is being trained is evidently given for its therapeutic value. Therapeutic use of work was viewed as part of the injured person's physical rehabilitation rather than vocational rehabilitation and therefore was not covered under the act ("Industrial rehabilitation," 1920). Thus, occupational therapy was cut off from many of its work-related programs by a political compromise over which it ultimately had little control. Work-related programs were not reestablished until 1943 when the Vocational Rehabilitation Act was changed to include coverage for medical services (Lassiter, 1972). In 1954, the Vocational Rehabilitation Act was further modified to include coverage for the training of rehabilitation personnel, including occupational therapists. In addition there were monies for research and demonstration projects (Lassiter, 1972). Among the demonstration projects were prevocational evaluation and training centers in which occupational therapists played a significant role. However, by the 1960s these projects became too expensive to continue, and the role of occupational therapy in work-related programs again went into a period of decline. Finally in the 1980s the interest returned. A position paper was written and a grant was funded to increase occupational therapists' awareness of the role of occupational therapy in work-related programs. Some of the current interests are assessment of work potential and aptitude skills, physical capacities assessment and work hardening, job evaluation, work experience, career exploration and job-seeking skills, independent living, and industrial consultation.

The level of occupational therapists' interest and opportunities in work-related programs has waxed and waned over the past 80 years. The fluctuations can be traced to politics and economics. When both were favorable or neutral, occupational therapists provided many examples of programs designed to help a person to gain or regain productive skills. However, when the politics and economics made it difficult for occupational therapists to provide such skill assessment and skill training, their activity in work-related programs decreased. The challenge will be to shape the political and economic factors in favor of occupational therapy if therapists want to maintain their role in helping people attain or regain productive skills.

Occupational Analysis

As illustrated thus far, the selection and discarding of media and methods in occupational therapy has not been accidental. Factors converge and diverge to increase or decrease the likelihood that a particular medium and its methods will be selected or discarded in the practice of occupational therapy. Culture sets the major parameters, but changes in society frequently alter the cultural set. Political and economic factors often work in combination. Political factors can be influenced by occupational therapists, but some events may occur over which therapists have little control. The results may be felt most keenly economically when reimbursement patterns result in changes in coverage of occupational therapy services. Technology may lead to dramatic changes in media or methods. Theoretical factors often introduce new media and methods into the treatment setting. Sometimes the new theory or model brings new media and methods with it; at other times just the explanation and the use of an existing medium or method changes. History often is used to explain the existence of media or methods when the origin has been lost through time. Research offers a better explanation for the use of media and methods but is more difficult to obtain.

All of these factors need to be considered when examining why certain media and methods appear in a clinic or practice setting. Can practicing occupational therapists explain why each medium or method is used in their practice setting? Is the explanation the best one, or is the explanation of history used by default? Perhaps a more systematic use of occupational or activity analysis should be promoted which includes the selection and discarding of factors as well as considerations such as range of motion, sensory stimulation, or amount of social interaction obtained.

Central to each of the factors are the concepts of interests and values. A culture, individuals, and professionals have interests and values. An interest is defined as a set that guides behavior in a certain direction or toward certain goals (Chaplin, 1975). A value is a social end or goal that is considered desirable to achieve (Chaplin, 1975).

In occupational therapy there seem to be three major areas to consider in interest and values. These are culture and society, the individual, and the profession. The eight factors that affect selection and discarding of media and methods can be organized under the cultural and social interest and values and professional interests and values. Under the *cultural and social* area are the cultural, social, economic, political, and technological factors. Under the *professional* are the theoretical, historical, and research factors. Under the *individual* are factors that must be determined by assessment of each individual. These are the roles performed by the individual and the functional abilities, skills, and capacities of the individual. When the three areas of cultural-social, individual, and professional interests and values are considered, there should be less chance of using media and methods that are out-of-date in society, not meaningful to the individual, and of questionable use to the profession.

Summary

This article presents and illustrates the major factors that influence the selection and discarding of media and methods in occupational therapy. The eight factors are the cultural, social, economic, political, technological, theoretical, historical, and research factors. The factors may operate in various combinations or alone to influence the use of a specific medium or method in practice. Therapists are encouraged to know these eight factors and in particular to be familiar with (a) what media and methods occupational therapists use, (b) why occupational therapists use those media and methods, (c) from where the media and methods come, (d) with whom the media and methods should be used in treatment, (e) how the media and methods are used, (f) when the media and methods are used, and (g) how much of the medium or method should be used. Educators, in particular, need to teach why a medium or method is used as well as how. Researchers need to provide more information as to why certain media and methods became part of our tool kit. Practitioners would be wise to follow the statement. If you know how, be sure you know why and be sure the why is consistent with the philosophy of occupational therapy.

References

Abbott, M. (1957). *A syllabus of occupational therapy procedures and techniques as applied to orthopedic and neurological conditions.* New York: American Occupational Therapy Association.

Adapted sand block. Part I. (1957). *American Journal of Occupational Therapy, 11,* 198.

Addams, J. (1900). Social education of the industrial democracy. *Commons, 5,* 17–28.

Addams, J. (1945). *Twenty years at Hull House, with autobiographical notes.* New York: Macmillan.

Barton, G. E. (1914). A view of invalid occupation. *Trained Nurse & Hospital Review, 52,* 327–330.

Bennett, R. L., & Driver, M. (1957). The aims and methods of occupational therapy in the treatment of the after-effects of poliomyelitis. *American Journal of Occupational Therapy, 11,* 145–153.

Blodgett, M. L. (1947). Sanding for exercise. *American Journal of Occupational Therapy, 1,* 6.

Borris, E. (1986). *Art and labor: Ruskin, Morris, and the craftsman ideal in America.* Philadelphia, PA: Temple University Press.

Chaplin, J. P. (1975). *Dictionary of psychology* (2nd ed.). New York: Dell.

Christiansen, C. H. (1981). Editorial: Toward resolution of crisis: Research requisites in occupational therapy. *Occupational Therapy Journal of Research, 1,* 115–124.

Clark, R. J. (1972). *The arts-and-crafts movement in America: 1876–1916.* Princeton, NJ: Princeton University Press.

Cynkin, S. (1979). *Occupational therapy: Toward health through activities.* Boston: Little, Brown.

Davis, E. U. (no date). *Just another biography.* Unpublished manuscript.

Di Sante, E. (1978). Technology transfer: From space exploration to occupational therapy. *American Journal of Occupational Therapy, 32,* 171–174.

Dorland's illustrated medical dictionary (26th ed.). Philadelphia, PA: W. B. Saunders, p. 809.

Dunton, W. R. (1917). *The growing necessity for occupational therapy.* New York: Teachers College. (In AOTA Archives, Moody Library, Galveston, TX).

Editorial: The 6th annual meeting. *Archives of Occupational Therapy, 1,* 419–427.

English, C. B. (1975). Computers and occupational therapy. *American Journal of Occupational Therapy, 29,* 43–47.

Favill, J. (1917). *Henry Baird Favill: 1960–1916.* Chicago: Rand McNally, p. 87.

Fiorentino, M. R. (1975). Occupational therapy: Realization to activation—1974 Eleanor Clarke Slagle lecture. *American Journal of Occupational Therapy, 29,* 15–21.

Forbes, E. S. (1951). Two devices for use in treating hemiplegics. *American Journal of Occupational Therapy, 5,* 49–51.

Gritzer, G., & Arluke, A. (1985). *The making of rehabilitation: A political economy of medical specialization, 1890–1980.* Berkeley, CA: University of California Press.

Gurney, G. W. (1959). Spring-squeeze sandblock. *American Journal of Occupational Therapy, 13,* 278.

Hall, H. J. (1905). The systematic use of work as a remedy in neurasthenia and allied conditions. *Boston Medical & Surgical Journal, 112,* 29–32.

Hall, H. J. (1910). Work-cure: A report of 5 years' experience at an institution devoted to the therapeutic application of manual work. *Journal of the American Medical Association, 54,* 12–14.

Hightower, M. D., et al. (1963). Grip sander. *American Journal of Occupational Therapy, 17,* 62–63.

Industrial rehabilitation—A statement of policies to be observed in the administration of the Industrial Rehabilitation Act. (1920). *FBVE Bulletin, 57.*

Jantzen, A. C. (1964). The role of research in occupational therapy. *Proceedings of the 1964 Annual Conference* (pp. 2–9). New York: American Occupational Therapy Association.

Johnson, J. A. (1983). The changing medical marketplace as a context for the practice of occupational therapy. In G. Kielhofner (Ed.), *Health through occupation: Theory and practice in occupational therapy* (pp. 163–177). Philadelphia, PA: F. A. Davis.

Kielhofner, G. (Ed.). (1985). *A model of human occupation: Theory and application.* Baltimore, MD: Williams & Wilkins.

Kielhofner, G., & Burke, J. P. (1983). The evolution of knowledge and practice in occupational therapy: Past, present and future (pp. 3–54). In G. Kielhofner (Ed.), *Health through occupation: Theory and practice in occupational therapy.* Philadelphia, PA: F. A. Davis.

Kornwolf, J. D. (1972). *M. H. Baillie Scott and the arts-and-crafts movement.* Baltimore, MD: Johns Hopkins Press.

Lassiter, R. A. (1972). History of the rehabilitation movement in America. In J. G. Cull & R. E. Hardy (Eds.), *Vocational rehabilitation: Profession and process* (pp. 5–58). Springfield, IL: Charles C Thomas.

Lears, T. J. J. (1981). *No place of grace: Antimodernism and the transformation of American culture: 1880–1920.* New York: Pantheon.

Levine, R. E. (in press-a). Guest editorial: Historical research: Ordering the past to chart our future. *Occupational Therapy Journal of Research.*

Levine, R. E. (in press-b). The influence of the arts-and-crafts movement on the professional status of occupational therapy. In W. Coleman (Ed.), *Written history monograph.* Rockville, MD: American Occupational Therapy Association.

Luther, J. (1902). The labor museum at Hull House. *Commons, 7,* 1–13.

Mathews, T. (1965). Reciprocal sanding device. *American Journal of Occupational Therapy, 19,* 354–355.

McNary, H. (1934). Anatomical considerations and technique in using occupations as exercise for orthopedic disabilities: III. Wrist and fingers. *Occupational Therapy Rehabilitation, 13,* 24–29.

Meyer, A. (1922). Philosophy of occupational therapy. *Archives of Occupational Therapy, 1,* 1–10. Reprinted as Chapter 4.

Morris, W. (Ed.). (1981). *American heritage dictionary of the English language.* Boston: Houghton Mifflin, p. 815.

Naylor, G. (1971). *The arts-and-crafts movement: A study of its sources, ideals, and influence on design theory.* Cambridge, MA: MIT Press.

Photographs of occupational therapy adapted equipment as developed in Veterans Administration and Army hospitals. (1947). Washington, DC: Department of Medicine & Surgery, Veterans Administration.

Shi, D. E. (1985). *The simple life: Plain living and high thinking in American culture.* New York: Oxford University Press.

Special courses in curative occupations and recreation. (1917, December). Chicago: Chicago School of Civics and Philanthropy Special Bulletin.

Svensson, V. W., & Brennan, M. C. (1954). Adapted weighted resistive apparatus. *American Journal of Occupational Therapy, 8,* 13.

20th biennial report of the board of public charities of the state of Illinois, July 1, 1906–June 30, 1908. Springfield, IL: Illinois State Journal Co., p. 58.

Upham, E. G. (1918a). Training of teachers for occupational therapy for the rehabilitation of disabled soldiers and sailors. *Federal Board for Vocational Education Bulletin, 6,* 1–76.

Upham, E. G. (1918b). Ward occupations in hospitals. *Federal Board for Vocational Education Bulletin, 25,* 1–57.

Wagner, C. (1904). *The simple life.* New York: Grosset & Dunlap.

West, M. (1904). The revival of handicrafts in America. *Bureau of Labor Bulletin, 55,* 1573–1622.

CHAPTER 48

Ethical Decision-Making Challenges in Clinical Practice

BEVERLY P. HOROWITZ

Changing health care environments, organizational charts, and occupational therapy department structure require practitioners to be effective problem solvers in fast-paced environments (Horowitz, 2001a, 2001b). Increased practice opportunities in school-based programs, home health care, and private practice also support increased professional autonomy and modified supervisory patterns and teamwork strategies. Simultaneously, demographic changes and increasing appreciation of the need to improve access to health care services challenges health care providers, including occupational therapists, to increase their understanding of diverse populations and to provide culturally competent care (Wells & Black, 2000). Professional education and clinical experience enables practitioners to amass resources, including clinical assessments and instruments to promote clinical reasoning for "best practice."

In today's health care environment practitioners face complex ethical problems and/or dilemmas, including the "business–administrative and community dimensions" often involved in ethical issues involving patient care (Purtilo, 1999, p. 28). Supportive peer relationships are optimal for effective problem solving to resolve ethical dilemmas, particularly when practitioners face problems that challenge their personal and/or professional values and professional integrity. However, organizational cultures in many of today's busy health care settings, with combinations of per-diem, part-time, and full-time staff, is not always conducive to cohesive departments or close collegial relationships, both of which are beneficial when practitioners face ethical problems.

Ethical decision-making in these environments requires practical problem-solving strategies to guide practitioners to evaluate all relevant information, define the presenting problem, determine tentative courses of action, and finally select and implement an ethical resolution (Darr, 1997; Purtilo, 1999; Scott, 1998).

One common ethical dilemma arises when providing health care services to uninsured individuals. Practitioners face conflicts between professional and ethical responsibilities to equitably support the health and well-being of our patients and the realities of health care business practices that typically require administrative review to ensure payment for services as a prerequisite for treatment. Often uninsured patients receive limited services, are transferred to alternative settings, or are denied non-emergency services. We face a different type of dilemma when we observe an experienced colleague whose personal problems are intruding upon their professional competence. What is our obligation to our colleagues, institutions, and patients? How do we respond? While these are dissimilar situations, each situation asks us to consider our individual and professional values and ethics, and presents a professional challenge.

Values and Ethics and Ethical Decision-Making

In our increasingly heterogeneous society, individuals have diverse personal beliefs and values and are influenced by internalized principles that guide their relationships with people (Wells & Black, 2000). These personal values, often coupled with cultural and religious perspectives, support concepts of morality, the guidelines and standards that protect our human values and accompany our social interactions (Horowitz, 1996; Purtilo, 1999).

Personal biases and prejudice, whether conscious or unconscious, similarly influence moral perspectives, our view of the world, and our ability to both understand and work with diverse populations. Prejudice and biases extend beyond the usual "isms" (e.g., racism, ageism, sexism) to attitudes related to parenting, sexual orientation, leisure, work ethics, and retirement. Reflection on our own values, perspectives, and biases enables us to understand personal values that are the basis of our morality (Diller, 1999; Horowitz, 1996, 2001a, 2001b).

Ethics is the systematic study of what may be called the "nature of morality" (Bailey & Schwartzberg, 1995, p. 2; Horowitz, 1996; Purtilo, 1999). It provides an organized framework to understand and discuss personal and social values, individual and social behavior, and methods for resolving conflicts between values and ethical principles in our daily lives. Religion, culture, family, and community influence individual values and moral principles; however, we are also influenced by our forbearers and history, including perspectives on morality, ethical principles, and ethical behavior. Deontologic and teleologic ethical theories are two theoretical approaches with particular relevance for health care practitioners (Horowitz, 2001a, 2001b, 1996; Purtilo, 1999). Deontology can be summarized as an absolutist duty-driven theory, associated with philosopher Immanuel Kant (1724–1804). It holds that behavior needs to be based upon moral obligation or "duty," and that one's conduct can be perceived as following correct or incorrect moral precepts, regardless of the consequences. In contrast, teleological theory, often identified with "utilitarianism," associated with John Stuart Mill and Jeremy Bentham, is less concerned with determining correct or incorrect conduct, and more concerned with the consequences of conduct and behavior (Purtilo, 1999; Rhodes, 1989).

These perspectives continue to reflect dialog on ethical behavior today, in both our personal and professional lives and provide a foundation for understanding ethical principles of fidelity, justice, beneficence, nonmaleficence, veracity, autonomy, and self-determination (Horowitz, 1996; Purtilo, 1999). Teleologic, or utilitarian theories, influence our thinking, when we focus our attention on the consequences of either individual or social behavior or policies, and seek actions that bring about the "best balance of benefits over burdens" for our patients and their families. In contrast, when we choose between two courses of action, and select one because we feel it to be morally correct, we are responding to deontologic ethical theory (Horowitz, 1996, 2001a, 2001b; Purtilo, 1999, p. 48).

However, how do we recognize ethical issues, challenges, and dilemmas? Ethical issues commonly face us. These issues present moral principles that may pose challenges to individual values, but do not necessarily pose a problem. This may include a concern regarding advance directives for one particular client (e.g., Do Not Resuscitate Orders), or a hospital admission policy that requires insurance documentation for entry into a rehabilitation program. They may also involve situations where we perceive threats to moral values, requiring systematic analysis and decision-making to determine a course of action. Ethical dilemmas are more complex ethical problems that cause ethical distress. Here, there is no one best course of action, rather a problem that involves conflicting values, where each possible action results in conflicting values, for example, a conflict between the principles of autonomy versus nonmaleficence, or fidelity versus beneficence (Horowitz, 2001a, 2001b; Purtilo, 1999).

Codes of Ethics, Legal Issues, and Social Responsibility

Society expects health care professionals to be of high moral standing with similar expectations of fiduciary provider–patient/client relationships, built upon trust, privacy, and confidence (Kutchins, 1991; Levy, 1976; Lo, 1995). Licensed health care professionals commonly are required to be of "good moral character" and maintain high professional standards, with legal sanctions for misconduct, establishing policy to codify this expectation (New York State Department of Education, 1993, p. 11). Health professionals are expected to: (1) Avoid misrepresentation, including implications for documentation; (2) Be faithful and honest in relationships with patients and colleagues; (3) Provide competent professional services to promote health and well-being; (4) Be cognizant of precautions to prevent harm; and (5) Provide patients with accurate information about treatment, including treatment options (American Occupational Therapy Association, 2000a; Hansen, 2001; Horowitz, 2001a; Lo, 1995).

Health care professional codes of conduct typically emulate the ancient physicians' Hippocratic Oath and codes of the professions of law, medicine, and clergy. They publicly enunciate shared values, historically represent a means of self-regulation, and acknowledge the importance of public trust in the health professions. In this tradition, the Occupational Therapy Code of Ethics (AOTA, 2000a) sets forth the following principles of occupational therapy:

1. Concern for the well-being of clients;
2. Avoid harm;
3. Respect for the rights of clients;
4. High standards of competence;
5. Compliance with policies of the profession and laws regulating practice;
6. Provide accurate information about occupational therapy services; and
7. High professional conduct.

These principles reflect shared professional values, including altruism; equality and impartiality; freedom, including professional independence and the commitment to freedom of choice for all people; justice; dignity; valuing each person's uniqueness; truthfulness; prudence; discipline; discretion; and vigilance (American Occupational Therapy Association Commission on Standards and Ethics, 1996; Horowitz, 1996). However, while these professional principles provide an ethical framework for practice, practitioners need to distinguish ethical problems and dilemmas from clinical, administrative, or legal issues, and determine appropriate approaches for differing problems and needs.

Practitioners generally have experience identifying and resolving clinical and administrative problems. Health care organizations have written operating procedures and supervisory personnel who provide administrative direction. Practitioners often have access to texts, journals, and monographs that address clinical reasoning and practice issues for persons with a range of diagnoses across the life span. Additionally, technological advances and the information explosion enable increasing numbers of practitioners to have ready access to varied computer databases, professional listserves and journals to obtain current information on best practice (Horowitz, 2001b).

There is a wealth of information available on ethical decision-making. However, occupational therapy practice focuses on clinical interventions to address client goals, often with a focus on promoting functional capability and occupational performance. Additionally, our health care environment requires practitioners to balance clinical–ethical considerations, organizational policies and expectations, third-party payer requirements, clinical demands, financial pressures, and personal and professional values (Crabtree, 1991; Darr,

1997, Hofland, 1994; Horowitz, 2001a, 2001b; Kyler-Hutchison, 1996; Scott, 1997). These pressures may ultimately affect clinical decision-making and interfere with collaborative treatment planning with clients and families (Haas, 1995). Like many disciplines, accredited occupational therapy programs are required to include course material that enables students to appreciate and understand ethical principles and relationships between ethics and practice (Accreditation Council for Occupational Therapy Education, 1998). Professional organizations, including the American Occupational Therapy Association, provide resources for practitioners to increase their knowledge of methods of resolving ethical dilemmas in practice (Accreditation Council for Occupational Therapy Education, 1998; American Speech-Language Hearing Association, 2001a, 2001b; Hansen, 2001; Scott, 1997). Occupational therapy practitioners are skilled analysts of human behavior and problem solvers, but have less experience and professional support to increase ethical decision-making capabilities in most practice settings.

Ethical problems arise when we find ourselves facing moral challenges. They commonly occur when we find ourselves in situations that force us to reflect upon our personal and professional beliefs, values, and responsibilities. Ethical dilemmas result when we perceive ourselves caught between conflicting values and ethical principles that require choices between competing "morally correct" solutions and courses of action (Purtilo, 1999, p. 72). One such dilemma may develop in the context of strong professional relationships with patients. For example, in the course of regular treatment a severely ill patient may choose to ask her therapist questions about her medical condition and prognosis instead of seeking this information from her physician. How should the therapist respond? What is her responsibility? Ethical principles instruct us to be honest and truthful and not provide false hope, or inaccurate information. However, the principle of beneficence simultaneously asks us to be concerned with "doing good," and the principle of nonmaleficence instructs us to prevent harm, including potential negative consequences of interventions. Crafting an appropriate ethical solution requires reflection on personal values and perceived conflicting ethical principles, and determination of alternative choices and available courses of action. Here, the challenge is to utilize broad-based clinical skills and clinical judgment to answer questions we can honestly answer, empower the patient to speak with her physician, and address those health care needs within our domain to maximize quality of life and well-being.

In other situations, ethical problems may have corresponding legal implications (Horowitz, 1996; Scott, 1997; Wenston, 1987). For example, ethical concepts regarding confidentiality need to be understood in the context of both professional ethics as well as the law. For example, therapists who inappropriately disclose confidential patient information regarding HIV may find themselves reported for violations of both the AOTA Code of Ethics as well as violations of state statutes (Kyler-Hutchison, 1995; Liang, 2000). Inappropriate disclosure of medical information regarding HIV status in some states can result in civil and criminal penalties (Liang, 2000). Additionally, conduct considered professionally unethical increasingly also violates criminal or licensure law. Specific examples are noted in The Occupational Therapy Code of Ethics in Principle 1, which prohibits exploitation of recipients of services "sexually, physically . . . or in any manner," and in Principle 5, which requires accurate representation of "qualifications, education, experience, training, and competence" (American Occupational Therapy Association, 2000a; Scott, 1997). Relationships and similarities between ethical standards and legal requirements are clear when state law delineates specific unprofessional conduct, as in New York State. Two examples of unprofessional conduct listed by New York State's Board of Regents include: "willful or grossly negligent failure to comply with substantial provisions of Federal, State, or local law . . ."; and "willfully making or filing a false report . . ."; or "practicing beyond the scope permitted by law . . ." corresponding to Principles 5 and 6 in AOTA's Code of Ethics, which commit occupational therapists to comply with all laws regulating practice, and to accurately document information about occupational therapy services (American Occupational Therapy Association, 2000a; New York State Department of Education, 1993, p. 30).

In addition to being knowledgeable about ethical practice, occupational therapy practitioners need to fully understand licensure requirements and their scope of practice, professional standards of practice, and requirements of varied accrediting agencies. We are expected to comply with the full range of laws, from Constitutional law to criminal law and administrative law (including regulations of federal agencies such as the Equal Opportunity Commission (EEOC), Centers for Disease Control (CDC), and Occupational Safety and Health Administration (OSHA). Additionally, we need to be knowledgeable about health care law, regulations, and policy, particularly those with direct impact upon practice (American Occupational Therapy Association, 2000b; Bailey & Schwartzberg, 1995; Horowitz, 2000; Liang, 2000; Scott, 1997). Major federal legislation with significant impact upon occupational therapy practice include: Public Law 94–142, PL 99–457, and PL 105–17 (special educational needs of disabled children and toddlers), the Omnibus Reconciliation Act of 1987 and 1990 (nursing home reform and services), Medicare and Medicaid regulations (rehabilitation services, including occupational therapy), and the Americans with Disabilities Act (ADA) (PL 101–336) (civil rights legislation for disabled persons in the areas of education), employment, public accommodations, transportation, and telecommunications (Bailey & Schwartzberg, 1995; Dunn, 2000). State insurance law and state Medicaid policy directly affect coverage of occupational therapy services for clients across the life span. Therapists involved in nontraditional practice need to be particularly cognizant of legal issues, including licensure regulations, malpractice law, laws and regulations regarding consultation, and contract law (Bailey & Schwartzberg, 1995; Horowitz, 1996; Kornblau, 1992; Scott, 1997).

Strategies for Ethical Decision-Making

Ethical problems and dilemmas can occur in everyday practice, in clinical or administrative settings, educational environments, or within professional relationships. Professional Codes of Ethics, such as AOTA's Code of Ethics, socialize and commit practitioners to shared values and responsibilities to guide professional conduct. They are optimally utilized in combination with a systematic approach to ethical decision-making. This process guides data gathering for problem identification, data analysis, determining an optimal course of action, and individual reflection on action outcomes. Ethical decision-making frameworks optimally include opportunities for self-reflection and feedback to guide the overall process, modify problem analysis, and conceptualize potential courses of action (Horowitz, 1996, 2001a, 2001b; Scott, 1998).

Purtilo's Six-Step Approach (Purtilo, 1999) provides one practical ethical decision-making strategy that addresses the needs of health care practitioners in varied contexts. It includes:

1. Data gathering and getting the story straight;
2. Problem identification;

3. Problem analysis utilizing ethical theory and principles;
4. Exploration of practical options;
5. Selecting and executing a course of action; and
6. Evaluation of the process and the outcome.

This six-step process organizes and structures the problem-solving process to prevent practitioners from allowing emotional reactions and time pressures to direct their behavior. Step 1 asks practitioners to gather all relevant information, determine the accuracy of the information they obtain, and the context in which information was gathered. In Step 2 the problem analysis process promotes self-questioning. It asks, What is the morally correct course of action? How does one maintain professional integrity within this situation? Who has primary responsibility for resolving this situation? Step 3 requires practitioners to utilize their knowledge of ethical principles, including teleologic (utilitarian) and deontologic approaches, to determine the kind of ethical problem or dilemma they face, including competing values and principles. Formulations of all possible, practical solutions, including anticipated consequences, follow in Step 4. At this point in the process, with data and analysis in hand, one needs to consider available options, selecting among those deemed most appropriate. Practitioners then need to act (Step 5) and initiate a response to the ethical problem or dilemma. While individuals may or may not successfully execute actions to resolve their dilemma, this structured ethical decision-making approach constructively increases information about the problem or dilemma, thereby reducing distress and potential "burnout." The last step (Step 6) is evaluative. It poses the questions: What went well? What could be done differently? How did this action affect you? Affect other people's perceptions of you? Are you empowered for future ethical decision-making (Purtilo, 1999)?

Ethical Decision-Making in Practice

In practice, ethical problems and/or dilemmas may occur in response to conflicts between values and ethical principles; ethical principles set forth within the AOTA Code of Ethics; and responsibilities to employers, patients/clients, our profession, and ourselves (American Occupational Therapy Association, 2000; Bailey & Schwartzberg, 1995; Kyler-Hutchison, 1996; Purtilo, 1999). We may observe an impaired friend and colleague unable to provide competent treatment, resulting in an ethical dilemma and personal conflict between being

faithful (fidelity) and the principle "do no harm" (nonmaleficence). Or, we find ourselves employed in a medical center with budget constraints; increasing demand for services; knowledgeable, inquiring consumers; and a waiting list of patients, from patients with acute head injuries to medically ill developmentally delayed children. The reality of scarce resources poses challenges to health care professionals, often with resulting conflicts between principles of justice and equity for needy patients, principles of fidelity (faithfulness) to colleagues and employers, and the principles of veracity (honesty) and beneficence (bringing about good) in relationships with patients and families.

Case Study

The following case study demonstrates the utility of a structured ethical decision-making approach. Occupational therapist Evelyn McNeil has recently become employed as a school-based practitioner in a suburban primary school in New York State. Ms. McNeil has a reputation as an expert clinician, and has experience in a wide range of pediatric rehabilitation settings, with children with chronic illness. She attends continuing education programs, including local workshops to increase clinical skills utilizing sensory integration evaluation procedures and treatment approaches. However, her knowledge about school-based practice is limited.

The Kennedy Elementary School, where she provides occupational therapy services, is a suburban primary school serving preschool children and students from grades 1 through 3. This neighborhood school is recognized as a model school and encourages interdisciplinary approaches between educators and therapists. Children served have varied diagnoses and problems; many are developmentally delayed. Parents are encouraged to volunteer within the classroom, and there are positive partnerships among the parent–teacher associations, faculty, and school administration.

Ms. McNeil works closely with teachers and parents and believes in the efficacy of sensory integrative treatment to promote educational and therapeutic goals for her young students. She promotes the benefits of occupational therapy, use of standardized sensory integration evaluation, and use of a sensory integration (SI) practice model to enable children with sensory modulation disorders to more appropriately respond to "environmental demands and be more successful learners" (Dunn, 2000, p. 35). Ms. McNeil also conducts in-service programs and writes guidelines for suggested classroom activities for children with a range of disorders and needs. In order to promote her strengths, she distributes business cards and in-service materials. These materials highlight her expertise as an occupational therapy specialist in pediatrics with advanced training and expertise in SI practice. Her success promoting occupational therapy has resulted in strong administrative support, a series of public relations stories on the occupational therapy program, and decisions to apply for grant funding to increase building space and equipment for optimal implementation of SI treatment. This competitive grant application requires Ms. McNeil to provide an updated curriculum vitae, including verification of licensure and her credentials as a pediatrics specialist with expertise in use of SI evaluation and treatment methodologies.

Are there ethical problems and potentially legal issues in this scenario? While occupational therapists can utilize a range of practice models, including the sensory integrative practice model, without advanced certification, occupational therapists can obtain certification by Sensory Integration International to document competence to administer and interpret the Sensory Integration Praxis Test (SIPT) (Sensory Integration International, 2001). Ms. McNeil does not have this certification, nor does she hold board certification in pediatrics from the American Occupational Therapy Association. Clearly, she appears to be indicating a level of expertise that she does not possess.

Misrepresenting credentials to colleagues and her employer is a breach of faith. The AOTA Code of Ethics (Principle 6) commits practitioners to the principle of veracity and states, "Occupational therapy personnel shall accurately represent their credentials, qualifications, education, experience, training, and competence." In addition to violating the spirit of Principle 6, Ms. McNeil disregarded Principle 7, which states, "Occupational therapy personnel shall treat colleagues and other professionals with fairness, discretion, and integrity," and the ethical principle of fidelity. This misrepresentation can potentially cause the Kennedy School administration significant embarrassment and professional harm given their support of her work and efforts to obtain funding for an enlarged treatment area to support her use of a sensory integration practice model. In addition in New York State, unsubstantiated claims of "professional superiority" are also considered unprofessional conduct (New York State Department of Education, 1993, p. 31).

The ethical problems presented in this case study were avoidable. Ms. McNeil worked diligently to promote occupational therapy and her program. However, she neglected ethical implications implicit in the words "specialist" and "expertise," and ramifications of her marketing strategy. Colleagues, employers, and consumers recognize and value practitioners who have achieved advanced clinical competencies (Scott, 1998). Advanced competencies and specialization typically denote additional training, certification through advanced professional examination, or completion of recognized continuing education programs. Thus, misuse of these words is confusing, particularly given recent efforts to enable occupational therapists to develop and receive acknowledgement of advanced competencies through the American Occupational Therapy Association's Board Specialty Certification Program in Pediatrics and the availability of certification from Sensory Integration International to document competence in administering the Sensory Integration and Praxis Text (American Occupational Therapy Association, 2000c; Sensory Integration International, 2002).

Today's demanding outcome-oriented health care programs focus on efficient, effective treatment approaches. Treatment programs are often short; client caseloads high. Evidence of continuing education is increasingly required to maintain licensure, to meet administrative employer requirements, or to demonstrate professional competency. School systems and school-based practitioners face different challenges, but also have limited resources; growing numbers of children with identified needs for occupational therapy services; and administrative, taxpayer, and consumer questions regarding outcomes.

Busy practitioners thus commonly focus their attention on clinical issues, often with less attention to the full meaning and consequences of other professional decisions. Small occupational therapy departments often promote practitioner autonomy and reduced routine on-site collegial communication and interactions. Pragmatic strategies to enable individual practitioners to integrate and apply their personal and professional values, and knowledge of ethical principles, including the AOTA Code of Ethics, for ethical decision-making are increasingly valuable. These strategies provide practical guidelines to analyze ethical problems and dilemmas in our changing world, empower decision-making and action, and encourage reflection on the relationships among practice, our core values and ethics, and professional social responsibilities and legal obligations.

References

Accreditation Council for Occupational Therapy Education. (1998). *Standards for an accredited education program for the occupational therapist.* Bethesda, MD: American Occupational Therapy Association.

American Occupational Therapy Association. (2000a). Occupational therapy code of ethics (2000). *American Journal of Occupational Therapy, 54,* 614–616.

American Occupational Therapy Association. (2000c). *The specialty certification programs in geriatrics, pediatrics, or neurorehabilitation.* Bethesda, MD: Author.

American Occupational Therapy Association. (2000b). *Standards of practice for occupational therapy.* Retrieved September 5, 2000, from www.aota.org/otsp.asp

American Occupational Therapy Association, Commission on Standards and Ethics. (1996). *1966 occupational therapy code of ethics reference guide.* Bethesda, MD: Author.

American Speech–Language Hearing Association. (2000a). *Code of Ethics.* Retrieved September 3, 2001, from www.professional.asha.org/library/code_of_ethics.htm

American Speech–Language Hearing Association. (2000b). *Standards and implementation for professional service programs in audiology and speech–language pathology* (Effective Jan. 1. 2002). Retrieved September 8, 2001, from www.professional.asha.org/contents.htm.#professionals

Bailey, D., & Schwartzberg, S. (Eds.). (1995). *Ethical and legal dilemmas in occupational therapy.* Philadelphia: FA Davis.

Crabtree, J. (1991). The effect of referral for profit on therapists and client's autonomy and fair competition. *American Journal of Occupational Therapy, 45,* 464–466.

Darr, K. (1997). *Ethics in health services management* (3rd ed.). Baltimore: Health Professions Press.

Diller, J. (1999). *Cultural diversity: A primer for the human services.* Albany: Wadsworth Publishing.

Dunn, W. (2000). *Best practice occupational therapy in community service with children and families.* Thorofare NJ: Slack.

Hansen, R. (2001). *Guidelines to the occupational therapy code of ethics.* Retrieved 2001 from www.aota.org/memhers/area2/links/lasp?

Haas, J. (1995, January/February). Ethical considerations of goal setting for patient care in rehabilitation medicine. *American Journal of Physical Medicine and Rehabilitation,* S16–S20.

Hofland, B. (1994). When capacity fades and autonomy is constricted: A client-centered approach to residential care. *Generations, 18,* 31–37.

Horowitz, B. (2001a, April). *Strategies for ethical decision-making.* Paper presented at the annual American Occupational Therapy Association Conference, Philadelphia, PA.

Horowitz, B. (2001b, October). *Professional ethics: It's academic.* Paper presented at the annual conference of the National Council of State Boards of Examiners for Speech–Language Pathology and Audiology, Pittsburgh, PA.

Horowitz, B. (1996). Ethical issues and gerontic occupational therapy practice. In O. Larson, R. Stevens-Ratchford, L. Pedretti, & J. Crabtree (Eds.), *ROTE: The role of occupational therapy with the elderly* (pp. 144–165). Rockville, MD: AOTA.

Kornblau, B. (1992). Legal issues in occupational therapy consultation. In E. Jaffe & C. Epstein (Eds.), *Occupational therapy consultation* (pp. 594–621). St. Louis: Mosby Yearbook.

Kutchins, H. (1991). The fiduciary relationship: The legal basis for social workers' responsibilities to clients. *Social Work, 36,* 106–113.

Kyler-Hutchison. P. (1996). Issues in ethics. In AOTA Commission on Standards and Ethics, *1996 occupational therapy code of ethics reference guide* (pp. 43–44). Bethesda: AOTA.

Levy, C. (1976). *Social work ethics.* New York: Human Sciences Press.

Liang, B. (2000). *Health law and policy.* Boston: Butterworth Heinemann.

Lo, B. (1995) *Resolving ethical dilemmas: A guide for clinicians.* Baltimore: Williams & Wilkins.

New York State Education Department, Office of Professional Credentialing. (1993). *Occupational therapy and occupational therapy assistant handbook.* Albany: Author.

Purtilo, R. (1999). *Ethical dimensions in the health professions* (3rd ed.). Philadelphia: Saunders.

Rhodes, M. (1989). *Ethical dilemmas in social work practice.* Milwaukee, Wisconsin: Family Service America.

Sensory Integration International. (2002). *Certification programs.* Retrieved January 9, 2002 from (www.sensory-int.com/certification.html).

Scott. R. (1997). *Promoting legal awareness in physical occupational therapy.* St. Louis: Mosby.

Scott, R. (1998). *Professional ethics: A guide for rehabilitation professionals.* St. Louis: Mosby.

Wells, S., & Black, R. (2000). *Cultural competency for health professionals.* Bethesda, MD: AOTA.

Wenston, S. (1987). Applying philosophy to ethical dilemmas. In G. Anderson & V. Glesnes-Anderson (Eds.), *Health care ethics* (pp. 22–33). Rockville, MD: Aspen Publishers.

Physical Agent Modalities

The American Occupational Therapy Association (AOTA) asserts that physical agent modalities (PAMs) may be used by occupational therapists and occupational therapy assistants in preparation for or concurrently with purposeful and occupation-based activities or interventions that ultimately enhance engagement in occupation (AOTA, 2008a, 2008b). AOTA further stipulates that PAMs may be applied only by occupational therapists and occupational therapy assistants who have documented evidence of possessing the theoretical background and technical skills for safe and competent integration of the modality into an occupational therapy intervention plan (AOTA, 2008b). The purpose of this paper is to clarify the appropriate context for use of PAMs in occupational therapy. It is the professional and ethical responsibility of occupational therapy practitioners to be knowledgeable of and adhere to applicable state laws.

Physical agent modalities are those procedures and interventions that are systematically applied to modify specific client factors when neurological, musculoskeletal, or skin conditions are present that may be limiting occupational performance. PAMs use various forms of energy to modulate pain, modify tissue healing, increase tissue extensibility, modify skin and scar tissue, and decrease edema or inflammation. PAMs are used in preparation for or concurrently with purposeful and occupation-based activities (Bracciano, 2008).

Categories of physical agents include superficial thermal agents, deep thermal agents, and electrotherapeutic agents and mechanical devices.

- *Superficial thermal agents* include but are not limited to hydrotherapy/whirlpool, cryotherapy (cold packs, ice), Fluidotherapy™, hot packs, paraffin, water, infrared, and other commercially available superficial heating and cooling technologies.

- *Deep thermal agents* include but are not limited to therapeutic ultrasound, phonophoresis, short-wave diathermy, and other commercially available technologies.

- *Electrotherapeutic agents* use electricity and the electromagnetic spectrum to facilitate tissue healing, improve muscle strength and endurance, decrease edema, modulate pain, decrease the inflammatory process, and modify the healing process. Electrotherapeutic agents include but are not limited to neuro-muscular electrical stimulation (NMES), functional electrical stimulation (FES), transcutaneous electrical nerve stimulation (TENS), high-voltage galvanic stimulation for tissue and wound repair (ESTR), high-voltage pulsed current (HVPC), direct current (DC), iontophoresis, and other commercially available technologies (Bracciano, 2008).

- *Mechanical devices* include but are not limited to vasopneumatic devices and continuous passive motion (CPM).

PAMs are categorized as preparatory methods (AOTA, 2008a) that also can be used concurrently with purposeful activity or during occupational engagement. Preparatory methods support and promote the acquisition of the performance skills necessary to enable an individual to resume or assume habits, routines, and roles for engagement in occupation.

The exclusive use of PAMs as a therapeutic intervention without direct application to occupational performance is not considered occupational therapy. When used, *PAMs are always integrated into a broader occupational therapy program* as a preparatory method for the therapeutic use of occupations or purposeful activities (AOTA, 2008a).

Occupational therapists and occupational therapy assistants must have demonstrated and verifiable competence in order to use PAMs in occupational therapy practice. The foundational knowledge necessary for proper use of these modalities requires appropriate, documented professional education, which includes continuing education courses, institutes at conferences, and accredited higher education courses or programs. Integration of PAMs in occupational therapy practice must include foundational education and training in biological and physical sciences. Modality-specific education consists of biophysiological, neurophysiological, and electrophysiological changes that occur as a result of the application of the selected modality. Education in the application of PAMs also must include indications, contraindications, and precautions; safe and efficacious administration of the modalities; and patient preparation, including the process and outcomes of treatment (i.e., risks and benefits). Education should include essential elements related to documentation, including parameters of intervention, subjective and objective criteria, efficacy, and the relationship between the physical agent and occupational performance.

Supervised use of the PAM should continue until service competency and professional judgment in selection, modification, and integration into an occupational therapy intervention plan is demonstrated and documented (AOTA, 2009).

The occupational therapist makes decisions and assumes responsibility for use of PAMs as part of the intervention plan. The occupational therapy assistant delivers occupational therapy services under the supervision of the occupational therapist. Services delivered by the occupational therapy assistant are selected and delegated by the occupational therapist (AOTA, 2009). When an occupational therapist delegates the use of a PAM to an occupational therapy assistant, both must comply with appropriate supervision and state regulatory requirements and ensure that preparation, application, and documentation are based on service competency and institutional rules. Only occupational therapists with service competency in this area may supervise the use of PAMs by occupational therapy assistants. Occupational therapy assistants may gain competency only in those modalities allowed by state and laws and regulations.

The *Occupational Therapy Code of Ethics and Ethics Standards (2010)* (AOTA, 2010) provides principles that guide safe and competent professional practice and that must be applied to the use of PAMs. The following principles from the *Code and Ethics Standards* are relevant to the use of PAMs:

Occupational therapy personnel shall:

- *Principle 1E:* provide occupational therapy services that are within each practitioner's level of competence and scope of practice (e.g., qualifications, experience, and the law).

- *Principle 1F:* use, to the extent possible, evaluation, planning, intervention techniques, and therapeutic equipment that are evidence-based and within the recognized scope of occupational therapy practice.

- *Principle 1G:* take responsible steps (e.g., continuing education, research, supervision, and training) and use careful judgment to ensure their own competence and weigh potential for client harm when generally recognized standards do not exist in emerging technology or areas of practice.

- *Principle 5F:* take responsibility for maintaining high standards and continuing competence in practice, education, and research by participating in professional development and educational activities to improve and update knowledge and skills.

- *Principle 5G:* ensure that all duties assumed by or assigned to other occupational therapy personnel match credentials, qualifications, experience, and scope of practice.

- *Principle 5H:* provide appropriate supervision to individuals for whom they have supervisory responsibility in accordance with AOTA official documents and local, state, and federal or national laws, rules, regulations, policies, procedures, standards, and guidelines. (AOTA, 2010)

References

American Occupational Therapy Association. (2008a). Occupational therapy practice framework: Domain and process (2nd ed.). *American Journal of Occupational Therapy, 62*, 625–683. http://dx.doi.org/10.5014/ajot.62.6.625

American Occupational Therapy Association. (2008b). Physical agent modalities: A position paper. *American Journal of Occupational Therapy, 62*, 691–693. http://dx.doi.org/10.5014/ajot.62.6.691

American Occupational Therapy Association. (2009). Guidelines for supervision, roles, and responsibilities during the delivery of occupational therapy services. *American Journal of Occupational Therapy, 63*, 797–803. http://dx.doi.org/10.5014/ajot.63.6.797

American Occupational Therapy Association. (2010). Occupational therapy code of ethics and ethics standards (2010). *American Journal of Occupational Therapy, 64*, S17–S26. http://dx.doi.org/10.5014/ajot.2010.64S17

Bracciano, A. G. (2008). *Physical agent modalities: Theory and application for the occupational therapist* (2nd ed.). Thorofare, NJ: Slack.

Authors

Alfred G. Bracciano, EdD, OTR, FAOTA
Scott D. McPhee, DrPH, OT, FAOTA
Barbara Winthrop Rose, MA, OTR, CVE, CHT, FAOTA

for

The Commission on Practice
Sara Jane Brayman, PhD, OTR/L, FAOTA, *Chairperson*
Adopted by the Representative Assembly 2003M37.
Edited by the Commission on Practice, 2007.

Revised by the Commission on Practice, 2012.
Debbie Amini, EdD, OTR/L, CHT, C/NDT, *Chairperson*
Adopted by the Representative Assembly Coordinating Council (RACC) for the Representative Assembly, 2012.

This revision replaces the 2008 document Physical Agent Modalities. Previously published and copyrighted 2008, by the American Occupational Therapy Association in the *American Journal of Occupational Therapy, 62*, 691–693.

Complementary and Alternative Medicine

The American Occupational Therapy Association (AOTA) asserts that complementary and alternative medicine (CAM) may be used responsibly by occupational therapists and occupational therapy assistants as part of a comprehensive approach to enhance engagement in occupation by people, organizations, and populations to promote their health and participation in life (AOTA, 2005; Giese, Parker, Lech-Boura, Burkhardt, & Cook, 2003). Occupational therapy is a holistic, client-centered practice that acknowledges the importance of context and environment in framing a client's occupational needs, desires, and priorities (AOTA, 2008). Because CAM is a culturally sensitive system used by nearly 40% of adults and 12% of children in the United States (Barnes, Bloom, & Nahin, 2008), it is important to acknowledge the ethical and pragmatic issues surrounding the use of CAM in occupational therapy practice. This position paper defines the appropriate use of CAM by occupational therapy practitioners[1] within the scope of occupational therapy practice.

Use

The U.S. Department of Health and Human Services reports that CAM is used in the United States by persons who are "seeking ways to improve their health and well-being or to relieve symptoms associated with chronic, even terminal, illnesses or the side effects of conventional treatments for them" (Barnes et al., 2008). CAM interventions most often are used for treatment of pain conditions by non-poor women ages 30–69 with significant levels of education beyond high school (Barnes et al., 2008). Similar to the holistic nature of occupational therapy practice, practitioners who use CAM also address the influence of the contexts on health status and collaborate with clients who demonstrate a desire for personal control over health outcomes (Cheung, Wyman, & Halcon, 2007). Clients who are living with and adjusting to life with chronic conditions such as back pain or a traumatic event such as domestic abuse may combine the holistic nature of CAM approaches with other intervention approaches to improve their ability to participate in occupations they need and want to perform.

Definition

The National Center for Complementary and Alternative Medicine (NCCAM) of the National Institutes of Health has identified five domains of CAM practice and defines *complementary and alternative medicine* as "a group of diverse medical and health care systems, practices, and products that are not presently considered to be part of conventional medicine" (NCCAM, 2010). The five domains of CAM practice are (1) alternative medical systems, (2) mind–body interventions, (3) biologically based treatments, (4) manipulative and body-based methods, and (5) energy therapies. By definition, *alternative medicine* is practiced *in place of* conventional medicine, while *complementary interventions* are accessed *in conjunction with* allopathic medical practices.

---

[1]When the term *occupational therapy practitioner* is used in this document, it refers to both occupational therapists and occupational therapy assistants (AOTA, 2006). *Occupational therapists* are responsible for all aspects of occupational therapy service delivery and are accountable for the safety and effectiveness of the occupational therapy service delivery process. *Occupational therapy assistants* deliver occupational therapy services under the supervision of and in partnership with an occupational therapist (AOTA, 2009).

The definition of CAM is dynamic. Practices contained within the definition of CAM change as clinical evidence supports their inclusion with conventional health practices, and novel approaches emerge (AOTA, 2005; Giese et al., 2003). The term *integrative medicine* is used for combined treatments from conventional medicine and CAM for which there is high-quality scientific evidence of safety and effectiveness (NCCAM, 2008).

Research

The NCCAM was established by Congress in 1998 through Title VI, Section 601, of the Omnibus Consolidated and Emergency Appropriations Act of 1999 (P.L. 105-277) as the federal government's lead agency for scientific research on CAM. The NCCAM mission is to investigate promising CAM products and practices with neutrality and scientific rigor to determine their safety and effectiveness, to train CAM researchers, and to provide information about CAM to professionals and the general public (NCCAM, 2008). Since its inception, the NCCAM has funded more than 1,200 research projects at scientific institutions across the United States and internationally.

The NCCAM has proposed a framework for setting research priorities that consists of four pillars: (1) scientific promise, (2) extent and nature of practice and use, (3) amenability to rigorous scientific inquiry, and (4) potential to change health practices (NCCAM, 2009). Key priority areas are currently non-mineral, non-vitamin, natural products and mind–body interventions such as yoga, tai chi, qi gong, guided imagery, meditation, deep-breathing exercises, and progressive relaxation (NCCAM, 2009). Studies to support the integration of CAM and conventional medicine, to encourage insurance coverage for CAM therapies, and to develop practice and referral guidelines are needed in addition to research about the safety and efficacy of CAM practices (Coulter & Khorsan, 2008; Herman, D'Huyvetter, & Mohler, 2006).

Access to information about CAM practices has been enhanced by a collaborative project between the National Library of Medicine and the NCCAM. These two government agencies have created *CAM on PubMed* (see http://nccam.nih.gov/research/camonpubmed/), a search option that automatically limits research citations to a CAM subset from the MEDLINE database and additional life science journals.

Use Within the Scope of Occupational Therapy Practice

Occupational therapy values engagement in occupations and promotes the health and participation of people, organizations, and populations through engagement in occupation (AOTA, 2008). *Occupations* are "activities . . . of everyday life, named, organized, and given value and meaning by individuals and a culture" (Law, Polatajko, Baptiste, & Townsend, 1997, p. 29). Occupations encompass activities of daily living (ADLs), instrumental activities of daily living, rest and sleep, education, work, play, leisure, and social participation (AOTA, 2008).

Occupational therapy practitioners may utilize CAM in the delivery of occupational therapy services when they are used as preparatory methods or purposeful activities to facilitate the ability of clients to engage in their daily life occupations. CAM approaches have been utilized in occupational therapy for several years and include but are not limited to guided imagery, massage, myofascial release, meditation, and behavioral relaxation training (AOTA, 1998; Brachtesende, 2005; Lindsay, Fee, Michie, & Heap, 1994; Scott, 1999). Yoga postures also have been used prior to engagement in ADLs to reduce reliance on pain medication and to promote relaxation for restorative sleep (Brachtesende, 2005).

Occupational therapy practitioners need to respect the use of CAM as part of the client's occupational performance habits, routines, or rituals and to understand that CAM practices may be embedded within particular cultures (Cassidy, 1998a, 1998b). In a study of patients with cardiac conditions in Hong Kong, the use of qi gong as a method for reducing stress added psychological benefit to the reduction of blood pressure when compared to progressive relaxation training alone (Hui, Wan, Chan,

& Yung, 2006). By collaborating with the client in the selection and application of specific CAM interventions, the occupational therapy practitioner supports and respects the client's autonomy and reasoned participation in decision-making. Outcome studies about engagement in occupation continue to be a priority for determining the efficacy and effectiveness of using CAM techniques during occupational therapy intervention.

To determine whether to use CAM in the delivery of occupational therapy services, occupational therapists must evaluate the client, develop an intervention based on the client's needs and priorities, and conduct outcomes measurement. The evaluation contributes to the understanding of the client's strengths, priorities, and current limitations in carrying out daily occupations. Evaluation and intervention address factors that influence the client's occupational performance, including how the client performs the daily life occupations, the demands of those occupations, and the contexts and environments within which those occupations are performed. As part of the evaluation and the intervention, the occupational therapy practitioner must determine whether the use of CAM is consistent with the client's cultural practices, priorities, and needs; is safe to use; and is an appropriate approach to facilitate the ability of the client to participate in daily life occupations and to promote health and participation. Selected assessments are used to measure the effectiveness of the outcomes of occupational therapy services and guide future therapeutic interventions with the client. The occupational therapy practitioner must measure whether the use of CAM results in positive outcomes for improving occupational performance.

Ethical Considerations, Continuing Competency, and Standards of Practice

The *Occupational Therapy Code of Ethics and Ethics Standards (2010)* (AOTA, 2010a) mandates safe and competent practice, holding occupational therapy practitioners responsible for maintenance of high standards of competence. Occupational therapy practitioners need to maintain continuing competency in CAM approaches just as they do with other areas of practice. Using CAM approaches may require additional training, competency examinations, certification, and regulatory knowledge (AOTA, 2010b). The use of specific CAM approaches may be subject to federal, state, and often local municipal regulations that govern practice, advertising, ethics, professional terminology, and training (AOTA, 2010c). It is the responsibility of occupational therapy practitioners to know and comply with applicable laws and regulations associated with the use of CAM approaches during occupational therapy intervention. Occupational therapy practitioners must abide by state regulations when billing for occupational therapy services that incorporate the use of CAM. Practitioners must distinguish between the incorporation of CAM techniques into occupational therapy practice and the use of CAM as a salutatory method that is separate from occupational therapy practice (AOTA, 2007, 2008).

Issues of client safety and health care worker safety are salient to all areas of occupational therapy practice. The use of CAM requires attention to client safety in consumer decision-making, client interventions, and professional education and training. The risks and benefits of CAM used in occupational therapy should be communicated to clients as standard practice in a client-centered, evidence-based approach to service provision.

Payment for Services

The NCCAM (2008) reports that U.S. adults annually spend $34 billion out-of-pocket on CAM products and services. CAM services, although often paid for privately, increasingly are covered by insurance companies and health maintenance organizations (Astin, Pelletier, Marie, & Haskell, 2000; Cleary-Guida, Okvat, Oz, & Ting, 2001; Wolsko, Eisenberg, Davis, Ettner, & Phillips, 2002). Factors that influence third-party payers to include selected CAM in health care policies include cost-effectiveness, consumer demand, demonstrated clinical efficacy, and state mandate (Pelletier & Astin, 2002; Pelletier, Astin, & Haskell, 1999).

Summary

Occupational therapy practitioners facilitate proficient and meaningful engagement in the significant occupations of life. CAM practices, systems, and products may be appropriately incorporated into occupational therapy practice to encourage a client's engagement in meaningful occupations. Scientific studies are needed to validate the safety and efficacy of CAM methods within occupational therapy practice. Advanced-level training and continuing education are important to acquire the knowledge and skill to utilize CAM methods, to address the concerns for patient safety and informed consent, and to meet the rigors of regulatory requirements.

References

American Occupational Therapy Association. (1998). OT perspective: Complementary care survey results. *OT Week, 12*(48), 4.

American Occupational Therapy Association. (2005). Complementary and alternative medicine (CAM). *American Journal of Occupational Therapy, 59,* 653–655.

American Occupational Therapy Association. (2006). Policy 1.41. Categories of occupational therapy personnel. In *Policy manual* (2009 ed.). Bethesda, MD: Author.

American Occupational Therapy Association. (2007). *Definition of occupational therapy practice for the AOTA Model Practice Act.* (Available from the State Affairs Group, American Occupational Therapy Association, 4720 Montgomery Lane, Bethesda, MD 20814)

American Occupational Therapy Association. (2008). Occupational therapy practice framework: Domain and process (2nd ed.). *American Journal of Occupational Therapy, 62,* 625–683.

American Occupational Therapy Association. (2009). Guidelines for supervision, roles, and responsibilities during the delivery of occupational therapy services. *American Journal of Occupational Therapy, 63,* 173–179.

American Occupational Therapy Association. (2010a). Occupational therapy code of ethics and ethics standards (2010). *American Journal of Occupational Therapy, 64*(Suppl.), S17–S26.

American Occupational Therapy Association. (2010b). Standards for continuing competence. *American Journal of Occupational Therapy, 64*(Suppl.), S103–S105.

American Occupational Therapy Association. (2010c). Standards of practice for occupational therapy. *American Journal of Occupational Therapy, 64*(Suppl.), S106–S111.

Astin, J. A., Pelletier, K. R., Marie, A., & Haskell, W. L. (2000). Complementary and alternative medicine use among elderly persons: One-year analysis of a Blue Shield Medicare supplement. *Journals of Gerontology Series A: Biological Sciences and Medical Sciences, 55*(1), M4–M9.

Barnes, P. M., Bloom, B., & Nahin, R. (2008, December 10). Complementary and alternative medicine use among adults and children: United States, 2007. *CDC National Health Statistics Report.* Retrieved January 6, 2010, from, http://nccam.nih.gov/news/camstats/2007/

Brachtesende, A. (2005). Using complementary and alternative medicine in occupational therapy. *OT Practice, 10*(11), 9–13.

Cassidy, C. M. (1998a). Chinese medicine users in the United States. Part I: Utilization, satisfaction, medical plurality. *Journal of Alternative and Complementary Medicine, 4*(1), 17–27.

Cassidy, C. M. (1998b). Chinese medicine users in the United States. Part II: Preferred aspects of care. *Journal of Alternative and Complementary Medicine, 4*(2), 189–202.

Cheung, C. K., Wyman, J. F., & Halcon, L. L. (2007). Use of complementary and alternative therapies in community-dwelling older adults. *Journal of Alternative and Complementary Medicine, 13*(9), 997–1006.

Cleary-Guida, M. B., Okvat, H. A., Oz, M. C., & Ting, W. (2001). A regional survey of health insurance coverage for complementary and alternative medicine: Current status and future ramifications. *Journal of Alternative and Complementary Medicine, 7*, 269–273.

Coulter, I. D., & Khorsan, R. (2008). Is health services research the Holy Grail of complementary and alternative medicine research? *Alternative Therapies in Health and Medicine, 14*(4), 40–45.

Giese, T., Parker, J. A., Lech-Boura, J., Burkhardt, A., & Cook, A. (2003). *The role of occupational therapy in complementary and alternative medicine* [White Paper, adopted by the AOTA Board of Directors June 22, 2003]. (Available from American Occupational Therapy Association, 4720 Montgomery Lane, Bethesda, MD 20814)

Herman, P. M., D'Huyvetter, K., & Mohler, M. J. (2006). Are health services research methods a match for CAM? *Alternative Therapies in Health and Medicine, 12*(3), 78–83.

Hui, P. M., Wan, M., Chan, W. K., & Yung, P. M. (2006). An evaluation of two behavioral rehabilitation programs, qigong versus progressive relaxation, in improving the quality of life in cardiac patients. *Journal of Alternative and Complementary Medicine, 12*(4), 373–378.

Law, M., Polatajko, H., Baptiste, W., & Townsend, E. (1997). Core concepts of occupational therapy. In E. Townsend (Ed.), *Enabling occupation: An occupational therapy perspective* (pp. 29–56). Ottawa, ON: Canadian Association of Occupational Therapists.

Lindsay, W. R., Fee, M., Michie, A., & Heap, I. (1994). The effects of cue control relaxation on adults with severe mental retardation. *Research in Developmental Disabilities, 15*, 425–437.

National Center for Complementary and Alternative Medicine. (2008). *Overview of NCCAM.* Retrieved January 6, 2010, from http://nccam.nih.gov/news/events/grants08/slides2.htm

National Center for Complementary and Alternative Medicine. (2009). *NCCAM priority setting—Framework and other considerations.* Retrieved January 6, 2010, from http://plan.nccam.nih.gov/ index.cfm?-module=paper2

National Center for Complementary and Alternative Medicine. (2010). *What is complementary and alternative medicine?* Retrieved January 6, 2010, from http://www.nccam.nih.gov/health/whatiscam/

Omnibus Consolidated and Emergency Appropriations Act of 1999, P.L. 105-277, Title VI, Section 601.

Pelletier, K. R., & Astin, J. A. (2002). Integration and reimbursement of complementary and alternative medicine by managed care and insurance providers: 2000 update and cohort analysis. *Alternative Therapies in Health and Medicine, 8*(1), 38–39, 42, 44.

Pelletier, K. R., Astin, J. A., & Haskell, W. L. (1999). Current trends in the integration and reimbursement of complementary and alternative medicine by managed care organizations (MCOs) and insurance providers: 1998 update and cohort analysis. *American Journal of Health Promotion, 4*, 125–133.

Scott, A. H. (1999). Wellness works: Community service health promotion groups led by occupational therapy students. *American Journal of Occupational Therapy, 53*, 566–574.

Wolsko, P. M., Eisenberg, D. M., Davis, R. B., Ettner, S. L., & Phillips, R. S. (2002). Insurance coverage, medical conditions, and visits to alternative medicine providers: Results of a national survey. *Archives of Internal Medicine, 162*, 281–287.

Additional Reading

Bausell, R. B., Lee, W. L., & Berman, B. M. (2001). Demographic and health-related correlates to visits to complementary and alternative medical providers. *Medical Care, 9*, 190–196.

Burkhardt, A., & Parker, J. (1998, November 26). OT perspective: Complementary care survey results. *OT Week, 12*(48), 4.

Carlson, J. (2003). *Complementary therapies and wellness: Practice essentials for holistic healthcare.* Upper Saddle River, NJ: Prentice Hall.

Eisenberg, D. M., Davis, R. B., Ettner, S. L., Appel, S., Wilkey, S., Van Rompay, M., et al. (1998). Trends in alternative medicine use in the United States, 1990–1997: Results of a follow-up national survey. *JAMA, 280*, 1569–1575.

Eisenberg, D. M., Kessler, R. C., Van Rompay, M. I., Kaptchuk, T. J., Wilkey, S. A., Appel, S., et al. (2001). Perceptions about complementary therapies relative to conventional therapies among adults who use both: Results from a national survey. *Annals of Internal Medicine, 13*, 344–351.

Kaboli, P. J., Doebbeling, B. N., Saag, K. G., & Rosenthal, G. E. (2001). Use of complementary and alternative medicine by older patients with arthritis: A population-based study. *Arthritis and Rheumatology, 45*, 398–403.

Ni, H., Simile, C., & Hardy, A. M. (2002). Utilization of complementary and alternative medicine by United States adults: Results from the 1999 National Health Interview Survey. *Medical Care, 40*, 353–358.

Rakel, D. P., Guerrera, M. P., Bayles, B. P., Desai, F. J., & Ferrara, E. (2008). CAM education: Promoting a salutogenic focus in health care. *Journal of Alternative and Complementary Medicine, 14*(1), 87–93.

Author

Terry Giese, MBA, OT/L, FAOTA

for

The Commission on Practice
Janet V. DeLany, DEd, MSA, OTR/L, FAOTA, *Chairperson*

Adopted by the Representative Assembly Coordinating Council (RACC) for the Representative Assembly. Revised by the Commission on Practice 2011.

Note. This revision replaces the 2005 document *Complementary and Alternative Medicine,* previously published and copyrighted in 2005 by the American Occupational Therapy Association in the *American Journal of Occupational Therapy, 59,* 653–655.

Telehealth

The purpose of this paper is to provide the current position of the American Occupational Therapy Association (AOTA) regarding the use of telehealth by occupational therapists and occupational therapy assistants[1] to provide occupational therapy services. This document describes the use of telehealth within occupational therapy practice areas, as described in the existing research. Additionally, occupational therapy practitioner[2] qualifications, ethics, and regulatory issues related to the use of telehealth as a service delivery model within occupational therapy are outlined. Occupational therapy practitioners are the intended audience for this document, although others involved in supervising, planning, delivering, regulating, and paying for occupational therapy services also may find it helpful.

Telecommunication and information technologies have prompted the development of an emerging model of health care delivery called *telehealth,* which involves health care services, health information, and health education. AOTA defines *telehealth* as the application of evaluative, consultative, preventative, and therapeutic services delivered through telecommunication and information technologies. Occupational therapy services provided by means of a telehealth service delivery model can be *synchronous,* that is, delivered through interactive technologies in real time, or *asynchronous,* using store-and-forward technologies. Occupational therapy practitioners can use telehealth as a mechanism to provide services at a location that is physically distant from the client, thereby allowing for services to occur where the client lives, works, and plays, if that is needed or desired (AOTA, 2010d). An overview of telehealth technologies is included in Appendix A. *Telerehabilitation* within the larger realm of telehealth is the application of telecommunication and information technologies for the delivery of rehabilitation services. Key terms related to telehealth and telehealth technologies are defined in Appendix B.

Use of Telehealth Within Occupational Therapy

Occupational therapy practitioners use telehealth as a service delivery model to help clients develop skills; incorporate assistive technology and adaptive techniques; modify work, home, or school environments; and create health-promoting habits and routines. Benefits of a telehealth service delivery model include increased accessibility of services to clients who live in remote or underserved areas, improved access to providers and specialists otherwise unavailable to clients, prevention of unnecessary delays in receiving care, and workforce enhancement through consultation and research among others (Cason, 2012a, 2012b). By removing barriers to accessing care, including social stigma, travel, and socioeconomic and cultural barriers, the use of telehealth as a service delivery model within occupational therapy leads to improved access to care and ameliorates the impact of personnel shortages in underserved areas. Occupational therapy outcomes aligned with telehealth include the facilitation of occupational performance, adaptation, health and wellness, prevention, and quality of life.

---

[1]The *occupational therapist* is responsible for all aspects of occupational therapy service delivery and is accountable for the safety and effectiveness of the occupational therapy service delivery process. The *occupational therapy assistant* delivers occupational therapy services under the supervision of and in partnership with the occupational therapist (AOTA, 2009).

[2]When the term *occupational therapy practitioner* is used in this document, it refers to both occupational therapists and occupational therapy assistants (AOTA, 2006).

Telehealth has potential as a service delivery model in each major practice area within occupational therapy. Note that given the variability of client factors, activity demands, performance skills, performance patterns, and contexts and environments, the candidacy and appropriateness of a telehealth service delivery model "should be determined on a case-by-case basis with selections firmly based on clinical judgment, client's informed choice, and professional standards of care" (Brennan et al., 2010, p. 33). See Appendix C for applications and evidence supporting the use of telehealth within occupational therapy practice areas.

Evaluation Using Telehealth Technologies: Tele-Evaluation

The traditional telephone system continues to be a low-cost alternative for effectively conducting interview assessments by various health care professionals (Cooper et al., 2002; Dreyer, Dreyer, Shaw, & Wittman, 2001; Winters, 2002), and advanced communication technologies have broadened the possibilities for conducting evaluations. Studies have described the use of telehealth in areas that are of concern to occupational therapy, such as evaluation and consultative services for wheelchair prescription (Barlow, Liu, & Sekulic, 2009; Schein, Schmeler, Brienza, Saptono, & Parmanto, 2008; Schein, Schmeler, Holm, Saptono, & Brienza, 2010; Schein et al., 2011), neurological assessment (Savard, Borstad, Tkachuck, Lauderdale, & Conroy, 2003), adaptive equipment prescription and home modification (Sanford et al., 2007), and ergonomic assessment (Baker & Jacobs, 2013).

Clinical reasoning guides the selection and application of appropriate telehealth technologies necessary to evaluate client needs and environmental factors. Therapists should consider the reliability and validity of specific assessment tools when administered remotely. Researchers have investigated the reliability of assessments such as the Functional Reach Test and European Stroke Scale (Palsbo, Dawson, Savard, Goldstein, & Heuser, 2007); the Kohlman Evaluation of Living Skills and the Canadian Occupational Performance Measure (Dreyer et al., 2001); and the FIM™, the Jamar Dynamometer, the Preston Pinch Gauge, the Nine-Hole Peg Test, and the Unified Parkinson's Disease Rating Scale (Hoffman, Russell, Thompson, Vincent, & Nelson, 2008) and found these tools to be reliable when administered remotely through telehealth technologies. In some cases, an in-person assistant, such as a paraprofessional or other support person, may be used to relay assessment tool measurements or other measures (e.g., environmental, wheelchair and seating) to the remote therapist during the evaluation process.

When choosing a telehealth model for conducting an evaluation, occupational therapists need to consider the client's diagnosis, client's preference, access to technology, and ability to measure outcomes when using that model. The occupational therapist may determine that an in-person evaluation is required for some clients. Because of the evolving knowledge and technology related to telehealth, occupational therapists should review the latest research to remain current about the appropriate use of telehealth technologies for conducting evaluations.

Intervention Using Telehealth Technologies: Teleintervention and Telerehabilitation

A telehealth model of service delivery may be used for providing interventions that are preventative, habilitative, or rehabilitative in nature. When planning and providing interventions delivered with telehealth technologies, Scheideman-Miller et al. (2003) reported that the appropriateness and maintenance of the technology and the sustainability of participation by the client are important factors to consider. As related to occupational therapy interventions, some factors to consider include technology availability and options for the occupational therapy practitioner and the client; the safety, effectiveness, sustainability, and quality of interventions provided exclusively through telehealth or in combination with in-person interventions; the client's choice about receiving interventions by means of telehealth technologies; the client's outcomes, including the client's perception of services provided; reimbursement; and compliance with federal and state laws, regulation, and policy, including licensure requirements (Cason & Brannon, 2011).

Consultation Using Telehealth Technologies: Teleconsultation

Teleconsultation is a virtual consultation that includes the

- Expert provider and client,

- Expert provider and local provider with the client present, or

- Expert provider and local provider without the client present.

Teleconsultation uses telecommunication and information technologies for the purpose of obtaining health and medical information or advice.

Teleconsultation has been used to overcome the shortage of various rehabilitation professionals across the United States. For example, an occupational therapist or prosthetist can remotely evaluate and adjust a client's prosthetic device using computer software with videoconferencing capability and remote access to a local clinician's computer screen despite the physical distance between the expert and client (Whelan & Wagner, 2011). Similarly, Schein et al. (2008) demonstrated positive outcomes associated with teleconsultation between a remote seating specialist and a local therapist for evaluating wheelchair prescriptions. The Veterans Health Administration is using teleconsultation for veterans with traumatic brain injuries in a process that involves interactive videoconferencing technology and Web-based management systems (Girard, 2007). In the practice area of pediatrics, Wakeford (2002) used videoconferencing technologies to consult on play performance in children with special needs.

Practitioners should contact state professional licensure boards in their state as well as in the state where the client is located for further clarification on policies related to teleconsultation before rendering services. Some states do have consultation and licensure exemption provisions, although application of the consultation and licensure exemption provisions to facilitate temporary (i.e., consultative) interstate occupational therapy practice using telehealth technologies has not been established (Cason & Brannon, 2011).

Monitoring Using Telehealth Technologies: Telemonitoring

Occupational therapy practitioners can use telehealth technologies to monitor a client's adherence to an intervention program, assist a client in progressing toward achieving desired outcomes, and track and respond to follow-up issues and concerns within a client's natural environments. For example, the Gator Tech Smart House (Mann & Milton, 2005) developed at the University of Florida provides an array of self-*monitoring* analysis and *reporting* technology (SMART) technologies that monitor and cue clients remotely. Examples include the SmartShoe (Naditz, 2009), which determines fall risk by analyzing walking behavior patterns in a client's own environment and sends the information to a remote site. Similarly, home exercise programs can be monitored remotely using a *haptic* (touch-sensitive) control interface to track a client's hand position while providing resistive forces remotely (Popescu, Burdea, Bouzit, & Hentz, 2000).

Tang and Venables (2000) used smartphones to deliver rehabilitation interventions remotely by using wireless Internet or Intranet access and by providing frequent prompts and cues regarding when and how to complete daily living occupations. Wireless technologies such as these are expanding opportunities for occupational therapy practitioners to implement interventions using telehealth technologies where clients live, work, and play and to provide services throughout the day rather than only within the occupational therapy clinic.

Appendix D provides case examples of how occupational therapy practitioners use telehealth technologies to support health and participation in occupations.

Practitioner Qualifications and Ethical Considerations

AOTA asserts that the same ethical and professional standards that apply to in-person delivery of occupational therapy services also apply to the delivery of services by means of telehealth technologies. Occupational therapy practitioners should refer to the *Occupational Therapy Code of Ethics and Ethics Standards (2010)* (AOTA, 2010a). As stated in this document, occupational therapy practitioners are responsible for ensuring their individual competence in the areas in which they provide services. In addition, Principle 1B of the *Code and Ethics Standards* states that "occupational therapy personnel shall provide appropriate evaluation and a plan of intervention for all recipients of occupational therapy services specific to their needs" (AOTA, 2010a, p. S19). This requirement reinforces the importance of careful consideration about whether evaluation or intervention through a telehealth service delivery model will best meet the client's needs and is the most appropriate method of providing services given the client's situation.

Clinical and ethical reasoning guides the selection and application of appropriate telehealth technology necessary to evaluate and meet client needs. Occupational therapy practitioners should consider whether the use of technology and service provision through telehealth will ensure the safe, effective, appropriate delivery of services. To determine whether providing occupational therapy by means of telehealth is in the best interest of the client, the occupational therapist must consider the following:

- Complexity of the client's condition

- Knowledge, skill, and competence of the occupational therapy practitioner

- Nature and complexity of the intervention

- Requirements of the practice setting

- Client's context and environment.

Additionally, the American Telemedicine Association's "A Blueprint for Telerehabilitation Guidelines" outlines important administrative, clinical, technical, and ethical principles associated with the use of telehealth (Brennan et al., 2010). Occupational therapy practitioners may use various educational approaches to gain competency in using telehealth technologies. They may gain an understanding about basic telehealth service delivery model and telehealth technologies as a part of entry-level education (Standard B.1.8; Accreditation Council for Occupational Therapy Education, 2012) or may participate in continuing educa-tion opportunities as clinicians to acquire expertise in this area (Theodoros & Russell, 2008). Examples of ethical considerations related to telehealth are outlined in Table 1.

The *Specialized Knowledge and Skills in Technology and Environmental Interventions for Occupational Therapy Practice* document (AOTA, 2010b) describes the knowledge and skills necessary for entry- and advanced-level practice in technology. Practitioners should have a working knowledge of the hardware, software, and other elements of the technology they are using and have technical support personnel available should problems arise (Schopp, Hales, Brown, & Quetsch, 2003). They should use evidence, mentoring, and continuing education to maintain and enhance their competency related to the use of a telehealth service delivery model within occupational therapy.

Supervision Using Telehealth Technologies

State licensure laws, institution-specific guidelines regarding supervision of occupational therapy students and personnel, the AOTA *Guidelines for Supervision, Roles, and Responsibilities During the Delivery of Occupational Therapy Services* (AOTA, 2009), and the *Occupational Therapy Code of Ethics and Ethics Standards (2010)* (AOTA, 2010a) must be followed, regardless of the method of supervision. Telehealth technologies may be used within those guidelines to the extent that they take into account the unique characteristics of telehealth supervision, to support students and practitioners working in isolated or rural areas (Miller, Miller,

Table 1. Ethical Considerations and Strategies for Practice Using Telehealth Technologies

ETHICAL CONSIDERATIONS	STRATEGIES FOR ETHICAL PRACTICE
Fully inform the client regarding the implications of a telehealth service delivery model versus an in-person service delivery model.	Occupational therapy personnel shall . . . "Establish a collaborative relationship with recipients of service including families, significant others, and caregivers in setting goals and priorities throughout the intervention process. This includes full disclosure of the benefits, risks, and potential outcomes of any intervention; the personnel who will be providing the intervention(s); and/or any reasonable alternatives to the proposed intervention." (Principle 3A) "Obtain consent before administering any occupational therapy service, including evaluation, and ensure that recipients of service (or their legal representatives) are kept informed of the progress in meeting goals specified in the plan of intervention/care." (Principle 3B)
Abide by laws and scope of practice related to licensure and provision of occupational therapy services using telehealth technologies.	"Occupational therapy personnel shall comply with institutional rules, local, state, federal, and international laws and AOTA documents applicable to the profession of occupational therapy." (Principle 5)
Adhere to professional standards.	Occupational therapy personnel shall . . . "Provide occupational therapy services that are within each practitioner's level of competence and scope of practice (e.g., qualification, experience, the law)." (Principle 1E) "Take responsible steps (e.g., continuing education, research, supervision, training) and use careful judgment to ensure their own competence and weigh potential for client harm when generally recognized standards do not exist in emerging technology or areas of practice." (Principle 1G) "Take responsibility for maintaining high standards and continuing competence in practice, education, and research by participating in professional development and educational activities to improve and update knowledge and skills." (Principle 5F) "Occupational therapy personnel shall comply with institutional rules, local, state, federal, and international laws and AOTA documents applicable to the profession of occupational therapy." (Principle 5)
Understand and abide by approaches that ensure that privacy, security, and confidentiality are not compromised as a result of using telehealth technologies.	Occupational therapy personnel shall . . . "Ensure that confidentiality and the right to privacy are respected and maintained regarding all information obtained about recipients of service, students, research participants, colleagues, or employees. The only exceptions are when a practitioner or staff member believes that an individual is in serious foreseeable or imminent harm. Laws and regulations may require disclosure to appropriate authorities without consent." (Principle 3G) "Maintain the confidentiality of all verbal, written, electronic, augmentative, and nonverbal communications, including compliance with HIPAA regulations." (Principle 3H)
Understand and adhere to procedures if there is any compromise of security related to health information.	Report any breach of security to an appropriate health privacy officer, or seek guidance of an independent legal counsel.

(Continued)

Table 1. Ethical Considerations and Strategies for Practice Using Telehealth Technologies *(Cont.)*

ETHICAL CONSIDERATIONS	STRATEGIES FOR ETHICAL PRACTICE
Assess the effectiveness of interventions provided through telehealth technologies by consulting current research and conducting ongoing monitoring of client response.	Occupational therapy personnel shall . . . "Refer to other health care specialists solely on the basis of the needs of the client." (Principle 1I) "Reevaluate and reassess recipients of service in a timely manner to determine if goals are being achieved and whether intervention plans should be revised." (Principle 1C) "Use, to the extent possible, evaluation, planning, intervention techniques, and therapeutic equipment that are evidence-based and within the recognized scope of occupational therapy practice." (Principle 1F)
Recognize the need to be culturally competent in the provision of services via telehealth, including language, ethnicity, socioeconomic and educational background that could affect the quality and outcomes of services provided.	Occupational therapy personnel shall . . . "Provide services that reflect an understanding of how occupational therapy service delivery can be affected by factors such as economic status, age, ethnicity, race, geography, disability, marital status, sexual orientation, gender, gender identity, religion, culture, and political affiliation." (Principle 4F) "Make every effort to facilitate open and collaborative dialogue with clients and/or responsible parties to facilitate comprehension of services and their potential risks/benefits." (Principle 3J)

Note. HIPAA = Health Insurance Portability and Accountability Act of 1996 (Pub. L. 104–191). Ethical principles are from AOTA's (2010a) *Occupational Therapy Code of Ethics and Ethics Standards (2010)*.

Burton, Sprang, & Adams, 2003; Hubbard, 2000). However, practitioners engaged in telehealth supervision should be cautious when relying on legal or other standards that were not necessarily established with telehealth supervision in mind. Factors that may affect the model of supervision and frequency of supervision include the complexity of client needs, number and diversity of clients, skills of the occupational therapist and the occupational therapy assistant, type of practice setting, requirements of the practice setting, and other regulatory requirements (AOTA, 2009). Supervision must comply with applicable state and federal practice regulations, state and federal insurance programs, relevant workplace policies, and the *Occupational Therapy Code of Ethics and Ethics Standards (2010)* (AOTA, 2010a).

Legal and Regulatory Considerations

Occupational therapy practitioners are to abide by state licensure laws and related occupational therapy regulations regarding the use of a telehealth service delivery model within occupational therapy (Cwiek, Rafiq, Qamar, Tobey, & Merrell, 2007). Given the inconsistent adoption and nonuniformity of language regarding the use of telehealth within occupational therapy, it is incumbent upon the practitioner to check a state's statutes, regulations, and policies before beginning to practice using a telehealth service delivery model. Typically, information may be found on state licensure boards' Web sites. The absence of statutes, regulations, or policies that guide the practice of occupational therapy by means of telehealth delivery should not be viewed as authorization to do so. State regulatory boards should be contacted directly in the absence of written guidance to determine the appropriateness of using telehealth technologies for the delivery of occupational therapy services within their jurisdictions. In addition, the policies and guidelines of payers should be consulted. At this time, occupational therapy practitioners are to comply with the licensure and regulatory requirements in the state where they are located and the state where the client is located (Cason & Brannon, 2011).

Occupational therapy practitioners are to abide by Health Insurance Portability and Accountability Act (HIPAA, 1996; Pub. L. 104–191) regulations to maintain security, privacy, and confidentiality of all records and interactions. Additional safeguards inherent in the use of technology to deliver occupational therapy services must be considered to ensure privacy and security of confidential information (Watzlaf, Moeini, & Firouzan, 2010; Watzlaf, Moeini, Matusow, & Firouzan, 2011). Occupational therapy practitioners are to consult with their practice setting's privacy officer or legal counsel or to consult with independent legal counsel if they are in independent or other practice outside of an institutional setting to ensure that the services they provide through telehealth are consistent with protocol and HIPAA regulations.

Funding and Reimbursement

It is the position of AOTA that occupational therapy services provided with telehealth technologies should be valued, recognized, and reimbursed the same as occupational therapy services provided in person. At this writing, Medicare does not list occupational therapy practitioners as eligible providers of services delivered through telehealth technologies. However, AOTA supports the inclusion of occupational therapy practitioners on Medicare's approved list of telehealth providers. The U.S. Department of Defense and Veteran's Health Administration use occupational therapy practitioners for select telehealth programming.

Opportunities for reimbursement exist through some state Medicaid programs; insurance companies; and private pay with individuals, school districts, agencies, and organizations. Medicaid reimbursement is available at the discretion of each state, because it is subject to specific requirements or restrictions within a state. It is recommended that occupational therapy practitioners contact their state Medicaid or other third-party payers to determine the guidelines for reimbursement of services provided through telehealth technologies.

When billing occupational therapy services provided by means of telehealth technologies, practitioners must distinguish the service delivery model, often designated with a *modifier* (Cason & Brannon, 2011). However, regardless of whether the services are reimbursed or the practitioner is responsible for completing paperwork related to billing, the nature of the service delivery as being performed through telehealth should be thoroughly documented.

Summary

Telehealth is a service delivery model that uses telecommunication technologies to deliver health-related services at a distance. Occupational therapy practitioners are using synchronous or asynchronous telehealth technologies to provide evaluative, consultative, preventative, and therapeutic services to clients who are physically distant from the practitioner. Occupational therapy practitioners using telehealth as a service delivery model must adhere to the *Occupational Therapy Code of Ethics and Ethics Standards (2010)* (AOTA, 2010a), maintain the *Standards of Practice for Occupational Therapy* (AOTA, 2010c), and comply with federal and state regulations to ensure their competencies as practitioners and the well-being of their clients.

Occupational therapy practitioners must give careful consideration as to whether evaluation or intervention through a telehealth service delivery model will best meet the client's needs and provide the most appropriate method of providing services given the individual's situation. Clinical and ethical reasoning guides the selection and application of appropriate telehealth technology necessary to evaluate and meet client needs.

References

Accreditation Council for Occupational Therapy Education. (2012). 2011 Accreditation Council for Occupational Therapy Education (ACOTE®) standards. *American Journal of Occupational Therapy, 66*(6, Suppl.), S6–S74. http://dx.doi.org/10.5014/ajot.2012.66S6

American Medical Association. (2011). *CPT 2012.* Chicago: Author.

American Occupational Therapy Association. (2006). Policy 1.44: Categories of occupational therapy personnel. In *Policy manual* (2009 ed., pp. 33–34). Bethesda, MD: Author.

American Occupational Therapy Association. (2009). Guidelines for supervision, roles, and responsibilities during the delivery of occupational therapy services. *American Journal of Occupational Therapy, 63,* 797–803. http://dx.doi.org/10.5014/ajot.63.6.797

American Occupational Therapy Association. (2010a). Occupational therapy code of ethics and ethics standards (2010). *American Journal of Occupational Therapy, 64*(6, Suppl.), S17–S26. http://dx.doi.org/10.5014/ajot.2010.64S17

American Occupational Therapy Association. (2010b). Specialized knowledge and skills in technology and environmental interventions for occupational therapy practice. *American Journal of Occupational Therapy, 64*(6, Suppl.), S44–S56. http://dx.doi.org/10.5014/ajot.2010.64S44

American Occupational Therapy Association. (2010c). Standards of practice for occupational therapy. *American Journal of Occupational Therapy, 64*(6, Suppl.), S106–S111. http://dx.doi.org/10.5014/ajot.2010.64S106

American Occupational Therapy Association. (2010d). Telerehabilitation. *American Journal of Occupational Therapy, 64*(6, Suppl.), S92–S102. http://dx.doi.org/10.5014/ajot.2010.64S92

Backman, C. L., Village, J., & Lacaille, D. (2008). The Ergonomic Assessment Tool for arthritis: Development and pilot testing. *Arthritis and Rheumatism, 59,* 1495–1503. http://dx.doi.org/10.1002/art.24116

Baker, N., & Jacobs, K. (2010). Tele-ergonomics: A novel approach to computer workstation ergonomic assessment and modification. In *Proceedings of the Human Factors and Ergonomics Society 54th Annual Meeting (2010)* (p. 36). Santa Monica, CA: Human Factors and Ergonomics Society.

Baker, N., & Jacobs, K. (2013). Tele-ergonomics. In S. Kumar & E. Cohn (Eds.), *Telerehabilitation* (pp. 163–174). London: Springer.

Barlow, I. G., Liu, L., & Sekulic, A. (2009). Wheelchair seating assessment and intervention: A comparison between telerehabilitation and face-to-face service. *International Journal of Telerehabilitation, 1,* 17–28. http://dx.doi.org/10.5195/ijt.2009.868

Bendixen, R., Horn, K., & Levy, C. (2007). Using telerehabilitation to support elders with chronic illness in their homes. *Topics in Geriatric Rehabilitation, 23,* 47–51.

Bendixen, R., Levy, C., Lutz, B. J., Horn, K. R., Chronister, K., & Mann, W. C. (2008). A telerehabilitation model for victims of polytrauma. *Rehabilitation Nursing, 33,* 215–220. http://dx.doi.org/10.1002/j.2048-7940.2008.tb00230.x

Bendixen, R., Levy, C., Olive, E., Kobb, R., & Mann, W. (2009). Cost-effectiveness of a telerehabilitation program to support chronically ill and disabled elders in their homes. *Telemedicine and e-Health, 15,* 31–38. http://dx.doi.org/10.1089/tmj.2008.0046

Brennan, D., Tindall, L., Theodoros, D., Brown, J., Campbell, M., Christiana, D., . . . Lee, A. (2010). A blueprint for telerehabilitation guidelines. *International Journal of Telerehabilitation, 2,* 31–34. http://dx.doi.org/10.5195/ijt.2010.6063

Brewer, B. R., Fagan, M., Klatzky, R. L., & Matsuoka, Y. (2005). Perceptual limits for a robotic rehabilitation environment using visual feedback distortion. *IEEE Transactions on Neural Systems and Rehabilitation Engineering, 13,* 1–11. http://dx.doi.org/10.1109/TNSRE.2005.843443

Bruce, C., & Sanford, J. A. (2006). Development of an evidence-based conceptual framework for workplace assessment. *Work, 27,* 381–389.

Cason, J. (2009). A pilot telerehabilitation program: Delivering early intervention services to rural families. *International Journal of Telerehabilitation, 1,* 29–38. http://dx.doi.org/10.5195/ijt.2009.6007

Cason, J. (2011). Telerehabilitation: An adjunct service delivery model for early intervention services. *International Journal of Telerehabilitation, 3,* 19–28. http://dx.doi.org/10.5195/ijt.2011.6071

Cason, J. (2012a). An introduction to telehealth as a service delivery model within occupational therapy. *OT Practice, 17*(7), CE1–CE8.

Cason, J. (2012b). Telehealth opportunities in occupational therapy through the Affordable Care Act. *American Journal of Occupational Therapy, 66,* 131–136. http://dx.doi.org/10.5014/ajot.2012.662001

Cason, J., & Brannon, J. A. (2011). Telehealth regulatory and legal considerations: Frequently asked questions. *International Journal of Telerehabilitation, 3,* 15–18. http://dx.doi.org/10.5195/ijt.2011.6077

Chumbler, N., Quigley, P., Sanford, J., Griffiths, P., Rose, D., Morey, M., . . . Hoenig, H. (2010). Implementing telerehabilitation research for stroke rehabilitation with community dwelling veterans: Lessons learned. *International Journal of Telerehabilitation, 2,* 15–21. http://dx.doi.org/10.5195/ijt.2010.6047

Cooper, R., Fitzgerald, S., Boninger, M. L., Cooper, R. A., Shapcott, N., & Cohen, L. (2002). Using telerehabilitation to aid in selecting a wheelchair. In R. Simpson (Ed.), *RESNA 2002 annual conference proceedings* (pp. 245–247). Minneapolis, MN: RESNA Press.

Cwiek, M. A., Rafiq, A., Qamar, A., Tobey, C., & Merrell, R. C. (2007). Telemedicine licensure in the United States: The need for a cooperative regional approach. *Telemedicine and e-Health, 13,* 141–147. http://dx.doi.org/10.1089/tmj.2006.0029

Darkins, A., Ryan, P., Kobb, R., Forster, L., Edmonson, E., Wakefield, B., & Lancaster, A. E. (2008). Care coordination/home telehealth: The systematic implementation of health informatics, home telehealth, and disease management to support the care of veteran patients with chronic conditions. *Telemedicine and e-Health, 14,* 1118–1126. http://dx.doi.org/10.1089/tmj.2008.0021

Diamond, B. J., Shreve, G. M., Bonilla, J. M., Johnston, M. V., Morodan, J., & Branneck, R. (2003). Telerehabilitation, cognition and user accessibility. *NeuroRehabilitation, 18,* 171–177.

Dreyer, N. C., Dreyer, K. A., Shaw, D. K., & Wittman, P. P. (2001). Efficacy of telemedicine in occupational therapy: A pilot study. *Journal of Allied Health, 30,* 39–42.

Federal Communications Commission. (2010). *Voice-over-Internet protocol.* Retrieved from www.fcc.gov/voip/

Forducey, P. G., Ruwe, W. D., Dawson, S. J., Scheideman-Miller, C., McDonald, N. B., & Hantla, M. R. (2003). Using telerehabilitation to promote TBI recovery and transfer of knowledge. *NeuroRehabilitation, 18,* 103–111.

Gallagher, T. E. (2004). Augmentation of special-needs services and information to students and teachers "ASSIST"—A telehealth innovation providing school-based medical interventions. *Hawaii Medical Journal, 63,* 300–309.

Germain, V., Marchand, A., Bouchard, S., Drouin, M. S., & Guay, S. (2009). Effectiveness of cognitive behavioural therapy administered by videoconference for posttraumatic stress disorder. *Cognitive Behaviour Therapy, 38,* 42–53. http://dx.doi.org/10.1080/16506070802473494

Girard, P. (2007). Military and VA telemedicine systems for patients with traumatic brain injury. *Journal of Rehabilitation Research and Development, 44,* 1017–1026. http://dx.doi.org/10.1682/JRRD.2006.12.0174

Gros, D. F., Yoder, M., Tuerk, P. W., Lozano, B. E., & Acierno, R. (2011). Exposure therapy for PTSD delivered to veterans via telehealth: Predictors of treatment completion and outcome and comparison to treatment delivered in person. *Behavior Therapy, 42,* 276–283. http://dx.doi.org/10.1016/j.beth.2010.07.005

Harada, N. D., Dhanani, S., Elrod, M., Hahn, T., Kleinman, L., & Fang, M. (2010). Feasibility study of home telerehabilitation for physically inactive veterans. *Journal of Rehabilitation Research and Development, 47,* 465–475. http://dx.doi.org/10.1682/JRRD.2009.09.0149

Harrison, A., Derwent, G., Enticknap, A., Rose, F. D., & Attree, E. A. (2002). The role of virtual reality technology in the assessment and training of inexperienced powered wheelchair users. *Disability and Rehabilitation, 24,* 599–606. http://dx.doi.org/10.1080/09638280110111360

Health Insurance Portability and Accountability Act, Pub. L. 104–191, 101 Stat. 1936 (1996).

Hegel, M. T., Lyons, K. D., Hull, J. G., Kaufman, P., Urguhart, L., Li, Z., & Ahles, T. A. (2011). Feasibility study of a randomized controlled trial of a telephone-delivered problem solving occupational therapy intervention to reduce participation restrictions in rural breast cancer survivors undergoing chemotherapy. *Psycho-Oncology, 20,* 1092–1101. http://dx.doi.org/10.1002/pon.1830

Heimerl, S., & Rasch, N. (2009). Delivering developmental occupational therapy consultation services through telehealth. *Developmental Disabilities Special Interest Section Quarterly, 32*(3), 1–4.

Hermann, V. H., Herzog, M., Jordan, R., Hofherr, M., Levine, P., & Page, S. J. (2010). Telerehabilitation and electrical stimulation: An occupation-based, client-centered stroke intervention. *American Journal of Occupational Therapy, 64,* 73–81. http://dx.doi.org/10.5014/ajot.64.1.73

Hoffman, H. G., Patterson, D. R., & Carrougher, G. J. (2000). Use of virtual reality for adjunctive treatment of adult burn pain during physical therapy: A controlled study. *Clinical Journal of Pain, 16,* 244–250. http://dx.doi.org/10.1097/00002508-200009000-00010

Hoffmann, T., Russell, T., Thompson, L., Vincent, A., & Nelson, M. (2008). Using the Internet to assess activities of daily living and hand function in people with Parkinson's disease. *NeuroRehabilitation, 23,* 253–261.

Hori, M., Kubota, M., Kihara, T., Takahashi, R., & Kinoshita, A. (2009). The effect of videophone communication (with Skype and webcam) for elderly patients with dementia and their caregivers. *Gan To Kagaku Ryoho, 36S,* 36–38. Retrieved from www.ncbi.nlm.nih.gov/pubmed/20443395

Hubbard, S. (2000, December 4 & 18). A case example of remote supervision. *OT Practice, 5,* 16–18.

Individuals With Disabilities Education Act Amendments of 1997, Pub. L. 105–117, 20 U.S.C. § 1400 *et seq.*

Kairy, D., Lehoux, P., Vincent, C., & Visintin, M. (2009). A systematic review of clinical outcomes, clinical process, healthcare utilization and costs associated with telerehabilitation. *Disability and Rehabilitation, 31,* 427–47. http://dx.doi.org/10.1080/09638280802062553

Kelso, G., Fiechtl, B., Olsen, S., & Rule, S. (2009). The feasibility of virtual home visits to provide early intervention: A pilot study. *Infants and Young Children, 22,* 332–340. http://dx.doi.org/10.1097/IYC.0b013e3181b9873c

Kim, J. B., & Brienza, D. M. (2006). Development of a remote accessibility assessment system through three-dimensional reconstruction technology. *Journal of Rehabilitation Research and Development, 43,* 257–272. http://dx.doi.org/10.1682/JRRD.2004.12.0163

Kim, J. B., Brienza, D. M., Lynch, R. D., Cooper, R. A., & Boninger, M. L. (2008). Effectiveness evaluation of a remote accessibility assessment system for wheelchair users using virtualized reality. *Archives of Physical Medicine and Rehabilitation, 89,* 470–479. http://dx.doi.org/10.1016/j.apmr.2007.08.158

Lewis, J. A., Boian, R. F., Burdea, G., & Deutsch, J. E. (2005). Remote console for virtual telerehabilitation. *Studies in Health Technology and Informatics, 111,* 294–300.

Lewis, J. A., Deutsch, J. E., & Burdea, G. (2006). Usability of the remote console for virtual reality telerehabilitation: Formative evaluation. *Cyberpsychology and Behavior, 9,* 142–147. http://dx.doi.org/10.1089/cpb.2006.9.142

Mann, W. C., & Milton, B. R. (2005). Home automation and SMART homes to support independence. In W. C. Mann (Ed.), *Smart technology for aging, disability, and independence* (pp. 33–66). Hoboken, NJ: Wiley.

Merians, A. S., Jack, D., Boian, R., Tremaine, M., Burdea, G. C., Adamovich, S. V., . . . Poizner, H. (2002). Virtual reality–augmented rehabilitation for patients following stroke. *Physical Therapy, 82,* 898–915.

Miller, T. W., Miller, J. M., Burton, D., Sprang, R., & Adams, J. (2003). Telehealth: A model for clinical supervision in allied health. *Internet Journal of Allied Health Sciences and Practice, 1*(2), 1–8.

Naditz, A. (2009). Still standing: Telemedicine devices and fall prevention. *Telemedicine and e-Health, 15,* 137–141. http://dx.doi.org/10.1089/tmj.2009.9989

Neubeck, L., Redfern, J., Fernandez, R., Briffad, T., Bauman, A., & Freedman, S. B. (2009). Telehealth interventions for the secondary prevention of coronary heart disease: A systematic review. *European Journal of Preventive Cardiology, 16,* 281–289. http://dx.doi.org/0.1097/HJR.0b013e32832a4e7a

Palsbo, S. E., Dawson, S. J., Savard, L., Goldstein, M., & Heuser, A. (2007). Televideo assessment using Functional Reach Test and European Stroke Scale. *Journal of Rehabilitation Research and Development, 44,* 659–664. http://dx.doi.org/10.1682/JRRD.2006.11.0144

Popescu, V. G., Burdea, G. C., Bouzit, M., & Hentz, V. R. (2000). A virtual-reality-based telerehabilitation system with force feedback. *IEEE Transactions on Information Technology in Biomedicine, 4,* 45–51. http://dx.doi.org/10.1109/4233.826858

Rand, D., Katz, N., & Weiss, P. L. (2009). Intervention using the VMall for improving motor and functional ability of the upper extremity in poststroke participants. *European Journal of Physical and Rehabilitation Medicine, 45,* 113–121.

Rand, D., Kizony, R., & Weiss, P. T. (2008). The Sony PlayStation II EyeToy: Low-cost virtual reality for use in rehabilitation. *Journal of Neurologic Physical Therapy, 32,* 155–163. http://dx.doi.org/ 10.1097/ NPT.0b013e31818ee779

Rand, D., Weiss, P. L., & Katz, N. (2009). Training multitasking in a virtual supermarket: A novel intervention after stroke. *American Journal of Occupational Therapy, 63,* 535–542. http://dx.doi.org/ 10.5014/ ajot.63.5.535

Sanford, J., Hoenig, H., Griffiths, P., Butterfield, T., Richardson, P., & Hargraves, K. (2007). A comparison of televideo and traditional in-home rehabilitation in mobility impaired older adults. *Physical and Occupational Therapy in Geriatrics, 25,* 1–18. http://dx.doi.org/10.1080/J148v25n03_01

Savard, L., Borstad, A., Tkachuck, J., Lauderdale, D., & Conroy, B. (2003). Telerehabilitation consultations for clients with neurologic diagnoses: Cases from rural Minnesota and American Samoa. *NeuroRehabilitation, 18,* 93–102.

Scheideman-Miller, C., Clark, P. G., Moorad, A., Post, M. L., Hodge, B. G., & Smeltzer, S. (2003, January). Efficacy and sustainability of a telerehabilitation program. In *Proceedings of the 36th Annual Hawaii International Conference on System Sciences* (pp. 11–21). Washington, DC: IEEE Computer Society.

Schein, R. M., Schmeler, M. R., Brienza, D., Saptono, A., & Parmanto, B. (2008). Development of a service delivery protocol used for remote wheelchair consultation via telerehabilitation. *Telemedicine and e-Health, 14,* 932–938.

Schein, R. M., Schmeler, M. R., Holm, M. B., Pramuka, M., Saptono, A., & Brienza, D. M. (2011). Telerehabilitation assessment using the Functioning Everyday with a Wheelchair-Capacity instrument. *Journal of Rehabilitation Research and Development, 48,* 115–124. http://dx.doi.org/10.1682/JRRD.2010.03.0039

Schein, R. M., Schmeler, M. R., Holm, M. B., Saptono, A., & Brienza, D. M. (2010). Telerehabilitation wheeled mobility and seating assessments compared with in person. *Archives of Physical Medicine and Rehabilitation, 91,* 874–878. http://dx.doi.org/10.1016/j.apmr.2010.01.017

Schmeler, M. R., Schein, R. M., McCue, M., & Betz, K. (2009). Telerehabilitation and clinical applications: Research, opportunities, and challenges. *International Journal of Telerehabilitation, 1,* 59–72. http://dx.doi.org/10.5195/ijt.2009.6014

Schopp, L. H., Hales, J. W., Brown, G. D., & Quetsch, J. L. (2003). A rationale and training agenda for rehabilitation informatics: Roadmap for an emerging discipline. *NeuroRehabilitation, 18,* 159–170.

Sheridan, T. B. (1992). Musings on telepresence and virtual presence. *Presence, 1,* 120–125.

Steel, K., Cox, D., & Garry, H. (2011). Therapeutic videoconferencing interventions for the treatment of long-term conditions. *Journal of Telemedicine and Telecare, 17,* 109–117. http://dx.doi.org/ 10.1258/ jtt.2010.100318

Tang, P., & Venables, T. (2000). "Smart" homes and telecare for independent living. *Journal of Telemedicine and Telecare, 6,* 8–14. http://dx.doi.org/10.1258/1357633001933871

Theodoros, D., & Russell, T. (2008). Telerehabilitation: Current perspectives. *Current Principles and Practices of Telemedicine and e-Health, 131,* 191–209.

Verburg, G., Borthwick, B., Bennett, B., & Rumney, P. (2003). Online support to facilitate the reintegration of students with brain injury: Trials and errors. *NeuroRehabilitation, 18,* 113–123.

Wakeford, L. (2002, November 25). Telehealth technology for children with special needs. *OT Practice, 7,* 12–16.

Watzlaf, V., Moeini, S., & Firouzan, P. (2010). VoIP for telerehabilitation: A risk analysis for privacy, security, and HIPAA compliance, Part I. *International Journal of Telerehabilitation, 2,* 3–14. http://dx.doi.org/ 10.5195/ijt.2010.6056

Watzlaf, V., Moeini, S., Matusow, L., & Firouzan, P. (2011). VoIP for telerehabilitation: A risk analysis for privacy, security, and HIPAA compliance, Part II. *International Journal of Telerehabilitation, 3,* 3–10. http:// dx.doi.org/10.5195/ijt.2011.6070

Weiss, P. L., & Jessel, A. S. (1998). Virtual reality applications to work. *Work, 11,* 277–293.

Whelan, L., & Wagner, N. (2011). Technology that touches lives: Teleconsultation to benefit persons with upper limb loss. *International Journal of Telerehabilitation, 3,* 19–22. http://dx.doi.org/10.5195/ijt.2011.6080

Winters, J. M. (2002). Telerehabilitation research: Emerging opportunities. *Annual Review of Biomedical Engineering, 4,* 287–320. http://dx.doi.org/10.1146/annurev.bioeng.4.112801.121923

Additional Resources

American Telemedicine Association's Telerehabilitation Special Interest Group/Resources, www.americantelemed.org/i4a/pages/index.cfm?pageid=3328

Center for Telehealth and e-Health Law (CTel), http://ctel.org/

International Journal of Telerehabilitation, http://telerehab.pitt.edu/ojs/index.php/telerehab

Journal of Telemedicine and Telecare, http://jtt.rsmjournals.com/

Rehabilitation Engineering Research Center for Telerehabilitation, www.rerctr.pitt.edu

Telehealth Resource Centers, www.telehealthresourcecenter.org/

Telemedicine and e-Health, www.liebertpub.com/TMJ

Authors

Jana Cason, DHS, OTR/L, FAOTA

Kim Hartmann, PhD, OTR/L, FAOTA

Karen Jacobs, EdD, CPE, OTR/L, FAOTA

Tammy Richmond, MS, OTR/L, FAOTA

for

The Commission on Practice

Debbie Amini, EdD, OTR/L, CHT, *Chairperson*

The COP would like to acknowledge the contributions of the authors of the 2010 Telerehabilitation
Position Paper:

Mark R. Schmeler, PhD, OTR/L, ATP

Richard M. Schein, PhD

Andrea Fairman, MOT, OTR/L, CPRP

Amanda Brickner, MOT, OTR/L

William C. Mann, PhD, OTR

Adopted by the Representative Assembly Coordinating Council (RACC) for the Representative Assembly, 2012.

Revised by the Commission on Practice 2012.

Note. This revision replaces the 2010 document *Telerehabilitation Position Paper,* previously published and copyrighted
2010 by the American Occupational Therapy Association in the *American Journal of Occupational Therapy, 64*(6, Suppl.),
S92–S102. http://dx.doi.org/10.5014/ajot.2010.64S92

Appendix A. Overview of Telehealth Technologies

Synchronous Technologies: Videoconferencing

Synchronous technologies enable the exchange of health information in *real time* (i.e., live) by interactive audio and video between the patient or client and a health care provider located at a distant site. Several options for videoconferencing are available; they include voice over the Internet protocol (VoIP) services, mobile videoconferencing systems, "plain old telephone service" (POTS), videoconferencing, and high-definition television (HDTV) technologies (see Table A1).

VoIP services use a computer, special VoIP phone, or traditional phone with adapter to convert voice into a digital signal that travels over the Internet (Federal Communications Commission, 2010). Integrated with video software, VoIP provides a mechanism for Internet-based videoconferencing. Similarly, mobile videoconferencing uses a mobile device (e.g., smartphone, electronic tablet) with videoconferencing capabilities to transmit audio and video over a wireless or cellular network. POTS videoconferencing primarily uses an analog telephone line or landline to support audio and video transmission through a videophone or specialized equipment connected to a television. HDTV videoconferencing requires an HD television, console, HD camera, remote control, and high-speed broadband connection at both locations. Unlike the technologies described above and marketed for consumer use, telehealth networks use high-end videoconferencing technologies (e.g., Polycom, Tandberg) and fiber-optic telephone lines (e.g., T1 lines) or high-speed Internet to connect sites.

Advantages of VoIP, mobile, POTS, and consumer HDTV technologies include service provision within the context where occupations naturally occur (e.g., home, work, community), minimal infrastructure requirements, and lower costs for equipment and connectivity (e.g., residential service plan, data plan). Disadvantages may include privacy, security, and confidentiality risks; lack of infrastructure (e.g., limited access to high-speed Internet/broadband; inadequate bandwidth for connectivity); recurring expense (e.g., residential service plan, data plan); diminished sound or image quality; and technological challenges associated with end-user experience and expertise with videoconferencing technology (Cason, 2011; see Table A1).

Asynchronous Technologies

Telehealth applications that are asynchronous, commonly referred to as "store-and-forward" data transmission, may include video clips, digital photographs, virtual technologies, and other forms of electronic communications. With *asynchronous technologies,* the provider and client are not connected at the same time. Potential applications for asynchronous telehealth technologies within occupational therapy include home assessments and recommendations for home modifications that are based on recorded data of the home environment; recommendations for inclusion of ergonomic principles and workstation modifications that are based on recorded data of the work environment; and secure viewing of video segments for evaluation and intervention purposes.

Technologies That May Be Synchronous or Asynchronous

Telemonitoring Technologies

Occupational therapy practitioners providing services through telehealth technologies can take advantage of *s*elf-*m*onitoring *a*nalysis and *r*eporting *t*echnology (SMART) to monitor a client's occupational performance within the home and community. SMART technologies that are wireless allow the occupational therapy practitioner to provide services within varied environments without restricting the client's movements within those environments. These technologies provide information that allows an offsite occupational therapy practitioner to assess performance and modify services and the environment and also enable occupational therapy practitioners to understand the real-life occupations and performance challenges of the client and to plan appropriate interventions. As a result, occupational therapy practitioners can tailor environmental accommodations for clients with physical limitations or can develop individualized technology-based cueing systems for clients with cognitive disabilities so that they can live more independently.

Virtual Reality Technologies

Virtual reality (VR) typically refers to the use of interactive simulations created with computer hardware and software to present users with opportunities to engage in environments that appear and feel similar to real-world objects and events (Sheridan, 1992; Weiss & Jessel, 1998). Although typical use of VR technologies does not constitute a telehealth service delivery model, live data (synchronous) streamed to a remote occupational therapy practitioner or recorded data (asynchronous) used by an occupational therapy practitioner to monitor and adjust a client's course of treatment would constitute the use of VR technologies within a telehealth service delivery model. Occupational therapy practitioners can use a telehealth service delivery model with VR technologies when conducting evaluations and providing interventions. A remote console telerehabilitation system (ReCon, Rutgers University, New Brunswick, NJ) incorporating VR technology provides occupational therapy practitioners with three-dimensional representations of the client's movements, VR-based exercise progress, and motor performance updates (Lewis, Boian, Burdea, & Deutsch, 2005; Lewis, Deutsch, & Burdea, 2006). Telehealth combined with VR has been used to provide feedback and information remotely as part of occupational therapy intervention (Merians et al., 2002), to distract people from physical pain, and to improve their adherence to therapeutic exercises (Hoffman, Patterson, & Carrougher, 2000).

Further, VR provided through telehealth technologies is effective in enabling people to compare the difference between their desired level of occupational engagement and their current functional status after a stroke (Brewer, Fagan, Klatzky, & Matsuoka, 2005; Merians et al., 2002; Rand, Katz, & Weiss, 2009; Rand, Weiss, & Katz, 2009), using virtual environments as part of the assessment and training of users of power wheelchairs (Harrison, Derwent, Enticknap, Rose, & Attree, 2002), and evaluating and determining home accessibility using three-dimensional construction of the architectural features of the environment (Kim & Brienza, 2006; Kim, Brienza, Lynch, Cooper, & Boninger, 2008).

Low-cost video capture gaming systems (e.g., Nintendo Wii, Sony Playstation's EyeToy and MOVE, XBOX-360 Kinect) were not developed specifically for rehabilitation, but they offer an easy-to-set-up, fun, and less expensive alternative to the expensive VR systems (Rand, Kizony, & Weiss, 2008). Although typical use of gaming systems does not constitute telehealth, live data (synchronous) streamed to a remote occupational therapy practitioner or recorded data (asynchronous) used by an occupational therapy practitioner to monitor and adjust a client's course of treatment would constitute a telehealth application of the devices.

Table A1. Telehealth Technologies

TECHNOLOGY TYPE	EXAMPLES	CONSIDERATIONS
Synchronous	• Voice over Internet protocol software • Mobile videoconferencing • Consumer high-definition television videoconferencing • "Plain old telephone service" • Videoconferencing • Telehealth network with commercial videoconferencing system • Virtual reality (VR) technologies (with live-streaming data to remote practitioner)	• Confidentiality (security, privacy) • Integrity (information protected from changes by unauthorized users) • Availability (information, services) • Cost–benefit ratio • Socioeconomic considerations • Leveraging existing infrastructure (equipment and personnel) • Technology connection requirements (e.g., broadband, T1 line) • Sound and image quality
Asynchronous	• Video recording devices • Cameras (photographs) • Devices enabling electronic communication • VR technologies (with store-and-forward data to remote practitioner)	• Equipment accessibility • Provider and end-user comfort, experience, and expertise with technology
Synchronous (interactive) or asynchronous (store-and-forward data)	• Telemonitoring technologies – Home monitoring systems/devices – Wireless sensors • VR technologies – Remote use of VR systems/devices	

Note. From "Telerehabilitation: An Adjunct Service Delivery Model for Early Intervention Services," by J. Cason, 2011, *International Journal of Telerehabilitation, 3*(1), p. 24. http://dx.doi.org/10.5195/ijt.2011.6071 Copyright © 2011 by Jana Cason. Adapted with permission.

Appendix B. Glossary

asynchronous—A method of exchanging health information whereby the provider and patient or client are not connected at the same time; commonly referred to as "store-and-forward" data transmission and may include video clips, digital photographs, virtual technologies, and other forms of electronic communications.

eHealth—A broad term encompassing health-related information and educational resources (e.g., health literacy Web sites and repositories, videos, blogs), commercial "products" (e.g., apps), and direct services delivered electronically (often through the Internet) by professionals, nonprofessionals, businesses, or consumers. May also be written as *e-Health* or *E-Health*; sometimes used interchangeably with *health informatics*.

haptic technology—A tactile feedback technology that takes advantage of a user's sense of touch by applying forces, vibrations, or motions upon the user.

health informatics—Use of information technologies for health care data collection, storage, and analysis to enhance health care decisions and improve quality and efficiency of health care services.

mHealth—The delivery of health-related information and services using mobile communication technology (e.g., smartphone, electronic tablet, or other mobile devices).

modifier—A modifier used in conjunction with a *Current Procedural Terminology* (American Medical Association, 2011) code to identify the type of technology used within a telehealth service delivery model. GT is the most common modifier; it indicates use of interactive audio and video telecommunications technology. The GQ modifier designates the use of asynchronous technologies; reimbursement for this modifier is limited.

privacy officer—A position or office that responds to concerns over the use of personal information, including medical data and financial information. It ensures adherence to regulations but is not limited to legislation concerning the protection of patient medical records (e.g., Health Insurance Portability and Accountability Act of 1996, Pub. L. 104–191).

protocol—A written document specifying standard operating policies and procedures for application of telehealth technologies in delivering services.

synchronous—A method of exchanging health information in real time (i.e., live) between the patient or client and a health care provider located at a distant site.

telehealth—The application of evaluative, consultative, preventative, and therapeutic services delivered through telecommunication and information technologies.

telehealth technologies—The hardware and software used in delivering services remotely by means of a telehealth service delivery model.

telemedicine—Medical services delivered through communication and information technologies.

telerehabilitation—The application of telecommunication and information technologies for the delivery of rehabilitation services.

virtual reality—A computer-simulated environment of the real world; can be coupled with telehealth technologies as part of a telehealth service delivery model.

Appendix C. Applications of Telehealth Within Occupational Therapy Practice Areas

Children and Youth

Evidence supports the use of a telehealth service delivery model to deliver appropriate early intervention (EI) and school-based services effectively and efficiently. EI services, mandated by Part C of the Individuals With Disabilities Education Act Amendments of 1997 (IDEA; Pub. L. 105–117), are designed to promote development of skills and enhance the quality of life of infants and toddlers who have been identified as having a disability or developmental delay (Cason, 2011). Telehealth technology supports delivery of EI services (Cason, 2009, 2011; Heimerl & Rasch, 2009; Kelso, Fiechtl, Olsen, & Rule, 2009).

Similarly, evidence supports the use of telehealth for the delivery of occupational therapy services within the school setting for evaluation and intervention (Gallagher, 2004) as well as for reintegration of students with traumatic injury following acute rehabilitation (Verburg, Borthwick, Bennett, & Rumney, 2003). Telehealth may be used within school-based interprofessional team models for wellness programming, including efforts to combat the obesity epidemic among children and for programming targeting prevention of violence among youth (Cason, 2012b). School-based occupational therapy services focus on helping children with disabilities participate in and, thus, benefit from the instructional program.

In addition to what has been stated, telehealth technology may provide another avenue for the occupational therapy practitioner to observe the child's level of participation in a school setting without risk of altering the setting by being physically present. This unobtrusive observation strategy can allow the occupational therapy practitioner to consult with the teacher and offer strategies to alter the child's level of participation (e.g., strategies to facilitate a child's use of self-regulation skills, encourage appropriate interaction with peers, or facilitate the child's physical participation in an instructional activity).

The potential benefit of this observation strategy is to ensure the maintenance of the day-to-day integrity of the classroom while providing the practitioner with an understanding of the specific sensory, cognitive, physical, and emotional demands placed on the child in the setting. This technology may also provide the ability to record observations that contribute to the therapist's data collection during evaluation; this information can then be used as a baseline from which to support Individualized Education Program teams in developing goals and objectives and measuring progress in the child's level of participation in the setting. In rural or large urban school districts, this technology can assist the occupational therapy practitioner with more efficiently supporting multiple campuses that may be located across large distances, thereby facilitating the interprofessional team process as well as reducing costs incurred to allow a practitioner the time and transportation resources to support multiple campuses.

Productive Aging

The growing number of older adults in the United States creates opportunities for occupational therapy practitioners to use telehealth to promote health and wellness, prevention, and productive aging while reducing health care costs. The use of telerehabilitation to remotely monitor and provide self-management strategies to older adults who are chronically ill and living in their homes has been found to decrease hospitalizations and nursing home stays (Bendixen, Levy, Olive, Kobb, & Mann, 2009). Interactive videoconferencing technologies promote health and aging in place among older adults (Bendixen, Horn, & Levy, 2007; Harada et al., 2010; Hori, Kubota, Kihara, Takahashi, & Kinoshita, 2009). The use of home monitoring devices such as self-monitoring analysis and reporting technology (SMART) enable occupational therapy practitioners to remotely monitor clients' occupational performance and provide recommendations for environmental modifications and interventions to support occupational performance (Mann & Milton, 2005).

Health and Wellness

Telehealth also supports health and wellness and prevention programming through assessment and management of obesity (Neubeck et al., 2009) and chronic diseases such as diabetes mellitus, congestive heart failure, and hypertension (Darkins et al., 2008; Steel, Cox, & Garry, 2011).

Mental Health

Opportunities exist for occupational therapy practitioners to use telehealth to promote participation and psychological and social functioning for clients within the home, at work, and in the community through engagement in meaningful occupations. Research demonstrates efficacy of telehealth as a delivery model for psychological and behavioral interventions among individuals with posttraumatic stress disorder (PTSD) and other mental health issues (Germain, Marchand, Bouchard, Drouin, & Guay, 2009; Gros, Yoder, Tuerk, Lozano, & Acierno, 2011).

Rehabilitation, Disability, and Participation

In the practice area of rehabilitation, disability, and participation, the use of a telehealth service delivery model promotes occupational performance, adaptation, participation, and quality of life for clients with polytrauma, neurological, and orthopedic conditions. Telehealth provides remote access to occupational therapy services through assessment of physical function and goal setting, integration of individualized exercise interventions, training in adaptive strategies such as environmental modifications and energy conservation, and consultation on durable medical and adaptive equipment (Chumbler et al., 2010; Sanford et al., 2007).

Published studies support the use of telehealth in improving functional outcomes with individuals with stroke (Chumbler et al., 2010; Hermann et al., 2010), survivors of breast cancer (Hegel et al., 2011), veterans with polytrauma (Bendixen et al., 2008), and individuals with traumatic brain injury (Diamond et al., 2003; Forducey et al., 2003; Girard, 2007; Verburg et al., 2003). Additional studies have used a telehealth service delivery model to evaluate activities of daily living and hand function in individuals with Parkinson's disease (Hoffman, Russell, Thompson, Vincent, & Nelson, 2008) and other neurological impairments (Savard, Borstad, Tkachuck, Lauderdale, & Conroy, 2003). Seating experts used telehealth to provide remote wheelchair prescription and consultation to individuals with neurological and orthopedic conditions (Barlow, Liu, & Sekulic, 2009; Schein, Schmeler, Holm, Saptono, & Brienza, 2010; Schein et al., 2011). In addition to positive clinical outcomes, evidence indicates a high level of practitioner and client satisfaction associated with a telehealth service delivery model (Kairy, Lehoux, Vincent, & Visintin, 2009; Steel et al., 2011).

Work and Industry

Schmeler, Schein, McCue, and Betz (2009) detailed the use of assistive technology via a telehealth service delivery model for clinical and vocational applications. Telehealth is also being used to support work through remote assessment and analysis of work spaces. Bruce and Sanford (2006) described using teleconferencing to complete remote assessments and discussed the need for a highly structured and comprehensive assessment tool to be able to complete remote assessments.

Backman, Village, and Lacaille (2008) developed the Ergonomic Assessment Tool for Arthritis (EATA) to evaluate the workplace for people with arthritis. The EATA was designed so that the worker could gather the data for the assessment without an expert visiting the workplace. Pilot testing of the method indicated that workers could successfully gather the necessary information for appropriate intervention identification (Baker & Jacobs, 2013). Baker and Jacobs (2010) developed a systematic two-step program, the Telerehabilitation Computer Ergonomics System *(tele-CES)*. This systematic program will allow ergonomically trained health professionals to (1) remotely assess the computer workstation and (2) on basis of the assessment, generate explicit, participant-specific workstation modification recommendations. The recommendations will be easily implemented; reduce pain, discomfort, and fatigue; and eliminate barriers to productivity.

Appendix D. Telehealth Case Examples

CASE DESCRIPTION	USE OF TELEHEALTH	OUTCOME
Lisa is a 70-year-old woman who has difficulty performing her daily occupations because of a stroke resulting in right-sided weakness. Although she had learned compensatory techniques for completing activities of daily living (ADLs), instrumental ADLs, and work, she still wants to increase the use of her right hand, particularly for tasks related to managing her farm. Lisa learned of a program in a nearby community using new technology that might be beneficial for people with hemiparesis; however, the clinic is 2 hours from her home.	Lisa meets with her occupational therapist in a clinic for the initial evaluation. During the evaluation, Lisa learns additional strategies for incorporating the use of her right hand to perform her farm work. She is fitted for a functional electrical stimulation orthosis that she can use at home once it is programmed in the clinic. Twice each week, Lisa meets with her occupational therapist by computer, using a Web camera and online video software. As Lisa continues to make progress, the occupational therapist instructs her in how to more effectively use her right hand for completion of ADLs and farm chores.	Lisa is able to make functional gains in using her right hand for everyday occupations. She reports that she is able to rely less on compensatory strategies and use her right hand more easily, especially while completing ADLs. Lisa achieved these outcomes with only two trips to the clinic and without therapist travel.
José is a 35-year-old administrative assistant working at an urban university. He has been employed in this position for 5 years. Recently, he began experiencing discomfort in his neck, shoulder, and back areas. He reported this discomfort, which he associated with computer work, to his immediate supervisor.	Josh scheduled an appointment with an occupational therapist who had expertise in ergonomic workstation evaluation. During his initial contact with the occupational therapist, he requested that because of his busy schedule, he would prefer to have his evaluation conducted through telehealth technology. The occupational therapist asked Josh to have photographs taken of him while working at his office computer workstation. The occupational therapist requested that the photographs be from multiple angles and then e-mailed to a secure platform, where the therapist would be able to review them. In addition, Josh was asked to keep a time log for a week into which he would input information on his activities along with when he experienced discomfort. A telephone consultation was arranged, during which the occupational therapist reviewed findings from the photographs along with the time log. Josh reported on the time log that he sat at his computer workstation 100% of the time during the work day. During this time, he multitasked by using a hand-held telephone while keying. It was observed from the photographs that Josh was using a notebook computer, which placed him in an awkward posture for computing.	Explicit workstation modification recommendations were provided by the occupational therapist by means of a telephone consultation with Josh. The recommendations included raising the notebook computer so that his head was not positioned in flexion or extension and that the monitor was about arm's length away (closed fist) and using a keyboard and mouse as input devices. An adjustable keyboard tray was recommended for the keyboard and mouse. On the basis of data from the time log, the occupational therapist encouraged Josh to change his work behaviors by taking regular stretch breaks every 20 minutes. A second telephone consultation occurred within 2 weeks. Josh reported that his supervisor ordered the external notebook computer accessories and that this new workstation arrangement had reduced his discomfort.

(Continued)

Appendix D. Telehealth Case Examples *(Cont.)*

CASE DESCRIPTION	USE OF TELEHEALTH	OUTCOME
Angela is a 10-year-old girl with a complicated medical history that includes spina bifida. She is significantly limited in her ability to be mobile in the home and community. Although she uses a basic power wheelchair to drive around town and attend her family activities, it is in poor condition and too small for her. Angela cannot adequately reposition herself or properly perform a weight shift because of decreased upper-extremity strength and range of motion.	Angela has trouble traveling and sitting for long distances. She and her mother meet with an occupational therapy generalist in person at a nearby clinic. Concurrently, an occupational therapist who has expertise in wheeled mobility participates in an occupational therapy session remotely using a videoconferencing system. The remote occupational therapist provides consultation to the local occupational therapist, Angela, and her mother about seating system frames, bases, and accessories; policy implications and funding mechanisms; and wheeled mobility and seating options.	After interviewing Angela and her mother and observing Angela navigate in her current chair, the remote occupational therapist recommends the appropriate power wheelchair and power seat functions. Upon approval from the insurance company, the remote occupational therapist uses the videoconferencing system to monitor the delivery, evaluate the fitting, and provide feedback and advice to Angela about use of the wheelchair within the community and home. Angela has benefited from services without the need to travel a long distance. The local practitioner gained additional knowledge about wheeled mobility and seating options.
Ethan is a 55-year-old self-employed entrepreneur who has severe depression, anxiety, and isolation after head and neck cancer resection surgery. The surgery left one side of his face disfigured. He plans to have reconstructive surgery in the future. Meanwhile, Ethan has difficulties with eating, fatigue, facial–body image, depression, and pain. He lives alone and over 50 minutes away from the hospital/outpatient therapy clinic. Ethan was seen by an occupational therapist in the hospital and prescribed outpatient occupational therapy for his physical and mental impairments. Due to travel distance to the outpatient therapy clinic and anxiety associated with being seen in public, Ethan is interested in the option to continue his therapy at home through secure videoconferencing technology.	Ethan completed a telehealth participation screening and initial occupational therapy evaluation during his hospital stay. It was determined that he would continue with occupational therapy twice a week via telehealth using secure videoconferencing software and a Web camera within his home environment. During the biweekly occupational therapy sessions delivered via telehealth technologies, focus is on establishing a therapeutic wellness plan and implementing compensatory eating techniques, pain management and relaxation techniques, stress management, and engagement in progressive physical activities. Ethan completes a home program and a daily journal sent to him by his occupational therapist through electronic communications technology.	Ethan is able to manage his physical and mental impairments and is able to leave his house to purchase groceries and complete other errands in his community. His pain is tolerable, and breathing and stamina have improved to allow 20–30 minutes of physical activity after 6 weeks of occupational therapy delivered through telehealth technologies. Ethan continues his daily journaling. The occupational therapist will follow up with Ethan via telehealth technologies weekly until reconstruction surgery and again after surgery to make sure Ethan continues his wellness plan.

Part VI. The Scholarship of Occupation-Based and Evidence-Based Practice

The particular objects for which the corporation is formed are as follows: the advancement of occupation as a therapeutic measure; for the study of the effect of occupation upon the human being; and for the scientific dispensation of this knowledge.

—National Society for the Promotion of Occupational Therapy (1917, p. 2)

The American Occupational Therapy Association (AOTA; 2007) envisions that as the occupational therapy profession enters its second century, it will be "a powerful, widely recognized, science-driven, and evidence-based profession . . . meeting society's occupational needs" (p. 614). The similarities between AOTA's *Centennial Vision* and the above incorporation statement of the National Society for the Promotion of Occupational Therapy at the inception of the profession in 1917 are striking. Both visions strongly emphasize occupation and science. These parallels were explored in-depth in Schwartz's (2009) seminal Eleanor Clarke Slagle Lecture, which highlighted that the scholarship of occupation is not a new concept.

Throughout occupational therapy's history, many of the profession's leaders advocated for practice to be informed by science (Ayres, 1963; Dunn, 2001; Dunton, 1918, 1934; Farber, 1989; Fiorentino, 1975; Forsyth, Summerfield Mann, & Kielhofner, 2005; Gillette, 1991; Licht, 1946; Nelson, 1996; Noble, 1937; Pollock, 1929; Reed, 1986; Rood, 1958; Smith, 1963; Stattel, 1956; Trombly, 1995 [see Chapter 11]). Most of the literature consistently called for research to include partnerships between the profession's scholars and practitioners. Table VI.1 provides a small sample of statements made during the first 50 years of the profession about the vital need for occupational therapy to establish a solid scientific base for practice. Exhibit VI.1 shows a still-valid outline of the relevance of statistics to occupational therapy published in 1929 (see Active Reflection VI.1).

Although the call to establish the science of occupational therapy has been expressed globally since the profession's earliest years, this invitation was not widely accepted. For many decades, a gulf between science and practice

prevailed (Ilott, 2012; Kielhofner, 2005; Lin, Murphy, & Robinson, 2010). However, in recent years this dichotomy has been more strongly challenged and several conceptual frameworks and practical guidelines for integrating scholarship into practice have been published (Fleming-Castaldy & Gillen, 2013; Forsyth et al., 2005; Ilott, 2003; Kielhofner, 2005; Lin et al., 2010; Sudsawad, 2005).

The richness of research material and its application to treatment techniques has been slow to seep to the therapy level.

—Rood (1958, p. 328)

Most significant to the advancement of the scholarship of practice in the United States has been the institution of a postbaccalaureate degree as the required educational level for occupational therapists and the concurrent establishment of educational standards for entry-level curricula to include the development of competencies for research and evidence-based practice (EBP; Accreditation Council for Occupational Therapy Education [ACOTE®], 2012).

Table VI.1. Historical Perspectives on the Scholarship of Practice

Decade	Representative Quote
1910s	"The patient should be carefully studied" (Dunton, 1918, p. 320). Dunton (1918) called for occupational therapy practitioners to devise "instruments or methods by which outcomes could be measured so that the work could be brought into accordance with the current scientific and systematic values of medicine."
1920s	"It was planned to use the same schedule so that the data derived therefrom might be compared and combined not only in state hospital systems and other state institutions but in all institutions where occupational therapy is used" (Pollock, 1929, p. 419). "In contrast, think of the time and money which has been expended on investigating the action of this or that drug, think of the discussions, many of them fruitless, which have waged round the use of hypnotism, suggestion, psychoanalysis, the action of endocrines etc., and yet a topic of the importance of occupation has never previously been considered worthy of an afternoon's discussion by any division of the Medico-Psychological Association. Why has this been so? In my opinion, it has been due to the fact that occupational therapy has been regarded from the utilitarian and economic point of view, and the curative aspect, if considered at all, has largely been lost sight of" (Henderson, Thomson, Brodie, & Robertson, 1925).
1930s	"Occupational therapy aims to furnish a scheme of scientifically arranged activities." (Kidner, 1932, p. 234). "It should be remembered that without a record of the data, the value of the work accomplished may be questioned since it is not available for the use of others unless put in proper written form" (Dunton, 1934, p. 328). "In order to fully emphasize its value in rebuilding and developing the personality, the approach of each therapist must be on a sound scientific basis. The continued application of occupational therapy must also be on this same basis. If the treatment and its reaction, successful or unsuccessful, of every patient is recorded carefully, no matter in what type of work or activity he is engaged, eventually there will be a sufficient collection of data to make possible the selection of the most appropriate application" (Noble, 1937, p. 107).
1940s	"The crying need today is for more statistical and general information regarding costs, case loads, types of cases treated and results based on the records we have kept. Scientific research is of equal importance" (Committee on Scientific Study and Research, 1941, p. 411). "Scientific method must be applied to occupational therapy if its continued acceptance is desired. The scientific method includes the orderly arrangement of significant facts in an attempt to establish causal relationships. When such relationships are checked by adequate controls truth is established." (Licht, 1946, p. 17).
1950s	"As each selected field of occupational therapy seeks to improve its clinical application, it is earnestly hoped that more questions will be the result" (Stattel, 1956, p. 198). "I have also great respect for Occupational Therapy as a research tool. It is under the test of Occupational Therapy that specific difficulties come to light, and an intelligent occupational therapist can go far in analyzing their scientific nature and significance" (Dott, 1958, p. 7). "The desire to verify and extend the implications drawn from such analyses has led occupational therapists to an interest in empirical research methods. Illustrative of this interest was the 1954 research symposium at which occupational therapists, psychologists, and physicians of national repute collaborated to outline promising research techniques and potentially fruitful areas for investigation" (Phillip, Helen, & James, 1959, p. 16).
1960s	"Occupational therapy has much face validity, testimonials as to its merits, acceptance as a form of treatment, but is it inclined, perhaps to engage in repetitive practice as against scrutinizing basic concepts and theoretical problems? Should it remain the handmaiden of psychiatry or should it take the longer and more difficult way to professional maturity by means of research, using the best consultative advice, training suitable individuals, re-orientating the training curricula and pressing for grants to carry out research projects? What are its limits and potentialities? And can it take on the task of scientific validation?" (Smith, 1963, p. 20).

Internationally, postbaccalaureate programs, professional associations, and national and local policies require occupational therapy practitioners to develop and apply competencies for EBP (Forsyth et al., 2005; Glegg & Holsti, 2010; Ilott, 2012; World Federation of Occupational Therapists, 2008). Those educated to engage in scientific inquiry and use evidence can contribute their acquired knowledge, skills, and attitudes to effectively bridge the gap between science and practice (Fleming-Castaldy & Gillen, 2013). Although the scholarship of practice and scholarly practice are sometimes equated, they do differ. *Scholarly practice* involves using the knowledge base of the profession or discipline in one's practice" (AOTA, 2009, p. 790, italics added). It is comprised of EBP, which

Exhibit VI.1. Principal Purposes of Statistics in Occupational Therapy

1. To furnish definite bases for comparison of related concurrent facts.
2. To enable comparisons to be made of data relative to the same class of phenomena compiled for different periods of time.
3. To reveal laws underlying phenomena that could not be determined by individual observations.
4. To show trends in phenomena that otherwise would be undiscoverable.
5. To reveal relations of cause and effect that otherwise would remain hidden.
6. To serve as a guide for administrative, legislative, social, and commercial action.
7. To reveal success or failure and thus become true indices of progress.

Note. From "The Need, Value, and General Principles of Occupational Therapy Statistics," by H. Pollock, 1929, *Occupational Therapy and Rehabilitation,* Vol. 7, p. 417.

includes scientific inquiry *and* theory (AOTA, 2009; Forsyth et al., 2005; Illot, 2004). The scholarship of practice is a component of the field's overall and multifaceted research. The multiple dimensions of scholarship in occupational therapy are clearly articulated in AOTA's (2009) official document, *Scholarship in Occupational Therapy,* which is outlined in Table VI.2.

Part VI provides seminal works that promote the advancement of scholarship in occupational therapy. Although diverse viewpoints are presented, all authors share a commitment to engagement in scholarly inquiry that can best inform occupation-based practice. Each work highlights the need for research that contributes to our knowledge base about the validity and efficacy of therapeutic occupation and the meaningfulness of occupation.

> *New therapists should be encouraged to continue research activity and undertake projects of suitable size to fit workload thus allowing research to become part of a normal working pattern and not slip into the realms of esoteric possibility that someone else may make into reality.*
> —Ravetz (1987, p. 255)

The first chapter contains Holm's oft-cited 2000 Eleanor Clarke Slagle Lecture. In this presentation, Holm critically examines occupational therapy's lack of evi-

Table VI.2. Scholarship in Occupational Therapy

Type	Description	Role of Practitioner in Scholarship
Scholarship of discovery	Engagement in original research that leads to the development or creation of new knowledge that contributes to expanding the knowledge base of the profession.	Contribute to the improved understanding of the constructs and processes of the profession (e.g., occupation and its therapeutic use) through participation in empirical and historical research and theory development and philosophical inquiry.
Scholarship of integration	Concerned with making creative connections both within and across disciplines to integrate, synthesize, interpret, and create new perspectives and theories.	Contribute to the improved understanding of the profession's theoretical base via transdisciplinary inquiry across a range of theories, practice areas, techniques, and methodologies.
Scholarship of application	Application of the knowledge generated by scholarship of discovery or integration to address real problems at all levels of society.	Establish evidence concerning the reliability, validity, and utility of an assessment tool or outcome measure and the efficacy of a specific intervention. Appropriately use assessments, outcome measures, or interventions on the basis of the strength of the evidence.
Scholarship of teaching and learning	The systematic study of teaching or learning and the public sharing and review of such work through professional forums.	Develop and use evidence in client education to support participation in meaningful occupations. Challenge occupational therapy educators to find better ways to prepare diverse students to be competent professionals who advance the profession. Empirically determine and apply better instructional methodologies to prepare students to meet the demands of a rapidly changing and increasingly complex health care environment.

Note. Adapted from "Scholarship in Occupational Therapy," by the American Occupational Therapy Association, 2009, *American Journal of Occupational Therapy,* Vol. 63, pp. 790–796. Copyright © 2009 by the American Occupational Therapy Association. Used with permission.

dence demonstrating that the profession's practices are valid or effective. The inability to provide data supportive of occupational therapy interventions presents several ethical dilemmas as practitioners provide services based on limited evidence. Holm begins her discussion by examining the changes that have occurred in the health care environment, which have affected how occupational therapy services are provided. Most significant has been the increased emphasis on the need to justify service through the provision of evidence that supports what occupational therapy practitioners do in daily practice. Holm asserts that this societal press for EBP is one to which practitioners must respond, if occupational therapy is to remain a viable profession.

Holm defines *EBP* and provides a clear overview of the standards used to measure the strength of evidence. Holm contends that a practitioner's confidence level in his or her clinical decisions should be congruent with the best current evidence available on the given intervention. Strength of evidence for occupational therapy intervention is examined along a five-level hierarchy (see Active Reflection VI.2). Concrete examples and realistic clinical scenarios highlight the implications of Holm's key points for everyday practice, emphasizing the relevance and need for "in-the-trenches" practitioners to use EBP. The critical difference between preferred practice and EBP is emphasized.

> *We need records and statistics to promote the advance of the profession and to establish a firm scientific basis for the various procedures we are using. I realize that this need is hard to satisfy. Scientific truth is established with great difficulty.*
> —Pollock (1929, p. 416)

Holm's stance that the acquisition of evidence to support best practices must be conducted in actual practice settings (and not in isolated ivory towers) is particularly important when one considers that other health care professionals are reporting evidence on their function-oriented practices (Gillen, 2013 [see Chapter 63]; Gutman, 1998; Langhammer & Stanghelle, 2011; Rensink, Schuurmans, Lindeman, & Hafsteinsdóttir, 2009; Wood, 1998). The existence of professional competition cannot be ignored (Clark, 2010). The resulting press for all occupational therapy practitioners to increase their research competencies to ensure our profession's survival is well supported throughout Holm's treatise.

To help practitioners develop and integrate these abilities with active clinical reasoning, Holm poses five

questions. She suggests that affirmative answers to these questions indicate positive steps toward EBP. Holm honestly addresses systemic and personal barriers to EBP, reframing them as sources of motivation. She concludes by challenging all occupational therapy practitioners to take the ethical step of advancing the profession by ensuring their practice is based on solid evidence. Holm's call for research remains timely as the societal demand for research to support what we do and how we do it justifiably persists (Fleming-Castaldy & Gillen, 2013).

As Owens (1964) argued a half-century ago,

> How much more do we now know then we knew then, as to why certain methods and certain devices are superior to others in the treatment of particular patients? Have we proved beyond reasonable doubt that this apparatus was wholly advantageous to the patient? That it was unrivalled by other means in achieving the specific aim of treatment? What steps are we taking to establish our premises on the firm ground of careful and critical research rather than on the sand of complacent surmise? NOT MUCH AND NOT ENOUGH must be our answer if we face the facts with honesty and courage. (pp. 1–2)

Since the publication of Holm's lecture on EBP, the hierarchical model she presented has become widely accepted with systemic reviews and randomized clinical trials (RCTs) being promoted as essential to the profession's research base (Dierette, Rozich, & Viau, 2009; Gutman, 2009a, 2009b; Ilott, 2012; Shaw & Shaw, 2011). EBP is globally expected of practitioners (Bennett & Bennett, 2000; Curtin & Jaramazovic, 2001; Cusick & McCluskey, 2000; Glegg & Holsti, 2010; Ilott, 2012), infused in the profession's codes of ethics (AOTA, 2010; Canadian Association of Occupational Therapists, 2007; College of

---

Active Reflection VI.2. Hierarchy of Evidence for Occupation-Based Practice

Consider the levels of evidence outlined in Table 49.1, and reflect on your knowledge of occupational therapy.

- Which foundational aspects of occupation-based practice may be difficult to quantify to attain the highest levels of evidence?
- What are the implications for the profession if key tools of practice (e.g., the conscious use of self, narrative reasoning) are not supported by high levels of scientific evidence?
- What are the research alternatives for determining the efficacy of the aspects of practice that do not lend themselves to an experimental design?

Occupational Therapists, 2010), and embedded in the curriculum of occupational therapy education programs (ACOTE, 2012; Cusick & McCluskey, 2000).

Calls for EBP using the highest level of evidence are prevalent in the literature (Dierette et al., 2009; Gutman, 2009a, 2009b; Shaw & Shaw, 2011). Despite broad-based endorsement of the EBP pyramid, concerns have been raised about the singular use of this hierarchy to support occupational therapy practice. The reality that occupation-based, client-centered practice requires more than the integration of empirical scientific studies must be acknowledged (Frantis, 2005; Hinojosa, 2007, 2013; Ilott, 2004; Reagon, Bellin, & Boniface, 2010; Turner, 2007). Worthy of consideration is the view that the hierarchical model's relegation of qualitative research to the lowest level of evidence diminishes the contributions of the dynamic, holistic, and humanistic nature of occupational therapy (Reagon et al., 2010; Tomlin & Borgetto, 2011). According to Sackett, Strauss, Richardson, Rosenberg, and Haynes (2000), *EBP* is "the integration of best research evidence *with clinical expertise and patient values*" (p. 1, italics added). Although Holm does incorporate these considerations in her discussion, the most lasting influence of her seminal lecture is the hierarchy of evidence she presented.

The development of a body of knowledge in a professional carries with it considerable personal responsibility for making both rationale (scientific) judgments and intuitive (artistic) decisions.
—Yerxa (1967, p. 2)

An exemplar of the critical discourse which the hierarchical model of evidence has generated is presented in this part's next chapter by Tickle-Degnen and Bedell. The authors reflect on their thought processes, which led them as scholars and practitioners to realize that the exclusive use of any model in occupational therapy was inappropriate given the complexity and variety of the phenomenon with which the field's practitioners work. They discuss their shared concerns about the potential impact of the widely accepted EBP hierarchy on clinical decision making, if these rankings are used exclusively to guide clinical decisions. Tickle-Degnen and Bedell assert that a sole reliance on the hierarchical model limits consideration of available valid information that is relevant to a needed decision. As a result, suboptimal decisions might be made by practitioners who use only the evidence provided in the standard five-level evidence pyramid.

Active Reflection VI.3. Patterns and Possibility

Review the literature to find an RCT about an area of occupational therapy that most interests you.
- What evidence does this work provide to guide your practice?
- What facets of the study's focus could be enhanced by the use of a heterarchical approach to inquiry?

Consider the population used in this RCT and identify methods that could be used to acquire information about participant patterns and possibility.

Describe how the knowledge you seek can be used to enhance the scholarship of practice.

Tickle-Degnen and Bedell note that the most recent definition of *evidence-based medicine* includes the integration of the best available evidence with established clinical expertise and client perspectives. Tickle-Degnen and Bedell contend that the lack of consideration of these factors and overreliance on the EBP pyramid negates qualitative research. They clearly articulate the value of knowledge beyond the causality and probability provided in this hierarchy to include the gathering and use of information about patterns (e.g., client perceptions, characteristics, contexts, occupational profiles) and possibility (e.g., available options, potential outcomes).

Tickle-Degnen and Bedell assert that causality, probability, patterns, and possibility are equally important; therefore, each should be considered when making clinical decisions. Through a realistic case example, they illustrate how using their inclusionary approach to assess, select, and use research information in a heterarchical (not hierarchical) manner can effectively inform clinical decision making. This inclusive, flexible, and multifaceted approach can support the scholarship of practice in multiple ways. It can be used to understand diverse sources of information beyond research and be readily applied to many types of clinical decisions, not just those related to intervention (see Active Reflection VI.3).

Through science, the therapeutic value of occupation can be predicted and explained, but purposefulness of an occupational process cannot be measured and explained through research. Thus, the purposefulness of occupation will always remain as our art.
—Gilfoyle (1984, pp. 578–579)

In Chapter 51, Lee and Miller expand on the stance that clinical decision making must be informed by multiple sources of knowledge. They contend that occupational therapy practitioners should not use definitions of *EBP* that have been put forth by experts in evidence-based medicine, because these definitions identify research as the sole source of evidence. Although Lee and Miller recognize the excellence of these definitions and the value of research, they argue that any definition of *EBP* used to guide occupational therapy practice must reflect the contextual nature of the occupational therapy process. As a result, the experiences, beliefs, values, and knowledge of the practitioner and client must be accepted as valuable sources of evidence and thereby included in the definition of *EBP* (see Active Reflection VI.4).

To support their assertion, Lee and Miller contrast the standardized procedures used in medicine with the highly contextual and dynamic nature of the occupational therapy process. Each discipline also views the role of the individual quite differently. Medicine places people receiving services in a passive recipient role, but occupational therapy considers each person to be unique and equal in a collaborative therapeutic relationship. The implications of these differences are clear. EBP in occupational therapy must recognize the variety of evidence brought by the person and practitioner to the clinical context.

Lee and Miller review and critique classical views about methods of judging evidence. They conclude that the methods of appraising belief can provide a unique classification for the different types of evidence that the therapeutic relationship brings to occupational therapy interventions. Lee and Miller provide thoughtful reflections on possible beliefs and perspectives of the person and practitioner that should be considered when evaluating the potential outcome of an occupational therapy intervention. They present an evidence matrix that summarizes the varieties of evidence methods and perspectives that should be considered during the occupational therapy process. An overview of the process of evidence-based, clinical decision making is provided in an illustration, with the authors emphasizing a dynamic approach to integrating evidence. Lee and Miller describe four strategies—(1) intrusion, (2) parsimony, (3) consensual validation, and (4) cross validation—that can be flexibly applied to diverse evidence, highlighting the continuous and often circular nature of evidence-based, clinical decision making.

> *We are dealing with persons, not cases, and with this firmly fixed in our minds we shall be more likely to find a solution. In reality these considerations should often have the first place in our minds and the medical picture the second.*
>
> —Varrier-Jone (1941, p. 368)

Active Reflection VI.4. The Contextualized Nature of Research

Reflect on the RCT that you analyzed in Active Reflection VI.3.
- What context was the focus of this study?
- What additional contextual information would be helpful to obtain to better inform practice in this area? Explain your reasoning.
- What are the benefits to occupational therapy in broadening the definition of *EBP* to include beliefs, perspectives, and contexts?

Lee and Miller's conclusion that all research paradigms and designs add value to the scholarship of practice and that the client's perspectives and experiences should be integrated into all clinical decisions is strongly supported in this part's next chapter. In this work, Hammell examines the congruence between qualitative research and client-centered practice. As she notes, qualitative research has become an increasingly accepted method of inquiry, because it contributes to occupational therapy's knowledge base about issues that are important and relevant to clients. Although qualitative research by its very nature is personal, creative, and fluid, Hammell cautions that standards must be met to ensure that studies are appropriate, relevant, and meaningful. However, the rigid rules that are used to design and critique quantitative studies do not apply to qualitative methods. Hammell addresses the lack of explicit guidance available to help consumers of research determine the strength, credibility, and usefulness of qualitative research. Because occupational therapy research is meant to inform the profession's theoretical base and improve its practice, critical scrutiny of all types of scholarly inquiry is required.

Hammell contends that qualitative research can be rigorous even though it is not prescriptive. She reflects on the assumptions that underlie qualitative inquiry and the assessment of its quality and identifies the criteria of authenticity and plausibility as most pertinent to evaluating qualitative research. Integrating the work of numerous qualitative theorists and researchers, Hammell presents an evaluative framework that includes 14 general points to consider to satisfy the standards of *authenticity* (i.e., reliability and trustworthiness) and *plausibility* (i.e., seemingly probable, relevant, and appropriate). She discusses every point and provides targeted questions to use to assess the quality of research according to each criterion. Potential researchers who actively reflect on these questions and apply this framework in the design of qualitative studies will ensure their research methods are appropriate and complete.

> **Active Reflection VI.5. The Quality of Qualitative Research**
>
> Review the literature to find a qualitative study about an area of occupational therapy that most interests you. Critique the authenticity and plausibility of this research using Hammell's evaluative framework.
> - Which criteria are met and which need to be strengthened to improve the credibility, trustworthiness, relevance, and usefulness of this study?

> **Active Reflection VI.6. Politics, Power, and Research**
>
> Consider the qualitative study that you analyzed in Active Reflection VI.5.
> - What are the political structures and power relationships evident in this study?
> - Did the researcher actively involve participants in the study design and implementation?
> If yes, explain how it strengthened the study. If no, describe the potential impact of the lack of participant involvement on the study.
> - Discuss how this study could be strengthened to be congruent with client-centered and occupation-based research.

Throughout her discussion, Hammell emphasizes the vital role of the research participant. She directly addresses the power issues that arise in traditional research paradigms. Hammell asserts that if occupational therapy practitioners and researchers are truly committed to the profession's client-centered approach, they must actively seek participant involvement throughout the research process (see Active Reflection VI.5).

> *Each must contribute at his own level so that the whole may be more complete, since each with different background and interests will see different facets of the same problem.*
>
> —Rood (1958, p. 328)

The need for occupational therapy researchers to partner with clients when establishing research agendas and designing and completing research studies is explored in depth in this part's final chapter. Hammell, Miller, Forwell, Forman, and Jacobsen challenge occupational therapy practitioners and researchers to acknowledge the reality that typically the profession's research is not conducted in a client-centered manner. This incongruence between occupational therapy's stated philosophy and actual practices disempowers clients and diminishes the value of the field's research. Conversely, Hammell et al. contend that research conducted in a collaborative manner is conceptually consistent with client-centered and occupation-based practice. Hence, it is better research with increased relevance and greater impact.

To help readers consciously reflect on how power differentials affect research studies, Hammell et al. compare and contrast traditional researcher-centered research with client-centered collaborative research. According to Hammell et al., the latter methodology realigns power as researchers and participants equally contribute their respective expertise. The resulting collaborative research ensures that studies are "informed by, and relevant to, clients' lives, values and priorities"

(Chapter 53). The authors support their argument with pertinent examples from the occupational therapy research literature and challenge the profession to focus identifying and removing barriers to collaborative research. Hammell et al. maintain that the research's politics and power dynamics must be addressed for occupational therapy research to move beyond the rhetoric of client-centered practice and actualize these foundational principles in practice (see Active Reflection VI.6).

> *Perhaps most significant for the future development of our body of knowledge is the increased awareness that the scientific attitude is not incompatible with concern for the client as a human being but may be one of the best foundations for acting on that concern.*
>
> —Yerxa (1967, p. 1)

Occupational therapy practitioners are ethically bound to actively seek and critically review new theoretical and scientific information and continuously and consciously integrate this acquired knowledge into their work to ensure the provision of client-centered, evidence-based, and occupation-based practice (AOTA, 2009, 2010; Fleming-Castaldy & Gillen, 2013; Kielhofner, 2005). Using empirical, qualitative, and theoretical research to guide practice is a professional responsibility (AOTA, 2009; Forsyth et al., 2005; Reed, 1986); therefore, a culture shift from a profession based on tradition to one informed by evidence is needed (Fleming-Castaldy & Gillen, 2013). To attain this goal, professional association resources, case-based workshops, small-group projects, expert facilitators, journal clubs, and the implementation of the clear steps and concrete strategies for implementing EBP provided by Lin et al. can be helpful. Appendix VI.A, "Guide to Evaluating Research Evidence: Guiding Questions," outlines Lin et al.'s guiding questions for the evaluation of quantitative research. Easily accessible resources to obtain and appraise evidence are provided in Appendix V.I.B. Conscious application of these suggestions and assertive use of the information provided in this part's chapters can foster effective collaborations among practitioners, theorists, and researchers to advance the scholarship of occupational therapy across practice settings and nations (Forsyth et al., 2005; Illot, 2012; Kielhofner, 2005; Lin et al., 2010).

> *Constantly the question must be put, 'Why did I fail?' and 'Why did I succeed?'*
>
> —Noble (1937, p. 107)

Active reflection on the critical discourses provided in this section and those provided in Part III, "Contextual Considerations for Engagement in Occupation and Participation," are needed to ensure the profession remains true to its ethos and does not marginalize the personal, cultural, social, and political contexts of occupational therapy (Papadimitriou, Magasi, & Frank, 2012; Peloquin, 2005 [see Chapter 62]). These considerations are essential to practice based on scholarship because the contemporary definition of *EBP* retains "the triad identified by the pioneers, namely research, patient choice, and practitioner wisdom . . . [and] also recognizes the criticality of the context, especially competing priorities, resource constraints and the myriad differences between settings, populations, countries, and people" (Ilott, 2012, p. 2).

Given the complexities of implementing scholarship-informed, client-centered, evidence-based, and occupation-based practice, the final part of this text includes seminal works on the challenges to and the opportunities for the envisioned future of the profession.

> *Therapists should themselves know more about their subject. As an interested observer for many years standing it has been a pleasure to see how our knowledge of occupational therapy has increased . . . . This is largely due to the interest and spirit of investigation which has actuated so many therapists. That such investigations will have value to those making them should be self-evident, but should there be a therapist who has not done some bit of research, if he or she will only do so I am sure that at its conclusion he or she will find that his or her knowledge and ability have increased and, therefore, his or her professional value.*
>
> —Dunton (1934, p. 328)

References

Accreditation Council for Occupational Therapy Education. (2012). 2011 Accreditation Council for Occupational Therapy Education (ACOTE®) standards. *American Journal of Occupational Therapy, 66*(Suppl.), S6–S74. http://dx.doi.org/10.5014/ajot.2012.66S6

American Occupational Therapy Association. (2007). AOTA's *Centennial Vision* and executive summary. *American Journal of Occupational Therapy, 61*, 613–614. http://dx.doi.org/10.5014/ajot.61.6.613

American Occupational Therapy Association. (2009). Scholarship in occupational therapy. *American Journal of Occupational Therapy, 63*, 790–796. http://dx.doi.org/10.5014/ajot.63.6.790

American Occupational Therapy Association. (2010). Occupational therapy code of ethics and ethics standards (2010). *American Journal of Occupational Therapy, 64*, S17–S26. http://dx.doi.org/10.5014/ajot.2010.64S17

Ayres, A. J. (1963). The development of perceptual–motor abilities: A theoretical basis for treatment of dysfunction [Eleanor Clarke Slagle Lecture]. *American Journal of Occupational Therapy, 17*, 221–225.

Bennett, S., & Bennett, J. (2000). The process of evidence-based practice in occupational therapy: Informing clinical decisions. *Australian Journal of Occupational Therapy, 47*, 171–180. http://dx.doi.org/10.1046/j.1440-1630.2000.00237.x

Canadian Association of Occupational Therapists. (2007). *Canadian Association of Occupational Therapists code of ethics.* Retrieved from http://www.caot.ca/default.asp?pageid=35

Clark, F. A. (2010). Power and confidence in professions: Lessons for occupational therapy. *Canadian Journal of Occupational Therapy, 77*, 264–269. http://dx.doi.org/10.2182/cjot.2010.77.5.2

College of Occupational Therapists. (2010). *Code of ethics and professional conduct.* Retrieved from http://www.cot.org.uk/homepage/publications/?l=l&ListItemID=393&ListGroupID=248.

Committee on Scientific Study and Research. (1941). Committee reports: Committee on Scientific Study and Research American Occupational Therapy Association. *Occupational Therapy and Rehabilitation, 20*(6), 409–412.

Cooper, A. (1941, Spring). Some reflections on occupational therapy. *Occupational Therapy,* pp. 9–12.

Curtin, M., & Jaramazovic, E. (2001). Occupational therapists' views and perceptions of evidence-based practice. *British Journal of Occupational Therapy, 64,* 214–222.

Cusick, A., & McCluskey, A. (2000). Becoming an evidence-based practitioner through professional development. *Australian Occupational Therapy Journal, 47,* 159–170. http://dx.doi.org/10.1046/j.1440-1630.2000.00241.x

Dierette, D., Rozich, A., & Viau, S. (2009). The Issue Is— Is there enough evidence for evidence-based practice in occupational therapy? *American Journal of Occupational Therapy, 63,* 782–786.

Dott, N. (1958). Twenty-fifth anniversary congress of the SAOT: Opening address. *Scottish Journal of Occupational Therapy, 32,* 6–8.

Dunn, W. (2001). The sensations of everyday life: Empirical, theoretical, and pragmatic considerations [Eleanor Clarke Slagle Lecture]. *American Journal of Occupational Therapy, 55,* 608–620.

Dunton, W. R. (1918). The principles of occupational therapy. *Public Health Nurse, 18,* 316–332. http://dx.doi.org/10.1097/00000446-195102000-00069

Dunton, W. R. (1934). The need for and value of research in occupational therapy. *Occupational Therapy and Rehabilitation, 13,* 325–328.

Farber, S. (1989). Neuroscience and occupational therapy: Vital connections [Eleanor Clarke Slagle Lecture]. *American Journal of Occupational Therapy, 43,* 637–646.

Fiorentino, M. (1975). Occupational therapy: Realization to activation [Eleanor Clarke Slagle Lecture]. *American Journal of Occupational Therapy, 29,* 15–21.

Fleming-Castaldy, R. P., & Gillen, G. (2013). The Issue Is—Ensuring that education, certification, and practice are evidence based. *American Journal of Occupational Therapy, 67,* 364–369. http://dx.doi.org/10.5014/ajot.2013.006973

Forsyth, K., Summerfield Mann, L., & Kielhofner, G. (2005). Scholarship of practice: Making occupation-focused, theory-driven, evidence-based practice as a reality. *British Journal of Occupational Therapy, 68,* 260–268.

Frantis, L. (2005). The Issue Is—Nothing about us without us: Searching for the narrative of disability. *American Journal of Occupational Therapy, 59,* 577–579. http://dx/doi.org/10.5014/ajot.59.5.577

Gilfoyle, E. (1984). Transformation of a profession [Eleanor Clarke Slagle Lecture]. *American Journal of Occupational Therapy, 38,* 575–584. http://dx.doi.org/10.5014/ajot.38.9.575

Gillen, G. (2013). A fork in the road: An occupational hazard. *American Journal of Occupational Therapy, 67,* 641–652. http://dx.doi.org/10.5014/ajot.2013.676002 Reprinted as Chapter 63.

Gillette, N. (1991). The Issue Is—Research directions for occupational therapy. *American Journal of Occupational Therapy, 45,* 563–565. http://dx.doi.org/10.5014/ajot.45.6.563

Glegg, S. M. N., & Holsti, L. (2010). Measures of knowledge and skills for evidence-based practice: A systematic review. *Canadian Journal of Occupational Therapy, 77,* 219–232. http://dx.doi.org/10.2182/cjot.2010.77.4.4

Gutman, S. (1998). The Issue Is—Domain of function: Who's got it? Who's competing for it? *American Journal of Occupational Therapy, 52,* 684–689. http://dx.doi.org/10.5014/ajot.52.8.684

Gutman, S. (2009a). From the Desk of the Editor—Why haven't we generated sufficient evidence? Part I: Barriers to applied research. *American Journal of Occupational Therapy, 63,* 235–237. http://dx.doi.org/10.5014/ajot.63.3.235

Gutman, S. (2009b). From the Desk of the Editor—Why haven't we generated sufficient evidence? Part II: Building our evidence. *American Journal of Occupational Therapy, 63,* 383–385. http://dx.doi.org/10.5014/ajot.63.4.383

Henderson, D. K., Thomson, A., Brodie, M., & Robertson, D. (1925). Occupational therapy: A series of papers. *Journal of Mental Science, 71,* 59–80. http://dx.doi.org/10.1192/bjp.71.292.59

Hinojosa, J. (2007). Becoming innovators in an era of hyperchange [Eleanor Clarke Slagle Lecture]. *American Journal of Occupational Therapy, 61,* 629–637. http://dx.doi.org/10.5014/ajot.61.6.629

Hinojosa, J. (2013). The evidence-based paradox. *American Journal of Occupational Therapy, 67*(2), e18–e23. http://dx.doi.org/10.5014/ajot.2013.005587

Ilott, I. (2003). Challenging the rhetoric and reality: Only an individual and systemic approach will work for evidence-based occupational therapy. *American Journal of Occupational Therapy, 57,* 351–354. http://dx.doi.org/10.5014/ajot.57.3.351

Ilott, I. (2004). Evidence-based practice forum: Challenges and strategic solutions for a research emergent profession. *American Journal of Occupational Therapy, 58,* 347–352.

Ilott, I. (2012). Evidence-based practice: A critical appraisal. *Occupational Therapy International, 19*(1), 1–6. http://dx.doi.org/10.1002/oti.1322

Kidner, T. B. (1932). Occupational therapy: Its aims and developments. *Occupational Therapy and Rehabilitation, 11,* 233–240.

Kielhofner, G. (2005). A scholarship of practice: Creating discourse between theory, research and practice. *Oc-*

cupational Therapy in Health Care, 19, 7–15. http://dx. doi.org/10.1300/J003v19n01_02

Langhammer, B., & Stanghelle, J. K. (2011). Can physiotherapy after stroke based on the Bobath concept result in improved quality of movement compared to the motor relearning programme? Physiotherapy Research International, 16, 69–80. http://dx.doi.org/10.1002/pri.474

Licht, S. (1946). The objectives of occupational therapy. Occupational Therapy and Rehabilitation, 25, 17–22. http://dx.doi.org/10.1177/000841744601300303

Lin, S. H., Murphy, S. L., & Robinson, J. C. (2010). The Issue Is—Facilitating evidence-based practice: Process, strategies, and resources. American Journal of Occupational Therapy, 64, 164–171. http://dx.doi.org/10.5014/ajot.64.1.164

National Society for the Promotion of Occupational Therapy. (1917). Certificate of incorporation. Clifton Springs, NY: Author.

Nelson, D. (1996). Why the profession of occupational therapy will flourish in the 21st century [Eleanor Clarke Slagle Lecture]. American Journal of Occupational Therapy, 51, 11–24. http://dx/doi.org/10.5014/ajot.51.1.11

Noble, M. O. (1937). The necessity for research work in occupational therapy. Occupational Therapy and Rehabilitation, 16, 107–110.

Owens, A. C. (1964). Editorial. Occupational Therapy, 27(2), 1–2.

Papadimitriou, C., Magasi, S., & Frank, G. (2012). Current thinking in qualitative research: Evidence-based practice, moral philosophies, and political struggles. OTJR: Occupation, Participation and Health, 32(Suppl. 1), S2–S5. http://dx.doi.org/10.3928/15394492-20111005-01

Peloquin, S. M. (2005). Embracing our ethos, reclaiming our heart. American Journal of Occupational Therapy, 59, 611–625. http://dx.doi.org/10.5014/ajot.59.6.611 Reprinted as Chapter 62.

Phillip, A., Helen, S., & James, N. (1959). Psychological attributes of occupational therapy crafts. American Journal of Occupational Therapy, 13(1), 16–22.

Pollock, H. (1929). The need, value, and general principles of occupational therapy statistics. Occupational Therapy and Rehabilitation, 7, 415–420.

Ravetz, C. (1987). The rights and responsibilities of qualification [Editorial]. British Journal of Occupational Therapy, 50, 255.

Reagon C., Bellin B., & Boniface, G. (2010). Challenging the dominant voice: The multiple evidence sources of occupational therapy. British Journal of Occupational Therapy, 73(6), 284–86. http://dx.doi.org/10.4276/030802210X12759925469069

Reed, K. L. (1986). Tools of practice: Heritage or baggage? [Eleanor Clarke Slagle Lecture]. American Journal of Occupational Therapy, 40, 597–605.

Rensink, M., Schuurmans, M., Lindeman, E., & Hafsteinsdóttir, T. (2009). Task-oriented training in rehabilitation after stroke: Systematic review. Journal of Advanced Nursing, 65, 737–754. http://dx.doi.org/10.1111/j.1365-2648.2008.04925.x

Rood, M. S. (1958). Every one counts. American Journal of Occupational Therapy, 5, 326–329.

Sackett, D. L., Strauss, S. E., Richardson, W. S., Rosenberg, W., & Haynes, R. B. (2000). Evidence-based medicine: How to practice and teach it. Edinburgh, Scotland: Churchill Livingstone.

Schwartz, K. B. (2009). Reclaiming our heritage: Connecting the founding vision to the Centennial Vision [Eleanor Clarke Slagle Lecture]. American Journal of Occupational Therapy, 63, 681–690. http://dx.doi.org/10.5014/ajot.63.6.681

Shaw, J., & Shaw, D. (2011). Evidence and ethics in occupational therapy. British Journal of Occupational Therapy, 74, 254–256. http://dx.doi.org/10.4276/030802211X13046730116650

Smith, N. M. (1963). WFOT Study Course 2: Transitional programmes in psychiatric occupational therapy. Occupational Therapy, 26(8), 20–23.

Stattel, F. (1956). Equipment designed for occupational therapy [Eleanor Clarke Slagle Lecture]. American Journal of Occupational Therapy, 10, 194–198.

Sudsawad, P. (2005). Concepts in clinical scholarship: A conceptual framework to increase usability to outcome research for evidence-based practice. American Journal of Occupational Therapy, 59, 351–355. http://dx.doi.org/10.5014/ajot.59.3.351

Tomlin, G., & Borgetto, B. (2011). Research pyramid: A new evidence-based practice model for occupational therapy. American Journal of Occupational Therapy, 65, 189–196. http://dx.doi.org/10.5014/ajot.2011.000828

Trombly, C. (1995). Occupation: Purposefulness and meaningfulness as therapeutic mechanisms [Eleanor Clarke Slagle Lecture]. American Journal of Occupational Therapy, 49, 960–972. http://dx.doi.org/10.5014/ajot.49.10.960 Reprinted as Chapter 11.

Turner, A. (2007). Health through occupation: Beyond the evidence. Journal of Occupational Science, 14, 9–15. http://dx.doi.org/10.1080/14427591.2007.9686578

Varrier-Jones P. C. (1941). The middle case: An unsolved problem in tuberculosis. *Lancet, 237,* 368–370. http://dx.doi.org/10.1016/S0140-6736(00)60820-6

World Federation of Occupational Therapists. (2008). *Occupational therapy entry-level qualifications position statement revised CM2008.* Retrieved from http://www.wfot.org/ResourceCentre.aspx

Wood, W. (1998). Nationally Speaking—It is jump time for occupational therapy. *American Journal of Occupational Therapy, 52,* 403–411. http://dx.doi.org/10.5014/ajot.52.6.403

Yerxa, E. (1967). Authentic occupational therapy [Eleanor Slagle Clarke Lecture]. *American Journal of Occupational Therapy, 21,* 1–9.

Appendix VI.A. Guide to Evaluating Research Evidence: Guiding Questions

- Was the design appropriate for the research study and for answering the research question?
- Was the sampling plan appropriate? Does the sampling technique affect whether the findings could be generalized to different groups in practice or in the population?
- Could the nonresponse rate or number of people who dropped out of the study affect the results and generalizability?
- Was the sample size adequate? Was the same size large enough for the statistical methods used and to ensure adequate power in determining the results?
- Was the statistical approach appropriate to answer the question?
- What were the results? Are the findings statistically significant?
- Are the findings clinically significant? How large were the treatment effects or effect size?
- Does the evidence pertain to my clinical situation? Are the populations or contexts in the study similar?
- Can the therapeutic intervention be implemented in my clinical setting (e.g., does it require special equipment or training)?

Note. Adapted from "Facilitating Evidence-Based Practice: Process, Strategies, and Resources," by S. H. Lin, S. L., Murphy, and J. C. Robinson, 2010, *American Journal of Occupational Therapy, Vol. 64,* p. 166. Copyright © 2010 by the American Occupational Therapy Association. Used with permission.

Appendix VI.B. Resources to Appraise Evidence

Resource	Description
CATmaker www.cebm.net/index.aspx?o=1216)	A free software tool to help create critically appraised topics (CATS).
Centre for Health Evidence www.cche.net/usersguides/main.asp	A subscription site providing information on core topics in evidence-based medicine and detailed guides on appraising research.
Cochrane Library www.thecochranelibrary.com/view/0/index.htmland	Free access to medical and other health care databases and extensive systematic reviews and meta-analyses.
Critical Appraisal Skills Programme www.phru.nhs.uk/Pages/PHD/resources.htm	Free appraisal tools and links resources in the United Kingdom.
Evidence-Based Medicine Toolkit www.ebm.med.ualberta.ca/	Free practice guidelines and evidence-based medicine tools.
Evidence-based occupational therapy www.otevidence.info/	An international occupational therapy website providing information, strategies, resources, and links for evidence-based practice and research.
OTDBASE www.otdbase.org/.	A subscription site providing online indexing and search service for over 20 international occupational therapy journals.
OTseeker www.otseeker.com	An open access data base of critically appraised randomized controlled trials and systemic reviews relevant to occupational therapy.
PubMed www.ncbi.nlm.nih.gov/pubmed/	A free site for searching more than 22 million citations with links to full-text content (fees may apply for content).
World Health Organization HINARI program www.who.int/hinari/en/.	An international open database of more than 8,000 informational resources available in 30 languages.

Note. From Ilott (2012) and Lin et al. (2010).

CHAPTER 49

Our Mandate for the New Millennium: Evidence-Based Practice

2000 ELEANOR CLARKE SLAGLE LECTURE

MARGO B. HOLM

The health-care environment of the past quarter-century went through numerous evolutionary processes that affected how occupational therapy services were provided. The last iterations of these processes included requests for the evidence that supported what we were doing. This year's Eleanor Clarke Slagle Lecture (a) examines the strength of the evidence associated with occupational therapy interventions—what we do and how we do it—(b) raises dilemmas we face with our ethical principles when some of our practices are based on limited evidence, and (c) proposes a framework of continued competency to advance the evidence base of occupational therapy practice in the new millennium.

If the next several patients you were to see asked you, "How do you know that what you do and how you do it really works?" would you be able to provide them with research evidence similar to that found in the pamphlets that come with your prescription medications? The evidence would include a summary of research on each occupational therapy intervention option you are considering. It would delineate the percentage of patients who benefited from each option and the percentage of those who did not. It would also clearly describe *what* each intervention consists of and *how* each is to be implemented for yielding the best outcomes for particular patient populations. Additionally, the data that support the recommended frequency and duration for each intervention would be included. It is unlikely that you could provide such evidence today. Will you be able to provide the evidence by 2010? As professionals, we have gone on record committing

ourselves to evidence-based practice in Principle 2.B of our *Occupational Therapy Code of Ethics*, which states, "Occupational therapy personnel shall fully inform the service recipients of the nature, risks, and potential outcomes of any interventions" (American Occupational Therapy Association [AOTA], 1994, p. 1037). *Can we meet this commitment?*

In this year's Slagle Lecture, I will use a common definition of evidence-based practice and discuss why it has meaning for the context in which our profession finds itself today. First, I will use a five-level measuring stick (see Table 49.1) to examine the strength of the evidence or the lack of evidence associated with occupational therapy interventions—*what* we do and *how* we do it—the same measuring stick that is also being used by referring physicians, educational services administrators, and health maintenance organization purchasers of services as they appraise our evidence. Second, I will raise throughout the lecture dilemmas that face us when we try to reconcile some of the principles in our Code of Ethics with the practice of occupational therapy based on limited evidence. Third, I will use the framework of continued competency to discuss what is needed to practice occupational therapy, based on research evidence, in the new millennium.

Evidence-Based Practice

As we are all aware, the health-care environment of the past quarter-century underwent numerous evolutionary processes that greatly affected *how* occupational therapy services were provided! For example, in many practice settings, we were confronted with prospective payment reimbursement, capitation models, reduced staffing ratios, and job losses. Additionally, we are now being judged by the functional outcomes our patients achieve. The fact that patient outcomes are improved

This chapter was previously published in the *American Journal of Occupational Therapy, 54*, 575–585. Copyright © 2000, American Occupational Therapy Association. Reprinted with permission. http://dx.doi.org/10.5014/ajot.54.6.575

Table 49.1. Hierarchy of Levels of Evidence for Evidence-Based Practice

Level	Description
I	Strong evidence from at least one systematic review of multiple well-designed randomized controlled trials
II	Strong evidence from at least one properly designed randomized controlled trial of appropriate size
III	Evidence from well-designed trials without randomization, single group pre–post, cohort, time series, or matched case-controlled studies
IV	Evidence from well-designed nonexperimental studies from more than one center or research group
V	Opinions of respected authorities, based on clinical evidence, descriptive studies, or reports of expert committees

Note. From "Evidence-Based Everything," by A. Moore, H. McQuay, & J.A.M. Gray (Eds.), 1995, *Bandolier, 1*(12), p. 1. Copyright © 1995 by Bandolier. Reprinted with permission.

with occupational therapy services is no longer sufficient to justify our services, unless we can also explain *what* we do and *how* we do it so that others can replicate our interventions and achieve similar outcomes with comparable patients with like needs, wants, and expectations. The emphasis on justifying our practice patterns has been reflected in the increasing numbers of requests for the research-based evidence that supports what we are doing.

So, what is evidence-based practice? It has been defined as "integrating individual clinical expertise" with the "conscientious, explicit and judicious use of current best evidence in making decisions about the care of individual patients" (Sackett, Rosenberg, Gray, Haynes, & Richardson, 1996, p. 71). Thus, in our Code of Ethics we have also affirmed our commitment to evidence-based practice in Principle 3.D, "Occupational therapy personnel shall perform their duties on the basis of accurate and current information" (AOTA, 1994, p. 1037). *Can we meet this commitment?*

Gray (1997) described the evolution of evidence-based practice as progressing from providing services as efficiently and cheaply as possible, to "doing things better," then to *"doing things right,"* and finally to "doing the right things" (p. 17). He has also proposed that evidence-based practice for the new millennium must focus on "doing the right things right" (p. 17). In other words, the necessary shift to the evidence-based practice of occupational therapy will require us to justify *why* we do *what* we do in addition to *how* we do it.

Of course, Gray's proposal implies that for any given patient population, we *know* what is "right" and, furthermore, that we *know* the "right" way to do what we do. Silverman (1998) put it another way: "How do we go about drawing a line between 'knowing' and 'doing' . . . and when do we know enough about the . . . consequences of our interventions to proceed with confidence" (p. 5)?

As occupational therapy practitioners, we have always used multiple sources of evidence, or "ways of knowing," to guide our "doing," including evidence derived from the oral tradition, our own beliefs and values, patient preferences, assessment data, the opinions of experts, and research evidence (Brown, 1999; Bury & Mead, 1998). Historically, our evidence resided within individual practitioners and was handed down from practitioner to practitioner; thus, it was not accessible to all. With the advent of occupational therapy textbooks and journals, opinions of experts and research evidence have been published and are now accessible to all. Although each source of evidence has inherent value for some aspect of our practice, no single source of evidence, or even all of them together, enables us to know enough to proceed to our "doing" with absolute confidence.

Information Overload and Hierarchies of Evidence

Our level of confidence in our clinical decisions should be based, in part, on the strength of the evidence we use. Fortunately, the evidence that is available has been expanding at an exponential rate; however, this expansion has created two problems: (a) There is too much evidence to sift through, and (b) the quantity of evidence does not equal quality of evidence. Shenk (1997) addressed the problem of expansion when he noted, "Just as fat has replaced starvation as [the] number one dietary concern, information overload has replaced information scarcity" (p. 29). An editorial in the *Journal of the American Medical Association (JAMA)* expressed concerns about the second problem: the quality of the evidence in which we may place our confidence. Rennie (1986) lamented that publication alone does not mean quality. The author noted wryly that there is

no study too fragmented, no hypothesis too trivial, no literature citation too biased or too egotistical, no design too warped, no methodology too bungled, no presentation of results too inaccurate and too contradictory, no analysis too self-serving, no argument too circular, no conclusion too trifling or too unjustified, and no grammar and syntax too offensive for a paper to end up in print. (p. 2391)

It is because of the glut of evidence and concerns about quality control that ranking systems, or hierarchies, were developed to rate the strength of the research designs being used to generate the evidence (Moore, McQuay, & Gray, 1995; Sackett, Haynes, & Tugwell, 1985; Sackett, Richardson, Rosenberg, & Haynes, 1997). These *hierarchies of evidence* were designed to help practitioners sort through the options and select the "current best evidence" available to guide decisions about *what* to do and *how* to do it for a particular patient or patient population.

Examples of Occupational Therapy Evidence

Although evidence hierarchies vary somewhat in their rigor, the rank order of the levels of evidence is similar, with the best evidence ranked at Level I and less convincing evidence ranked at lower levels (see Table 49.1). Each level represents the research strategies that were used to structure the investigations. At the top of the hierarchy are those designs deemed (a) least vulnerable to bias, (b) more generalizable, and (c) more likely to yield patient outcomes that can confidently be attributed to the intervention being studied (see Table 49.1). Therefore, if it is current, and available, you want the "best" evidence, which is a Level I research design. The evidence hierarchy, or measuring stick, that I will use has five levels (Moore et al., 1995). At the top of the hierarchy, or Level I, are studies in which we, and those we must convince about the efficacy and effectiveness of occupational therapy, should have the most confidence. They are also the studies that we must strive to plan, implement, and publish.

Level I Evidence

Level I studies are defined as "strong evidence from at least one systematic review of multiple well-designed randomized controlled trials" (Moore et al., 1995, p. 1). Level I systematic reviews usually take one of two forms: (a) meta-analytic studies or (b) systematic reviews. Both methods (a) require adherence to rigorous procedures, with well-defined study criteria for inclusion, and (b) are usually restricted to studies that use randomized controlled clinical trials. Additionally, both methods use statistical analyses to evaluate the data from each study and the studies in total.

So, what does this mean for everyday practice? Picture yourself in this scenario: You work on a neurorehabilitation unit and a new medical resident asks you, "Why does my patient need both a physical therapy exercise program and occupational therapy? What evidence do you have that cooking tasks, adapted checkers games, and those other things you do make any difference in upper-extremity motor performance?" An appropriate response would be the provision of *current best evidence* in the form of a Level I study. Occupational therapy researchers Lin, Wu, Tickle-Degnen, and Coster (1997) carried out a meta-analytic study of 17 articles, including four articles on studies of patients with neurological impairments. They found that in studies designed to improve the motor performance of patients with neurological impairments, the outcomes were significantly better when the patients' exercises were embedded into everyday tasks than when the patients only performed rote exercises. This study is just one example of evidence that you can use to support *what* we do and *how* we can do it to yield improvements in patients with neurological impairments and upper-extremity motor deficits.

What about Level I current best evidence for other areas of practice? A meta-analytic study of the efficacy of sensory integration treatment was recently conducted by an occupational therapy researcher (Vargas & Camilli, 1998). This rigorous meta-analysis of 22 studies considered every possible influence on the outcomes of sensory integration treatment, including (a) adherence to sensory integration treatment criteria, (b) total treatment hours, (c) diagnosis and age, (d) design and sampling, (e) number of outcomes and measurement categories, (f) professional affiliation of the researchers, (g) geographic location of the studies, and (h) publication years. The results of the study, however, provide us with a stark reminder of the difference between preferred practice and evidence-based practice.

Many therapists prefer to use a sensory integration approach to intervention with both children and adults. But *current* best evidence, namely those studies published since 1983, indicated "an absence of sensory integration effects in recent studies and the equivalence of sensory integration and alternative treatments," neither of which yielded improvement in the sensory–perceptual area (Vargas & Camilli, 1998, p. 197). In other words, the experimental groups' outcomes following sensory integration interventions were no better than those of the control groups that received no treatment, regardless of the outcome being measured. When compared with alternative types of treatment, outcomes of the sensory integration groups were equivalent but not very effective. Although we may *prefer* to ignore the findings of this study, our actions would be in conflict with Principle 2.B of our Code of Ethics in which we commit to "fully inform the service recipients of the nature, risks, and potential outcomes of any interventions" (AOTA, 1994, p. 1037), especially if their effectiveness is in question. Tickle-Degnen (1998) developed excellent sample dialogues for communicating mixed or nonsupportive evidence about proposed interventions to patients.

The failure of these studies to demonstrate the superiority of sensory integration techniques over no treatment does not negate the possibility that (a) the outcome measures were insensitive to the changes produced, (b) the wrong outcomes were measured, or (c) the effects were obscured by the application of sensory integration techniques to inappropriate populations. Another possibility is that the statistical power, or sample size, may have been inadequate. Ottenbacher and Maas (1999) pointed out that often the effect sizes in our studies, or the magnitude of the difference between the experimental and contro l groups, indicate that our interventions do yield clinically worthwhile differences. However, we often do not have large enough samples to reject the null hypotheses, and therefore we conclude wrongly that our interventions are not effective (Mulligan, 1998; Ottenbacher & Maas, 1999; Vargas & Camilli, 1998).

Just as our practices change over time, so too should the evidence base of our practice. It will be important to revisit the evidence to see whether new sensory integration interventions being used in clinics and promoted in workshops, new measures such as those related to the family's perspective suggested by Cohn and Cermak (1998), or larger sample sizes can provide better support for *what* we do and *how* we do it when using sensory integration interventions.

Now, put yourself into this second scenario: The budget administrator in your hospital is questioning the use of life skills groups with a chronic mental health population. You do a computer search, and using the Cochrane Database of Systematic Reviews (www.update-software.com/cochrane/cochrane-frame.html), you find a review entitled, "Life Skills Programmes for People With Chronic Mental Illness" (Nicol, Robertson, & Connaughton, 1999). The review examined life skills programs that focused on interpersonal skills, self-care, time management, financial management, nutrition, and household skills as well as use of community re-

sources. Unfortunately, only two randomized clinical trials were found that met the criteria, and both were conducted more than 15 years ago. Even though evidence was sparse and not what one would call current, it was the best evidence available, and the reviewers proceeded to conclude that:

> there is next to no evidence that life skills training programmes are of value to those with serious mental illnesses . . . [and] until such time as any evidence of benefit is available it is questionable whether recipients of care should be put under pressure to attend such programmes. (Nicol et al., p. 10/21)

The reviewers went on to state, "If life skills training is to continue as a part of rehabilitation programmes a large, well designed, conducted and reported pragmatic randomized trial is an urgent necessity" (p. 2/21), but then they added, "There may even be an argument for stating that maintenance of current practice, outside of a randomize d trial, is unethical" (p. 2/21).

Providing this current best evidence for life skills training with a chronic mental health population to any budget administrator could pose a threat or an opportunity. The threat comes if only the reviewers' *conclusions* are noted, namely that occupational therapy life skills groups are ineffective for chronic mental health populations at best and unethical at worst. If we provide no new evidence that counteracts the findings of the Cochrane reviewers, then it could be implied that we are in tacit agreement with the recommendation. If we take this stance, however, the threat could be generalized to other settings or populations in which life skills programs are used. We then would have to ask ourselves the next logical question: "If there is no evidence that life skills programs make any difference with chronic mental health populations (with whom they have been used since time immemorial), what evidence is there that life skills programs are effective with developmental disability or traumatic brain injury populations?" Our opportunity lies in responding to the reviewers' *recommendation* to design, carry out, and report the findings from a large, randomized controlled trial, a design that is also known as a Level II study in our evidence hierarchy. This is the next level of evidence.

Level II Evidence

The evidence needed to confirm or reject the Cochrane database findings about life skills programs is not found in the ivory towers of universities but, rather, in occupational therapy clinics and community-based practices. The study suggested by the Cochrane reviewers was a Level II research design, which consists of "strong evidence from at least one properly designed randomized controlled trial of appropriate size" (Moore et al., 1995, p. 1). For example, to conduct a randomized controlled trial in a clinic, this would mean that after a practitioner has collected baseline performance data on a patient, any patient who meets the criteria already established for participation in a life skills program would be randomly assigned to one of three groups: (a) a control group or attention group (no occupational therapy), (b) an alternative therapy group (e.g., a social work group that talks about life skills), or (c) an occupational therapy life skills group. Typically, randomized clinical trials include large numbers of participants. These participants can be accrued either slowly over time at one site or more quickly through collaboration among multiple clinical sites. The latter, multisite studies can dampen the spirits of even the most enthusiastic of researchers because of scheduling problems, budgeting issues, and philosophical differences. The problems with randomized control trials at single or multiple sites can be ove rcome by planning carefully, educating therapists in systematic data collection methods, ensuring that research intervention protocols are delivered in a standardized manner, and monitoring adherence to research procedures.

The common argument against doing randomized trials is the belief that patients who are randomized to the control or placebo conditions will not benefit or progress if they do not participate in occupational therapy treatment, for example, the sensory integration interventions or life skills groups. However, Portney and Watkins (1993) noted that:

> in situations where the efficacy of a treatment is being questioned because current knowledge is inadequate, it may actually be more ethical to take the time to make appropriate controlled comparisons than to continue clinical practice using potentially ineffective techniques. (p. 29)

Three examples of Level II randomized controlled occupational therapy clinical trials, which accurately followed intent-to-treat principles—in other words, carried out their statistical analyses on the basis of the number of participants that entered the study, not only those who completed it—were published in *JAMA* (Ray

et al., 1997), *Lancet* (Close et al., 1999), and the *Journal of the American Geriatrics Society (JAGS)* (Cummings et al., 1999). These studies examined the impact of occupational therapy interventions on falls reduction among nursing home residents and community-based frail older adults. In the large multicenter nursing home study published in *JAMA*, the proportion of recurrent fallers in the experimental facilities was significantly less ($p = .03$) than in the control facilities (Ray et al., 1997). In addition to the physician and nursing components, the occupational therapy interventions consisted of wheelchair positioning and maintenance and resident and staff instruction on safe transfers.

In the study of community-based older adults with a history of falls published in *Lancet,* the experimental group had significantly fewer falls ($p = .05$) at the 12-month follow-up than the control group. The experimental group had received a home visit and a follow-up phone call by an occupational therapist that focused on home safety and modification of the home environment (Close et al., 1999).

In the study published in the *JAGS*, community-based older adults who presented to hospital emergency rooms after falls were randomly assigned to either a post–acute event occupational therapy intervention group or a control group. The occupational therapy intervention consisted of home safety recommendations, education, and minor home modifications. At the 12-month follow-up, the risk of falling, the risk of recurrent falls, and the odds of being admitted to a hospital were significantly lower in the occupational therapy group than in the control group (Cummings et al., 1999).

These three studies provide strong Level II evidence of the efficacy of occupational therapy for falls reduction among nursing home residents and community-based frail older adults. These are but three examples of Level II studies that you can provide to nursing home administrators, outpatient rehabilitation coordinators, or emergency room physicians as supporting evidence that *what* we do and *how* we do it can make a significant positive difference to older adults at risk for falling.

Level III Evidence

However, what happens when Level I and Level II studies are not available? According to Gray (1997), "The absence of excellent evidence does not make evidence-based decision making impossible; in this situation, what is required is the best *evidence available,* not the best evidence possible" (p. 61). For example, picture yourself in this third scenario: The new physiatrist at your rehabilitation facility came from a setting where the occupational therapists used Bobath axial rolls for patients with stroke who had hemiplegia and shoulder subluxation, and she writes specific orders for their use. You are not convinced that the axial rolls work very well, and you prefer the type of sling that you have been using for the past 10 years—the same one that your physical disabilities professor preferred. In addition, the axial rolls seem to increase your patients' shoulder pain. Even though you found no Level I or Level II studies in your literature search, you located four studies that meet Level III criteria (Brooke, Lateur, Diana-Rigby, & Questad, 1991; Hurd, Farrell, & Waylonis, 1974; Williams, Taffs, & Minuk, 1988; Zorowitz, Idank, Ikai, Hughes, & Johnston, 1995).

Level III studies derive their "evidence from well-designed trials without randomization, single group pre–post, cohort, time series or matched case-controlled studies" (Moore et al., 1995, p. 1). Although you are pleased to find that the best evidence available indicated that the Bobath axial roll made no difference, or even increased shoulder displacement (Zorowitz et al., 1995), you also find that the sling that you prefer fared no better. In fact, you find that the evidence for use of an axial roll, a sling, or a wheelchair trough for reducing shoulder displacement is mixed at best, and some of the most recent evidence indicates that the sling you prefer actually increases vertical asymmetry (Brooke et al., 1991). At that moment, Principle 1.C of our Code of Ethics comes to mind—"occupational therapy personnel shall take all reasonable precautions to avoid harm to the recipient of services" (AOTA, 1994, p. 1037)—only now its relevance has new meaning. You have learned two lessons from your search: (a) You are appalled to learn that your preferred intervention may have done harm, and (b) you have learned that although you are not from a state that requires continuing education for licensure, the relevance of one aspect of our Code of Ethics (Principle 3.C) is now clearer: "Occupational therapy personnel shall take responsibility for maintaining competence by participating in professional development and educational activities" (AOTA, 1994, p. 1037).

Next, imagine that you are an occupational therapy practitioner employed by a skilled nursing facility. You frequently encounter new residents who qualify for rehabilitation services because of a 3-day hospital stay. However, because they have a primary diagnosis of dementia of the Alzheimer type and severe memory impairments, their ability to benefit from any rehabilitation is frequently challenged. A Level III study combining occupational therapy compensatory strategies and behavioral techniques featured in *JAGS* (Rogers et al., 1999) may have the type of evidence you are looking for. The study found that during a 1-week occupational therapy skill intervention condition using compensatory strategies and a structured environment, the residents with dementia significantly increased the proportion of time they engaged in self-dressing and significantly decreased their disruptive behaviors compared with the usual care. During the 3-week occupational therapy habit training condition that followed, residents were able to maintain their gains. Additionally, during both occupational therapy intervention conditions, the use of labor-intensive physical assists decreased significantly. A Level III study such as this can be used to provide fiscal intermediaries with supporting evidence that *what* we do and *how* we do it can benefit even nursing home residents who are severely disabled and cognitively impaired.

The next Level III study could be helpful if you find yourself in the following scenario: You work for a private therapy company that provides services to several group homes for adults with developmental disabilities. The owner of the homes tells you that he had been "surfing the Net" and had found the Cochrane Database Systematic Review on the ineffectiveness of life skills groups. Given the conclusions of the reviewers, he wants to know what evidence you have that indicates that the life skills groups you are implementing are effective. You tell him that you also read the review and point out that applying the findings from the Cochrane review to his clients might not be in their best interest because the participants in the studies described in the review had chronic mental illness and were in hospital-based programs—a population very different from his community-based clients with developmental disabilities. You explain that since reading the review, you have been using the methods and outcomes described in a Level III study by Neistadt and Marques (1984), whose participants also had developmental disabilities. You then show him the data you have collected over the past 3 months, documenting the specific life skills groups each client in his facilities has participated in as well as their outcomes. You note that all clients have made gains.

A fourth example of a Level III study pertains to school-based practice and pediatrics wherein occupational therapy practitioners are frequently associated with *fine motor* skills training. This association with fine motor skills is not surprising, though, because when you use the key words fine motor to search through the 10 million journal articles indexed in MEDLINE, 1 of the 10 subject headings you are presented with, and the only profession, is *occupational therapy*. A Level III intervention study by Case-Smith et al. (1998) found that preschoolers with fine motor delays who received direct occupational therapy services improved their fine motor skills and related functional performance significantly, and the rate of gain was greater than that of their peers who had no fine motor delays (p. 788). The next time you need to convince your educational services administrator about the benefits that occupational therapy can offer to preschool populations with fine motor delays, bring this supporting evidence, along with a Level IV study by McHale and Cermak (1992).

Level IV Evidence

According to Moore et al. (1995), Level IV studies consist of "evidence from well-designed non-experimental studies from more than one center or research group" (p. 1). Sometimes our inquiry into the need for, or effectiveness of, an intervention begins with a multisite descriptive study. The Level IV study by McHale and Cermak (1992) described the time allocated to fine motor activities and tasks in six elementary school classrooms. Minute-by-minute data collection indicated that 30 percent to 60 percent of the day was dedicated to fine motor tasks, with writing tasks predominating. This study provides the context and relevance of occupational therapy interventions for preschoolers with fine motor delays—preschoolers who will soon become elementary school students.

Level V Evidence

The lowest level of the hierarchy of evidence is Level V, which is defined as "opinions of respected authorities, based on clinical evidence, descriptive studies or reports of expert committees" (Moore et al., 1995, p. 1). Unlike Level IV descriptive studies, Level V studies do not need to be from multiple centers or research groups. Studies that use qualitative designs are also identified as Level V studies. One such study published recently in the *Occupational Therapy Journal of Research (OTJR)* (Bye, 1998) involved in-depth interviews of therapists who worked with terminally ill patients. For a profession that is used to facilitating functional gains in patients rather than in preparing them for death, this Level V study provides a framework for guiding the practice of occupational therapy in end-of-life care. The study had as its core aim "Affirming Life: Preparing for Death" (Bye, 1998, p. 8). Interventions focused on "building against loss," achieving "normality within a changed reality," regaining "cli-

ent control" over daily routines and activities, providing "supported and safe" environments, and finding "closure in some aspects of their lives" (p. 8). It is Level V studies like this one that enable researchers to describe and probe aspects of our practice that cannot be accomplished with Level I and Level II studies and simultaneously pave the way for future research. Level V evidence also can help us define new programs that have the potential to benefit populations not typically associated with rehabilitation or occupational therapy and point the way to new areas of inquiry and program development.

Also included in Level V evidence are the opinions of respected authorities. Although all the other examples of evidence I have cited were based on research, or from external sources, Level V evidence allows for the evidence *residing within the practitioner*. When we use opinion-based evidence, we are grounding our clinical reasoning and therapeutic decisions and actions in the advice of experts, established practices, continuing education information, or reference texts by known leaders in the field (Brown, 1999; Bury & Mead, 1998). It is not unusual for fieldwork students, entry-level practitioners, and practitioners changing practice areas to rely primarily on the opinions of master practitioners, supervisors, or therapists with specialty certification. It is also not unusual for us to continue to provide interventions that are based on the wisdom of the "form in the file drawer," which represents established practices that have "always been done that way."

When we use Level V evidence based on clinical experience and expertise to guide decision-making with our patients, we must be aware of how our own values, beliefs, and biases influence our decisions. In a study of physicians' perceptions of their patients' preferences, patients were asked to rate four preferred courses of action for a life-threatening illness, and their physicians were asked to predict their patients' preferences as well as to state their preferences for themselves. Unfortunately the physicians' predictions of their patients' preferences more closely matched their own preferences than those of their patients (Schneiderman, Kaplan, Pearlman, & Teetzel, 1993). It is because of the potential power associated with clinical expertise that ethicists Lidz and Meisel (1983) remind us that we must not view the decision-making process with patients as one of merely persuading the patient to accept what we believe to be the proper course.

However, it is precisely our clinical experience, clinical expertise, and clinical reasoning that Sackett et al. (1996) referred to in their definition of evidence-based practice when they speak of "*integrating individual clinical expertise* [italics added]" with the "use of current best evidence in making decisions about the care of individual patients" (p. 71). I would like to emphasize that if we are to practice evidence-based occupational therapy, evidence can only be used to inform clinical expertise, not replace it, and clinical expertise must be used in conjunction with the best available evidence, not substituted for it (Bury & Mead, 1998; Sackett et al., 1996).

We have made a commitment in our Code of Ethics to "collaborate with service recipients or their surrogate(s) in determining goals and priorities throughout the intervention process" (AOTA, 1994, p. 1037). It is in the fulfillment of this commitment that patient and practitioner together must consider the evidence before them and make informed decisions about the occupational therapy interventions that will best meet the patient's needs, wants, and expectations. *Can we meet this commitment?*

Collective Evidence

I have applied a five-level measuring stick to some of our evidence and cited examples of evidence associated with each level. But what about the strength of our collective evidence as a scholarly profession? To get a snapshot of the bigger picture, I applied the same hierarchy to all articles published in *OTJR* for the past 5 years (1995–1999). I chose the *OTJR* because it is "devoted to the advancement of knowledge through scientific methods" (Abreu, Peloquin, & Ottenbacher, 1998, p. 757). As you can see in Table 49.2, over the past 5 years, the preponderance of the evidence in our research journal was at Level V, which is defined as "opinions of respected authorities, based on clinical evidence, descriptive studies or reports of expert committees" (Moore et al., 1995, p. 1). Obviously, a journal must receive manuscripts before they

can be published. As our collective research competence improves, so will the levels of evidence that we are able to generate and submit for publication.

Evidence-Based Practice and Continued Competency

At graduation, more than one class has heard the speaker say something similar to, "Half of what we taught you will not be true in 5 years. Unfortunately, we do not know which half" (Sackett et al., 1997, p. 38). Therefore, a commitment we have made to ourselves and to our service recipients in our Code of Ethics is to "take responsibility for maintaining competence by participating in professional development and educational activities" (AOTA, 1994, p. 1037). The importance of continued competency to occupational therapy practitioners was confirmed in a recent report entitled "Continued Competency in Occupational Therapy: Recommendations to the Profession and Key Stakeholders" by the National Commission on Continued Competency in Occupational Therapy (NCCCOT) (Mayhan, Holm, & Fawcett, 1999). From a survey of a stratified random sample of 550 of the 88,885 occupational therapists and 550 of the 33,512 occupational therapy assistants in the database of the National Board for Certification in Occupational Therapy (response rate = 33 percent), the NCCCOT found that more than 85 percent of the respondents endorsed the importance of continued competency for occupational therapy practitioners. Members of the NCCCOT also conducted in-depth interviews with representatives of other stakeholders in the future of our profession. These stakeholders included employers, payers, institutional and individual private accreditation program representatives, consumer advocates, and health policy analysts. These stakeholders shared the common perception that our continued competency is important to consumer protection and that individual occupational therapy practitioners have "the primary and ultimate responsibility for assuring their own continued competency" (Mayhan et al., 1999, p. 54).

Although we must be able to demonstrate competency in the core functions delineated in our *Standards of Practice* (AOTA, 1998) and the functions associated with the professional roles we fulfill (AOTA, 1993), we must also develop competence in research skills. Because of the changes in clinical practice as well as the changes in the evolving evidence base of occupational therapy, if we do not develop the research skills necessary to make use of the current best evidence for our patients, the result will be a progressive decline in our clinical competency.

Table 49.2. Hierarchy of Evidence Applied to Articles Published in the *Occupational Therapy Journal of Research*, 1995–1999

Level	Design	Number of Articles
I	Systematic reviews, meta-analytic studies	1
II	Randomized controlled trials	6
III	Trials without randomization	21
IV	Nonexperimental studies from more than one center	11
V	Opinions of respected authorities, descriptive studies	41

Note. Based on hierarchy by Moore, McQuay, and Gray (1995).

In a special issue of *the American Journal of Occupational Therapy (AJOT)* devoted to professional competence, Abreu et al. (1998) led off their article with a prediction that in a practice environment that is continually changing, the survival of the profession depends, in part, on the "capacity of therapists to achieve competence in scientific inquiry and research" (p. 751). Then, using the levels of research competence identified by the American Occupational Therapy Foundation (1983) and Mitcham (1985), they explicated descriptors of the associated knowledge, skills, and attitudinal research competencies for practitioners at the beginning, intermediate, and advanced levels of occupational therapy research. What is necessary for continued competence in research and for our professional survival is for all of us to increase the number and level of our research competencies—not just to "maintain competence" as is the wording in our Code of Ethics but, rather, to improve our competence. *Can we meet this challenge?*

How Do I Become an Evidence-Based Practitioner?

At the *individual* level, each of us could fulfill all the research competencies identified by Abreu et al. (1998) and still not be an evidence-based practitioner, unless we also use the evidence and use it appropriately. This means that even if the evidence is clear and we decide that we can easily fit it into our preferred practice patterns, if it is not appropriate or acceptable to the patient, it is not evidence-based practice for that patient. As individuals, we must examine our practices to determine whether we are "integrating individual clinical expertise" with the "conscientious, explicit and judicious use of current best evidence" (Sackett et al., 1996, p. 71) by asking ourselves five questions. If we can answer affirmatively to any of the questions, we are making the right moves toward evidence-based practice.

Question 1: Do I Examine What I Do by Asking Clinical Questions?

The process of evidence-based practice begins by identifying the interventions that we use frequently in our practices with particular populations of patients, or for particular problems in performance, and then posing questions. Richardson, Wilson, Nishikawa, and Hayward (1995) identified the anatomy of a clinical question as having four parts: (a) the patient, population, or problem; (b) the intervention, which may include frequency and duration; (c) the outcome of interest; and (d) the comparison intervention. An example of a clinical question using this format might be: (a) In patients who have sustained a cerebrovascular accident, (b) does the use of a resting splint on the affected hand for 3 hours each day (c) reduce tone and increase function (d) compared with no splinting?

Question 2: Do I Take Time to Track Down the Best Evidence to Guide What I Do?

To answer your clinical question, you must track down the evidence. This involves computer searches with key words and syntax that will efficiently locate the best evidence as well as hand searches (Booth & Madge, 1998). Typical databases you might search are MEDLINE, CINAHL, the Cochrane Database of Systematic Reviews, the ACP Journal Club, Evidence-Based Medicine, DARE, ERIC, PsycLit, and OT SEARCH. In addition to published articles, OT SEARCH includes manuscripts that have not been published but provide evidence that should be considered. You will also need to conduct hand searches of appropriate journals because not all articles on a specific topic will automatically show up in a database search and because not all journals are indexed. In addition to electronic and journal resources, there are human resources who can help you, and reference librarians should be at the top of the list. Additionally, researchers in related disciplines can be helpful because they may have access to important unpublished data, or they may be able to put you in touch with their colleagues who have been conducting studies relevant to the evidence you are trying to track down.

Question 3: Do I Appraise the Evidence or Take It at Face Value?

To appraise the evidence, of course, includes everything you hated about any research course you took, or why you may have avoided taking any. Appraising the evidence requires that you analyze each section of an article and apply the evidence hierarchy to determine at which level the study meets the established criteria. Article analysis is central to evidence-based practice, but it can also be very difficult. One of the structured article review instruments, such as those found on the Web sites of The Cochrane Collaboration, the University of Alberta, Mc Master University, and York University, can help you get started, or you can develop a review tool based on the 1993–1994 *JAMA* article series entitled, "User's Guide to the Medical Literature." When you get to the section of the article that includes the statistics, get out the snacks and bring up Trochim's data analysis

Web site at Cornell University to reduce your anxiety and start you on your way to understanding the numbers before you (Trochim, February 20, 2000).

Question 4: Do I Use the Evidence to Do the Right Things Right?

One way to use the evidence before you is to develop a clinical guideline for your practice and format it according to the six "rights" identified by Graham (1996): Is "the right person, doing the right thing, the right way, in the right place, at the right time, with the right result" (p. 11)? The clinical guideline for "doing the right things right" is developed by using the evidence you locate to delineate the six "rights":

1. Who is the *right* person to implement the intervention? What level of competence is required? Is special certification required? Can an occupational therapy assistant implement the intervention?
2. What is the *right* thing to do? What does the evidence tell you? Does the patient agree?
3. What is the *right* way to implement the intervention? Does the evidence suggest a protocol or specifications that must be met? Can the patient's dignity and privacy be maintained equally in all contexts in which the intervention could be implemented? Does the frequency or duration of the intervention make a difference?
4. What is the *right* place in which to implement the intervention? Is the home better than the clinic? Is the clinic better than the classroom? Is equipment required that dictates where the intervention must take place?
5. What is the *right* time to provide the intervention? Does time since onset of disability or admission to rehabilitation services make a difference? Does delaying the intervention make a difference? Does the time of day make a difference? Does time until, or since, discharge make a difference?
6. What is the *right* result? Did the intervention do what it was intended to do? Is the patient satisfied with the result? Are you satisfied with the result? After you have implemented the evidence-based guideline, ask yourself Question 5.

Question 5: Do I Evaluate the Impact of Evidence-Based Practice?

To assess the impact of the evidence-based clinical guideline you developed in response to Question 4, you would begin with a chart audit to determine whether the guideline was actually used and, then, whether it was used as intended. Finally, patient outcomes, cost-effectiveness, patient satisfaction, and therapist satisfaction must also be considered. The impact of the latter, therapist satisfaction with evidence-based practice, is pivotal, especially given the barriers to evidence-based practice.

Barriers and Motivation for Evidence-Based Practice

As Law and Baum (1998) noted in an issue of the *Canadian Journal of Occupational Therapy* dedicated to evidence-based practice, there are many barriers to its practice at both the system level and the individual level. The barriers cited include lack of administrative support, lack of access to research evidence, lack of skill in finding the evidence, lack of skill in interpreting the evidence, and lack of time. These barriers were reiterated in a Level V study of Canadian therapists' perceptions of evidence-based practice (Dubouloz, Egan, Vallerand, & von Zweck, 1999). The authors found that although therapists perceived evidence-based practice as a way of looking for understanding of the interventions they used, it also generated feelings of inadequacy related to research skills. Additionally, there were attitudinal barriers in that the therapists perceived that the evidence they would find might threaten the ways they preferred to practice.

Gray (1997) suggested a formula that we might find helpful as we seek to identify factors that will influence our performance of evidence-based practice (see Figure 49.1). He perceived that the performance of evidence-based practice is directly influenced by motivation multiplied by competence divided by the barriers we need to overcome. Many factors in the context in which we practice today can be barriers to us; however, I am choosing to reframe them under motivation. Therefore, legislation, regulation, prospective payment system for skilled nursing facilities, capitations on reimbursement, new patient populations, new practice environments, new collaborations, and a new episodic reimbursement system for rehabilitation hospitals and exempt rehabilitation units can all be entered into the formula as motivation. I perceive them as motivators because they provide for us the impetus to describe, exam-

$$\text{Performance} = \frac{\text{Motivation} \times \text{Competence}}{\text{Barriers}}$$

Figure 49.1. Factors affecting the performance of evidence-based practice (Gray, 1997, p. 7).

ine, and publish the evidence derived from what we do and how we do it. Also under motivation add the principles in our Code of Ethics that require us, for ethical practice, to "collaborate with service recipients," "fully inform . . . [them] of the nature, risks, and potential outcomes of any intervention," and "avoid harm" to them as well as to "perform . . . duties on the basis of accurate and current information" and "take responsibility for maintaining competence" (AOTA, 1994, p. 1037).

At a minimum, competence in this formula refers to competence in searching for, appraising, and applying existing evidence in everyday practice. For professional survival, however, we must be able to generate, publish, and make accessible to all the evidence that we now have to search for. This requires that we learn to gather evidence systematically in our practices as well as learn the know ledge, skills, and attitudes associated with occupational therapy research at the beginning, intermediate, or advanced levels of competence (Abreu et al., 1998).

Although one could dwell on barriers in the work environment and in the laws, regulations, and reimbursement systems, the barrier over which we have most influence is our own attitudes. On the basis of the findings of the Canadian study (Dubouloz et al., 1999), we have been alerted ahead of time that it may not be the external barriers but, rather, our own attitudinal barriers that may hinder the practice of evidence-based occupational therapy in the United States in the new millennium.

However, there are four encouraging examples of our movement toward evidence-based practice in the United States. Perhaps in response to the evidence-based practice initiatives of our Canadian and British colleagues, the new *Standards for an Accredited Educational Program for the Occupational Therapist* developed by the Accreditation Council for Occupational Therapy Education (ACOTE) require that occupational therapist graduates be able to "provide evidence-based effective therapeutic intervention related to performance areas" (ACOTE, 1999, p. 579). Furthermore, the AOTA Executive Board passed a motion that an evidence-based panel be formed to review and evaluate research that relates to *The Guide to Occupational Therapy Practice* (Moyers, 1999, 2000) in order to make the document evidence based. Additionally, the *AJOT* Associate Editor for Evidence-Based Practice, Linda Tickle-Degnen, instituted the Evidence-Based Practice Forum in which she guides practitioners through some aspect of evidence-based practice.

The best practice example, however, is from the notice in the *Coverage Policy Bulletin* of Aetna US Healthcare in which coverage of cognitive rehabilitation was recently announced. Although the studies were not Level I or Level II studies, the evidence was convincing. It states in the bulletin:

> The efficacy of cognitive therapy so far has been measured by its objective influence on function and the subjective value of these changes to the individual. Although current evidence supports cognitive therapy as a promising approach, definitive conclusions regarding its efficacy must await large-scale, well-conducted, controlled trials. (Aetna US Healthcare, 2000)

We can provide that evidence!

Conclusion

Eleanor Clarke Slagle was a proponent of habit development. Therefore, I will suggest two new habit patterns that we need to develop if we are to address proactively the realities of our professional exigencies. Each suggested habit pattern is followed by a question.

Habit 1: Evidence-Based Practice Now

Although the evidence for *what* we do and *how* we do it may be difficult to find, we have an obligation to become competent in, and make a habit of, searching for the evidence, appraising its value, and presenting it to those we serve in an understandable manner.

Question 1. After reading this lecture, could you provide your next several patients with a summary of the research evidence on the occupational therapy intervention options you are considering for them so that together you could make the best decisions?

Habit 2: The Evidence Base of Occupational Therapy in the New Millennium

We also have an obligation to improve our research competencies, to develop the habit of using those competencies in everyday practice, and to advance the evidence base of occupational therapy in the new millennium. Only then can we be sure that as we seek to do the "right things right," we are fulfilling our ethical responsibility to perform our "duties on the basis of accurate and current information" (AOTA, 1994, p. 1037). I will close by asking you to think ahead one decade.

Question 2. If in the year 2010 you stand accused of practicing occupational therapy based on research, will there be enough evidence to convict you?

Acknowledgments

I thank the following colleagues for their hearty critiques of my thinking and of the Slagle manuscript: Lynette S. Chandler, PhD, PT; Denise Chisholm, MS, OTR/L; Louise Fawcett, PhD, OTR/L, FAOTA; Sharon Gwinn, MS, OTR/L; Tamara Mills, OTR/L; Sharon Novalis, MSOT, OTR/L; Varick Olson, PhD, PT; Beth Skidmore, OTR/L; Ronald G. Stone, MS, OTR/L; George Tomlin, PhD, OTR/L; and especially to my mentor, Joan C. Rogers, PhD, OTR/L, FAOTA, ABDA.

References

Abreu, B., Peloquin, S. M., & Ottenbacher, K. (1998). Competence in scientific inquiry and research. *American Journal of Occupational Therapy, 52,* 751–759. http://dx.doi.org/10.5014/ajot.52.9.751

Accreditation Council for Occupational Therapy Education. (1999). Standards for an accredited educational program for the occupational therapist. *American Journal of Occupational Therapy, 53,* 575–582. http://dx.doi.org/10.5014/ajot.53.6.575

Aetna US Healthcare. Cognitive rehabilitation. *Coverage Policy Bulletin.* Retrieved March 6, 2000, from http://www.aetnaushc.com/cpb/data/CPBA0214.htm

American Occupational Therapy Association. (1993). Occupational therapy roles. *American Journal of Occupational Therapy, 47,* 1087–1099. http://dx.doi.org/10.5014/ajot.47.12.1087

American Occupational Therapy Association. (1994). Occupational therapy code of ethics. *American Journal of Occupational Therapy, 48,* 1037–1038. http://dx.doi.org/10.5014/ajot.48.11.1037

American Occupational Therapy Association. (1998). Standards of practice for occupational therapy. *American Journal of Occupational Therapy, 52,* 866–869. http://dx.doi.org/10.5014/ajot.52.10.866

American Occupational Therapy Foundation. (1983). The Foundation—Research competencies for clinicians and educators. *American Journal of Occupational Therapy, 37,* 44–46.

Booth, A., & Madge, B. (1998). Finding the evidence. In T. Bury & J. Mead (Eds.), *Evidence-based health care: A practical guide for therapists* (pp. 107–135). Woburn, MA: Butterworth-Heinemann.

Brooke, M., Lateur, B., Diana-Rigby, G., & Questad, K. (1991). Shoulder subluxation in hemiplegia: Effects of three different supports. *Archives of Physical Medicine and Rehabilitation, 72,* 582–586.

Brown, S. J. (1999). *Knowledge for health-care practice: A guide for using research evidence.* Philadelphia: Saunders.

Bury, T., & Mead, J. (1998). *Evidence-based health care: A practical guide for therapists.* Woburn, MA: Butterworth-Heinemann.

Bye, R. A. (1998). When clients are dying: Occupational therapists' perspectives. *Occupational Therapy Journal of Research, 18,* 3–24.

Case-Smith, J., Heaphy, T., Marr, D., Galvin, B., Koch, V., Ellis, M. G., & Perez, I. (1998). Fine motor and functional performance outcomes in preschool children. *American Journal of Occupational Therapy, 52,* 788–800. http://dx.doi.org/10.5014/ajot.52.10.788

Close, J., Ellis, M., Hooper, R., Glucksman, E., Jackson, S., & Swift, C. (1999). Prevention of falls in the elderly trial (PROFET): A randomised controlled trial. *Lancet, 353,* 93–97.

Cohn, E. S., & Cermak, S. A. (1998). Including the family perspective in sensory integration outcomes research. *American Journal of Occupational Therapy, 52,* 540–546. http://dx.doi.org/10.5014/ajot.52.7.540

Cummings, R. G., Thomas, M., Szonyi, G., Salkeld, G., O'Neill, E., Westbury, C., & Frampton, G. (1999). Home visits by an occupational therapist for assessment and modification of environmental hazards: A randomized trial of falls prevention. *Journal of the American Geriatrics Society, 47,* 1397–1402.

Dubouloz, C.-J., Egan, M., Vallerand, J., & von Zweck, C. (1999). Occupational therapists' perceptions of evidence-based practice. *American Journal of Occupational Therapy, 53,* 445–458. http://dx.doi.org/10.5014/ajot.53.5.445

Graham, G. (1996, June). Clinically effective medicine in a rational health service. *Health Director, 11–12.*

Gray, J.A.M. (1997). *Evidence-based health care: How to make health policy and management decisions.* New York: Churchill Livingstone.

Hurd, M. M., Farrell, K. H., & Waylonis, G. W. (1974). Shouldersling for hemiplegia: Friend or foe? *Archives of Physical Medicine and Rehabilitation, 55,* 519–522

Law, M., & Baum, C. (1998). Evidence-based occupational therapy. *Canadian Journal of Occupational Therapy, 65,* 131–135.

Lidz, C. W., & Meisel, A. (1983). *Informed consent and the structure of medical care. In Making health-care decisions: The ethical and legal implications of informed consent in the patient–practitioner relationship* (Vol. 2). Washington, DC: U.S. Government Printing Office.

Lin, K., Wu, C., Tickle-Degnen, L., & Coster, W. (1997). Enhancing occupational performance through occupationally embedded exercise: A meta-analytic review. *Occupational Therapy Journal of Research, 17,* 25–47.

Mayhan, Y. D., Holm, M. B., Fawcett, L. C. (Eds.) & National Commission on Continued Competency in Occupational Therapy. (1999). *Continued competency in occupational therapy: Recommendations to the profession and key stakeholders.* Gaithersburg, MD: National Board for Certification in Occupational Therapy.

McHale, K., & Cermak, S. A. (1992). Fine motor activities in elementary school: Preliminary findings and provisional implications for children with fine motor problems. *American Journal of Occupational Therapy, 46,* 898–903. http://dx.doi.org/10.5014/ajot.46.10.898

Mitcham, M. D. (1985). *Integrating research competencies into occupational therapy: A teaching guide for academic and clinical educators.* Rockville, MD: American Occupational Therapy Foundation.

Moore, A., McQuay, H., & Gray, J. A. M. (Eds.). (1995). Evidence-based everything. *Bandolier, 1*(12), 1.

Moyers, P. A. (1999). The guide to occupational therapy practice. *American Journal of Occupational Therapy, 53,* 247–322. http://dx.doi.org/10.5014/ajot.53.3.247

Moyers, P. A. (2000). Letters to the editor—Author's response. *American Journal of Occupational Therapy, 54,* 113–114.

Mulligan, S. (1998). Patterns of sensory integration dysfunction: A confirmatory factor analysis. *American Journal of Occupational Therapy, 52,* 819–828.

Neistadt, M. E., & Marques, K. (1984). An independent living skills training program. *American Journal of Occupational Therapy, 38,* 671–676.

Nicol, M. M., Robertson, L., & Connaughton, J. A. (1999). Life skills programs for people with chronic mental illness. *Cochrane Database of Systematic Reviews, 3: The Schizophrenia Group.* Retrieved January 26, 2000, from http://www.update-software.com/cochrane.htm

Ottenbacher, K. J., & Maas, F. (1999). Quantitative Research Series—How to detect effects: Statistical power and evidence-based practice in occupational therapy research. *American Journal of Occupational Therapy, 53,* 181–188. http://dx.doi.org/10.5014/ajot.53.2.181

Portney, L. G., & Watkins, M. P. (1993). *Foundations of clinical research: Applications to practice.* Norwalk, CT: Appleton & Lange.

Ray, W. A., Taylor, J. A., Meador, K. G., Thapa, P. B., Brown, A. K., Kajihara, H. K., Davis, C., Gideon, P., & Griffin, M. R. (1997). A randomized trial of a consultation service to reduce falls in nursing homes. *Journal of the American Medical Association, 278,* 557–562.

Rennie, D. (1986). Guarding the guardians: A conference on editorial peer review. *Journal of the American Medical Association, 256,* 2391–2392.

Richardson, W. S., Wilson, M. C., Nishikawa, J., & Hayward, R. S. (1995). The well-built clinical question: A key to evidence-based decisions. *ACP Journal Club, 123,* A-12.

Rogers, J. C., Holm, M. B., Burgio, L. D., Granieri, E., Hsu, C., Hardin, J. M., & McDowell, B. J. (1999). Improving morning care routines of nursing home residents with dementia. *Journal of the American Geriatrics Society, 47,* 1049–1057.

Sackett, D. L., Haynes, R. B., & Tugwell, P. (1985). How to read a clinical journal. In D. L. Sackett, R. B. Haynes, & P. Tugwell (Eds.), *Clinical epidemiology: A basic science for clinical medicine* (pp. 285–322). Boston: Little, Brown.

Sackett, D. L., Richardson, W. S., Rosenberg, W., & Haynes, R. B. (1997). Critically praising the evidence. In D. L. Sackett, W. S. Richardson, W. Rosenberg, & R. B. Haynes (Eds.), *Evidence-based medicine: How to practice and teach EBM* (pp. 38–156). New York: Churchill Livingstone.

Sackett, D. L., Rosenberg, W. M., Gray, J. A. M., Haynes, R. B., & Richardson, W. S. (1996). Evidence-based medicine: What it is and what it isn't. *British Medical Journal, 312,* 71–72.

Schneiderman, L. J., Kaplan, R. M., Pearlman, R. A., & Teetzel, H. (1993). Do physicians' own preferences for life-sustaining treatment influence their perceptions of patients' preferences? *Journal of Clinical Ethics, 4,* 28–32.

Shenk, D. (1997). *Data smog.* San Francisco: Harper Edge.

Silverman, W. A. (1998). *Where's the evidence?: Debates in modern medicine.* New York: Oxford University Press.

Tickle-Degnen, L. (1998). Quantitative Research Series—Communicating with clients about treatment outcomes: The use of meta-analytic evidence in collaborative treatment planning. *American Journal of Occupational Therapy, 52,* 526–530. http://dx.doi.org/10.5014/ajot.52.7.526

Trochim, W. (February 20, 2000). *What is the research methods knowledge base.* Retrieved from http://trochim.human.cor-nell.edu/kb/index.htm

Vargas, S., & Camilli, G. (1999). A meta-analysis of research on sensory integration treatment. *American*

Journal of Occupational Therapy, 53, 189–198. http://dx.doi.org/10.5014/ajot.53.2.189

Williams, R., Taffs, L., & Minuk, T. (1988). Evaluation of two support methods for the subluxated shoulder in hemiplegic patients. *Physical Therapy, 68,* 1209–1213.

Zorowitz, R. D., Idank, D., Ikai, T., Hughes, M. B., & Johnston, M. V. (1995). Shoulder subluxation after a stroke: A comparison of four supports. *Archives of Physical Medicine and Rehabilitation, 76,* 763–771.

CHAPTER 50

Heterarchy and Hierarchy: A Critical Appraisal of the "Levels of Evidence" as a Tool for Clinical Decision Making

LINDA TICKLE-DEGNEN AND GARY BEDELL

One day the two authors of this paper were having a "quick conversation" that started with one of us (Linda) asking for advice about a research study that fell within the expertise of the other (Gary). As is often the case with quick conversations, the topic transformed and soon we were engaged in a more lengthy and gradually intensifying dialogue about a different topic: in this case, the role of *levels of evidence* in clinical reasoning. The term levels of evidence refers to a ranking scale that is used in evidence-based practice as a tool for determining the quality of information coming from research evidence (e.g., Holm, 2000 [see Chapter 49]; Law & Philp, 2002; Sackett, Strauss, Richardson, Rosenberg, & Haynes, 2000). We discovered that we both had worried about the inflexible ranking of research studies according to the standard levels of evidence model, and had worried even more about the possible effects of this model on clinical decision making in rehabilitation if the model were put into practice in an exclusive manner. As we sorted and clarified our thoughts, we came to the conclusion that the basis of these worries was that in actuality we as practitioners do not think in an inflexible or exclusionary manner about any source of information, *nor should we* given the complexity of human responses, the realities of practice resources, and the wide variety and quality of different forms of information available to us. If practitioners were to use exclusively the standard levels of evidence model in their selection and use of information, they would be making suboptimal decisions based upon less information than that which was relevant, valid, and available for making the decisions. This creates a paradox in that the very model that is intended to support

the use of best evidence in decision making, in fact fails to support the formation of a best decision, and may even hinder it, if applied rigidly and exclusively.

By no means are we the only ones to worry about the problems of a model that restricts the use of information from a vast pool of important and available information. Writers across health practice disciplines have had similar worries. Sackett et al. (2000), in their recent revision of a foundational text of evidence-based medicine responded to some of these worries by revising their original description of evidence-based medicine, which had focused on using information from research studies as the primary source of information. The revision gave evidence-based medicine a more encompassing focus that included "the integration of best research evidence with clinical expertise and patient values." Under this new description, all three information elements have equal status in clinical decision making. Although this revision begins to address some of the concerns, it does not address specifically the problem of the rigid and exclusive use of the standard levels of evidence model for selecting and using evidence from research studies. In this respect, Law and Philp (2002) have voiced a common concern of occupational therapists that the standard levels help to rank evidence from quantitative research designs yet do not help to rank evidence from qualitative designs. This concern is an important one and applies not only to the failure of the levels with respect to qualitative designs, but also with respect to many quantitative designs.

The purpose of this paper is to argue for a method of including all relevant, valid, and available research evidence for making clinical decisions. We limit our discussion to research evidence because the levels of evidence model typically applies to research rather than other forms of information. Furthermore, we discuss only research evidence related to the goal of choosing appropriate therapeutic interventions for clients because the levels of evidence model typically used in occupational therapy is one that evaluates evidence with this goal in mind. However, we recognize that our discussion is relevant for understanding how all forms of information, not merely research evidence, come together into several types of clinical decisions, not merely ones related to choosing interventions.

It is our position that the standard levels of evidence model is not inherently wrong for certain purposes in evidence-based practice. Rather it is wrong when applied in a manner that excludes the use of all relevant, valid, and available research evidence for clinical decision making. This paper is offered with the intent to address a recent challenge from the Editor's Desk in *The American Journal of Occupational Therapy* (Ottenbacher, Tickle-Degnen, & Hasselkus, 2002). The editorial asked the following questions:

> What is the best evidence for occupational therapy? Can best evidence come not only from large randomized controlled trials, but also from other types of study designs, such as single-subject, quasi-experimental, correlational, narrative analysis, ethnographic, and phenomenological designs? (pp. 248–249)

We hope to reframe the argument about best evidence in occupational therapy and to invite the readership to join the discussion. We begin with a critical appraisal of the standard levels of evidence model used in rehabilitation and end with suggestions for an approach that moves away from overzealous exclusion of research studies and toward a more inclusionary approach. We favor a flexible, multifaceted approach to assessing, selecting, and using research evidence. Information goals in clinical practice are *heterarchical* in organization rather than *hierarchical* (see Austin & Vancouver, 1996, for a relevant review). There are multiple information goals that are better treated as forming a network. As opposed to the standard levels of evidence model in which a single overriding goal guides the retrieval and use of information, in a heterarchical approach there is a network of goals which function in parallel.

A Description of the Standard Levels of Evidence Model

The standard levels of evidence model is a ranking of research studies along two dimensions that are inte-

grated into one ranking scale (e.g., Holm, 2000; Law & Philp, 2002; Sackett et al., 2000). One dimension is the internal validity of the research design for answering questions of causation (Cook & Campbell, 1979). For example, studies that are well designed randomized controlled trials (RCT) or meta-analytic syntheses of these types of trials have high internal validity because they have controlled for nonintervention factors that may affect the results of the study. The well-designed RCT provides a strong demonstration that research participants' outcomes are *caused* by having received or not received a tested intervention, not caused by other factors, such as biased assignment of participants to intervention and comparison groups. Studies that have some control over nonintervention factors in their designs, such as quasi-experiments or case-control studies, have intermediate levels of internal validity. Studies that have low internal validity are ones that have designs, such as case reports, in which there were no controls for factors other than the intervention that may affect the results. These studies provide less definitive, evidence for the intervention causing changes in the research participants, although, as we argue in a later section, they may provide valid evidence of another form.

The second dimension integrated into the ranking scale of the standard levels of evidence model is statistical conclusion validity (Cook & Campbell, 1979). Statistical conclusion validity has to do with confidence about *probabilities* of effectiveness in a population. Research studies that can show with high confidence the degree to which the intervention is likely to be effective in the larger clinical population have high statistical conclusion validity. These studies, which fall at the top of the ranking scale, have large sample sizes and reliable, valid measures. Studies that cannot provide a confident estimation of the degree to which the intervention is likely to be effective in the larger clinical population, because of small sample size or poor reliability of measurement or inappropriate data analysis, have low statistical conclusion validity and fall at the bottom of the ranking scale.

The standard levels of evidence model contains a single ranking system that integrates these two dimensions of study validity. Designs that have both high internal and statistical conclusion validity, such as RCTs with large sample sizes, receive the top ranking. Intermediate ranks are assigned to studies that have high validity on one dimension but compromised validity on another dimension (with a lowered internal validity driving the ranking down more heavily than a lowered statistical conclusion validity). And studies that have low validity on both dimensions receive the lowest ranking.

A Limitation of the Standard Levels of Evidence Model

The standard model is useful for selecting and using high quality research evidence for the clinical information goal of learning about probabilities of an intervention's causal effect in the clinical population as a whole. This type of information is very important in choosing and communicating about intervention evidence. If the only available studies are ones that fall lower in the standard ranking system, the practitioner must be cautious about her or his claims to others about intervention causing beneficial outcomes and the probability of that effect. If relevant top-ranking studies are available, then the practitioner can be more confident in making these claims to clients, managers, and funding agencies.

But there is more to choosing and communicating about an intervention than simply understanding its probability of causing a beneficial outcome in a population. Practitioners are concerned not only with causality and probability, but also with *patterns* and *possibility* when it comes to selecting an intervention. Quantitative and qualitative studies that do not provide information about causality or about the probability of effects occurring in the population as a whole are excluded or devalued by the standard levels of evidence model. However, these studies may provide relevant and valid intervention-related information about (a) patterns, in the form of associations and profiles, of client attributes, perceptions, occupations, and contexts, and (b) the range of possible intervention strategies and outcomes. Pattern and possibility information may come from quantitative descriptive, observational, and correlational designs, and qualitative narrative analysis, ethnographic, and phenomenological designs. The seeking of causality, probability, pattern, and possibility information are equal status information goals with respect to choosing an intervention. In addition, a single research study can have a higher quality status for providing valid evidence about one type of information (e.g., causality) while having a lower quality status for providing valid evidence about another type of information (e.g., pattern). The organization of research information into a single hierarchy of levels may provide a solution to the "best" evidence for answering a certain information need (e.g., causality information), yet will not provide a solution to the "best" interven-

tion choice. A better model for organizing information is a heterarchy in which it is understood that goals are organized in a multidimensional web of linkages.

An Illustration

How might the search for, evaluation of, and use of research evidence be organized in a heterarchical model? In client-centered practice, this organization begins with the client's needs and goals. The occupational therapy practitioner, who is the primary retriever and conduit of information, works with the client to (1) identify the research information needs of the client and the practitioner, (2) translate these needs into a search for relevant types of research evidence, (3) evaluate the quality of these different types of retrieved research evidence in relation to the specific information needs of the client and practitioner, (4) synthesize the information from research studies, (5) synthesize research evidence with patient preferences and practitioner expertise, (6) make a decision about what to do, and (7) try out the intervention and revise accordingly.

We offer as illustration a hypothetical case in which a young man named John wants to get and retain a satisfying job. John is diagnosed with HIV/AIDS and has difficulty managing his symptoms, medications, and daily life routines. The occupational therapy practitioner works with John and identifies a set of research information needs and then translates them into clinical questions that guide the research retrieval process. John and the practitioner have identified that they need answers to the questions listed below. The questions are categorized broadly, and not necessarily mutually exclusively, in to ones of possibility, pattern, causality, and probability:

1. *What is possible?* What is the range of interventions that have been used with people similar to John who would like to get and retain a job? What is the range of outcomes that people similar to John have experienced while participating in these interventions?

2. *Is there a pattern?* Are there patterns of satisfaction and dissatisfaction that people similar to John feel with certain intervention strategies, intensities, or contexts? Are there patterns of daily life routines in people similar to John that predict a successful versus unsuccessful response to intervention?

3. *Is there causality?* Does a self-management intervention strategy (Gifford, Laurent, Gonzales, Chesney,

& Lorig, 1998) lead to improvements in management of symptoms, medication, and daily life routines in people similar to John? Do improvements in management of symptoms, medication, and daily life routines lead to positive job outcomes in people similar to John?

4. *What is the probability?* How common is it for people similar to John to be able to learn to manage their symptoms, medications, and daily life routines? Is it likely that people similar to John will have positive job outcomes following a selfmanagement intervention?

For answering question sets 1 and 2 above, both qualitative and quantitative studies can provide "best" evidence and must be judged according to the degree to which they provide meaningful and deep description of possibilities and patterns, as opposed to the degree to which they provide controls related to causal inference purposes. For answering question sets 3 and 4, quantitative studies are likely to involve designs and procedures that are relevant, however, it is not necessarily only the randomized control trial that provides the best evidence. For example, in set 3, single subject designs can offer clarity in terms of tracking small increments in change over time. In set 4, large population surveys with random selection of participants may be the best evidence.

Once research studies are retrieved and evaluated for their informational value, the practitioner works with John in an iterative, flexible manner to synthesize the research findings, then take this synthesis and integrate it with information related to John's preferences and the practitioner's prior experience and expertise into a "big picture" of the intervention options for John. From here, they make tentative decisions about intervention, try them out, and revise as needed.

Future Directions

Our illustration of John is underdeveloped. Suppose that John is African-American, lives in New York City, has a prior history of substance abuse, is easily fatigued, experiences periodic bouts of depression, and has a supportive extended family. The use of research evidence becomes more challenging the more details we know about John. There will be little if any evidence about people who were exactly like John and living in John's circumstances. Practitioners must know how to take research evidence that may not be closely applicable to the specific client or to the specific context of intervention,

integrate it, communicate about it, and then decide with the client what they will do to meet the client's needs. In this paper, we have not developed models for evaluating possibility and pattern information. Furthermore, we have not addressed how to evaluate and weigh evidence from a study as it applies to the needs of a particular client (applicability) or to the resources of the intervention setting (feasibility), though others have provided preliminary guidelines (Sackett et al., 2000; Tickle-Degnen, 2002). Nor have we addressed how to weigh information from research findings, client preferences, and practitioner expertise as decisions are made.

The hypothetical case of John illustrates the gaps we have in our current models for evaluating and using research evidence. From a heterarchical perspective, we must have multiple and linked methods for evaluating the informational value of different forms of research evidence. In their clinical reasoning, practitioners synthesize complex information in a flexible manner. Evidence-based practice must build models, based upon this natural process, that help practitioners to evaluate and synthesize research evidence from multiple studies then integrate it with information coming from other sources in a manner that is useful and practical for clinical decision making. We hope that others enter this discussion to express opinion and insight either in the venue of the Evidence-Based Practice Forum or through letters to the editor.

References

Austin, J. T., & Vancouver, J. B. (1996). Goal constructs in psychology: Structure, process, and content. *Psychological Bulletin, 120,* 338–375.

Cook, T. D., & Campbell, D. T. (1979). *Quasi-experimentation: Design and analysis issues for field settings.* Chicago: Rand McNally.

Gifford, A. L., Laurent, D. D., Gonzales, V. M., Chesney, M. A., & Lorig, K. R. (1998). Pilot randomized trial of education to improve self-management skills in men with symptomatic HIV/AIDS. *Journal of Acquired Immune Deficiency Syndrome and Retrovirology, 18,* 136–144.

Holm, M. B. (2000). The 2000 Eleanor Clarke Slagle Lecture: Our mandate for the new millennium: Evidence-based practice. *American Journal of Occupational Therapy, 54,* 575–585. http://dx.doi.org/10.5014/ajot.54.6.575 Reprinted as Chapter 49.

Law, M., & Philp, I. (2002). Evaluating the evidence. In M. Law (Ed.), *Evidence-based rehabilitation: A guide to practice* (pp. 97–107). Thorofare, NJ: Slack.

Ottenbacher, K. J., Tickle-Degnen, L., & Hasselkus, B. R. (2002). From the desk of the editor—Therapists awake! The challenge of evidence-based occupational therapy. *American Journal of Occupational Therapy, 56,* 247–249. http://dx.doi.org/10.5014/ajot.56.3.247

Sackett, D. L., Strauss, S. E., Richardson, W. S., Rosenberg, W., & Haynes, R. B. (2000). *Evidence-based medicine:* *How to practice and teach EBM* (2nd ed.). Edinburgh, Scotland: Churchill-Livingstone.

Tickle-Degnen, L. (2002). Communicating evidence to clients, managers, and funders. In M. Law (Ed.), *Evidence-based rehabilitation: A guide to practice* (pp. 221–254). Thorofare, NJ: Slack.

CHAPTER 51

The Process of Evidence-Based Clinical Decision Making in Occupational Therapy

CHRISTOPHER J. LEE AND LINDA T. MILLER

There is a need for occupational therapy to conceive of evidence-based practice in a way that reflects the contextualized nature of occupational engagement. In occupational therapy, we should resist following the lead of experts in evidence-based medicine, such as Sackett and his colleagues (Rosenberg & Donald, 1995; Sackett, Rosenberg, Gray, Haynes, & Richardson, 1996; Sackett, Straus, Richardson, Rosenberg, & Haynes, 2000), who advocate that clinical decision-making must be based on systematic appraisal of the best research evidence. Instead, we argue here that evidence-based clinical decision-making in occupational therapy should encompass the diverse variety of evidence brought to the clinical context by both the client and therapist.

The following definitions of evidence-based practice are excellent examples of those espoused by medicine. Rosenberg and Donald (1995, p. 1122) define evidence-based practice as "the process of systematically finding, appraising, and using contemporaneous research findings for clinical decision." Similarly, Sackett et al. (1996, p. 71) describe evidence-based practice as "the conscientious, explicit, and judicious use of current best evidence in making decisions about the care of individual patients." Both of these definitions reflect a core belief that evidence-based practice entails systematic appraisal of the best research evidence. More recently, Sackett et al. (2000, p. 1) refer to evidence-based medicine as "the integration of best research evidence with clinical expertise and patient values." Although this definition acknowledges the expertise of the clinician and the values of the patient, it still clings to research as the only source of evidence. We propose that the values, beliefs, knowledge, and experiences of the clinician and client be recognized, in addition to research, as valuable sources of evidence in the clinical decision-making process.

Although the core belief about evidence-based medicine is beginning to acknowledge the expertise of the clinician and the values of the patient, it does not adequately reflect the highly contextualized and dynamic nature of occupational therapy. The practice of occupational therapy is an individualized activity shaped by a unique client-therapist relationship; it is not a static outcome that can be achieved by following a rigid procedure. Furthermore, as noted by Tickle-Degnen and Bedell (2003 [see Chapter 50]), the use of a single, invariant hierarchy of research evidence serves to depreciate the information provided by research methods other than randomized clinical trials. There are many kinds of research, and each variety can provide important insights into the nature of occupational performance.

Occupational therapy is highly contextualized, and evidence-based practice should reflect the different kinds of evidence that clients as well as therapists bring to the therapeutic process. When describing evidence-based practice in occupational therapy, it is important to emphasize that rehabilitation is a dynamic process. Unlike medical interventions, which can be described as standardized procedures, occupational therapy interventions are often more aptly described as dynamic *processes*. Indeed, the *Occupational Therapy Practice Framework: Domain and Process* (American Occupational Therapy Association [AOTA], 2002) clearly identifies occupational therapy as a dynamic process. To further delineate the distinction between medical practice and occupational therapy practice, consider the role of the patient or client. Medical procedures are frequently pharmacological or surgical in nature, with the patient playing a passive or receptive role. In

This chapter was previously published in the *American Journal of Occupational Therapy, 57*, 473–477. Copyright © 2003, American Occupational Therapy Association. Reprinted with permission. http://dx.doi.org/10.5014/ajot.57.4.473

contrast, the rehabilitation client plays a participatory role in the dynamic therapy process. Therefore, we argue that effective evidence-based practice in occupational therapy should acknowledge the diverse kinds of evidence brought to the clinical context by both the client and therapist.

Methods of Evidence

In his classic paper on the sources of evidence that serve to substantiate belief, Peirce (1877) presents four general methods of appraising belief that he identifies as the method of tenacity, the *method of authority,* the *a priori method,* and the method of science. In the clinical context, each of these methods introduces a different kind of evidence into the therapeutic process.

The method of tenacity refers to the unwavering acceptance of an idea because it is what one already believes; it is the continuing adherence to a belief on the basis of its longstanding acceptance. As Peirce (1877) comments, such "a steady and immovable faith yields great peace of mind" (p. 7). But this method of sustaining a belief requires considerable resolution and the ability to dismiss contrary opinion and evidence. As Peirce notes, "the social impulse is against it. . . . Unless we make ourselves hermits, we shall necessarily influence each other's opinions" (p. 8).

The method of authority refers to the uncritical acceptance of an idea because it is advocated by a respected individual, group, or institution. In large part, the method of authority perpetuates common beliefs in a culture. As Peirce (1877) notes, "It is mere accident of their having been taught as they have, and of their having been surrounded with the manners and associations they have, that has caused them to believe as they do and not far differently" (p. 10).

The *a priori* method refers to the acceptance of an idea because it is consistent with reason; that is, it is an idea that "we find ourselves inclined to believe" (Peirce, 1877, p. 10) because it seems to make sense. Although the *a priori* method "is far more intellectual and respectable from the point of view of reason than either of the others" (p. 10), it remains the case that what one person is inclined to believe as reasonable is not necessarily the same as what another person is inclined to believe. As Peirce notes, it "is always more or less a matter of fashion" (p. 11) to determine whether a conclusion is agreeable to reason.

The fourth method described by Peirce (1877) is science. Peirce viewed science as a method of overcoming the "accidental and capricious element" (p. 11) in the other methods. However, in contemporary accounts, science is no longer attributed such a degree of objectivity. For instance, in his influential historical analysis of science, Kuhn (1970) argues that "an apparently arbitrary element, compounded of personal and historical accident, is always a formative ingredient of the beliefs espoused by a given scientific community at a given time" (p. 4). Furthermore, Kuhn notes that "few philosophers of science still seek absolute criteria for the verification of scientific theories" (p. 145) because "no theory can ever be exposed to all possible relevant tests" (p. 145). Thus, in considering science as a method of appraising belief, it is important to acknowledge the provisional nature of scientific evidence.

The methods of appraising belief described by Peirce (1877) provide a useful classification of the different kinds of evidence that may be introduced into the therapeutic process by the client and therapist. An account of the variety of client beliefs is given in the next section of the paper, followed by an account of the variety of therapist beliefs. These beliefs affect the therapeutic process; they represent the kinds of evidence warranting consideration when appraising the potential therapeutic benefit of an intervention in occupational therapy.

Client Perspective

In terms of client beliefs held on the basis of tenacity, a client with osteoarthritis, for example, may be quite emphatic in expressing her dislike for swimming pools each time a therapist suggests that she consider participating in a therapeutic aquatics program. The tenacity with which the client maintains an unwavering disdain for swimming pools is an important piece of evidence to consider in appraising the potential therapeutic benefit of an aquatics program. A second illustration of the consequence of beliefs held on grounds of tenacity stems from the fact that some beliefs are cornerstones of a client's construction of self. Consider a client for whom being independent is of utmost importance and central to his view of himself. In order to maintain his perception of personal independence, the client may underestimate the number of times he has fallen in his home when asked in an interview or in completing a questionnaire. Although evidence of a self-presentation bias, such as a misreporting of falls, can be difficult for a therapist to discover, it is important to recognize that a client's highly persistent beliefs about himself or herself pervade his or her perspective of therapeutic goals and outcomes.

In terms of beliefs held on the basis of authority, a peer with related experiences can be a compelling source of information affecting therapeutic goals and outcomes. For instance, a peer who uses a walker can represent an authoritative source of evidence about the utility of a particular type of walker, and a peer's negative evaluation of a walker can be a barrier to its use by the client despite the recommendations of the therapist.

Consider as well an example of the *a priori* method: A client is reluctant to use a walker as recommended by her therapist, preferring to use a cane. She reasons that a cane is better for her to use because it is lighter in weight and seems to offer her as much support as the walker. Although such reasoning is not rigorous, the conclusion is reasonable to the client.

Finally, scientific findings reported in the media, including the Internet, can be taken by clients as a valid basis of belief. Media reports of scientific research are intended to be compelling for the audience, and it is conceivable for a brief account of the treatment of rheumatoid arthritis in yesterday's news to affect a client's beliefs about the treatment of his or her arthritis. In sum, these examples indicate that clients bring to therapy a variety of beliefs that can be important sources of evidence to consider when appraising the eventual therapeutic benefit of an intervention.

Therapist Perspective

Therapists also demonstrate the varieties of belief described by Peirce (1877). In terms of beliefs held on the basis of tenacity, occupational therapists share a set of core beliefs about practice. Kanny (1993) identified seven core values that occupational therapists use to guide clinical decisions. These values include, for instance, an unselfish concern for the welfare of others, an affirmation of the intrinsic uniqueness of each person, and a valuing of self-direction in the pursuit of meaningful goals. Occupational therapists also hold the fundamental belief that the engagement in occupation is a vital component of health and well-being. Obviously, these professional beliefs have a substantial effect on therapeutic goals and outcomes. Insomuch as the core beliefs underlying occupational therapy are different than those of other health professions, it is reasonable for occupational therapists to hold a somewhat different conception of evidence-based practice than other health professionals.

Therapists demonstrate beliefs that are based on authority when practices are modelled in accord with the ideas of clinical specialists or individuals highly regarded for their expertise on particular issues. Institutional guidelines or mandates may also serve as a source of authority for therapists insomuch as they establish the set of common practices at a particular institution.

In clinical practice, the *a priori* source of evidence refers to the use of clinical experience to inform practice. Clinical experience is an important repository of information gained from working with other clients, and it represents an appropriate place to begin the process of accruing evidence.

Lastly, science encompasses a diverse variety of peer-reviewed research relevant to occupation. We believe that all research has the potential to contribute to a fuller understanding of occupational performance, and no one kind of research can be judged universally to be the best source of evidence.

In many discussions of research methods, randomized clinical trials, systematic reviews of randomized clinical trials, and meta-analyses of randomized clinical trials are ranked as providing the highest quality of evidence (e.g., Egan, Dubouloz, von Zweck, & Vallerand, 1998; Greenhalgh, 1997; Law & Philip, 2002; Lloyd-Smith, 1997; Porter & Matel, 1998; Sackett et al., 2000; Taylor, 1997). However, many research questions are aptly addressed by research methods other than randomized clinical trials (Tickle-Degnen & Bedell, 2003 [see Chapter 50]). For example, investigations of the subtle complexity of a client's personal experiences are facilitated by qualitative methods, and studies informing the appropriate use of standardized assessments are well served by descriptive and correlational methods. To state universally that experimental methods, such as randomized clinical trials, represent the highest quality of evidence disregards the multifaceted nature of clinical practice and depreciates the diverse variety of research in occupational therapy.

In sum, the conception of evidence-based practice as a systematic appraisal of the best evidence does not reflect the diverse kinds of evidence brought to the clinical context by clients and therapists. If occupational therapy is truly a contextualized activity shaped by a unique client–therapist relationship, then the full variety of client and therapist beliefs, as summarized in the evidence matrix presented in Table 51.1, should be considered in the course of goal setting and in anticipating the eventual therapeutic benefit of an intervention.

The process of evidence-based clinical decision making in occupational therapy is illustrated in Figure 51.1. The figure shows how the evidence gathered from the client, the therapist, and research inform clinical ac-

Table 51.1. Evidence Matrix: Varieties of Evidence Classified by Method and Perspective

	Perspective	
Method*	**Client**	**Therapist**
Tenacity	Personal Beliefs & Convictions	Professional Values
Authority	Personal Experts	Clinical Experts
A Priori	Personal Reasoning & Experience	Clinical Reasoning & Experience
Science	Publicized Science	Research Literature

*From Peirce (1877).

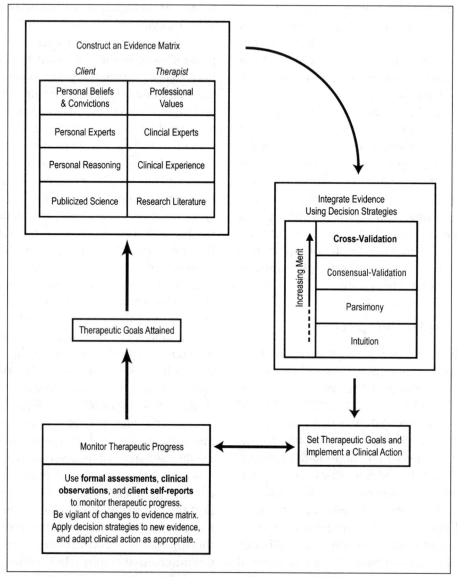

Figure 51.1. The evidence-based occupational therapy process.

tion and, subsequently, how clinical evidence informs modifications to the course of clinical action. Further, the process clearly demonstrates how the evidence cumulated with respect to each individual client becomes integrated into the therapist's repertoire of clinical ex-

perience with the potential to affect future decision making. To this point, we have considered the elements of constructing an evidence matrix; the integration of evidence using decision strategies and the monitoring of therapeutic progress are examined below.

Integrating Evidence Using Decision Strategies

We have suggested that in order to make appropriate decisions in clinical practice, it is necessary to integrate multiple pieces of evidence in a way that recognizes the contextualized nature of clinical practice. This necessitates a dynamic approach to integrating evidence. Each client–therapist relationship provides a unique matrix of evidence. Evidence can conflict, and it may be necessary to consider new evidence as therapy progresses. The four strategies described below, referred to as *intuition, parsimony, consensual-validation,* and *cross-validation,* have sufficient flexibility to be applied to a diverse variety of evidence.

Decisions made on intuition are those based on what feels right or seems reasonable. Such decisions are frequently difficult to justify because of their subjective nature, despite the fact that they may reflect extensive clinical experience.

Parsimony is a strategy for choosing among alternative interventions. The principle of parsimony is a general heuristic stating that if two propositions are equally tenable the simpler one is preferable. Thus, in deciding between two or more interventions of equal potential benefit, the principle of parsimony holds that the simpler intervention should be employed. In judgments of parsimony, simpler means requiring fewer assumptions. Thus, in deciding between two interventions, it is the one whose imputed benefit is based on fewer assumptions that is preferable.

For example, consider the following two hypothetical interventions aimed at improving the legibility of a child's handwriting. The first intervention involves activities for hand strengthening and activities for improving hand coordination. The second intervention emphasizes "sky writing" letters in the air in addition to hand strengthening and hand coordination activities. Both interventions assume that strength and coordination are important aspects of handwriting skill, but the second intervention makes the additional assumption that writing letters in the air facilitates the development of handwriting skill. In the situation where these two interventions appear to be equally effective, the principle of parsimony would hold that the first intervention is to be preferred. In other words, one begins with the simpler explanation of handwriting skill and switches to the more assumption-burdened explanation only when warranted by a clear demonstration that it is a more effective intervention.

A third decision strategy is consensual-validation; it reflects a belief that as more persons concur with a particular conclusion, the more likely it is to be valid. In clinical practice, consensual-validation often takes the form of informal consultation with colleagues who serve as a sounding board for clinical reasoning. In the research process, consensual-validation is provided by a formal mechanism of peer review. In general, consensual-validation is preferable to intuition or parsimony as a strategy for decision making. Although consensual-validation should not be construed as providing objectivity, it does result in decisions that have greater acceptability to others.

Arguably, the most justifiable decisions are those based on multiple sources of evidence and multiple decision strategies. Thus, in assimilating a diverse array of evidence, it is important to look for cross-validation in different sources of evidence as well as between the conclusions afforded by intuition, parsimony and consensual-validation. The concept of cross-validation is not novel; it has long been advocated as an approach to substantiating the validity of evidence. For example, Campbell and Fiske (1959) proposed the multitrait–multimethod matrix as an approach to validating evidence in which validity is strengthened by demonstrating convergence of findings across a variety of methodological and measurement approaches. The rationale of cross-validation rests on the premise that convergence of findings across multiple and varied sources of evidence indicates that the findings are not spurious, but rather are impervious to methodological variation. Consequently, decisions based on cross-validation are less likely to be influenced by bias or subjective interpretation.

Monitoring Therapeutic Progress

In the process of setting therapeutic goals, it is important that one or more measures be taken prior to intervention and periodically throughout the course of intervention to provide evidence of change as a function of the intervention. Such evidence can take the form of formal assessments or evaluations, informal clinical observations, and client self-reports, with a combination of these methods considered to be most valid on the premise of cross-validation. Further, one should be vigilant of changes to the evidence matrix over time, especially client and therapist beliefs and expectations pertaining to the progress and outcome of therapy. In these respects, it is important that evidence continue to be gathered throughout the clinical process to facilitate the best possible treatment.

With the eventual attainment of therapeutic goals, the process of evidence-based clinical decision making circles back upon itself. A therapist's observations, measures, and explanations of the therapeutic progress of one client contribute to the evidence matrix of future clinical practice by becoming part of clinical experience. Furthermore, this information offers a basis for preparing more formal commentaries on clinical practice for contribution to professional journals, and especially when cumulated across clients, the process of evidence-based clinical decision making provides a basis for integrating a program of research within clinical practice. In the longer term, such contributions to the literature of occupational therapy serve to develop clinical experience to a point of clinical expertise, providing an authoritative basis for other therapists to model therapeutic practices.

Conclusion

Occupational therapy has evolved its own professional values and beliefs. In our opinion, the approach of evidence-based medicine, as advocated by experts such as Sackett and his colleagues (Rosenberg & Donald, 1995; Sackett et al., 1996; Sackett et al., 2000), depreciates the core values and beliefs of occupational therapy. In contrast, we believe that the process of evidence-based clinical decision making described in this paper embraces occupational therapy's professional values and beliefs. There is no doubt that research evidence is essential to the practice of occupational therapy. But in our opinion, we should resist accepting the relative infrequency of randomized clinical trials evaluating occupational therapy interventions as a weakness in the scientific grounding of occupational therapy practice. Rather, the relative infrequency of randomized clinical trials may simply reflect the limited relevance and applicability of this design to occupational therapy practices and interventions. We argue that evidence-based occupational therapy should encompass a diverse variety of evidence, and it should value all research paradigms and designs as having the potential to inform clinical practice. Evidence-based occupational therapy should integrate a client's beliefs with the therapist's experiences and draw on pertinent expertise and research. As clearly stated in the *Occupational Therapy Practice Framework: Domain and Process* (2002), "clients bring knowledge about their life experiences and their hopes and dream" (p. 615) to the clinical context. The client's knowledge and experiences should be explicitly integrated into the process of evidence-based clinical decision making in occupational therapy; otherwise, we neglect "occupational therapy's unique focus on occupation and daily life activities and the application of an intervention process that facilitates engagement in occupation to support participation in life" (p. 609).

References

American Occupational Therapy Association (2002). Occupational therapy practice framework: Domain and process. *American Journal of Occupational Therapy, 56,* 609–639. http://dx.doi.org/10.5014/ajot.56.6.609

Campbell, D., & Fiske, D. (1959). Convergent and discriminant validation by the multitrait-multimethod matrix. *Psychological Bulletin, 54,* 81–105.

Egan, M., Dubouloz, C.-J., von Zweck, C., & Vallerand, J. (1998). The client-centred evidence-based practice of occupational therapy. *Canadian Journal of Occupational Therapy, 65,* 136–143.

Greenhalgh, T. (1997). *How to read a paper: The basics of evidence-based medicine.* London: BMJ Publishing Group.

Kanny, E. (1993). Core values and attitudes of occupational therapy practice. *American Journal of Occupational Therapy, 47,* 1085–1086. http://dx.doi.org/10.5014/ajot.47.12.1085

Kuhn, T. S. (1970). *The structure of scientific revolutions* (2nd ed.). Chicago: University of Chicago Press.

Law, M., & Philip, I. (2002). Evaluating the evidence. In M. Law (Ed.), *Evidence-based rehabilitation: A guide to practice.* Thorofare, NJ: Slack.

Lloyd-Smith, W. (1997). Evidence-based practice and occupational therapy. *British Journal of Occupational Therapy, 60,* 474–478.

Peirce, C. S. (1877). The fixation of belief. *Popular Science Monthly, 12,* 1–15.

Porter, C., & Matel, J. L. S. (1998). Are we making decisions based on evidence? *Journal of the American Dietetic Association, 98,* 404–407.

Rosenberg, W., & Donald, A. (1995). Evidence-based medicine: An approach to clinical problem-solving. *BMJ, 310,* 1122–1126.

Sackett, D. L., Rosenberg, W. M., Gray, J. A., Haynes, R. B., & Richardson, W. S. (1996). Evidence-based medicine: What it is and what it isn't. *BMJ, 312,* 71–72.

Sackett, D. L., Straus, S. E., Richardson, W. S., Rosenberg, W., & Haynes, R. B. (2000). *Evidence-based medicine: How to practice and teach EBM* (2nd ed.). Edinburgh, Scotland: Churchill Livingstone.

Taylor, M. C. (1997). What is evidence-based practice? *British Journal of Occupational Therapy, 60,* 470–473.

Tickle-Degnen, L., & Bedell, G. (2003). Evidence-Based Practice Forum—Heterarchy and hierarchy: A critical appraisal of the "levels of evidence" as a tool for clinical decision making. *American Journal of Occupational Therapy, 57,* 234–237. http://dx.doi.org/10.5014/ajot.57.2.234 Reprinted as Chapter 50.

CHAPTER 52

Informing Client-Centred Practice Through Qualitative Inquiry: Evaluating the Quality of Qualitative Research

KAREN WHALLEY HAMMELL

Introduction

Although qualitative research methods have only recently been included in occupational therapy curricula, they are being embraced by those researchers who recognise both their utility in exploring many of the issues that are of relevance and importance to clients and the profession and their congruence with client-centred philosophy (Hammell 2001).

If qualitative research is to provide convincing evidence on which to base practice, it must be capable of withstanding critical scrutiny regarding the quality and relevance of the researchers' work (Kuzel and Engel 2001). Agencies that fund health-related research require guidance on how to evaluate qualitative research (Devers 1999) and practitioners need sufficient information from which to evaluate the strength and plausibility of the evidence reported, yet little explicit guidance has been provided within the occupational therapy literature to assist in this process of evaluation. Further, it has been proposed that because occupational therapists espouse a client-centred orientation to practice (College of Occupational Therapists [COT] 2000), the research base that informs practice should itself reflect a client-centred orientation, demonstrating efforts to include clients as collaborators throughout the research process (Hammell 2001).

The procedure for critiquing qualitative research is not one of judging a rigid adherence to rules or specific prescriptive criteria (Hasselkus 1995) but is a process of weighing the various elements of the research in an effort to determine their appropriateness given the purpose and context of the study (Hasselkus 1991).

Although qualitative research entails an inherently creative process, this cannot preclude the rigour of both research process and reporting. Whilst radical postmodernists argue that evaluative criteria reflect a form of academic oppression and a desire to impose conformity on diversity (Rosenau 1992), occupational therapy research is undertaken for the benefit of clients and with the goal of informing theory and improving practice. It is therefore incumbent upon the profession to evaluate all inquiry with attention to how dependably it might achieve these goals (Kuzel and Engel 2001).

Popay and Williams (1998) outlined several ways in which qualitative research could contribute to the pursuit of evidence-based health care: probing 'taken for granted' practices, exploring organisational culture, evaluating complex policy initiatives, understanding client or provider behaviours and exploring client experiences and perspectives. This paper examines a framework of general guidelines with which to evaluate the quality of those forms of qualitative inquiry undertaken to explore client perspectives and experiences, advocating for research to be undertaken and reported according to principles that are rigorous but not prescriptive. Those forms of qualitative research that explore organisational cultures, social processes or practices (for example, institutional ethnographies or discourse analyses) require different evaluative criteria and will not be the subject of this paper.

Epistemology and Methodology: Assumptions About Knowledge and Inquiry

Qualitative research is sometimes presented as 'a basket of technical tools, devoid of the epistemological and theoretical basis that underpin its claims to be a legitimate means of generating knowledge' (Popay and Williams 1998, p35). It is important that any discussion of ways to evaluate the quality of qualitative research does not focus solely on technical questions of research design and data adequacy while ignoring issues of epistemology. Qualitative research is not solely a collection of methods that serves to supplement or provide an alternative to quantitative methods. Rather, qualitative inquiry reflects a set of philosophical assumptions. Evaluation of research methods must therefore be undertaken in the context of the underlying paradigms that inform them.

A paradigm is a set of basic beliefs or assumptions. Research paradigms define for researchers what falls within and outside the limits of legitimate inquiry and are epistemological and methodological in nature (Guba and Lincoln 1994).

Epistemological assumptions concern theories of knowledge: beliefs about the type of knowledge that we can acquire and the reliability of claims to knowledge. For example, qualitative researchers believe that it is never possible to be objective, detached or devoid of values so that all researchers—irrespective of methodology used—will perceive and interpret reality differently, based on their backgrounds and experience. They also contend that human behaviour can only be understood in social context; that behaviour goes beyond what is observed, incorporating subjective meanings, values and perceptions. Their research methods therefore seek to explore subjective experience, giving credence to people's beliefs, value systems and the meanings with which they interpret their experiences (Hammell and Carpenter 2000). Indeed, qualitative research seeks to accord equal status to lay knowledge and negate the tendency within health services for providers to see themselves as having 'knowledge' (superior) while clients have 'beliefs' (inferior) (Good 1994). These are issues of both epistemology and power.

Methodological assumptions are concerned with how the researcher can go about finding out whatever it is that he or she believes can be known, based upon prior epistemological assumptions (Guba and Lincoln 1994).

How might epistemological and methodological assumptions influence research methods and claims to knowledge? The quality of life of disabled people is often said to have been 'measured' using tools devised by researchers. This reflects an epistemological assumption that researchers can be objective and value-free and thus design research instruments that are universal and uncontaminated by contextual factors. However, research has demonstrated that the quality of a life can

only be assessed by the person whose life it is because it is both person and context specific. Thus, Dale (1995, p1133) contended that any claims by health professionals to have measured the 'improvement in quality of life experienced by a patient, using current tools, cannot be true. Therefore associated literature is false and of no value to either the patient or the health professional.' These are epistemological and methodological arguments.

Simply undertaking a few unstructured interviews does not constitute qualitative research. Qualitative research—like quantitative research—is not a collection of methods for data collection and analysis but a reflection of deeper philosophical issues concerning claims to knowledge and beliefs about how human beings can be studied. These assumptions underlie assessments of the quality of research.

Evaluating Research

Criteria for assessing the quality, rigour and merit of quantitative research are well established and include strategies supporting reliability, internal and external validity and generalisation. Krefting (1991) observed that 'too frequently, qualitative research is evaluated against criteria appropriate to quantitative research and is found to be lacking' (p214). This is not due to any inherent inadequacy in qualitative research but, rather, to the inappropriate imposition of criteria developed for a different form of inquiry. Clearly, any attempt to assess quantitative research by qualitative criteria would be equally inept (Carpenter and Hammell 2000).

Given the pluralistic nature of qualitative inquiry, not all qualitative research can be evaluated using the same criteria or strategies. As Sandelowski (1986) noted, the term 'qualitative research' is imprecise and refers to many dissimilar research methods. Lincoln and Guba (1985) proposed four criteria for evaluating qualitative research which have been adopted by many researchers: credibility, transferability, dependability and confirmability. Cautious of advocating seemingly prescriptive categories, Carpenter and Hammell (2000) proposed using the criteria of authenticity and plausibility suggested by Atkinson (1990) to evaluate qualitative research undertaken within the rehabilitation professions.

Authenticity

'Authenticity' pertains to the reliability and trustworthiness of the research process: evaluating the role played by the researchers' biographical position (for example, gender, education, ethnicity, age and social class) and degree of engagement with the subject matter and participants, which are factors that affect data collection, analysis and sensitivity to differing theoretical perspectives (Strauss and Corbin 1990). Authenticity also pertains to the relevance of the study: the importance of the topic and the potential contribution of the study to the literature (Hammersley 1992).

Further, Marshall and Rossman (1989) stressed the need for the explicit demonstration of how the research data tied into a body of theory. Sandelowski (1986) proposed that a qualitative study was credible or authentic 'when it presents such faithful descriptions or interpretations of a human experience that the people having that experience would immediately recognise it from those descriptions or interpretations as their own' (p30). For the study to be regarded as authentic, the researcher must provide a data base that enables the reader to determine whether the findings from one situation could reasonably be applied to another situation that is sufficiently similar (Robson 1993).

Plausibility

'Plausibility'—seeming probable but not proved—is concerned with determining whether 'the findings of the study, whether in the form of description, explanation, or theory, "fit" the data from which they are derived' (Sandelowski 1986, p32). Fundamentally, a careful reader should be able to determine whether the analysis, interpretations and conclusions drawn from the data are plausible. This focuses on whether the method of sampling is relevant and appropriate, whether the sample relates to the group of which they are members and whether a bias occurred due to either sampling or access. Plausibility may be assessed by determining whether the researcher obtained sufficient data and whether any degree of triangulation was used. Plausibility may also be assessed through consideration of the proportion of data that has been taken into account in the process of analysis and interpretation: whether data have been selectively extracted to fit a chosen theoretical or interpretive framework. An audit (decision) trail should enable the reader to determine the adequacy of the research process and, further, to assess whether interpretations flow from the data rather than being imposed on the data (Robson 1993).

Mays and Pope (1995, p110) observed: 'As in quantitative research, the basic strategy to ensure rigour in qualitative research is systematic and self-conscious research design, data collection, interpretation, and com-

Table 52.1. Framework of Guidelines for Evaluating Qualitative Research (see Baxter and Eyles 1997, Carpenter and Hammell 2000)

– The appropriateness of the study, methodology and methods
– Literature review
– Study participants
– Data collection: methods
– Data collection: process and documentation
– Length of time spent in fieldwork
– Reflexivity and the researcher role
– Attention to power relations
– Presenting participants' perspectives
– Data analysis and theoretical constructs
– Relating current findings to existing theory
– Respondent validation
– Study conclusions
– Ethical implications: representation and publication

munication.' Drawing upon the work of a large number of qualitative researchers and theorists (notably Baxter and Eyles 1997), this paper proposes a framework of 14 general criteria that might satisfy the imperative for authenticity and plausibility and which will serve as possible reference points (or 'anchor points' [Baxter and Eyles 1997]) both for those who undertake and write about qualitative research and for those who read and use the subsequent reports (see Table 52.1).

Framework of Guidelines

The Appropriateness of the Study, Methodology and Methods

The methodology and methods employed in any research reflect particular epistemological assumptions concerning how claims to knowledge might be justified. The terms 'methods' and 'methodology' are not interchangeable. The term methodology refers to the philosophical and theoretical aspects of the approaches employed to develop knowledge: a theory of how research should or ought to proceed given the nature of the issue it seeks to address. Research methods are the actual techniques and strategies employed to acquire knowledge and manipulate data (Harding 1987, Jary and Jary 1991, Cancian 1992, Maynard 1994). Thus, 'The methodological question cannot be reduced to a question of methods: methods must be fitted to a pre-determined methodology' (Guba and Lincoln 1994, p108). Methodological questions, in turn, are determined by epistemological assumptions.

Some points to consider (applicable to both quantitative and qualitative methodologies):

- What prompted the study and was its purpose clearly stated (Law et al 1998)?
- Is information provided concerning the potential usefulness or clinical relevance of the study?
- Does the chosen methodology 'fit' the research issue and is the study design justified and appropriate for the study issue?

If researchers state that they have used a specific approach—for instance, grounded theory or phenomenology—there should be evidence that they followed the very specific guidelines that characterise and define it and that they are familiar with the original literature that underpins and informs the chosen approach (Hasselkus 2000, Eva 2001). Otherwise, these declarations have neither foundation nor meaning.

- Who prompted the study? Was this a researcher-driven project? Was it prompted by consumer or client-identified concerns (Oliver 1999)? Was it initiated by a company or institution with a particular economic or philosophical stake in the issue (Brechin and Sidell 2000)? Weaver et al (2001), for example, generated an agenda for future spinal cord injury research based on input from consumers and care providers.

Evidence-based occupational therapy must take account of client choice, reflecting clients' experiences and values (Mead 1998, Canadian Association of Occupational Therapists et al 1999, COT 2000). It is argued that the research undertaken to generate such evidence should be ethically consistent with this practice philosophy (Hammell 2001). 'By involving participants in formulating research questions and by asking them for feedback on data collections and interpretations, researchers are more likely to investigate questions that are relevant to participants' lives' (Kirsch 1999, p12). Therefore, did the researchers study an issue that clients would care about (Frankel 1999)?

Literature Review

Some points to consider:

- Was the study justified with reference to the literature?
- Did previous work expose gaps in current knowledge? And does this support the need for the present study (Law et al 1998)?
- Was all relevant literature surveyed and used as background to the study? If the literature review was limited in its scope, was this limitation justified? Were

limits imposed by the researchers' personal ideologies or biases?

For example, in electing to fit chronic illness into a feminist framework, Wendell (1996) drew on literature generated exclusively by female theorists, ignoring work by leading disability theorists. This separated disabled women from cutting-edge disability theory (Barnes 1998) and appeared to support the notion that sexism can and should be eradicated while ableism remains intact. Further, by supporting a simplistic dichotomy of genders that divides the population into two apparently homogeneous groups, Wendell (1996) discredited the experiences of those whom 'queer' theorists describe as 'transgendered', for example, hermaphrodites, transvestites and transsexuals (Ingraham, 1994; Namaste, 1994; Stein and Plummer, 1994). In some instances, however, an innovative perspective using a particular body of literature can serve to challenge 'thinking as usual' and shed new insights on a particular issue.

Study Participants

Some points to consider:

- Was the sampling method appropriate and relevant?
- Was sampling random or purposeful and did this match the purpose and nature of the study?

Sampling may be 'theoretical', in which a sample is initially drawn to include as many factors as possible that might affect variability of behaviour and experience. Groups may be selected 'purposively', for example on the basis of age, geography, culture, sexual orientation or gender, to reveal salient experiences relevant to the research question or to test, modify and perhaps challenge the analysis. Choosing participants in a range of settings enhances the representativeness within the population and the potential to apply the findings to other settings (generalisability).

- How was the participant group determined and recruited? (Was it a representative group or selected on the basis of access [Carpenter and Hammell 2000]?)
- How many people participated, and what were their levels and types of participation (Law et al 1998)?
- Are there clear descriptions of the participants and the setting? (With sufficient detail to determine whether the findings might apply to other similar settings [generalisability] [Robson 1996]?) A description of the participants reveals who was allowed to speak and who was not (Baxter and Eyles 1997).

- What were the characteristics of those who declined to participate? (Were the reasons for declining provided? This may give some idea about the perceived relevance of the research to those invited to participate.)
- What determined the sample size? (This is usually determined by 'data saturation', a recurrent patterning of themes and issues [Bertaux 1981]. It cannot, therefore, be precisely determined in advance.)
- How was informed consent obtained? And to what did they consent (Barnitt and Partridge 1999)? If appropriate, was consent negotiated with the participants as the study evolved (Wendland and Hammell 2000)?
- What were the ethical considerations, for example, regarding confidentiality (Barnitt and Partridge 1999, Wendland and Hammell 2000)? Was approval obtained from a formal ethics committee?

Data Collection: Methods

Some points to consider:

- Were multiple methods used? Were these choices justified? Did they address the same or different questions (Baxter and Eyles 1997)? 'Triangulation' is based on the premise that comparison and convergence of perspectives from two or more different methods of data collection or sources helps to confirm the data and examine all aspects of a phenomenon.

Triangulation may be undertaken in four ways (Law et al, 1998; Brechin and Sidell, 2000). Triangulation by data or sources involves multiple informants, to corroborate, illuminate or elaborate the phenomenon (Marshall and Rossman, 1989). The range of data may be sourced, for example, by time, work shift, space or person (for example, different family members or members of couples [Krefting, 1991]). Triangulation by methods incorporates multiple ways of collecting data, for example, using interviews, participant observation, official documents and/or personal diaries. These must all be appropriate to the study and the participant group. The purpose is not to identify the 'truth' (because qualitative researchers recognise that no single truth or perspective exists) but to identify rival accounts and encourage a more reflexive analysis of the data.

Triangulation may be undertaken using various *theories*, employing different perspectives to discover different ways of thinking about or approaching the issue. Triangulation may also occur by using multiple *investigators*, or peer review, to produce a diversity of perspectives, prompting deeper reflection and analysis. However, if investigators share, for example, the same educational or professional training, social class, gender, 'race' and sexual orientation, they tend also to share a world-view and may be inclined to corroborate rather than challenge assumptions (Collins, 1991; Hammell, 2001). The aim of peer review is not to establish a gold standard but to critique interpretations and expose preconceptions (Hasselkus, 1991). This is not unproblematic. If there are unequal power relations between the researchers (for example, in a student/supervisor relationship), one may defer to the other's perspective (Baxter and Eyles, 1997). Some qualitative researchers argue that assessing interrater reliability is an important method for ensuring rigour. Research suggests that experienced researchers will identify similar themes within the data but will 'package' these differently, congruent with their own theoretical orientation (Armstrong et al., 1997). Consistency of coding and interpretation may reflect shared 'thinking as usual' and does not necessarily support the status of any findings (Armstrong et al., 1997). 'Member checking' may also be undertaken by the participants and their peer group (Law et al., 1998; Hammell, 2001).

- What are the implications of any discrepancies that arise from different data sources? How are these explored and interpreted (Baxter and Eyles, 1997)? (There is little merit in undertaking triangulation unless these tensions are both exposed and explored.)

Data Collection: Process and Documentation

Some points to consider:

- What were the methods for collecting data and were the methods appropriate to the research purpose?
- Was the data collection process flexible, responding to emerging themes or new questions or issues?
- How were the interviews conducted? Were the interviews interactive and sensitive to the language and concepts used by study participants? Were the questions reframed and expanded or was their scope progressively narrowed (Krefting 1991)? Did the interviews allow for the identification and discussion of opposing viewpoints (Gliner 1994)? Who undertook the interviews?

Did the research process reinforce hierarchies of power: researcher -> assistant -> participant (Gorelick 1991, Kelly et al., 1994)? And how will this be accounted for in terms of positionality and reflexivity vis-à-vis the participants, the data and the analysis? If assistants were used, why were they used? (For example, was this due to language issues or to researchers' priorities regarding time use [Carpenter and Hammell, 2000]?).

- How were the data recorded? Were audio tapes used? Who transcribed these? (This pertains to issues of power and of proximity to the data.) Were field-notes maintained? When were these recorded and what was included? Was a diary used to record ideas, theories or problems (Carpenter and Hammell, 2000)?
- What was the researcher's level of participation? (For example, passive observation, full participation or assistance [Law et al., 1998]?)
- What was the participants' level of participation? For example, were they used solely as sources of data ('data fodder'; Barnitt and Partridge, 1999, p258) or involved as co-researchers and co-writers (for example, Rebeiro and Allen, 1998; Rebeiro et al., 2001)? The level of participant involvement may be dependent upon their own time constraints and desire for further active inclusion and this may be noted by the researcher.

Length of Time Spent in Fieldwork

This provides some insight into the thoroughness of the data-gathering process and the quality of the researchers' access to the setting. Some points to consider:

- What factors determined the length of fieldwork? Does it appear that sufficient time was spent to achieve data saturation and to develop familiarity with the setting? Does this inspire confidence that interpretations were not threatened by premature closure of analysis (Lincoln and Guba 1985) or does it appear that participant numbers and duration of fieldwork were determined in advance, irrespective of emerging findings?

Reflexivity and the Researcher Role

Qualitative researchers treat all data as the products of dynamic interaction. The experience and background of the researcher are used as resources and, like all dimensions of the research process, require critical reflection. Either ignored or denigrated as 'bias' within quantitative inquiry, the researcher's background is placed in the foreground within qualitative inquiry to demonstrate that preconceptions, values and positioning have been interrogated and not taken for granted. Thus, reflexivity pertains to the need for a critical examination of the ways in which the researcher and the research process shaped the research relationship, data collection and data analysis. Some points to consider:

- Is the researchers' role critically examined? (Is there a critical analysis of the researchers' biographical and philosophical positioning?)

Biographical positioning refers (for example) to the professional status, education, gender, ethnicity, social class, age, disability and sexual orientation of the researcher and the researched. These dimensions of biography reflect differentials of power in society and thus also in the research relationship (England 1994, Carpenter and Hammell 2000). Philosophical positioning pertains to the researcher's commitment to a certain frame of reference, for example, feminist theory, action research or the social model of disability (Hammell 2000). The researcher's theoretical outlook shapes the research and should be made explicit (Johnson 2000).

- What was the impact of the research process on data collection? (Was it perceived by the participants to be too time consuming? Too intrusive? What was the impact of the presence of the observer [Brannen 1993]?)

Attention to Power Relations in the Research Process

Traditionally, the researcher controls the research design, defines the parameters of the theoretical framework and decides how the study is conducted, analysed, written up and disseminated (Bhavnani, 1993; Barnes et al., 1999). This sits uncomfortably with client-centred philosophy and thus also with the Code of Ethics and Professional Conduct for Occupational Therapists (COT 2000). It is not possible to erase power differentials, but how does the researcher attempt to contest them (Acker et al 1991, Yoshida et al 1998, Kirsch 1999)? Some points to consider:

- How does the researcher contest power imbalances? (For example, in the relationships between the researcher and the researched and between the data and the theory [Oakley, 1981; Lather, 1991; Punch, 1994].)
- How were the participants involved in identifying the research question and in developing the research design (Lather, 1991; Yoshida et al., 1998; Kirsch, 1999)?
- Were interviews interactive? (Including self-disclosure, answering questions and providing information [Oakley, 1981].) Sequential interviews help to build relationships and enable greater depth in probing participants' perspectives (Lather, 1991).
- How were interpretations and meanings negotiated (rather than imposed) and conclusions and recommendations determined?

- How was agreement achieved concerning the location of published findings (Yoshida et al., 1998)?

Presenting Participants' Perspectives

Some points to consider:
- Do verbatim quotes appear in the report? (This is an opportunity to enable participants to speak for themselves.)
- How were these selected?
- Do they support the researcher's interpretations?

Given that the researcher controls:
- whose voices are presented (and whose are not)
- the context in which they are presented
- how many quotes are presented
- whether dissenting views are presented/permitted (Kirsch 1999, Oakley 1999), how were these decisions made (Carpenter and Hammell 2000)?

Data Analysis and Theoretical Constructs

Some points to consider:
- How did the findings 'emerge from the data' (Law et al., 1998)? (Or was this part of the rhetoric of research—did theory appear in reality to have submerged or coopted the data [Ribbens and Edwards, 1998]?)
- What procedures were used for analysis? How were concepts refined and relationships between concepts clarified? Does the researcher outline the rationale for transforming data to themes or codes? Was the process systematic?
- How plausible are the linkages between data and theory? Are the interpretations justified? (Were they justified for all cases or for selected cases?) If research assistants collected the data, it must be made explicit that the data were interpreted by those without direct connection with the research setting.
- What proportion of the data was taken into account? (How well did the analysis succeed in incorporating all the observations? Are the themes inclusive of all the data [Law et al., 1998]? If not, how and why were selections made? For example, did the researcher extract only the data that fitted preconceived ideas or favoured ideologies [Carpenter and Hammell, 2000]?)

Armstrong et al (1997, p605) noted that 'all analysis is a form of interpretation . . . in which the researchers' own views have important effects'. While this tends to be overlooked or, indeed, denied by quantitative researchers, qualitative researchers acknowledge that analysis is informed by their positioning and will self-consciously explore this relationship.
- Does the analysis take into account and add to the existing knowledge (the theoretical context)?
- Was the analysis sensitive to the language and perspectives of the study participants? (Or were these subsumed into the constructs and ideology brought by the researcher [Mauthner and Doucet, 1998]?)

Popay et al. (1998) claimed: 'Research concerned with the appropriateness of care and with understanding the basis of lay and professional behaviour and action must privilege subjective meaning or lay knowledge if it is to provide good evidence to inform practice and policy' (p. 344, emphasis added).
- Were alternative explanations explored? (Participant researchers, team review and peer examination may enhance plausibility of interpretations [Kirsch, 1999].)
- Is an audit/decision trail provided so that readers can follow the research and reasoning process? The audit or decision trail illustrates the reasoning process and should provide sufficient information for readers to gauge the plausibility of analysis and whether the interpretations arose from or were imposed upon the data (Robson, 1993; Law et al., 1998).

Relating Current Findings to Existing Theory

Many qualitative researchers advocate for an intellectually engaged form of analysis that moves beyond simply identifying and describing themes within individual studies (unfortunately still a common practice in occupational therapy research) to discussing the meaning of the data, exploring how study findings relate to, contest or further existing theories (Maynard, 1994; Secker et al., 1995; Frank, 1997; Hammell and Carpenter, 2000; for examples, see Carpenter, 1994; Corring and Cook, 1999; Peachey-Hill and Law, 2000).

Frank (1997) observed that while the development of categories and domains is an essential step in qualitative research, themes or categories are not an end in themselves. The data should then be analysed in terms of theory: 'a process by which data are recontextualized in the world of social thought' (Frank, 1997; p. 85). Kuzel and Engel (2001, p129) believed 'that it is impossible to derive an interpretation without some reference to assumed facts, values, theories; this stock of knowledge is what brings meaning to experience'. To judge the worth of qualitative research demands consideration of the theoretical position—the stock of knowledge—from which the researcher operated and the degree of fit with the purposes of the research (Kirsch, 1999). Some points to consider:

- Was the theoretical perspective underpinning the study clearly stated (Law et al 1998)?
- Do the findings support or contest existing theories or concepts (Marshall and Rossman, 1989; Shepard et al., 1993; Peters, 1996)?
- Has the researchers' use of theory stifled innovation (Baxter and Eyles, 1997)? (Adherence to a particular theoretical orientation may either sharpen sensitivity to participants' perspectives or shape and silence their voices [Parr, 1998].)
- What are the implications of the findings for occupational therapy theory and practice (Law et al., 1998)?

Respondent Validation

Both qualitative research and client-centred practice seek to explore phenomena from the participant's perspective; view individuals as inseparable from their contexts and environments; seek to understand clients' values and beliefs; and respect clients' knowledge (Popay et al., 1998; Hammell and Carpenter, 2000; Hammell, 2001). However, qualitative research is not inevitably client centred. Without a commitment to realigning power and incorporating consumer views and values into the research process, qualitative research may be experienced as being at least as disempowering, exploitative and irrelevant as other forms of research (Fonow and Cook, 1991; Oliver, 1992; Ward and Flynn, 1994; Lawson, 1995; Bonnell, 1999; Oakley, 1999). Some points to consider:

- How were the participants or their peers given the opportunity to clarify interpretations and review and comment on categories and themes derived during data analysis (Yoshida et al., 1998; Bonnell, 1999; Hammell, 2001)? (For example, by reviewing written transcripts and through follow-up meetings or focus groups; Lather, 1991; Opie, 1992; Olesen, 1994; Kirsch, 1999; Carpenter and Hammell, 2000; Hammell, 2000.)

This is not to seek confirmation or consensus so much as a commentary on the plausibility of the interpretations and theoretical framework (Borlund, 1991; Opie, 1992; Baxter and Eyles, 1997). Differences in perspective should be documented and discrepant viewpoints noted to enable a reader to determine whether the researcher has imposed a viewpoint that is at odds with the participants' own understandings (Borlund, 1991; Carpenter and Hammell, 2000). Participants do not have privileged

access to 'the truth' (Hammersley, 1992; Opie, 1992) but they do have privileged access to their own perspectives (Baxter and Eyles, 1997). Kirsch (1999) argued that participants have the right to have their interpretations presented, especially when there is disagreement with the interpretations and meanings imposed by the researcher. Are representations perceived as faithful to the experiences of the participants (Sandelowski, 1986; Krefting, 1991)? Does the researcher account for the participants' viewpoints as well as those of the researcher?

- Are the participants comfortable with how their experiences will be used (Stacey, 1991; Scott, 1999; Johnson, 2000)? (For example, have researchers avoided stereotype? Have they employed theories with which participants disagree [Borlund, 1991; Maynard, 1994]? Disability researchers, for example, have found that not all disabled people share their own perspectives concerning the merits of the social model of disability that is often used to interpret their lives [Stone, 1997; Wirz and Hartley, 1999].)

It is pertinent to note that participants may be at least as well informed as their researchers (Mead 1998, Needham and Oliver 1998).

Study Conclusions

Some points to consider:

- What did the study conclude and are the conclusions justified in relation to the data collected and consistent with the findings? Do the conclusions account for all the data? And, importantly, do the data account for all the conclusions?
- Do the conclusions help to clarify the theory? Do they add to theory development and future clinical practice? (that is, are they relevant and useful [Law et al., 1998]?)
- Do the conclusions relate back to the literature?
- What are the implications of the findings and how might the findings be used?

As Popay et al (1998, p349) claimed: 'In the context of HSR [health services research], qualitative research should have some clear implications for policy and practice.'

Ethical Implications: Representation and Publication

Some points to consider:

- How are participants and their experiences represented? (For example, are health care providers represented as 'experts' and clients as passive and dependent recipients of care [Carpenter and Hammell, 2000]? Has the researcher sought to avoid appropriation, exploitation and stereotype [Bhavnani, 1993; Brannen, 1993; Kirsch, 1999]?)

- Where are the findings presented? Where are they not? (Whose interests inform these choices [Kelly et al., 1994; Carpenter and Hammell, 2000; Hammell, 2000]? Despite claims to client-centredness, occupational therapy researchers tend to publish and present their research findings in those fora that will speak to their own peers and further their own careers rather than ensuring access for the groups from which the study participants were drawn [Barnes, 1992; Oliver, 1992; Shakespeare, 1996].)
- Was the researcher explicit about both the purpose of the research and the researchers' agenda (Barnitt and Partridge, 1999)?
- How and to whom is accountability established (Carpenter and Hammell, 2000)?
- Whose point of view is used to represent the findings? (If participants disagreed with researchers, are their perspectives presented [Opie, 1992; Riger, 1992; Altheide and Johnson, 1994]?)
- Does the research narrow the gap between 'lay' and 'expert' knowledge (Brechin and Sidell, 2000)? (Service users need research evidence with which to inform their own choices; it is the basis for informed consent [Mead, 1998; Needham, 2000; Hammell, 2001]. This also encourages researchers to report their findings in language that is clear and accessible rather than élitist and exclusionary [Hooks, 1989; Said, 1994].)

Discussion

The framework outlined in this paper is intended to serve two purposes. First, it is hoped that recourse to a set of guidelines such as those offered here will act as prompts or stimuli for qualitative researchers to consider and adopt, commensurate with the nature and purpose of each research project. Not every suggestion will be appropriate to every study (indeed, many will not). However, it is proposed that each of the 14 suggested guidelines should be considered and evaluated as the research is planned and adopted where *appropriate to the study*. Second, the guidelines are intended to assist occupational therapy practitioners to evaluate the quality of qualitative research as this is reported and, hence, its value and relevance in informing an evidence-based practice.

While it is unquestionably difficult to represent a qualitative research study adequately in those professional journals that have established word limits to suit the more succinct reporting style of quantitative researchers (whose data are reduced to statistics), this is not impossible. Some qualitative researchers circumvent this constraint by writing several papers that address different aspects or dimensions of the research and findings; others accomplish clarity and comprehensiveness within a single article (for excellent examples of papers which meet at least 11 of the 14 proposed criteria within the space limitations of a single journal article, see: Carpenter, 1994; Pollock et al., 1997; Corring and Cook, 1999; Rebeiro and Cook, 1999; Evans, 2000).

Conclusion

It is important to reiterate that although there can be no mandatory rules for gauging the merits of qualitative research, there needs to be a framework that enables a judgement to be made concerning the plausibility and authenticity of research designs and subsequent published accounts (Baxter and Eyles, 1997; Carpenter and Hammell, 2000). This is especially important for research undertaken into issues of health and social care, where research can—and should—have consequences for those people we study.

The 14 criteria outlined in this paper are general and may be satisfied in different ways, congruent with the nature and purpose of each study. This paper draws upon the work of many qualitative research theorists in suggesting various strategies that might be used to ensure the rigour of qualitative research design and the integrity of qualitative research reports. These strategies should be used where appropriate to the nature of the study, demonstrating that decisions can be justified and that the research methods reflect the epistemological assumptions underpinning the methodology.

The goal must be to achieve a high standard of qualitative research which will have meaning and relevance to the groups that occupational therapists study, contribute to the knowledge base of the profession and demonstrate the potential of qualitative research to inform the client-centred, evidence-based practice of occupational therapy.

Acknowledgements

This paper is based on a presentation at the 2nd International Qualitative Evidence-Based Practice Conference at Coventry University, 14–16 May 2001. I am grateful to my anonymous reviewers for their insightful and helpful comments on the first draft of this paper.

References

Acker J, Barry K, Esseveld J (1991) Objectivity and truth: problems in doing feminist research. In: M Fonow, J Cook, eds. *Beyond methodology: feminist scholarship as lived research.* Bloomington, IN: Indiana University, 133–53.

Altheide DL, Johnson JM (1994) Criteria for assessing interpretive validity in qualitative research. In: N Denzin, Y Lincoln, eds. *Handbook of qualitative research.* Thousand Oaks, CA: Sage, 485–98.

Armstrong D, Gosling A, Weinman J, Marteau T (1997) The place of interrater reliability in qualitative research: an empirical study. *Sociology, 31*(3), 597–606.

Atkinson P (1990) *The ethnographic imagination: textual constructions of reality.* London: Routledge.

Barnes C (1992) Qualitative research: valuable or irrelevant? *Disability, Handicap and Society, 7*(2), 115–24.

Barnes C (1998) Book review: The rejected body. Feminist philosophical reflections on disability, by S Wendell. *Disability and Society, 13*(1), 145–47.

Barnes C, Mercer G, Shakespeare T (1999) *Exploring disability. A sociological introduction.* Cambridge: Polity Press.

Barnitt R, Partridge C (1999) The legacy of being a research subject: follow-up studies of participants in therapy research. *Physiotherapy Research International, 4*(4), 250–61.

Baxter J, Eyles J (1997) Evaluating qualitative research in social geography: establishing 'rigour' in interview analysis. *Transactions of the Institute of British Geographers, 22*(4), 505–25.

Bertaux D (1981) From the life history approach to the transformation of sociological practice. In: D Bertaux, ed. *Biography and society.* Beverley Hills: Sage, 29–45.

Bhavnani K-K (1993) Tracing the contours: feminist research and feminist objectivity. *Women's Studies International Forum, 16*(2), 95–104.

Bonnell C (1999) Gay men: drowning (and swimming) by numbers. In: S Hood, B Mayall, S Oliver, eds. *Critical issues in social research: power and prejudice.* Buckingham, Open University Press, 111–23.

Borlund K (1991) 'That's not what I said': interpretive conflict in oral narrative research. In: SB Gluck, D Patai, eds. *Women's words: The feminist practice of oral history.* New York: Routledge, 63–75.

Brannen J (1993) Research notes: The effects of research on participants: findings from a study of mothers and employment. *Sociological Review, 41*(2), 328–46.

Brechin A, Sidell M (2000) Ways of knowing, In: R Gomm, C Davies, eds. *Using evidence in health and social care.* London: Sage and The Open University, 3–25.

Canadian Association of Occupational Therapists, the Association of Canadian Occupational Therapy University Programmes, the Association of Canadian Occupational Therapy Regulatory Organisations and the Presidents' Advisory Committee (1999) Joint position statement on evidence-based occupational therapy. *Canadian Journal of Occupational Therapy, 66*(5), 267–69.

Cancian FM (1992) Feminist science: methodologies that challenge inequality. *Gender and Society, 6*(4), 623–42.

Carpenter C (1994) The experience of spinal cord injury: the individual's perspective—implications for rehabilitation practice. *Physical Therapy, 74*(7), 614–29.

Carpenter C, Hammell KW (2000) Evaluating qualitative research. In: KW Hammell, C Carpenter, I Dyck, eds. *Using qualitative research: a practical introduction for occupational and physical therapists.* Edinburgh: Churchill Livingstone, 107–19.

College of Occupational Therapists (2000) *Code of ethics and professional conduct for occupational therapists.* London: COT.

Collins PH (1991) Learning from the outsider within. The sociological significance of Black feminist thought. In: MM Fonow, JA Cook, eds. *Beyond methodology: feminist scholarship as lived research.* Bloomington, IN: Indiana University Press, 35–59.

Corring D, Cook J (1999) Client-centred care means that I am a valued human being. *Canadian Journal of Occupational Therapy, 66*(2), 71–82.

Dale AE (1995) A research study exploring the patient's view of quality of life using the case study method. *Journal of Advanced Nursing, 22,* 1128–34.

Devers KJ (1999) How will we know 'good' qualitative research when we see it? Beginning the dialogue in health services research. *Health Services Research, 34,* 1153–88.

England K (1994) Getting personal: reflexivity, positionality and feminist research. *Professional Geographer, 46*(1), 80–89.

Eva G (2001) Multiple voices, multiple paths (Letter). *British Journal of Occupational Therapy, 64*(2), 107.

Evans R (2000) The effect of electronically-powered indoor/outdoor wheelchairs on occupation: a study of users' views. *British Journal of Occupational Therapy, 63*(11), 547–53.

Fonow MM, Cook JA (1991) Back to the future. A look at the second wave of feminist epistemology and methodology. In: MM Fonow, JA Cook, eds. *Beyond methodology: feminist scholarship as lived research.* Bloomington, IN: Indiana University Press, 1–15.

Frank G (1997) Is there life after categories? Reflexivity in qualitative research. *Occupational Therapy Journal of Research, 17*(2), 84–98.

Frankel RM (1999) Standards of qualitative research. In: BF Crabtree, WL Miller, eds. *Doing qualitative research.* 2nd ed. Thousand Oaks, CA: Sage, 333–46.

Gliner JA (1994) Reviewing qualitative research: proposed criteria for fairness and rigor. *Occupational Therapy Journal of Research, 14*(2), 78–90.

Good BJ (1994) *Medicine, rationality and experience.* Cambridge: University of Cambridge Press.

Gorelick S (1991) Contradictions of feminist methodology. *Gender and Society, 5*(4), 459–77.

Guba EG, Lincoln YS (1994) Competing paradigms in qualitative research. In: N Denzin, Y Lincoln, eds. *Handbook of qualitative research.* Thousand Oaks, CA: Sage, 105–17.

Hammell KW (2000) Representation and accountability in qualitative research. In: KW Hammell, C Carpenter, I Dyck, eds. *Using qualitative research: a practical introduction for occupational and physical therapists.* Edinburgh: Churchill Livingstone, 59–71.

Hammell KW (2001) Using qualitative research to inform the client-centred evidence-based practice of occupational therapy. *British Journal of Occupational Therapy, 64*(5), 228–34.

Hammell KW, Carpenter C (2000) Introduction to qualitative research in occupational and physical therapy. In: KW Hammell, C Carpenter, I Dyck, eds. *Using qualitative research: a practical introduction for occupational and physical therapists.* Edinburgh: Churchill Livingstone, 1–12.

Hammersley M (1992) *What's wrong with ethnography?* London: Routledge.

Harding S (1987) Introduction: Is there a feminist method? In: S Harding, ed. *Feminism and methodology.* Bloomington, IN: Indiana University Press, 1–14.

Hasselkus BR (1991) Qualitative research: not another orthodoxy. *Occupational Therapy Journal of Research, 11*(1), 3–7.

Hasselkus BR (1995) Beyond ethnography: expanding our understanding and criteria for qualitative research. *Occupational Therapy Journal of Research, 15*(2), 75–84.

Hasselkus B (2000) Critically reading qualitative research. TriJoint Congress (Abstracts). *Canadian Journal of Occupational Therapy, 67,* S145.

Hooks B (1989) *Talking back. Thinking feminist, thinking black.* Boston: South End Press.

Ingraham C (1994) The heterosexual imaginary: feminist sociology and theories of gender. *Sociological Theory, 12*(2), 203–19.

Jary D, Jary J (1991) *The Harper Collins dictionary of sociology.* New York: Harper Collins.

Johnson K (2000) Interpreting meanings. In: R Gomm, C Davis, eds. *Using evidence in health and social care.* London: The Open University and Sage, 65–85.

Kelly L, Burton S, Regan L (1994) Researching women's lives or studying women's oppression? Reflections on what constitutes feminist research. In: M Maynard, J Purvis, eds. *Researching women's lives from a feminist perspective.* London: Taylor and Francis, 27–48.

Kirsch GE (1999) *Ethical dilemmas in feminist research. The politics of location, interpretation and publication.* Albany, NY: State University of New York Press.

Krefting L (1991) Rigor in qualitative research: the assessment of trustworthiness. *American Journal of Occupational Therapy, 45*(3), 214–22.

Kuzel AJ, Engel JD (2001) Some pragmatic thoughts about evaluating qualitative health research. In: J Morse, J Swanson, A Kuzel, eds. *The nature of qualitative evidence.* London: Sage, 114–38.

Lather P (1991) *Getting smarter: feminist research and pedagogy with/in the postmodern.* London: Routledge.

Lawson V (1995) The politics of difference: examining the quantitative/qualitative dualism in post-structuralist feminist research. *Professional Geographer, 47*(4), 449–57.

Lincoln YS, Guba EG (1985) *Naturalistic inquiry.* Beverley Hills, CA: Sage.

Law M, Stewart D, Letts L, Pollock N, Bosch J, Westmorland M (1998) *Guidelines for critical review of qualitative research.* Available at http://www.fhs.mcmaster.ca/rehab/ebp/ Accessed on 14.11.2000.

Marshall C, Rossman GB (1989) *Designing qualitative research.* Newbury Park, CA: Sage.

Mauthner N, Doucet A (1998) Reflections on a voice-centred relational method. In: J Ribbens, R Edwards, eds. *Feminist dilemmas in qualitative research: public knowledge and private lives.* London: Sage, 119–146.

Maynard M (1994) Methods, practice and epistemology: the debate about feminist research. In: M Maynard, J Purvis, eds. *Researching women's lives from a feminist perspective.* London: Taylor and Francis, 10–25.

Mays N, Pope C (1995) Rigour and qualitative research. *British Medical Journal, 311,* 109–12.

Mead J (1998) Clinical effectiveness: another perspective to evidence-based healthcare. In: T Bury, J Mead, eds. *Evidence-based healthcare: a practical guide for therapists.* Oxford: Butterworth-Heinemann, 26–42.

Namaste K (1994) The politics of inside/out: queer theory, poststructuralism and a sociological approach to sexuality. *Sociological Theory, 12*(2), 220–31.

Needham G (2000) Research and practice: making a difference. In: R Gomm, C Davis, eds. *Using evidence in health and social care.* London: The Open University and Sage, 131–51.

Needham G, Oliver S (1998) Involving service users. In: T Bury, J Mead, eds. *Evidence-based healthcare: a practical guide for therapists.* Oxford: Butterworth-Heinemann, 85–103.

Oakley A (1981) Interviewing women: a contradiction in terms. In: H Roberts, ed. *Doing feminist research.* London: Routledge, 30–61.

Oakley A (1999) People's ways of knowing: gender and methodology. In: S Hood, B Mayall, S Oliver, eds. *Critical issues in social research: power and prejudice.* Buckingham: Open University Press, 134–70.

Olesen V (1994) Feminisms and models of qualitative research. In: NK Denzin, YS Lincoln, eds. *Handbook of qualitative research.* London: Sage, 158–74.

Oliver M (1992) Changing the social relations of research production? *Disability, Handicap and Society, 7*(2),1, 101–14.

Oliver S (1999) Users of health services: following their agenda. In: S Hood, B Mayall, S Oliver, eds. *Critical issues in social research: power and prejudice.* Buckingham: Open University Press, 139–53.

Opie A (1992) Qualitative research, appropriation of the 'other' and empowerment. *Feminist Review, 40,* 52–69.

Parr J (1998) Theoretical voices and women's own voices. In: J Ribbens, R Edwards, eds. *Feminist dilemmas in qualitative research: public knowledge and private lives.* London: Sage, 87–102.

Peachey-Hill C, Law M (2000) Impact of environmental sensitivity on occupational performance. *Canadian Journal of Occupational Therapy, 67*(5), 304–13.

Peters DJ (1996) Qualitative inquiry. Expanding rehabilitation medicine's research repertoire: a commentary. *American Journal of Physical Medicine and Rehabilitation, 75*(2), 144–48.

Pollock N, Stewart D, Law M, Sahagian-Whalen S, Harvey S, Toal C (1997) The meaning of play for young people with physical disabilities. *Canadian Journal of Occupational Therapy, 64*(1), 25–31.

Popay J, Rogers A, Williams G (1998) Rationale and standards for the systematic review of qualitative literature in health services research. *Qualitative Health Research, 8*(3), 341–51.

Popay J, Williams G (1998) Qualitative research and evidence-based health care. *Journal of the Royal Society of Medicine, 91*(Suppl. 35), 32–37.

Punch M (1994) Politics and ethics in qualitative research. In: NK Denzin, YS Lincoln, eds. *Handbook of qualitative research.* London: Sage, 83–97.

Rebeiro KL, Allen J (1998) Voluntarism as occupation. *Canadian Journal of Occupational Therapy, 65*(5), 279–85.

Rebeiro K, Cook JV (1999) Opportunity, not prescription: an exploratory study of the experience of occupational engagement. *Canadian Journal of Occupational Therapy, 66*(4), 176–87.

Rebeiro KL, Day DG, Semeniuk B, O'Brien MC, Wilson B (2001) Northern Initiative for Social Action: An occupation-based mental health programme. *American Journal of Occupational Therapy, 55,* 493–500.

Ribbens J, Edwards R (1998) *Feminist dilemmas in qualitative research: public knowledge and private lives.* London: Sage.

Riger S (1992) Epistemological debates, feminist voices. Science, social values and the study of women. *American Psychologist, 47,* 730–40.

Robson C (1993) *Real world research: a resource for social scientists and practitioner-researchers.* Blackwell: Oxford.

Rosenau PM (1992) *Post-modernism and the social sciences: insights, inroads, and intrusions.* Princeton, NJ: Princeton University Press.

Said E (1994) *Representations of the intellectual.* New York: Vintage.

Sandelowski M (1986) The problem of rigor in qualitative research. *Advances in Nursing Science, 8*(3), 27–37.

Scott P (1999) Black people's health: ethnic status and research issues. In: S Hood, B Mayall, S Oliver, eds. *Critical issues in social research: power and prejudice.* Buckingham: Open University Press, 80–93.

Secker J, Wimbush E, Watson J, Milburn K (1995) Qualitative methods in health promotion research: some criteria for quality. *Health Education Journal, 54,* 74–87.

Shakespeare T (1996) Rules of engagement: doing disability research. *Disability and Society, 11*(1), 115–19.

Shepard KF, Jensen GM, Schmoll BJ, Hack LM, Gwyer J (1993) Alternative approaches to research in physical therapy: positivism and phenomenology. *Physical Therapy, 73,* 88–97.

Stacey J (1991) Can there be a feminist ethnography? In: SB Gluck, D Patai, eds. *Women's words. The feminist practice of oral history.* New York: Routledge, 111–19.

Stein A, Plummer K (1994) 'I can't even think straight': 'queer' theory and the missing sexual revolution in sociology. *Sociological Theory, 12*(2), 178–87.

Stone E (1997) From the research notes of a foreign devil: disability research in China. In: C Barnes, G Mercer, eds. *Doing disability research.* Leeds: The Disability Press, 207–27.

Strauss A, Corbin J (1990) *Basics of qualitative research.* Newbury Park, CA: Sage.

Ward L, Flynn M (1994) What matters most: disability, research and empowerment. In: MH Rioux, M Bach, eds. *Disability is not measles. New research paradigms in disability.* North York, Ont: L'Institut Roeher, 29–48.

Weaver FM, Guihan M, Pape T, Legro M, LaVela S, Collins E, Langbein E, Goldstein B (2001) Creating a research agenda in SCI based on provider and consumer input. *SCI Psychosocial Process, 14*(2), 77–88.

Wendell S (1996) *The rejected body: feminist philosophical reflections on disability.* New York: Routledge.

Wendland T, Hammell KW (2000) Understanding another life: using qualitative research in undergraduate education. In: KW Hammell, C Carpenter, I Dyck, eds. *Using qualitative research: a practical introduction for occupational and physical therapists.* Edinburgh: Churchill Livingstone, 97–106.

Wirz SL, Hartley SD (1999) Challenges for universities of the North interested in community based rehabilitation. In: E Stone, ed. *Disability and development.* Leeds: The Disability Press, 89–106.

Yoshida K, Willi V, Parker I, Self H, Carpenter S, Pfeiffer D (1998) Disability partnerships in research and teaching in Canada and the United States. *Physiotherapy Canada,* Summer, 198–205.

Chapter 53

Sharing the Agenda: Pondering the Politics and Practices of Occupational Therapy Research

Karen R. W. Hammell, William C. Miller, Susan J. Forwell, Bert E. Forman, and Brad A. Jacobsen

Introduction

Although occupational therapists have been challenged to acknowledge the political nature of their work (1,2), little attention has yet been given to either the politics or practices of occupational therapy research (3–5). Research practices have been critiqued, however, by critical disability theorists, who have stated that: "in the way it has been conceived, organised and conducted, as well as in the nature and use of results, traditional disability research in . . . rehabilitation . . . has been carried out by representatives of professional groups with little or no consultation with, or involvement of, disabled people themselves (other than as research subjects)" [(6), p. 152]. Clearly, this appraisal sits uncomfortably with the collaborative, client-centred philosophy that is said to underpin occupational therapy's practices (7), and merits consideration of the degree to which occupational therapy researchers engage in collaborative research with disabled people.

The term disabled people, used throughout this paper, is employed by critical disability theorists to signify that people who have impairments are disabled by social and political responses to their differences (8). Of importance to occupational therapists, and to the subject matter of this paper, is the understanding that to "disable" is to "deprive of power" (9). Thus, people with impairments—who may have considerable abilities—do not "have" disabilities, although they may be disabled (3). Importantly, if people who have impairments are deprived of power, they may be disabled by the research process.

Client-centred practice is an approach to practice fundamentally concerned with realigning power and with ensuring that occupational therapy is informed by, and relevant to, clients' lives, values, and priorities (7,10). Research is one of occupational therapy's practices, yet there has been little discussion about how client-centred philosophy influences occupational therapy research such that research is informed by, and relevant to, clients' lives, values, and priorities. Client-centred practice is usually discussed in terms of clinical practice, although no rationale has been offered to justify the exclusion of research practice from this overarching philosophy. On the contrary, it has been argued that occupational therapy's espoused commitment to client-centred practice ought to include the practice of research (4) and, further, that collaborative—or participatory—research is conceptually compatible with both client-centred practice and with occupation-based practice (11).

Disability theorists contend that research undertaken collaboratively by consumers and researchers increases both the relevance of research and its impact (12,13), and may help to bridge the gulf—or theory/practice gap—between the worlds of academe and of clinical practice (14). Moreover, it has been suggested that if researchers and disabled people pool their expertise, there is the potential to achieve better research (15).

Because legislation in several countries now requires health and social service providers to ensure that clients have direct input into the evaluation of services, collaborative research is becoming both an ethical and a legal requirement in these jurisdictions (3,16). In the United Kingdom, for example, occupational therapy researchers are expected to work collaboratively and to involve consumers at all stages of the research process (17). In North America, some funding agencies invite disabled people to collaborate in identifying issues that require research, and actively involve them in reviewing grant applications to ensure the relevance of research and the potential value of anticipated outcomes (18).

Pollard et al. (2) observe: "There is a growing awareness in occupational therapy of the need to address the political contexts in which practice, education and research take place" (p. xvii). The current political context in which occupational therapy research takes place is one of increasing demands for meaningful consumer participation (3,16). However, in 2000, Townsend et al. (19) observed that few occupational therapy researchers were involved in collaborative research. In an effort to appraise the degree to which occupational therapy researchers have engaged in collaborative research with disabled people, a comprehensive review of the occupational therapy peer-reviewed journals (1999–2009) was undertaken using the CINAHL database. Only 18 articles (out of 4290) were found to describe collaborative research undertaken by occupational therapists with clients or consumer groups (unpublished data). This would seem to suggest that occupational therapy's client-centred rhetoric is not reflected in the profession's research practices. Because occupational therapy practices are said to be framed within a collaborative, client-centred philosophy (7) the purpose of this paper is to foster reflection on the collaborative, client-centred practices of occupational therapy research and to encourage occupational therapists to enable meaningful client participation in the occupation of research.

Whose Research Agenda?

Occupational therapists have discussed client-centred practice for over two decades and have defined this as practice that emanates from the client's perspective (7). Because research is one of occupational therapists' practices, there would seem to be an obvious answer to the question: Whose perspectives should inform the agenda for occupational therapy research? However, disabled people claim that research agendas are usually determined not by those who are the espoused beneficiaries of research, but by academics, clinicians, and funding bodies (20). This is an expression of power, for as McKnight [(21), p. 31] observed: "there is no greater power than the right to define the question". Although the imperative for occupational therapy to be evidence-based continues to energize the profession's interest in research, critics contend that much of the rehabilitation evidence-base itself is flawed because it has been developed from research undertaken with-

out consideration of the issues that matter to disabled people (22,23). Moreover, Macfarlane (16) claims that collaborative research with service users "highlights the distortion—rather than the neutrality—of research conducted from a supposedly objective distance" (p. 203).

It has been claimed that those people who know what it is like to live with a specific condition "will have a good idea of which research questions are worth asking, and when a research question should be framed differently" [(24), p. 724]. It is difficult for researchers to know whether their questions are worth asking, or which questions are worth asking, if they do not ask. However, evidence suggests that study participants often strive to provide this sort of valuable information, by "writing in the margins".

Attempting to Influence the Agenda: Writing in the Margins

Many researchers who have used quantitative surveys have noted the tendency for respondents to write comments in the margins of their questionnaires in apparent attempts to describe the context for their responses and to provide relevant information about important questions the researchers failed to ask (25,26). This may suggest that those who are the subjects of research desire more input into the research process than they are often permitted, and that they may be attempting to influence the research agenda such that it addresses their priorities and needs and those issues they perceive to be important, so that research is more client-centred.

For example, Clayton et al. (25) employed a quantitative survey to enable the refinement of a model to guide the development of health-related interventions for people with multiple sclerosis. Acknowledging that questionnaires have inherent limits, because they only obtain answers to those questions the researchers deem worth asking, the researchers discovered that fully one-quarter of their respondents had added comments to the margins of the questionnaire, often despite considerable writing difficulties. Primarily, the respondents wished to describe the context for their answers to the standardized questions and to explain important and relevant issues about which the researchers had failed to enquire: "You didn't ask but I thought I would tell you" (p. 516).

In another study, Warms et al. (26) used a quantitative survey to gain insight into the experience of living with chronic pain for people with spinal cord injury or amputation. Over half their respondents wrote comments on the survey forms, which sometimes extended for several pages. "Respondents critiqued the research questions, the methods of gathering data, and the focus of the research in general" (p. 250), with several stating, "This is what you should be asking . . ." (p. 249). Drawing from their experience of living with pain and impairment, many respondents outlined what "needs to be known" (p. 250). Advice included "critiques of what was being asked, how it was asked, and ways to obtain better results", while some participants "expressed concern that the questionnaire did not ask what was important to them" (p. 250). Indeed, some felt the survey questions revealed a lamentable lack of knowledge on the part of the researchers. These critiques are important, because by challenging the relevance of the research questions these disabled people contested the value of the research findings. However, because researchers often employ assistants to process their quantitative findings, they may be unaware of the valuable qualitative data that has been written to them in their margins.

In an effort to foreground the perspectives of some of the participants in our own studies, the following section highlights instances in which they have endeavoured to insert their perspectives and assert their agendas. Two contrasting methodologies are presented to illustrate different approaches to research and to enacting our profession's espoused client-centred principles.

Example 1. Dictating the Agenda: Researcher-Centred Research

A quantitative study was undertaken (by KRWH) to explore the relationship between perceived levels of social support and levels of anxiety and depression among people with either severe traumatic brain injury (TBI) or spinal cord injury (SCI), and their partners. The research, which was planned in a traditional colonial manner—without any input from people with either TBI or SCI—used two standardized interviews to capture data that could be converted to a quantitative score and analysed statistically. [Study details published previously (27,28)]. However, it was apparent that the participants' spontaneous comments provided data that were more instructive than their responses to the standardized questions, and the researcher jotted these comments in the margins of the questionnaires.

In response to the study's questions concerning daily social interactions, a man who had been a successful architect before he sustained a severe TBI stated: "Your questions are making me feel like a reject from society." This not only confirmed that research is neither a neutral activity nor one without consequences for those whom we choose to study, but also suggested that without input from disabled people, issues may be approached in ways that may be offensive or irrelevant. The research did not expose the reasons why his social interactions were so limited because these types of questions were not part of the standardized script, and it was therefore impossible to determine how his restricted life could have been enhanced. Indeed, by maintaining a firm grasp on power, the researcher significantly restricted and pre-scripted the parameters of knowledge that could be learned from the study participants.

In response to a question concerning community living, the wife of a man who had sustained an SCI blurted out: "They thought at the Spinal Centre that the important thing was to be able to transfer. He still can't—but it doesn't matter. He's happy and I'm happy. There are more important things." This was a profound statement, but one that remained unexplored because the research agenda was not focused on issues of importance to the research participants but on issues predetermined by the researcher. Clearly, this participant was trying to convey something she felt was important and a pertinent dimension of knowledge was lost because the researcher did not explore the things that might make life happy after a severe traumatic injury, but stuck, instead, to the standardized script. Regrettably, despite occupational therapy's espoused allegiance to practising in a client-centred manner, this example of research practice remains unexceptional, even in the twenty-first century.

It is important to note that the nagging concerns about power, which arose during this study, were not necessarily the consequence of using quantitative research methods. Qualitative methods do not inevitably ensure equality, but can reinforce the status quo of power just as effectively as quantitative methods (29). Power dynamics cannot change unless researchers work conscientiously to change them.

Example 2. Sharing the Agenda: Collaborative Research

People with SCI (18,30) and researchers (31) have identified fatigue as an issue of priority for research. In an attempt to enhance the relevance and usefulness of research by working in partnership with people living with SCI (3,18,32,33–35), and in an effort to enact occupational therapy's client-centred principles (7), a study into the experience of fatigue following SCI was planned, undertaken, analysed, and reported by a collaborative research team of occupational therapy academics, and peer counsellors from the British Columbia Paraplegic Association.

Seeking a Client-Centred Approach to Data Collection

The focus-group method was chosen by the team to enable participants to define their priorities, explore those issues they deemed important, assert their perspectives, and develop their analysis of a common experience (36,37). Because focus groups can enable a high level of participant involvement (37) and are a relatively non-hierarchical research method (38,39) they hold considerable promise as a client-centred research method. By virtue of the number of research participants, focus groups have the potential to shift the balance of power towards the participants and away from the researcher, to enable participants to assert their own agendas and to develop the themes most important to them (39). Within the group context it may be easier for research participants to challenge researchers' views or assertions and even to change the direction or focus of the research (39). Importantly, working with groups can place demands for accountability on researchers because the group dynamic cultivated within the focus group is likely to produce expectations for action (40). However, without a sincere commitment to sharing power with group participants, focus groups can be as hierarchical and researcher-driven as any other research method. (A full description of this research, including its purpose, process, outcome, and planned action, are reported elsewhere) (41,42).

Asserting and Inserting Agendas

Although it is possible that some people might feel constrained by a group research method and be unable to express their opinions, we found that the focus-group format fostered discussion and enabled participants to raise concerns that had not been anticipated by the research team. Several focus-group participants spontaneously expressed frustration with previous research in which they had been involved, which they felt lacked both relevance and a commitment to action. For example, they were frustrated with medical research that had enquired whether the pain they experienced was burning or tingling yet had failed to ask about the impact of pain on their lives. Moreover, after participating in pre-

vious research they had not received any feedback concerning the research findings or the actions planned by the researchers to address these findings. This prompted participants in one focus group to question what research accomplishes, and for whom. They complained:

"It gets frustrating . . . it is just all these studies"; "Studies study, but what have you learned?"; "It is tiring"; "It is not only tiring, it is a waste of money"; "Did anything come of it?"

Focus group leader: "So, . . . much more research needs to be grounded in the self-expressed needs of the community?"

"And actually followed through on"; "So that it has some use".

There was a clear expectation on the part of these participants that researchers are responsible for ensuring that research yields meaningful results and actions, an expectation compatible with client-centred practices.

Congruent with the suggestion that focus groups can enable participants to assert perspectives that may differ from those of researchers (39), the participants in one group insisted that fatigue was a symptom of a more profound problem, and challenged the researchers on the underlying premise of the research itself:

"It's okay to talk about fatigue, but that word—throw that word aside. Really, it's like you're getting bent on a word. . . . A major part of why you go through what you go through is because you feel hopeless, feel tired";

"I think it's a symptom of something bigger than what we're talking about here. . . . I'm going to throw your whole thing out of the water. . . . I don't think fatigue is really what we're looking at";

"I don't either. I agree".

The participants' insights informed subsequent efforts to develop and appraise appropriate interventions to address the relationships they identified between fatigue, pain, depression, and a sense of helplessness or hopelessness, thereby broadening and deepening the original research focus on fatigue (42). One participant also suggested an insightful direction for future research: "Maybe a research project for another time could be: If 60% of people with spinal cord injury experience this fatigue [and] 40% don't, Why? What's going on here?"

Power, Politics, and Research

Critical disability theorists have long observed that irrespective of whether researchers employ qualitative or quantitative methods, the power of the researcher is enshrined in their control over the research design, process, analysis, and dissemination of research findings (20,32). Because research participants do not always receive feedback from researchers, they may be unable to learn what conclusions have been drawn from the research or what actions will be undertaken in light of the study findings (43,44). It should not be surprising, therefore, that although some people find participation in research to be empowering and rewarding, others have reported that the research process can be disempowering and claim that the absence of tangible results provokes anger and frustration (45).

It is also important to note that research is not an entirely altruistic endeavour, but one that can yield rich rewards for researchers, enabling students to attain degrees and academics to accumulate papers and conference presentations, and achieve peer recognition, promotion, research grants, and tenure (3,46).

Critics observe that research is a political occupation, either reinforcing or countering existing power differentials (40,47). Indeed, Foucault (48) viewed knowledge and power as so inseparable that he termed this relationship power/knowledge. Therefore, to contemplate the practice of research—the generation of knowledge—is inevitably to confront issues of power.

Power, Politics, and Occupational Therapy Research

Power is integral to the occupation of research. Identifying a research question and data collection method, analysing data, and disseminating knowledge all require choices, and these choices are informed by perspectives, values, and priorities. At all these decision points, power resides in control (49), with power either shared with participants, or monopolized by researchers. Although critical disability theorists have long claimed that "central to the problem of rehabilitation is the failure to address the issue of power" [(50), p. 104], occupational therapists have only recently begun to engage seriously with theoretical analyses of power (2,3). Moreover, occupational therapists have not subjected the politics of their research practices to significant critical analysis (4,5) despite espousing a client-centred orientation to practise fundamentally concerned with power (3,51). It is helpful, therefore, to draw from the work of postcolonial theorists, who have paid considerable attention both to power and to the occupation of research.

Critical Theory and Research

Postcolonial theory is a form of critical theory specifically concerned with empowerment of the dispossessed, the establishment of minorities' rights, and with achieving just and equitable relationships among people (52,53). In particular, postcolonial theorists examine how marginalized and disempowered people (those who are considered to be "inferior" on the basis of normative judgements about physical ability and appearance, colour, behaviour, etc.) are represented, marginalized, and disempowered by those wielding more power. Thus, it has been suggested that critical post-colonial perspectives should inform disability research (3).

When a research issue is defined by the researcher, the research process is controlled by the researcher, and the findings are analysed and disseminated according to the researcher's perspectives and priorities, this reflects a colonial methodology (54). Post-colonial theorists claim that researchers must develop an awareness not only of "who speaks, from where, and for whom" [(55), p. 89], but also of whose perspectives are discounted, suppressed, or unacknowledged. These are political choices. However, they do not occur in a vacuum, but in a political context (2), with client-centred aspirations challenged by the competing demands of funding agencies, institutional stakeholders, and career aspirations (3).

Enabling Meaningful Participation in Research

Evidence-based practice and client-centred practice are claimed to be the two most influential paradigms in current health-care practice (56). To reflect their client-centred philosophy and to ensure the relevance and usefulness of research evidence, occupational therapists need to identify effective means of including consumers in research to ensure it addresses the values and priorities of those whom research has traditionally been "about." As a first step, for example, some researchers have sought to identify the research priorities of people with specific diagnoses in an effort to develop a research agenda addressing issues of importance to clients (e.g. 33). This enables research to achieve a client-centred focus, even if the research process itself is not collaborative. Expanding this process to ascertain the research priorities of clinicians might also be a means to address occupational therapy's current theory/practice gap.

How might the practice of occupational therapy research better reflect the client-centred, collaborative ethos claimed to underpin the occupational therapy profession (7)? As in all client-centred practices, client-centred research builds on the premise that everyone's contributions have equal value (57) and is characterized by meaningful and reciprocal partnerships in all phases of the research process, a nonhierarchical approach to power, mutual respect for the equally valuable yet different knowledge, skills, and perspectives contributed by all team members, an openness to learning by all parties (by being unthreatened and constantly challenged by ideas and perspectives contributed by other team members and research participants), and a commitment to translate research results into meaningful action (14,33,58,59). Greenwood and Levin (58) note that community research partners "contribute urgency and focus to the [research] process, because it centers on problems they are anxious to solve" (p. 96). Thus, collaboration with those people traditionally used solely as research "subjects" demands a high standard of accountability. Collaborative research presents unique challenges, due to the politics of organizations (policies, procedures, and practices) and the politics of professionalism (60), the time-consuming nature of research, and the need to achieve a balance of expertise and sufficient funding to ensure participants are compensated equitably. Although considerable debate within the occupational therapy profession has focused on institutional barriers to client-centred clinical practice, little attention has centred on either the institutional or professional barriers to client-centred research practice. However, issues involved in overcoming barriers to collaborative research are now beginning to be discussed in the occupational therapy literature [e.g. 11,61], and exemplars of client-centred occupational therapy research are increasingly to be found in the literature [e.g. 62,63].

Recent research demonstrates that disabled people's organizations want to be engaged actively in shaping research agendas (12) and to be involved as partners in designing, implementing, disseminating, and evaluating research of relevance to their priorities and needs (13). Moreover, disabled people are identifying those factors that they perceive as constituting barriers to their participation in research with academics (13). If the occupational therapy profession is seriously committed to collaborative, client-centred practices, concerted attention could usefully focus on how barriers to client participation in the occupation of research might be identified, addressed, and overcome.

Conclusion

Evidence demonstrates that occupational therapy research practices do not consistently reflect the client-centred ethos said to underpin the profession. Moreover, little attention has been paid to the politics of occupational therapy research, or to the institutional and professional environments in which research is undertaken. Examples in this paper suggest that research participants wish to influence agendas to make research more relevant to their needs and priorities.

Power dynamics cannot change unless researchers work conscientiously to change them. By enabling clients to share in establishing research agendas, and by engaging in collaborative research, occupational therapists are more likely to develop evidence-based theories and interventions that are informed by, and relevant to, clients' lives, values, and priorities.

Acknowledgements

The authors greatly appreciate the time, effort, and input of the participants in both the studies cited in this paper. They acknowledge their sincere appreciation of Dr Andrea Townson, who was a valued member of the research team, and of their research assistant Bobby Lee. They also acknowledge the Canadian Institutes of Health Research Institute of Aging who provided a New Investigator salary award for Dr Miller.

Sponsorship

The focus group research discussed in this paper was funded by a Michael Smith Foundation for Health Research, Disability Health Research Network grant.

Declaration of interest: The authors report no conflicts of interest. The authors alone are responsible for the content and writing of the paper.

References

1. Law M. The environment: A focus for occupational therapy. *Can J Occup Ther* 1991;58:171–80.
2. Pollard N, Sakellariou D, Kronenberg F. Preface. In: Pollard N, Sakellariou D, Kronenberg F, editors. *A political practice of occupational therapy.* Edinburgh: Churchill Livingstone Elsevier; 2009. p xvii.
3. Hammell KW. *Perspectives on disability and rehabilitation: Contesting assumptions; challenging practice.* Edinburgh: Churchill Livingstone Elsevier; 2006.
4. Hammell KW. Reflections on . . . a disability methodology for the client-centred practice of occupational therapy research. *Can J Occup Ther* 2007;74:365–9.
5. Finlayson M. Developing our science. *Can J Occup Ther* 2007;74:363.

6. Thomas C. *Female forms: Experiencing and understanding disability.* Buckingham: Open University Press; 1999.

7. Canadian Association of Occupational Therapists. *Enabling occupation: An occupational therapy perspective.* 2nd ed. Ottawa: Author; 2002.

8. Swain J, French S, Cameron C. *Controversial issues in a disabling society.* Buckingham: Open University Press; 2003.

9. Chambers. *Chambers' twentieth century dictionary.* Edinburgh: Chambers; 1972.

10. Law M, Baptiste S, Mills J. Client-centred practice: What does it mean and does it make a difference? *Can J Occup Ther* 1995;62:250–7.

11. Letts L. Occupational therapy and participatory research: A partnership worth pursuing. *Am J Occup Ther* 2003; 57: 77–87.

12. Priestley M, Waddington L, Bessozi C. New priorities for disability research in Europe: Towards a user-led agenda. ALTER: *European J Disabil Res* 2010;4:239–55.

13. Priestley M, Waddington L, Bessozi C. Towards an agenda for disability research in Europe: Learning from disabled people's organisations. *Disabil Society* 2010;25:731–46.

14. White GW, Suchowierska MA, Campbell M Developing and systematically implementing participatory action research. *Arch Phys Med Rehabil* 2004;85:(4 Suppl. 2):S3–12.

15. Ward L, Flynn M. What matters most: Disability, research and empowerment. In: Rioux MH, Bach M, editors. *Disability is not measles: New research paradigms in disability.* North York, ONT: L'Institut Roeher; 1994. p 29–48.

16. Macfarlane S. Opening spaces for alternative understandings in mental health practice. In: Allen J, Briskman L, Pease B, editors. *Critical social work: Theories and practices for a socially just world.* 2nd edn. Crows Nest, NSW, Australia: Allen & Unwin; 2009. p 201–13.

17. Ilott I, White E. 2001 College of Occupational Therapists' Research and Development Strategic Vision and Action Plan. *Br J Occup Ther* 2001;64:270–7.

18. White GW, Nary DE, Froehlich AK. Consumers as collaborators in research and action. *J Prev Interv* 2001;21:15–34.

19. Townsend E, Birch D, Langley J, Langille L. Participatory research in a mental health clubhouse. *Occup Ther J Res* 2000;20:18–29.

20. Barnes C, Mercer G, Shakespeare T. *Exploring disability: A sociological introduction.* Cambridge: Polity; 1999.

21. McKnight J. Professionalised service and disabling help. In: Brechin A, Liddiard P, Swain J, editors. *Handi-cap in a social world.* Sevenoaks, UK: Hodder & Stoughton; 1981:24–33.

22. Basnett I. Health care professionals and their attitudes toward and decisions affecting disabled people. In: Albrecht GL, Seelman KD, Bury M, editors. *Handbook of disability studies.* London: Sage Publications; 2001. p 450–67.

23. Glasby J, Beresford P. Who knows best? Evidence-based practice and the service user contribution. *Critic Soc Pol* 2006;26:268–84.

24. Goodare H, Lockwood S. Involving patients in clinical research: Improves the quality of research. *BMJ* 1999;319:724–5.

25. Clayton DK, Rogers S, Stuifbergen A. Answers to unasked questions: Writing in the margins. *Res Nurs Health* 1999;22:512–22.

26. Warms CA, Marshall HM, Hoffman AJ, Tyler EJ. There are a few things you did not ask about my pain: Writing on the margins of a survey questionnaire. *Rehabil Nurs* 2005;30:248–56.

27. Hammell KW. Psychosocial outcome following spinal cord injury. *Paraplegia* 1994;32:771–9.

28. Hammell KW. Psychosocial outcome following severe closed head injury. *Int J Rehabil Res* 1994;17:319–32.

29. Bhopal K. Gender, "race" and power in the research process. In: Truman C, Mertens D, Humphries B, editors. *Research and inequality.* London: UCL Press; 2000. p 67–79.

30. Hart KA, Rintala DH, Fuhrer MJ. Educational interests of individuals with spinal cord injury living in the community: Medical, sexuality, and wellness topics. *Rehabil Nurs* 1996;21:82–90.

31. Fawkes-Kirby TM, Wheeler MA, Anton HA, Miller WC, Townson AF, Weeks CAO. Clinical correlates of fatigue in spinal cord injury. *Spinal Cord* 2008;46:21–5.

32. Barnartt S, Altman B. Exploring theories and expanding methodologies: Where we are and where we need to go. *Res Soc Sci Disabil* 2001;2:1–7.

33. Abma TA. Patient participation in health research: Research with and for people with spinal cord injuries. *Qual Health Res* 2005;15:1310–28.

34. Stone E, Priestley M. Parasites, pawns and partners: Disability research and the role of non-disabled researchers. *Br J Sociol* 1996;47:699–716.

35. White GW. Consumer participation in disability research: The golden rule as a guide for ethical practice. *Rehabil Psychol* 2002;47:438–46.

36. Kitzinger J. Focus groups with users and providers of health care. In: Pope C, Mays N, editors. *Qualitative research in health care.* 2nd ed. London: BMJ; 2000. p 20–9.

37. Morgan DL. *Focus groups as qualitative research.* London: Sage Publications; 1988.

38. Kitzinger J, Barbour RS. Introduction: The challenge and promise of focus groups. In: Barbour RS, Kitzinger J, editors. *Developing focus group research: Politics, theory and practice.* London: Sage Publications; 1999. p 1–20.

39. Wilkinson S. How useful are focus groups in feminist research? In: Barbour RS, Kitzinger J, editors. *Developing focus group research: Politics, theory and practice.* London: Sage Publications; 1999. p 64–78.

40. Baker R, Hinton R. Do focus groups facilitate meaningful participation in social research? In: Barbour RS, Kitzinger J, editors. *Developing focus group research: Politics, theory and practice.* London: Sage Publications; 1999. p 79–98.

41. Hammell KW, Miller WC, Forwell SJ, Forman BE, Jacobsen BA. Fatigue and spinal cord injury: A qualitative analysis. *Spinal Cord* 2009;47:44–9.

42. Hammell KW, Miller WC, Forwell SJ, Forman BE, Jacobsen BA. Managing fatigue following spinal cord injury: A qualitative exploration. *Disabil Rehabil* 2009;31:1437–45.

43. Kitchin R. The researched opinions on research: Disabled people and disability research. *Dis Soc* 2000;15:25–47.

44. Northway R. Disability, nursing research and the importance of reflexivity. *J Adv Nurs* 2000;32:391–7.

45. Barnitt R, Partridge C. The legacy of being a research subject: Follow-up studies of participants in therapy research. *Physio Res Int* 1999;4:250–61.

46. Hall BL. From margins to center? The development and purpose of participatory research. *Am Sociol* 1992;23:15–28.

47. Mohanty CT. Under Western eyes: Feminist scholarship and colonial discourses. In: Williams P, Chrisman L, editors. *Colonial discourse and postcolonial theory.* New York: Columbia University Press; 1994. p 196–220.

48. Foucault M. *Power/knowledge.* New York: Pantheon Books; 1980.

49. Brown M, Gordon WA. Empowerment in measurement: "Muscle", "voice" and subjective quality of life as a gold standard. *Arch Phys Med Rehabil* 2004;85:(4 Suppl 2): S13–20.

50. Oliver M. *Understanding disability: From theory to practice.* Basingstoke, UK, Macmillan; 1996.

51. Cockburn L, Trentham B. Participatory action research: Integrating community occupational therapy practice and research. *Can J Occup Ther* 2002;69:20–30.

52. Said EW. *Orientalism,* London: Routledge; 1979.

53. Young RJC. *Postcolonialism,* Oxford: Oxford University Press; 2003.

54. Ryen A. Colonial methodology? In: Truman C, Mertens D, Humphries B, editors. *Research and inequality.* London: UCL Press; 2000. p 67–79.

55. Childs P, Williams P. *An introduction to post-colonial theory.* London: Prentice-Hall; 1997.

56. Ford S, Schofield T, Hope T. What are the ingredients for a successful evidence-based patient choice consultation?: A qualitative study. *Soc Sci Med* 2003;56:589–602.

57. Nolan M, Hanson E, Grant G, Keady J. *User participation in health and social care research.* Maidenhead: Open University Press; 2007.

58. Greenwood DJ, Levin M. Reconstructing the relationships between universities and society through action research. In: Denzin NK, Lincoln YS, editors. *Handbook of qualitative research.* 2nd ed. Thousand Oaks, CA: Sage Publications; 2000. p 85–106.

59. Turnbull AP, Friesen BJ, Ramirez C. Participatory Action Research as a model for conducting family research. *J Assoc Persons Severe Handicaps* 1998;23:178–88.

60. Braye S. Participation and involvement in social care. In: Kemshall H, Littlechild R, editors. *User involvement and participation in social care: Research informing practice.* London: Jessica Kingsley; 2000. p 9–28.

61. Taylor RR, Braveman B. Hammel J. Developing and evaluating community-based services through participatory action research: Two case examples. *Am J Occup Ther* 2004;58:73–82. http://dx.doi.org/10.5014/ajot.58.1.73

62. Ripat JD, Redmond JD, Grabowecky BR. The Winter Walkability project: Occupational therapists' role in promoting citizen engagement. *Can J Occup Ther* 2010;77:7–14.

63. Rebeiro K. How qualitative research can inform and challenge occupational therapy practice. In: Hammell KW, Carpenter C, editors. *Qualitative research in evidence-based rehabilitation.* Edinburgh: Churchill Livingstone Elsevier; 2004. p 89–102.

Part VII. Envisioning the Future of Occupation-Based Practice

Our practice in the future should be evaluated not only on the basis of measurable scientific outcomes but also by what it contributes to individual human dignity and a sense of mastery and self-respect.

—Yerxa (1980, p. 534)

In the above quote, Yerxa (1980) puts forth a vision of the profession's future that will require practitioners to pursue the art of occupational therapy, along with its science. Her view is consistent with many of the authors of prior chapters, who emphasized that it is essential for the art of occupational therapy to be actualized in practice. *Artful practice* includes the conscious use of self and the skilled application of occupation, as guided by theories that are consistent with the profession's core values, founding principles, desired goals, and established domain of concern (Hinojosa, 2013; Mosey, 1996). As evident in Part I, "Occupational Therapy's Heritage: Historical and Philosophical Foundations for Occupation-Based Practice," both the art and science of occupational therapy were critical to the profession's founding. However, as thoughtfully examined in several chapters, the influence of historical movements, sociopolitical forces, and health care system trends has often constrained this art and, at times, threatened its viability.

> *The average hospital suffers from occupational blindness.*
>
> —Tracy (1921, p. 397)

From occupational therapy's early struggles to define itself to the reductionist fallout from the field's allegiance to the medical model, our profession has faced many challenges and weathered several paradigm shifts throughout its first century of growth (Schemm, 1994; Shannon, 1977; West, 1984). Concerns voiced in the 1990s about the disparities between reimbursement-driven practice and the provision of client-centered, occupation-based practice remain relevant today as the profession realizes the challenges and opportunities afforded by current health care reform (Burke & Cassidy, 1991; Fisher & Friesema, 2013; Howard, 1991).

The emergence of professional competition and active infringement on occupational therapy's domain of concern also underscore the need for the profession to retain its art (Clark, 2011; Gutman, 1998; Wood, 1998). As others embrace the use of occupation as a primary tool of practice, the absence of this art in the American Occupational Therapy Association's (AOTA's; 2007) *Centennial Vision* statement can give external audiences a constrained view of the profession. The *Centennial Vision's* aspiration for occupational therapy to be widely recognized as powerful and able to meet society's occupational needs on the basis of evidence and driven by science is a worthy goal (Clark, 2007). However, a myopic focus on scientific evidence does injustice to the art of our practice (Peloquin, 1989). For occupational therapy to fully attain its goal of being widely recognized as *the* profession to globally meet occupational needs, the art of occupational therapy must become as celebrated as it science.

> *Occupational therapy is a client-centered health profession concerned with promoting health and well-being through occupation.*
>
> —World Federation of Occupational Therapists (2010, p. 1)

Our profession has a strong history of striving to balance the art and science of practice (Law, 2002; Peloquin, 1989; Schemm, 1994; Wood, 1995). The authors in this part provide thoughtful insights into this discourse. They examine the profession's past and current realities that presently influence the field and will affect its future. They stress the need for practitioners to sustain a commitment to occupational therapy's founding beliefs, which emphasize the value of the therapeutic relationship and the use of occupation throughout the occupational therapy process. Several also accentuate the realistic need for occupational therapy practitioners to become politically astute and market savvy to ensure the profession remains viable, now and in its next century. It is my hope that active reflection on the issues raised by the authors of these pivotal works will inspire readers to fully embrace and actively use the art *and* science of occupational therapy to enable occupational well-being and full participation for all.

> *Remember, if you think of work merely as employment and not as a real calling, you will fail in rendering help to those to whom you minister.*
> —Slagle (1930, p. 276)

Part VII begins with an exploration of the value of the profession's history to contemporary occupational therapy practice. In this classic 1981 Presidential Address, Johnson examines the "old" values of humanism, caring, and the therapeutic relationship, and the "new" directions of science, logic, and depersonalization. She examines the conflict between being humanistic and caring while striving to meet demands to be scientific and objective, expressing concern that the profession is moving toward reductionism and away from holism. A historical review of the characteristics of the founders of occupational therapy and the evolution of the profession up to 1981 is provided. As Johnson notes, there was substantial growth in the profession during this time period with respect to the types of clients served, settings in which occupational therapy practitioners provided service, and the field's repertoire of tools of practice. However, she cautions that this growth may have sacrificed depth for breadth.

Johnson challenges practitioners to question their work, so they can maintain holistic values while developing knowledge and skills in a scientific sense. She calls for increased professional support for entry-level therapists, administrators, researchers, and educators to ensure they are able to meet the challenges of their roles. Increased research is also needed to substantiate the value of occupational therapy by developing a solid, unifying theoretical foundation. Personal poignant examples highlight Johnson's presentation, emphasizing the depth of meaning inherent in these professional values and considering the complexities of occupational therapy practice. She concludes that combining the old values of humanism and holism with the new values of science, research, and knowledge will enable occupational therapy practitioners to acquire new competence and attain professional unity.

In the years since Johnson's address, attaining her vision for powerful new directions for the profession has been seriously limited by the aforementioned conflict between the foundational values of occupational therapy and those of reimbursement-driven practice that highly values and rewards productivity. In the next chapter, Schwartz offers a way to effectively deal with the challenges, demands, and frustrations of reimbursement-driven systems of care. She presents the *excellence perspective* as a way to ensure quality of care as well as efficient care. The excellence perspective is contrasted with the *efficiency perspective,* which emphasizes productivity. The history of the efficiency perspective is presented, and its introduction to health care management is examined. Adopting the efficiency perspective in health care resulted in a change from a humanistic emphasis to a business administration focus. The incongruence between a business model and the provision of humanistic health care presents a dilemma as to how to achieve quality and efficiency. Schwartz proposes the excellence perspective as an alternative to the efficiency perspective, stating that if one stresses excellence as his or her primary goal, productivity also will be enhanced.

> *Plant the idea in hospital executives and let it germinate. True, a seed is often lost because of the weedy growth about it. However, the best plants are found where the first sowing is followed by steady and quiet cultivation based upon a confidence in the value of the seed sown.*
> —Tracy (1921, p. 399)

Because leadership is a critical factor in successful implementation of the excellence perspective, Schwartz identifies ways that leaders can shape organizations in which members strive for excellence. A case study that exemplifies the characteristics of the excellence perspective, including leaders who epitomize the leadership qualities fundamental for success, is provided. The excellence perspective can be used as a guide for program innovation, as it is congruent with occupational therapy's concern for quality patient care and with the health care system's emphasis on productivity. Practitioners must develop leadership skills and knowledge of management to be able to explicate consumer needs and design and implement programs on the basis of excellence.

Schwartz's call for leaders to "articulate the profession's contribution and introduce new ideas that can lead practice" (p. 737) is effectively answered in this part's next two chapters, which eloquently present thought-provoking viewpoints on occupational therapy in the 21st century. American and Canadian perspectives on dreams, dilemmas, and decisions for occupational therapy practice in this century are respectfully presented by Yerxa and Polatajko. In Chapter 56, Yerxa puts forth the assumption that the 21st century will have several unique characteristics that will be important to occupational therapy practitioners and the consumers of our services. These characteristics—increase in chronicity; knowledge of human purpose; complexity of daily living; awareness of demands from the environments in which people live and work; emphasis on personal power, autonomy, self-direction, and self-responsibility; and a new conceptualization of health as people's capacities to achieve goals through a repertoire of skills—are briefly described. A clear link between each characteristic and the philosophy and unique body of knowledge of occupational therapy is provided. On the basis of this congruence and occupational therapy practitioners' ability to effectively meet the needs reflected in each of the identified characteristics, Yerxa asserts that the 21st century will begin a millennium of occupation.

Our field is varied, our opportunities are large.
—Shaw (1928, p. 206)

Yerxa strongly emphasizes the value of authentic occupational therapy and reflects on the potential of occupational science to enrich and broaden practice. Implications for the future of occupational therapy are discussed, and the need for practitioners to establish their priorities in the "millennium of occupation" is examined. She calls for the profession to accentuate the potential of people with disabilities, with practitioners serving as advocates and allies for individuals and their families. Yerxa concludes that the knowledge, skills, and values of occupational therapy practitioners, as founded in the profession's early philosophical base, will enable us to ensure that people with chronic illnesses and disabilities will perceive themselves as whole and capable and develop the skills they need to achieve competency and autonomy. Social barriers to this self-definition will be removed, enabling all people to thrive and live with purpose.

Polatajko continues this theme of viewing people with disabilities in a "new light" in the 21st century, thus requiring occupational therapy to shift its emphasis. She envisions a future world in which the concept of handicap will be eliminated through the creation of an environment in which individuals with different abilities and disabilities can live meaningful lives with dignity. In this new world, occupational therapy's focus will change from reducing impairments to preventing handicaps through empowerment. Definitions of *handicap, impairment,* and *disability* are provided and contrasted. The relationship of occupation to these concepts is examined, and the basic assumptions and core values of occupational therapy are reviewed.

Polatajko urges practitioners to translate rhetoric into action. She puts forth her vision for the profession, emphasizing the full potential of occupation. Unequivocally embracing the power of occupation can ensure that occupational therapy attains a leadership position in the 21st century. Adopting occupation as the core concept of our profession and entrenching occupation into our professional value system is essential for achieving the ultimate goal of practice: the empowerment of occupational competence. Polatajko concludes that occupational therapy practitioners are uniquely positioned to eliminate handicaps for all by enabling occupational competence during the next millennium.

The services throughout the country be alert to create and exploit new opportunities in treatment and prevention.
—Mirrey & Johnson (1969, p. 17)

Yerxa's and Polatajko's dreams for occupational therapy in the 21st century share many commonalities with the profession's imagined future that have been articulated in the past. Almost 50 years ago, Wilma West presented her visionary Eleanor Clarke Slagle Lecture, which has remained startlingly relevant. In this lecture, West puts forth a call for social activism, community-based practice, and research to ensure that occupational therapy practitioners respond proactively to change. Since West gave this address—when the golden anniversary of our profession was celebrated—the nuclear age, bipartisanship, and federal–state alliances of which she spoke have been replaced by the age of terrorism, political divisiveness, and state antipathy toward the federal government. However, many of her points remain pertinent as the profession approaches its centennial. West's call to move beyond the profession's traditional, limited identification with the medical model to a broad conceptualization of *health,* which includes prevention of illness and disability, maintenance and promotion of well-being, and the facilitation of normal growth and development, is striking in its timeliness. Her identification of a role for occupational therapy practitioners as health agents in community-based settings and her argument that we must aggressively adapt and redesign our roles to be viable in a changing society and an evolving health care system remains contemporary almost a half century later.

West's stance that occupational therapy practitioners must advocate for equal access to comprehensive health care resonates in the ongoing debate about the Patient Protection and Affordable Care Act (2010) and its implementation. Her discussion of developing pediatric health care services, Head Start, and the community mental health movement provides an interesting historical perspective for readers. West's vision for the practice possibilities afforded by these initiatives has been realized in pediatrics but remains unfulfilled in other practice domains. The decades of legislation following the 1960s resulted in mandates for occupational therapy services in early intervention and school-based practice, enabling practitioners to seize the opportunities West describes. However, West's fear that the profession would remain wedded to a traditional medical model has continued to limit practice in other areas. The rich potential she saw for occupational therapy practitioners in community-based prevention, health promotion, and intervention programs was largely ignored in the ensuing decades since her lecture. Instead of expanding exponentially as West envisioned, the profession's presence in mental health settings has diminished greatly, although exceptions do exist. Progressive practitioners have exemplified the active agency that West called for and collectively advanced community-based occupational therapy practice (Metropolitan District of New York, 2009; Swarbrick & Pratt, 2006). West's discussion of the importance of membership in a professional association to attain unity in the field is also demonstrated by these leaders.

> *There is so much to do, but the great growth and the encouragement experienced during the past few years should enable occupational therapists to look forward with confidence and hope to the future; a future which holds wonderful promise of further achievements and of the general adoption of the principles and practice for which the American Occupational Therapy Association stands.*
>
> —Kidner, 1922, p. 502

West concluded her Eleanor Clarke Slagle Lecture with the hope that a future generation of occupational

---

Active Reflection VII.1. Professional Association Membership

West reflected on the role of a professional association in shaping the future of the field and advocated for unified efforts among members to attain shared objectives. Since West's time, numerous legislative acts have passed that have been formative in the growth of the profession, most through AOTA's concerted efforts. However, the majority of occupational therapy practitioners are not AOTA members.

- What deters practitioners from joining AOTA?
- What AOTA benefits can be promoted to increase membership?
- What actions can AOTA members and leaders take to help practitioners recognize they are collectively responsible for shaping the future of the profession via membership in their professional association?

---

therapy practitioners would look back and see a profession that was dynamically sharing a professional consciousness and collective responsibility. Current practitioners now have the opportunity to fulfill this dream. As West noted, societal trends are unmistakable and irreversible, so it is up to all practitioners to be mutually responsible and assume new roles and adopt new practices in response to these changes. Occupational therapy's recommitment to its core values, as evidenced in the *Occupational Therapy Practice Framework* (3rd ed.; *Framework;* AOTA, 2014; see Appendix A), now provides the shared vision that West had aspired for the profession. Applying the *Framework* can help current and future occupational therapy practitioners seize the opportunities put forth by West almost half a century ago. West also expressed hope that one day a "better definition" of our profession would be developed. The *Framework* provides a holistic view of our profession that I think would please West. The six primary domains (i.e., mental health; productive aging; children and youth; health and wellness; work and industry; rehabilitation, disability, and participation) put forth in AOTA's (2007) *Centennial Vision* as framing occupational therapy education, practice, research, and policies in the 21st century are also highly consistent with West's vision for the profession (see Active Reflection VII.1).

One of West's principal aspirations for occupational therapy was that its practitioners would move from traditional roles in medical settings to creating new roles as health agents serving diverse communities. The vital contribution occupational therapy makes to community-based practice is well supported in the literature (Scaffa & Reitz, 2014). In Chapter 59, Leclair challenges occupational therapy practitioners to broaden their community perspective to include community development. Leclair observes that typical community-based practice remains focused on the unique occupations of the individual, without consideration of the shared occupations of a community. Although use of an individualized approach in a person's natural setting has great value, Leclair proposes that a community development approach can enable sustainable change within a community that is beneficial to all members. By having community members define their mutual concerns and desires, determine their priorities, set their objectives, and build on their local resources and joint capacities, occupational therapy practitioners can forge effective partnerships to develop self-sustaining programs that meet communities' central occupational needs.

Leclair's focus on the community as a client is consistent with the *Framework* and international practice guidelines that identify the client of occupational therapy services as inclusive of groups, communities, and populations (AOTA, 2014; World Federation of Occupational Therapists, 2010). To help practitioners move from a micro-level (i.e., the individual) approach to a macro-level (i.e., the community) approach, Leclair discusses the literature that defines *occupation* to include the concepts of *shared occupations* and *co-occupations*. She describes the limitations of existing categorizations of occupation that do not address the collective occupations of communities and the challenges of applying current occupation-based models to communities. Leclair reviews community development models and calls for collaborative partnerships between occupational therapy scholars and practitioners to develop and test occupation-based models for community development. Because the benefits of collective participation in shared or interconnected occupations can exceed those attained by one-to-one occupational therapy, expansion of the field's practice and scholarship into community development is warranted. Practitioners who partner with communities to develop occupation-based programs can foster social change, enable occupational well-being, and advance occupational justice (see Active Reflection VII.2).

The real success of the movement often depends upon the faith of the launchers. If occupational therapy be 'tried' with a feeling of possible failure, the odds will be against it. There is no success in doubt, there is no success in fear, there is no success in division of purpose. Convince yourself of the value of occupational therapy, and then establish its use.

—Tracy (1921, p. 399)

Active Reflection VII.2. Macro-Level Thinking for Community Development

Moving from an individualized micro-level approach to a population-based macro-level one is essential for community development practice. To foster this shift in mindset, think about the common characteristics of people who live in your home community and their shared occupations.

- Do these fit into the definitions of *occupation* that are provided in Table 59.1?
- What collective or interconnected occupations are missing from these definitions?
- How would you categorize these mutually shared occupations?

Reflect on your community's resources for collective participation in shared or interconnected occupations.

- Are there sufficient opportunities for community members to engage in occupations together? Describe one area where you think an occupational therapy practitioner could partner with community members to develop a program to meet an unmet occupational need of your community.

The advancement of the occupational therapy profession into new domains of practice has historically required practitioners to move beyond their traditional modes of practice and established ways of thinking. As Fearing notes in Chapter 60, change is inevitable. However, not all respond to change in the same way. Some people serve as the catalyst for change, others embrace change when it occurs with enthusiasm, and others view change with apprehension and avoid it. Fearing discusses the power of personal, professional, and organizational contexts to influence the ability to change. She encourages practitioners to actively reflect on how personal experiences, values, relationships, occupations, and life choices contribute to the development of strategies to manage change. By recognizing the uniqueness of our own stories and those of our clients, we can develop partnerships that consider personal contexts, foster hope, and enable desired change.

Fearing contends that change is embedded in our professional context. She analyzes how seemingly incremental actions and small events can contribute to tipping points that result in substantial change. Practitioners' graduated use of occupation with clients can foster transformative changes in their lives, and an understanding of tipping points throughout one's professional career can create contexts that welcome change. Fearing examines how changes implemented by individuals gain momentum when other people join this process. Her examples of the resulting commitment to use contemporary theory in practice, advocate for clients, and engage in peer mentoring exemplify how embracing change in current professional contexts can best prepare practitioners for the future.

Because organizational contexts may thwart desired and needed change, Fearing acknowledges the struggle client-centered practitioners face in overmanaged practice environments. However, she does not accept the inevitability of a disconnect between occupational therapy's values and objectives and those of organizations. Rather, Fearing proposes practitioners use their collective power to transform organizational contexts to create healthy workplaces. The impact of choice (or lack thereof) on personal, professional, and organizational change is well articulated by Fearing. Her call to act authentically and consciously when responding to change is particularly relevant in our era of hyperchange (Hinojosa, 2007). Given that the future is unknown, Fearing advocates a transformative leadership approach to imposed change and scenario planning to create a desired future that imagines possibilities.

> *There is certainly something wrong when we become satisfied with things as they are and no longer strive for something new. Can any one of us be sure that this does not apply to her? It is not long since there was only a handful of occupational therapists in Great Britain, struggling to prove that they possessed something which was of value to the patient. Now the profession has been established and is fast spreading into new spheres—undreamed of until recently. In order to keep pace with new developments, the therapist must remain eager to learn. She is of no value . . . if her ideas are not up to date or if she is not willing to learn.*
>
> —Bramwell (1952, p. 6)

An envisioned reality in which the healing potential of occupation is valued is put forth in Chapter 61. In her seminal treatise, Pierce declares that a time of congruence has arrived that can result in the emergence of a powerful occupation-based profession. This congruence is the result of two major forces converging. The first is the exponential growth in our field's knowledge about occupation. The second force is society's increased valuation of functional outcomes. The reality that other professions have noticed the potential of the latter is indisputable. The danger of others imitating occupational therapy practice and claiming our profession's area of expertise cannot be ignored. Pierce challenges occupational therapy practitioners to face this competition by simply being the best at what we do. We must expeditiously translate our sub-

stantial knowledge about occupation into the realization of superior, occupation-based practice.

To effectively achieve this outcome, Pierce proposes that the profession must build three bridges to bring the full potential of occupation to fruition. She describes these bridges—a generative discourse on the use of occupation in practice, practice demonstration sites, and effective education—in a straightforward, realistic manner. To help practitioners forge these bridges, Pierce provides three conceptual tools. These tools, including the dimensions of power, sources of therapeutic power, and the occupational design process, are explored in depth. Their congruence with the core values of occupational therapy is highly evident. The efficacy of using this occupation design approach considers the complexities of the person's occupational experience and the uniqueness of the therapeutic process, and is clearly supported by the literature and practice examples. Pierce's discussion about how the subjective and contextual dimensions of the occupational experience interact with the elements of the occupational design process to produce the therapeutic power of occupation highlights the unique knowledge base of our profession. All occupational therapy practitioners must fluently articulate and actively use this uniqueness in daily practice. This reality and responsibility cannot be ignored.

> *When I was in active practice, during the war, the nurse, physiotherapists and I found that many of our endeavors fell short of what was needful. Often patients we had worked hardest for just failed to make the grade—drifted into chronic invalidism. Then we called in the O.Ts. They had their dual approach—the psychological stimulus to do pleasing things within the patients' capacity; and the physical 'know how' of duly advancing gradations. And then we achieved full rehabilitation with the patient, the focus and this therapeutic team gathered round him, harmoniously cooperating to achieve his full potential.*
>
> —Dott (1967, pp. 4–6)

Pierce stressed the need for occupational therapy to "critically examine and recreate its traditions in theory and practice if it is to live up to its potential" (p. 784). This necessity is eloquently addressed in Chapter 62. In this moving Eleanor Clarke Slagle Lecture, Peloquin synthesizes the profession's historical and philosophical foundations to describe the ethos of occupational therapy. Because an ethos is comprised of beliefs to guide practitioners, Peloquin contends that a recommitment to the distinctive values, sentiments, and thoughts of occupational therapy is required to meet current practice challenges. She explores these ethological beliefs as reflected in the profession's seminal literary works. The result blends ideas and images into five guiding beliefs that highlight (1) temporal, environmental, and situational aspects of occupation; (2) healing potential of occupation; (3) use of occupational engagement to co-create lives; (4) affirming power of caring and helping; and (5) effective use of the art and science of practice.

Peloquin's analysis includes numerous inspirational statements from the founders of occupational therapy and former Slagle lecturers. Although these words resonate with Peloquin's message that the ethos of occupational therapy is the rock of the profession, the intrusive impact of medical and business models on our field cannot be ignored. Thus, she thoughtfully examines the disintegrative impact of these forces on practice and the resulting depersonalization that occurs. Peloquin reframes the disheartening contexts of current practice and uses them as motivators to reclaim occupational therapy's heart. Rather than bemoaning current realities, practitioners must face adversity by recommitting to the profession's ethos. Peloquin confidently asserts that our reaffirmation to be artists, scientists, and pathfinders who reach for hearts and hands to co-create lives and enable occupations that heal will ensure our profession's future.

> *You have a unique opportunity for service in that you can adapt your materials and your technique to meet the individual need. To you the hospital patient is not primarily a 'fracture,' a 'chest case' or a 'neurosis;' but a human being who must be helped back to normality, given confidence, new interests, and a new job if necessary. More than any other hospital workers, you have it in your power to open windows through which people can look at life with fresh hope and fresh vision.*
>
> —Hilton (1942, p. 196)

Peloquin's call to embrace the ethos of occupational therapy and reclaim the heart of the profession is echoed in this text's final chapter, which includes Gillen's Eleanor Clarke Slagle Lecture. In his thought-provoking thesis, Gillen builds on Peloquin's point that we must be conscious of the diminishment of our field when we stray too far from occupational therapy's core

---

Active Reflection VII.3. Reclaiming the Heart of Practice

Reflect on your personality, assets, and limitations.
- What character strengths will assist you in remaining true to the ethos of occupational therapy in an ever-changing health care system?
- What personal shortcomings may make it difficult to integrate the art and science of practice to reach hearts as well as hands?
- What resources are available to help you work on your limitations and strengthen your assets to become a pathfinder, enable occupations that heal, and co-create lives?
- How can you forge your professional life to advance the ethos of occupational therapy in potentially disheartening environments?

---

beliefs. Integrating an extensive literature review, he supports his points by describing methods used to treat impaired motor control and assess cognition over the course of the profession's history. Framing his lecture according to a classic story plot, Gillen examines the field's evolution from its initial normalcy of active doing to a fascination with approaches that seemed more sophisticated and scientific. As Gillen notes, the decision to replace interventions that engaged the client in actual doing with applied techniques that relegated the person to a passive recipient was a dramatic departure from our core values and founding principles.

The frustrating outcome of this shift has been abandonment of occupation-based approaches and loss of confidence in our role as providers of *occupational* therapy. Gillen describes the resulting role blurring, dual encroachment, and professional envy that occurs when occupational therapy practice is more representative of other professions than our own. The exciting decades of research on motor control interventions that support the validity and efficacy of occupation-based approaches is countered in a most sobering manner by the reality that non–occupational therapy researchers are the prime authors of these works. Gillen's review of key studies that embrace our professed and philosophical occupational therapy methods and their parallels with our historical literature is enlightening, exciting, and disconcerting. If others are eager to adopt approaches that were fundamental to occupational therapy until the 1960s, and brand them as "contemporary" and "cutting edge," why do reductionist practices still prevail in our field? (see Active Reflection VII.3).

Similar concerns are raised by Gillen with respect to the approaches typically used by occupational therapy practitioners to assess cognition. The widespread use of non-occupation-based, contrived, two-dimensional tools in occupational therapy practice ignores the complexities of dual tasks in a three-dimensional world and the impact of novelty on testing. The critical need for occupational therapy practitioners to use performance-based measures with ecological validity is articulated well by Gillen. Fortunately, occupational therapy scholars have developed cognitive assessments that effectively meet these criteria; however, they are not the norm in our field, but they are standard practice in other disciplines. Despite these concerns, Gillen maintains hope that our profession can use the knowledge acquired from its forays away from our founding principles to inform our return to them. He poses several key points for occupational therapy practitioners to consider as we forge ahead to ensure that *occupation* is recognized and celebrated as the essence of occupational therapy (see Active Reflection VII.4).

> *During our transformation, our value system will change; however, we must not let external demands dictate those changes. Rather, we should change because we continue to seek the truth of our values. Professional values grow from the search for truth, and during our transformation we must act on the values of our history, and we must continue to seek the meaning and truth of our present.*
>
> —Gilfoyle (1984, p. 577)

Gillen's conclusion that occupational therapy needs to journey back to its roots in order to map its future brings this text full circle and back to the text's first part on historical and philosophical foundations. The tremendous current and future potential of occupational therapy, as envisioned by the authors of this text's chapters and other leading occupational therapy scholars, is

---

Active Reflection VII.4. Taking the Right Fork

Yerxa (1967) advised that "professional authenticity in occupational therapy means that the occupational therapist in every professional act defines the profession" (p. 8).
- What actions can you take to ensure that your responses to those considerations put forth by Gillen at the conclusion of his Eleanor Clarke Slagle Lecture accurately reflect authentic occupational therapy? Consider the factors for providing occupational therapy at its best listed in Exhibit VII.1.
- How will you ensure that your daily practice effectively encompasses the art and science of occupational therapy to be best practice?

---

exhilarating. Because many in our field have renewed their commitment to fundamental beliefs about the therapeutic power of occupation, we now have a fortified foundation for the fulfillment of these visions. It is hoped that the chapters selected for this text sustain the readers' commitment to our profession's founding principles as they face the inevitable challenges of practice today and throughout the 21st century. Occupational therapy practitioners who uphold our profession's heritage by holistically using occupation in a manner meaningful to a person and relevant to his or her contexts will contribute greatly to society, enabling all people to be self-directed, engage in occupational roles, and fully participate in life. This was the vision of the founders of occupational therapy in the early 20th century, and it is the ongoing promise of our profession as we proceed through our next century (see Exhibit VII.1).

> *The rapidly changing, complex world of today creates new and increasing demands upon and expectations for the professionals. The development and maintenance of a vitality essential to the existence of a profession and to the fulfillment*

Exhibit VII.1. Occupational Therapy at Its Best

Occupational therapy is at its best when it
- Is evidence-based and client-centered,
- Enables choice and control,
- Acknowledges the power of engagement in occupation,
- Recognizes the force of the environment as a means of intervention,
- Has a broad intervention focus,
- Measures out comes of participation, and
- Focuses on occupations important to each person within his or her environment.

Note. Adapted from "Participation in the Occupations of Everyday Life," by M. Law, 2002, *American Journal of Occupational Therapy, 56,* 640–649. Copyright © 2002, American Occupational Therapy Association. Adapted with permission.

of its obligations to society is inextricably bound to its philosophy of education and those processes directed toward attaining professional competency.
—Fidler (1966, p. 1)

References

American Occupational Therapy Association. (2007). AOTA's *Centennial Vision* and executive summary. *American Journal of Occupational Therapy, 61,* 613–614. http://dx.doi.org/10.5014/ajot.61.6.613

American Occupational Therapy Association. (2014). Occupational therapy practice framework: Domain and process (3rd ed.). *American Journal of Occupational Therapy, 68*(Suppl. 1), S1–S48. http://dx.doi.org/10.5014/ajot.2014.682006 Reprinted as Appendix A.

Bramwell, D. B. (1952). International Congress of Occupational Therapy. *Scottish Journal of Occupational Therapy, 14,* 6.

Burke, J., & Cassidy, J. (1991). Disparity between reimbursement-driven practice and humanistic values of occupational therapy. *American Journal of Occupational Therapy, 45,* 173–176. http://dx.doi.org/10.5014/ajot.45.2.173

Clark, F. (2007). *AOTA's* Centennial Vision: *What it is, why it is right.* Retrieved from www.aota.org/News/Centennial/Updates/41919.aspx?FT=.vnd.ms-powerpoint

Clark, F. (2011). High-definition occupational therapy's competitive edge: Personal excellence is the key [Presidential Address]. *American Journal of Occupational Therapy, 65,* 616–622. http://dx.doi.org/10.5014/ajot.2011.656001

Dott, N. (1967). Chairman's opening remarks. *Scandinavian Journal of Occupational Therapy, 69,* 4–6.

Fidler, G. (1966). Conceptual framework for professional education. *American Journal of Occupational Therapy, 20,* 1–8.

Fisher, G., & Friesema, J. (2013). Health Policy Perspectives—Implications of the Affordable Care Act for occupational therapy practitioners providing services to Medicare recipients. *American Journal of Occupational Therapy, 67,* 502–506. http://dx.doi.org/10.5014/ajot.2013.675002

Gilfoyle, E. (1984). Transformation of a profession [Eleanor Clarke Slagle Lecture]. *American Journal of Occupational Therapy, 38,* 575–584. http://dx.doi.org/10.5014/ajot.38.9.575

Grady, A. P. (1992). Nationally Speaking—Occupation as a vision. *American Journal of Occupational Therapy, 46,* 1062–1065. http:/dx.doi.org/10.5014/ajot.46.12.1062

Gutman, S. (1998). The domain of function: Who's got it? Who's competing for it? *American Journal of Occupational Therapy, 52,* 684–689.

Hilton, I. (1942). An open letter to members of the A.O.T. *Occupational Therapy, 3/4,* 196.

Hinojosa, J. (2007). Becoming innovators in an era of hyperchange [2007 Eleanor Clarke Slagle Lecture]. *American Journal of Occupational Therapy, 61,* 629–637. http://dx.doi.org/10.5014/ajot.61.6.629

Hinojosa, J. (2013). The Issue Is—The evidence-based paradox. *American Journal of Occupational Therapy, 67,* e18–e23. http://dx.doi.org/10.5014/ajot.2013.005587

Howard, B. (1991). How high do we jump? The effect of reimbursement on occupational therapy. *American Journal of Occupational Therapy, 45,* 875–881.

Kidner, T. B. (1922). Editorial. *Archives of Occupational Therapy, 1,* 499–502.

Law, M. (2002). Participation in the occupation of everyday life. *American Journal of Occupational Therapy, 56,* 640–649. http://dx.doi.org/10.5014/ajot.56.6.640

Metropolitan District of New York. (2009, January). MNYD Mental Health Task Force. *NYSOTA News,* p. 12.

Mirrey, L. M., & Johnson, B. (1969). The green paper. *Occupational Therapy, 32*(1), 17.

Mosey, A. C. (1996). *Psychosocial components of occupational therapy.* New York: Raven Press.

Patient Protection and Affordable Care Act, Pub. L. No. 111–148, § 3502, 124 Stat. 119, 124 (2010).

Peloquin, S. (1989). Sustaining the art of practice in occupational therapy. *American Journal of Occupational Therapy, 43,* 219–226.

Scaffa, M., & Reitz, M. (Eds.). (2014). *Occupational therapy in community-based practice settings* (2nd ed.). Philadelphia: F. A. Davis.

Schemm, R. L. (1994). Looking Back—Bridging conflicting ideologies—The origins of American and British Occupational Therapy. *American Journal of Occupational Therapy, 48,* 1082–1088. http://dx.doi.org/10.5014/ajot.48.11.1082

Shannon, P. (1977). The derailment of occupational therapy. *American Journal of Occupational Therapy, 31,* 229–234.

Shaw, C. (1928). Occupation as an aid to recovery. *Occupational Therapy and Rehabilitation, 8*(3), 199–206.

Slagle, E. C. (1930). Address to graduates. *Occupational Therapy and Rehabilitation, 9,* 271–276.

Swarbrick, P., & Pratt, C. (2006). Consumer-operated self-help services: Roles and opportunities for occupational therapists and occupational therapy assistants. *OT Practice, 11*(5), CE1–CE8.

Tracy, S. E. (1921). Getting started in occupational therapy. *Trained Nurse and Hospital Review, 67*(5), 397–399.

West, W. L. (1984). A reaffirmed philosophy and practice of occupational therapy for the 1980s. *American Journal of Occupational Therapy, 38,* 15–23. http://dx.doi.org/10.5014/ajot.38.1.15

Wood, W. (1995). Weaving the warp and weft of occupational therapy: An art and science for all times. *American Journal of Occupational Therapy, 49,* 44–52. http://dx.doi.org/10.5014/ajot.49.1.44

Wood, W. (1998). Nationally Speaking—Is it jump time for occupational therapy? *American Journal of Occupational Therapy, 52,* 403–411. http://dx.doi.org/10.5014/ajot.52.6.403

World Federation of Occupational Therapists. (2010). *Statement on occupational therapy.* Retrieved from http://www.wfot.org/aboutus/aboutoccupationaltherapy/definitionofoccupationaltherapy.aspx

Yerxa, E. (1967). Authentic occupational therapy [1966 Eleanor Clark Slagle Lecture]. *American Journal of Occupational Therapy, 21,* 1–9.

Yerxa, E. (1980). Occupational therapy's role in creating a future climate of caring. *American Journal of Occupational Therapy, 34,* 529–534.

CHAPTER 54

Old Values–New Directions: Competence, Adaptation, Integration

JERRY A. JOHNSON

One of the truly exciting and stimulating benefits that derives from being president of an organization like the American Occupational Therapy Association is the opportunity to be exposed to the problems and concerns of 20,000–25,000 people and to be involved in the resolution of some of those issues. It is an incredible experience, and one can never be quite so provincial or so quick to render judgment after having held such a position.

One of the privileges of no longer serving as president is the opportunity to reflect upon the experience and its meaning for my life. For me, that has meant devoting a considerable amount of time exploring the values of our profession, the directions in which the profession seems to be headed, my values, and the way that I want to spend the remainder of my life.

So, when invited to make this presentation, I accepted immediately. The topic seemed so natural in relation to my thoughts about our profession and about me, and it offered an opportunity to address issues of personal concern and professional interest. When it was time to write, however, the process was slow and arduous. Concepts that seemed clear were, upon examination, ambiguous. Connections between and among competence, adaptation, and integration were more tenuous than I had assumed. Concepts were supported by beliefs and anecdotal experience, rather than by hard scientific evidence.

In the final analysis, it was my own internal conflict that made writing difficult. The title of this presentation, "Old Values–New Directions," epitomized a conflict between the old, enduring values of humanism, caring, belief in the individual, and concern for the cli-

ent, and the new values and new directions pointing toward science, rigor, objectification, logic, analysis, dehumanization, and depersonalization. This conflict seems to represent a decision: a choice between being humanistic and caring, or being scientific and objective.

Thus my challenge today is to discuss this conflict, not because I have answers, but in the hope that clarification of the issues surrounding the conflict may help us find a satisfactory means of resolving it. I believe that the conflict is serious, that it has the potential to divide our profession, with one group opting for the old values and the comfortable, traditional approaches to practice, and the other seeking to move in the direction of scientific advancement. Intuitively, I feel that the creativity and sensitivity that are generally characteristic of occupational therapists offer hope for resolution of the conflict. However, we must be consciously aware of our fears as well as of our aspirations if we are to succeed in our endeavors.

To address this complex matter of conflict, I will first give you my interpretations of the concepts to be addressed. Then I will discuss values and their meaning for us as professionals. Next, I will review the "discovery" and evolution of occupational therapy as it occurred factually and conceptually. Finally, I will describe the nature of the conflicts, as I understand them, and offer some general thoughts about their resolution.

Definition of Terms

I will explain my interpretations of each of the words contained in the title of my presentation so that there will be a common understanding of the context within which I use each concept.

For the terms *old* and *values*, I have opted for the interpretation that suggests our values have been in existence for a long time and are familiar or known from the past. As such they have intrinsic worth, exist as social principles, and are held in high esteem.

New directions, when contrasted with *old values*, suggests that we are dealing with a phenomenon that has not existed before or has only recently been observed, experienced, and made manifest. *Direction* is defined as the way a person or thing faces or points, or a line or point toward which a moving person or thing goes. Thus the term *new directions* suggests that we are facing a particular way, a way that is new and unfamiliar and that may change our course by replacing the more comfortable and enduring values that we esteem.

Definitions of *competence, adaptation,* and *integration* offer interesting possibilities for interpretation within the context of a potential shift in our direction. *Competence* is defined as being fit or able, or as having capacities equal to expectations or requirements. When expectations or requirements shift, *adaptation,* or change, is necessary if we are to conform to new or revised circumstances, and if we are to achieve a better adjustment to a different environment. *Integration* suggests that the parts can be brought together and made whole, or renewed.

In summary, we confront the possibility of a change in our directions, a change that is currently perceived in our literature as moving toward science and reductionism and away from humanism and holism. However, competence, adaptation, and integration suggest that there may be hope for satisfactory resolution of the conflict between old values and new directions. This is the context from which I will speak today.

The Meaning of Values

The literature about professions and professionalization suggests that professionals conceptualize certain problems, or perplexing questions, that are of primary concern to members of their profession. Resolution of these problems becomes the focus of the profession's attention and energy and determines actions to be taken by its members in every sphere of practice, education, research, political activity, decision-making, and other endeavors. These problems, or questions, significantly affect the standards for content of educational programs, as well as the organization, location, and structure of the profession's services. They are influential in attracting and recruiting prospective students and may influence the degree to which there is high attrition or "burn-out" at certain levels of professional achievement or practices. These problems, or perplexing ques-

tions, frequently reflect the values of the profession's members and may heavily influence the directions of the profession.

The directions that our profession has taken seem to be predicated on values, rather than on the basis of problems or perplexing questions. Our literature consistently reflects some of our values:

1. The value of the individual as a total person (1);
2. The value of purposeful activity (2), the value of occupation (3) in producing change and recovery;
3. The value of goal-oriented activity designed for a given individual's skills and abilities (3);
4. The value of permitting patients to choose meaningful activities (1)—activities that might, as Susan Tracy suggested, run parallel to the activity or occupation in which they would have been normally engaged (4);
5. The value of seeing the individual interacting within the framework of the environment (5); and
6. The value we place upon ourselves, our feelings, and our interactions with the patient/client as vital, integral, and caring components of the therapeutic process.

Rarely do occupational therapists do things *to* clients; rather, we engage in a collaborative process *with* them. Each party assumes responsibility and understands that the ultimate goal is for clients to achieve the fullest degree of responsibility for their lives of which they are capable.

These values appear throughout our literature. Although the language has changed, their meaning to us as occupational therapists has not. These are our espoused values (6), and the assumptions upon which they rest are that life is more than mere existence and that health is more than the absence of disease. For us, as therapists, health is a dynamic state of being that is reflected in the behaviors of people who have optimized their resources and who are living their lives fully, creatively, and expressively.

In my experience it seems that people are attracted to a profession because that profession, in its practice, demonstrates actions and behaviors that reflect its values, values that probably are common to and shared by both individuals in the profession and the profession itself.

As I considered this, I reflected on the experiences that brought me into occupational therapy as well as the experiences that reinforced my values and belief in the inherent and potential powers of our profession.

I was the older of two children; my father was a lawyer; my mother, a school teacher. About the time I was 4 or 5, my father became an active alcoholic. His addiction rapidly worsened, and within a very short time span, our lives seemed to shift dramatically while many of our resources went into alcohol. It finally became necessary for my mother to seek employment. Divorce was out of the question both because of the prejudices of the time and because alimony was not permitted under state laws.

As his drinking patterns increased in severity, so did violence. Many nights I ran to town—barefooted, in my pajamas—to get the police to come stop the threats or the fighting—hoping that no one would be killed or seriously injured before I could return home with help. The police would attempt to reason with my father and to calm him; if that failed, he was sometimes whipped soundly. If that approach, too, failed, he would be taken to jail to sober up. It then became my responsibility to go to his cell to bargain with him: If we would let him come home, would he stay sober?

During one of these visits I saw a woman in a cell who was very psychotic. She had been jailed because there was no place to restrain her, no drugs to sedate her, and she had to be declared insane by the court before she could be transferred to a distant state hospital for treatment.

Later, during my college years, I spent two summers with the American Friends Service Committee in institutional service units. The purpose of these units was twofold:

1. To promote understanding among people by having representatives of varied races and religions work for a common goal, which was
2. To improve treatment of the mentally ill in state hospitals.

I spent one summer in a Texas hospital and another summer in a hospital in Ohio. In both hospitals I was assigned to wards with the most disturbed, paranoid, suicidal, or homicidal patients. Most of them had been hospitalized for a long time; few had any contacts with family or friends.

Treatment consisted of insulin or electric shock, isolation in empty cells, restraints—which usually meant being chained to a bench—or occasional beatings. There were no occupational therapists to come to the wards, and generally, the patients could not leave the wards.

We used games, discussion, and behavior modeling to bring about change, and I realized our effectiveness only after returning to visit later. During that visit one of the patients described to me, in exquisite detail, what it meant to her when I took a crayon and paper in for her to use while I talked with her when she was disturbed and shackled to a bench.

As I thought about these and other experiences, I realized how strongly developed my sense of value was about humane treatment and concern for the individual patient. So, as I reviewed the literature in preparing this presentation, it was not surprising to find these and similar values occurring repeatedly. This led me to believe that others had had similar experiences. In retrospect, many of the values we have that relate to caring may well come from experiences in state hospitals and other long-term care facilities where there was only the staff to care about patients and in which sometimes caring was the only treatment medium available.

I suspect that many of you selected occupational therapy as your career choice because you, too, found that your values could be reinforced and channeled in satisfying ways through the therapist/client relationship. We care—and we believe in what we do. This I know from personal experience as well as from visits with so many of you during my terms as president.

To summarize this discussion of values and their meaning for us, I believe that competent, thoughtful, caring people are drawn to a profession like occupational therapy for several reasons:

1. Commitment to the conceptual, perplexing questions that the profession addresses (which in my earlier experience related primarily to humane care of the ill and disabled);
2. Shared concern for the values espoused by and seen in a profession's practice, particularly as that practice reflects attempts to resolve specific questions; and
3. Opportunity to commit one's creativity, energies, and life to resolution of problems that matter—that make a difference in the quality of life and the quality of the environment.

The commitment to our values is deep and strong, but there may be pitfalls for us as professionals if values are not expressed within a context of scientific thought. So let us move to a discussion of the "discovery" and evolution of occupational therapy and see how our values fit into a larger scheme.

The "Discovery" and Evolution of Occupational Therapy

The concepts and observations upon which our profession was founded were formulated when medicine and related sciences lacked knowledge and tools to understand or eliminate the causes of many illnesses, diseases, and social problems. Many illnesses, such as tuberculosis or mental illness, required prolonged hospitalization or institutionalization. Problems such as abject poverty resulted in placements in poor farms. These conditions resulted in decreased or impaired activity and often necessitated removal of the "sick" or impoverished individual from home and family.

Physicians, having limited knowledge and without the technology available today, had to develop and systematically use their powers of observation and judgment. In the absence of diagnostic tests, they relied upon intuition to connect scientific or systematic observations and empirical evidence with limited knowledge to make a diagnosis. (The term *empirical evidence* as used herein refers to reliance on practical experience without reference to scientific principles; empiricism is the dependence of a person on his or her own experience and observation, disregarding theory, reasoning, and science. At times it may be necessary to rely upon one's experience and observations because there are no scientific principles to explain the phenomenon.) It was necessary to diagnose and treat within a broad context and to look for external (to the body) or environmental causes and cures. It was acknowledged that microbes or germs produced illness or disease, but many physicians believed that external stress, produced perhaps by work or other environmental conditions, created the conditions in which germs or microbes were triggered into action.

Consequently, focus on a broad spectrum of interrelationships led to the following conclusions:

1. A relation existed between the environment and a person's state of health;
2. Recovery from illness or depression was influenced by activity; and
3. More specifically, when certain conditions were present, improvement occurred following engagement in activity or occupation.

It was thus hypothesized that activity, or occupation, and improvement in one's medical condition were related. Most members of society, lacking disciplined skill in observation and trust in their intuitive powers, would likely describe the same phenomenon as "busy work."

Our founders were physicians, architects, social workers, secretaries, teachers of arts and crafts, nurses, and of course, the first occupational therapists. Each brought a different perspective and came from a unique background and orientation, yet each observed the effects of occupation in their individual environments and believed in its curative powers. In some ways, this gathering of "specialists" represented the context in which systems theory has been most effective—that is, in situations when a group of specialists representing different perspectives and backgrounds meet to consider the resolution of complex problems.

The individuals who gave life to our profession were visionaries, persons with strong convictions and the courage to uphold and support their convictions. The men who participated in our "discovery" were humanists as well as scientists, exerting leadership to change the course of illness and medical care. Female founders were also unique: educated and dedicated professionals, exerting leadership to change social conditions and to promote healing—people who opted for a life that did not conform to the expectations of women as held by society at that time. These pioneers had competence, discipline, and the determination to succeed.

They seemed to share similar characteristics: the ability to define problems broadly and to organize an effective response to such problems; the ability to act and to reflect upon what they learned from their actions, thereby modifying their behaviors as necessary; the ability to transmit their goals and the rationale underlying these goals to others. They also had power—power granted not by the sanction of society but power that comes from within: intuitive power; power created by belief and conviction, as they are honed by knowledge and observation; the power of disciplined minds and compassionate spirits. These qualities are demonstrated in their writing, their decisions, their interactions with others, and, most importantly, in their legacy to us. Their lives were devoted to bringing about change in the human condition. Their experience convinced them that occupation was the vehicle by which such change could be made possible.

Rene Dubos, whose life has been devoted to study of the interrelationships between living organisms and their environment, suggests that great discoveries are often intuitive and occur when surprising outcomes result from an observed phenomenon (7).

Robert Merton, the noted sociologist of science from Columbia University, "has shown in his writings that almost all major ideas arise more than once, independently, and often virtually at the same time." (8) Our professional literature reflects the concepts expressed by Dubos and Merton.

In this sense, our founders made not only a surprising discovery when they observed that occupation influenced recovery from illness, but they also translated that discovery into action by forming the National Society for the Promotion of Occupational Therapy.

At this point an interesting turn occurred. Once occupational therapy was identified, the demand for services quickly followed. The literature that I reviewed became silent about the scientific aspects of this great "discovery."

World War I was followed by legislation mandating occupational therapy services in rehabilitation. The depression brought with it demands for retraining the unemployed. World War II, followed by the Korean War, the Vietnam War, and the "wars" on poverty, stroke, heart disease, cancer, and other disabling conditions, created a great demand for occupational therapists (9). We responded.

Our tools, techniques, and values were quickly adapted to new categories of clients. We moved into many new environments to provide services: hospitals, rehabilitation centers, community mental health centers, private practice, community treatment centers, physicians' offices, nursing homes, home health, well-baby clinics, and school systems. We managed by training aides and volunteers or by becoming consultants and by supervising others.

Not only did we move into new environments, but we also adapted our repertoire of tools. We used arts and crafts, splinting and orthotics, therapeutic use of self, prevocational exploration, neurodevelopmental and kinesiological theories and techniques, activities of daily living, and more recently, exercise routines previously used in physical therapy.

Sensory-integrative therapy emerged, but it came primarily from a research base. Its adherents used a test (the Southern California Sensory Integrative Test) designed to diagnose and treat certain deficits. Treatment programs oriented to specific problems were planned and an attempt was made to formulate and organize both diagnosis and treatment into a theoretical framework.

Change, "meeting needs," and adaptation have been a way of life for us. We have been responsive to society's demands and to the needs of our clients. Indeed, those needs and demands have had priority over the needs of the profession and of its members.

We met the ever-changing challenges for delivery of services and created many jobs. This ensured the survival of our profession, the importance of which cannot be minimized. We adapted well and our efforts have without question produced a significant result: a greater demand for occupational therapists than we have ever been able to supply.

This growth was not accomplished without a price, however, and today we are beginning to pay that price.

The conditions under which our profession rapidly developed were such that demand for services quickly increased and has continued unabated. There was little time for our founders' visions to be nurtured, expanded, or understood intellectually or conceptually—rather, there was demand that the ideas, the convictions, the values be put into action immediately.

Part of the price we now pay is that our directions frequently seem to be predicated not upon the observations and concepts of our founders but upon external sources and influences: the influence of medicine, the perceived power of the federal government, sources of reimbursement for treatment, and limited vision and lack of confidence in our potential, as reflected in a narrow concept of practice and cluttered professional education programs specifying breadth rather than depth. Argyris and Schon, in *Theory and Practice: Increasing Professional Effectiveness,* state that factors such as these reflect the demands or expectations of special interest groups but that they are external to the nature of professional practice and education (6).

With each new direction we have taken, the shortage of qualified personnel has increased. To respond to the problem of personnel shortages, we have experimented and continue to experiment with a variety of ways to recruit, certify, and retread personnel for entry into our profession. Some plans have been creative and innovative; others were taken in anticipation of government action (if we fail to act, the government will). Attempts to "fill the gap" have been an obsession with us.

Abraham Maslow is reported to have once said that "If the only tool you have is a hammer you tend to see every problem as a nail" (10). We seem to have taken this approach, believing that if we can just recruit enough students, provide amnesty for enough persons who have "dropped out," or promote enough COTAs to OTRs, our problems will be solved.

Dubos proposes an interesting perspective that seems applicable to our situation. As a proponent of adaptation, he warns that, if adaptation is carried too far, without awareness of the consequences, the desired change may be harmful rather than helpful. He illustrates this point by describing how the body adapts to air pollution on a short-term basis, but develops chronic bronchitis or emphysema if the stress of short-term adaptive processes must continue indefinitely. In crowded social environments, individuals put on blinders and no longer perceive the crowd; in so doing, however, they sacrifice a certain quality of interpersonal life (7).

Dubos provided this additional description. He related that Pasteur once taught the physiology of architecture at the Ecole des Beaux Arts in Paris. To demonstrate the importance of good ventilation, he conducted the following experiment. He placed a bird in a bell jar in which the oxygen was not renewed so that it gradually diminished. The bird adapted by decreasing its activity and remaining almost immobile. Pasteur then removed the bird and replaced it with a new one, abruptly introducing it to an atmosphere low in oxygen. The new bird began to move about and promptly died. Not only did this demonstration illustrate the importance of good ventilation, but it also demonstrated that we unconsciously adapt to unfavorable circumstances, but only if they occur slowly (7).

The principles of human adaptation presented by Dubos can be applied to professions as well as to people. We have adapted over time to medical and social need and demand but without recognizing the consequences of our adaptive behavior. Some of these consequences as they now confront us are listed below.

First, we have not considered the impact of introducing new therapists, who are still maturing and are educated only at the baccalaureate level, into the stress-producing environments that exist today. We have had time to acclimate ourselves and have acquired some of the requisite knowledge, skills, and tools through experience, but new therapists are often introduced to the environment abruptly.

Second, our sole focus on meeting needs of the disabled and of society has led to the neglect of the importance of fostering, nurturing, and supporting people who move into more demanding, challenging, and often lonely positions as administrators, clinical specialists, researchers, and curriculum directors. One has only to see the number of vacancies for curriculum directors or researchers to understand the nature of the problem. When therapists move into these positions, almost every segment of our profession wants and needs something from them: participation in a task

force, continuing education opportunities, membership on or chairing a committee. Yet, as a profession, we offer little support to people in these positions.

Clinical or entry-level therapists sell a commodity that is primarily patient oriented: skill in diagnosing certain kinds of problems relating to performance; a treatment procedure, methodology, or technique; a splint or an adaptive device. The commodity that a researcher, a faculty member, or an administrator sells is an idea, a concept. Regardless of the commodity that we offer, however, we need documentation of its worth, its value, its potential dangers, and the conditions under which it is most effective. We have been so busy selling the commodity that we have neglected the work that must be done to substantiate the value of that commodity. The more we move up and extend our contacts, the more documentation for support is required.

My personal experience and explorations lead me to suggest that people in general, people as professionals, and professions composed of people, all need to be nurtured. Many forms of sustenance are required to strengthen and prepare or to renew and revitalize us, especially in times of rapidly changing conditions and high stress, both of which are found in abundance today.

Finally, the third consequence of our overadaptation to society's needs and demands is reflected in the fact that we have defined our problem as one of insufficient human resources at the entry level—or lack of nails—rather than defining conceptual problems and perplexing questions. A theoretical framework cannot emerge from the problem of insufficient personnel. Nor does the availability of jobs attract thoughtful persons who want to commit themselves, their energies, and their resources to a career.

The absence of well-defined theories limits our scope, our focus, and our research. It puts us in the position of relying on such things as role-delineation studies—studies of past performance and activity to support our endeavors. These studies do not provide a base of knowledge to support us. The absence of a solid theoretical foundation also causes us to overemphasize old values and their "rightness." It leads, I believe, to our condemnation of medicine for its lack of humanitarianism, its dehumanizing approach, its reductionism—because this further justifies our position.

So, as our evolution has brought us face-to-face with society's expectations for research and of the need for scientific support (or at least examination) of our therapeutic rationale and procedures, *we* fall back on old values and seek to defend our positions.

We face a painful conflict, and we are ill prepared for the new directions with their implications for change in our lives. The tragedy is that we are also ill prepared to defend our services and our education.

How, then, has our conceptual development progressed, and what hope is there for us?

A review of our literature suggests that conceptual development was initiated by our founders. It then was generally dormant until Dr. Reilly, in 1961 (see Chapter 7), translated the vision and "discovery" of our founders into a hypothesis:

That man, through the use of his hands as they are energized by mind and will, can influence the state of his own health.

She attributed this hypothesis to our founders and said of it:

"The splendor of its vision goes far beyond rating it as an idea conceived once in a lifetime or even once in a century. Rather, it falls in the class of one of those great beliefs which has advanced civilization. Its magnificence lies in the optimistic vote of confidence it gives to human nature. It implies that there is a reservoir of sensitivity and skill in the hands of man which can be tapped for his health. It implies the rich adaptability and durability of the central nervous system which can be influenced by experiences. And more than all this, it implies that man, through the use of his hands, can creatively deploy his thinking, feelings and purposes to make himself at home in the world and to make the world his home." (p. 2)

Dr. Reilly continues: "For a profession organized around this hypothesis it sets few limits to its growth. It merely endows a group with the obligation to acquire reliable knowledge leading to a competency to serve the belief. Because this is a hypothesis about health, it requires that this knowledge be made available for the guidance of physicians and that it be made applicable to a wide range of medical problems."

Reilly concluded her lecture with a suggestion that the hypothesis would begin its proof when we identified the drive in Man for occupation and would continue as we shaped our services to fill that need. We

"belong," she said, "to a profession that requires the mind to look at the history of man's achievements throughout civilization. It requires the spirit to respond to the wonders of what man has accomplished with his hands." (11)

Consider for a moment the beauty and power of Reilly's statement—and the potential that it offers to each of us as we join with our clients to assist them in fulfilling this potential in their lives. This is our heritage, our legacy, our challenge. It gives us a direction that can be sought regardless of the environment in which we work. It offers tremendous potential for channeling our values into productive outcomes. It requires no distinction of age or category of disease. It is universal.

This hypothesis, too, lay dormant for a period of time, although work in related areas was progressing.

Most recently, in the fall of 1980, Kielhofner et al. published a series of four articles in which a model of human occupation emanating from Reilly's hypothesis was proposed (12). It is suggested in this model that occupation, or function, is central to human life and that the occupational therapist is uniquely qualified to address deficits or problems causing dysfunction. The purpose of occupational therapy is to facilitate the transition of persons with illnesses or disabilities from a state of dependency and dysfunction to or toward a state of full participation and meaningful function in the environments in which they live. Consequently, we address the problems or deficits unique to each individual as well as the social system in which he or she functions and lives.

We have targeted for ourselves a level of performance that is high indeed: an approach to holistic treatment that requires consideration of many complex factors, frequently crossing interdisciplinary lines to understand and grasp the principles of:

1. Normal development in all spheres throughout the life span;
2. Pathology and its relation to function and dysfunction;
3. Adaptation and change;
4. Learning and acquisition of competence;
5. Integrative processes; and
6. Human interaction within the context of the environment.

We now add to this list of requirements an understanding of the principles of occupational behavior and general systems theory. And, as if this is not enough, we must also understand research—because it is by and through research that we determine whether or not our theoretical constructs have substance and produce the results that we claim. The knowledge acquired from research and its findings may enable us to explain, with some degree of assurance, how, under what conditions, and when therapeutic intervention is effective. It makes possible prediction, with some degree of certainty, to say when and with whom our methods of intervention will be beneficial. It may even lead to some degree of control over factors that produce or aggravate disability and dysfunction.

Research can be viewed as a form or system of communication, for it is the language of scientists and of critical thinkers. When persons from other disciplines examine and understand the methods by which we have critically evaluated and analyzed what we do, they can have confidence in what we say we produce or accomplish.

I believe that the works of Reilly and Kielhofner et al. (as well as that of Ayres, although in a slightly different context) are significant contributions to the conceptual development needed by our profession. This work is very rudimentary, but it begins to formulate the conceptual questions to be addressed, uniquely, by our profession. It also offers potential for drawing the separate and disparate parts of our profession together under one conceptual umbrella and for connecting these parts not only to each other but to the whole.

We have identified for ourselves a goal that is extremely complex and of enormous magnitude for we must have knowledge to understand the cause of dysfunction, to diagnose dysfunction as it affects performance and occupation, to identify and establish the appropriate program and process for specific individuals that will result in adaptation and ultimately integration, to bring about change in society and in technology so that both share responsibility for adapting to the needs of humans—and all living things on this earth.

Without question, this goal, this sense of direction, offers a service needed by society now and one that will be needed in ever increasing ways as technology expands. As Dubos said, the most tragic problem confronting industrialized nations is that society is increasingly unable to provide people with a function that has a profound meaning for their lives.

How, then, can we pursue this goal—and make it a reality rather than a vision or a set of values for people who want to do good things?

Thoughts for the Future

I have no certain answers for us, but I can share with you some of my thoughts, my tentative suggestions. I, like you, have intuitive feelings, beliefs, and some empirical evidence from my observations and practice that suggest we have the potential to offer "A sufficiently vital and unique service for medicine to support and society to reward." (11) Ideally, this will be a stimulus for our most creative thinking so that, together, we can find appropriate answers for us and for our profession.

First, it is important to recognize the conflict that confronts us: our desire to retain values that have been an integral part of our profession and, on the other hand, our recognition of the importance of science and research—accompanied by our fears about the directions in which science and research may take us. The potential changes have frightening implications for us—professionally and personally. None of us can help but wonder, "What will happen to me in this process of change?" Will there be a place for me to continue working, and how will I fit? What will happen to my program, my patients, my students, my job?" These questions must be addressed.

Second, I believe that we must redefine the problems that our profession is to address. We must have a sense of direction, a series of perplexing questions to which we, as a profession, commit ourselves. The problem is not one of a shortage of people; it is a shortage of ideas, of concepts, of critically defined questions and problems that attract people, that captivate their imaginations and tap their creativity, that use their intellectual capacity, that say to them, "Here is a problem, a perplexing question of great social value and individual meaning. Join us. Become an occupational therapist and help us find answers." Saving lives is important—but what is the redeeming value of saving lives if they cannot be lived with dignity and meaning?

This has been brought home to me through two recent experiences. In the first instance, I was driving home one day and, as I turned a corner near my house, I saw an older woman sitting on the ground, near the corner. She waved, and I waved back. A moment later it occurred to me to stop and walk back to see about her. She greeted me with obvious relief and said, "I thought no one would ever stop." She had stumbled and fallen and could not get up by herself. After asking about injuries, I helped her get to her feet, and we talked a bit. As I started to leave, she asked if I knew how old she was. "Oh, perhaps 60," I replied. "No," she laughed,

"I'm 96." Then she stood tall and straight, looked down at me, and said, "I take a walk every day—but today I stumbled on something I didn't see and fell." Being a bit shaken at her age, my fear of potential injury to her, and not knowing quite what to do, I asked if she would like me to walk home with her.

"Oh, no," she replied, with tears welling in her eyes and a look of terror crossing her face, "I live with my daughter, and if I can't walk by myself, she'll put me in a nursing home—I don't want to be put away." How tragic that people must devote their energies and spend their last years struggling to avoid being put away.

In the second experience, I have, with my family, watched helplessly as a rapidly progressive nervous system degeneration has deprived my mother of her ability to use her body, to communicate, to function.

Medical science and humanistic, caring physicians have literally saved her life but neither the art nor the science of medicine has freed her of the indignity of her illness: incontinence; total loss of speech and ability to form words with her lips; contractures, rigidity, and spasticity in her hands, arms, trunk, and body that prohibit other forms of communication except through limited signs and signals; difficulties with eating, chewing, swallowing, and even keeping the food in her mouth. She is totally dependent on the sensitivity, awareness, and understanding of others to comprehend and respond to every need that she has; her sharp, alert, functioning mind is locked inside a useless body. She knows all that goes on; she hears, sees, cries, laughs, thinks, and feels—but our ability to comprehend is so limited.

I have watched as caring family and friends come to visit. Interaction is so limited and so uncomfortable that sometimes we come in twos or threes and end up talking to each other as though mother is not there. Or we are afraid, perhaps of tiring her or perhaps of our own discomfort and helplessness—and so we move into another room to sit and talk.

I, too, share this sense of helplessness and know how difficult it is to "treat" the members of one's family. I recognize the limitations of my own knowledge of the art and science of our practice. Still, this experience has given me a new appreciation for the potential of our profession as well as a greater realization of the complexity of the issues that we seek to address.

In addition to identifying the problems, the perplexing questions, to which we address ourselves, we must develop plans and strategies, or "road maps," to guide us as we commit ourselves and our resources to the process of seeking answers. It is necessary to recognize that each set of questions may produce some answers, but answers will also create new questions. Our search may be unending.

Third, we should set aside our condemnations of medicine and science, our contempt for basic research and reductionism. Instead, we should focus our energies and resources on those things *we* need to do. As I have learned to recognize and read the messages my own body sends to my unaware mind, I increasingly recognize that my anger is not usually about something "out there," but is a result of my frustration, pain, or anxiety about my own feelings of inadequacy, or impotence, my inability to accomplish or fulfill personal needs or certain expectations. We can learn, wisely, from the experiences of others, and avoid their pitfalls, but let us use our energies creatively and constructively to fulfill our purposes.

Fourth, I believe that we need to recognize and acknowledge the power of knowledge. We work in environments where one is measured against standards of knowledge and where power, emanating from knowledge, resides with those who have knowledge. Our own professional goals, as they are implicitly reflected in our values, require a high level of achievement, knowledge, and experience. We need to recognize the value that knowledge, of itself, has, how it can support *all* of us, and how it can nurture and open doors for us.

It is easy to be frightened by knowledge—by those who are perceived as being knowledgeable. My graduate students are frightened of my knowledge and of the control over their lives that it may give me. I, in turn, am frightened at their knowledge of clinical practice— and fearful of exposing my ignorance. It is only when we both acknowledge our fears and know that we can each make a unique contribution to strengthen the totality of our mutual experience that we move forward together.

Fifth, we need to acknowledge the validity of our professional value system. These values are expressed in the total context of our lives: How we care for ourselves and each other, how we treat our environment, and how we behave toward our colleagues, our friends, our families, and all the other creatures and living things that inhabit this earth we call home. We value freedom to make choices; independence to exercise those decisions; physical ability to come and go as we please; health; the warmth and meaning of home, friends, and privacy; the opportunity to engage intellect and creativity in meaningful activity; and the inherent spirituality and dignity that enables us to appreciate love and beauty—in all its forms.

Each of us, as professionals and as individual members of society, must retain and support our values. We value people, and their right to dignity. We value their desire to integrate themselves into life to the extent possible for them—and we seek to help them enter the mainstream of life: to shop in markets, to attend movies, to listen to the music of great symphonies, to see and feel the beauty of ballet, to work, to play, to watch, to feel. Government should not have to be responsible for bringing about such attitudes; we should accept that responsibility because it is just and right for us to do so, because we believe that every human being has the right and the responsibility to participate in life to the extent he or she is capable and desires to do so.

Still, we must also recognize some of the limitations inherent in acting on values alone or without the requisite knowledge base. A healthy respect for knowledge enables us to translate values into action effectively, thereby increasing our chances of producing lasting results.

Finally, we need to put our fears of specialization to rest. Dubos says that most of the great discoveries have been intuitive and have come from phenomenologists: people who see a problem as a whole without looking at its inner mechanisms or detailed parts (7). The discovery itself usually comes in the form of a surprise, an unexpected outcome of an event, observation, or experiment. As I said earlier, occupational therapy was just such a discovery—the observation that patients and clients who engaged in activity or occupation seemed to recover.

However, Dubos states that the great discovery alone may not be sufficient. There must also be people who are logicians and analysts, people who are committed to understanding and explaining how, when, and under what conditions the unexpected outcome, the surprise occurs. This process has two parts at work in occupational therapy. One is that of looking at the whole organism in relation to its environment. This is a complicated relationship, according to Dubos, that requires a complex response by the organism. The complexity of this problem (which Dubos calls adaptation, and we call occupational therapy) "may well require development of a new scientific approach because existing scientific methodologies may not be applicable to its resolution. . . . This new science would have to learn to predict the total organism's response to very complex situations." (7)

The second part of this process is an examination of the individual and of his or her deficits and assets, followed by a plan that promotes improved function through reduction of deficits and strengthening of assets. In this and other instances, Dubos stresses the importance of the reductionist approach to provide explanations. Further, both Dubos and general systems theorists emphasize the relevance, and indeed critical importance, of bringing specialists from many areas together to solve problems. The science of adaptation, says Dubos, "must be viewed from the perspectives of medicine, technology, architecture, and social life because not only must humans adapt to new conditions, but technology and environments must also be adapted to human needs."(7)

The discovery of our founders and the work of Reilly, Kielhofner et al.; and of Ayres and others provide the sketchy outlines of a model that may ultimately provide a unifying theoretical or conceptual force in our profession, integrating under one umbrella our concepts and treatment approaches in areas as diverse as pediatrics and gerontology as disparate as physical dysfunction, sensory integration, and psychiatry; and even providing a coherent, logical place for hand specialists, feeding specialists, and activity specialists. We need generalists *and* specialists, for each has a contribution to make. The potential contribution of each increases the value of the whole if appropriate connections and linkages can be established through research and theory development.

Our traditional values, when supplemented and supported by knowledge, offer us the potential to become a powerful presence in our society—powerful in that we provide a resource that enables individuals to live their lives as they want, to become what they want to be.

I believe that we do not have to sacrifice our old values for new ones but that we can merge the old and the new, thereby strengthening each. Our old values, when combined with the new, emphasizing science and knowledge, can forge powerful new directions for our profession. In so doing, we will acquire new competence. The process of adaptation will bring about change, but integration can provide us with a unity and wholeness that we have not yet achieved.

Perhaps, as we think of old values and new directions, of the concepts and meaning of competence, adaptation, and integration, we should heed the advice of Pericles when he spoke to the Athenians:

Fix your eyes on the greatness of your profession as you have it before you day by day; fall in love with her, and when you feel her greatness, remember that her greatness was won by people with courage, with knowledge of their duty, and with a vision that all things are possible. (13)

Acknowledgments

The author gratefully acknowledges the guidance and direction given by Fanny B. Vanderkooi and Florence M. Stattel as she entered the occupational therapy profession, as well as the contributions of Ann P. Grady, Gail Fidler, Donna King, Elizabeth J. Yerxa, the faculty and students at Washington University, and other friends and colleagues for their intellectual stimulation and challenge, friendship, and support of her personal, conceptual, and professional development.

References

1. Yerxa EJ: Authentic occupational therapy. *Am J Occup Ther 21:* 6, 1967.
2. Ayres AJ: Occupational therapy for motor disorders resulting from impairment of the central nervous system. *Rehab Lit* October 1960.
3. Wiest A: *Activity Book for the Ill, Convalescent, and Disabled of All Kinds as Well as the Hand of the Physician,* Stuttgart: Ferdnand Emke, Anje Ruil, Am J Occup Ther 21: 280–324, 1967.
4. Tracy S: *Studies in Invalid Occupations,* Boston: Whitcomb and Burrows, 1910.
5. Yerxa EJ: *The Present and Future Audacity of Occupational Therapy,* unpublished paper presented at Washington University, St. Louis, MO, October 1980.
6. Argyris C, Schon D: *Theory in Practice: Increasing Professional Effectiveness,* San Francisco: Jossey Books, Pub., 1980.
7. Dubos R, Escandi JP: *Quest: Reflections on Medicine, Science, and Humanity,* New York: Harcourt, Brace, Jovanovich, 1979.
8. Merton RK: On the shoulders of giants, quoted in Gould SJ: *The Panda's Thumb,* New York: W.N. Norton & Co., 1980.
9. Johnson JA: Commitment to action. *Am J Occup Ther 30:* 135–148, 1976.
10. Maslow A: *Quest,* May–June, 1977.
11. Reilly M: Occupational therapy can be one of the great ideas of 20th century medicine. *Am J Occup Ther 16:* 1–9, 1962. Reprinted as Chapter 7.
12. Kielhofner G, et al.: A Model of Human Occupation, Parts 1–4, *Am J Occup Ther 34:* 572–581; 34: 657–670; 34: 731–737; 34: 777–788, 1980.
13 Quotation from Hislop H: The not-so-impossible dream, *Phys Ther 55:* 1069–1080, 1975.

CHAPTER 55

Creating Excellence in Patient Care

KATHLEEN BARKER SCHWARTZ

Occupational therapists today are working in health-care organizations that operate from an efficiency perspective. That is, administration's goals are concerned with increasing efficiency in order to succeed financially. Experts argue that this approach can put quality at risk (Snoke, 1987; Starr, 1988). This paper proposes an alternative approach—the excellence perspective—as a way to address quality and at the same time sustain productivity.

The chapter traces the evolution of the efficiency perspective and provides a critique of this approach as applied to health-care organizations. It examines the historical origins of the excellence perspective and describes its use in business and its potential for health care. To illustrate how the excellence perspective can be successfully applied to health, a case study of an inpatient unit in a large teaching hospital in northern California is presented.

The Efficiency Perspective and Health-Care Management

The efficiency perspective originated in industry with principles introduced by Frederick Winslow Taylor in the early 1900s (Copley, 1923). Taylor declared that "scientific management" would enhance productivity by increasing worker performance and increase profitability by reducing labor costs (Taylor, 1919). A critical feature of scientific management was the creation of a class of managers who were guided primarily by concerns for efficiency and profit (Hoxie, 1916). In response to Taylor's ideas, labor unions argued that if scientific management took hold, the craftsman would

This chapter was previously published in the *American Journal of Occupational Therapy, 44,* 816–821. Copyright © 1990, American Occupational Therapy Association. Reprinted with permission. http://dx.doi.org/10.5014/ajot.44.9.816

lose his autonomy and become little more than an animated tool of management (Montgomery, 1984).

Taylor's ideas did take hold. Indeed, scientific management ideology provides the foundation for the efficiency perspective in management today (Drucker, 1954). A basic assumption of this perspective is that resources are finite and must be carefully controlled in order to achieve productivity. Control of scarce resources such as time, money, and staff is accomplished through a hierarchical organizational structure in which formal authority is delegated to managers who are responsible for monitoring efficiency and profitability (Perrow, 1970).

Although the efficiency perspective has exerted considerable influence in industry and business since 1920, the perspective has taken much longer to permeate health-care management. Although there is evidence to show that the doctrine of scientific management was preached to doctors as well as to businessmen (Haber, 1964), there is little data to show that the efficiency perspective was influential in the formative years of American hospitals.

Health-care institutions were not identified with the business concern of profitability in the early years of the 20th century. The health-care system at that time consisted of either charity or voluntary hospitals whose goals were humanitarian in nature (Starr, 1982). In many instances, doctors had authority over both the administrative and the clinical aspects of hospital care and thus fulfilled the roles of technical expert and manager. This was in contrast to industry where the skilled worker, or "doer," became separated from the manager, or "thinker" (Reich, 1983). One prominent Chicago physician evidently was mindful of events in industry when he warned his colleagues, "If we wish to escape the thralldom of commercialism, if we wish to avoid the fate of the tool-less workers, we must control the hospital" (Holmes, 1906, p. 320).

Indeed it was a shift in control and purpose that brought the efficiency perspective to health-care organizations. By 1970, the humanitarian emphasis had shifted to a concern for the best way to run hospitals as businesses (Drucker, 1973). The health-care industry expanded from hospitals into rehabilitation centers, outpatient services, nursing homes, and community programs. Accompanying this expansion was growth in the private insurance industry and in federal insurance programs through Medicare and Medicaid. The physician–manager role eroded and governance became separated from clinical management. Hospital administrators with master's degrees in business administration took over the business functions of hospitals, guided by the efficiency perspective.

The efficiency perspective has been justified on the grounds that health care in the United States is big business, and therefore health-care organizations should be run according to a business model, which emphasizes efficiency. Given modern concerns about rising costs in health care, the need for the efficiency perspective was deemed obvious: This approach enables management to focus on the goals of productivity and cost control.

Differences between business and health care, however, raise questions as to the goodness of fit with the efficiency perspective. One important difference lies in the mission of the organization. In business, profits are the top priority. In health care, quality patient care is the predominant goal. Some for-profit health-care facilities do exist, but a large proportion of health-care institutions remain nonprofit. Even the nonprofit facilities, however, have begun to shift their emphasis away from quality and toward cost reduction as a result of the cost-containment movement.

This shift in focus has highlighted a growing conflict between practitioner and administrator. Differing professional orientations place the administrator trained from a business perspective on the side of efficiency and the practitioner trained from a humanistic perspective on the side of quality. Whereas the administrator focuses on the efficient use of funds and increased productivity, the health-care practitioner desires freedom to act in the full interests of the patient and resources to provide the most advanced treatment ("Balancing Health Care Costs," 1988).

One way to address this dilemma of efficiency versus quality is to reframe the question: Can all organizations achieve quality as well as efficiency? Some management theorists argue that this is possible, if organizations use the excellence perspective.

The Excellence Perspective and Health-Care Management

The origins of the excellence perspective can be traced to the work of Mary Parker Follett (Follett, 1924; Fox & Urwick, 1973). Follett articulated her management philosophy in the first part of the 20th century, at the same time that scientific management was gaining popularity. She proposed that businesses would be effective only when they created an environment that stimulated each member to make his or her fullest contribution. Indeed, she argued that the strength of an organization depended on its ability to create a "working unit," in which shared values and common interests could evolve (Follett, 1987). Follett proposed that the best way to create organizational environments that fostered such working units was through shared decision-making and participative governance, a position in direct opposition to the authoritarian approach advocated by Taylor.

Follett's interest in creating an environment in which people could contribute fully was probably due in part to her own experience as a woman. She was also influenced by the idealistic leanings of several of her instructors at Harvard and by her professional experience as the founder of a group of community centers called the Roxbury League (Cabot, 1934; Crawford, 1971). The prescience of Follett's vision has recently been acknowledged (Mullins, 1979; Parker, 1984). March (1965) claimed Follett was ahead of her time: Her ideas did not fit in with the management wisdom of her age, an age dominated by the efficiency perspective.

Contemporary management theorists challenge the efficiency perspective. They argue that it has not helped American business, which is suffering from declines in product quality and in productivity (Reich, 1983). They urge that we move away from the concern of efficiency and toward a focus on excellence (Peters & Austin, 1985; Peters & Waterman, 1982). They claim that if one emphasizes excellence as the primary goal, then productivity is not sacrificed but, rather, is enhanced (Walton, 1985).

Studies of successful businesses that exemplify the excellence perspective show several common elements (Deal & Kennedy, 1982; Waterman, 1987). A key element is the definition of a vision that can guide the direction and activities of an organization. This vision should be shared, that is, the organization's members must value its mission. Leadership is a critical factor (Kouzes & Posner, 1989). It is the leader with a vision who helps shape the organization. Leaders create an environment that fosters collaboration, one that encourages and recognizes the contributions of all members. Case studies show that organizations committed to a shared goal, with leaders who direct the organization's resources toward that goal, create an environment that achieves quality and productivity (Posner, Kouzes, & Schmidt, 1985).

Since the first writings on this management perspective were published, much interest has been expressed, as has some criticism. Questions arise as to how an organization creates a vision, which is a vague concept at best. How does an organization convince its members to work toward a shared goal? How does one become the kind of leader who can shape an environment that enables members to achieve excellence and productivity? Recent writings by organizational theorists who support this perspective have attempted to answer these questions (Bradford & Cohen, 1984).

For example, Kouzes and Posner (1989) used data from their research based on 1,372 questionnaires and interviews to describe how leaders bring forth the best in themselves and others. The authors discussed the concept of vision, which they said is not mysterious and which can be defined as mission, goal, purpose, or simply the desire to make something happen that will contribute to quality. Kouzes and Posner described the ways that effective leaders create an environment in which members want to achieve excellence: (a) they enable others to see the possibilities a vision holds; (b) they are willing to take risks and experiment with new ideas; (c) they enable others to act and therefore to feel strong, capable, and committed; (d) they lead by example, through actions that support their words; and (e) they encourage others through genuine acts of caring. The authors' book is replete with descriptions of acts of leadership that contributed to excellence in performance. Examples are cited from both the public sector and private industry.

Deal, Kennedy, and Spiegel (1983) addressed the specific application of the excellence perspective to health-care institutions. They asserted that although this perspective is not abundant in health care, some organizations do exemplify excellence. As examples, they described a prestigious urban teaching hospital and a community rehabilitation facility. Although these organizations differ in size (large versus small), mission (acute care versus long-term care), and financial status (nonprofit versus for profit), they share certain elements. Deal et al. found each organization was

committed to being the best. For one, this meant the best teaching hospital; for the other, the best rehabilitation facility. This vision was shared by all members and shaped by leaders who committed the necessary resources to achieve this goal. Individual contributions were encouraged and recognized. Within the rehabilitation facility, the occupational therapy department was well respected for its contribution to excellence. Its members were encouraged to contribute and, in fact, developed several patient-care programs. The director of occupational therapy had recently been promoted to vice president; at that level she anticipated having a greater opportunity to further her vision of excellence in patient care (D. Robinson, personal communication, October 30, 1982).

Case Study

The Asian and Pacific American Psychiatric Inpatient Program at San Francisco General Hospital in San Francisco, California, opened in 1980. It later served as the model for the development of four other inpatient programs to serve Latinos, Blacks, women, and patients with AIDS-related psychiatric illnesses. These five programs, designed to provide culturally sensitive psychiatric care to minority and ethnic patients, were recently awarded a certificate of significant achievement by the American Psychiatric Association (American Psychiatric Association, 1987).

It all began when Francis Lu, MD, participated in a 1979 National Institute for Mental Health conference on ethnic and minority curriculum development. Out of that conference grew his idea about how to provide the best culturally sensitive care to ethnic and minority patients. Lu envisioned an Asian-focus unit in which patients of that ethnic background would come together with professionals of the same background. He believed that acutely disturbed patients could benefit from services provided by professionals who spoke the same language and understood cultural values and beliefs. This view is supported by experts who argue that successful treatment can only occur when the professional comes to understand the patient's story, that is, the way a person views himself or herself in the world (Coles, 1989; Taylor, 1989).

Dr. Lu laid the groundwork for this idea through discussions with the hospital's administration. The department of psychiatry at San Francisco General Hospital is a joint undertaking of the city and county of San Francisco and the University of California, San Francisco. Lu persuaded the administration that his idea would assist the hospital to better address the needs of San Francisco's diverse population. He proposed that a core group of mental health professionals who shared a similar vision could provide more effective diagnosis and treatment. He argued that for the same cost as traditional treatment, higher quality care would be achieved. No special grants or funding were requested; however, Lu did gain administrative support for the concept of a focus unit as well as a commitment to provide funds for recruitment. Leaders in the Asian community were approached, and they expressed their support for the idea. According to the 1980 census, 21.3 percent of San Francisco's residents are Asian American.

The unit began with two professionals of Asian origin, Lu and one nurse. The staff grew to consist of a program director, a senior attending physician, nurses, social workers, and an occupational therapist—all of Asian descent. Those who came to work on the unit did so because they shared the vision of an Asian-focus patient care unit. The unit offered professionals the opportunity to contribute their knowledge of Asian languages and culture. Once the vision was established, the professionals shaped the unit's direction and goals. The goals were (a) to provide culturally sensitive psychiatric care, (b) to provide multi-disciplinary training opportunities, and (c) to develop a body of research to improve both patient care and education.

The way patient treatment was conducted was determined by the developing unit's vision and goals. The staff employed treatment approaches most likely to provide excellent patient care that was culturally sensitive. An ethnomedical approach to diagnosis and treatment was viewed as more consistent with the unit's goal than the traditional biomedical model. This ethnomedical approach not only focuses on diagnosis and precipitating incident but explores information regarding previous life and stresses in the home country; the escape experience and refugee events; and language, cultural, financial, and racial problems encountered in the United States. The staff also explores beliefs the patient might hold about illness, for example, the belief that disease is caused by an excess or deficiency of yin and yang. This approach provides treatment based on an understanding of the patient's perceived symptoms and difficulties (Lee, 1985).

The milieu is designed to make patients comfortable. Rice and tea are routinely served with meals. Ethnic newspapers, books, and music tapes are available. Family members are allowed to bring home cooked food during their visits. Great importance is placed on family involvement and linkages with the community once the person is discharged. Evelyn Lee, EdD, became program director in 1982. Lu described Dr. Lee as a charismatic and caring leader who has energetically directed the unit toward its mission to provide psychotic and severely depressed Asian American patients with an environment that understands their pain and their cultural background (F. Lu, personal communication, November 30, 1989).

Lisa Lai, OTR, was hired in 1982 as the unit's occupational therapist. Lai has relied on general principles of occupational therapy coupled with creativity and her knowledge of Asian language and culture. Occupational therapy treatment uses occupation that is both meaningful and purposeful; Lai uses an approach to treatment that takes into account both patients' functional needs and their values and beliefs. For example, the cooking group features recipes from various Asian and Pacific countries. Support for treatment that addresses both the meaning and the purpose of occupation has been a growing theme in the professional literature (Yoder, Nelson, & Smith, 1989). Lai asserts that treatment that combines professional expertise with a sensitivity to the language and values of patients can result in major changes in patients' status and responsiveness to treatment (L. Lai, personal communication, November 30, 1989).

In summary, the Asian-focus unit exemplifies many of the characteristics of the excellence perspective. It began with an idea, a vision, that would join others in the pursuit of excellence in patient care. This vision represents the shared values and beliefs of the professionals within the unit. Its leaders epitomize the leadership qualities of the excellence perspective: They have enabled others to see the possibilities of their vision, they have experimented with new ideas, and they have encouraged professionals within the unit to make individual contributions. They lead through example and encourage through caring. Development of the Asian-focus unit was hard work; it took several years to achieve the cohesion it has now. Its evolution required patience, a commitment of resources from the administration, and energy and understanding from the professionals within the unit. Recruitment has been and remains an issue. The unit must attract and retain competent professionals with an Asian background and language capability who share the same sense of mission. Although the program has gained national recognition for its innovative approach, there is a feeling expressed by some within the facility that the program promotes a segregated approach to treatment, one that separates patients as well as staff. This belief assumes that the focus units maintain a separate mission from the rest of the organization. Another viewpoint, however, is that the focus units simply offer one way to achieve the overall mission of the hospital, which is to provide quality patient care for the residents of San Francisco. Further research is planned to document the effectiveness of the focus unit in patient treatment (Lee & Lu, 1989).

Discussion

One might ask, if the excellence approach leads to higher-quality patient care, why is it not used by more health-care organizations? The answer, in part, is that people act in ways that are most comfortable. As this paper has shown, the efficiency perspective is predominant in health care. Efficiency has become the primary goal; quality patient care is a secondary goal. Common wisdom dictates that if one focuses on efficiency, one gets productivity and reasonable patient care. Excellence in patient care has been presumed to be something that could only be achieved at a financial risk. Research has contributed to disproving this assumption, but common wisdom dies hard. We must also examine the nature of leadership in health-care organizations. Administrators tend to be conservative, particularly in a climate that is so heavily focused on cost containment and short-term financial performance. The majority of leaders using the excellence perspective are from organizational cultures noted for being more innovative, such as high technology. Finally, there can be little energy for innovation in an environment where the vision is survival. Only when one replaces that vision with one of excellence can energy be freed for making changes that can contribute to quality patient care as well as to productivity.

Implications for Occupational Therapy

As this case study has shown, health-care professionals were the leaders in developing a program to achieve quality patient care. Because many administrators are preoccupied with finances, it will probably fall to health professionals to continue to lead the focus on excellence. Occupational therapists can contribute to this effort by developing ideas to increase the quality of services within our domain.

As the profession of occupational therapy plans for its future, one vision that emerges is that of the multifaceted occupational therapist, a person who is a competent clinician, a supporter of and contributor to research, and a strong manager–leader (Directions for the Future, 1990). This vision says we can no longer afford to have occupational therapists who are knowledgeable only about patient evaluation and treatment. Instead, we need people who are able to articulate the profession's contribution and introduce new ideas that can lead practice. This requires leadership ability and management knowledge. Occupational therapists can use the excellence perspective as a guide to program innovation. It is a perspective that fits with the occupational therapist's concern for quality patient care and the administration's concern for productivity.

Acknowledgments

I express my appreciation to the staff and patients of the Asian and Pacific American Psychiatric Inpatient Program at San Francisco General Hospital, San Francisco, California. In particular I would like to cite the assistance of Francis Lu, MD, Assistant Clinical Professor of Psychiatry, University of California, San Francisco; Evelyn Lee, EdD, Assistant Clinical Professor of Psychiatry, University of California, San Francisco; Lisa Lai, OTR, Staff Occupational Therapist, San Francisco General Hospital; and Judy Levin, OTR Senior Occupational Therapist, San Francisco General Hospital.

References

American Psychiatric Association. (1987, Oct 16). *Six exceptional programs for the mentally ill share hospital and community awards.* News release.

Balancing health-care costs and quality. (1988, June). *Occupational Therapy News*, p. 3.

Bradford, D. L., & Cohen, A. R. (1984). *Managing for excellence.* New York: Wiley.

Cabot, R. (1934). Mary Parker Follett: An appreciation. *Radcliffe Quarterly, 18*, 81.

Coles, R. (1989). *The call of stories.* Boston: Houghton Mifflin.

Copley, F. B. (1923). *Frederick W Taylor: Father of scientific management.* New York: Harper & Brothers.

Crawford, D. (1971). Mary Parker Follett. In D. Crawford (Ed.), *Notable American women 1607–1950* (pp. 639–641). Cambridge, MA: Belknap Press.

Deal, T. E., & Kennedy, A. A. (1982). *Corporate cultures.* Reading, MA: Addison–Wesley.

Deal, T. E., Kennedy, A. A., & Spiegel, A. H. (1983). How to create an outstanding hospital culture. *Forum, 26,* 21–34.

Directions for the Future. (1990, January). Meeting of the American Occupational Therapy Association, San Diego, CA.

Drucker, P. F. (1954). *The practice of management.* New York: Harper & Row.

Drucker, P. F. (1973). *Management: Tasks, responsibilities, practices.* New York: Harper & Row.

Follett, M. P. (1924). *Creative experience.* New York: Longmans, Green.

Follett, M. P. (1987). Freedom and coordination. Lectures in business organization. In A. Brief (Ed.), *Ancestral books in the management of organizations.* New York: Garland.

Fox, M., & Urwick, L. (Eds). (1973). *Dynamic administration: The collected papers of Mary Parker Follett.* London: Pitman.

Haber, S. (1964). *Efficiency and uplift.* Chicago: University of Chicago Press.

Holmes, B. (1906). The hospital problem. *Journal of the American Medical Association, 38,* 320.

Hoxie, R. F. (1916). *Scientific management and labor.* New York: D. Appleton.

Kouzes, J., & Posner, B. (1989). *The leadership challenge.* San Francisco: Jossey–Bass.

Lee, E. (1985). Inpatient psychiatric services for Southeast Asian refugees. *Southeast Asian Mental Health.* Washington, DC: National Institute for Mental health.

Lee, F., & Lu, F. (1989). Assessment and treatment of Asian American survivors of mass violence. *Journal of Traumatic Stress, 2,* 93–120.

March, J. (Ed.). (1965). *Handbook of organizations.* Chicago: Rand McNally.

Montgomery, D. (1984). *Worker's control in America.* London: Cambridge University Press.

Mullins, L. (1979). Approaches to management. *Management Accounting, 57,* 15–18.

Parker, L. D. (1984). Control in organizational life: The contribution of Mary Parker Follett. *Academy of Management Review, 9,* 736–745.

Perrow, C. (1970). *Organizational analysis.* Monterey, CA: Brooks/Cole.

Peters, T., & Austin, N. (1985). *A passion for excellence: The leadership difference.* New York: Random House.

Peters, T., & Waterman, R. (1982). *In search of excellence: Lessons from America's best-run companies.* New York: Harper & Row.

Posner, B. Z., Kouzes, J. M., & Schmidt, W. H. (1985). Shared values make a difference. *Human Resource Management, 24,* 293–309.

Reich, R. B. (1983). *The next American frontier.* New York: Times Books.

Snoke, A. W. (1987). The hospital administrator. *Hospital Topics, 65,* 23–29.

Starr, P. (1982). *The social transformation of American medicine.* New York: Basic.

Starr, P. (1988, March 20). Increasingly, life and death issues become money matters. *New York Times,* p. E1.

Taylor, F. W. (1919). *The principles of scientific management.* New York: Harper & Brothers.

Taylor, S. E. (1989). *Positive illusions.* New York: Basic.

Walton, R. E. (1985). From control to commitment in the workplace. *Harvard Business Review, 63,* 77–84.

Waterman, R. H. (1987). *The renewal factor.* New York: Bantam.

Yoder, R. M., Nelson, D. L., & Smith, D. A. (1989). Added-purpose versus rote exercise in female nursing home residents. *American Journal of Occupational Therapy, 43,* 581–586.

CHAPTER 56

Dreams, Dilemmas, and Decisions for Occupational Therapy Practice in a New Millennium: An American Perspective

ELIZABETH J. YERXA

Humankind is poised to take a giant step into the 21st century. Will the year 2000 bring a great leap forward into a more humane, healthy, enlightened global community, or will it begin a downward spiral, toward an irretrievable loss of the dream for a good life? Scientists, philosophers, public policy makers, optimists, and pessimists are debating their visions of the future, looking into crystal balls filled with light or darkness.

Assumptions

As I enter this debate I bring a set of assumptions. The 21st century will possess characteristics that are of great importance to occupational therapists and the persons we serve.

First, the next century will begin an *era of chronicity* beyond that which the world has ever known. The population of persons with impairments will increase markedly, as will the number of persons at risk. This era of chronicity will result from the successes of medical technology, the aging of the populace, and the preservation of biological life on an unprecedented scale (Robinson, 1988).

Second, *new knowledge* emanating from the sciences, philosophy, literature, and the arts will affirm the significance of the uniqueness, individuality, and wholeness of each person (Edelman, 1992; Thelen, 1990). This new knowledge will enlighten scientists about lifespan development and the evolution of our species. Research, at last, will emphasize human purpose, action, goal-directedness, interests, curiosity, and consciousness, as well as the joy, despair, or boredom that persons experience when they engage in their daily rounds of activity (Csikszentmihalyi, 1975).

Third, daily life will increase in *complexity* (Toffler, 1981). Successful accomplishment of the activities of daily living will be much more challenging because of increased urbanization, the diversity of cultures interacting, the multiplicity of social role expectations, high technology, and the difficulty of educating children for competency in an instantaneously changing environment.

Fourth, the future will bring an *increased emphasis on personal power, autonomy, self-direction, and self-responsibility,* with a decrease in the influence of traditional paternalistic political and social systems. Persons will demand to control their own destinies and to participate in the decisions that affect them.

Fifth, the 21st century will see a *new conceptualization of health,* a shift away from the old idea that health means the absence of disease, pathology, or impairments. The new idea of health is reflected, for example, in Pörn's (in press) philosophy. He defined health as persons' capacities to achieve their goals and purposes through possession of a repertoire of skills.

Sixth, the new era will bring an *increased awareness of attending to the demands of the environments in which persons actually live and work.* Persons will learn such skills as mathematical computation, not by classroom drills and tests divorced from the pulsating rhythms of life, but in the real world of the supermarket, office, and shopping mall.

Research has demonstrated not only that transferring skills from the academic environment to the real world is difficult but that the skills learned are different (Lave, 1988). Thus learning a skill in a classroom might develop competency for schoolwork but not for the challenges of daily life.

Dreams

Within this context of the future, being an optimist and an occupational therapist (and the two characteristics usually do go together), I have a dream. My most audacious dream is that the 21st century will begin the millennium of occupation. Occupation, as engagement in self-initiated, self-directed, adaptive, purposeful, culturally relevant, organized activity, speaks to my assumptions about the future in compelling ways. The era of chronicity requires that some profession, recognize and reclaim the potential of persons with chronic conditions or at risk of developing them, so that these persons can achieve their purposes and so that social barriers to their self-definition will be removed. I nominate occupational therapy as that profession.

The new understanding emanating from the sciences about individuality and wholeness needs to be synthesized with the 70 years of knowledge about human activity, development, learning, and evolution that are embedded in the rich history of occupational therapy. We knew it all the time! For example, we knew that infants are driven by their unique curiosity to explore the world, learn from their experiences, and thus shape their nervous systems (Reilly, 1974). Engagement in occupation cannot be divorced from the meaning it possesses for the person.

The increased complexity of daily life for all persons demands a profession that knows a great deal about daily routines and how persons manage and thrive in their environments. My global travels have shown that occupational therapists everywhere focus on engagement in daily life, regardless of other differences in practice. Alvin Toffler (1981), the futurologist, proposed that all persons, not just those with impairments, will need "life organizers" (p. 377) to help them deal with the complexity of daily life in the 21st century. I nominate occupational therapists to be tomorrow's life organizers, using our knowledge of activities of daily living to help persons get their lives together in a complex world.

As for the increased emphasis on autonomy and personal responsibility, occupational therapists have always involved patients or other participants in formulating and carrying out their programs. In fact, authentic occupational therapy cannot take place unless the patient becomes his or her own agent of competency via occupation. Many other health-care professionals do not know how to help the patient do this because they are trained in an old paternalistic model of acute care. In his book, *Medicine at the Crossroads,* Konner recommended that physicians adopt a "new model" of the physician–patient bond called the "patient as colleague" (1993, p. 14) model, in which the physician and patient exchange views and plan treatment or prevention together. Occupational therapists who have used a similar approach for decades can catalyze change in the entire health-care system through their skill and example. In this way more persons will take responsibility for their own health.

A vision of health as the possession of a repertoire of skills to achieve one's own purposes fits with occupational therapy's traditional emphasis on skill, mastery, and competence that can be attained regardless of pathology or impairment. It also suggests that occupation that develops skills can prevent illness and influence health by developing competency and making life worth living. This view of health is compatible with Reilly's (1962) (see Chapter 7) great hypothesis that human beings, through the use of their hands as energized by mind and will, can influence the state of their own health. Such a perspective on health implies that every human being has resources that can be reclaimed through occupational therapy (Montgomery, 1984).

Research demonstrating that persons need to learn skills in the environments in which their skills will be used supports occupational therapists who create a "just right challenge" (p. 251) from the environment so that the person can make an adaptive response (Robinson, 1977). It also supports the importance of providing occupational therapy in the home, community, supermarket, shopping mall, workplace, or school, not in artificial environments such as clinics or hospitals. I opened my eyes to the importance of the real-life environment when I provided occupational therapy to children with cerebral palsy in a home program after 2 years of similar work in a hospital. Not only was it easier for children to learn skills when the skills did not have to be transferred to a different environment (as was necessary in the hospital), but as an occupational therapist, I could experience the challenges of their daily lives and employ them in increments that assured both a just-right challenge and a high probability of success (Burke, 1977).

Biological evolution, in all creatures, advances in relation to real environmental challenges, not *before* such challenges occur (Jordan, 1991). Nature does not plan ahead; only when an organism is faced with a real environmental challenge can it adapt. Occupational therapists who provide service in real-life environments are not only practical but are employing the most sophisticated form of intervention supported by neurobiology, evolutionary biology, and anthropology.

Decisions and Dilemmas

What implications do these perspectives of the future hold for occupational therapy practice? Arnold Beisser (1988), a physician who became almost totally paralyzed as a result of poliomyelitis, described his experience as follows:

> More important [than the physical helplessness] was being *separated from so many of the elemental routines that occupied people*. . . . I no longer felt connected with the familiar roles I had known in family, work, sports. *My place in the culture was gone*. (pp. 166–167) [Italics added]

Occupational therapists will need to establish their priorities for practice in the millennium of occupation. I recommend a decision in favor of the vital, fundamental issues that are most important to the person and society: survival, work, contribution, participation, delight in one's own actions. Focus on these will influence health through development of a repertoire of skills that reconnects persons to the elemental routines of their culture, restoring their place in the world. The dilemma is that the organization of the U.S. health-care system provides most of its resources for acute care, modalities, and techniques in an artificial environment that values short-term, measurable, physical changes and is not prepared to address these fundamental issues. As a result, the experiences recorded by articulate persons with disabilities—Lewis Puller (1991), Robert Murphy (1990), Arnold Beisser (1988), and Andre Dubus (1991)—as well as our research on persons with disabilities living in the community (Burnett & Yerxa, 1980)—show major unmet needs for help in dealing with such elemental issues as skills for living in the community, being part of one's culture, and having something satisfying to do. These authors and our research subjects did not mention occupational therapy in connection with their difficulties in daily living or their need to develop a new repertoire of skills at home or at work. If occupational therapy was mentioned at all it was as a minor aspect of acute care in the hospital.

The era of chronicity cries out for practice founded on an optimistic view of persons, their resources, and potential; one that emphasizes what is right, such as intrinsic motivation, rather than what is wrong, such as organ impairment. In spite of the Americans With Disabilities Act of 1990 (Public Law 101–336), persons with disabilities are too often stigmatized as second-class citizens or disposable persons. Unfortunately, this social attitude is so pervasive that persons with disabilities may be denied many social opportunities or internalize the stigma themselves, leading to depression and denial. This is a major dilemma. In the future world of genetic engineering and probable euthanasia, persons with disabilities are at risk of being eliminated as they were in Nazi Germany. Through new knowledge of occupation practiced by occupational therapists, these persons will be able to achieve their own purposes and to contribute to the variety and richness of society. Occupational therapists who are allies and advocates for persons with disabilities will help change society's attitudes from "those people are inferior" to "these people are fundamentally human, just like the rest of us." Through occupation this profession will reaffirm its commitment to persons with chronic conditions, a commitment initially made by Adolph Meyer (1922) (see Chapter 2) and Eleanor Clarke Slagle (1922) (see Appendix D).

A final implication is that occupational therapy practice will be enriched and broadened by new interdisciplinary knowledge of occupation, which some of us have named *occupational science*. Tomorrow's world needs a profession that views persons as both unique and whole, who create themselves through engagement in activity as driven by their interests and curiosity. Thus occupation, rather than being trivial, will be seen as the essential connector between the developing human organism and its environment, a creator of unique neural networks, motor patterns, and life-affirming mastery.

Science and philosophy's new interest in the wholeness of human beings belies the specialism that has permeated society and medicine. Persons have been divided into minds and bodies to fit into specialists' categories of mental health and physical disabilities. One of the greatest strengths of occupational therapy education has been its insistence on preparing students to look at persons as having not only muscles and joints but feelings, perceptions, families, communities, and unique patterns of daily activity. Ours is one of the few health professions that is educated to think this way, whose practitioners can serve anyone who needs to develop skills in the presence of a challenge labeled physical, psychiatric, developmental, or environmental. Our science and clinical experiences will help reconnect the human mind and body. Strengthening our generalist outlook with new knowledge will make our profession much more adaptable to the changing conditions of tomorrow's world environment. Evolutionary biology has taught us that specialists such as dinosaurs perish when their environment changes, whereas generalists such as cockroaches and human beings survive and prosper (Jordan, 1991).

A dilemma is created by the U.S. health-care system's low priority on providing resources for those labeled mentally ill and the resulting attrition in the numbers of occupational therapists adopting such practice. New knowledge of occupation that relates to skill, adaptation to changing circumstances, temporality, management and organization of the environment, and obtaining satisfaction through one's own action has a great deal to offer persons who are given psychiatric diagnostic labels. The millennium of occupation will reaffirm the commitment to improving the life opportunities of all persons regardless of diagnostic labels, because it is the right thing to do in a compassionate society and because occupational therapists have the knowledge and skill to make it happen. In the millennium of occupation, occupational therapists will enable human beings as whole persons to be reconnected with their culture through skills. Persons with disabilities will no longer be endangered or be isolated on islands of abnormality, but will perceive themselves as skilled, competent, and capable of mastery. The era of chronicity will be answered by the millennium of occupation. Health will ultimately be perceived not as the absence of impairment but as possession of a repertoire of skills to achieve one's own purposes. Robert Murphy (1990), an anthropologist paralyzed by a spinal cord tumor, at the end of his "journey into the world of the disabled," said that

> the essence of the well-lived life is the defiance of negativity, inertia and death. Life has a liturgy that must be continually celebrated and renewed; it is a feast whose sacrament is consummated in the paralytic's breaking out from his prison of flesh and bone, and in his quest for autonomy. (p. 230)

Occupational therapists, in the new millennium of occupation, can provide a key to the prison and tools for the quest for autonomy.

References

Americans With Disabilities Act of 1990 (Public Law 101–336). 42 U. S. C., § 12101.

Beisser, A. (1988). *Flying without wings: Personal reflections on being disabled*. New York: Doubleday.

Burke, J. P. (1977). A clinical perspective on motivation: Pawn versus origin. *American Journal of Occupational Therapy, 31,* 254–258.

Burnett, S., & Yerxa, E. J. (1980). Community-based and college-based needs assessment of physically disabled persons. *American Journal of Occupational Therapy, 34,* 201–207.

Csikszentmihalyi, M. (1975). *Beyond boredom and anxiety: The experience of play in work and games*. San Francisco: Jossey-Bass.

Dubus, A. (1991). Broken vessels. *Essays by Andre Dubus*. Boston: David R. Godine.

Edelman, G. (1992). *Bright air, brilliant fire. On the matter of mind*. New York: Basic.

Jordan, W. (1991). *Divorce among the gulls: An uncommon look at human nature*. San Francisco: North Point.

Konner, M. (1993). *Medicine at the crossroads*. New York: Pantheon.

Lave, J. (1988). *Cognition in practice*. New York: Cambridge University Press.

Meyer, A. (1922). The philosophy of occupational therapy. *Archives of Occupational Therapy, 1,* 1–10. Reprinted as Chapter 4.

Montgomery, M. A. (1984). Resources of adaptation for daily living: A classification with therapeutic implications for occupational therapy. *Occupational Therapy in Health Care. 1,* 9–33.

Murphy, R. F. (1990). *The body silent*. New York: Norton.

Pörn, I. (In press). Health and adaptedness. *Theoretical Medicine*.

Puller, L. B. (1991). *Fortunate son. The autobiography of Lewis B. Puller, Jr*. New York: Grove Weidenfeld.

Reilly, M. (1962). Occupational therapy can be one of the great ideas of 20th-century medicine. *American Journal of Occupational Therapy, 16,* 1–9. Reprinted as Chapter 7.

Reilly M. (1974). *Play as exploratory learning*. Beverly Hills, CA: Sage.

Robinson, A. (1977). Play: The arena for acquisition of rules for competent behavior. *American Journal of Occupational Therapy, 31,* 248–253.

Robinson, I. (1988). The rehabilitation of patients with long-term physical impairments: The social context of professional roles. *Clinical Rehabilitation, 2,* 339–347.

Slagle, E. C. (1922). Training aids for mental patients. *Occupational Therapy and Rehabilitation, 1,* 11–14.

Thelen, E. (1990). Dynamical systems and the generation of individual differences. In J. Colombo & J. W. Fagan (Eds.), *Individual differences in infancy: Rehability, stability, and prediction*. Hillsdale, NJ: Erlbaum.

Toffler, A. (1981). *The third wave*. New York: Bantam.

CHAPTER 57

Dreams, Dilemmas, and Decisions for Occupational Therapy Practice in a New Millennium: A Canadian Perspective

HELENE J. POLATAJKO

My dreams for occupational therapy in the new millennium are predicated on what I imagine the world will be like in that millennium. Although I would like to believe that the world will be free of war, disease, illness, indeed all sources of human misery, I do not believe that to be the destiny of humanity. Rather, I believe that there will always be some phenomena that will result in less-than-ideal situations for humankind. Whether these phenomena will result in disability or handicap, however, is another issue.

I Dream of a World Free of Handicap

In my dream, the world will be free of handicap in the new millennium. Free not because we have learned to rehabilitate those with disabilities but because we have learned to create an environment that allows those with different abilities to live with dignity. Free not because we have allowed those with disabilities to end their lives but because we have enabled those with different abilities to have meaningful lives. Free not because we have learned to prevent disability but because we have learned to eliminate handicap. In other words, I dream of a world that honors, respects, and values differences, a world that enables living with different abilities.

Before I go on describing my dream and its implications for occupational therapy, let me clarify how I am using the terms *disability* and *handicap* and how they relate to each other. In attempting to establish an international classification for the long-term functional and social consequences of disease, the World Health Organization (WHO) identified three distinct and independent classifications: impairment, disability, and

handicap. *Impairment* is defined as "any loss of psychological, physiological, or anatomical structure or function resulting from any cause" (1980, p. 27). *Disability* is defined as "any restriction or lack (resulting from an impairment) of ability to perform an activity in the manner or within the range considered normal for a human being" (p. 28). *Handicap* is "a disadvantage for a given individual, resulting from an impairment or disability, that limits or prevents the fulfillment of a role that is normal (depending on age, sex, and social and cultural factors) for that individual" (p. 29). In the vernacular of occupational therapy, handicap is a disadvantage that limits or prevents occupational role performance. Although WHO considers these classifications to be independent, there is, as apparent from the WHO definitions, a causal relationship among them (see Figure 57.1). It should be noted, however, that not all impairment leads to disability, nor does all disability lead to handicap. Indeed, because handicap is viewed as a disadvantage, and disadvantage is a social construct, disability must be seen as neither a necessary nor a sufficient condition for the creation of a handicap. In my dream the world will be free of handicaps because of occupational therapy—not the occupational therapy we know now, but the occupational therapy that surely must evolve because *occupation* is a powerful idea. To quote Thomas Jefferson, "It is neither wealth nor splendour, but tranquility and occupation, which give happiness" (cited in Foley, 1967, p. 399).

The great psychologist Hebb (1966) noted long ago that "living things must be active" (p. 248); that the

This chapter was previously published in the *American Journal of Occupational Therapy, 48,* 590–593. Copyright © 1994, American Occupational Therapy Association. Reprinted with permission. http://dx.doi.org/10.5014/ajot.48.7.590

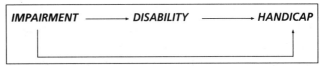

Figure 57.1. World Health Organization disablement model.

need for activity and the avoidance of boredom, the result of inactivity, are important determinants of human behavior. Recently, two courageous young persons, one Canadian and one American, provided dramatic personal testimony of the vital importance that activity or the lack of it, has in determining human behavior.

In Canada, a 25-year-old woman caught national media attention when she fought the legal system for the right to refuse life-sustaining treatment. Having spent $2\frac{1}{2}$ years in a hospital bed because of a disease that resulted in the permanent loss of all her independent function, including respiration, Nancy B. pleaded for the right to die. She told the judge that a life without the ability to do is not worth living ("Woman makes plea," 1991). She won her case. On February 13, 1992, Nancy B. died.

In the United States, 29-year-old Larry McAfee had a motorcycle accident that left him unable to walk, eat, or even breathe independently. After a year of intensive rehabilitation, out of finances, Larry was also doomed to a life in a hospital bed where, he said, "I used to just lie there on my back, being just so bored" (Schindehette & Wescott, 1993, p. 85). Two years later, "broken in spirit after being warehoused in a series of institutions, McAfee fought for the legal right to shut off his life-sustaining respirator" (Schindehette & Wescott, 1993, p. 85). Larry McAfee won his case. However, he is alive and well and living in the first independent-care home in the state of Georgia. While engaged in his fight to die, he discovered that he had options other than boredom, that in an environment that enabled occupation he could have an active, meaningful life. But Larry McAfee warned, "if ever I have to return to an institution, then I prefer death" (Schindeherte & Wescott, p. 86).

I Dream of a World Where Occupation Is a Powerful Idea

My dream for occupational therapy in the 21st century is that we will not only know unequivocally that occupation is a powerful idea but also choose to act on that idea, for "any powerful idea is absolutely fascinating and absolutely useless until we choose to use it" (Bach, 1988, p. 119).

Occupational therapy is in an exciting, transitional phase—a paradigm shift, as Kielhofner has described it (1992). If we make the right decisions now, if we frame the emerging paradigm well, I believe that the occupationaln therapy of the future will be quite different from the one we know today.

The occupational therapy we know now fails to realize the full potential of occupation. As Kielhofner (1992) and numerous others have pointed out, practice today is heavily influenced by the medical model. Practice is focused, primarily, on reducing impairment through the therapeutic use of purposeful activity. To quote Henderson et al. (1991), "the use of purposeful activity is the core of occupational therapy" (p. 370). In Canada, a similar emphasis on the therapeutic use of activity prevails. The definition of occupational therapy adopted by our national association begins with "Occupational therapy is the art and science which utilizes the analysis and application of activities" (Canadian Association of Occupational Therapists [CAOT], 1991, p. 140).

I Dream of a Discipline Focused on Occupation

In my dream, the occupational therapy of the future will realize the full potential of occupation. Practice will be grounded firmly in an occupational model. The focus of practice will shift from reducing impairment through purposeful activity to preventing handicap through occupational enablement.

My dream is predicated on two developments in our discipline, both called for by Ann Grady in her presidential address at the 72nd Annual Conference of the American Occupational Therapy Association. Grady asked occupational therapists to revisit and reaffirm the concepts and visions held by the founders of the discipline, to "reaffirm the idea that being meaningfully occupied provides direction for individuals and that successful engagement in the activity leads to individual satisfaction and promotes health and well-being" (1992, p. 1062), and to "provide the leadership needed to continue developing knowledge based on our founders' vision and to find myriad ways to apply that knowledge to the challenges of practice in the 21st century" (p. 1065).

For my dream to come true, we, as occupational therapists must:
- Affirm that occupation is a powerful idea
- Adopt occupation as the core concept
- Entrench occupation in our value system
- Become experts in enabling occupation.

My dream is that our continued study of occupation will make it possible, in the new millennium, for us to move beyond the rhetoric of the day and translate our values into action.

In my 1992 Muriel Driver Lecture, I articulated what I and a group of colleagues believe to be the core values of occupational therapy (see Appendix 57.A). I elaborate on these briefly below and describe what I think it means to translate these into action as we embrace occupation as the core concept of our discipline. (For a more extensive discussion, see Polatajko, 1992.)

The values statement concerns itself with the core elements of this discipline. The first two, the individual and human life, are shared with all health-care disciplines. The third, occupation, distinguishes occupational therapy from the rest. Occupational therapists view humans as occupational beings with a basic need to do.

Translating the Rhetoric Into Action

Translating these values into action means, first of all, acknowledging some basic assumptions about occupation.

Occupation is a basic survival need. Occupation is essential to the well-being of every person much in the same way that sleep and food are; occupational deprivation, like sleep deprivation or food deprivation, results in serious mental and physical deterioration of the person and may even result in death—often at the individual's own hand.

Occupation is an extremely complex, multilevel, *multi-faceted construct.* Occupation has cognitive, affective, physical, and environmental attributes and is individually determined; therefore, the study of occupation requires the investigation of the occupation, the person performing that occupation, the environmental context, and their interaction.

Occupational competence is the result of a goodness of fit among the person, the occupation, *and the environment.* Competence is defined as adequacy or sufficiency, answering all the requirements of an environment (Pridham & Schutz, 1985). That is, the occupational competence of any given person is determined by the interaction among the skills necessary to perform the occupation, the abilities of the person, and the demands of the environment in which the occupation is to be performed (see Figure 57.2).

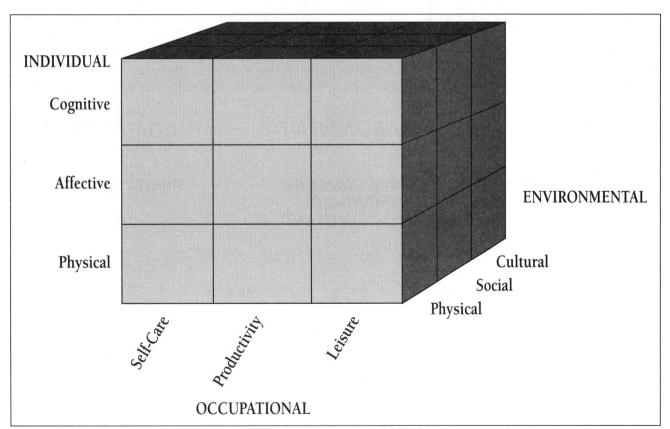

Figure 57.2. Occupational competence model.

Note. Reprinted with permission from Polatajko, H. J. (1992). Naming and framing occupational therapy: A lecture dedicated to the life of Nancy B. *Canadian Journal of Occupational Therapy, 59,* 189–200. Reprinted with permission of CAOT Publications.

Translating these values into action also means that:

Practice is client driven. The client's right to autonomy is taken seriously, and the client is understood to be a prosumer (defined by Toffler [1981, p. 11] as a fusion of producer and consumer) of occupational therapy services, keenly interested in exercising choice over the services that he or she accepts and accepting only those services that can be tailored to meet his or her needs.

Practice is founded on an ideology of empowerment (as defined by Rappaport, 1981). The role of occupational therapist is understood to be one of enhancing possibilities for persons to control their own lives at both a personal and a social level.

The ultimate goal of practice is wholly and solely the enablement of occupational competence. The purpose of practice is to alter the person's ability, the occupation, or the environment so that the person can achieve the necessary balance between ability and the environmental demands to enable occupational competence (see Figure 57.3).

Practice is context focused. Given the ideology of empowerment and the nature of occupation, services must be oriented toward, if not provided in, the person's context, that is, his or her physical, social, and cultural environment.

Practitioners take on many roles in enabling occupational competence. The traditional roles of hands-on clinician, administrator, researcher, and educator are not always adequate to enable occupational competence. Often, particularly when competence requires environment changes, new forms of practice are necessary, such as program designer, consultant, public educator, lobbyist, policy maker, and social critic.

Practitioners use many and any tools. Activity is only one of many tools used to enhance occupational competence. Practitioners use a variety of tools to enable clients; these may include technology, assistive devices, environmental adaptation, attitudinal shift, family education, social education, and policy change.

The domain of concern of the discipline is occupation. The body of knowledge of the discipline is centered on occupation. Scholarly inquiry is focused on understanding the phenomenon of occupation and the determinants of occupational competence. Given the complex nature of occupation, the study of occupation is multidisciplinary and multimethodological.

Occupational therapists are experts in occupation. As my dream comes true there will be a great deal of change for occupational therapy (see Figure 57.4). These changes will present all occupational therapists—present practitioners, administrators, researchers and educators alike—with dilemmas that each of us will have to resolve for ourselves and that the profession will have to resolve as a whole.

As my dream comes true there will be a great deal of change that will create dilemmas, not only for occupational therapists, but for the world in general. Once the

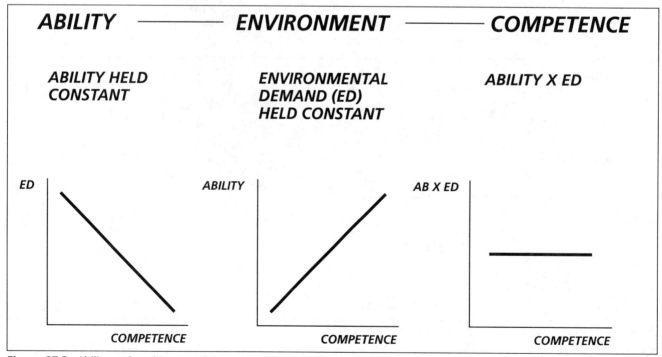

Figure 57.3. Ability and environment interaction.

OT. . .	Will no longer be. . .	But. . .
Ideology	Treatment	Empowerment
Model	Medical	Enabling
Goal	Impairment Reduction	Occupational Competence
Function	To Cure	To Enable
Role	Clinician	Multifaceted
Setting	Institution	Occupational Context
Hallmark	Activity	Occupational Perspective
Activity	**THE Means**	**THE End**

Figure 57.4. Changes for occupational therapy in the coming millennium.

central importance and power of occupation is realized, it will necessitate a shift in such basic notions as quality of life and human rights. This shift has already begun, as shown by the cases of Nancy B. and Larry McAfee.

I believe that mine is not an impossible dream. Rather, I believe that we, as a discipline, are uniquely poised to make this dream come true—to lead the way in health care. Steven Lewis, former Ambassador of Canada to the United Nations, speaking at the CAOT conference in June 1991, said:

> There is no other discipline that is so eclectic, so far ranging and whose core principles are at the very heart of where the health care system is going. . . . You are the only health profession that has fully embraced the concepts of health promotion, prevention, community-based care and the individual as centre to the process. ("Perspectives '91," 1991, p. 11)

As with all change, this change will be experienced with some hesitation, discomfort and, I hope, excitement. But when my dream comes true, I believe that occupational therapists will be instrumental in helping the world to enable all to achieve occupational competence and therefore eliminate handicap.

References

Bach, R. (1988). *One*. New York: Dell.

Canadian Association of Occupational Therapists. (1991) *Canadian occupational therapy guidelines for client-centered practice*. Toronto: Author.

Foley, J.P. (1967). *The Jeffersonian cyclopedic comprehensive collection of the views of Thomas Jefferson*. New York: Russel & Russel.

Grady, A.P. (1992). Nationally Speaking—Occupation as vision. *American Journal of Occupational Therapy, 46,* 1062–1065.

Hebb, D.O. (1966). *A textbook of psychology*. Philadelphia: Saunders.

Appendix 57.A

Occupational Therapy Values Statement

Occupational Therapy Values
As Occupational Therapists, We value

- The individual
- Human life
- Occupation.

About the individual,
We believe that humans are occupational beings, that

- Every individual has intrinsic dignity and worth.
- Every individual has the right to autonomy.
- Each individual is a unique whole.
- Each individual has abilities and competencies.
- Each individual has the capacity for change.
- Individuals are social beings.
- Individuals shape and are shaped by their environment.

About human life,
We believe that all human life has value, that

- The value of human life is based on meaning, not perfection.
- Quality of life is as valued as quantity.

About occupation,
We believe that occupation is a basic human need, that

- Occupation is an essential component of life.
- Occupation gives meaning to life.
- Occupation organizes behavior.
- Occupation has developmental and contextual dimensions.
- Occupation is socioculturally determined.

(Conceptual Framework Think Tank, 1992)

University of Western Ontario–Occupational Therapy

Adapted from H. J. Polatajko (1992). Naming and framing occupational therapy: A lecture dedicated to the life of Nancy B. *Canadian Journal of Occupational Therapy, 59,* 193. Adapted with permission of CAOT Publications.

Henderson, A., Cermak, S., Coster, W., Murray, E., Trombly, C., & Tickle-Degnen, L. (1991). Occupational science is multidimensional. *American Journal of Occupational Therapy, 45,* 370–372.

Kielhofner, G. (1992). *Conceptual foundations of occupational therapy.* Philadelphia: Davis.

Perspectives '91—Taking the initiative. (1991). *National, 8*(5), 11.

Polatajko, H.J. (1992). Naming and framing occupational therapy: A lecture dedicated to the life of Nancy B. *Canadian Journal of Occupational Therapy, 59,* 189–200.

Pridham, K.R., & Schutz, M.E. (1985). Rationale for a language for naming problems from a nursing perspective. *Image: The Journal of Nursing Scholarship, XVII*(4), 122–127.

Rappaport, J. (1981). In praise of paradox: A social policy of empowerment over prevention. *American Journal of Community Psychology, 9*(1), 1–25.

Schindehette, S., & Wescott, G. (1993, January 18). *Deciding not to die. People,* pp. 85–86.

Toffler, A. (1981). *The third wave.* Toronto: Bantam.

Woman makes plea to end life. (1991, November 29). *The Globe and Mail,* Section A, p. 4.

World Health Organization. (1980). *International classification of impairments, disabilities and handicaps (ICIDH).* Geneva, Switzerland: Author.

CHAPTER 58

Professional Responsibility in Times of Change

1967 ELEANOR CLARKE SLAGLE LECTURE

WILMA L. WEST

W e are now convened for the final day of a conference in celebration of the 50th anniversary of our professional life. Behind us lie five decades of individual and group endeavor—endeavor to develop a profession, to define and refine a service, to improve an image and extend its acceptance, to recruit others to our ranks and train them for perpetuation of our ideals, to research new and better ways of accomplishing our goals.

At this milestone in our history, one could be tempted to look back through the years and analyze the functional relationship between endeavors and accomplishments. Such stock-taking would surely yield an inventory of assets in many areas of effort in which we might feel mutual pride. It would also, however, show liabilities for which we remain collectively responsible. Still other accounts might appear as outstanding or receivable, thus implying the necessity for continued effort in the commitment to further progress. Depending on the perspective and purpose of the individual doing the analysis, this measure of our first 50 years might be impressive, discouraging, or inconclusive with respect to net accomplishment.

Santayana has warned that "He who neglects history will be condemned to repeat it." However, awareness and understanding of effort input with reference to success or failure of outcome are most functional when new approaches are being brought to the solution of old problems. If, on the other hand, changing or new conditions prevail and hence a different set of problems is presented, there is diminishing value in more than brief review of the methods of other people and times. The example of the inadequacy of conventional defenses in a nuclear age is the obvious one, but professional personnel in medical and educational fields today face a dilemma equal to that of the military in recognizing that old ways of solving problems are no longer adequate.

Let us turn, then, from any comfortable reflection on our past to the infinitely more exciting exercise of projecting our future. Wisely approached, this can be as scientific as a retrospective analysis and surely it is a more dynamic course if we wish to have a part in determining our future rather than merely accepting one on assignment or default of others.

One cannot be in the practice of any of the health professions today without being keenly aware of the many forces shaping his future roles and responsibilities. Nor can he neglect his duty to examine the implications of these forces in three dimensions: for himself as a professional person, for the profession of which he is a member, and for the professional organization which represents and promotes his individual and group interests. In brief, the questions currently confronting us are: What is happening in both our immediate and larger worlds? and, What does this mean to us?

The general stage for this discussion may be set by an analogy from another field that is strikingly similar to that of medicine. Francis Keppel, former commissioner of the Office of Education, Department of Health, Education, and Welfare, says that America is entering a third revolution in education. In the first revolution, education of the masses was achieved by the establishment of the public school system. Later, equality of education for all people became the rallying cry for school reform. Now the astounding advances in technology demand specialized and high-quality education for all regardless of race, creed, or social class.[1]

Today this country is well into a similar multistaged reorganization of health and medical care in which equal availability and high quality of health services are sought for all people. The bipartisan endorsement of providing services to meet two of man's most fundamental needs—for education and health care—has removed the question from the arena of welfare and politics and placed it in the larger domain of basic human development.

Whether one agrees with these trends wholly, partially, reluctantly, or not at all, one fact is virtually undeniable today: comprehensive health care, among others of man's needs, is beyond individual attainment for far too many people. If we accept this fact, we can accept the organization of increasingly costly and complex programs designed to reduce disease and disability among victims of economic disparity and to raise the health standards of our country as a whole.

"Governmental involvement (then) in the financing and organization of health services is here to stay and there is every indication that it will increase."[2] I submit, however, that governmental participation and individual responsibility are neither incompatible nor mutually exclusive. In fact, we must go even further in pursuit of a rationale that is in tune with both our changing times and a high standard of personal and professional integrity. I therefore tend to agree with another commentator on this subject who has said that "placing health in the category of the rights of man involves the transformation of a social desire into a moral imperative."[3] This imperative has been stated as follows by the New York Academy of Medicine: "That *all people* should have . . . *equal opportunity* to obtain a *high quality* of *comprehensive health care.*"

It is difficult to see how anyone could mount an argument against the humanitarian elements of this high goal. In the sense that the primary orientation of the professions is to the community interest, there *must* be concern for all people on the basis of equal opportunity and with a standard of the highest possible quality that it is within our ability to provide. Implications of most of the key phrases in this all-encompassing objective are clear. However, the last dimension—comprehensive health care—bears elaboration because it is with reference to this focus that we will examine how our profession can best adapt its philosophy and practice to future requirements.

At our annual conference in Minneapolis last year, the theme was "Dimensions of Change." Many of us, I am sure, recall the message of several thoughtful speakers who helped us read signs among today's maze of medical plans and programs that are as complex and confusing as the newest multistory interchange of highways around our large cities. I hope we also recall the repeated emphasis on *health,* as well as illness, on *prevention* of disease and disability, in addition to seeking the cures not yet discovered, on *maintenance and promotion of well-being,* not just being satisfied that there is an "absence of infirmity,"[4] on *continuity of care,* in lieu of only episodic attention to emergency conditions, and on *comprehensive health services* that must replace the diagnostic or categorical approach of conventional medicine.

The trends in these directions are unmistakable. They are also irreversible. To recognize them, however, is only the first step. We must also interpret their meaning for each of our specialty areas and aggressively adapt or redesign our roles to provide a more viable future service.

No one person can or should do this for all facets of his profession. Each must, however, do it for his own focus of interest and with all the professional outlook and insight he can muster. I can best relate these changing trends and their implications to the field of pediatrics, with which I have been most closely involved in recent years. I shall attempt to do so in the general framework of comprehensive health care for children and, more specifically, with reference to selected groups which present us with some very challenging opportunities to develop a preventive role for our profession. I shall conclude with some thoughts on the implications of these and other changes for the profession as a whole.

Comprehensive Health Care for Children

What is meant by comprehensive health care for children? This is a term that is variously defined, but on the conceptual level, I prefer the following statement to all others that I have read: "By comprehensive, we mean a constellation of health services that focuses on the patient as an individual human being rather than as a collection of assorted organ systems, some of which are diseased."[5] On the practical level, we believe this ideal must be translated into programs which include health supervision in the various parameters of growth and development and the regular use of specific devices for screening deficits and dysfunctions. Comprehensive health care for children, we feel, is committed to enhancing normal development as insurance against disease or, failing that objective, to the earliest possible casefinding of those conditions which have their origin in prenatal causes or in the disabling illnesses of infancy and the preschool years.

Both the number and scope of programs designed to provide health care for children are greater today than ever before. The idea behind them, however, is hardly a new one. For it was in 1890 in France that the first nursing conferences and milk stations were established to provide preventive health services for lower socio-economic segments of the child population. At that time the motive was to reduce the enormously high infant and preschool child mortality, but from these early beginnings, clinic services of similar types have developed throughout the world. In the United States, the milk stations of the World War I era subsequently became known as well-baby clinics and today, in many areas, are called child health conferences.

It is interesting to trace the broadening philosophy of these forerunners of modern comprehensive health care for children. Because such enterprises were designed to provide health supervision of well children, one of their primary functions was to screen children for evidence of abnormality or illness that might warrant referral for care.

A classic text on preventive medicine and public health[6] tells us that the child health conference was originally necessary because a large segment of the population was unable to pay for health supervision. However, it also goes on to point out that even today such services cannot be transferred to the private practitioner. The reason, the authors state, is that education and training of medical students is still largely oriented to the patient with cellular pathology, with the result that many practitioners today have limited interest in and knowledge of the principles and techniques of health supervision of growing children. Furthermore, child health personnel even in recent years have been largely preoccupied with the development of treatment and training programs for handicapped children.

And so, it seems, have occupational therapists in pediatrics. Thus we, too, have been slow to develop a role in prevention that might greatly enhance our total professional contribution to health care. Although our traditional commitment to medicine and our orientation to illness and treatment are understandable, our greater development of a preventive role, which is "an integral part of all medical practice, wherever it may be and under whatever auspices"[7] is long overdue.

There is even a sense of urgency to the situation that cannot be escaped. Consider for example the number and diversity of settings in which new health-care programs for children are constantly being developed. The well-child clinics or child health conferences that have already been mentioned are standard services of state and local health departments, but they are only one of several locales where continuing health supervision of children is assuming ever greater importance.

Probably the best known among others that I will discuss here are the Head Start programs that have received extensive publicity in the brief 2 years since their inception. Although the initial focus of these efforts was on enrichment of experience in preparation for school, a spin-off benefit of major importance has been identification and treatment of health deficits. It is of significance to us that the range of these deficits goes far beyond the dental and nutritional problems inevitable in the target populations and includes a high incidence of retarded or deviant physical and psychosocial development. As we well know, the chances for remediation of many such problems are infinitely better at age 3 or 4 than at beginning school age which, until now, has provided our earliest large-scale screening opportunity.

Another very new program of the Office of Economic Opportunity which was launched late this past summer could provide an even richer locus for occupational therapy in a preventive role. This is the development of Parent and Child Centers that is currently taking place in 36 American communities to provide services for disadvantaged families who have preschool children. A prime objective of these centers will be the use of techniques and processes both to prevent deviations and deficits and to stimulate development to the maximum potential. Among the skills and experience sought for staff are the ability to recognize and understand the developmental stages of young children and prescribe a plan for progress to meet each child's individual needs.[8]

To pediatric occupational therapists who have been concerned with the larger objective of optimal child growth and development as well as with restoration of impaired function, the possibilities inherent in these new centers must indeed be exciting. Think, for example, of the broad range of activities that could be used to provide multisensory input directed to the development of intellectual, emotional, social, and physical skills. The graded and guided use of activities for such purposes is so integral a part of occupational therapy that this would seem to be a most fitting application of our skills to plan, elicit, interpret, and modify both performance and behavior.

There are other groups of children for whom health surveillance could provide either prevention or earlier treatment. Sparked by the increasing prevalence of day-time employment of both parents or the absence of one parent and employment of the other, day care facilities have become a way of life for thousands of young American children. The larger of these, the day care centers, are units with seven to 75 or more children, a staff of one or more persons, and an organized program. In these settings today, ages of children usually range upwards from $2\frac{1}{2}$ years, this being the minimum age for most children to participate in group play or other organized activities. What an opportunity there is here to prevent, restrict, or retard development of problems we now see only when they are entrenched and disabling, often to a severe degree.

A final example is a group of children which has received special attention during the past year and is already providing the occupational therapist with a role in screening, evaluation, and programming as well as in treatment. This is the group served by the Children and Youth projects sponsored by the Children's Bureau.

Organized in areas of economic and social disruption, these projects are designed to provide comprehensive health care for large numbers of children who, under existing circumstances, have only marginal opportunity to develop a healthy mind and body. Now, however, a broad range of health professionals is being assembled to provide services which should greatly improve their future outlook.

Included in the authorized core staff for children and youth projects is an occupational therapist whose job description reads quite differently from the specifications for other pediatric roles. If a few of these promising new positions can be filled by therapists with vision as well as skill, there are few limits on the extent to which they will be permitted to develop a broader role. For example: in New York City, two pediatric neurologists on a children and youth project added an occupational therapist to assist them in screening for neurological deficits; in Dallas and in Denver, pediatricians directing diagnostic clinics use their therapists to evaluate motor performance and behavior adjustment and to participate in programming based on team findings and recommendations; and in several other areas of the country, therapists are involving children in activities which permit assessment in numerous areas of function and providing selected experiences to promote development of neuromuscular, emotional, and intellectual competencies of children.

These, then, are some of the programs made possible by the federal-state alliance to extend and improve health services for increasing numbers of people. They require of all professions a careful appraisal of changes that may be necessary as we jointly seek creative and workable solutions to both old and new problems. Although we have centered attention on one specialty of our profession, it is intriguing to think about how the number and kinds of changes in pediatrics today will inevitably, in time, affect every other age group and specialty field of occupational therapy.

Furthermore, there are equally radical changes occurring simultaneously in patterns of delivering health and medical services to all people. Witness, for example, the burgeoning community mental health programs and consider the implications of trends in that specialty of our profession. Are there not elements here, paralleling the new kinds of community-based services in pediatrics, which are dictating programs concerned with the maintenance and promotion of health as well as the treatment of illness? And hence, are there not here, too, strong indications for increased emphasis on the preventive role of occupational therapy?

Of course there are, and many progressive occupational therapists in both these and other specialties of our profession have already taken steps to keep pace with trends that require new or expanded roles. Furthermore, they have done so with such effectiveness that they have created roles and functions that greatly improve the image of our profession. In a sense, therefore, my commentary only reflects what I consider to be the best abroad in practice today, with a few thoughts on where, how, and why it seems particularly urgent that we intensify our efforts in these directions and at this time. I fear, however, that there are yet too many among us who do not sufficiently appreciate current trends and who therefore are not lending their efforts to hasten and make credible more functional roles throughout the profession. The platform at a general session of our annual conference and assured publication in our professional journal lend temptation to speak frankly to one's colleagues. And, the occasion of a golden anniversary provides a good point at which to cross the treacherous terrain of prophecy and hazard a glimpse of where our best future directions may lie. He who does so will always run the chance of suggesting some wrong turns, but he who does not has missed both an opportunity and a responsibility to share with others his views on areas of mutual concern.

We Are Committed to Our Profession as a Whole

I would like, now, to discuss some ramifications of these thoughts in terms of the profession as a whole rather than in the framework of any one or more specialty areas of practice. For, regardless of our individual concerns with separate fields, it is to the whole profession that we are jointly committed to and for which we must cooperatively work. My remaining remarks will explore some of the reasons why it seems important that this be so.

What is the relevance to us as a professional group of the changes I have discussed, of other changes that are taking place in patterns of providing health services, and of the implications these have for traditional and transitional roles in our profession? Is it enough that there is a growing number of clinicians in each of our specialty fields who are continually sharpening conventional skills and also developing new ones? Can we rely on the work of a small but increasing number of researchers among us to confirm the scientific basis of our practice? Does the greater sophistication of today's authors sufficiently raise the level of our professional literature? Will the growing number of our members who are obtaining graduate degrees insure a higher quality of performance in the future? Are changes that are being effected by the more progressive among our educators adequate to the preparation of tomorrow's therapists? In short, will the leadership of these and other significantly contributing individuals suffice? Indeed, should it have to?

Decidedly not. What is absent from this kind of thinking is the concept of group responsibility—responsibility for awareness and interpretation of those changes which affect any part of our profession, and responsibility for whatever group action is appropriate to facilitate or hasten adjustment to change. Thus, although we clearly recognize that "All occupations are dependent on the individual contributions" of those who practice them, we must also realize that "the effectiveness of an occupation is not gauged by individual efforts alone; the total efforts of occupational members working together with some degree of cooperation must also be considered. The public image of an occupation, then, is in part individual and in part collective. . . . Moreover, the goals of an occupation are only in a limited sense individual, for the individual responsibility of practitioners and a consciousness of the aims of the occupation are very much a function of collective action."9

There are, of course, many terms for the kind of collective action here referred to. Among them is what I shall call professional consciousness and responsibility. This is an attribute that we in occupational therapy have to a quite considerable degree. It has served us well in the 50 years of our professional development to date, primarily, I believe, because we have used it more in the sense of professional responsiveness to public interest and need than for purposes of protecting or promoting our constituent individuals and groups. These two major purposes of a profession— meeting external obligations to society on the one hand, and internal loyalties to members on the other—may often be in conflict. That they have not created serious problems or dichotomies for us up to this time may be viewed as a mixed blessing, for readings in the sociology of development of the professions make it clear that it is only a matter of time until they do. Factors which may have delayed this apparently inevitable process include our extremely small size and the relative homogeneity of a profession with only incompletely developed specialties.

Trend Toward Decreased Professional Unity

With the passage of time, however, we are experiencing both an increase in size and a proliferation of special skills among our members. As these two dimensions grow, we become increasingly subject to the influence of factors which will tend to decrease professional unity and promote segmentation in accordance with divergent interests and strengths as they develop among us. Although it will undoubtedly create some problems, this trend is by no means undesirable. On the contrary, it usually brings with it both an improved service, which results from increased knowledge and skill of specialists, and a growing professional influence which can be used to improve the status of those who provide that service.

There are signs that the era of segmentation is already upon us; witness for example, the increasing number of special interest meetings and concurrent sessions scheduled at this year's annual conference. While neither deploring the problems nor lauding the advantages an increase in this trend will bring, I hope that we will retain an attitude of general professional consciousness and concern for as long as we exist. Conviction of the need for this lies in the belief that "the chief factor. . . . in the accomplishments of any profession is the unified, aggressive efforts of its members."10

Numerous theories have been put forth to explain why persons pursuing an occupation come together and associate in a formal manner. These include everything from the likely initial motivation for exchange with those doing the same work, to such presently accepted objectives as raising standards of competence, formulating codes of ethics, improving education, undertaking protective and promotional activities, and many others. The activities of associations as major interest groups which participate in planning and policy decisions on matters of concern to them are generally thought of as a development of recent years undertaken to counter the influence of governmental regulations on professional activities; in fact, however, these date back at least three centuries when, as one writer says, "it was characteristic of the times that powers and duties of so extensive a nature were granted to vocational associations that they may be regarded as organs of the state."[11] Thus they are illustrative of the influence a well-organized profession can have on public decisions and policies.

I make no case for our professional association to aspire to this degree of power. I do, however, believe that both as individuals and as a professional group we should be assuming a far more frequent and contributing part in the planning of health services. It will, in fact, be mandatory that we do so if, as I said earlier, we are to have a part in shaping our own development.

Izutsu believes that "it is not too late to achieve positions of leadership that will determine the future" of our profession.[12] However, he also lists several steps that we must take if we are to remain equal to changing patterns in the organization and delivery of health services. Among these are the development of leaders not only to plan for therapy but to think in the broad spectrum of social planning; training of therapists in public health principles and procedures; and exposure, in our training, to community-oriented settings and other health team members in lieu of training primarily in hospital settings.

Professionally, We Often Resist Change

I do not suppose any of us knows, with any degree of certainty, the ideal future course for our profession. We do, however, see many signs that it must keep changing if it is to stay abreast of the larger world of which it is a part. Change is seldom easy or comfortable. Yet there is little about the world in which we live today that is more characteristic of it than the continual and fast-moving changes which transcend every aspect of our lives.

Although each of us makes the necessary adaptation to these changes as they affect our personal concerns and activities, we are slower as a group to adjust our professional directions and developments to that which is new. We are often, in fact, resistant to the suggested need for change and all that it implies in the necessity for new learning and the establishment of new roles and functions. We are also reluctant to explore new potentials, to experiment, to take an occasional risk.

From Therapist to Health Agent

Increasingly, today, I believe we should identify with the field of health services, thus broadening our traditional, more limited identification with medicine. We should enlarge our concept from that of being a therapist to one of functioning as a health agent with responsibility to help ensure normal growth and development. We should think more about roles in prevention as well as in treatment and rehabilitation, about socioeconomic and cultural as well as biological causes of disease and dysfunction, and about serving health needs of people in many other settings than the hospital.

One occasion on which this was expressed in a very effective way by a number of our colleagues was the conference on research in occupational and physical therapy held last February in Puerto Rico. In one of the discussion groups, there was studied avoidance of the term "patient," which many felt limited their concern to illness, and a plea for consideration of health as only one aspect of the developmental process of man which should not be isolated from other factors impinging on life. This kind of thinking and discussion culminated in the group's consideration of its topic in the framework of what they called "the continuum of health services which reflect the needs of man in his environment."[13]

A broad frame of reference? Admittedly, but it is also entirely in keeping with our traditional philosophy of concern for the person rather than just his disability. For us, therefore, the idea possesses what might be called "instant validity." It now needs rapid if not instant implementation.

We are living today in a world that is vastly different from that when occupational therapy began. It matters not so much that it has taken 50 years to reach this day, as that the next 50 see more, and more rapid, progress than the last. It matters less that we are still struggling to define our profession than that we build a broader base for the better definition that will one day be written. It matters most of all that we recognize the responsibility of the profession to change with changing demands for its services, to adapt via new approaches, to assume different roles, to develop the preparation for them, and to recruit in a new mold rather than by recasting the prototype of an earlier time.

On the eve of her retirement from active work in our national organization, Eleanor Clarke Slagle was paid the following tribute:

> Those of us who have been privileged to follow the winding trail of those years know of struggles, of courage in facing criticism, of disappointments and rewards, of patient waiting, persistent faith, and devoted work. The questing youth of our profession accepts both with commendation and condemnation what has been so painstakingly accomplished through this quarter century. But when they too can look back over an equal span of service in this field, they, and occupational therapy, will still be moving to the measure of the thought of Eleanor Clarke Slagle.[14]

That "equal span of service" has now passed so we, too, are looking back over the second quarter of a century which immediately precedes the present day. It seemed fitting that we do so in the context of both our practice to which she gave so much, and our professional association which she helped to organize, served as an officer in four capacities, and directed as its executive for many years. I, for one, hold to much that she obviously held high among her goals for the profession. Among those goals, I feel sure, was one related to the need for professional responsibility at all times. In times of change such as these, that need and our response to it will be of great importance in determining the next 50 years of our professional life. At the turn of the 21st century, when yet another generation looks back on these times, they may they see that ours was a dynamic posture of professional consciousness and responsibility.

References

1. Keppel, Francis, *The Necessary Revolution in American Education.* New York: Harper and Row (1966).

2. Burns, Evalina, "Policy Decisions Facing the United States in Financing and Organizing Health Care," *Public Health Reports,* 81, No. 8 (August 1966).

3. Dearing, W. P., "Prepaid Group Practice Medical Care Plans," *Public Health Reports,* 77, No. 10 (October 1962).

4. Preamble to the Constitution of the World Health Organization.

5. Kissick, William L., "Trends in the Utilization of Rehabilitation Manpower," *Manpower Utilization in Rehabilitation in New York City,* New York: New York City Regional Interdepartmental Rehabilitation Committee (September 1966).

6. Sartwell, P.E., Ed., *Maxcy-Rosenau Preventive Medicine and Public Health,* 9th ed. New York: Meredith Publishing Co. (1965).

7. Freeman, Ruth B., "Impact of Public Health on Society," *Public Health Reports,* 76, No. 4 (April 1961).

8. *Criteria for Parent and Child Centers,* Washington, D.C.: Office of Economic Opportunity (July 19, 1967).

9. Vollmer, Howard M. and Mills, Donald L., *Professionalization,* Englewood Cliffs, New Jersey: Prentice-Hall, Inc. (1966).

10. Stinnett, T. M., "Accomplishments of the Organized Teaching Profession," *The Teacher and Professional Organizations,* Washington, D.C.: The National Education Association (1956).

11. Carr-Saunders, A. M. and Wilson, P. A., "The Rise and Aims of Professional Associations," *The Professions,* Oxford: The Clarendon Press (1933).

12. Izutsu, Satoru, "The Changing Patterns of Patient Care" (A Position Paper) *Research Conference in Occupational Therapy and Physical Therapy,* New York: American Physical Therapy Association (1967).

13. Group Report, "Research in Patient Care," *Proceedings of the Research Conference in Occupational Therapy and Physical Therapy,* New York: American Physical Therapy Association (To be published).

14. "In the Past, Pride—In the Future, Faith," A Documentary of the Heritage, Growth, and Outlook of the American Occupational Therapy Association. Produced by the Association for its 41st Annual Conference, New York, New York (October 21, 1958).

CHAPTER 59

Reexamining Concepts of Occupation and Occupation-Based Models: Occupational Therapy and Community Development

LEANNE L. LECLAIR

ommunity development is "the process of organizing and/or supporting community groups
in their identification of important concerns
and issues, and in their ability to plan and implement
strategies to mitigate their concerns and resolve their
issues" (Labonte, 2007, p. 90). A community development approach responds to community-identified
needs, building local resources and capacities and
self-sustaining programs that foster change within
the community and potentially beyond (Laverack &
Labonte, 2000). Community development is different from community-based approaches. The distinction lies in who identifies the issues or concerns and
who holds the decision-making power (Labonte). In a
community-based approach, professionals or agencies
define the problem and develop strategies to remedy
the problem. The professionals or agencies may involve
local community members and groups to assist in solving the problem; however, the decision-making power
lies primarily with the professionals, agencies, and/or
program funder. For example, home care programs and
services use a community-based approach to provide
specific services to individuals living in the community that meet criteria established by policy makers.
Community-based approaches are important, but they
are not community development, which attempts to
support community groups in resolving concerns as
group members define them. Community development, like community-based approaches, does not focus only on health issues; it may also focus on issues
and initiatives that promote the social and economic
development of a community.

The term *community* has been defined in many ways.
However, according to Labonte (2007), when working
in community development, the community must
self-identify as a group with a common interest.

> We all belong to multiple communities at any
> given time. The essence of being a community
> is that there is something that is "shared." We
> cannot really say that a community exists until
> a group with a shared identity exists (Toronto
> Department of Public Health, 1994, p. 2).

A growing body of literature supports the role of occupational therapists in community development (Algado
& Cardona, 2005; Banks & Head, 2004; Bass-Haugen,
Henderson, Larson, & Matuska, 2005; Christiansen & Townsend, 2004; Lauckner, Pentland, & Patterson, 2007; Restall & Ripat, 2008; Restall, Ripat, &
Stern, 2003; Scaletti, 1999; Townsend, Cockburn, Letts,
Thibeault, & Trentham, 2007; Trentham, Cockburn, &
Shin, 2007; Wilcock, 2006). In the most recent guidelines for Canadian practice, Townsend, Beagen, et al.
(2007) broadened occupational therapy client categories to include communities, recognizing that occupational therapists have a unique contribution to make to
the health and well- being of communities. Townsend,
Cockburn, et al. called on occupational therapists to
engage in enabling social change at the macro-level using a community development approach. "Outcomes
of interest to occupational therapists in enabling social
change may be to advance occupational rights" (p. 155)
through occupational justice.

Occupational justice is a term that has emerged in
the occupational therapy literature over the past decade. It speaks to the occupational nature of all human
beings and the right of all individuals to participate in
meaningful and purposeful occupations (Townsend &

Wilcock, 2004). However, if occupational therapists wish to pursue occupational justice at the macro-level, "they need to build on their abilities in working cooperatively and in partnership with communities" (Pollard, Sakellariou, & Kronenberg, 2008, p. 27), concepts that are in keeping with community development. The purpose of this paper is to explore the challenges that both the definitions and categorizations of occupation and the application of occupation-based models of practice pose to occupational therapy practice in community development.

Key Issues

Definitions and Categorizations of Occupation

It is important to acknowledge that while our professional title has included occupation from the beginning, the focus on occupation in practice has wavered over the years. For several decades, the profession lost sight of its roots in occupation, working within the reductionistic, biomedical paradigm (Dickie, 2008). However, in the late 1970s, the profession again began to acknowledge occupation as the foundation of occupational therapy, and discourse about the definition and nature of *occupation* persists today (Dickie). Definitions of core concepts are the foundation of a profession's research and practice and shape its traditions through their emphasis and

values (Pierce, 2001). Currently, there is no consensus on a universal definition of *occupation* within the profession of occupational therapy. However, the literature is replete with richly textured and diverse explanations of the concept (Watson & Fourie, 2004).

Table 59.1 provides an overview of several definitions of occupation cited in the occupational therapy literature. Many definitions share the idea that occupation is experienced by the individual and is subjective. Some definitions assert the idea that value and meaning are also derived from cultural context and that participation in occupation benefits not only the individual but the communities in which they live, work, and play. Polatajko, Backman, et al. (2007) explored the characteristics of human occupation. They indicated that "the who of occupation may not only be a single person, but pairs, groups, communities, populations and even societies" (p. 40).

Shared or collective occupations?

Wilcock's (2006) definition of *occupation* in Table 59.1 supports the idea of shared occupation. Similarly, Doble and Caron (2008) suggested that individuals have the need "to engage in occupations with others who share common experiences, interests, values or goals" (p. 187). Eakman (2007) examined the social complexity of occupation, exploring occupation as a phenome-

Table 59.1. Definitions of *Occupation*

Author	Definition
Canadian Association of Occupational Therapists (1997)	Occupation is groups of activities and tasks of everyday life, named, organized, and given value and meaning by individuals and a culture; occupation is everything people do to occupy themselves, including looking after themselves (self-care), enjoying life (leisure), and contributing to the social and economic fabric of their communities (productivity) (p. 34).
McLaughlin-Gray (1997)	Occupation is perceived as "doing" by the individual, is goal-directed, carries meaning for the individual, and is repeatable (p. 16).
Golledge (1998)	Occupations are the daily living tasks that are part of an individual's lifestyle (p. 102).
Christiansen, Baum, & Bass-Haugen (2005)	Occupation is engagement in activities, tasks, and roles for the purpose of productive pursuit, maintaining one's self in the environment, and for purposes of relaxation, entertainment, creativity, and celebration (p. 548).
Kielhofner (2008)	Occupation is the doing of work, play, or activities of daily living within a temporal, physical, and sociocultural context that characterizes much of human life (p. 5).
Wilcock (2006)	Occupation provides the mechanism for social interaction and societal development and growth, forming the foundation of community, local, and national identity because individuals not only engage in separate pursuits, they are able to plan and execute group activity to the extent of national government or to achieve international goals for individual, mutual, and community purposes (p. 9).

non that may be co-constructed by individuals who are mutually engaged. Zemke and Clark (1996) described the idea of co-occupations of social beings, which by definition are occupations that involve at least two active participants, for example, infant and caregiver interactions. Segal (1998, 1999) also studied the idea of shared occupations, focusing her work on families. Family occupations occur when the whole family is engaged in an occupation together, for example, partaking in a family meal. However, the level of engagement in the occupation may not be equal among family members and their purpose and experiences may differ (Segal, 1998).

The notion that occupations can be shared among individuals, groups, and communities is not widely recognized or developed in the occupational therapy literature. Trentham et al. (2007) discussed the use of community development strategies to enable engagement in shared occupations. They emphasized the importance of supporting individuals' engagement in shared occupations "such as planning, learning, and skill building in a group context" (p. 62) to influence individual and community health. Christiansen and Townsend (2004) discuss shared occupations as being central to successful community living. Polgar and Landry (2004) discussed community participation in occupation. They described communities as "groups of people acting collectively in a desired or needed occupation" (p. 210). The community comes together in the performance of a common or collective occupation. For example, an occupational therapist using a community development approach to promote the health of a community of older adults could facilitate the planning of a community forum to bring together community members to identify their concerns and priorities for action. Each individual may have a different reason for participation in the community occupation and a different approach to participation. However, by identifying and focusing on common issues, community members declare a shared purpose and work together when acting on a particular goal. At the community forum, community members may identify that an issue of central concern is that they lack a place to congregate outdoors in their community. The community members may decide that they would like to develop a green space where they can engage in meaningful activities and contribute to the community. They may express an interest in developing a community garden for all to enjoy. The community garden can serve various purposes for the community members. Some individu-

als may enjoy the occupation of gardening, while others would like to spend time in the garden socializing or exercising. For some, the planning and organization of the community garden provides them with meaningful occupation. However, all partake in the shared occupation of building a community garden. Participation as a collective enables groups of people to fulfill certain functions and meet needs that they would be unable to achieve individually. "Participation in collective doing and interconnected occupations provides members with a sense of purpose, with a source of motivation and drive, and with an appreciation of their ability to share in shaping their communities" (Polgar & Landry, p. 211).

When working within a community development approach, the idea of shared occupation becomes fundamental to the process. The occupational therapist supports engagement in shared occupations and may take on various roles in the process. He or she may assist in bringing together different organizations that can contribute to building the community garden. For example, the municipal government may be able to offer assistance with procuring land for the garden; a garden nursery in the community may be able to donate plants; another business may be able to donate benches. The role the occupational therapist plays in the community development process will vary depending on the needs and capacities of the community. At times, the occupational therapist may take on a leadership role and at other times, he or she may serve as a facilitator in the community development process while other community members take on a leadership role.

Categorization of occupation

The Canadian Association of Occupational Therapists' (CAOT) definition, like other definitions of occupation, suggests that occupation can be categorized into three main areas: self-care, productivity, and leisure. However, the categorization of occupations is often problematic (Christiansen & Townsend, 2004; Dickie, 2008; Hammell, 2004, 2009). While it would seem that the categories fit some areas of practice, they do not appear to be universal. Occupational therapists working in community development may find categorizing occupations into self-care, productivity, and leisure does not fit with their practice; these categories and definitions may not be relevant to the collective occupations of a community. Christiansen and Townsend propose occupational categories that contribute to the success of communities, including social sanctions, cultural rituals, shared history, art, magic and religion, volunteerism, work, and sustainable practices. However, there has been very little discussion or debate in the occupational therapy literature about the occupational nature of communities. Without a greater understanding of the nature of community occupation, categorization is dubious. As occupational therapy continues to evolve and emerge in different areas of practice, such as community development, the profession needs to examine the categorization of occupation and its application to all clients (e.g., individuals, groups, communities).

Occupational Therapy Models of Practice

A core concept of occupational therapy models is client-centred practice. Townsend and Wilcock (2004) emphasized the link between the collaborative and inclusive nature of community development with "occupational therapy's social vision of client-centred approaches for enabling empowerment through occupations" (p. 77). Traditionally, the development of client-centred practice in occupational therapy has focused primarily on working with individuals. However, efforts to frame client-centred practice beyond the individual are emerging. For example, the Client-Centred Strategies Framework (Restall et al., 2003) provides strategies that occupational therapists can use when working in various contexts, including community or-

ganizing and coalition advocacy, both in keeping with a community development approach. Recently, Restall and Ripat (2008) explored occupational therapists' application of the strategies proposed in the Framework to their practice. A key finding of the study revealed that occupational therapists felt they lacked the knowledge and skills needed to practice community organizing and coalition advocacy. While the focus of their study was on the application of client-centred strategies in these areas, it speaks to the lack of exposure and experience therapists feel they have in community development approaches.

Occupational therapists working in community development may draw on several different models or approaches commonly used by other professionals working in this area of practice to inform their process. Table 59.2 provides an overview of the Community Development Continuum Model (Jackson, Mitchell, & Wright, 1989) and Rothman and Tropman's (1987) Taxonomy of Community Development. Occupational therapists have used the Community Development Continuum Model to frame practice in community development (Scaletti, 1999; Trentham et al., 2007). This model identifies five stages that link individual and social change (Townsend, Cockburn, et al., 2007). Scaletti proposed an approach that occupational therapists can use when working with this model in child

Table 59.2. Community Development Models

Community Development Continuum Model (Jackson et al., 1989)	Taxonomy of Community Development (Rothman & Tropman, 1987)
Developmental casework • develops the capacity of individuals to make informed decisions and advocate for their own needs	Locality development • process-oriented, stressing consensus and cooperation and aimed at building community capacity, group identity, and a sense of community
Mutual support • focuses on strengthening relationships with family, friends, and neighbours and forming new supports for self-help or mutual aid	Social planning • task-oriented, focused on rational and empirical problem solving, usually by an outside expert, with the goal of providing goods and services to people who need them
Issue identification and campaigns • deals with issues that move beyond the personal to a social, political, or community level	Social action • both task and process oriented, seeks the redistribution of power and resources for a disadvantaged segment of the population with the aim of changing policies of formal organizations
Participation and control of services • people in the community attempt to exercise greater control by joining groups or forming new organizations	
Social movements • through creating and joining social movements, participants seek some fundamental change in decisions that affect their lives and in the way those decisions are made • may be cooperative or confrontational	

and adolescent mental health. Another widely recognized community development framework used by occupational therapists is Rothman and Tropman's three models: locality development, social planning, and social action. "Each model is characterized by particular assumptions about where to start and where to focus in enabling change in micro- and macro-level structures" (Townsend, Cockburn, et al., p. 163). Trentham et al. used Rothman and Tropman's taxonomy and the Community Development Continuum Model "to link their work with individuals to broader community development objectives" (p. 57). They provided suggestions of how an occupational perspective might fit within these models.

The elements that distinguish occupational therapy's contributions from those of other professionals are our focus on occupation and our use of occupation-based models of practice when working with clients. Yet, many models in occupational therapy focus on individuals (Thibeault & Hebert, 1997). Hammell (2009) stated that "current theories of occupation provide little space for consideration of the importance of fostering interdependence or of contributing to the well-being of others" (p. 11). Lawlor (2003) suggested that theoretical and research models are needed to capture the essence of socially occupied beings doing something with someone else that matters.

Application of occupation-based models in community development

The Canadian Model of Occupational Performance and Engagement (CMOP–E) (Polatajko, Davis, et al., 2007) and the Person-Environment-Occupation Model (PEO) (Law et al., 1996), like other occupation-based models of practice, pose a challenge for practitioners working in community development. The language and concepts of the CMOP–E are similar to those of the PEO. Like the PEO, the CMOP–E categorizes occupation into self-care, productivity, and leisure, a categorization that does not necessarily fit with the collective occupations that are the focus of a community development approach. The CMOP–E and the PEO address the cognitive, affective, and physical performance components of the person. These performance components are not easily translated to a community. For example, how would one describe or evaluate the cognitive, affective, or physical abilities of a community? The environmental components of the CMOP–E and the PEO are an important part of a community development approach because often the community is seeking to change en-

vironmental aspects; however, the physical, social, cultural, and institutional environments of a community can be quite different from those of an individual. Both models refer to the client's occupational performance, and, more recently, the CMOP–E has included occupational engagement. What are a community's occupational performance or engagement issues and how does an occupational therapist identify them?

There are very few examples of the application of occupation-based models of practice to communities in the occupational therapy literature. Watson and Wilson (2003) discuss the application of the concept of person-environment-occupation at a community level. They suggest that occupational therapists "offer a unique approach to assessing community needs, assets and resources by conducting task analysis of population characteristics (i.e., persons), environments (i.e., performance contexts), and community actions (i.e., tasks and activities) that support or hinder health" (Watson & Wilson, p. 158). While the constructs of person-environment-occupation may be applicable to community clients, occupational therapists must conceptualize the constructs in a different way than is outlined in the PEO or CMOP–E. However, thinking about the constructs in relation to communities is an important first step in developing occupation-based models of practice that will support occupational therapists work in community development.

Wilcock (1998) introduced the Ecological Sustainability Model of Health as a tool for occupational therapists to promote healthy relationships between people and their environments. She refers to it as an "occupation-focused ecosustainable community development approach" (2006, p. 222). This model requires a focus on eco-sustainability when participating in community development, which Wilcock (2006) argues should be part of all community development activities. Algado and Cardona (2005) applied the model in their work with Guatemalan refugees and suggested that occupational therapists can use human occupation to restore balance in the natural environment while also contributing to community development. While this model has some application for occupational therapists working in community development, it has not been widely used or cited in the occupational therapy literature.

Several authors have explored the gap that exists between theory and practice (Forsyth, Summerfield, & Kielhofner, 2005; Kielhofner, 2005; Lee, Taylor, Kielhofner, & Fisher, 2008). Kielhofner (2005) proposed that those who will ultimately use theory in practice should be involved in its generation. He emphasized cooperative efforts in which practitioners and academics work together to advance theory and practice. Therefore, future development of occupation-based models that pertain to community development practice should be "derived from the experiences of occupational therapists currently working in community development" (Lauckner et al., 2007, p. 323) in partnership with scholars who share an interest in this area. Occupational therapists are encouraged to participate in research that contributes to the evolution of existing occupation-based models that would allow for their broader application to community development.

Conclusion

In order for occupational therapy to articulate clearly its role in community development, greater heed needs to be given to our understanding of the application of our definitions and categorizations of occupation and occupation-based models of practice to community development. Given some of the current issues outlined in this paper, occupational therapists need to ask themselves about the nature of their work with communities. Are we enhancing participation in shared occupations? How might we categorize the community's occupations? Are we using occupation-based models of practice when working in community development? In an effort to advance the profession in community development, occupational therapy researchers and practitioners working with communities, along with their community partners, need to continue to explore and expand on the definition of shared occupation, categorizations of community occupations, and the development of occupation-based models of practice that can be used when working in community development.

Key Messages

- More critical discussion and debate is needed to further our understanding of collective or shared occupations.
- Occupational therapy needs to examine the categorization of occupation and its applications to all clients (e.g., individuals, groups, communities).
- There is a need for occupation-based models of practice that support occupational therapists working in community development.

Acknowledgements

I would like to thank Dr. Marcia Finlayson for her support and comments on various drafts of this paper, and the many colleagues and students who have challenged me to think critically about community development and occupational therapy practice.

References

Algado, S. S., & Cardona, C. E. (2005). The return of the corn men: An intervention project with a Mayan community of Guatemalan retornos. In F. Kronenberg, S. S. Algado, & N. Pollard (Eds.), *Occupational therapy without borders: Learning from the spirit of survivors* (pp. 336–350). Toronto, ON: Elsevier Churchill Livingstone.

Banks, S., & Head, B. (2004). Partnering occupational therapy and community development. *Canadian Journal of Occupational Therapy, 71*, 5–7.

Bass-Haugen, J., Henderson, M. L., Larson, B. A., & Matuska, K. (2005). Occupational issues of concern in populations. In C. H. Christiansen, C. M. Baum, & J. Bass-Haugen (Eds.), *Occupational therapy: Performance, participation, and well-being* (3rd ed., pp. 167–182). Thorofare, NJ: Slack Incorporated.

Canadian Association of Occupational Therapists. (1997). *Enabling occupation: An occupational therapy perspective*. Ottawa, ON: Author.

Christiansen, C., Baum, C., & Bass-Haugen, J. (Eds.). (2005). *Occupational therapy: Performance, participation and well-being* (3rd ed.). Thorofare, NJ: Slack Incorporated.

Christiansen, C. H., & Townsend, E. (Eds.). (2004). *Introduction to occupation: The art and science of living*. Upper Saddle River, NJ: Prentice Hall.

Dickie, V. (2008). What is occupation? In E. B. Crepeau, E. S. Cohn, & B. A. B. Schell (Eds.), *Willard and Spackman's occupational therapy* (11th ed., pp. 15–21). Philadelphia: Lippincott Williams & Wilkins.

Doble, S., & Caron, J. S. (2008). Occupational well-being: Rethinking occupational therapy outcomes. *Canadian Journal of Occupational Therapy, 75*, 184–190.

Eakman, A. (2007). Occupation and social complexity. *Journal of Occupational Science, 14*, 82–91.

Forsyth, K., Summerfield, L. M., & Kielhofner, G. (2005). Scholarship of practice: Making occupation-focused, theory-driven, evidence-based practice a reality. *British Journal of Occupational Therapy, 68*, 260–268.

Golledge, J. (1998). Distinguishing between occupation, purposeful activity and activity, part 1: Review and explanation. *British Journal of Occupational Therapy, 61*, 100–105.

Hammell, K. W. (2004). Dimensions of meaning in the occupations of daily life. *Canadian Journal of Occupational Therapy, 71*, 296–305.

Hammell, K. W. (2009). Sacred texts: A sceptical exploration of the assumptions underpinning theories of occupation. *Canadian Journal of Occupational Therapy, 76*, 6–13.

Jackson, T., Mitchell, S., & Wright, M. (1989). The community development continuum. *Community Health Studies, 13*(1), 66–73.

Kielhofner, G. (2005). A scholarship of practice: Creating discourse between theory, research and practice. *Occupational Therapy in Health Care, 19*(1/2), 7–16.

Kielhofner, G. (2008). *Model of human occupation: Theory and application* (4th ed.). Baltimore: Lippincott Williams & Wilkins.

Labonte, R. (2007). Community, community development, and the forming of authentic partnerships: Some critical reflections. In M. Minkler (Ed.), *Community organizing and community building for health* (2nd ed., pp. 88–102). New Brunswick, NJ: Rutgers University Press.

Lauckner, H., Pentland, W., & Patterson, M. (2007). Exploring Canadian occupational therapists' understanding of and experiences in community development. *Canadian Journal of Occupational Therapy, 74*, 314–325.

Laverack, G., & Labonte, R. (2000). A planning framework for community empowerment goals within health promotion. *Health Policy and Planning, 15*, 255–262.

Law, M., Cooper, B., Strong, S., Stewart, D., Rigby, P., & Letts, L. (1996). The Person–Environment–Occupation model: A transactive approach to occupational performance. *Canadian Journal of Occupational Therapy, 63*, 9–23.

Lawlor, M. C. (2003). The significance of being occupied: The social construction of childhood occupations. *American Journal of Occupational Therapy, 57*, 424–434. http://dx.doi.org/10.5014/ajot.57.4.424

Lee, S. W., Taylor, R., Kielhofner, G., & Fisher, G. (2008). Theory use in practice: A national survey of therapists who use the Model of Human Occupation. *American Journal of Occupational Therapy, 62*, 106–117.

McLaughlin-Gray, J. (1997). Application of the phenomenological method to the concept of occupation. *Journal of Occupational Science, 4*, 5–17.

Pierce, D. (2001). Untangling occupation and activity. *American Journal of Occupational Therapy, 55*, 138–146. http://dx.doi.org/10.5014/ajot.55.2.138

Polatajko, H., Backman, C., Baptiste, S., Davis, J., Eftekhar, P., Harvey, A., . . . Connor, A. (2007). Human occupation in context. In E. Townsend & H. Polatajko (Eds.), *Enabling occupation II: Advancing an occupational therapy vision for health, well-being, & justice through occupation* (pp. 37–61). Ottawa, ON: CAOT Publications ACE.

Polatajko, H., Davis, J., Stewart, D., Cantin, N., Amoroso, B. Purdie, L., & Zimmerman, D. (2007). Specifying the domain of concern: Occupation as core. In E. Townsend & H. Polatajko (Eds.), *Enabling occupation II: Advancing an occupational therapy vision for health, well-being, and justice through occupation* (pp. 13–36). Ottawa, ON: CAOT Publications ACE.

Polgar, J. M., & Landry, J. E. (2004). Occupations as a means to individual and group participation in life. In E. Townsend & C. H. Christiansen (Eds.), *Introduction to occupation: The art and science of living* (pp. 197–220). Upper Saddle River, NJ: Prentice Hall.

Pollard, N., Sakellariou, D., & Kronenberg, F. (2008). Political competence in occupational therapy. In N. Pollard, D. Sakellariou, & F. Kronenberg (Eds.), *A political practice of occupational therapy* (pp. 21–38). Edinburgh, UK: Elsevier.

Restall, G., & Ripat, J. (2008). Applicability and clinical utility of the client-centred strategies framework. *Canadian Journal of Occupational Therapy, 75*, 288–300.

Restall, G., Ripat, J., & Stern, M. (2003). A framework of strategies for client-centred practice. *Canadian Journal of Occupational Therapy, 70*, 103–112.

Rothman, J., & Tropman, J. (Eds.). (1987). *Strategies of community organization*. Itasca, IL: F. E. Peacock Publishers.

Scaletti, R. (1999). A community development role for occupational therapists working with children, adolescents and their families: A mental health perspective. *Australian Occupational Therapy Journal, 46*, 43–51.

Segal, R. (1998). The construction of family occupations: A study of families with chidren who have Attention Deficit/Hyperactivity Disorder. *Canadian Journal of Occupational Therapy, 65*, 286–292.

Segal, R. (1999). Doing for others: Occupations within families with children who have special needs. *Journal of Occupational Science, 6*(2), 1–8.

Thibeault, R., & Hebert, M. (1997). A congruent model for occupational therapy in health promotion. *Occupational Therapy International, 4*, 271–293.

Toronto Department of Public Health. (1994). *Making communities*. Toronto, ON: Department of Public Health.

Townsend, E., Beagan, B., Kumas-Tan, Z., Versnel, J., Iwama, M., Landry, J., . . . Brown, J. (2007). Enabling: Occupational therapy's core competency. In E. Townsend & H. Polatajko (Eds.), *Enabling occupation II: Advancing an occupational therapy vision for health, well-being, and justice through occupation* (pp. 87–133). Ottawa, ON: CAOT Publications ACE.

Townsend, E., Cockburn, L., Letts, L., Thibeault, R., & Trentham, B. (2007). Enabling social change. In E. Townsend & H. Polatajko (Eds.), *Enabling occupation II: Advancing an occupational therapy vision for health, well-being, and justice through occupation* (pp. 153–171). Ottawa, ON: CAOT Publications ACE.

Townsend, E., & Wilcock, A. (2004). Occupational justice and client-centred practice: A dialogue in progress. *Canadian Journal of Occupational Therapy, 71*, 75–87.

Trentham, B., Cockburn, L., & Shin, J. (2007). Health promotion and community development: An application of occupational therapy in primary health care. *Canadian Journal of Community Mental Health, 26*(2), 53–69.

Watson, D., & Wilson, S. A. (2003). *Task analysis: An individual approach* (2nd ed.). Bethesda, MD: AOTA Press.

Watson, R., & Fourie, M. (2004). Occupation and occupational therapy. In R. Watson & L. Swartz (Eds.), *Transformation through occupation* (pp. 19–32). London: Whurr Publishers.

Wilcock, A. A. (1998). *An occupational perspective of health.* Thorofare, NJ: Slack.

Wilcock, A. A. (2006). *An occupational perspective of health* (2nd ed.). Thorofare, NJ: Slack.

Zemke, R., & Clark, F. (Eds.). (1996). *Occupational Science: The evolving discipline.* Philadelphia: F. A. Davis.

CHAPTER 60

Change: Creating Our Own Reality

VIRGINIA G. FEARING

I have been a closet Muriel Driver Lecturer for years. Let me explain. Never dreaming that I might one day actually stand here, yearly I have challenged myself to identify a Muriel Driver Lecture topic that seemed timely and worth pursuing. In all the years of eagerly anticipating the topic chosen by the Muriel Driver Lecturer, my closet topic of the year has never come close to the one that was actually delivered. Nevertheless, this private game has enriched my professional life, often leading down paths of inquiry that sometimes resulted in publication and always generated reflection. Thank you, Muriel Driver, for the inspiration, and CAOT for the opportunity, this one time, to have *my* topic of the year and the *actual* lecture congruent.

In recognition of this, the 75th anniversary of the Canadian Association of Occupational Therapists I have chosen the topic *Change: Creating our own Reality*. I will explore change in relation to three topics: the power of context, the importance of choice, and finally how creating our own reality keeps bringing us 'back to the future', the theme for this year's congress.

Change, as Stephen Hawking reminds us, is the one constant we have in our lives. This constancy includes surges of change, which Toffler described as waves (1981), washing in one after, and on top of, the other. The first wave, agricultural, changed us around 8,000 BC from hunter-gatherers to farmers. The second wave, industrial, saw a migration starting in the 1700s from farms to industry. The third wave, information, began in the mid 1950's when people began to be valued for their brains, and for the first time, more than half of the workforce consisted of white collar workers (Harris, 1998). The fourth wave, that of knowledge, has already arrived. Weiner and Brown (1997) describe their per-

ception of the coming economy as the 'emotile economy'. The word emotile is a combination of emotional, that is, heightened concern for personal well-being, and motile described as fast-moving, portable, and non-fixed. In an attempt to help us think about and understand our changing world and prepare for the future, many people have written in a variety of ways about these changing eras (Harris, 1998; Picard-Greffe, 1994; Wacker & Taylor, 2000; Weiner & Brown, 1997) which are occurring more and more rapidly.

We are a product, not of individual waves, but of the complex result of the impact of each succeeding wave on the others. The wave analogy is a good one. We can visualize in some cases being lifted off our feet and slammed, stunned, onto shore, wondering what hit us, and in other cases riding the crest of the wave with exhilaration. Chilton (1995) exhorted us to "wade in deep and risk riding the waves of change to unknown lands. . . ." We are, she said ". . .well equipped to ride these waves" (p. 184). Some of us seek waves; some of us try to avoid them and, of course, some of us make waves. Whether sought or not, we know that the waves of change are washing over us with increasing speed (Chilton, 1994, 1995; Finlayson, 2000; Madill 1986; Madill, Cardwell, Robinson, & Brintnell, 1986). We labour to keep our bearings, our sense of self in the present, while at the same time heading for unknown shores and our potential future.

The Power of Context

Although the power of context includes global, national and environmental change, I will focus on personal, professional and organization change contexts.

Personal

In the context of person, the most dramatic and exciting change that is occurring around us is the transformation through many stages and over time, of tiny dependent infants into toddlers, teenagers, adults, older adults, and eventually seniors. We are not only biologically changing as we and our families age, but we are also changing within the context of our relationships, our environments and our occupations. This developing process involves thinking, feeling and doing within the context of a changing world. Because occupational therapists believe that each person's story unfolds in a unique and personal manner, we recognize that over time individuals develop personal repertoires of strategies to use in managing change. Effective or not, these personal strategies are part of each individual's daily living in a changing world. Working, partnering, parenting, educating, cooking, cleaning, worrying, learning, playing, we live and work and play in a rich broth of complex, changing demands and interfaces. It is easy to lose track of who we are and what is important to us. Rushing through our lives, as we tend to do, we may never have slowed down enough to name the values we wish to live by. However surely many of us have experienced the unease which accompanies a disconnection between what we are doing and what we believe to be the right thing to do. Whether we reflect on it or not, how we view ourselves changes as we build the story of our lives through the choices we make. Who we are within ourselves is the base-camp from which we venture forth. Our bodies know that what makes it possible to lift one foot to take a step forward is the fact that the other foot is placed firmly on the ground. Who we are matters. Let me give you a personal example.

My mother remembered with strong feelings, the first car that came to her area—and the fact that, being a girl, she was forced to stand aside and watch her brother have that breathtaking first ride. Always willing, eager for new experiences, before her death she had traveled by horse, plane, car, train, boat, canoe, camel and mule (this last to the bottom of the Grand Canyon and back). She knew who she was at the age of five—someone so eager to see the world that she felt impelled to climb into a strange, noisy machine and travel at the breathtaking speed of 20 miles an hour. She never forgot that injustice and the lost opportunity that she, the adventurer, was not allowed to ride in the first car in town because she was a woman. "I am so proud of my girls", she said toward the end of her life, "they just get into cars and go where they want to go", something we take for granted, a mere one generation later.

Whatever is important to us, we spend lifetimes negotiating, bargaining, manipulating, searching for the opportunity and the right to be who we are in the face of all kinds of well-meaning advice, and spoken and unspoken expectations from others who want us to be who they are or think we should be. Individuals bring personal context to every interaction. Understanding this, we realize as occupational therapists that it is foolish to hope we will change another person by telling them what to do or how to be.

Nevertheless we are all connected. Your triumphs are mine, as are your joys and sorrows, just as mine are yours. We tremendously influence each other by operating from a position of 'we', rather than 'I'. Competition, judgment, criticism, and control fall by the wayside as we focus on making space for each other as individuals-in-context. In doing so we create vital connections, enable change, and become stronger ourselves.

Professional

Our professional context is occupation, of course. People and organizations bring to us their issues-in-context related to occupation. We are deeply invested in assisting others not only to do what matters to them but also to figure out what that is. Change is a core concept of our profession. It is the essence of adaptation (Breines, 1989) and of learning. People come to us because we are occupational therapists and they need or want to know a different way of doing things in their lives.

We are trained to break daily living tasks down into component parts, so that our clients can re-master the whole task by addressing it incrementally. We have become conditioned to believing that change is incremental. In fact change is not necessarily incremental. In his book, *The tipping point: How little things can make a big difference*, Gladwell (2000) examines sudden and unexpected change. He describes how ideas and behaviours often spread like outbreaks of infectious disease, giving as an example, the single un-repaired broken window as signal that this neighborhood is no longer a crime free area. We are exquisitely sensitive to changes in context (Gladwell, 2000). The smallest event can become the tipping point that drives us, pell-mell, in another direction than we had been going or planning to go. We recognize this tipping point in the saying, "That was the straw that broke the camel's back". Sometimes when morale takes a nosedive, the tipping point can be traced back to some small event—something said or done, or not said or done, that was the final straw. Catastrophic life decisions can be made because one small event blocks the vision of a future that seemed, until that moment, attainable.

Of course, the tipping point can be in the positive direction. Lorne Kimber, describes in his story contained in Haslam's book (2000), *Heroes next door: The courage to come back*, how an occupational therapist in 1983 believed that he, Kimber could become computer literate. This therapist signed him up for a computer course and 18 years later Kimber speaks with gratitude and affection of this intervention. He has never looked back. "I may have MS", he whispers, "but MS doesn't have me". This therapist's intervention was a very positive tipping point in the direction of his future. Being believed in, heard, valued—all create potential positive tipping points, just as not being believed in, not being heard and not being valued can create negative ones.

As occupational therapists we are often working right out there at the tipping point where people can either become discouraged, cope, or be transformed. Working as we do with so many people, we can become sensitized to potential tipping points and our role in enabling a positive direction, in this way preventing, wherever possible, catastrophic decisions based on a moment of chaos.

In my position as Professional Practice Director, I have come to believe that a therapist's first job is a tipping point. It is confirmation, or not, of this profession as a life-long choice. Another tipping point, I believe, is an experienced therapist's first efforts to use modern theory. How can we enable that positive first experience so that clinicians can experience the power and practicality of good theory? Groups can have tipping points. Implementing current theory in practice is an example. Among a group of therapists, change can creep along, and creep along until suddenly there is a critical mass of people actually understanding and using theor y in practice, not just saying that they are. At that tipping point change can become explosive, contagious, exhilarating. We can enable these positive changes by learning when, where, and how to provide needed support so that individuals and groups do not have to struggle alone to keep up with progressing practice. An example of the power of providing support to front-line clinicians is the joint initiative between the School of Rehabilitation Sciences, UBC and Vancouver Hospital. The addition of an occupational therapy research scientist based at the hospital has become part of how we do business. His expertise, his presence, and his energy have provided a very positive tipping point to therapists already committed to evidence-based practice.

Another example of a tipping point is the responses we receive to our advocacy for clients, as advocates are created through the experience of making a difference.

That is, when we are successful in advocating for others, we are more likely to continue to do so. As occupational therapists, it is important to understand ways in which tipping points may come about.

Understanding change and the importance of our responses to change will help us create healthy workplaces and learning environments. At our best we create contexts for clients and for ourselves, that make a positive difference to what happens at that tipping point. It is important that we use our energies to understand change and also to be awake to the effects of change around us.

Here is one example where it would be easy to focus on the physical change and miss the personal and interpersonal changes that resulted. *Popular Mechanics* in 1949 predicted that computers in the future might weigh less than 1.5 tons! In the early 1970's, the personal computer still did not exist. 30 years later, 5-year old children mentor their parents on using the personal computer to gain information. Parents, in turn, mentor their children on evaluating the information that is obtained, creating an understanding and expectation among children that all knowledge does not come from authority and trickle down through hierarchy. Titles, hierarchy and control are often associated with controlling information, (sometimes withholding it, sometimes spinning it). In the face of new generations who have such easy access to information and to each other, we can expect that our titles, hierarchy, and control will not last. 150 occupational therapy staff have e-mail access to me, and to the Vice-President, and to the CEO as well. With today's technological tools available to us, we are no longer dependent on hierarchy for information. As a result, the old parental model of mentorship where experience mentored inexperience no longer fits our professional world. We all have knowledge and skills of value to others. The fact that I have worked for a hundred years doesn't matter at all, unless I remain actively open to interactive mentoring, a combination of both mentoring and being mentored. My value as a professional is based on how I practice in the present and especially how I am preparing to practice in the future. The challenge we all face is to remain open to learning and to create learning opportunities. Rapidly developing knowledge within our own profession and all around us is changing how we do business and surely how we will do business in the future.

Organizational

In terms of organizational context, many of us work or have worked in industrial age organizations that are trying to modernize by downsizing, re-engineering, reorganizing, amalgamating, decentralizing, project management, department management, program management, matrix management, too much management. Directly or indirectly, we are given to understand that wherever we are at the moment, it must be changed, often, we perceive, without regard to preserving, even acknowledging our strengths or engaging us in visualizing the future we could create together. Sometimes we respond by blazing a trail to the oppor tunity that ever y change creates. Sometimes we respond by blaming others, citing poor communication, and general lack of trust, and by doing so we place ourselves in a passive position. We have been 'done to' again. This becomes our reality. Even that person who remains in active mode, watching the waves and seeing trouble approaching, may be labeled 'resistant to change' or 'troublemaker' for calling an alert, if the alert cannot be communicated in a way that is understood by others. The present move toward autonomous practitioners is a case in point.

In keeping with the knowledge era, we are recruiting our brightest and best therapists, then expecting them to use their fine brains within industrial era organizations that are structured and managed to maintain a hierarchical approach to decision making and thinking in general. Therapists struggle to live their client-centred values in practices that are boxed within a controlling and closed environment. We are at risk for losing these therapists from our profession wherever the autonomous practitioner change wave is crashing into the old organizational management wave. This disconnect is particularly painful for occupational therapists because we are trained to provide leadership, to resolve issues, to be client-centred. Personally and professionally we live our values in organizations that may not be ready for us.

Whether we realize it or not, however, we are ready for them. I know it is a daunting thought, but we are the organization (Fearing & Ferguson-Paré, 2000; Levine, Locke, Searles, & Weinberger, 2001). If we want healthy workplaces, we will create them by being healthy ourselves. Naming values we expect to live in our workplaces, advocating for and contributing to healthy environments, always working to build connections among people and ideas, we can lead change when we choose to do so. We can play an important role in transforming our workplaces.

More and more of us are choosing to create our own organizations through private practice, in some cases brilliantly demonstrating how a viable organization can be client-centred while at the same time valuing and supporting continuous learning and innovation. Organizations, whether private or public, operate in a world where our individual and collective approaches to personal, professional, and organizational change are critically important.

The Importance of Choice

Change We Do Not Choose

Change in itself is simple; it is our response to change that may be complex. Change comes in two basic ways. Let me give you a simple example: I did not choose to have my hair turn grey although I have chosen to remain grey. The change-we-do-not-choose we can consider 'weather', as in, stormy or sunny weather (Flower, 1997a). Weather comes whether we wish it to or not. We all have 'weather' in our personal and professional lives and most of us know we can protect against weather but we can't stop it. However, we do have choice as to how we react to weather. Anyone who has lived in tornado country knows you can't stop tornados. We have no choice there. However, we do have choices about our response to the tornados. These choices range from herding everyone to the basement to piling into the car and trying to chase the funnel down. Within the same person, these responses may change. I have personally gone to the basement and also followed a tornado. It depended on what I was thinking, or not thinking, at the time. It is hard to predict our future response to weather. For example, we may be cautious and endure organizational chaos for years and suddenly find ourselves in the middle of a storm created by the risks we have taken by calling attention, in one way or another, to the lack of leadership. At any point we may make a move, whether carefully thought out or not, that better aligns our values and our actions. There can be repercussions that might include leaving the organization or alternatively, becoming stronger by experiencing the power of acting from authenticity. One voice can make a difference.

Sometimes we think we have no choice because we can see no options or possibilities. Part of our role as occupational therapists is to connect people to their potential futures. ". . .there is no more powerful example of leadership than giving people the chance to change their beliefs about what is possible" (Gilpin, 1998, p. 57). It is important to remember that our response to change is a choice, although we may not have chosen the change itself.

Change We Choose

There is also change we do choose. Education, accomplishment, and life circumstances can lead to choosing a different life direction. Sometimes we choose by doing nothing. This can be the result of fear. We manage fear differently. Some of us turn it into choice, energy and action, and others of us become helpless, depressed and paralyzed (Jeffers, 1987; Johnson, 1998). The advice to *Feel the fear and do it anyway* (Jeffers, 1987) is easier to act on in some situations than others and may require more skills and resources than we currently have. Choosing to do nothing may be the result of inertia, or recognition at some level that this is not important in the scheme of things.

What may appear to be a choice to do nothing, can in fact, be a stage of change. Boulter and Webb, in a 2001 pre-CAOT Congress workshop called *Understanding the Change Process in Clients*, brought to our attention the Transtheoretical Model of Change (Cancer Prevention Research Centre, 2001). The core constructs of this model include stages of change, ordered along a continuum from pre-contemplation, to contemplation, to preparation, to action and then to maintenance. This model, which focuses on the decision-making of the individual, helps us understand that people can be engaged in change long before it becomes apparent to others. With this model, thinking about losing weight is a stage of change, as is trying and failing several times, stages of change that may not be readily observable by others. Someone labeled resistant to change may in fact be in pre-contemplation, contemplation, even preparation mode. My point here is *not* that we are either in one stage or another—life is not that simple—but rather, that change is not always visible. We are always making choices within the contexts of the lives we live and those lived around us.

Choosing Our Response

Our power lies in having a choice in change and also in realizing that we have a choice in our responses to imposed change. Sometimes it takes a serious disruption in our personal, professional or organizational lives to force reflection and choice regarding how to be in the future. We can learn from the work being done regarding adversity. What at first may appear to be catastrophic can be the tipping point that leads to becoming active in creating a meaningful future. McMillan (1999) refers to several ways adversity can cause benefit.

The first way adversity may be beneficial, McMillan (1999) calls "What doesn't kill you makes you stronger", or stress inoculation. Many of us have at one time or another experienced increased confidence from having navigated tough situations successfully, or perhaps just survived. This is reflected in the saying, "Strong timber does not grow with ease, the stronger the wind, the stronger the trees" (Gilpin, 1998, p. 31). The second way is "heeding the wake-up call" indicating that the adverse event was interpreted as a warning to make significant changes. That first heart attack may be perceived as a wake up call to a healthier lifestyle. The third way is "People aren't so bad after all", a phenomenon regularly reported in the newspapers, as survivors of disaster marvel at experiencing the goodness of others who have come to their assistance. The final way adversity can cause benefit is what McMillan (1999) calls "Transformation through interpretation", that is, finding meaning. Transforming grief at the loss of a child in an accident into energy spent working to prevent similar events is one example. It helps to have a positive attitude to life in general and to be open to the possibility of change leading to transformation.

Transformation and Choosing Change

In a 1995 paper from Italy called *The importance of inner transformation in the activity process*, Piergrossi & Gibertom describe activities as "vehicles for emotional movement" (p. 37), which enrich function. They call attention to the inner transformation that occurs along with the external action of doing activities. Here the word transformation refers to the linkages formed between what we do, what memories this evokes in us, and how it becomes part of our story and our relationships. Mastering any challenge, whether it is rock-climbing, ice skating, navigating by scooter, or in some cases simply feeding oneself can become an epic in the story of one's life and the basis of a sense of competence and confidence.

Townsend (1997) suggests that the "potential to transform ourselves and society . . . lies in occupation" (p. 20). Transformation in this case refers to opportunities to choose and engage in occupations for the purposes of directing and changing personal or social aspects of life, in order to realize dreams and goals.

Can doing things differently cause a shift in perspective? Can a shift in perspective cause us to do things differently? Consider the possibility of transformation being a significant shift of perspective or point-of-view within a person, accompanied by a different way of

769

feeling about self. This transformation is recognized by others as a different way of doing and being in the world.

Believing as I do that occupational therapy is leadership in action, it is useful to see what leadership literature has to teach us about change and transformation. Modern leadership literature is exciting reading, as old-style controlling leadership is replaced with an enablement model described by Greenleaf (1998) as the leader-as-servant. This is the leader people choose to follow. Through that leader they waken not only to their own potential but also to the joy and satisfaction of acting in concert with their potential. Senge (in Jaworski, 1996) reflects that Jaworski in his personal and engaging book, *Synchronicity: The inner path of leadership*, takes the servant-as-leader idea another step, suggesting that ". . . the fundamental choice that enables true leadership in all situations . . . is the *choice to serve life*" (p. 2), that is, allowing life to unfold. This is transformative leadership, such a different approach than controlling leadership, and requiring far more skills and especially self-knowledge. Transformative leadership makes space for others to experience significant changes in perspective.

As occupational therapists, we are deeply involved in assisting others who are facing extraordinar y change. Remember that these change waves are in addition to the life changes that we are all experiencing. Lacking an understanding of the complexity of the change process, it is too easy to label others in our minds, or worse, on health records, regarding our perception of their ability to change: Resists change, unrealistic, unmotivated, non-compliant, un-cooperative. What an arrogant approach to use. It is a reflection of blindness regarding the complexity of change and its meaning in our individual and collective lives.

Reflecting on our roles as occupational therapists will lead us to avoid limiting other peoples' realities. When I tell you your dream or plan is unrealistic, you know that I do not understand transformation or the power of the human spirit in general, and yours in particular. Limiting your spirit because of limitations in my own is surely a form of aggression and can result in damage. You may choose not to be damaged, but what a lot of energy it can take, often at that tipping point when hope is all that keeps us going. As Margaret Somerville (2000) said, "Hope is our connection, as both individuals and societies, to the future," and ". . . hope is the oxygen of the human spirit; without it our spirit dies, whereas with it, it can survive even appalling suffering"

(p. xiv). Every time I hear someone say, "She, or he, has unrealistic expectations," I want to shout, "WELL, WHO DOESN'T?" Expectations are about hope and hope is our connection to the future.

What are barriers to making choices? It is easy to lose sight of possibilities when trying to cope with what is. For example, we are in the midst of an information explosion and resulting overload. Just keeping up with e-mail can be a challenge. Wacker & Taylor (2000) tell us that "By the start of the second decade of the twenty-first century, the information available to the average individual at any given point in time will be a hundred thousand times what it is today" (p. 13). We will not need faster access to information. What we will need is the space and time to think (Jensen, 2000). We need it now.

Whether as therapist or client, as we experience pressure from multiple and often conflicting demands, it is easy to blame others. We may label what does not suit us as 'lack of communication' and 'lack of trust'. It is a common reaction to feeling out of control. In fact many of us are finding it difficult to sort and focus on what is important among too much information and too many demands. That out-of-control sense contributes to fear, which feeds on rumour, that highly effective method of spreading distorted information.

"You begin to realize," Jenson (2000) *wrote, "that resistance to change is often misdiagnosed. Large numbers of people—more than most of us care to admit—need new tools and skills if they are to work in a world filled with infinite choices. Yet because of our ability to think our way out of most any situation, we assume the difficulties along the way must be the result of people digging in their heels. Please don't confuse choice overload with resistance to change" (p. 31).*

Part of what we can do for our clients and for each other, is to help sort out what will make a difference to the future we are working toward; then we can work toward the skill changes necessary to get there. Skill change, whether developmental, adaptive, or reactive is part of our everyday lives. Changing, as we are, in a changing world, we are constantly learning new skills. The lack of necessary skills can be a barrier to change. We are 'people with varying abilities', a descriptor chosen under the guidance of occupational therapist Pam Andrews, by the Accessibility Committee at Vancouver Hospital. We are "people with varying abilities" rather than people segregated and labeled as "disabled" and by inference, "non-disabled." As people with varying abilities our skill changes and rates of change vary too.

Two people learning to navigate stairs safely may be challenged in different ways. In one case by new bifocals, which make it difficult to keep the feet in focus; in the other case by negotiating the same stairs when riding a mountain bike. Both people require concentration, balance and control of different kinds. These skill changes come about through trial and error, risk-taking, coaching, and practice. Changing of skills is important although I would argue that it is not transformation, unless it causes a significant change in perspective. Transformative change occurs from the inside out, although the catalyst to a change in perspective may be from the outside in. By removing barriers, encouraging, listening, believing, and sharing, the servant-leader enables transformation. The servant-leader makes space for transformation but cannot lead it.

Because we work with people as they navigate their way through challenges to daily living, we are uniquely positioned to assist organizations and individuals not simply to survive change, but rather to choose change, or a response to change that has meaning. We are experienced and confident in enabling people to address issues of immediate impor tance to them through adaptation, modification, learning and relearning. Change is more than that. It can be transformation.

Creating Our Own Reality Over Time

If we want a healthy future we have to create it ourselves. Whether personally, professionally, or organizationally, we work in the present to create a future that engages us in life. Sometimes surviving the moment requires full attention and leaves little thought or energy for the future. Surviving the moment may include living in the past, or perhaps reflecting on it. The paradox of time (Wacker & Taylor, 2000) as a context is that if I live in the present (or past), I may not have a future. If I live only in the future, I do not have a present. One of the arts of occupational therapy is in the occupations we choose to engage people in the present to use what they have learned in the past, in order to create a future that makes life worth living. As occupational therapists, we are in the business of assisting others to use their power to create their personal futures, which they carry within themselves. Sounds easy, doesn't it? The challenge is to be able to visualize what those futures might look like so that reasoned choices can be made.

Once we know what we want our future to look like, we can make choices that will get us there. Wayne Gretzky, hockey player, does not go to where the puck *is*, he goes to where it is going to be.

We can learn from the work done by the Royal Dutch Shell Group who, 'rather than relying on forecasts (which are invariably wrong), . . . does its planning for the future through the use of decision scenarios' (Jaworski, 1996, p. 140). They are using scenario planning not only to respond to the future, but also to help shape it. Let me give you one example of scenario planning, as reported by Jaworski. Initiated to help South Africa make its transition from an apartheid society to a representative democracy, and led by a member of the Shell Group, a leadership team working with key players in South Africa in the early 1990s developed four scenarios. These scenarios were named after birds. In the first scenario, called Ostrich, the government buried its head in the sand and did not call a free election. The second scenario, Lame Duck, involved prolonged transition in which no one was satisfied. Icarus, who, you may remember flew too close to the sun and fell to the ground, proposed that a black government would come to power and try to satisfy all promises made during the campaign (as other governments we can think of have done), thereby crashing the economy. The fourth scenario, Flamingoes (who rise slowly and fly together), concerned a coalition government. This process of scenario planning, public discussion, and choice helped shaped South Africa's future.

Scenario planning consists of identifying choices to be made to create the future we wish to live and involves reflecting on what is, envisioning what could be, and choosing how we wish to use our personal and collective power. It is not about passively waiting or blaming others. "The point of scenario spinning is to help us 'suspend our disbelief ' in all possible futures, so that we can see the possibilities with clear eyes" (Flower, 1997b, p. 59). Creating a future includes visualizing possibilities and recognizing potential for transformation from accomplishment, as well as from loss and/or chaos. To do this we understand that the power of achieving mastery is an internal experience that can influence many other activities. Gilpin (1998) in his book, *Unstoppable people: How ordinary people achieve extraordinary things*, reminds us that "We move relentlessly in the direction of our thoughts" (p. 41). Regardless of the positions we hold, we must ask ourselves over and over again, what can I do to enable this client, student, staff person, committee, organization, community to identify a meaningful future and to master the thinking, feeling and doing skills necessary to get there. As occupational therapists we make a difference, not only in the skills for daily living today but also in the skills for daily living tomorrow and in the future.

Conclusion

This year we celebrate 75 years of the Canadian Association of Occupational Therapists professional leadership. We are fortunate to have the vigorous and proactive support of CAOT. The climate of respect and collaboration we create together, the support we extend to others and receive ourselves contributes to positioning us where we can individually and collectively lead change and have a wonderful time doing it. At the same time that we celebrate 75 years, we look forward to the future when we will celebrate 100 years. I believe we are on the right track. As Mark Twain pointed out "Even if you are on the right track, you will get run over if you just sit there."

What do we want our personal, professional, and organizational contexts to look like in 2026? Grounded in theory that drives client-centred occupational therapy practice, we will be increasingly open to the rich learning to be gained from and with other disciplines, other approaches, and our clients. Our theory will mature to reflect our growing understanding of people making choices within the context of changing circumstances. We will be hyper-vigilant in our search for sound innovations and we will value the innovators. We will nurture the radical in each of us. We will rethink our approach to 'therapeutic relationships', focusing on building connections in the universe, rather than keeping distances. We will learn to use dialogue as a way of thinking together rather than from positions (Isaacs, 1999). We will teach therapists explicit skills for advocacy and negotiation. We will measure meaning, rather than, or perhaps along with, measuring change. We will learn from clients about the meaning of our goal setting processes in their lives, and how we can be more effective. Perhaps someone will develop a better way to classify occupation than self-care, productivity, and leisure.

In 2026, our recognition of the importance of choice will demonstrate 25 more years of actively seeking possibilities, leading research and professional development, and supporting each other through tipping points that can lead to positive transformation. Sometimes, where change is concerned, the best we can do is to be part of preparing a future so that others can have what we know in our hearts was, and is, our right too. We will be making choices that make space for occupa-

tional therapists of the future to be who they are in 50 years, in 2051.

Since our professional context is daily living, everything we experience or read has the potential to enlighten us regarding our roles as occupational therapists. Learning will become a way of being. "Learning is the gate, not the house" (Munenori, 1999). We will continue to create our own reality. We will not only recognize and value the skill of maintaining balance, our own and that of our clients, but we will live it. Balance will not be viewed as a set of scales that has equal parts such as work on one side and play on the other but rather the kind of balance that comes from being centred so that we act from a stable base. From that stable base, we will gain a keen sensitivity to rhythm— knowing when to move and when to let go. What we do, then, will flow from that stable base of knowing who we are as individual people. Knowing who we are as occupational therapists, that is, focused on enabling others to create a meaningful person–occupation–environment fit, has provided the stable base we needed as a profession to move forward with confidence. Our professional stable base is occupation and related theory.

In 2026, although our profession will be different than it is now, we will be positioned where we have chosen to be. Leadership in everyday occupational therapy practice occurs brilliantly, fluently, and frequently where therapists understand and live the potential of their roles in regard, not just to adaptation, but also to transformation. We are client-centred when we recognize and consider the power of individual and shared context. We are client-centred when we make space for and honour client choice. We are client-centred when we value the future we are creating individually and together. When we are truly awake to our potential as people through whom achievement occurs, we perceive possibilities rather than limitations. This is a circular process. The very process of enabling others changes who we are. Enabling others is leadership. It is occupational therapy.

Acknowledgements

The author wishes to thank Geraldine Moore, Editor, CAOT for her warm and knowledgeable support; Pam Andrews, for library support and encouragement; Shirley Salomon, for critically reading the content; the occupational therapists at Vancouver Hospital, a part of the Vancouver/Richmond Health Board, for their inspiration and patience. The author is particularly indebted to the many occupational therapists across Canada who participated in dialogue over the years and who regularly demonstrate that miracles occur at the frontline when sufficient supports are provided. As always, a special thank you to Harold and Paul Fearing for being who you are.

References

Breines, E. B. (1989). Development, change and continuity theories: An analysis. *Canadian Journal of Occupational Therapy, 56,* 109–112.

Cancer Prevention Research Center. (2001, January). *Transtheoretical Model.* Retrieved January 21, 2001 from http://www.uri.edu/research/cprc/transtheoretical.htm.

Chilton, H. (1994). National Perspective: Agenda for a credible future. *Canadian Journal of Occupational Therapy, 61,* 187–188.

Chilton, H. (1995). National Perspective: Partners in practice: Riding the waves of change. *Canadian Journal of Occupational Therapy, 62,* 183–187.

Fearing, V. G., & Ferguson-Paré, M. (2000). Leadership in daily practice. In V. G. Fearing, & J. Clark (Eds.). *Individuals in context: A practical guide to client-centred practice.* Thorofare, NJ: Slack.

Finlayson, M. (2000). National Perspective: Are you ready to dance with opportunity? *Canadian Journal of Occupational Therapy, 67,* 286–290.

Flower, J. (1997a). *Habits of mind for turbulent times.* Retrieved May 12, 2001 from http://www.well.com/user/bbear/change.html

Flower, J., (1997b). *Spinning the future.* Retrieved May 12, 2001 from http://www.well.com/user/bbear/change.html

Gilpin, A. (1998). *Unstoppable people: How ordinary people achieve extraordinary things.* London, UK: Random House.

Gladwell, M. (2000). *The tipping point: How little things can make a big difference.* New York: Little, Brown.

Greenleaf, R. K. (1998). In L.C. Spears (Ed.). *Insights on leadership: Service, stewardship, spirit, and servant-leadership.* Toronto, ON: John Wiley & Sons.

Harris, J. (1998). *The learning paradox: Gaining success and security in a world of change.* Toronto, ON: Macmillan.

Haslam, G. (2000). *Heroes next door: The courage to come back.* Vancouver, BC: Coast Foundation Society.

Isaacs, W. (1999). *Dialogue and the art of thinking together.* New York: Doubleday.

Jaworski, J. (1996). *Synchronicity: The inner path of leadership.* San Francisco, CA: Berrett-Koehler.

Jeffers, S. (1987). *Feel the fear and do it anyway.* Toronto, ON: Random House

Jensen, B. (2000). *Simplicity: The new competitive advantage in a worlds of more, better, faster.* Cambridge, MA: Perseus.

Johnson, S. (1998). *Who moved my cheese?* New York: G. P Putnam's Sons.

Levine, R., Locke, C., Searls, D., & Weinberger, D. (2001). *The cluetrain manifesto: The end of business as usual.* Cambridge, MA: Perseus.

MacKenzie, G. (1996). *Orbiting the giant hairball: A corporate fool's guide to surviving with grace.* Toronto, ON: Penguin Books.

Madill, H. M. (1986). National Perspective: Change: Crisis or challenge? *Canadian Journal of Occupational Therapy, 53,* 125–128.

Madill, H. M., Cardwell, M. T., Robinson, I. M., & Brintnell, E. S. (1986). Old themes, new directions—Occupational therapy in the 21st century. *Canadian Journal of Occupational Therapy, 53,* 38–44.

McMillen, J.C. (1999). Better for it: How people benefit from adversity. *National Social Work, 44,* 455–467

Munenori, (1999). In K. Kheng-Hor (Ed.), *The way of the samurai for millennium executives.* Malaysia: Pelanduk Publications.

Picard-Greffe, H. (1994). Muriel Driver Memorial Lecture: Back to the future. *Canadian Journal of Occupational Therapy, 61,* 243–249.

Piergrossi, J. C. & Gibertoni, C. (1995). The importance of inner transformation in the activity process. *Occupational Therapy International, 2* 36–47.

Senge, P. (1996). Introduction In J. Jaworski. *Synchronicity: The inner path of leadership.* San Francisco, CA: Berrett-Koehler.

Somerville, M. (2000). *The ethical canary: Science, society and the human spirit.* Toronto, ON: Penguin.

Toffler, A., (1981). *The third wave.* New York: Bantam Books.

Townsend, E. (1997). Occupation: Potential for personal and social transformation. *Journal of Occupational Science, 4,* 18–26.

Wacker, W. & Taylor, J. (2000). *The visionary's handbook: Nine paradoxes that will shape the future of your business.* New York: Harper

Weiner E. & Brown, A. (1997). *Insider's guide to the future.* USA: Boardroom.

CHAPTER 61

Occupation by Design: Dimensions, Therapeutic Power, and Creative Process

DORIS PIERCE

Two forces are converging, creating conditions both challenging and potentially fruitful for occupational therapy. The profession's knowledge base describing occupation is growing exponentially. At the same time, functional outcomes of intervention are being increasingly valued within the health-care environment. Other professions imitate and claim our areas of expertise in the most flattering and dangerous ways. To benefit from the convergence of these forces, occupational therapy must expeditiously translate understanding of occupation into powerful occupation-based practice. Three bridges must be built: a generative discourse, demonstration sites, and effective education.

The occupational design approach offers important conceptual tools with which to rapidly build these bridges to powerful practice. Described here are subjective and contextual dimensions of occupational experience; elements of the occupational design process; and how these factors produce therapeutic power through the appeal, intactness, and accuracy of interventions.

Within occupational therapy, there is explosive growth in our understanding of occupation, the field's primary modality (American Occupational Therapy Association [AOTA], 1995; Clark et al., 1991; Kielhofner, 1992; Nelson, 1997; Primeau, 1996; Schkade & Schultz, 1992; Yerxa et al., 1989; Zemke & Clark, 1996). Simultaneously, the health-care system is increasingly valuing functional, or occupational, outcomes. A potential time of congruence is approaching if occupational therapy can expeditiously translate an expanding knowledge of occupation into powerful occupation-based practice.

Occupational therapy is already responding to the stronger emphasis on functional outcomes in health care by moving away from medical model, compo-nent-based practice and toward more whole, top–down, occupation-based practice (Coster, 1998; Law, 1998). Other professions are also responding. They honor the validity of occupation in the most flattering and dangerous ways by imitating our focus and claiming it as their own area of expertise (Wood, 1998). In the face of aggressive competition for our traditional areas of practice, the key to our success is simple: just be the best at what we do. We must use occupation in the most powerful therapeutic ways possible. We must consistently target functional occupational patterns as outcomes. And, we must be eloquent about our unique clinical perspective.

When occupational science first made its promise to occupational therapy that basic research into typical occupations would enhance therapeutic efficacy (Clark et al., 1991; Yerxa et al., 1989), some doubted (Mosey, 1992). How would a scattershot of various studies into occupation effectively move the field forward? In critical need of research on clinical issues, could we afford investment of time and energy in basic research? These are good, tough questions. The usefulness to occupational therapy of basic research into occupation could be relatively limited if it is not complemented by specific strategies to bring this knowledge into practice.

To bring the full potential of occupation to bear in the lives of clients requires three critical bridges: a generative discourse regarding occupation-based practice, demonstration sites, and effective education. Building such bridges requires new conceptual tools. The occupational design approach described here offers the following concepts to support the translation of basic knowledge of occupation into practice applications: the subjective and contextual dimensions of occupational experience, occupational design process, and three sources of therapeutic power in occupation-based interventions. Before exploring these new concepts, let us look more closely at the three bridges, or the three creative loci in the life of the profession where knowl-

This chapter was previously published in the *American Journal of Occupational Therapy, 55,* 249–259. Copyright © 2001, American Occupational Therapy Association. Reprinted with permission. http://dx.doi.org/10.5014/ajot.55.3.249

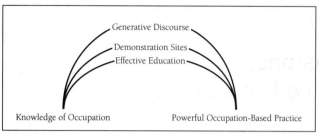

Figure 61.1. Three bridges required to rapidly translate knowledge of occupation into powerful occupation-based practice.

Note. From *Occupation by Design* by D. Pierce, 2003. Philadelphia: F. A. Davis. Reprinted with permission from publisher.

edge of occupation can be most forcefully and rapidly applied to enhance the power of practice (see Figure 61.1).

Three Bridges to Build: Translating Knowledge of Occupation Into Powerful Occupation-Based Practice

Bridge: A Generative Discourse on the Use of Occupation in Practice

The first bridge needed is an active discourse regarding the relation between theories and research describing typical occupations and their application in practice. This discussion must go on in public and private ways, from scholarly publications to the mind of the therapist during intervention. The discourse must be highly productive of useful new concepts. That is, we must be able to talk the talk of how occupation is used in practice frequently, fluently, and in a way that spurs a rapid evolution of innovative practice thinking.

We require language for articulating how the translation from knowledge to practice occurs. The most obvious explanation of how we use knowledge of occupation in practice is that by understanding occupation more fully, therapists are better prepared to use and interpret it in working with clients. The meaning of this statement, however, is not particularly transparent. Similarly, reasoning from a depth of background in how humans experience occupation is not a simple form of clinical thinking. Basing day-to-day practice on the study of occupation as it occurs in typical and atypical conditions is a demanding, theoretical, action-oriented, and fluid style of intervention. It is difficult to describe.

Generative discourse has already begun to produce an occupation-based practice language. For example, one clarifying concept that has emerged is the distinc-

tion between the use of occupation as the means of intervention versus the end of intervention (Cynkin, 1995; Gray, 1998 [see Chapter 10]; Trombly, 1995 [see Chapter 11]). Current research on functional outcomes and the development of top–down assessments will also provide new language to practice (Coster, 1998). Drawing heavily from anthropology is a fruitful strategy for importing humanistic theories to describe human experience, as is demonstrated by clinical reasoning and narrative research (Clark, 1993; Clark, Carlson, & Polkinghorne, 1997; Mattingly & Fleming, 1994). As this generative discourse about the use of knowledge of occupation in practice grows, occupational therapy will find the more technical, static structures of frames of reference a poor fit. The language of occupation-based practice will be more dynamic and reflective. A flourishing, generative discourse on the use of occupation in practice is an essential bridge for putting our knowledge of occupation to work, ultimately to enhance the efficacy of intervention.

Bridge: Practice Demonstration Sites

The field requires a thousand bridges in the form of practice demonstration sites that explore, create, model, and disseminate how it is that knowledge of occupation can be effectively brought to bear in different types of practice. This is where occupational therapy must walk the walk of occupation in practice.

Demonstration sites that are productive of new concepts regarding occupation-based practice will be marked by four indicators. They will depend on insightful clinical reasoning based in the study of occupation. Powerful intervention will be provided through custom-designed, naturalistic occupational experiences. Collaborative identification of desired, functional occupational patterns will provide the goals of intervention. And, lastly, these sites will be successful in communicating within the system of health care and establishing a sufficient referral and reimbursement base.

These programs already exist (Clark et al., 1997; Jackson, Carlson, Mandel, Zemke, & Clark, 1998). It is critically important that the field benefit from the accumulating expertise at such exemplary sites through publication of their successes. Descriptions of these programs are important to our shared sense of the potential variety and number of powerful, occupation-based, life-enhancing programs possible. In these changing and competitive times in health care, the bridge of successful practice demonstration sites is critical to the profession's survival.

Bridge: Educating Sophisticated Practitioners to Use Knowledge of Occupation in Practice

The field requires educational programs that have been specifically constructed with a focus on teaching effective occupation-based practice (Yerxa, 1998). Presently, students enter the field with cultural values that give higher status to technical, medical knowledge than to the highly theoretical yet commonsense knowledge of how what we do shapes who we are. If uninfluenced, these values produce graduates who respect the knowledge base of other professions more than they do their own. Students require much more rigorous education regarding occupation. The profession can no longer afford to give lip service to occupation in the curriculum while handing over the largest portion of the student's study time to component-focused and physiological knowledge.

Reprioritizing and shifting the balance of curriculum content so that students will emerge with the necessary skills for effectively applying an understanding of occupation in practice will deeply challenge occupational therapy education. Hard decisions will be required: Less anatomy and more ethnography of disability? less infant reflexes and more family theory? For some educators, these are shocking ideas. But the curriculum is not infinitely expandable. Too often, students enter the field feeling overwhelmed by their fragmented understanding of many different knowledge bases. It is the responsibility of educators, not students, to resolve the tough issues in our knowledge base in order to offer centrally integrating concepts.

To accomplish such a rapid refocusing of mission in our educational programs will require several efforts from educators: clear recognition that teaching specific intervention techniques will not provide a lasting education in today's fast-changing health-care environment; faculty development around knowledge of occupation in practice; commitment to preparing students with insight into occupational experience and its use in intervention; and reconfiguration of curricular structures. In this process, education will draw on the conceptual language springing from the generative discourse on occupation-based practice as well as from conceptual discoveries at demonstration sites. Students prepared in this way will be innovative, entrepreneurial, and drawn to sites at which exemplary practice is taking place.

The graduate who brings a deep preparation in occupation's use in practice will be able to not only walk the walk of occupation-based intervention, but also talk the walk. That is, graduates will be able to explain why their occupation-based interventions are effectively designed for a specific person with a specific goal. Such a sophisticated graduate will be ready to adapt interventions to a variety of persons, disabilities, and settings. She or he will use the language of occupation's therapeutic power in a way that is compelling, understandable to others, and anchored in everyday experience. Not only will graduates prepared in an occupation-focused curriculum use more powerful interventions, but they also will be more eloquent about why such an approach is effective.

Bridge-Building Tools: Dimensions of Occupation, Sources of Therapeutic Power, and Occupational Design Process

As stated, in order to thrive the profession requires three bridges to move knowledge of occupation into powerful applications in practice: a generative discourse, demonstration practice sites, and education that focuses on occupation-based intervention to produce sophisticated practitioners. In this effort, the following conceptual tools should prove useful: an understanding of the dimensions of occupational experience, language articulating the sources of therapeutic power in occupation-based interventions, and a process for design of therapeutic occupations.

Dimensions of Occupation: Sources of Therapeutic Power

To use occupation most effectively in practice, the therapist must understand its dimensions sufficiently to be able to conceptualize their occurring effects as they unfold during therapy. Here, I offer six primary dimensions of occupation (three subjective, three contextual) and the occupational design process. I will describe how these concepts translate into three primary sources of therapeutic power in occupation-based interventions (Pierce, 1997a, 1998, in press; Zemke & Pierce, 1994) (see Figure 61.2).

The important point here is not that these are the definitive dimensions of occupation or the final statement regarding the sources of its therapeutic power in practice. Other categories could have been constructed to describe occupation and its application, although many of the same concepts would surely have been included. The value of the occupational design approach presented here is that it broadly describes both the

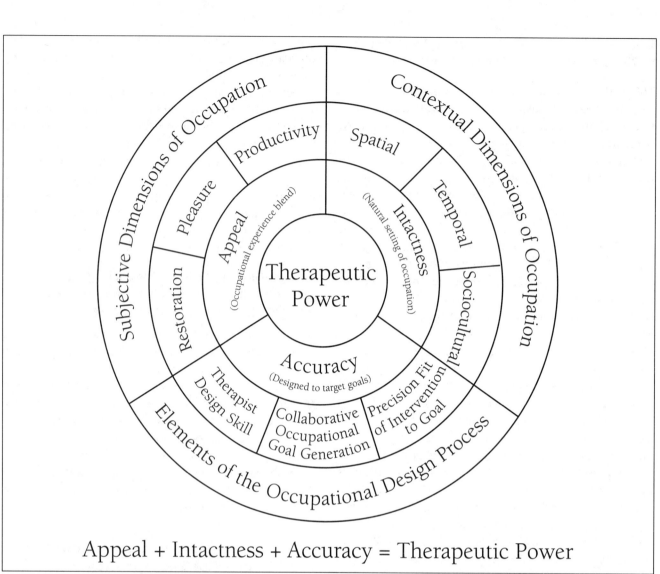

Figure 61.2. The occupational design approach: Conceptual tools for building occupation-based practice.

Note. From Occupation by Design by D. Pierce, 2003. Philadelphia: F. A. Davis. Reprinted with permission from publisher.

complex whole of a person's occupational experience and the elements of the therapeutic process in order to provide the therapist with conceptual sources of therapeutic power upon which she or he can easily reflect before, during, and after intervention.

Appeal: Designing with productivity, pleasure, and restoration. Appeal is the degree to which the client finds the therapeutic occupation desirable in terms of the levels of productivity, pleasure, and restoration he or she experiences (Pierce, 1997a, 1998). Designing intervention that has high appeal requires a knowledge base in how humans typically experience occupations along these subjective dimensions. This depth of knowledge must be matched by the therapist's skills for creating an informed perspective on the uniqueness of each client, especially

through observation and interview. Interventions that blend pleasure, productivity, and restoration in a careful mix that is most likely to be appealing to that person at that time can then be created collaboratively.

Beyond work, play, and self-care. Since the beginning of the profession, occupational therapists have thought of occupation within familiar categories provided by our western cultural history, such as work, play, leisure, and self-care. These commonsense categories (Geertz, 1983) carry great wisdom, tapping essential differences in human activity. As occupational scientists have begun to examine these categories more closely, however, they appear to be simplistic, value laden, decontextualized, and insufficiently descriptive of subjective experience (Pierce, 1997b; Primeau, 1996). There is an important place for these historical terms, certainly. Yet, they are not fully adequate to support masterful design of interventions based in knowledge of occupation.

By moving beyond the old categories, we can begin to examine how the subjective experience of occupation is made up of a unique mix of pleasure, productivity, and restoration. These three characteristics echo the familiar activity classes of play, work, and rest found in the occupational therapy literature. However, the radical difference is in the inclusive nature of the word *and*. In this approach, pleasure, productivity, and restoration are not categories among which one must choose to describe an occupation. Rather, they are three characteristics that exist simultaneously, to some degree, in all occupational experience. Every occupational experience is a blend of the three. This blending is central to the art of therapy to produce the most appealing therapeutic occupation for a client.

Productivity's contribution to the appeal of an occupation. Humans love to be productive. Give us a game, a goal, a project, or an inspiring product to build and we are off and running. Productivity seems to be central to our nature, perhaps built in by its support of our evolutionary success. Productivity extends beyond work to include the goal-focused dimension of all occupations. It often yields great personal satisfaction. To tap productivity in powerful intervention design, therapists must acquire a knowledge base that addresses productivity in theoretical and descriptive depth. Topics that might be included in such study are the history of industrialization and the Protestant work ethic (Gellner, 1988); the tie of work and identity (Christiansen, 1999); pride of craftsmanship (Cross, 1990; Dickie, 1998); the nature of unpaid work, such as housework and caregiving (Hasselkus, 1991; Primeau, 1992); typical career progressions and retirement (Healy, 1982); the dynamics of stress (Keller, Shiflet, & Bartlett, 1994); games and sports (Harris & Park, 1983); learning; and self-actualization (Maslow, 1954). If a client appears to be motivated by a therapeutic occupation high in the experience of productivity, the therapist can then draw on this knowledge of productivity's elements to design an intervention with a satisfying outcome and clear goal achievement.

Pleasure's contribution to the appeal of an occupation. Occupational therapists have always operated from an intuitive understanding of what is pleasurable in intervention. Making intervention pleasurable is a key to engagement. Perhaps this is why we still retain our use of play, crafts, cooking, and other usually pleasurable activities in our intervention repertoires, despite our difficulties in fitting such activities into medical settings. Because they are pleasurable, they are effective (Pierce, 1997b).

Pleasure is nearly the opposite of goal-focused productivity. Pleasure is process-focused. Pleasure is the degree of enjoyment a person experiences in an occupation. Influenced by our productivity-oriented society, occupational therapy has neglected research into pleasure in intervention, focusing instead on the seriousness and respectability of the study of purposefulness and intervention outcomes. It is natural when entering into a contract with clients to assist them in reaching certain goals that we should be primarily concerned with the productivity of that effort. Yet, the efficacy of our intervention also depends on its pleasure. Pediatric occupational therapists are especially aware of this and, so, depend heavily on play (Parham & Fazio, 1996). Even for those clients who can complete interventions through a determined commitment to outcomes, the addition of pleasure to the intervention has beneficial effects on mood, health, and recovery. Areas of understanding that would support a therapist's creative use of the pleasurable dimension of occupation to enhance the appeal of intervention include sensory and limbic system processing (Guyton, 1991; Martin, 1996), arousal (Fisher, Murray, & Bundy, 1991), thrill-seeking activities, play across the life span (Cohen, 1987; Cross, 1990; Rubin, 1980), crafts and hobbies (Fidler & Velde, 1999), comedy and humor (Huizinga, 1950), the link between highly physical activity and endorphins (Davis, 1984), and aesthetics (Goodman, 1951). Applying a developed understanding of pleasure to intervention design is bound to enhance the appeal, and thus the efficacy, of interventions.

Restoration's contribution to the appeal of occupation. Restoration is the subjective aspect of occupational experience that restores our energy levels and ability to continue to engage in our daily lives. Restoration is the most neglected and poorly understood of the three subjective dimensions of occupation. Though therapists may speak often about restoring persons, this is unlikely to slow the pace and demand of intervention. Despite Meyer's (1922; see Chapter 4) seminal description of rest as a primary occupation to be considered by the emerging field of occupational therapy, little has evolved from this idea in subsequent occupational therapy literature.

An understanding of the restorative dimension of occupation must be based in an appreciation of the basic, life-giving occupation of sleep (Coren, 1996; Hobson,

1989; Pierce, 1997b). Indeed, sleep is one occupation without which we would soon die. Because culture has long construed sleep as a ceasing of consciousness, occupational therapy has followed suit by being concerned solely with waking occupations. However, research from the relatively new specialty of sleep medicine is changing the conceptualization of sleep from unconsciousness to a different form of consciousness (Carskadon & Dement, 1994; Moorcroft, 1989). To grasp the patterns that exist in the round of daily activity, that round must be viewed in its full 24-hour circadian rhythm (Moore-Ede, Sulzman, & Fuller, 1982). Sleep quality affects neural plasticity, healing, immune function, cognitive capacities, physical abilities, and mood (Coren, 1996; Pierce, 1997b). As an occupation, sleep is fascinating. It shows clear neurophysiological fluctuations, developmental changes, and susceptibility to environmental influence and disruption (Bliwise, 1994; Schnelle, Alessi, Ouslander, & Simmons, 1993; Sheldon, Spire, & Levy, 1982). Disturbances in this occupation are specifically named as medical diagnoses, such as sleep apnea (Carskadon & Dement, 1994). Many of our clients have undiagnosed sleep problems due to respiratory disorders, neurophysiologic disorganization, medications, disruptive sleep environments, shift work, poorly managed schedules, or extended stays in intensive care units. Until occupational therapists understand enough about sleep to assure that it is providing an adequate base for other occupations, efficacy in treating waking occupational patterns will not reach its full potential.

Waking occupations that are highly restorative are also important to intervention. For a client who is very disorganized, depleted, or discouraged, intervention may need to be not highly productive, but highly restorative. Clinical judgment is required to discern what occupations a specific person may experience as restorative. People find waking restoration in different ways: quiet-focus occupations, such as needlework or woodworking; being in nature; viewing art; listening to music; quiet and solitude; socializing; a physical workout; self-care activities; or prayer and meditation. Of course, eating and drinking are also essential to restoration, though they can be done in ways that range from highly restorative to barely maintaining physiologic function. Occupational therapy is only at the beginning of exploring this important dimension in designing powerful, appealing intervention.

Masterful design of appealing intervention. Designing appealing intervention, and thus enhancing interven-

tion power, requires a sophisticated understanding of the productive, pleasurable, and restorative dimensions of the subjective experience of occupation. Taken one at a time, the importance of each of the three dimensions' contribution to the appeal of an occupation in intervention is easily argued. The true potency of using an occupational design approach lies, however, in the carefully blended combination of the three. High appeal is one source of therapeutic power. As such, appeal is a tool for the rapid building of the three bridges to strong occupation-based practice: a generative discourse, demonstration sites, and effective education.

Intactness: Designing With Spatial, Temporal, and Sociocultural Context

Intactness is the degree to which a therapeutic occupation occurs in the usual spatial, temporal, and sociocultural conditions in which it would usually occur for that client if it were not being used as intervention (Pierce, 1997a, 1998). Intactness can also be thought of as the naturalization of therapeutic occupation through the use of typical context. In the client's own settings, the challenges, barriers, adaptations, and potential problem solutions are more clearly evident than they can be in virtual and unfamiliar environments, such as the clinic. In the customary context, the objects, cues, and complete sequences involved in an occupation of concern are physically real to both the therapist and the client. The client is not required to reason from a simulated experience to the real challenge encountered later in full context. The custom-fit nature of a client's usual settings increases the generalizability and validity of the intervention.

In keeping with the individualistic western culture from which it springs, occupational therapy has traditionally focused more on the intraindividual characteristics of occupation than on the contextual dimensions. For this reason, it is likely that enhancing appeal through design with pleasure, productivity, and restoration will come more easily to therapists than will designing for intactness through the use of the client's typical context. Strengthening the intactness of intervention is likely to shift intervention toward enhanced understandability for clients, greater holism, more community-based interventions, and increased efficacy.

Spatial context as an element of intactness. In occupational therapy, the spatial dimension of occupation that is beyond immediate physiology has been little explored, with some exceptions in the areas of tools, adaptive devices, and architectural adaptations (Trombly, 1989; Wilcock, 1998; Zemke & Horger, 1995). To effectively use the spatial context of occupation in intervention, occupational therapists require a more sophisticated appreciation of how spaces and objects support, shape, and inhibit individual experience (Holohan, 1986; Pierce, 2000; Rowles, 1991).

The most primary spatial aspect of human occupation is our embodiedness (Frank, 1986). Evolution has shaped the human with unique capacities to interact with the physical world: the upright pelvis, the senses, the hand, and the fertile and ceaseless conceptualizations of the neocortex. We experience our lives from within a framework of human neurophysiology: sensation, perception, ideation, and movement (Ayres, 1985). Occupational therapists are masters at understanding how occupational experience is shaped by human embodiedness, especially as it is affected by disability.

Human cultural adaptation is marked by the innumerable physical objects involved in our behavior (Hodder, 1989). A rich material culture is central to our nature as occupational beings. We survive and express ourselves through our objects: clothing, crops, vehicles, shelters, tools, toys, foods, medicines, communication devices, written materials, and aesthetic and ritual objects (Dickie & Frank, 1996). Ethnic traditions are marked by unique material culture and the action routines that support it, passed down through generations. Spaces, tools, and products can express identity: People often become deeply attached to them (Csikszentmihalyi & Rochberg-Halton, 1981). The qualities of the spaces in which people work and live, including the light, sound, size, smell, and perceptions of safety or threat there, are not abstractions to them (Holohan, 1986). They are places full of personal meaning and cultural symbols (Altman & Low, 1992; Rowles, 1991). Mapping and interpreting novel spaces begins the moment people encounter them (Evans, 1980; Kaplan & Kaplan, 1981; Neisser, 1991). Routines are overlaid on familiar spaces, enabling us to reach for toothbrush and then toothpaste in their usual spots without pausing as we think about other things. It is not within an abstract space, but within a familiar and experientially patterned place that humans engage in most of their occupations.

Using the spatial dimension to enhance the intactness of occupation-based intervention requires the therapist to comprehend spatial experience from the client's perspective. How is embodiedness affecting experience? What are the usual spaces in which occupations of interest in the intervention occur, and how are the routines mapped over those environments? What objects are of importance in the occupational pattern of the client in terms of function, identity, and personal meaning? What do the spaces and objects tell the therapist about the client? Are there barriers in cherished places that may be disrupting desired occupational patterns? How are the client's typical occupational patterns laid out within home, workplace, or neighborhood? By developing such insights into the spatial dimension of a client's daily experience, the therapist can design powerfully intact therapeutic occupations.

Temporal context as an element of intactness. Occupational therapists deal constantly with the temporal structures of human occupation in intervention, yet the occupational therapy literature on the temporality of human experience is extremely limited. The most basic temporal pattern of our occupations is the circadian rhythm (Moore-Ede et al., 1982; Swaab, Fliers, & Partiman, 1985). Entrained to the light, we move in a general synchrony of fluctuations in energy level and the relatively predictable round of activities required to meet our physiological needs, such as sleeping and eating meals. With the advent of electric lighting, the predominant pattern of rising with the sun and going to bed with the dark loosened somewhat, but most people continue in the same light–dark-driven pattern that has presumably regulated human occupation since the beginning of time (Coren, 1996; Pierce, 1997b).

The temporality of the life span is also basic to our experience of occupation. In western cultures we see birth as a beginning and death as an ending to our mortal existence. This linear and finite view of time poses existential challenges for the individual's construction of an optimal occupational pattern over a lifetime. Some cultures see time in a more cyclic way, emphasizing the repeating patterns of similar events (Hall, 1983). The temporality of physiological and personal maturation also impose a general developmental shape on the occupational patterns of persons at different ages (Pierce, 2000; Royeen, 1994). Occupational therapists are commonly trained in developmental theories descriptive of life patterns across the life span. Such theories, however, are extradisciplinary and do not focus on changes in occupational experience with age.

Within these broad circadian and developmental templates, people construct a unique occupational pattern each day, orchestrating and completing a series of occupations (Clark, 1993; Segal & Frank, 1998). Within situational constraints, we manage the pace, duration, sequence, and timing of each occupation (Zerubavel, 1981). Habits and routines emerge from repeated patterns, simplifying management of the sequences (Zemke, 1994). Depending on the quality of engagement, time can feel like it is moving quickly or slowly. Memory allows reflection on the temporal patterns of our occupations and planning ahead in anticipation of their sequences and orchestration. Narratives are constructed and reconstructed to package experience in valued, storied configurations (Clark, 1993; Larson & Fanchiang, 1996). The cumulation of these daily patterns of experience over days or years can yield skill, adaptation, identity, and insight.

Using temporality to provide more powerfully intact intervention will require the therapist to reflect on the client's usual temporal experience of the occupation being used in intervention or being targeted as an outcome. By matching the pace, sequence, timing, circadian rhythm, and developmental structures of a therapeutic occupation to those most natural to the client, the power of the intervention is enhanced. Therapists tend to be intuitive about doing this, scheduling, for example, activities of daily living training for mornings and feeding sessions at mealtimes. However, by bringing this dimension of occupation in intervention more cogently to mind, it can be used, improved, researched, and taught more effectively than it can be while remaining on a more intuitive level of clinical action.

Sociocultural context as an element of intactness. The sociocultural dimension of occupational context is fairly well-understood in occupational therapy compared with the temporal and spatial dimensions of occupational context. Occupational therapy has drawn strongly from the social sciences, especially anthropology, since the time of Reilly (1974), appropriating such informative key concepts as relationship, family, kinship, community, class, race, ethnicity, gender, stigma, values, ritual, symbol, adaptation, narrative, history, economics, and politics. Skillful use of these conceptual aspects of the sociocultural context is critical to the impact of occupation-based intervention.

A fairly concrete aspect of the sociocultural dimension of occupation is the degree to which it is interactive. A unique class of occupations, called co-occupations, can occur only in interaction with a partner (Pierce, 1997a). Teaching, caregiving, and playing tennis are examples of co-occupations. Some occupations occur as shared or parallel experiences, such as watching television with others. Occupations can also occur in complete solitude.

A critical aspect of the sociocultural dimension of occupation in intervention is power relations (Foucault, 1980). Recognizing status and power dynamics between the client and others, such as the therapist, family members, other service providers, insurers, and institutions, is important to negotiating systems of care and advocating effectively for a client. Feminist theory can also make important contributions here, explicating the power relations that lie in the social construction of gender (Smith, 1987). Intact intervention requires that the client feel, at minimum, the degree of power over the therapeutic occupation that he or she would if the therapist were not involved. Significant intervention gains targeting the most important goals of a client can only be accomplished by letting go of the directive expert viewpoint and adopting a learning–collaborative view of intervention (Law, 1998; Rosa & Hasselkus, 1996).

Shared social and cultural expectations also shape our use of space and time. There is public space and private space, public time and private time (Hall, 1976, Zerubavel, 1981). Spaces can be crowded or empty of other people. Time can be social or solitary. Interpersonal space and timing of interactions are highly expressive of our identities in relation to others through eye contact, distance, touch, action synchrony, and turn taking (Hall, 1976). The complex symbolic meanings of places is passed down in the history of culture. Holidays, the 7-day week, and the workweek–weekend cycle strongly shape our occupational patterns through the established calendar (Zerubavel, 1981). Each culture has its own unique customs for constructing, valuing, and using the space and time within which its members experience occupations.

In terms of the sociocultural dimension, therapists are generally both insightful and intuitive in constructing intervention that is natural and well designed for and with individual clients. The founders of the field were attuned to such sociocultural concepts as habit training and return to a productive worker role after disability (Slagle, 1922; Quiroga, 1995). The framework of occupational behavior (Reilly, 1974) imported many informative social science concepts into the profession's literature that enhanced understanding of the sociocultural dimension. More and more, awareness of diversity is being drawn on to enhance intervention. In regard to the spatial, temporal, and sociocultural contexts of occupation, it is in designing within the sociocultural dimension that occupational therapy interventions are most powerfully intact.

Designing contextually intact therapeutic occupations. By understanding the contextual dimensions of occupational experience, the therapist can design occupation-based intervention that is more effective through its intactness. Of course, because of institutional and pragmatic constraints, it is not possible to consistently enact intervention in perfectly intact context. Intervention must approximate intactness to the degree feasible. And, being attuned to intactness, the therapist will be ready to move toward intactness in both small and large ways when opportunities arise. Questioning and seeking out the most intact temporal, spatial, and sociocultural conditions for each therapeutic occupation is a direct avenue to more powerful intervention. Thus, the idea of spatially, temporally, and socioculturally intact intervention contributes another useful tool for rapidly building bridges to strong occupation-based practice.

Accuracy: Designing to Target Client Goals Effectively

Accuracy is the degree to which the therapeutic occupation precisely targets collaboratively developed occupational goals. A good illustration of the variable degrees of accuracy that can occur is to consider the way in which group interventions can sometimes fit the goals of some clients in the group better than it does others. The accuracy of occupation-based interventions depends on therapist design skill, collaborative generation of occupational goals, and precision fit of the intervention to the goal.

Therapist design skill. Occupational therapists require highly sophisticated design skills. The average workday of an occupational therapist is a series of high challenges to design skill (Pierce, in press). An essential process of successful occupational therapy is consistently producing creative solutions to fit the life problems and goals of individual clients, doing this thinking much of the time during complex action.

As other professions have discovered, to produce graduates who can consistently design effective and creative outcomes that fit client needs, it is necessary to be explicit and deliberate in teaching these skills. Architects in training learn the process of design through the studio method (Boyer & Mitgang, 1996; Koberg & Bagnall, 1991; Schön, 1987). In addition to other classes, architecture students share a studio in which assigned design problems are worked on under the supervision of an experienced architect. Discussions, frequent group critiques, and formal design juries are used to develop the students' abilities to explicitly discuss the phases and strategies of the creative process in which they are engaged (Jones, 1981; Straub, 1978; Wade, 1977). Consumers are expected to give input throughout the development of architectural designs.

Engineering's educational approach focuses on successful problem solving, although the creative process itself has received little explicit attention in engineering curricula until recently (Fogler & LeBlanc, 1995). While immersed in content, such as physics or electrical theory, engineering students are simply presented with challenging problems to solve outside of class. The World Solar Car Race, for instance, is a now-famous engineering school problem. Engineers are especially skilled at planning and implementing large, multitask projects.

In medical education, problem-based learning is being used to enhance students' abilities to address the puzzles of daily practice through learning situations that emphasize self-directed and small group work on cases (Boud & Feletti, 1991; Royeen, 1995). The common features of the three professions' educational approaches are the students' engagement in constructed challenges, the requirement of creative thinking, and learning contexts that approximate practice settings.

Informed by the educational strategies of architecture, engineering, and medicine, occupational therapy can become better at educating practitioners in skillful occupational design. Of these three examples of professional education, architecture's studio approach provides the strongest match to occupational therapy because both professions emphasize process, an arts aesthetic, consumer involvement, and the ability to reflect on and discuss the creative thinking required for effective practice (Koberg & Bagnall, 1991; Mattingly & Fleming, 1994; Pierce, in press). Drawing on the curricular strategies of other professions, occupational therapists can be equipped with highly developed design skills of self-motivation, problem analysis, idea generation and selection, complex implementation, and process evaluation. Such sophisticated design skills can equip graduates to consistently create accurate, and thus therapeutically powerful, occupation-based interventions.

Collaborative occupational goal generation. Highly accurate interventions must target occupational patterns as the end, or goal, of intervention and create those goals in collaboration with the client. An occupational pattern is an observable shape or regularity in the recurrences of similar occupations in a person's life (Pierce,

1997a, 1997b; Zemke & Pierce, 1994). Therapists, clients, and caregivers frequently identify occupational patterns as goals; for example, a school-based intervention goal could be for a student to independently use the lunchroom. To target broad, functional occupational patterns as an end of intervention, a substantial knowledge of typical occupational patterns across the life span is essential. The therapist must understand how the targeted occupational patterns are a part of identity, social acceptance, function, and health.

Trombly (1995; see Chapter 11), Gray (1998; see Chapter 10), and Cynkin (1995) described the use of occupation and activity as the means and ends of intervention. Setting occupational pattern goals with clients is using occupation as the end of intervention. Top–down, or occupation-focused, assessments contribute significantly to occupational therapists' ability to target occupational patterns as ends of intervention (Coster, 1998). If the intervention accurately targets an occupational outcome desired by the client, even the most mechanistic approach to intervention can be considered occupation-based. To set occupational goals that are well fit to the client requires strong collaborative goal-setting skills (Law, 1998; Rosa & Hasselkus, 1996). For this, a willingness of the therapist to release the powerful position of expert decision-maker is essential. Highly developed abilities to interview, observe, and assist in prioritizing the client's and caregivers' needs are also required.

Precision fit of intervention to goal. Precision fit is simply a measure of how well the therapeutic occupation directly addressed the goals. The fit of the intervention to the goals can be weakened by many conditions common to intervention settings: limitations to intervention flexibility, such as standard protocols; inadequate time for intervention planning; attempting intervention in unsuitable environments or without adequate materials; or serving clients with diverse goals through group interventions. Even under such conditions the therapist can more effectively create therapeutic occupations that provide a powerful match to the client's needs by reflecting on the precision of the fit. This is hardly a new concept for occupational therapy, although it bears repeating.

Fitting a therapeutic occupation to client need is as old as the field. What is new here is the idea of reflecting on the *degree* of fit. Questioning whether an occupation-based intervention is being used is an ongoing theme of discussion in the profession (Wood, 1998). Less common is the questioning of *how well* the occupation used met a particular client's goals, what inter-

fered in that effort, and what activity or setting might have fit the targeted goals better. Reflecting on the preciseness of fit after an intervention is a valuable form of productive dreaming about ideal intervention. Used consistently, such reflection will yield growth for the therapist and enhanced efficacy for clients.

Accuracy: Therapist design skill, collaborative goals, and precision fit. Accuracy will boost the therapeutic power of any intervention. Powerful effects are produced by combining highly developed design skills, collaborative goals as the ends of intervention, and a therapeutic occupation that is precisely fit to those goals. Occupational therapists are the consummate professionals in this holistic approach to intervention. Thus, to the previous conceptual tools of appeal and intactness is now added a third important tool for making the bridge from knowledge of occupation to strong occupation-based practice—accuracy.

A Field's Translation: From Knowledge of Occupation to Designing for Therapeutic Power

The present is, paradoxically, both a fruitful and a dangerous time of congruence between our expanding knowledge base regarding occupation and the increased valuing of functional outcomes in health care. Occupational therapy must critically examine and recreate its traditions in theory and practice if it is to live up to its potential for providing clients with powerful interventions based on a deep understanding of occupational experience. To match the pace of change in health care, the profession must deliberately and rapidly build bridges between theoretical research on occupation and the powerful use of occupation in practice. A generative discourse around occupation-based practice, demonstration sites, and effective education are the bridges that are needed. Offered here are new conceptual tools for these bridge-building efforts: the subjective and contextual dimensions of occupation and the design process through which they can be translated into therapeutic occupations high in occupational appeal, intactness, and accuracy.

Acknowledgment

The ideas I present here are an outgrowth of years of discussion with Ruth Zemke, PhD, OTR, FAOTA, of the University of Southern California. Few are so fortunate in their colleagues.

References

Altman, I., & Low, S. M. (1992). *Place attachment*. New York: Plenum.

American Occupational Therapy Association. (1995). Position paper: Occupation. *American Journal of Occupational Therapy, 49,* 1015–1018.

Ayres, A. J. (1985). *Developmental dyspraxia and adult onset apraxia*. Torrance, CA: Sensory Integration International.

Bliwise, D. L. (1994). Normal aging. In M. H. Kryger, T. Roth, & W. C. Dement (Eds.), *Principles and practices of sleep medicine* (pp. 26–39). Philadelphia: Saunders.

Boud, D., & Feletti, G. (1991). *The challenge of problem-based learning*. New York: St. Martin's.

Boyer, E., & Mitgang, L. (1996). *Building community: A new future for architecture education and practice*. Princeton, NJ: Carnegie Foundation for the Advancement of Teaching.

Carskadon, M. A., & Dement, W. C. (1994). Normal human sleep: An overview. In M. H. Kryger, T. Roth, & W. C. Dement (Eds.), *Principles and practices of sleep medicine* (pp. 16–25). Philadelphia: Saunders.

Clark, F. (1993). Occupation embedded in a real life: Interweaving occupational science and occupational therapy, 1993 Eleanor Clarke Slagle Lecture. *American Journal of Occupational Therapy, 47,* 1067–1078. http://dx.doi.org/10.5014/ajot.47.12.1067

Clark, F., Azen, S., Zemke, R., Jackson, J., Carlson, M., Mandel, D., Hay, J., Josephson, K., Cherry, B., Hessle, C., Palmer, J., & Lipson, L. (1997). Occupational therapy for independent-living older adults: A randomized controlled trial. *Journal of the American Medical Association, 278,* 1321–1326.

Clark, F., Carlson, M., & Polkinghorne, D. (1997). The Issue Is—The legitimacy of life history and narrative approaches in the study of occupation. *American Journal of Occupational Therapy, 51,* 313–317.

Clark, F. A., Parham, D., Carlson, M. E., Frank, G., Jackson, J., Pierce, D., Wolfe, R. J., & Zemke, R. (1991). Occupational science: Academic innovation in the service of occupational therapy's future. *American Journal of Occupational Therapy, 45,* 300–310. http://dx.doi.org/10.5014/ajot.45.4.300

Cohen, D. (1987). *The development of play*. New York: New York University Press.

Coren, S. (1996). *Sleep thieves*. New York: Free Press.

Coster, W. (1998). Occupation-centered assessment of children. *American Journal of Occupational Therapy, 52,* 337–344.

Cross, G. (1990). *A social history of leisure since 1600*. State College, PA: Venture.

Csikszentmihalyi, M., & Rochberg-Halton, E. (1981). *The meaning of things: Domestic symbols and the self*. New York: Cambridge University Press.

Cynkin, S. (1995). Activities. In C. Royeen (Ed.), *The practice of the future: Putting occupation back into therapy* (pp. 7-1–7-52). Bethesda, MD: American Occupational Therapy Association.

Davis, J. (1984). *Endorphins*. Garden City, NJ: Dial Press.

Dickie, V. (1998). Households, multiple livelihoods, and the informal economy. *Scandinavian Journal of Occupational Therapy, 5,* 109–118.

Dickie, V., & Frank, G. (1996). Artisan occupations in the global economy: A conceptual framework. *Journal of Occupational Science: Australia, 3,* 45–55.

Evans, G. (1980). Environmental cognition. *Psychological Bulletin, 88,* 259–287.

Fidler, G. S., & Velde, B. P. (1999). *Activities: Reality and symbol*. Thorofare, NJ: Slack.

Fisher, A. G., Murray, E. A., & Bundy, A. C. (1991). *Sensory integration: Theory and practice*. Philadelphia: F. A. Davis.

Fogler, H. S., & LeBlanc, S. E. (1995). *Strategies for creative problem solving*. Englewood Cliffs, NJ: Prentice Hall.

Foucault, M. (1980). *Power/knowledge: Selected interviews and other writings 1972–1977*. New York: Pantheon.

Frank, G. (1986). On embodiment: A case study of congenital limb deficiency in American culture. *Culture, Medicine, and Psychiatry, 10,* 189–219.

Geertz, C. (1983). *The interpretation of cultures*. New York: Basic.

Gellner, E. (1988). *Plough, sword, and book: The structure of human history*. Chicago: University of Chicago Press.

Goodman, N. (1951). *The structure of appearance*. Cambridge, MA: Harvard University Press.

Gray, J. M. (1998). Putting occupation into practice: Occupation as ends, occupation as means. *American Journal of Occupational Therapy, 52,* 354–364. http://dx.doi.org/10.5014/ajot.52.5.354 Reprinted as Chapter 10.

Guyton, A. C. (1991). *Basic neuroscience*. Philadelphia: Saunders.

Hall, E. T. (1976). *The hidden dimension*. New York: Anchor Books, Doubleday.

Hall, E. T. (1983). *The dance of life: The other dimension of time*. New York: Anchor Books, Doubleday.

Harris, J., & Park, R. (1983). *Play, games, and sports in cultural contexts*. Champaign, IL: Human Kinetics.

Hasselkus, B. R. (1991). Ethical dilemmas in family caregiving for the elderly: Implications for occupational therapy. *American Journal of Occupational Therapy, 45,* 206–212. http://dx.doi.org/10.5014/ajot.45.3.206

Healy, C. (1982). *Career development.* Newton, MA: Allyn & Bacon.

Hobson, J. A. (1989). *Sleep.* New York: Scientific American Library.

Hodder, I. (1989). *The meaning of things: Material culture and symbolic expression.* Boston: Unwin-Hyman.

Holohan, C. J. (1986). Environmental psychology. *Annual Review of Psychology, 37,* 381–407.

Huizinga, J. (1950). *Homo ludens: A study of the play element in culture.* Boston: Beacon.

Jackson, J., Carlson, M., Mandel, D., Zemke, R., & Clark, F. (1998). Occupation in lifestyle redesign: The well elderly study occupational therapy program. *American Journal of Occupational Therapy, 52,* 326–336. http://dx-.doi.org/10.5014/ajot.52.5.326

Jones, J. C. (1981). *Design methods: Seeds of human futures.* New York: Wiley.

Kaplan, S., & Kaplan, R. (1981). *Cognition and environment: Functioning in an uncertain world.* New York: Praeger.

Keller, S., Shiflet, S., & Bartlett, J. (1994). Stress, immunity, and health. In R. Glaser & J. Kielcolt-Glaser (Eds.), *Handbook of human stress and immunity* (pp. 217–244). New York: Academic.

Kielhofner, G. (1992). *Conceptual foundations for occupational therapy.* Philadelphia: F. A. Davis.

Koberg, D., & Bagnall, J. (1991). *The all new universal traveler: A soft-systems guide to creativity, problem-solving, and the process of reaching goals.* Los Altos, CA: William Kaufmann.

Larson, E. A., & Fanchiang, S. P. C. (1996). Nationally Speaking—Life history and narrative research: Generating a humanistic knowledge base for occupational therapy. *American Journal of Occupational Therapy, 50,* 247–250. http://dx.doi.org/10.5014/ajot.50.4.247

Law, M. (Ed.). (1998). *Client-centered occupational therapy.* Thorofare, NJ: Slack.

Martin, J. H. (1996). *Neuroanatomy: Text and atlas.* Norwalk, CT: Appleton & Lange.

Maslow, A. (1954). *Motivation and personality.* New York: Harper and Row.

Mattingly, C., & Fleming, M. (1994). *Clinical reasoning: Forms of inquiry in a therapeutic practice.* Philadelphia: F. A. Davis.

Meyer, A. (1922). The philosophy of occupation therapy. *Archives of Occupational Therapy, 1,* 1–10. Reprinted as Chapter 4.

Moorcroft, W. H. (1989). *Sleep, dreaming, and sleep disorders.* New York: University Press of America.

Moore-Ede, M. C., Sulzman, F. M., & Fuller, C. A. (1982). *The clocks that time us.* Cambridge, MA: Harvard University Press.

Mosey, A. C. (1992). The Issue Is—Partition of occupational science and occupational therapy. *American Journal of Occupational Therapy, 46,* 851–853. http://dx.doi.org/10.5014/ajot.46.9.851

Neisser, U. (1991). Two perceptually given aspects of the self and their development. *Developmental Review, 11,* 197–209.

Nelson, D. L. (1997). Why the profession of occupational therapy will flourish in the 21st century, 1996 Eleanor Clarke Slagle Lecture. *American Journal of Occupational Therapy, 51,* 11–24. http://dx.doi.org/10.5014/ajot.51.1.11

Parham, L. D., & Fazio, L. (Eds.). (1996). *Play in occupational therapy for children.* St. Louis, MO: Mosby.

Pierce, D. (1997a). Sources of power in therapeutic applications of object play with young children at risk for developmental delays. In L. D. Parham & L. Fazio (Eds.), *Play in occupational therapy practice.* St. Louis, MO: Mosby.

Pierce, D. (1997b). The neurologic base of primary occupational patterns: Productivity, pleasure, and rest. In C. B. Royeen (Ed.), *AOTA Self-Paced Clinical Course: Neuroscience foundations of occupation* (pp. 1–28). Bethesda, MD: American Occupational Therapy Association.

Pierce, D. (1998). The Issue Is—What is the source of occupation's treatment power? *American Journal of Occupational Therapy, 52,* 490–491. http://dx.doi.org/10.5014/ajot.52.6.490

Pierce, D. (2000). Maternal management of the home as a developmental play space for infants and toddlers. *American Journal of Occupational Therapy, 54,* 290–299. http://dx.doi.org/10.5014/ajot.54.3.290

Pierce, D. (2003). *Occupation by design.* Philadelphia: F. A. Davis.

Primeau, L. A. (1992). A woman's place: Unpaid work in the home. *American Journal of Occupational Therapy, 46,* 981–988. http://dx.doi.org/10.5014/ajot.46.11.981

Primeau, L. A. (1996). Work and leisure: Transcending the dichotomy. *American Journal of Occupational Therapy, 50,* 569–577.

Quiroga, V. A. M. (1995). *Occupational therapy: The first 30 years 1900 to 1930.* Bethesda, MD: American Occupational Therapy Association.

Reilly, M. (1974). *Play as exploratory learning.* Beverly Hills, CA: Sage.

Rosa, S., & Hasselkus, B. (1996). Connecting with patients: The personal experience of professional helping. *Occupational Therapy Journal of Research, 16,* 245–260.

Rowles, G. D. (1991). Beyond performance: Being in place as a component of occupational therapy. *American Journal of Occupational Therapy, 45,* 265–271. http://dx.doi.org/10.5014/ajot.45.3.265

Royeen, C. B. (1994). The human life cycle: Paradigmatic shifts in occupation. In C. Royeen (Ed.) *The practice of the future: Putting occupation back into therapy* (pp. 1–24). Bethesda, MD: American Occupational Therapy Association.

Royeen, C. B. (1995). A problem-based learning curriculum for occupational therapy education. *American Journal of Occupational Therapy, 49,* 338–346.

Rubin, K. H. (1980). *New directions for child development: Children's play.* San Francisco: Jossey-Bass.

Schkade, J. K., & Schultz, S. (1992). Occupational adaptation: Toward a holistic approach for contemporary practice, part 1. *American Journal of Occupational Therapy, 46,* 829–837. http://dx.doi.org/10.5014/ajot.46.9.829

Schnelle, J. F., Alessi, C. A., Ouslander, J. G., & Simmons, S. F. (1993). Noise and predictors of sleep in a nursing home environment. In J. L. Albarede, J. E. Morley, T. Roth, & B. J. Vellas (Eds.), *Facts and research in gerontology, Vol. 7: Sleep disorders in the elderly* (pp. 89–99). New York: Springer.

Schön, D. (1987). *Educating the reflective practitioner.* San Francisco: Jossey-Bass.

Segal, R., & Frank, G. (1998). The extraordinary construction of ordinary experience: Scheduling daily life in families with children with attention deficit disorder. *Scandinavian Journal of Occupational Therapy, 5,* 141–147.

Sheldon, S., Spire, J., & Levy, H. (1982). *Pediatric sleep medicine.* Philadelphia: Saunders.

Slagle, E. C. (1922). Training aids for mental patients. *Archives of Occupational Therapy, 1,* 11–19.

Smith, D. E. (1987). *The everyday world as problematic.* Boston: Northeastern Press.

Straub, C. C. (1978). *Design process and communications: A case study.* Dubuque, IA: Kendall/Hunt.

Swaab, D. F., Fliers, E., & Partiman, T. S. (1985). The suprachiasmatic nucleus of the human brain in relation to sex, age, and senile dementia. *Brain Research, 342,* 37–44.

Trombly, C. (1989). *Occupational therapy for physical dysfunction* (3rd ed.). Baltimore: Williams & Wilkins.

Trombly, C. A. (1995). Occupation: Purposefulness and meaningfulness as therapeutic mechanisms, 1995 Eleanor Clarke Slagle lecture. *American Journal of Occupational Therapy, 49,* 960–972. Reprinted as Chapter 11.

Wade, J. W. (1977). *Architecture, problems, and purposes.* New York: Wiley.

Wilcock, A. (1998). *An occupational perspective of health.* Thorofare, NJ: Slack.

Wood, W. (1998). Nationally Speaking—It is jump time for occupational therapy. *American Journal of Occupational Therapy, 52,* 403–411. http://dx.doi.org/10.5014/ajot.52.6.403

Yerxa, E. J. (1998). Occupation: The keystone of a curriculum for a self-defined profession. *American Journal of Occupational Therapy, 52,* 365–372.

Yerxa, E. J., Clark, F., Frank, G., Jackson, J., Parham, D., Pierce, D., Stein, C., & Zemke, R. (1989). An introduction to occupational science: A foundation for occupational therapy in the 21st century. *Occupational Therapy in Health Care, 6*(4), 1–18.

Zemke, R. (1994). Habits. In C. Royeen (Ed.), *The practice of the future: Putting occupation back into therapy* (pp. 1–24). Bethesda, MD: American Occupational Therapy Association.

Zemke, R., & Clark, F. (1996). Preface. In R. Zemke & F. Clark (Eds.), *Occupational science: The evolving discipline* (pp. vii–xviii). Philadelphia: F. A. Davis.

Zemke, R., & Horger, M. (1995). Hands: Tools for crafting human adaptation. In C. Royeen (Ed.), *Hands on: Practical interventions for the hand* (pp. 1–36). Bethesda, MD: American Occupational Therapy Association.

Zemke, R., & Pierce, D. (1994). [Data set on occupational event log: Student sample]. Unpublished raw data.

Zerubavel, E. (1981). *Hidden rhythms: Schedules and calendars in social life.* Los Angeles: University of California Press.

CHAPTER 62

Embracing Our Ethos, Reclaiming Our Heart

2005 ELEANOR CLARKE SLAGLE LECTURE

SUZANNE M. PELOQUIN

This lecture holds familiar themes drawn from sentiments, values, and thoughts found in occupational therapy literature and elucidated through images, fables, and stories with human interest. In essence, this work is a historical and philosophical attempt to cast light on the ethos of occupational therapy. It is my hope to illuminate our ethos—the beliefs that guide us—and to do so in such a way that a fresh perspective on current challenges is possible. In the end, I will set before you this idea that asks affect and will to join with thought: To advance into the future embracing the ethos that has characterized occupational therapy since its inception is to reclaim the profession's heart.

I prepared for this day with a synthesis of my prior work, gathering new ideas to lift those thoughts to higher ground. In the process, an insight emerged. Over the years, many of you have told me that my work strikes a resonating chord, some of you naming that chord soulful, others philosophical, and still others poetic or lyrical. I believe that you discerned in my writing glints of an ethos that always has resonance, and your discernment sealed my choice of topic.

Any hope to cast light on an ethos is large enough to give one pause. This effort is but a start. I've read widely, thought deeply, and sifted many works for the beliefs that guide us. From dauntingly many iterations, I've culled themes well-worn and ethological. I've chosen words with care, seeking fidelity to our forebears and a quintessence that endures. The guiding beliefs that I propose are but my take on many other takes, here now for your taking, remaking, or leaving altogether.

The Meaning of a Professional Ethos

Dictionary definitions of the term ethos include these: a person's character or disposition; an individual's moral nature; the characteristic spirit or prevailing sentiment of a group; the genius—that extraordinary and distinctive capacity or aptitude—of a people or institution; the guiding beliefs, standards, or ideals that pervade and characterize a group; the spirit that motivates the ideas or practices of a community; the complex of fundamental values that permeate or actuate major patterns of thought and behavior (Simpson & Weiner, 1989).

A profession's ethos is thus an interlacing of sentiment, value, and thought that captures its character, conveys its genius, and manifests its spirit. An ethos carries beliefs so fundamental and sound that they endure, both transcending and supporting the particularities of shifting paradigms. The idea of a professional ethos kindles hope that one can apprehend and articulate a profession's character. Physician Larry Churchill (1975) said that ethological beliefs are "often loosely identified, seldom find articulate form, and generally operate inconspicuously in the routines of a given community" (p. 31). Physical therapist Christine Stiller (2000) understood a professional ethos as core beliefs held in a dynamic that responds to change. Nurse Anthony Tuckett (1998) said that an ideal ethos has moral integrity in addressing both what one ought to do and how one ought to be. Each thought a profession's ethos discoverable.

Metaphors reveal its functions. An ethos serves as touchstone against which individuals strike their actions to know their worth. As inner voice, an ethos inspires individuals and calls them back when they stray too far. An ethos sets a profession's course in ever-changing times. It is bare-bones plot in a heroic tale. Bold standard raised in a milling crowd, an ethos leads those with diverse roles and views to say, "That's right!" The pull of an ethos is unbroken, sometimes undertow in currents less

This chapter was previously published in the *American Journal of Occupational Therapy, 59*, 611–625. Copyright © 2005, American Occupational Therapy Association. Reprinted with permission. http://dx.doi.org/10.5014/ajot.59.6.611

ideal. Its confluence of sentiment, value, and thought yields guiding beliefs, both vital and lasting.

It is important at the outset to distinguish our profession's ethos from other more familiar of its characterizations. Intimations of the profession's character, genius, and spirit nest in key documents of the American Occupational Therapy Association. The official definition, for example, describes occupational therapy's unique purpose, focus, and populations (American Occupational Therapy Association [AOTA], 2004). The philosophical statement reveals our grasp of the nature of persons and of occupation (AOTA, 1979). The *Code of Ethics* sets guidelines for moral practice and relationships, linking them to cherished principles (AOTA, 1994). The core values and attitudes paper culls values from our documents and uses nursing's language to cast them as commitments (AOTA, 1993). *The Guide to Occupational Therapy Practice* describes to a broad audience the scope and actions of our therapy (Moyers, 1999). The *Occupational Therapy Practice Framework* lays out the domain and process of our work (AOTA, 2002). Singly and collectively these documents draw from, organize, standardize, or recognize aspects of our ethos. They reflect its contours and honor its substance. Even together, however, they neither constitute nor state our ethos.

Also drawing from and leading back to our ethos is discourse about the profession's paradigms, models, and legitimate tools—hallmarks of our knowledge and interventions. Especially close to the ethos are discussions of the art, science, and ethics of the profession and thoughts about our culture and integrative values (Hansen, 2003; Hasselkus, 2002, Hubbard, 1991; Kielhofner 1997; Mosey, 1981; Reed & Sanderson, 1999; Rogers, 1983; Shannon, 1977; West, 1984; Wilcock, 1998; Wood, 1995, 2004; Yerxa, 1967). Not yet within our literature, however, is there an exposé of the guiding beliefs that serve as ethos.

Absent from easy access, therefore, is the ground on which Robert K. Bing (1986) suggested we stand when he said this: "Where we will find comfort, safety, and stability is in those decades-old fundamentals and principles developed by our founders and practiced by our pioneers . . . our beliefs, our values—they form the rock upon which we must stand" (p. 670). The rock is there; we need only cast light on it.

The Ethos of Occupational Therapy

The early decades of the 20th century shaped the context from which our ethos emerged. Physician Sidney Licht (1967) shared a glimpse of those times from his lived experience. A loaf of bread cost a nickel, then. Eggs were 40 cents a dozen. A man who bought a 5 cent beer could eat all the hard-boiled eggs he wanted. There was neither radio nor television. Milk was brought to homes 7 days a week by horse-drawn wagons. Toast was made atop a gas range. Houses were heated with wood or coal, and neither electric refrigeration nor supermarkets existed. It cost a penny to send a postcard, a penny more to mail a letter. All telephones were black. Street lights were turned on by men called lamplighters; there were no traffic lights or parking meters. Ford's touring car sold for $360.00.

A recently industrialized society rued the effects of machines that maimed bodies at an alarming rate. Arts and crafts societies emerged against the monotony and lost autonomy of factory work. Sanitation was poor. Social workers such as Jane Addams saw the ill effects of city life among poor immigrants and offered community activities in neighborhood settlement houses. Engineers such as the Gilbreths advanced techniques to make people and machines more efficient. War was in the news. The ways through which neighboring countries supported their soldiers prompted readiness to do the same here.

In 1917, our profession's founding year, Binet proposed the IQ test; Dewey endorsed learning by doing. Many condemned the failure of hospitals to ready patients for return to society. Inhumane conditions for mental illness earned public exposure, and the National Committee for Mental Hygiene, launched by former patient Clifford Beers, sought better treatment. Human behavior was examined in the lights of inner purpose and environmental cause. Philosophers spoke of holism, common sense, and practical consequences (Peters, 1953; Roback, 1952). I've but skimmed the wellspring from which our ethos emerged.

Early supporters of the use of occupation, the founders of the Society for the Promotion of Occupational Therapy, and early occupational workers drew from this context and their experiences a common understanding: Occupation could help. In discussing the power of occupation and a therapy built around it, they reiterated central themes with visionary zeal. From their discussions, five beliefs emerged with guiding potential, each a confluence of sentiment, value, and thought. Each had the capacity to shape character, establish reputation, and carry the profession's spirit across changing times. Each became part of our ethos.

Because each ethological belief captures a distinct and equally important dimension of occupation or occupational therapy, each relates to the others existentially rather than sequentially or hierarchically. The end result is a complex of guiding beliefs, an ethos. It is this: (1) time, place, and circumstance open paths to occupation; (2) occupation fosters dignity, competence, and health; (3) occupational therapy is a personal engagement; (4) caring and helping are vital to the work; and (5) effective practice is artistry and science. Taken together, these beliefs capture that which we profess—declare and affirm—in the world.

I offer a sampling of each of these early beliefs and, on this golden anniversary of the first Eleanor Clarke Slagle Lecture in 1955, follow each sampling with thoughts from Slagle lecturers who extended them across time. These thoughts complement kindred ideas taken from all such lectures and showcased during today's prelecture time. If they evoke others from your memory, I am pleased.

Time, Place, and Circumstance Open Paths to Occupation

One guiding belief is that time, place, and circumstance open paths to occupation, challenges notwithstanding. Situated in life circumstances of all kinds, persons *occupy* time and place (Reed & Sanderson, 1999). Adolf Meyer (1922; see Chapter 4), a neuropathologist and champion of the profession, saw time's path to occupation. Sharing his philosophy of occupational therapy when professor of psychiatry at Johns Hopkins University, he said: "Man learns to organize time and he does it in terms of *doing* things . . . and one of the things he does we call work and occupation—we might call it the ingestion and proper use . . . of time with its successions of opportunities" (pp. 9–10).

Meyer (1922) cited philosopher Pierre Janet, noting that proper use of time is "the realization of reality, bringing the very soul of man out of dreams of eternity to the full sense and appreciation of actuality." Our role as occupation workers, Meyer said, consists of "giving opportunities rather than prescriptions" (p. 7). If a person's use of time was a doing, it was also and more essentially a becoming, a realization of the soul (Peloquin, 1990, 1997a; Wilcock, 1998). Meyer continued, "The awakening to a full meaning of time as the biggest wonder and asset of our lives and the valuation of opportunity and performance as the greatest measure of time; those are the beacon lights of the philosophy of the occupation worker" (p. 9).

Watching groups of mentally ill patients engaged in handwork, Meyer (1922) saw "a pleasure in achieve-

ment, a real pleasure in the use and activity of [one's] hands and muscles and a happy appreciation of time" (pp. 3–4). He said that valuing time led to a "conception of mental illness as problems of living" rather than as only problems with thinking, or diseases, or disorders of constitution (p. 4).

Taking a complementary if pragmatic view, Allan Cullimore (1921), chief of Educational Service in Letterman Hospital in San Francisco, spoke of time's worth. He applauded occupational therapy's real work as therapeutic agent, cautioning against busy work. "Occupational therapy planned to kill time," he said, "stands in the same relation to the real occupational therapy as that of first aid to medical treatment based on examination and careful diagnosis" (p. 537). "Occupations must lead somewhere," Cullimore said, "and the patient must want to follow" (p. 538). Time and circumstance, we note, open paths to occupation. Place and circumstance do so as well.

Many places of the time called for occupations: hospitals for the insane; wards in general hospitals, from pediatric to psychopathic to orthopedic; hospital workshops; sanitaria for the treatment of tuberculosis; tents and army barracks; schools for defectives; institutions for the blind; convalescent homes; and private dwellings. Meyer's (1922) philosophy included harmonic engagement with place: "Our conception of man is that of an organism that maintains and balances itself in the world of reality and actuality by being in active life and active use . . . and acting its time in harmony with its own nature and the nature about it" (p. 5). He supported an "orderly rhythm in the atmosphere" of mental hospitals, using among disturbed patients the habit training approach to life tasks—dressing, eating, working, playing—developed by Eleanor Clarke Slagle (Meyer).

Other early practitioners saw occupation at the interface of place and circumstance. Susan Tracy (1913), nurse and early practitioner, wrote, "The occupation room provides a new environment. It takes the patient away from his individual apartment and from the living rooms of the institution which may be filled with the suggestion of invalidism. It presents a cheerful atmosphere of quiet activity and a satisfying sense of something worthwhile being accomplished" (p. 4).

Discussions of helpful atmospheres led to the making of places that grew them. Thomas Kidner (1923), Canadian architect and founder, published designs for recreation halls, workshops, and theaters to accommodate occupations. A few years later, Louis Haas (1927), director of Men's Therapeutic Occupations at Bloomingdale Hospital in White Plains, New York, published more designs, noting reciprocal ties between occupation and place: "In occupational therapy," he said, "any corner that would hold a couple of chairs was at first considered a place in which this treatment could be given. . . . The treatment itself was used as a means of transforming, not only the patient, but the very inadequate floor spaces and unsightly walls, into more inspiring surroundings" (p. 285). Many instances of environmental transformations appear in our literature (Carlova & Ruggles, 1946; Slagle, 1938).

Thoughts about occupation's emergence from time, place, and circumstance have endured. In her Slagle lecture, Anne Fisher (1998) made the connection succinctly and well. She said: "The term occupation conveys the powerful essence of our profession—enabling people to seize, take possession of, or occupy the spaces, time, and roles of their lives" (p. 511). Some 30 years earlier, Gail Fidler (1966) had said in her lecture, "Man's innate drive to fulfill his needs for self-identity and realization through productive transactions with his object and interpersonal world is and has been the cornerstone of occupational therapy" (p. 8). Our ethos, in part, is this: Time, place, and circumstance open paths to occupation. Guided by this belief, occupational therapy practitioners are pathfinders.

Occupation Fosters Dignity, Competence, and Health

Another guiding belief is that occupation fosters dignity, competence, and health. Founder William Rush Dunton, Jr. (1919) conveyed his belief in the healing role of occupation in a creed that prefaced a book on wartime work, known as reconstruction therapy. He wrote:

> That occupation is as necessary to life as food and drink. That every human being should have both physical and mental occupation. That all should have occupations which they enjoy. . . . That sick minds, sick bodies, sick souls, may be healed through occupation. (p. 17)

Almost 10 years earlier, Robert Carroll (1910), a physician in Asheville, North Carolina, had noted the worth of occupation in terms of dignity and competence, confidently proposing a "Law of Work" and asserting that "work truly is life." He said:

> The greatest influence, the true and lasting benefit in work as a therapeutic agent, rests in the

moral uplift, the great mastering of self which comes when one is taught to work right, when one knows the joy and forgets the burden of doing, when self-mastery displaces indulgence, when doubt of one's strength is replaced by faith. (p. 2034)

Whether endorsed as moral creed or scientific law, the belief was this: Occupation fosters dignity, competence, and health. Meta Anderson (1920) thus said that occupational therapy "should inspire the feeling of pleasure and self-respect which comes from being useful, and the feeling of power which comes from progressive daily achievement" (p. 326). Most poignant is her story, told in the language of the day:

> An official was visiting the work of the feebleminded in a certain school. The teacher reported the good work done by the various schoolchildren. When she had finished, a low grade girl member of the class tugged at her sleeve and said, "Tell him that I cleaned the garbage can." She had cleaned the garbage can and had done it very well. She beamed over the praise given to her after she had called attention to her accomplishment. She had been useful and her joy was unbounded. (p. 326)

One soldier gave this testimonial to occupation: "I got a new vision of life. . . . [I] saw the dignity of labor made new and interesting, and even more powerful because of the handicap" (Cooper, 1918, pp. 24–25).

Belief in the healing power of occupation—in its capacity to help individuals become hale and whole—has endured. What bolder affirmation than that in the Slagle lecture of Mary Reilly (1962): "The hypothesis that I presented for evidence of proof was that man, through the use of his hands, as they are energized by mind and will, can influence the state of his own health. I asked if this were a kind of idea that America could subscribe to and to that I replied with a resounding yes" (p. 8). Our ethos, in part, is this: Occupation fosters dignity, competence, and health. Guided by this belief, occupational therapy practitioners enable occupations that heal.

Occupational Therapy Is a Personal Engagement

A third guiding belief holds that occupational therapy is a personal engagement. Engagement—the commitment to involve and occupy oneself and be bound by mutual promise—was thought necessary for patient and therapist alike. George Barton (1920), an architect and founder informed by nursing courses and his own disability, clarified the aim of occupational work:

> Not in the making of a product, but in the making of a MAN, of a man stronger physically, mentally, and spiritually than he was before, for just as his body can be strengthened by carefully graded exercise from week to week, as his mind can be strengthened and be improved in the same way, so also may his spirit be reborn in greater strength and purity by the effort for, and the realization of his triumph over disability and despair. (p. 308)

Such engagement and cocreation were essentially and deeply personal.

Also personal were responses among patients such as those ill from tuberculosis. These touched Bayard Crane (1919), a physician in Rutland, Massachusetts. He said, "In them pain will create outcry or fright. Monotony will produce depression, discouragement, or desperation. Uselessness will break down initiative and ambition" (p. 63). Crane sought occupational workers who could "help meet the individual patient more on his own terms. . . . I am pleading" he said, "for a method which aims to further individualize with the temperament of each patient. . . . It is an attempt to instill in the treatment enspiring [*sic*] influences created by diversion, by occupation of mind, by stimulation of flagging interests, and by reeducation of faith and self-confidence" (p. 64). The need for occupational workers to engage as and with persons was clear.

Charlotte Moodie (1919), nurse and director of Social Service at Grace Hospital in Detroit, described patients who were engaged:

> Here, in his wheelchair we find Joe, recovering from a fractured thigh, busily engaged in carving a breadboard or bookrack. Close by, lying flat on his back is Max, a bright cheery young chap . . . tuberculosis of the spine . . . ties him to his bed. He is now making a wool sweater by means of which Miss Tracy calls "rake knitting." In the women's ward is Mrs. Schuster making a basket, something she has always wanted to do. (p. 314)

This scene of patients much engaged evokes the image of a practitioner who had explored capacity, interest,

and meaning, inspired confidence and courage, and personally engaged.

Years earlier, Tracy (1913) had described the requisite engagement, noting that occupational nurses "are constantly being impressed with the fact that the technical and mechanical part of their work is but one aspect of their professional duty, that a broader conception must be attained—a sense of obligation to minister to the individual as well as to the disease" (p. 9) and to be "thoughtful of the deeper needs of her patient" (p. 11). Therapeutic obligation included deep consideration.

Meyer (1922; see Chapter 4) spoke of the integrity implicit in such engagement: "It takes rare gifts and talents and rare personalities to be real pathfinders in this work. There are no royal roads; it is all a problem of being true to one's nature and opportunities and of teaching others to do the same with themselves" (p. 7). Being true and real were important. Equally vital to the engagement were other ways of being endorsed by Kidner (1929) in an address to graduating students:

> May you realize in increasing measure the value of certain spiritual things which are the real making of life, but which we call by many common names. Kindness, humanity, decency, honor, and good faith—to give these up under any circumstances whatever, would be a loss greater than any defeat, or even death itself. (p. 385)

Perceptions of occupational therapy as a personal engagement have endured. Elizabeth Yerxa (1967) spoke eloquently of this view in her Slagle lecture:

> We cannot really help clients unless *we are there;* that is we feel, we encounter, we take time, we listen and we *are* ourselves. . . . Personal authenticity as an occupational therapist means that the therapist allows himself to feel real emotion as he enters into mutual relation with the client. . . . Philosophically, we do not see man as a "thing" but as a being whose choices allow him to discover and determine his own Being. Our media, our emphasis upon the client's potentials, the necessity for him to act and the mutuality of our relationship with him provide a milieu in which his suffering can be translated into the resolve to become his true self. (p. 8)

Our ethos, in part, is this: Occupational therapy is a personal engagement—a mutual commitment to involve and occupy the self and be bound by promise. Guided by this belief, occupational therapy practitioners cocreate daily lives.

Caring and Helping Are Vital to the Work

A fourth guiding belief within our ethos is that caring and helping are vital to the work. Herbert Hall (Hall & Buck, 1915), physician and early practitioner, spoke with deep feeling of any individual left idle or bereft. He said, "Put yourself in that man's place—imagine the despair and the final degeneration that must sap at last all that is brave and good in life" (p. viii).

Ora Ruggles (Carlova & Ruggles, 1946), reconstruction aide during World War I, enacted the empathy endorsed by Hall. She explained the caring effects of such empathy: "I don't see what's missing. I see what's there. I see real manhood. I see great courage. I see tremendous strength. I see true spirit. That's what gives me courage, strength, and spirit. I gain as much or more as the men I try to help" (p. 76). She said that she had made a great discovery, simple, yet so effective: "It is not enough to give a patient something to do with his hands," she said. "You must reach for the heart as well as the hands. It's the heart that really does the healing" (p. 69). Early practitioners sought to develop traits that shaped such caring. Moodie (1919) valued, "above all, infinite patience, the ability to teach and to criticize without causing offense or discouragement, the power of inspiring confidence in others, and last but not least an optimistic temperament and a sense of humor" (p. 314).

Hall (1922a) described the nature of our helping: "Occupational therapy . . . attempts to restore the general effectiveness of people who have become incapacitated through illness and who are not able to make satisfactory progress by their own unguided efforts" (p. 163). Respect for personal dignity was central to such helping. Susan Wilson (1929), chief occupational therapist at Brooklyn State Hospital, said that "the patient's every moment is carefully supervised," but "the treatment must not become too paternal, killing the patient's sense of responsibility for his own person" (p. 191). Similarly, Crane (1919) characterized our therapy as one which "makes the patient a creator, a doer" (p. 64).

Affirmations of our caring have endured. In her 1980 Slagle lecture, Carolyn Baum called us back to this belief at a time when health delivery systems had turned less caring. She said:

Occupational therapy harnesses will and gives the individual control through activity. That is human, that is care. We are respected by physicians and the health care system for that caring . . . through our professional relationships we reach out and with empathy to show that we care, hoping that from this caring the person will find his own strength. (p. 515)

And exhortations to help have endured, as June Sokolov (1957) reminded us in her lecture:

In this role of helping people to achieve commonly held objectives, nothing is more rewarding than our deepening awareness of human strength and frailty. One learns to hold aloft the ideal, to expect from people the most and the best of which they are capable yet to respect human frailty and hence to treasure the least of the offerings. (pp. 18–19)

Affirming respect for dignity in our helping, Jerry Johnson (1973) said in her Slagle, "The client and the therapist participate in a collaborative process . . . whereby the therapist provides an experiential learning environment in which the client can initiate or participate in occupational performance meaningful to him" (p. 3). Our ethos, in part, is this: Caring and helping are vital to our work. Guided by this belief, occupational therapy practitioners reach for hearts as well as hands (Peloquin, 2002a).

Effective Practice Is Artistry and Science

A fifth guiding belief is that effective occupational therapy is at once artistry and science. The interpersonal art is part of our ethos. A patient told Ruggles (Carlova & Ruggles, 1946), "You're an artist in the greatest medium of all. You're an artist in people" (p. 92). Slagle (1927), in her management roles, saw art's necessity among occupational workers. She said:

For, if lacking in this—in understanding, in give and take, in spiritual vision of the "end problem" of all too many cases, the craftsman may make some initial showing, but the work will eventually flag and be largely a failure. (p. 126)

Supporting such artistry and vision, physician Addison Thayer (1908) of Portland, Maine, told a colleague using occupation, "It is not so much the work as the way you inspire the person to take it up" (p. 1486).

Artistry of the apt intervention is also part of the ethos. As an example, an anonymous piece in *The Modern Hospital* read in 1922, "Every OT worker of experience has seen hard, rebellious men and women soften and become teachable under the influence of quiet work . . . which may carry over into the machine life a new sense of humanity, a growing love of creative accomplishment" (p. 374). When Tracy (1921) personified occupational therapy as a wise woman walking swiftly through hallways to her patients, she included artful interventions:

> A young house painter who has fallen hurt from a staging and is pretty badly hurt. . . . Next, a psychopathic patient in a bed held in a restraining jacket. . . . Third, a man who repairs furniture. Only one of his hands are [*sic*] available at present. Then a three-year-old baby with a new arm in place of one crushed by an automobile. Occupational Therapy sets down her basket—There is something interesting for each person. (Tracy, 1921, p. 398)

Belief in the value of our art, in its interpersonal and interventional aspects, has endured. Geraldine Finn (1972) argued for both in her Slagle lecture, saying,

> It is this process of creative thinking which is required of us, as occupational therapists, in order to interpret our knowledge about human performance . . . and human relations . . . in the service of maintaining the health of a community. It is necessary for us to begin to think creatively about our particular understanding of man's needs and to start to build new images around this knowledge. (p. 63)

Science has been of equal value Hall (1922b) called occupational therapy "the science of prescribed work" (p. 245). Elizabeth Upham (1918), director of the art department at Milwaukee Downer College, framed it more deeply as "the science of healing by occupation" (p. 13). Calling for records and statistics in occupational therapy, Horatio Pollock (1929), director of the Statistical Bureau of the New York Department of Mental Hygiene, regarded occupational therapy "as a scientific effort for the restoration to health of the mentally and physically ill" (p. 416).

Barton's (1915) scientific hypotheses, thought extreme, included one that any medicine of the day listed in *materia medica* books had an occupational equivalent. If doctors prescribed benzol as a leucotoxin, he said, occupational therapists could engage the same patient in canning work so that benzine fumes could yield the same effect (Barton, 1915). Signs of scientific pursuit were everywhere. Harry Mock (1919), a lieutenant colonel, supported the Walter Reed way of noting motion gained. He included a photograph of a soldier flexing to view his measurements. The caption read, "Visualizing results encourages the patient" (p. 13).

Belief in science as part of our ethos has endured. In the first Slagle lecture, Florence Stattel (1956) said this: "We have been given a wonderful professional heritage of courage and wisdom and as we continue to extend our hand to benefit mankind, may we continue to believe and search for further knowledge" (p. 194). Our long-standing belief in science has grown to recognize a discipline of occupational science well-represented by the Slagle lectures of Florence Clark (1993) and Ruth Zemke (2004).

The idea of an integrated practice based on art and science permeates cases published in our early years. One is representative:

> Private J. was studying law when he was drafted. . . . He was wounded by shrapnel in his left arm and a stiff, flexed elbow had resulted. Reading law books would hardly benefit his condition but J. was interested also in making mission furniture out of old boxes and lumber. . . . Using his left hand chiefly, he soon became adept at hammering, sawing, planing, and other movements which necessitated a certain amount of flexion and extension of the elbow joint. Every week the amount of motion in the joint was measured and a careful record made. When J. saw by actual measurement that his range of motion in this joint was increasing, he was indeed happy and redoubled his efforts. Practically full joint movement had been restored when he was finally discharged. (Mock, 1919, p. 14)

Beliefs about practice as artistry *and* science have endured. Joan Rogers' (1983; see Chapter 41) Slagle lecture discussed our reasoning as a confluence of science, art, and ethics. In the very next lecture, Elnora Gilfoyle (1984) noted kinship in art and science: "Imagination," she said, "is the common quality in both science and art" (p. 578). She elaborated:

> In science, imagination organizes experiences into concepts, and in art imagination allows us to enter into the human experiences. Science offers explanations and rational knowledge, whereas art carries an awareness of intuitive knowledge. Science of therapy is a creation to explain, and the art of therapy is a creation to relate. (p. 578)

Our ethos, in part, is this: Effective practice is artistry and science. Guided by this belief, occupational therapy practitioners are distinctly artists and distinctly scientists, both at the same time, all the time (Collins & Porras, 1994).

The Guiding Power of Our Ethos

Consider the guiding potential of our ethos: (1) time, place, and circumstance open paths to occupation; (2) occupation fosters dignity, competence, and health; (3) occupational therapy is a personal engagement; (4) caring and helping are vital to the work; and (5) ffective practice is artistry and science. Each belief is expressive, persuasive, and thoughtful. Each evokes the best of who we are; each plumbs the depth of what we do. Together they afford us this view: We are pathfinders. We enable occupations that heal. We cocreate daily lives. We reach for hearts as well as hands. We are artists and scientists at once. This is our character; this is our genius; this is our spirit.

Ours is an ethos of engagement—a commitment to involve and occupy ourselves and be bound by mutual promise. Were we to distill the complex of our guiding beliefs into one brief account, our ethos might be this: Engagement for the sake of persons and their occupational natures. We engage so that others may also engage (Moyers, 1999).

Formed in the youth of our profession, our ethos calls to mind a clear-sighted youth from *The Little Prince*. Antoine de Saint-Exupéry (1943) there argued that as many individuals mature, they lose their capacity to imagine, discern deeply, and thus understand. Remembering a childhood drawing, he said:

> I showed my masterpiece to the grown-ups, and asked them whether the drawing frightened them. But they answered "Frighten? Why

should anyone be frightened by a hat?" My drawing was not a picture of a hat. It was a boa constrictor digesting an elephant. But since the grown-ups were not able to understand it, I made another drawing: I drew the inside of the boa constrictor, so that the grown-ups could see it clearly. . . . The grown-ups' response, this time, was to advise me to lay aside my drawings of boa constrictors from the inside or the outside, and devote myself instead to geography, history, arithmetic and grammar. That is why, at the age of six, I gave up what might have been a magnificent career as a painter. (p. 4)

Similar experiences pull many from their imaginative capacities. Devoting themselves to routine matters, they weaken their powers of discernment. But when the 6-year-old in this story matured, he used his childhood drawing to predict the quality of understanding that he might expect from others. He explained:

> I have lived a great deal among grown-ups. I have seen them intimately, close at hand. . . . Whenever I met one of them who seemed to me at all clear-sighted, I tried the experiment of showing him my Drawing Number One, which I have always kept. I would try to find out, so, if this was a person of true understanding. But whoever it was, he, or she, would always say: "That is a hat." Then I would never talk to that person about boa constrictors, or primeval forests, or stars. . . . I would talk to him about bridge, and golf, and politics, and neckties. And the grown-up would be pleased to have met such a sensible man. (de Saint Exupéry, 1943, p. 5)

De Saint Exupéry clung to the clear-sightedness of his youth. He preserved his imaginative capacities while considering grown-up matters. Similarly, we might hold close the clarity, imagination, and perspective of our ethos as we consider matters grown up in our profession.

Challenges to the Integrative Ethos

We mostly agree that in spite of rich contributions to our development, views from medical and business models can wither our health care, educational, and scholarly aims. Among those views are an emphasis on rational fixing, a reliance on method and protocol, a drive for efficiency and profit (Peloquin, 1993a). Embrace of such views could lead to these beliefs, each true in its way but stark in its omission: Time, place, and circumstance produce profit margins. Performance fixes dysfunction. Therapy is a detached transaction. Problem solving is essentially the work. Effective practice is best-researched protocol.

Complaints from many sectors of our profession discern in such beliefs a disregard (Peloquin, 1993a). Consider this: If time, place, and circumstance produce profit margins, paths to occupation can get blocked. If performance fixes dysfunction, quests for dignity, competence, and health can be thwarted. If occupational therapy is a transaction, personal engagement can get lost. If problem solving is key, caring can matter less. If effective practice is best-researched protocol, artistry can seem esoteric. In this way, one might mistakenly think organizational profit opposed to professed aims, therapeutic purpose at odds with personal meaning, technical efficiency preempting human presence, competent solutions more prized than caring actions, and scientific reasoning sounder than artful intuition. Such polarized thought is not surprising in view of Churchill's (1975) argument that ethological norms, typically integrative and complex, are vulnerable to dualisms. Polarized thought can temporarily disintegrate an ethos.

A practitioner's felt-experience of a disintegrating trend is a sense of juggling, a struggle to stand in place with some views held but briefly, a stretch to keep tossed items safe but still within reach. Pressed to disregard functions that they deem valuable, practitioners feel deep consequences in every realm of practice. We've named one *depersonalization*.

Depersonalization evokes a radical image in its removal of persons. When personal care is hollowed from health delivery, practitioners feel the assault, and those seeking care are devastated (Peloquin, 1993b). René Magritte rendered the angst well in a work called *The Therapist*. A seated and caped figure sits squarely under a slivered moon and flattened hat. Face and chest are gone, replaced by emptiness. Doubtful that this therapist could find paths to occupation. The promise of engagement is slim. Caring expressions seem improbable, helping unlikely. Depersonalization mutes our call to engage for the sake of persons and their occupational natures. It spawns disheartening times, places, and circumstances. The realities and dangers of depersonalization permeate cultural images. As forms of art, they help us discern de Saint-Exupéry's boa consuming the elephant. And we should be frightened by this hat.

We must ask: Is our ethos the problem? Is its interlacing of sentiment, value, and thought outdated fancy to be put aside? I think not. I propose instead a reframing of disheartening contexts in the clear light of our ethos. Listen to the Parable of Two Frogs (author unknown, 1999):

> A group of frogs were hopping contentedly through the woods, going about their froggy business, when two of them fell into a deep pit. All of the other frogs gathered around the pit to see what could be done to help their companions. When they saw how deep the pit was, they agreed that it was hopeless and told the two frogs that they should prepare themselves for their fate, because they were as good as dead. . . .

> The two frogs continued jumping with all their might, and after several hours of this, were quite weary. Finally, one of the frogs took heed to the calls of his fellow frogs. Exhausted, he quietly resolved himself to his fate, lay down at the bottom of the pit, and died. The other frog continued to jump as hard as he could, although his body was wracked with pain and he was quite exhausted.

> Once again, his companions began yelling for him to accept his fate, stop the pain and just die. The weary frog jumped harder and harder and, wonder of wonders, finally leaped so high that he sprang from the pit.

> Amazed, the other frogs celebrated his freedom and then, gathering around him asked, "Why did you continue jumping when we told you it was impossible?" The astonished frog explained to them that he was deaf, and as he saw their gestures and shouting, he thought they were cheering him on. What he had perceived as encouragement inspired him to try harder and to succeed against all odds.

We too can reframe disheartening contexts. Our ability to do so rises from the capacity for resilience that Susan Fine (1990) described in her Slagle lecture. She asked, "Who rises above adversity?" (p. 493). I say that we do.

We acknowledge an enormous cleft of land in Arizona, a dangerously deep pit and obstacle to circumvent, but reframe it positively as the Grand Canyon. Likewise, we can reframe challenges to our ethos as calls for its reclamation. The challenges can cheer us on.

A Fresh Perspective on Current Challenges

Five reflections follow, each framing a current challenge in light of a guiding belief. Together they suggest actions so grounded in our ethos that they promise reclamation of our heart. Let me explain. Dictionary definitions of the term *heart* yield a more fulsome meaning than we sometimes suppose. Heart is the seat of feeling but is also the seat of understanding and thought. It is the depths of soul or spirit. Heart is the source of life and its vital principle; heart is one's disposition, temperament, and character; heart is courage; it is the source of human ardor, enthusiasm, or energy; heart is the innermost part of anything (Simpson & Weiner, 1989). Because the full-bodied meaning of *heart* is so like that of ethos connotationally and metaphorically, an embrace of the profession's ethos seems an embrace of our heart.

We Are Artists *and* Scientists

Guided by the belief that effective practice is artistry *and* science, we are artists and scientists at once (Collins & Porras, 1994). Honoring our ethos, we strive toward integrative practices (Peloquin, 1994, 2002a). Gestalt visions grounded our ethos in it origins, images of whole persons possessed of mind, body, *and* spirit; hands *and* hearts; physical *and* mental health. How can we reclaim those? For one, we can prompt the imagination that drives our science and art. Consider a beach scene. Sand and water come together at seaside, quite distinct but dynamically related. Seaside *is* because of land and ocean. Grains of sand and waves of sea together make seaside. Seaside would not *be* if one were gone.

More images may fire our gestalt capacities. A nesting doll holds others within itself. A dance evokes rhythmic moves, some made in tandem. Woodland streams send many-sourced waters in shared directions. A butterfly draws one form from another. A symphony makes harmony from differing sounds. A tapestry brings warp and weft to pleasing patterns (Baum, 1980; Wood, 1995). A cyclist pedals two wheels smoothly and at once. Yin-yang magatamas show goodness of fit in

neatly opposed designs. Each image disrupts our dichotomies. Each prompts integrative thought.

Add to such imagery the question asked by William James (1947) about whether we walk more essentially with the right or the left leg. Clearly we need both. And if we drift to polar thinking, we might consider ski poles, together lending support and balance. Can we not imagine cosupportive synergies drawn from science *and* art (Peloquin, 1994)? If so, we can see intervention, education, and inquiry as venues for the integration of competence *and* caring, professional purpose *and* personal choice, productivity *and* self-actualization, problem solving *and* collaboration, evidence *and* meaning. That perspective captures our ethos.

Even in the business world, James Collins and Jerry Porras (1994) endorsed the "genius of the and" noting that "a highly visionary group will aim to be distinctly yin and distinctly yang, both at the same time, all the time" (p. 45). When, in light of our ethos, we envision and enact our belief that effective practice is artistry and science, we realize a vital principle of our profession. And in doing so we reclaim our heart.

We Are Pathfinders

Guided by the belief that time, place, and circumstance open paths to occupation, we are pathfinders. But how can we find paths to occupation in managed care and other disintegrating environments? We must first see overly managed systems as polarized. Management—skillful handling and control—is a distinct part of good care, but even in the realm of horse training, where the term *management* originated, experts suggest this broader view:

> We shall have to give up our inclination to control our horse by force. Instead we shall have to try to learn to respect the way that he wants to do things. . . . And, instead of trying to impose on our particular animal the idea of what he should be able to achieve, we must first seek to learn what his capabilities really are . . . we shall have to add to our analytical capability an equal capacity for intuitive thought. . . . Without this, our relationship with our horse will be one of spiritual warfare instead of harmony and beauty. (Hassler, 1994, p. 16)

Strife occurs in health systems when control preempts care. Without harmonious relationships and respect for choice, management fails (Curtin, 2003). If we had galloping costs, unbridled excesses, and runaway procedures, these called for taming. But they did not warrant the split vision that has made an oxymoron of managed care (Peloquin, 1996). To see the split is to discern the missing care. And that discernment opens paths for its return.

In his reflections about educational systems, Gordon Davies (1991) asked a hard question of those on governing boards with control: "Are we helping to create an environment" he asked, "in which teaching and learning are honored and can flourish?" (p. 58). He saw in governance a pathfinding role. He heard a call to engender restlessness throughout the system, disturb complacency, and insist that rules be broken for the sake of learning (Davies). Likewise we might ask, "Are we making environments in which occupation can flourish?" Our activists, theorists, and innovators have asked. They have seen their pathfinding roles. They cause restlessness and disturb complacency as they challenge oppressive policy, affirm occupation as central, and make new practice sites—in clubhouses, workplaces, and community centers—for the sake of occupation.

Others make paths in quiet ways. Practitioners nest kindness, choice, and respect in approved interventions, working within payment rules to enhance performance. They foster dignity. Practitioners working in cramped spaces share big and courageous ideas that help clients remake their lives. They foster competence. Practitioners with huge caseloads in rushed circumstances craft cogent letters that extend occupational therapy. They foster health. Blocked as some may be from real occupation, they feel its steady pull. They heed its innermost call for dignity, competence, and health. They shape circumstances that hasten its return. Their efforts call to mind the words of Nkosi Johnson (Wooten, 2004), an African child and activist who died of AIDS at the age of 12: "Do all you can with what you have in the time you have in the place you are" (Norris, 2004).

If health care environments seem disintegrative, they are not unique. Educators face a press for what Kerry Walters (1991) called a vulcanization of students, a Spock-like penchant for rational problem solving that stunts affective growth. Technologies proliferate, some putting interpersonal ken and harmony at risk. Through confluent models that foster learning with, about, and for whole persons, occupational therapy educators grow human potential and blaze trails to

occupation (Peloquin, 2002b). Scholars face cut-throat trends to earn grant funds for institutional gain. Some are pushed toward discontinuous projects that neither flow from preferred inquiry nor grow the profession's work (Mosey & Abreu, 1998). Through mindfulness, integrative methods, and a compass set on occupation, scholars make pathways back to our ethos (Abreu, Peloquin, & Ottenbacher, 1998).

Practitioners who honor occupation in disintegrating environments are pathfinders. When, challenges of all kinds notwithstanding, we affirm the belief that time, place, and circumstance open paths to occupation, we enact the courage of our profession. And we reclaim our heart.

We Reach for Hearts as Well as Hands

Guided by the belief that caring and helping are vital to our work, we reach for hearts as well as hands. Nine decades after he first said them, Hall and Buck's (1915) words still ring clear: "Put yourself in that man's place—imagine the despair" (p. viii). Depersonalized contexts in our times can fire such imagination and stoke our wills. Listen to Alfie Kohn (1990):

> No imported solution will dissolve our problems of dehumanization and coldness. No magical redemption from outside of human life will let us break through. The work that has to be done is work, but we are better equipped for it than we have been led to believe. To move ourselves beyond ourselves, we already have what is required. We are human and we have each other. (pp. 267–268)

How are we equipped to move ourselves beyond ourselves? Stories from the autobiography of Ora Ruggles point to our capacity for empathy (Peloquin, 1995). At its core a disposition toward fellowship, empathy is a turning toward another not just to solve a problem but to care and to help. Ora's turning enabled her reaching, made clear in her work with a girl named Edith (Peloquin, 1995).

Ora launched a program at Olive View sanatorium, knowing that a board of directors would inspect her work before granting space or funds. She first intervened with Edith, a teen with spinal tuberculosis so severe that she lay arched and prone in a Bradford Frame. Ora found a mirror that let Edith see her hands; she built her a worktable. Noting Edith's flair for style and skill at sewing, she nurtured her potential as a dress designer and suggested doll clothes as a start. Edith produced fine work.

When county board members visited Edith, Ora heard a woman nicknamed "Hawkeye" regret time spent on such a "hopeless case." Ora said, "No one is hopeless who wants to be helped, and there's nobody in this place who wants to be helped more than Edith does. That's why I'm working with her and that's why I'm going to continue working with her." She smiled at Edith. "And that's why she's going to get well" (Carlova & Ruggles, 1946, p. 168). Hawkeye said that such sentiment was fine, but the board sought clear results.

Edith was to have shin bone segments grafted to her unstable spine. She yearned to pay for her surgery but doubted such income from doll clothes. Ora considered the situation. She made stylized figures from pipe cleaner and suggested that Edith clothe and group these to show rhythm and life. Edith caught on, creating ballets, skaters on a pond. Other patients joined in, making backgrounds and bases. The doll clothes sold readily in Los Angeles, and Edith's share of the profits funded her surgery.

At the next visit of the board, a physician reviewed Ora's work, and even Hawkeye was impressed. They approved a workshop that Ora helped design. Edith was discharged. She attended a fashion design school, became a well-known dress designer, supported her family, and funded patients at Olive View. The story is a tribute to Edith's spirit. It tells of Ora's empathy and good management sense.

John Gums (1994) would applaud the work of Ruggles, whose reaching for hearts and hands spread fellowship broadly. Gums said:

> Every human being is born with the capacity to empathize. Most medical professionals, through their training, are taught to squeeze out that natural ability. Rediscovering it later in our professional life is a goal we should all have. Evidence suggests that to do so, emphasis must be placed on consideration of human life. (p. 251)

The rediscovery of empathy is not an add-on task to juggle alongside others, but more like the act of a cyclist turning the wheels of competence and caring at once. Elsewhere I've suggested that empathy is a considered way of being brought to our doing, no matter what that doing is (Peloquin, 1995). Being present to another in time is not the same as having lots of time. Consider interactions during checkout at a grocery store. In a few minutes, some cashiers forge real connections. We have much more time than most cashiers, and we connect well through our doing. And if being present admittedly *takes* energy, it paradoxically restores it, unlike the drain toward emptiness of depersonalization.

When, in light of our ethos, we affirm to ourselves and to others that caring and helping are vital to our work, when we empathically dispose ourselves toward that end, we share the ardor of the profession. In doing so, we reclaim the profession's heart.

We Cocreate Daily Lives

Guided by the belief that occupational therapy is a personal engagement, we cocreate daily lives. But how can we engage in cocreation when so much pulls us elsewhere? Media messages say that a clock has filled our souls. We wear time-machines strapped to our bodies. We're out of sorts without them. We tick with the many things that we must do. We stay wound up and out of touch with ourselves and others; we buzz within. We race with time, hoping to beat it. While seeking a control that eludes us, we turn from healthy rhythms of occupation and relationship. We loathe the idea of getting behind, or worse, of getting worn, ugly, and old. We have nearly forgotten what it means to engage with the world and connect with others (Peloquin, 1990).

If we hope to engage—to involve and occupy ourselves and others and be bound by mutual promise—we must expand our views of time. Consider the book *Cheaper by the Dozen*, about Frank Gilbreth, honorary member of the Society for the Promotion of Occupational Therapy. Gilbreth's son described his father's passion for efficiency. Fully clothed and sitting on the carpet, Gilbreth taught his 12 children the most expedient way to bathe while extending the life of the soap. If we see time only as a commodity, we have split his larger vision. Gilbreth's son, Frank Jr. (1948) shared what we have missed:

> Someone once asked Dad: "But what do you want to save time *for*? What are you going to do with it?
>
> "For work, if you love that best," said Dad. "For education, for beauty, for art, for pleasure."
>
> He looked over the top of his pince-nez. "For mumblety-peg if that's where your heart lies." (p. 237)

We mark time; we count units of productivity because we must. But only if we engage with the world will we find where our hearts lie. And only if we engage with others can we help them find what they love best.

Most media messages that commodify time differ from a sense of time's wonder, like that of our forebears, found in the story of *The Velveteen Rabbit* (Williams, 1978). The Rabbit, new to a young boy's nursery, asked the Skin Horse, a kindly older toy, a question that we too ask:

> "What is REAL?" asked the Rabbit one day. . . . "Does it mean having things that buzz inside you and a stick-out handle?"
>
> "Real is not how you are made," said the Skin Horse. "It's a thing that happens to you. When a child loves you, then you become Real."
>
> "Does it hurt?" asked the Rabbit.
>
> "Sometimes," said the Skin Horse, for he was always truthful. "When you are Real you don't mind being hurt."
>
> "Does it happen all at once, like being wound up," he asked, "or bit by bit?"
>
> "It doesn't happen all at once," said the Skin Horse. "You become. It takes a long time. That's why it doesn't often happen to people who break easily, or have sharp edges, or who have to be carefully kept. Generally, by the time you are Real, most of your hair has been loved off, and your eyes drop out and you get loose joints and are very shabby. But these things don't matter at all, because once you are Real you can't be ugly, except to people who don't understand." (pp. 16–17)

When engaged and real, Yerxa (1967) said that "we feel, we encounter, we take time, we listen and we are ourselves" (p. 8). A modern-day story reveals such engagement.

> I sustained a severe, complicated injury to my right dominant hand. . . . I was prescribed occupational therapy treatment. . . . As at many previous sessions, I was seated across from Karen (the occupational therapist), prepared to begin my treatment. However, this time was different. I gazed down at my right hand resting on the tabletop and suddenly regarded it in a totally different light than ever before—I became aware that I was permanently disfigured. . . .

> Overwhelmed by this realization, tears welled in my eyes, and I whispered, "It's so ugly."

> Without missing a beat, Karen . . . explained that my emotions were a normal reaction to my injury . . . reassured me that this was a normal response and that we could discuss the process during therapy sessions . . . she assured me that I wasn't alone; we would work through it together. When Karen finished, I was utterly speechless. Karen had given voice to my despair. . . . For the first time since the accident, I felt as if someone could truly empathize with my plight. (Ponsolle-Mays, 2003, pp. 246–247)

The storyteller, Michelle Ponsolle-Mays (2003), later became an occupational therapist. She wrote, "And when I now use my right hand to help someone with an activity, what I see is no longer ugly—it is my personal swan" (p. 247). To the extent that we engage with others so that they can create their daily lives, we become real.

As part of our mutual promise, we can also engage as professional citizens, speaking for persons and their occupational natures. That voice—raised to secure meaningful pursuits for all—can be the defining character of our organizations (Sullivan, 1999). Professional citizenship will balance market forces if we hold what Harold Perkin (1989) called "the professional social ideal," a commitment to society as a fellowship rather than only as a marketplace in which persons become consumers and profit matters most (Peloquin, 1997b). Only then will we integrate social justice and economic solvency to shape real reform (Perkin, 1989). Only then will profit support real profession.

When, in light of our ethos, we commit to the personal engagement of occupational therapy, when we engage with others so that they might seize their daily lives, we practice real occupational therapy. We share the innermost core of the profession, and we reclaim our heart.

We Enable Occupations That Heal

Guided by the belief that occupation fosters dignity, competence, and health, we enable occupations that heal. When asked to see what we do as performance that fixes dysfunction, we might recall Meyer's (1922; see Chapter 4) vision of our dual beacon lights of performance *and* opportunity. Ours is a unique perspective. We see everyday activities as a making of lives and worlds, a broader and deeper view than that of mere performance or function, and one steeped in opportunity. Philosopher Elaine Scarry (1985) noted the world-making function of persons:

> As one maneuvers each day through the realm of tablecloths, dishes, potted plants, ideological structures, automobiles, newspapers, ideas about families, streetlights, languages, city parks, one does not at each moment actively perceive the objects as humanly made; but if one for any reason stops and thinks about their origins, one can with varying degrees of ease recognize that they have human makers. (p. 312)

The image of someone in the act of making is one in which human being—its character, heart, and spirit—flows into personal doing. The difference between doing and making is one of substance and not semantic. Human making is a creation, our humane engagement a cocreation (Peloquin, 1997a).

Consider activities of daily living. We name hair care grooming, but we can see it as an act of making oneself presentable, attractive, or even likeable. What we call cooking we could easily call the making of a meal nested within larger makings—of hearth, home, or tradition. What we call work is more deeply the making of a living, a family, a reputation, a community, a society. Wherever it falls in Abraham Maslow's (1970) scheme of need, health, and hope, we see human making in daily tasks (Peloquin, 1997a). We see occupations as vital links to dignity, competence, and health. That perspective can lift our clever line, *Occupational therapy, skills for the job of living,* to higher and more healing ground where living is more than a job. And from there we might say, *Occupational therapy, making daily lives* (Peloquin, 2002a). That perspective captures our ethos.

In her poem, Janet Petersen (1976) casts even simple occupations as expressions of the human spirit:

> There is a shouting SPIRIT deep inside me:
> TAKE CLAY. It cries,
> TAKE PEN AND INK,
> TAKE FLOUR AND WATER,
> TAKE A SCRUB BRUSH,
> TAKE A YELLOW CRAYON
> TAKE ANOTHER'S HAND
> AND WITH ALL THESE SAY YOU,
> SAY LOVING. (p. 61)

Through occupations such as these, the human spirit emerges, manifesting itself in small and large ways. Its emergence graces photographs of individuals seized by occupation (Menashe, 1980).

Practice stories revere this spirit. Therapist Betty Baer (2003) introduced us to a Vietnam veteran with a high-level spinal cord injury and from a remote part of Texas; he called himself a "Mountain Man." Betty wrote:

> J. was self-conscious about the hole left in his throat from the tracheotomy. He thought that an Indian choker necklace would be a good way to cover up the hole. Unfortunately, he was unable to make this himself, even with the best of OT compensatory techniques and gadgets. Since I had a little experience with beadwork, we decided that he would create the design and I would be his "hands"—following his directions to produce the choker necklace. We thought this would be a good experience. It was important for J. to direct his care—why not direct his creativity as well?
>
> This was a big challenge for both of us. It was difficult for him to put into words the steps of the activity his hands knew how to do so well. It was challenging for me to follow his instructions, and not just improvise on the knowledge of beadwork that I already possessed.
>
> To our mutual amazement, the choker . . . looked great. J. wore it with pride and received many compliments. This activity not only transformed a handful of beads into a necklace, but it also transformed J.'s role from a passive patient to active teacher. It was a truly wonderful OT/patient experience . . . one I will never forget. (p. 5)

When, in spite of constraints, practitioners make their interventions meaningful, lively, and even fun, they infuse therapy's purposive aims with its capacity to encourage and inspire. Acting on the belief that occupation fosters dignity, competence, and health, we embrace the spirit of the profession. As we enable healing occupations, we reclaim our heart.

Conclusion

We can stand on the rock that is our ethos and from there proclaim our view: Time, place, and circumstance open paths to occupation. Occupation fosters dignity, competence, and health. Occupational therapy is a personal engagement. Caring and helping are vital to the work. Effective practice is artistry and science. Our profession takes this stand for the sake of persons and their occupational natures. We engage—we involve and occupy ourselves and commit to mutual promise—so that others may also engage. This is our character; this is our genius; this is our spirit.

Mihaly Csikszentmihalyi (1993), a modern-day friend of occupational therapy, offered thoughts to guide a profession through this millennium. His thoughts reverberate with our ethos. "You are a part of everything around you," he said. "You shall not deny your uniqueness. You are responsible for your actions. You shall be more than what you are" (pp. 289–290).

The reflective part of this lecture began with de Saint-Exupéry's story, to which I now return. Here, a wise fox shares goodbyes with the little prince:

> "Goodbye," [the little prince] said.
> "Goodbye," said the fox. "And now here is my secret, a very simple secret; it is only with the heart that one can see rightly; what is essential is invisible to the eye."
> "What is essential is invisible to the eye," the little prince repeated, so that he would be sure to remember. (1947, p. 87)

The ethos of occupational therapy restores our clear-sightedness so that we see what is essential: We are pathfinders. We enable occupations that heal. We cocreate daily lives. We reach for hearts as well as hands. We are artists and scientists at once. If we discern this in ourselves, if we act on this understanding every day, we will advance into the future embracing our ethos of engagement. And we will have reclaimed a magnificent heart.

Acknowledgments

My thanks go to those who preceded me in the Slagle tradition; those who nominated and introduced me; those who shared stories, images, or songs; those who helped find resources; those who warmed seeds of this work in Texas, California, Pennsylvania, and Oklahoma; those who gave me PowerPoint hints; those who gentled my prelecture mix into being; those who helped me today. I also thank those who have taught me, read me, challenged me, and worked beside me. You have all encouraged me. I especially thank each of you for being here—family, friends, teachers, students, and colleagues—because without an audience, a lecture hardly exists. Unlike interactive lectures that fill my days, this is a reading. I hope that you still feel included.

References

Abreu, B., Peloquin, S. M., & Ottenbacher, K. (1998). Competence in scientific inquiry and research. *American Journal of Occupational Therapy, 52,* 751–759. http://dx.doi.org/10.5014/ajot.52.9.751

American Occupational Therapy Association. (1979). Resolution C, 531-79. The philosophical base of occupational therapy. *American Journal of Occupational Therapy, 33,* 785.

American Occupational Therapy Association. (1993). Core values and attitudes of occupational therapy practice. *American Journal of Occupational Therapy, 47,* 1085–1086. http://dx.doi.org/10.5014/ajot.47.12.1085

American Occupational Therapy Association. (1994). Occupational therapy code of ethics. *American Journal of Occupational Therapy, 48,* 1037–1038. http://dx.doi.org/10.5014/ajot.48.11.1037

American Occupational Therapy Association. (2002). Occupational therapy practice framework: Domain and process. *American Journal of Occupational Therapy, 56,* 609–639. http://dx.doi.org/10.5014/ajot.56.6.609

American Occupational Therapy Association. (2004). Definition of occupational therapy practice for the AOTA Model Practice Act. (Available from the State Affairs Group, AOTA, Bethesda, MD.)

Anderson, M. L. (1920). Mental reconstruction through occupational therapy. *Modern Hospital, 14,* 326–327.

Anonymous. (1999). Parable of two frogs. *The Lord's grace. General stories of God's grace.* Retrieved February 23, 2004, from http://lordsgrace.com/stories

Anonymous. (1922). What David Belasco said. *Modern Hospital, 18,* 373–374.

Baer, B. (2003). The mountain man and the bead lady. *Revista OT,* April, 5.

Barton, G. E. (1915). Occupational therapy. *Trained Nurse and Hospital Review, 54,* 138–140.

Barton, G. E. (1920). What occupational therapy may mean to nursing. *Trained Nurse and Hospital Review, 64,* 304–310.

Baum, C. M. (1980). The 1980 Eleanor Clarke Slagle Lecture—Occupational therapists put care in the health system. *American Journal of Occupational Therapy, 34,* 505–516.

Bing, R. K. (1986). The subject is health: Not of facts but of values. *American Journal of Occupational Therapy, 40,* 667–671. http://dx.doi.org/10.5014/ajot.40.10.667

Carlova, J., & Ruggles, O. (1946). *The healing heart.* New York: Messner.

Carroll, R. S. (1910). The therapy of work. *JAMA, 54,* 2032–2035.

Churchill, L. R. (1975). Ethos and ethics in medical education. *North Carolina Medical Journal, 36,* 31–33.

Clark, F. (1993). The 1993 Eleanor Clarke Slagle Lecture—Occupation embedded in a real life: Interweaving occupational science and occupational therapy. *American Journal of Occupational Therapy, 47,* 1067–1078. http://dx.doi.org/10.5014/ajot.47.12.1067

Collins, J. C., & Porras, J. (1994). *Built to last. Successful habits of visionary companies.* New York: Harper Collins.

Cooper, G. (1918). Re-weaving the web: A soldier tells what it means to begin all over again. *Carry On, 1,* 23–26.

Crane, B. T. (1919). Occupational therapy. *Boston Medical and Surgical Journal, 181,* 63–65.

Csikszentmihalyi, M. (1993). *The evolving self: A psychology for the third millennium.* New York: Harper Collins.

Cullimore, A. R. (1921). Objectives and motivation in occupational therapy. *Modern Hospital, 17,* 537–538.

Curtin, L. (2003). Ethics in management. A relationship ethos might help. *Journal of Clinical Systems Management, 5,* 8–9.

Davies, G. K. (1991). Teaching and learning: What are the questions? *Teaching Education, 4,* 57–61.

de Saint-Exupéry, A. (1943). *The little prince.* New York: Harcourt Brace Jovanovich.

Dunton, W. R., Jr. (1919). *Reconstruction therapy.* Philadelphia: Saunders.

E. E. (1921). Occupational therapy. *Hospital Progress, 2,* 265.

Fidler, G. S. (1966). Learning as a growth process: A conceptual framework for professional education. *American Journal of Occupational Therapy, 20,* 1–8.

Finn, G. (1972). The occupational therapist in prevention programs. *American Journal of Occupational Therapy, 26,* 59–66.

Fine, S. B. (1990). The 1990 Eleanor Clarke Slagle Lecture. Resilience and human adaptability: Who rises above adversity? *American Journal of Occupational Therapy, 45,* 493–503.

Fisher, A. G. (1998). The 1998 Eleanor Clarke Slagle Lecture—Uniting practice and theory in an occupational framework. *American Journal of Occupational Therapy, 52,* 509–521. http://dx.doi.org/10.5014/ajot.52.7.509

Gilbreth, F. B. (1948). *Cheaper by the dozen.* New York: Thomas Y. Cromwell.

Gilfoyle, E. (1984). The 1984 Eleanor Clarke Slagle Lecture—Transformation of the profession. *American Journal of Occupational Therapy, 38,* 575–584. http://dx.doi.org/10.5014/ajot.38.9.575

Gums, J. (1994). Empathy to apathy: A consequence of higher education? *Pharmacotherapy, 14,* 250–251.

Haas, L. J. (1927). The next step in occupational therapy development. *Occupational Therapy and Rehabilitation 6,* 283–302.

Hall, H. J. (1922a). American Occupational Therapy Association. *Archives of Occupational Therapy 1,* 163–165.

Hall, H. J. (1922b). Science so-called. *Modern Hospital, 18,* 558–559.

Hall, H. J., & Buck, M. M. (1915). *The work of our hands.* New York: Moffat, Yard.

Hansen, R. A. (2003). Ethics in occupational therapy. In E. B Crepeau, E. C. Cohn, & B. A. Boyt Schell (Eds.), *Willard and Spackman's occupational therapy* (pp. 953–961). Philadelphia: Lippincott Williams & Wilkins.

Hasselkus, B. R. (2002). *The meaning of everyday occupation.* Thorofare, NJ: Slack.

Hassler, J. K. (1994). *Beyond the mirror—The study of the mental and spiritual aspects of horsemanship.* Quarryville, PA: Goals Unlimited.

Hubbard, S. (1991). Towards a truly holistic approach to occupational therapy. *British Journal of Occupational Therapy, 54,* 415–418.

James, W. (1947). *A new name for some old ways of thinking.* New York: Longmans, Green.

Johnson, J. (1973). The 1972 Eleanor Clarke Slagle Lecture—Occupational therapy: A model for the future. *American Journal of Occupational Therapy, 27,* 1–7.

Kidner, T. B. (1923). Planning for occupational therapy. *Modern Hospital, 21,* 414–428.

Kidner, T. B. (1929). Address to graduates. *Occupational Therapy and Rehabilitation, 8,* 379–385.

Kielhofner, G. (1997). *Conceptual foundations of occupational therapy.* Philadelphia: Davis.

Kohn, A. (1990). *The brighter side of human nature.* New York: Basic.

Licht, S. (1967). The founding and the founders of the American Occupational Therapy Association. *American Journal of Occupational Therapy, 21,* 269–277.

Maslow, A. H. (1970). *Religions, values and peak experiences.* New York: Viking.

Menashe, A. (1980). *Inner grace. Photographs by Abraham Menashe.* New York: Alfred A. Knopf.

Meyer, A. (1922). The philosophy of occupational therapy. *Archives of Occupational Therapy, 1*, 1–10.

Mock, H. E. (1919). Curative work. *Carry On, 1*, 12–17.

Moodie, C. S. (1919). The value of occupational therapy to the nursing profession. *Hospital Social Service Quarterly, 1*, 313–315.

Mosey, A. C. (1981). *Occupational therapy: Configuration of a profession*. New York: Raven.

Mosey, A., & Abreu, B. A. (1998, April). *Research as a tool rather than an end of inquiry*. Short course presented at the American Occupational Therapy Association Annual Conference & Expo, Baltimore.

Moyers, P. (1999). The guide to occupational therapy practice. *American Journal of Occupational Therapy, 53*, 247–322. http://dx.doi.org/10.5014/ajot.53.3.247

Norris, M. (Interviewer). (2004, December 1). *All Things Considered* [Radio broadcast]. Washington, DC: National Public Radio.

Peloquin, S. M. (1990). Time as a commodity: Reflections and implications. *American Journal of Occupational Therapy, 45*, 147–154.

Peloquin, S. M. (1993a). The patient–therapist relationship: Beliefs that shape care. *American Journal of Occupational Therapy, 47*, 935–942. http://dx.doi.org/10.5014/ajot.45.2.147

Peloquin, S. M. (1993b). The depersonalization of patients: A profile gleaned from narratives. *American Journal of Occupational Therapy, 47*, 830–837. http://dx.doi.org/10.5014/ajot.47.9.830

Peloquin, S. M. (1994). Occupational therapy as art and science: Should the older definition be reclaimed? *American Journal of Occupational Therapy, 48*, 1093–1096. http://dx.doi.org/10.5014/ajot.48.11.1093

Peloquin, S. M. (1995). The fullness of empathy: Reflections and illustrations. *American Journal of Occupational Therapy, 49*, 24–31.

Peloquin, S. M. (1996). The Issue Is—Now that we have managed care, shall we inspire it? *American Journal of Occupational Therapy, 50*, 455–459. http://dx.doi.org/10.5014/ajot.50.6.455

Peloquin, S. M. (1997a). The spiritual depth of occupation: Making worlds and making lives. *American Journal of Occupational Therapy, 51*, 167–168. http://dx.doi.org/10.5014/ajot.51.3.167

Peloquin, S. M. (1997b). Should we trade person-centered service for a consumer-based model? *American Journal of Occupational Therapy, 51*, 612–615. http://dx.doi.org/10.5014/ajot.51.7.612

Peloquin, S. M. (2002a). Reclaiming the vision of *Reaching for Heart as Well as Hands*. *American Journal of Occupational Therapy, 56*, 517–526. http://dx.doi.org/10.5014/ajot.56.5.517

Peloquin, S. M. (2002b). Confluence: Moving forward with affective strength. *American Journal of Occupational Therapy, 56*, 69–77.

Perkin, H. (1989) *The third revolution: Professional elites in the modern world*. London and New York: Routledge.

Peters, R. S. (Ed.). (1953). *Brett's history of psychology*. New York: Macmillan.

Petersen, J. (1976). *A book of yes*. Niles, IL: Argus.

Pollock, H. M. (1929). The need, value, and general principles of occupational therapy statistics. *Occupational Therapy and Rehabilitation, 8*, 415–420.

Ponsolle-Mays, M. (2003). My ugly duckling. In D. R. Labowitz (Ed.), *Ordinary miracles. True stories about overcoming obstacles and surviving catastrophes* (pp. 246–247). Thorofare, NJ: Slack.

Reed, K. L., & Sanderson, S. N. (1999). *Concepts of occupational therapy*. Philadelphia: Lippincott Williams & Wilkins.

Reilly, M. (1962). Occupational therapy can be one of the great ideas of 20th century medicine. *American Journal of Occupational Therapy, 16*, 1–9. Reprinted as Chapter 7.

Roback, A. A. (1952). *History of American psychology*. New York: Library Publishers.

Rogers, J. C. (1983). The 1983 Eleanor Clarke Slagle Lecture—Clinical reasoning: The ethics, science, and art. *American Journal of Occupational Therapy, 37*, 606–616. Reprinted as Chapter 41.

Scarry, E. (1985). *The body in pain: The making and unmaking of the world*. New York: Oxford University Press.

Shannon, P. (1997). The derailment of occupational therapy. *American Journal of Occupational Therapy, 31*, 229–234.

Simpson, J. A., & Weiner, E. S. C. (Eds.). (1989). *The Oxford English dictionary*. Oxford: Clarendon Press.

Slagle, E. C. (1927). To organize an "OT" department. *Occupational Therapy and Rehabilitation, 6*, 125–130.

Slagle, E. C. (1938). From the heart. *Occupational Therapy and Rehabilitation, 16*, 343–345.

Sokolov, J. (1957). Therapist into administrator. Ten inspiring years. *American Journal of Occupational Therapy, 11*, 13–19.

Stattel, F. M. (1956). Equipment designed for occupational therapy. *American Journal of Occupational Therapy, 10*, 194–198.

Stiller, C. (2000). Exploring the ethos of the physical therapy profession in the United States: Social, cultural, and historical influences and their relationship to education. *Journal of Physical Therapy Education, 14,* 7–15.

Sullivan, W. M. (1999). What is left of professionalism after managed care? *Hastings Center Report, 29,* 7–13.

Thayer, A. (1908). Work cure. *JAMA, 51,* 1485–1486.

Tracy, S. E. (1913). *Studies in invalid occupation.* Boston: Whitcomb and Barrows.

Tracy, S. E. (1921). Getting started in occupational therapy. *Trained Nurse and Hospital Review, 67,* 397–399.

Tuckett, A. G. (1998). An ethic of the fitting: A conceptual framework for nursing practice. *Nursing Inquiry, 5,* 220–225.

Upham, E. (1918). Rehabilitation of disabled soldiers and sailors—Teacher training for occupational therapy. *Training of teachers for occupational therapy for the rehabilitation of disabled soldiers and sailors.* Washington, DC: Federal Board for Vocational Education: Government Printing Office.

Walters, K. S. (1991). Critical thinking, rationality, and the vulcanization of students. *Journal of Higher Education, 61,* 448–467.

West, W. (1984). A reaffirmed philosophy and practice of occupational therapy for the 1980s. *American Journal of Occupational Therapy, 38,* 15–23.

Wilcock, A. A. (1998). Reflections on doing, being, and becoming. *Canadian Journal of Occupational Therapy, 65,* 248–256.

Williams, M. (1978). *The velveteen rabbit or how toys become real.* New York: Avon.

Wilson, S. C. (1929). Habit training for mental cases. *Occupational Therapy and Rehabilitation, 8,* 189–197.

Wood, W. (1995). Weaving the warp and weft of occupational therapy: An art and science for all times. *American Journal of Occupational Therapy, 49,* 44–52. http://dx.doi.org/10.5014/ajot.49.1.44

Wood, W. (2004). The heart, mind, and soul of professionalism in occupational therapy. *American Journal of Occupational Therapy, 58,* 249–257. http://dx.doi.org/10.5014/ajot.58.3.249

Wooten, J. (2004). *We are all the same.* New York: Penguin.

Yerxa, E. J. (1967). The 1966 Eleanor Clarke Slagle Lecture—Every one counts. *American Journal of Occupational Therapy, 12,* 1–9.

Zemke, R. (2004). The 2004 Eleanor Clarke Slagle Lecture—Time, space, and the kaleidoscopes of occupation. *American Journal of Occupational Therapy, 58,* 608–620.

CHAPTER 63

A Fork in the Road: An Occupational Hazard?

2013 ELEANOR CLARKE SLAGLE LECTURE

GLEN GILLEN

Good evening and welcome! I am thrilled to be at this podium and just as thrilled to be resuming my life an hour from now! This honor has been overwhelming in a good way, as you can imagine and, also as you can imagine, stressful. I have to thank my colleagues at Columbia University for consistently reminding me over the past year that this is an honor, not a punishment. In all seriousness, however, I am particularly touched to be delivering this lecture in San Diego. The last time I was in this city was the day after I completed my mental health fieldwork about 5 miles from where we are now. That was about 25 years ago, and it was the final hurdle to completing my bachelor's degree in occupational therapy at New York University. The occupational therapists who worked in the unit that I trained on that summer firmly embraced and applied Mary Reilly's occupational behavior frame of reference. I feel lucky that I was thoroughly trained in her approach and had the chance to read her 1961 Slagle lecture (Reilly, 1962; see Chapter 7) multiple times that summer.

My Thesis

My thesis today is relatively straightforward. I (well, we, because it takes a village to put these lectures together) chose the title *A Fork in the Road: An Occupational Hazard?* for several reasons. As a relatively young profession, occupational therapy has made tremendous strides in its growth and will only continue to do so. However, there have been times on our professional journey when we have begun to lose sight of and confidence in our methods, including intervention and

assessment approaches, which I will discuss. These proverbial "forks in the road" during our profession's development may have led us away from our professed and philosophical occupational therapy methods.

Similarly, these forks in the road have resulted in hazards such as "professional blurring," "dual encroachment," and "professional envy," which I will discuss. Finally—exciting, albeit frustrating—the incredible volume of research that has been conducted over the past decades has only served to solidify the validity and effectiveness of our professed and philosophical occupational therapy methods. Exciting? Yes—our profession's philosophical base and methods are being supported by a variety of scientific methods. Frustrating? Yes—many of these methods are no longer called *occupational therapy*, and many occupational therapists do not seem to even be using them.

Framework: Voyage and Return

I am going to frame this lecture and my ideas around a classic story plot. Although literary scholars disagree on the final count, clearly only a finite number of story plots can be used to describe and summarize the books we read, movies we watch, television programs we watch, and stories we tell. Christopher Booker (2004), an English journalist and author, published the book *The Seven Basic Plots: Why We Tell Stories*. His text is a Jungian-influenced analysis of stories and their psychological meaning. His seven identified basic plots, with examples, include

1. Overcoming the monster: *Jack and the Beanstalk, Frankenstein,* and *Jaws*
2. Rags to riches: *Cinderella and Aladdin*
3. The quest: *Don Quixote* and *Raiders of the Lost Ark*

This chapter was previously published in the *American Journal of Occupational Therapy, 67,* 641–652. Copyright © 2013, American Occupational Therapy Association. Reprinted with permission. http://dx.doi.org/10.5014/ajot.2013.676002

4. Comedy: *The Marriage of Figaro* and Shakespeare's comedies
5. Tragedy: *The Picture of Dorian Gray* and *King Lear*
6. Rebirth: *A Christmas Carol* and *It's a Wonderful Life*
7. Voyage and return (the plot I focus on): *Gulliver's Travels, Robinson Crusoe, Alice in Wonderland,* the *Wizard of Oz* and, in my opinion, our journey as an occupational therapy profession.

Examples of steps in the voyage-and-return plot include (Booker, 2004):

- *From normalcy to falling into the other world:* Normalcy is our usual, customary, traditional, normal functioning as a profession. I define *other worlds* as not just our attempts to be influenced by, but our adoption of and substitution of, other professions' approaches and techniques. The obvious hazard is professional role blurring and loss of professional identity.

- *Fascination with puzzling and unfamiliar things:* Even in past Slagle lectures, we have called our own interventions "commonplace" (Reilly, 1962, p. 1) and "unsophisticated" (Hollis, 1979, p. 499). When I first began as a full-time academician, I was lamenting with a seasoned colleague about why our students are still reporting not seeing occupation practiced in the clinics. She responded by saying that occupation appears to not be sophisticated. She also added, "It's not sexy!" If we feel that the tools of our trade are both commonplace and unsophisticated (and, I suppose, if we're not feeling sexy), it makes sense that we would seek out seemingly more sophisticated techniques and approaches. However, it does not guarantee that these approaches are more effective or even in line with our profession's philosophy. We begin to envy our colleagues in other professions, and further professional blurring continues.

- *Frustration:* Although I am only in the clinic 1 day a week, most of my day is about problem solving and celebrating the small successes one would expect to see on an acute neurology unit. However, there are everyday frustrations in clinics across the country that we all know as well. Why is this not working? How can I make clients better, and how can I do this faster? Why are they trying to do what I do? Why doesn't everyone know my role here?

- *Thrilling escape and return to normalcy:* It might not be thrilling, but our return to normalcy is imperative. I am going to argue that to move forward, we may have to take a few steps back to get to where we want to be.

Methods

I use two practice areas based on my expertise in neurorehabilitation to support my stance: (1) our evolved approaches to cognitive assessment and (2) our evolved approaches for people with performance limitations secondary to impaired motor control. These are just two examples. If these are not areas that are part of your practice, please reflect on your own areas of practice as I continue and think about common themes. I believe the voyage-and-return plot line can be applied to many areas of practice, such as working with hand injuries, working with mental health challenges, working in pediatrics, and so forth. I do want to be clear that this lecture is not about a specific area of practice; rather, I am using specific areas of practice to discuss our development as a profession. To document the plot of the story of our profession's development in these areas, I have reviewed the *Archives of Occupational Therapy,* 1922–1924; *Occupational Therapy and Rehabilitation,* 1925–1951; the *American Journal of Occupational Therapy,* 1947–present; the Eleanor Clarke Slagle lectures, 1955–present; *Willard and Spackman's Occupational Therapy,* Editions 1–11; and all editions of selected specialty textbooks, including *Occupational Therapy: Practice Skills for Physical Dysfunction* and *Occupational Therapy for Physical Dysfunction.* (And yes, the much discussed and touted balance of work, rest, and play has been a myth for me this year.)

Our Normalcy

Because my research for this lecture goes back to the early 1900s, that is my starting point. What is our normalcy in the area of working with our clients with performance limitations secondary to impaired motor control? Our unique contribution to all areas of practice was quite clear at this early time. We were, and still should be, the leaders in the actual doing and the actual practice (Meyer, 1922; see Chapter 4).

Normalcy and Motor Control Interventions

The first documented case study in our journals that described occupational therapy interventions for motor control deficits after stroke was in Volume 1, Issue 1, of the *Archives of Occupational Therapy* in 1922. Occupational therapist Evelyn Lawrence Collins (1922) described being invited by Mrs. Slagle to do home care on the Lower East Side of Manhattan. She described her case as a woman bedridden after a "paralytic stroke" and the woman's neighbor describing that "she can't do nothing; she has only got one hand" (p. 36). Collins went on to give a short description of what we now mistakenly call a "contemporary" approach to motor control rehabilitation. Remember, this article was published in 1922. She described engaging the affected hand using a bilateral activity as the means to remediate hand function. The activity of creating three small purses had all the makings of what we have recently rediscovered and proven: Repetitive and purposeful activity has the powerful potential to remediate motor function.

As I continued to review our profession's literature, I found that the occupational therapy approach to remediating motor control continued to be solidified and consistent across the life course. Occupational therapy interventions for this population were described as bilateral crafts (Collins, 1922); toy making for "uncomplicated paralysis" (Dean, 1922, p. 216); tool use, working looms, making rugs (Bowman, 1923); using a metronome during typing training (Spackman, 1947); engaging lower functioning clients in activity by unweighting the upper limb using a suspension sling (Covalt, Yamshon, & Nowicki, 1949; Spackman, 1947); project making (Suckle & Thompson, 1949); activities that provide graded resistance (Covalt et al., 1949); remedial games (Boeshart & Blau, 1951); an activity-based approach based on choosing selected activities (e.g., adapted games, filing, bilateral activities) determined by impairment level (Press, 1951); toy training (Robinault, 1953); bilateral activities such as sanding and wood working; and, again, using a suspension sling (Hopkins, 1963).

How then can we describe our normalcy? The words that we as an occupational therapy profession have historically used to describe this area of practice have one thing in common: They are primarily words of action. They include *practicing, doing, active, activity, repetitive, life related, skill building,* and *relearning* (Brunyate, 1947; Meyer, 1922 [see Chapter 4]; Spackman, 1947).

Fork in the Road

In reality, our normalcy and consistency in this area of practice lasted from about 1922 to the late 1950s or early 1960s, as noted earlier. So, just about 40 years. As the world changed dramatically around this time, our language and documented approaches took a dramatic turn as well—a proverbial fork in the road. Remember, we had been concerned that our approaches were commonplace, unsophisticated and, yes, not sexy. Booker

(2004) described this point in the plot as a having a fascination for unfamiliar things. We began to get, perhaps, overfocused on sets of techniques that may have looked more sophisticated and important than our normalcy. Instead of being just influenced by others' approaches, we in fact took an adoption approach and, if you will, a replacement approach. To illustrate, take a look at how our approach to remediating motor control impairments across the life course changed from the third to the fourth edition of Willard and Spackman's (1963, 1971) *Occupational Therapy* (Table 63.1).

As the left column of the table clearly indicates, we were still clearly focused on being the profession that engaged clients in the actual doing and the actual practice. Action words and everyday living were highlighted. Our approach was clear; we were remediating motor control in the context of using everyday activities (Hopkins, 1963). After that, our language and description of occupational therapy abruptly and dramatically changed (Huss, 1971), as indicated in the right column.

In fact, the third edition of Willard and Spackman's (1963) *Occupational Therapy* was a transitional volume and confusing at times. This edition was consistent with our sense of normalcy with the exception of an added last and new chapter on neuromuscular integration. This chapter was described as a framework derived from the biological sciences, neurology, physiology, phylogeny, and ontogeny as it related to occupational therapy. It was the initial description in our textbooks of sets of techniques to be applied to our clients and—with one exception, Margaret Rood—exclusively approaches that did not stem from occupational therapy. To summarize

Table 63.1. Changing Descriptions of Occupational Therapy for Clients With Impaired Motor Control Across the Life Course

Willard and Spackman's (1963) Occupational Therapy, 3rd Edition	Willard and Spackman's (1971) Occupational Therapy, 4th Edition
Cut meat	Ice
Wash and dry dishes	Tap
Open and hold an umbrella	Rub
Carry a tray of dishes	Brush
Finger paint	Stretch
Feed and wash with the affected extremity	Pattern
Suspend or unweight the arm during activity	Compress
Use of rolling pin	Wrap
Use of carpet sweeper	Inhibit
Etc.	Facilitate

and to be a bit facetious, we transitioned from having our clients brush their hair and teeth so that they might relearn motor control and maximize participation to having us, the therapists, brush over muscle–tendon units so that we could facilitate a muscle contraction. We abruptly switched from our patients actively doing (third edition; Willard & Spackman, 1963) to our patients being somewhat passive recipients of our services (fourth edition; Willard & Spackman, 1971).

Our normalcy in this area has been lost over the years. Even in our own textbooks we incorrectly refer to our traditional approaches as total approaches developed by other disciplines such as neurosurgery, physiatry, physical therapy, psychiatry, neurophysiology, and so forth. This was not our tradition. It was never our normalcy. In our current language (American Occupational Therapy Association [AOTA], 2008), these techniques and total approaches would be categorized as preparatory, which relegates activity and occupation to an afterthought.

Following this path led to a dramatic shift away from our core values and occupational therapy principles. We clearly moved away from the actual doing and the actual practice as described by Adolf Meyer in 1922 to a culture in which our primary role was to "do to" our clients. At the same time Mary Reilly (1962; see Chapter 7) was delivering the most often-quoted sentence in any Slagle lecture to date, which, as you know, contains the key phrase "man through the use of his hands" (p. 1), we started to take the stance that the therapist's hands are the key to recovery. To make a point, I do not want to be taken the wrong way with regard to the use of our hands. My clinical appointment is in acute neurology, and I am clear on the importance of well-honed hands-on skills for the purposes of safety, task completion, comfort, and reassurance.

Frustration

In the voyage-and-return plot, the next plot point is frustration (Booker, 2004). Did we choose the correct fork? At this point in our profession's journey, our reliance on the techniques and approaches of our colleagues from other professions has outlasted our own occupational therapy approach by at least a decade—50 years compared with our 40 years of normalcy. The currency and efficacy of these techniques and approaches we have dubbed "traditional" has been called into question for at least 2 decades by scholars and scientists from our field and others, and this questioning continues (Butler & Darrah, 2001; Damiano,

2007; Horak, 1991; Kollen et al., 2009; Mathiowetz & Haugen, 1994).

Confusion over our role may persist when professional blurring, professional envy, and dual-sided encroachment occur. Here is an example of this professional blurring or, perhaps, professional envy. Although the following two studies (like all studies) have limitations, and their methods may vary, the message is, I believe, a powerful one and, yes, a frustrating one. Smallfield and Karges (2009) aimed to classify occupational therapy intervention for stroke survivors on an inpatient rehabilitation unit. They discovered that more sessions were spent on prefunctional activities rather than on functional activities. In fact, almost 66% of sessions were not related to function. They further stated that "occupational therapists use prefunctional activities that aim to improve performance skills and body structures more often than occupation-based activities that incorporate meaningful activities into therapy sessions" (p. 412). How can that be?

In contrast, our colleagues in physical therapy performed a similar study to describe physical therapy interventions for people with stroke undergoing inpatient rehabilitation (Jette et al., 2005). They documented that fewer than 20% of interventions were classified as prefunctional and more than half would be classified as interventions related to areas of occupation using the language in our current practice framework (AOTA, 2008). Granted, most were in the focused category of functional mobility. I hope you can see my concern and point regardless.

In his 1996 Slagle lecture, David Nelson (1997) spoke of his concern that people from other professions are coming late to the table and claiming credit for some of the great ideas of occupational therapy. I agree wholeheartedly. Although I was never a popular kid, I am very proud to be part of a profession that seems to have won the "most-popular" contest. Have you looked around and listened for the past decade? It seems as though so many of our colleagues in other disciplines want to be us. Their current chosen methods (both in practice and in writing) are quickly morphing into our traditional occupational therapy. We know that imitation is the sincerest form of flattery—okay, I am flattered, but more so, frustrated.

It is hard, however, to stand our ground and defend our own practice when the same argument may be made against us. We cannot defend our scope of practice if we do not practice what and how we preach. How can we challenge our colleagues' use of our modalities if in many cases we are not being seen using them ourselves (reflect back on the findings of Smallfield & Karges, 2009) and if we freely use theirs? I would identify this problem as a dual encroachment related to scope of practice.

In her 2000 Slagle lecture, Margo Holm charged us with a mandate for the new millennium: evidence-based practice, which is consistent with our *Centennial Vision* (AOTA, 2007). Wow! We have a ton of data to sort through. I mean this in a good way. The past decade has resulted in an explosion of research to help us guide our practice. My colleagues and I just completed a project for AOTA focused on defining effective interventions to improve occupational performance for people with motor deficits after stroke. We reviewed almost 5,000 abstracts, and multiple papers met our strict inclusion criteria. This review was limited to the past several years and included literature both from occupational therapy and from our colleagues in other disciplines as long as a change in occupational performance was noted. For the first time in my career as an occupational therapist, I was over-whelmed by the sheer amount of evidence that was generated. On the basis of this current evidence-based review, if I was going to summarize which interventions are effective in improving occupational performance, I would de-

scribe them as *practicing, doing, active, activity, repetitive, life related, skill building,* and *relearning.*

Yes, these words should look familiar; earlier, I described that our profession's professed philosophy and approach is being further validated from a science perspective. This validation is to be celebrated! It is what we had previously been doing for years.

Further descriptions of these approaches include task-oriented approach, task-specific training, repetitive task practice, task-related training, massed practice, high intensity, active, and real-world focused. Occupational therapy is truly an art and science. However—again, frustratingly—these approaches are not being called occupational therapy.

I show some parallels in Figure 63.1. On the left side are descriptions of specific tasks that come from our own early literature as described earlier, including early editions of our journals and early editions of Willard and Spackman's *Principles of Occupational Therapy,* as discussed earlier. On the right side are examples of tasks used in both adult and pediatric rigorous evidence-based protocols that have documented improved occupational performance using a variety of methods: quantitative, qualitative, self-report, significant-other report, and so forth (Gordon, Schneider, Chinnan, & Charles, 2007; Taub et al., 1994). These parallels are not

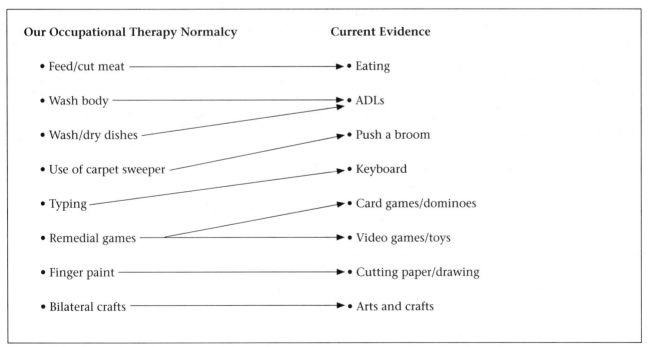

Our Occupational Therapy Normalcy   **Current Evidence**

- Feed/cut meat ———————————————————→ • Eating
- Wash body —————————————————————→ • ADLs
- Wash/dry dishes
- Use of carpet sweeper ———————————→ • Push a broom
- Typing —————————————————————————→ • Keyboard
- Remedial games ————————————————→ • Card games/dominoes
- Finger paint ——————————————————→ • Video games/toys
- Bilateral crafts —————————————————→ • Cutting paper/drawing
- Arts and crafts

Figure 63.1. Comparison of occupational therapy's normalcy and current evidence-based practice.

Note. ADLs = activities of daily living.

difficult to find if you go back far enough in our literature, but they are pretty far back at this point.

Furthermore, and a further reason to celebrate, many of the techniques and principles we developed and documented as a profession decades ago are now considered cutting edge and, my favorite misnomer, "contemporary." In the first edition of *Principles of Occupational Therapy,* Brunyate (1947) discussed treating a child with cerebral palsy, stating that "the child can practice picking up the glass a number of times" (p. 284) and reminding us that "repetitive use will gradually teach control" (p. 276). This concept is one of the most basic motor learning principles used to guide practice today. We now use the seemingly more sophisticated terms of *blocked practice* and *repetitive task practice* (Schmidt & Lee, 2011). Clare Spackman (1954) also reminded us that "relearning the desired skills requires practice all day long everyday" (p. 214). Suggested time? Sixteen hours per day! We now called this *massed practice,* which is a foundation of constraint-induced movement therapy, without doubt effective for a subset of our clients.

Over the years, some of the "traditional" approaches used have shied away from resistive activities. We were early proponents of using resistive activities (Brunyate; 1947; Covalt et al., 1949), consistent with current understanding that weakness after acquired brain injury is a crucial factor to consider to improve occupational performance (Ada, Dorsch, & Canning, 2006).

We have been unweighting severely hemiparetic limbs to promote early use and motor control for decades (Covalt et al., 1949; Spackman, 1947). We did this using deltoid aids and inexpensive counterbalance slings (Urquhart, 1975). Now, seemingly more sophisticated versions of unweighting limbs using expensive robotics are considered contemporary and cutting edge.

On the basis of current research, the efficacy of occupational therapy in motor recovery is based on a triad: early intervention, task-oriented training, and repetition of therapies. New and emerging research continues to demonstrate that the use of this triad, which highlights repetitive practice of real-world activities (our normalcy), not only has the potential to improve motor function and occupational performance, it also has the powerful potential to remodel and reorganize people's brains. Task-specific training sessions spent "simply" playing games, performing simulated office work, doing housekeeping chores, practicing walking, or practicing how to open and close a door or drawer (our normalcy) has resulted in use-dependent cortical changes. This involvement in everyday activities

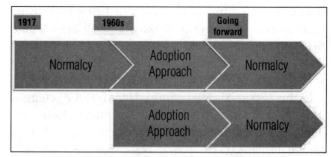

Figure 63.2. Timeline related to our involvement in motor control training and cognitive assessment. The top timeline represents occupational therapy's involvement in the area of motor control. The bottom timeline represents occupational therapy's involvement in the area of cognitive assessment.

- Increases gray matter in sensory and motor areas both ipsilateral and contralateral to the affected limb and to the bilateral hippocampi,
- Strengthens motor cortical areas and associated descending cortical connections,
- Increases contralesional and ipsilesional cortical activation on functional MRI, and
- Increases areas of activation to the cerebellum and mid-brain (Young & Tolentino, 2011).

As a clinician, this is the icing on the cake; as a researcher and someone who wants occupational therapy to achieve its *Centennial Vision* (AOTA, 2007)—that is, to be a "powerful, widely recognized, science-driven, and evidence-based profession" (p. 613)—I find it fascinating, exciting and, if I may, sexy as well! Let's never again call our techniques unsophisticated.

Just to review our journey related to motor control, our early involvement related to motor control training was clear from the inception of the profession. It was only around the 1960s when our professed methods took a dramatic shift in favor of our colleagues' methods (see Figure 63.2). I will talk about moving forward soon.

Cognitive Rehabilitation and Assessment: Our Normalcy?

I want to switch gears and use another area of practice as an example to describe our voyage before summarizing. Our involvement in the arena of cognitive rehabilitation, which is better described for our purposes as improving occupational performance for those with cognitive deficits, is not as clear. I use cognitive assessment as my specific example. Our involvement in this practice area definitely came later than working with people with performance deficits secondary to motor impairments. You can argue that it is a newer field, and I agree; however, the earliest attempts at rehabilitating people with cognitive deficits date back to the First World War (Boake, 1989). In our professional journals, the first papers concerning cognition did not appear until the mid-1960s. Our first official statement on cognition and occupational therapy was approved in 1991 (AOTA, 1991). Not until the fourth edition of Willard and Spackman's *Occupational Therapy* (Gilfoyle & Grady, 1971) was cognition addressed. This volume contained the first list of instruments recommended for use by occupational therapists for clients with a variety of diagnoses that result in cognitive–perceptual–motor dysfunction or delays. Included on this list (with the one exception of A. Jean Ayres, who delivered the Slagle lecture in 1963) were assessments developed exclusively by our colleagues in other disciplines (educational psychology, psychology, neuropsychology, etc.). These tools, even at face value, had limited resemblance to what was the normalcy of original and authentic occupational therapy—another proverbial fork in the road and, using Booker's (2004) plot points, an early fascination with unfamiliar things.

It may be interesting to note that our shift in motor control approaches was happening at the same time as our adoption of others' cognitive assessment approaches. The time line on top in Figure 63.2 represents our journey related to motor control. The time line on the bottom represents our journey related to our involvement in cognitive rehabilitation. Note the lack of early history and the early adoption of our colleagues' approaches. Indeed, these times were turbulent, and science was advancing at a startling rate. We were unsure of our seemingly unsophisticated methods and adopted what appeared to be a more advanced and sophisticated approach.

Our literature continued to support the almost exclusive use of the assessment approaches of our colleagues in other disciplines. This support continued through multiple editions of Willard and Spackman's *Occupational Therapy* and continued to be solidified when the first several editions of our specialty texts were published and the same or similar tools were recommended. What continued to solidify what I will call *an adopted approach to cognitive assessment* was further blurred when many of our colleagues in our profession began to develop instruments that exclusively included test items similar to those on instruments developed by our colleagues in other disciplines.

Our normalcy related to cognitive assessment can be described using the following descriptors: originally and primarily adopted from other disciplines, not occupation based, contrived, novel, two dimensional in a three-dimensional world, tested in an 8.5- × 11-inch space, and pen and paper or table top based. There are many concerns related to the exclusive use of this level of measurement when our focus is on occupational performance. Our client's lives and occupations are quite complicated. Engagement in occupation requires the ability to use multiple cognitive processes, motor skills, and language skills simultaneously. In addition, on top of all that, we need to regulate our emotions. Life and occupation are not about a simplistic cognitive manipulation.

Concerns Regarding Our Normalcy

One major concern is that this style of measurement does not take into account the well-documented dual-task paradigm. A *dual-task paradigm* is a procedure in research that requires a person to perform two tasks simultaneously to compare performance with single-task conditions. If Task 1 is stepping over obstacles and Task 2 is memorizing a grocery list, one may have a relatively high level of performance when performing the tasks in isolation. When one is then asked to step over obstacles while memorizing, one of three performance changes will most likely be noted: degraded performance in Task 1, in Task 2, or in both tasks.

To fully experience the dual-task paradigm, simply think about all the times you were rushing to work and got behind somebody who was walking and texting. Think about that person's walking speed. The research is clear. Dual-task measures are more accurate at discriminating cognitive impairment than traditional (single) measures (Holtzer, Burright, & Donovick, 2004). The dual-task research is very controlled to ensure that one is doing only two tasks at once. Again, this is still not everyday life. Life is not controlled. It does not take place in a quiet, well-lit room that is free of distractions. It requires not only dual tasking but multitasking, many times with external time pressures that must also be managed. Even tasks such as dressing that appear so simplistic or, as we have called them, unsophisticated rely on a dynamic interplay of multiple neural networks and cognitive–perceptual processes to be successful (Árnadóttir, 2011). There is nothing simple about it.

The next concern is novelty. I have reviewed survey research to document the cognitive assessments most commonly used by occupational therapists and reviewed the items included to evaluate cognition (Koh, Hoffman, Bennett, & McKenna, 2009; Korner-Bitensky, Barrett-Bernstein, Bibas, & Poulin, 2011; Menon-Nair, Korner-Bitensky, & Ogourtsova, 2007). Item examples include block designs, design drawing or copying, draw a man, butterfly puzzles, gesture copying, pegboard designs, cancellation tasks, memorizing a number string, and making trails. Although novelty testing may be important for our high-level clients with executive dysfunction, it puts many of our clients at a disadvantage. We know this from our own lives and because this paradigm has been in the literature for more than a decade. Performance of novel tasks requires increased attentional control, compromises secondary task performance (i.e., memory), renders one unable to use proceduralized control or "autopilot," and decreases overall task performance (Beilock, Wierenga, & Carr, 2002).

Finally, in terms of concerns, the concept of ecological validity or variants thereof can be found in the psychology literature dating back to 1943 (Schmuckler, 2001). *Ecological validity* typically refers to whether one can generalize from observed behavior in testing to natural behavior in the world. I have a more pragmatic definition: So what? What does it really mean if one cannot count backward from 100 by 7s or draw two intersecting pentagons? What does that tell us about occupational performance?

At least two conditions determine whether a tool is ecologically valid (Chaytor & Schmitter-Edgecombe, 2003):

1. *Verisimilitude,* the degree to which the cognitive demands of the test theoretically resemble the cognitive demands in the everyday environment ("functional cognition"); identifies difficulty in performing real-world tasks
2. *Veridicality,* the degree to which existing tests are empirically related to measures of everyday functioning (requires a statistical analysis).

To satisfy the first condition, that is, that the demands of the assessment theoretically resemble everyday demands, we need to move away from block designs, design drawing and copying, draw a man, butterfly puzzles, gesture copying, pegboard designs, cancellation tasks, memorizing a number string, making trails, and so forth and back to what makes us unique—that is, performance-based cognitive assessments using real-world tasks in the correct environmental context. Satisfying the second condition of ecological validity, that is, a statistical relationship with measures of everyday function, will most likely not occur if we continue on our current path. For more than 30 years, scholars and researchers have been concerned about the clear lack of a relationship between this level of cognitive measurement and daily functioning (Bouwens et al., 2008; Burgess et al., 2006; Heaton & Pendleton, 1981), thus highlighting the need for direct observation (both standardized and nonstandardized) of everyday activities: our true normalcy.

True Normalcy

In addition to 30 years of documenting this weak relationship between cognitive testing and real-world functioning, there has been a 30-year dialogue by our colleagues in other professions about what to do about it. Here again is why we should celebrate. We, the profession of occupational therapy, developed some of the first cognitive assessments that used occupation and occupational analysis to document how cognition supported or limited participation in everyday occupations. No more guessing. We should continue to be the leaders in the area of occupation and performance-based assessment. In the area of mental health, 37 years ago Sara Brayman and colleagues developed and published the Comprehensive Occupational Therapy Evaluation (Brayman, Kirby, Misenheimer, & Short, 1976). Many of the behaviors included on this scale were identified by A. Jean Ayres 60 years ago. Almost 30 years ago, Claudia Allen, who delivered the Slagle lecture in 1987, developed the first version of the Routine Task Inventory (Allen, 1985).

The first occupation-based cognitive assessment in the area of neurorehabilitation was developed by an Icelandic master's-degree student at the University of Southern California in 1985.

Gudrun Árnadóttir was way ahead of her time and almost 30 years ago tried to get us neurotherapists to return to our roots of occupation in this area of practice with the Árnadóttir OT–ADL Neurobehavioral Evaluation, now known as the ADL-focused Occupation-based Neurobehavioral Evaluation (A–ONE; Árnadóttir, 1990, 2011). Soon after that Carolyn Baum, who delivered the Slagle lecture in 1980, and her colleagues developed and published the Kitchen Task Assessment (Baum & Edwards, 1993), which continued to evolve into the Executive Function Performance Test (Baum et al., 2008). In the same time frame, Anne Fisher, who delivered the Slagle lecture in 1998, developed and published the Assessment of Motor and Process Skills (AMPS; Fisher, 1992; Fisher & Jones, 2011) and subsequently the School AMPS (Atchison, Fisher, & Bryze, 1998; Fisher, Bryze, & Atchison, 2000), both measures of occupational performance and performance skills and the gold standard in terms of the sophistication of its psychometric properties (Fisher, 1993).

Frustration

So, we have an almost 40-year history of solving the problem of identified limitations in typical cognitive assessment by creating occupation-based assessments. These tools are completely appropriate to use with our clients throughout the life course who are living with performance deficits secondary to cognitive deficits. However, the next question is, Are we using them in practice? In too many instances, the answer appears to be "no" on the basis of published survey research (Koh et al., 2009; Korner-Bitensky et al., 2011; Menon-Nair et al., 2007) and, I will add, experience. Again, our journey related to this area of practice is colored by an early adoption of the approach to assessment used by our colleagues in other disciplines. Because of this, our journey is also colored by professional blurring and again dual encroachment. I want to read a couple of quotes to you:

- "Predictions based on neuropsychological test data tend to be more accurate if the particular tasks utilized during testing closely match or simulate the individual's everyday and vocational demands" (Sbordone, 2001, p. 199).
- "The ecological validity of neuropsychological testing can be extended by observing the patient's approach to tasks in the assessment environment and by observing the patient in his or her normal activities" (Bennett, 2001, p. 237).
- "The importance of reliable behavioural observations, made in more ecologically valid environments than purely the consulting room is stressed" (Manchester, Priestley, & Jackson, 2004, p. 1067).

None of these quotes are from occupational therapists. They are quotes in the literature from our colleagues in other disciplines. Again, imitation is the sincerest form of flattery. However, I guess our colleagues can say the same about us. Again, I hope you see my concern.

Our colleagues in other disciplines are now developing assessments that use items that clearly represent the authentic use of occupation in an attempt to be a more valid and accurate measure of everyday cognition. Si-multaneously, we continue to use (and develop) assessments that can best be described as novel, contrived, and having little to do with occupation and everyday life (Koh et al., 2009; Korner-Bitensky et al., 2011; Menon-Nair et al., 2007).

Here is the current reality. We have already designed, developed, and aggressively tested the psychometric properties of our performance-based cognitive assessments and performance-based assessments in general. We do not need to scramble to create them. We simply need to adopt our own tools and return to our own philosophy, our normalcy. We need to celebrate our decades of work as a profession. Although I referred to some of these tools earlier, there are too many to name in one article. Most are readily available and just awaiting adoption. These tools cover the life course and highlight our unique contribution to this interprofessional area of practice.

Return to Normalcy

The last point in Booker's (2004) voyage-and-return plot is return to normalcy. This return is imperative. I have used the fork in the road to describe our professional journey. As stated earlier, in my opinion it is pretty clear we need to journey back to move forward. We need to reclaim what we do and realize that nobody does occupation better than we do.

How do we hasten this return back to our normalcy? At the return plot point in Booker's (2004) text, he challenged us to consider this quote: "At this point the real question posed by the whole adventure is: How far have they learned or gained from their experience? Have they been fundamentally changed?" (p. 106).

I argue that we have been changed because of our professional journey. We have changed for the better and have already begun the journey back to our philosophical roots. I envision a time in our immediate future when practitioners not only respect but use the sophisticated and effective tools of our trade.

Many of the heroes and heroines in voyage-and-return plots return for the better and have been changed for the good. Descriptors in these plots include returning wiser, more developed, and evolved; having a deeper understanding; having expanded knowledge and awareness; returning back to the familiar (our normalcy); returning as a better person (I will add practitioner, educator, and researcher); having learned something from the journey; and, most important, having a clear future.

How do we hasten our return? Again, time is of the essence. The good news is this should not be difficult. We have already done the work. We must now simply embrace it. Some considerations are as follows:

- How much time is spent on impairment-level and preparatory interventions that are not occupation based? Practitioners, I challenge you to consider your practice in terms of the actual percentage of time spent in occupation. I encourage you to reflect on this and, with your peers, implement a plan to consistently increase this percentage over the next months. By the way, I have no problem with preparatory activities. I do have a concern over how they may be being overused.

- A related issue is whether we are using authentic occupations in the clinic or catalog-purchased contrived activities. Practitioners, this change needs to occur now. I will tell you this is not only doable, it is also less expensive! We have generated a body of research emphasizing the use of real, familiar, and age-appropriate objects and occupations.

- We need to move away from "therapists doing to" and back to a model of "clients doing"—back to the actual practice and the actual doing we discussed in 1922 and that, again, are now being called cutting edge and contemporary. Everything old is new again.

- Do we look like occupational therapists? If we visited each other's clinics, how often would we see authentic occupations being used? We need to practice what we preach. If we do not, we are on unsteady ground to protect what we do. At the same time, we need to stop encroaching on our colleagues' approaches and methods.

- There is nothing wrong with being influenced by our colleagues in other professions. However, let us learn from our mistakes and, going forward, maintain our confidence that our approach is effective, artistic, scientific, reimbursable, and evidence based. Let us not repeat our mistakes of replacing our approach by adopting others' techniques.

- Let's stop trying to convince ourselves and our colleagues that we can predict occupational performance from non–occupation-based assessments.

- In terms of assessment, the time to embrace performance-based assessments is today, if not yesterday. As stated, these tools are already developed and available. Some argue that we do not have time to use them. I would argue back not only that they are time savers but that we do not have time not to use them to maintain our professional identity.

- How much information should we include in entry-level texts and programs related to potentially outdated approaches to assessment and intervention that are not historically ours and have not shown the ability to predict or improve occupational performance? How much curriculum time and testing should we spend on this material?

To be a science-driven and evidence-based profession that is globally connected (AOTA, 2007) and, may I add, reimbursable, we need to move away from having our clients spell the word *world* backward and move back to engagement in real-world tasks.

In summary, we are at a critical point in our voyage and development. As never before, our philosophical approach, the art and science that is occupational therapy, and our normalcy are clearly being supported by our scientific methods. Again, we need to celebrate it! But, more important, we need to embrace it and integrate it. Let's all promise to go back to work as change agents embracing our roots, celebrating the amazing work and the accomplishments of our young profession. Let's get excited to go back to our clinics, our classrooms, and our laboratories and put the occupation back in occupational therapy.

References

Ada, L., Dorsch, S., & Canning, C. G. (2006). Strengthening interventions increase strength and improve activity after stroke: A systematic review. *Australian Journal of Physiotherapy, 52,* 241–248. http://dx.doi.org/10.1016/S0004-9514(06)70003-4

Allen, C. K. (1985). *Occupational therapy for psychiatric diseases: Measurement and management of cognitive disabilities.* Boston: Little, Brown.

American Occupational Therapy Association. (1991). Occupational therapy services management of persons with cognitive impairments. *American Journal of Occupational Therapy, 45,* 1067–1068. http://dx.doi.org/10.5014/ajot.45.12.1067

American Occupational Therapy Association. (2007). AOTA's *Centennial Vision* and executive summary. *American Journal of Occupational Therapy, 61,* 613–614. http://dx.doi. org/10.5014/ajot.61.6.613

American Occupational Therapy Association. (2008). Occupational therapy practice framework: Domain and process (2nd ed.). *American Journal of Occupational Therapy, 62,* 625–683. http://dx.doi.org/10.5014/ajot.62.6.625

Árnadóttir, G. (1990). *The brain and behavior: Assessing cortical dysfunction through activities of daily living.* St. Louis, MO: Mosby.

Árnadóttir, G. (2011). Impact of neurobehavioral deficits on activities of daily living. In G. Gillen (Ed.), *Stroke rehabilitation: A function-based approach* (3rd ed., pp. 456–500). St. Louis, MO: Mosby.

Atchison, B. T., Fisher, A. G., & Bryze, K. (1998). Rater reliability and internal scale and person response validity of the School Assessment of Motor and Process Skills. *American Journal of Occupational Therapy, 52*, 843–850. http:// dx.doi.org/10.5014/ajot.52.10.843

Ayres, A. J. (1963). The development of perceptual–motor abilities: A theoretical basis for treatment of dysfunction (Eleanor Clarke Slagle Lecture). *American Journal of Occupational Therapy, 27*, 221–225.

Baum, C. M., Connor, L. T., Morrison, T., Hahn, M., Dromerick, A. W., & Edwards, D. F. (2008). Reliability, validity, and clinical utility of the Executive Function Performance Test: A measure of executive function in a sample of people with stroke. *American Journal of Occupational Therapy, 62*, 446–455. http://dx.doi.org/10.5014/ajot.62.4.446

Baum, C., & Edwards, D. F. (1993). Cognitive performance in senile dementia of the Alzheimer's type: The Kitchen Task Assessment. *American Journal of Occupational Therapy, 47*, 431–436. http://dx.doi.org/10.5014/ajot.47.5.431

Beilock, S. L., Wierenga, S. A., & Carr, T. H. (2002). Expertise, attention, and memory in sensorimotor skill execution: Impact of novel task constraints on dual-task performance and episodic memory. *Quarterly Journal of Experimental Psychology, 55*, 1211–1240. http://dx.doi.org/10.1080/02724980244000170

Bennett, T. L. (2001). Neuropsychological evaluation in rehabilitation planning and evaluation of functional skills. *Archives of Clinical Neuropsychology, 16*, 237–253.

Boake, C. (1989). A history of cognitive rehabilitation of head-injured patients, 1915–1980. *Journal of Head Trauma Rehabilitation, 4*, 1–8. http://dx.doi.org/10.1097/00001199-198909000-00004

Boeshart, L. K., & Blau, L. (1951). Remedial games as an occupational therapy modality in the treatment of physical disabilities. *American Journal of Occupational Therapy, 5*, 47–48.

Booker, C. (2004). *The seven basic plots: Why we tell stories.* New York: Continuum.

Bouwens, S. F., van Heugten, C. M., Aalten, P., Wolfs, C. A., Baarends, E. M., van Menxel, D. A., & Verhey, F. R. (2008). Relationship between measures of dementia severity and observation of daily life functioning as measured with the Assessment of Motor and Process Skills (AMPS). *Dementia and Geriatric Cognitive Disorders, 25*, 81–87. http://dx.doi.org/10.1159/000111694

Bowman, M. (1923). Report of the round table on crafts for the physically disabled. *Archives of Occupational Therapy, 2*, 467–474.

Brayman, S. J., Kirby, T. F., Misenheimer, A. M., & Short, M. J. (1976). Comprehensive occupational therapy evaluation scale. *American Journal of Occupational Therapy, 30*, 94–100.

Brunyate, R. W. (1947). Occupational therapy for patients with cerebral palsy. In H. S. Willard & C. S. Spackman (Eds.), *Principles of occupational therapy* (pp. 274–287). Philadelphia: J. B. Lippincott.

Burgess, P. W., Alderman, N., Forbes, C., Costello, A., Coates, L. M. A., Dawson, D. R., . . . Channon, S. (2006). The case for the development and use of "ecologically valid" measures of executive function in experimental and clinical neuropsychology. *Journal of the International Neuropsychological Society, 12*, 194–209. http://dx.doi.org/10.1017/S1355617706060310

Butler, C., & Darrah, J. (2001). Effects of neurodevelopmental treatment (NDT) for cerebral palsy: An AACPDM evidence report. *Developmental Medicine and Child Neurology, 43*, 778–790. http://dx.doi.org/10.1017/S0012162201001414

Chaytor, N., & Schmitter-Edgecombe, M. (2003). The ecological validity of neuropsychological tests: A review of the literature on everyday cognitive skills. *Neuropsychology Review, 13*, 181–197. http://dx.doi.org/10.1023/B:NERV.0000009483.91468.fb

Collins, E. L. (1922). Occupational therapy for the homebound. *Archives of Occupational Therapy, 1*, 33–40.

Covalt, D. A., Yamshon, L. J., & Nowicki, V. (1949). Physiological aid to the functional training of the hemiplegic arm. *American Journal of Occupational Therapy, 3*, 286–288.

Damiano, D. (2007). Pass the torch, please. *Developmental Medicine and Child Neurology, 49*, 723. http://dx.doi.org/10.1111/j.1469-8749.2007.00723.x

Dean, A. H. (1922). Report of the round table on woodwork and their finishings. *Archives of Occupational Therapy, 3*, 215–218.

Fisher, A. G. (1992). *Assessment of Motor and Process Skills* (Research ed. 6.1). Unpublished test manual, Colorado State University, Occupational Therapy Department.

Fisher, A. G. (1993). The assessment of IADL motor skills: An application of many-faceted Rasch analysis. *American Journal of Occupational Therapy, 47*, 319–329.

Fisher, A. G. (1998). Uniting practice and theory in an occupational framework (Eleanor Clarke Slagle Lecture). *American Journal of Occupational Therapy, 52*, 509–521. http:// dx.doi.org/10.5014/ajot.52.7.509

Fisher, A. G., Bryze, K., & Atchison, B. T. (2000). Naturalistic assessment of functional performance in school settings: Reliability and validity of the School AMPS scales. *Journal of Outcome Measurement, 4,* 491–512.

Fisher, A. G., & Jones, K. B. (2011). *Assessment of Motor and Process Skills: Development, standardization, and administration manual* (7th ed., revised). Ft. Collins, CO: Three Star Press.

Gilfoyle, E. M., & Grady, A. P. (1971). Cognitive–perceptual–motor behavior. In H. S. Willard & C. S. Spackman (Eds.), *Occupational therapy* (4th ed., pp. 401–479). Philadelphia: J. B. Lippincott.

Gordon, A. M., Schneider, J. A., Chinnan, A., & Charles, J. R. (2007). Efficacy of a hand-arm bimanual intensive therapy (HABIT) in children with hemiplegic cerebral palsy: A randomized control trial. *Developmental Medicine and Child Neurology, 49,* 830–838. http://dx.doi.org/10.1111/ j.1469-8749.2007.00830.x

Heaton, R. K., & Pendleton, M. G. (1981). Use of neuropsychological tests to predict adult patients' everyday functioning. *Journal of Consulting and Clinical Psychology, 49,* 807–821. http://dx.doi.org/10.1037/0022-006X.49.6.807

Hollis, L. I. (1979). Remember (Eleanor Clarke Slagle Lecture). *American Journal of Occupational Therapy, 33,* 493–499.

Holm, M. B. (2000). Our mandate for the new millennium: Evidence-based practice (Eleanor Clarke Slagle Lecture). *American Journal of Occupational Therapy, 54,* 575–585. http://dx.doi.org/10.5014/ajot.54.6.575

Holtzer, R., Burright, R. G., & Donovick, P. J. (2004). The sensitivity of dual-task performance to cognitive status in aging. *Journal of the International Neuropsychological Society, 10,* 230–238. http://dx.doi.org/10.1017/ S1355617704102099

Hopkins, H. H. (1963). Cerebral vascular accidents and hemiplegia. In H. S. Willard & C. S. Spackman (Eds.), *Occupational therapy* (3rd ed., pp. 240–252). Philadelphia: J. B. Lippincott.

Horak, F. B. (1991). Assumptions underlying motor control for neurological rehabilitation. In *Contemporary management of motor control problems: Proceedings of the II–STEP Conference.* Alexandria, VA: Foundation for Physical Therapy.

Huss, A. J. (1971). Sensorimotor treatment approaches. In H. S. Willard & C. S. Spackman (Eds.), *Occupational therapy* (4th ed., pp. 373–400). Philadelphia: J. B. Lippincott.

Jette, D. U., Latham, N. K., Smout, R. J., Gassaway, J., Slavin, M. D., & Horn, S. D. (2005). Physical therapy interventions for patients with stroke in inpatient rehabilitation facilities. *Physical Therapy, 85,* 238–248.

Koh, C. L., Hoffmann, T., Bennett, S., & McKenna, K. (2009). Management of patients with cognitive impairment after stroke: A survey of Australian occupational therapists. *Australian Occupational Therapy Journal, 56,* 324–331. http:// dx.doi.org/10.1111/j.1440-1630.2008.00764.x

Kollen, B. J., Lennon, S., Lyons, B., Wheatley-Smith, L., Scheper, M., Buurke, J. H., . . . Kwakkel, G. (2009). The effectiveness of the Bobath concept in stroke rehabilitation: What is the evidence? *Stroke, 40,* e89–e97. http:// dx.doi.org/10.1161/STROKEAHA.108.533828

Korner-Bitensky, N., Barrett-Bernstein, S., Bibas, G., & Poulin, V. (2011). National survey of Canadian occupational therapists' assessment and treatment of cognitive impairment post-stroke. *Australian Occupational Therapy Journal, 58,* 241–250. http://dx.doi. org/10.1111/j.1440-1630.2011.00943.x

Manchester, D., Priestley, N., & Jackson, H. (2004). The assessment of executive functions: Coming out of the office. *Brain Injury, 18,* 1067–1081. http://dx.doi.org/1 0.1080/02699050410001672387

Mathiowetz, V., & Haugen, J. B. (1994). Motor behavior research: Implications for therapeutic approaches to central nervous system dysfunction. *American Journal of Occupational Therapy, 48,* 733–745. http://dx.doi. org/10.5014/ajot.48.8.733

Menon-Nair, A., Korner-Bitensky, N., & Ogourtsova, T. (2007). Occupational therapists' identification, assessment, and treatment of unilateral spatial neglect during stroke rehabilitation in Canada. *Stroke, 38,* 2556–2562. http://dx.doi.org/10.1161/STROKEAHA.107.484857

Meyer, A. (1922). The philosophy of occupation therapy. *Archives of Occupational Therapy, 1,* 1–10. Reprinted as Chapter 4.

Nelson, D. (1997). Why the profession of occupational therapy will flourish in the 21st century (Eleanor Clarke Slagle Lecture). *American Journal of Occupational Therapy, 51,* 11–24. http://dx.doi.org/10.5014/ ajot.51.1.11

Press, V. R. (1951). A proposed classification and activity list for spastic hemiplegias. *American Journal of Occupational Therapy, 5,* 251–256.

Reilly, M. (1962). Occupational therapy can be one of the great ideas of 20th century medicine (Eleanor Clarke Slagle Lecture). *American Journal of Occupational Therapy, 16,* 1–9. Reprinted as Chapter 7.

Robinault, I. P. (1953). Occupational therapy technics for the preschool hemiplegic: Toys and training. *American Journal of Occupational Therapy, 7,* 205–207.

Sbordone, R. J. (2001). Limitations of neuropsychological testing to predict the cognitive and behavioral functioning of persons with brain injury in real-world settings. *NeuroRehabilitation, 16,* 199–201.

Schmidt, R. A., & Lee, T. D. (2011). *Motor control and learning: A behavioral emphasis* (5th ed.). Champaign, IL: Human Kinetics.

Schmuckler, M. A. (2001). What is ecological validity? A dimensional analysis. *Infancy, 2,* 419–436. http://dx.doi.org/10.1207/S15327078IN0204_02

Smallfield, S., & Karges, J. (2009). Classification of occupational therapy intervention for inpatient stroke rehabilitation. *American Journal of Occupational Therapy, 63,* 408–413. http://dx.doi.org/10.5014/ajot.63.4.408

Spackman, C. S. (1947). Occupational therapy for patients with physical injuries. In H. S. Willard & C. S. Spackman (Eds.), *Principles of occupational therapy* (pp. 174–300). Philadelphia: J. B. Lippincott.

Spackman, C. S. (1954). Occupational therapy for patients with physical disabilities, part 1. In H. S. Willard & C. S. Spackman (Eds.), *Principles of occupational therapy* (2nd ed., pp. 168–255). Philadelphia: J. B. Lippincott.

Suckle, H. M., & Thompson, C. V. (1949). Occupational therapy in the treatment of neurosurgical patients. *American Journal of Occupational Therapy, 3,* 1–3.

Taub, E., Crago, J. E., Burgio, L. D., Groomes, T. E., Cook, E. W., 3rd, DeLuca, S. C., & Miller, N. E. (1994). An operant approach to rehabilitation medicine: Overcoming learned nonuse by shaping. *Journal of the Experimental Analysis of Behavior, 61,* 281–293. http://dx.doi.org/10.1901/jeab.1994.61-281

Urquhart, K. (1975). Inexpensive counterbalance arm sling. *American Journal of Occupational Therapy, 29,* 360–361.

Willard, H. S., & Spackman, C. S. (Eds.). (1963). *Occupational therapy* (3rd ed.). Philadelphia: J. B. Lippincott.

Willard, H. S., & Spackman, C. S. (Eds.). (1971). *Occupational therapy* (4th ed.). Philadelphia: J. B. Lippincott.

Young, J. A., & Tolentino, M. (2011). Neuroplasticity and its applications for rehabilitation. *American Journal of Therapeutics, 18,* 70–80. http://dx.doi.org/10.1097/MJT.0b013e3181e0f1a4

APPENDIX A

OCCUPATIONAL THERAPY PRACTICE

FRAMEWORK:
Domain & Process
3rd Edition

Contents

Preface S1
   Definitions S1
   Evolution of This Document S2
   Vision for This Work S3
Introduction S3
Domain S4
   Occupations S5
   Client Factors S7
   Performance Skills S7
   Performance Patterns S8
   Context and Environment S8
Process S9
   Overview of the Occupational Therapy Process S10
   Evaluation Process S13
   Intervention Process S14
   Targeting of Outcomes S16
Conclusion S17
Tables and Figures
   Table 1. Occupations S19
   Table 2. Client Factors S22
   Table 3. Performance Skills S25
   Table 4. Performance Patterns S27
   Table 5. Context and Environment S28
   Table 6. Types of Occupational Therapy
     Interventions S29
   Table 7. Activity and Occupational Demands S32
   Table 8. Approaches to Intervention S33
   Table 9. Outcomes S34
   Exhibit 1. Aspects of the Domain of Occupational
     Therapy S4
   Exhibit 2. Process of Occupational Therapy
     Service Delivery S10
   Exhibit 3. Operationalizing the Occupational
     Therapy Process S17
   Figure 1. Occupational Therapy's Domain S5
   Figure 2. Occupational Therapy's Process S10
   Figure 3. Occupational Therapy Domain
     and Process S18
References S36
Authors S40
Acknowledgments S40
Appendix A. Glossary S41
Appendix B. Preparation and Qualifications of Occupational
   Therapists and Occupational Therapy Assistants . . . S47

Copyright © 2014 by the American Occupational Therapy Association.

When citing this document the preferred reference is: American Occupational Therapy Association. (2014). Occupational therapy practice framework: Domain and process (3rd ed.). *American Journal of Occupational Therapy, 68*(Suppl. 1), S1–S48. http://dx.doi.org/10.5014/ajot.2014.682006

PREFACE

The *Occupational Therapy Practice Framework: Domain and Process,* 3rd edition (hereinafter referred to as "the *Framework*"), is an official document of the American Occupational Therapy Association (AOTA). Intended for occupational therapy practitioners and students, other health care professionals, educators, researchers, payers, and consumers, the *Framework* presents a summary of interrelated constructs that describe occupational therapy practice.

Definitions

Within the *Framework, occupational therapy* is defined as

the therapeutic use of everyday life activities (occupations) with individuals or groups for the purpose of enhancing or enabling participation in roles, habits, and routines in home, school, workplace, community, and other settings. Occupational therapy practitioners use their knowledge of the transactional relationship among the person, his or her engagement in valuable occupations, and the context to design occupation-based intervention plans that facilitate change or growth in client factors (body functions, body structures, values, beliefs, and spirituality) and skills (motor, process, and social interaction) needed for successful participation. Occupational therapy practitioners are concerned with the end result of participation and thus enable engagement through adaptations and modifications to the environment or objects within the environment when needed. Occupational therapy services are provided for habilitation, rehabilitation, and promotion of health and wellness for clients with disability- and non–disability-related needs. These services include acquisition and preservation of occupational identity for those who have or are at risk for developing an illness, injury, disease, disorder, condition, impairment, disability, activity limitation, or participation restriction. (adapted from AOTA, 2011; see Appendix A for additional definitions in a glossary)

When the term *occupational therapy practitioner* is used in this document, it refers to both occupational therapists and occupational therapy assistants (AOTA, 2006). Occupational therapists are responsible for all aspects of occupational therapy service delivery and are accountable for the safety and effectiveness of the occupational therapy service delivery process. Occupational therapy assistants deliver occupational therapy services under the supervision of and in partnership with an occupational therapist (AOTA, 2009). Additional information about the preparation and qualifications of occupational therapists and occupational therapy assistants can be found in Appendix B.

Evolution of This Document

The *Framework* was originally developed to articulate occupational therapy's distinct perspective and contribution to promoting the health and participation of persons, groups, and populations through engagement in occupation. The first edition of the *Framework* emerged from an examination of documents related to the *Occupational Therapy Product Output Reporting System and Uniform Terminology for Reporting Occupational Therapy Services* (AOTA, 1979). Originally a document that responded to a federal requirement to develop a uniform reporting system, the text gradually shifted to describing and outlining the domains of concern of occupational therapy.

The second edition of *Uniform Terminology for Occupational Therapy* (AOTA, 1989) was adopted by the AOTA Representative Assembly (RA) and published in 1989. The document focused on delineating and defining only the occupational performance areas and occupational performance components that are addressed in occupational therapy direct services. The third and final revision of *Uniform Terminology for Occupational Therapy* (AOTA, 1994) was adopted by the RA in 1994 and was "expanded to reflect current practice and to incorporate contextual aspects of performance" (p. 1047). Each revision reflected changes in practice and provided consistent terminology for use by the profession.

In Fall 1998, the AOTA Commission on Practice (COP) embarked on the journey that culminated in the *Occupational Therapy Practice Framework: Domain and Process* (AOTA, 2002b). At that time, AOTA also published *The Guide to Occupational Therapy Practice* (Moyers, 1999), which outlined contemporary practice for the profession. Using this document and the feedback received during the review process for the third edition of *Uniform Terminology for Occupational Therapy,* the COP proceeded to develop a document that more fully articulated occupational therapy.

The *Framework* is an ever-evolving document. As an official AOTA document, it is reviewed on a 5-year cycle for usefulness and the potential need for further refinements or changes. During the review period, the COP collects feedback from members, scholars, authors, practitioners, and other stakeholders. The revision process ensures that the *Framework* maintains its integrity while responding to internal and external influences that should be reflected in emerging concepts and advances in occupational therapy.

The *Framework* was first revised and approved by the RA in 2008. Changes to the document included refinement of the writing and the addition of emerging concepts and changes in occupational therapy. The rationale for specific changes can be found in Table 11 of the second edition of the *Framework* (AOTA, 2008, pp. 665–667).

In 2012, the process of review and revision of the *Framework* was initiated again. Following member review and feedback, several modifications were made to improve flow, usability, and parallelism of concepts within the document. The following major revisions were made and approved by the RA in the Fall 2013 meeting:

- The overarching statement describing occupational therapy's domain is now stated as "achieving health, well-being, and participation in life through engagement in occupation" to encompass both domain and process.
- *Clients* are now defined as persons, groups, and populations.
- The relationship of occupational therapy to organizations has been further defined.
- *Activity demands* has been removed from the domain and placed in the overview of the process to augment the discussion of the occupational therapy practitioner's basic skill of activity analysis.
- *Areas of occupation* are now called *occupations.*
- *Performance skills* have been redefined, and Table 3 has been revised accordingly.
- The following changes have been made to the interventions table (Table 6):
  ○ *Consultation* has been removed and has been infused throughout the document as a method of service delivery.
  ○ Additional intervention methods used in practice have been added, and a clearer distinction is made among the interventions of *occupations, activities,* and *preparatory methods and tasks.*
  ○ *Self-advocacy* and *group interventions* have been added.
  ○ *Therapeutic use of self* has been moved to the process overview to ensure the understanding that use of the self as a therapeutic agent is integral to the practice of occupational therapy and is used in all interactions with all clients.
- Several additional, yet minor, changes have been made, including the creation of a preface, reorganization for flow of content, and modifications to several definitions. These changes reflect feedback received from AOTA members, educators, and other stakeholders.

Vision for This Work

Although this revision of the *Framework* represents the latest in the profession's efforts to clearly articulate the occupational therapy domain and process, it builds on a set of values that the profession has held since its founding in 1917. This founding vision had at its center a profound belief in the value of therapeutic occupations as a way to remediate illness and maintain health (Slagle, 1924). The founders emphasized the importance of establishing a therapeutic relationship with each client and designing a treatment plan based on knowledge about the client's environment, values, goals, and desires (Meyer, 1922). They advocated for scientific practice based on systematic observation and treatment (Dunton, 1934). Paraphrased using today's lexicon, the founders proposed a vision that was occupation based, client centered, contextual, and evidence based—the vision articulated in the *Framework*.

INTRODUCTION

The purpose of a *framework* is to provide a structure or base on which to build a system or a concept (*American Heritage Dictionary of the English Language*, 2003). The *Occupational Therapy Practice Framework: Domain and Process* describes the central concepts that ground occupational therapy practice and builds a common understanding of the basic tenets and vision of the profession. The *Framework* does not serve as a taxonomy, theory, or model of occupational therapy.

By design, the *Framework* must be used to guide occupational therapy practice in conjunction with the knowledge and evidence relevant to occupation and occupational therapy within the identified areas of practice and with the appropriate clients. Embedded in this document is the profession's core belief in the positive relationship between occupation and health and its view of people as occupational beings. Occupational therapy practice emphasizes the occupational nature of humans and the importance of occupational identity (Unruh, 2004) to healthful, productive, and satisfying living. As Hooper and Wood (2014) stated,

> A core philosophical assumption of the profession, therefore, is that by virtue of our biological endowment, people of all ages and abilities require occupation to grow and thrive; in pursuing occupation, humans express the totality of their being, a mind–body–spirit union. Because human existence could not otherwise be, humankind is, in essence, occupational by nature. (p. 38)

The clients of occupational therapy are typically classified as *persons* (including those involved in care of a client), *groups* (collectives of individuals, e.g., families, workers, students, communities), and *populations* (collectives of groups of individuals living in a similar locale—e.g., city, state, or country—or sharing the same or like characteristics or concerns). Services are provided directly to clients using a collaborative approach or indirectly on behalf of clients through advocacy or consultation processes.

Organization- or systems-level practice is a valid and important part of occupational therapy for several reasons. First, organizations serve as a mechanism through which occupational therapy practitioners provide interventions to support participation of those who are members of or served by the organization (e.g., falls prevention programming in a skilled nursing facility, ergonomic changes to an assembly line to reduce cumulative trauma disorders). Second, organizations support occupational therapy practice and occupational therapy practitioners as stakeholders in carrying out the mission of the organization. It is the fiduciary responsibility of practitioners to ensure that services provided to organizational stakeholders (e.g., third-party payers, employers) are of high quality and delivered in an efficient and efficacious manner. Finally, organizations employ occupational therapy practitioners in roles in which they use their knowledge of occupation and the profession of occupational therapy indirectly. For example, practitioners can serve in positions such as dean, administrator, and corporate leader; in these positions, practitioners support and enhance the organization but do not provide client care in the traditional sense.

The *Framework* is divided into two major sections: (1) the *domain,* which outlines the profession's purview and the areas in which its members have an established body of knowledge and expertise, and (2) the *process,* which describes the actions practitioners take when providing services that are client centered and focused on engagement in occupations. The profession's understanding of the domain and process of occupational therapy guides practitioners as they seek to support clients' participation in daily living that results from the dynamic intersection of clients, their desired engagements, and the context and environment (Christiansen

& Baum, 1997; Christiansen, Baum, & Bass-Haugen, 2005; Law, Baum, & Dunn, 2005).

Although the domain and process are described separately, in actuality they are linked inextricably in a transactional relationship. The aspects that constitute the domain and those that constitute the process exist in constant interaction with one another during the delivery of occupational therapy services. In other words, it is through simultaneous attention to the client's body functions and structures, skills, roles, habits, routines, and context—combined with a focus on the client as an occupational being and the practitioner's knowledge of the health- and performance-enhancing effects of occupational engagements—that outcomes such as occupational performance, role competence, and participation in daily life are produced.

Achieving health, well-being, and participation in life through engagement in occupation is the overarching statement that describes the domain and process of occupational therapy in its fullest sense. This statement acknowledges the profession's belief that active engagement in occupation promotes, facilitates, supports, and maintains health and participation. These interrelated concepts include

- *Health*—"a state of complete physical, mental, and social well-being, and not merely the absence of disease or infirmity" (World Health Organization [WHO], 2006, p. 1).
- *Well-being*—"a general term encompassing the total universe of human life domains, including physical, mental, and social aspects" (WHO, 2006, p. 211).
- *Participation*—"involvement in a life situation" (WHO, 2001, p. 10). Participation naturally occurs when clients are actively involved in carrying out occupations or daily life activities they find purposeful and meaningful. More specific outcomes of

occupational therapy intervention are multidimensional and support the end result of participation.

- *Engagement in occupation*—performance of occupations as the result of choice, motivation, and meaning within a supportive context and environment. Engagement includes objective and subjective aspects of clients' experiences and involves the transactional interaction of the mind, body, and spirit. Occupational therapy intervention focuses on creating or facilitating opportunities to engage in occupations that lead to participation in desired life situations (AOTA, 2008).

Domain

Exhibit 1 identifies the aspects of the domain, and Figure 1 illustrates the dynamic interrelatedness among them. All aspects of the domain, including occupations, client factors, performance skills, performance patterns, and context and environment, are of equal value, and together they interact to affect the client's occupational identity, health, well-being, and participation in life.

Occupational therapists are skilled in evaluating all aspects of the domain, their interrelationships, and the client within his or her contexts and environments. In addition, occupational therapy practitioners recognize the importance and impact of the mind–body–spirit connection as the client participates in daily life. Knowledge of the transactional relationship and the significance of meaningful and productive occupations form the basis for the use of occupations as both the means and the ends of interventions (Trombly, 1995). This knowledge sets occupational therapy apart as a distinct and valuable service (Hildenbrand & Lamb, 2013) for which a focus on the whole is considered stronger than a focus on isolated aspects of human function.

OCCUPATIONS	CLIENT FACTORS	PERFORMANCE SKILLS	PERFORMANCE PATTERNS	CONTEXTS AND ENVIRONMENTS
Activities of daily living (ADLs)*	Values, beliefs, and spirituality	Motor skills	Habits	Cultural
Instrumental activities of daily living (IADLs)	Body functions	Process skills	Routines	Personal
Rest and sleep	Body structures	Social interaction skills	Rituals	Physical
Education			Roles	Social
Work				Temporal
Play				Virtual
Leisure				
Social participation				

*Also referred to as *basic activities of daily living (BADLs)* or *personal activities of daily living (PADLs)*.

Exhibit 1. Aspects of the domain of occupational therapy. All aspects of the domain transact to support engagement, participation, and health. This exhibit does not imply a hierarchy.

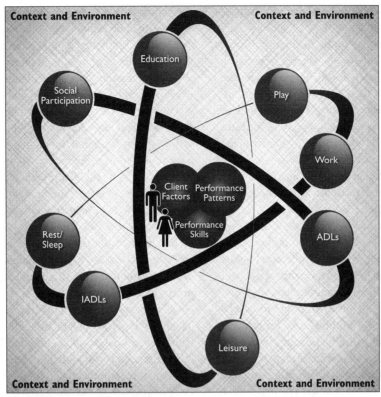

Figure 1. Occupational therapy's domain.
Note. ADLs = activities of daily living; IADLs = instrumental activities of daily living.

The discussion that follows provides a brief explanation of each aspect of the domain. Tables included at the end of the document provide full descriptions and definitions of terms.

Occupations

Occupations are central to a client's (person's, group's, or population's) identity and sense of competence and have particular meaning and value to that client. Several definitions of *occupation* are described in the literature and can add to an understanding of this core concept:

- "Goal-directed pursuits that typically extend over time, have meaning to the performance, and involve multiple tasks" (Christiansen et al., 2005, p. 548).
- "The things that people do that occupy their time and attention; meaningful, purposeful activity; the personal activities that individuals choose or need to engage in and the ways in which each individual actually experiences them" (Boyt Schell, Gillen, & Scaffa, 2014a, p. 1237).
- "When a person engages in purposeful activities out of personal choice and they are valued, these clusters of purposeful activities form occupations

(Hinojosa, Kramer, Royeen, & Luebben, 2003). Thus, occupations are unique to each individual and provide personal satisfaction and fulfillment as a result of engaging in them (AOTA, 2002b; Pierce, 2001)" (Hinojosa & Blount, 2009, pp. 1–2).

- "In occupational therapy, occupations refer to the everyday activities that people do as individuals, in families and with communities to occupy time and bring meaning and purpose to life. Occupations include things people need to, want to and are expected to do" (World Federation of Occupational Therapists, 2012).
- "Activities . . . of everyday life, named, organized, and given value and meaning by individuals and a culture. Occupation is everything people do to occupy themselves, including looking after themselves . . . enjoying life . . . and contributing to the social and economic fabric of their communities" (Law, Polatajko, Baptiste, & Townsend, 1997, p. 32).
- "A dynamic relationship among an occupational form, a person with a unique developmental structure, subjective meanings and purpose, and the

resulting occupational performance" (Nelson & Jepson-Thomas, 2003, p. 90).

- "Occupation is used to mean all the things people want, need, or have to do, whether of physical, mental, social, sexual, political, or spiritual nature and is inclusive of sleep and rest. It refers to all aspects of actual human doing, being, becoming, and belonging. The practical, everyday medium of self-expression or of making or experiencing meaning, occupation is the activist element of human existence whether occupations are contemplative, reflective, and meditative or action based" (Wilcock & Townsend, 2014, p. 542).

The term *occupation,* as it is used in the *Framework,* refers to the daily life activities in which people engage. Occupations occur in context and are influenced by the interplay among client factors, performance skills, and performance patterns. Occupations occur over time; have purpose, meaning, and perceived utility to the client; and can be observed by others (e.g., preparing a meal) or be known only to the person involved (e.g., learning through reading a textbook). Occupations can involve the execution of multiple activities for completion and can result in various outcomes. The *Framework* identifies a broad range of occupations categorized as activities of daily living (ADLs), instrumental activities of daily living (IADLs), rest and sleep, education, work, play, leisure, and social participation (Table 1).

When occupational therapy practitioners work with clients, they identify the many types of occupations clients engage in while alone or with others. Differences among persons and the occupations they engage in are complex and multidimensional. The client's perspective on how an occupation is categorized varies depending on that client's needs and interests as well as the context. For example, one person may perceive doing laundry as work, whereas another may consider it an IADL. One group may engage in a quiz game and view their participation as play, but another group may engage in the same quiz game and view it as education.

The ways in which clients prioritize engagement in selected occupations may vary at different times. For example, clients in a community psychiatric rehabilitation setting may prioritize registering to vote during an election season and food preparation during holidays. The unique features of occupations are noted and analyzed by occupational therapy practitioners, who consider all components of the engagement and use them effectively as both a therapeutic tool and a way to achieve the targeted outcomes of intervention.

The extent to which a person is involved in a particular occupational engagement is also important. Occupations

can contribute to a well-balanced and fully functional lifestyle or to a lifestyle that is out of balance and characterized by occupational dysfunction. For example, excessive work without sufficient regard for other aspects of life, such as sleep or relationships, places clients at risk for health problems (Hakansson, Dahlin-Ivanoff, & Sonn, 2006).

Sometimes occupational therapy practitioners use the terms *occupation* and *activity* interchangeably to describe participation in daily life pursuits. Some scholars have proposed that the two terms are different (Christiansen & Townsend, 2010; Pierce, 2001; Reed, 2005). In the *Framework,* the term *occupation* denotes life engagements that are constructed of multiple activities. Both occupations and activities are used as interventions by practitioners. Participation in occupations is considered the end result of interventions, and practitioners use occupations during the intervention process as the means to the end.

Occupations often are shared and done with others. Those that implicitly involve two or more individuals may be termed *co-occupations* (Zemke & Clark, 1996). Caregiving is a co-occupation that involves active participation on the part of both the caregiver and the recipient of care. For example, the co-occupations required during parenting, such as the socially interactive routines of eating, feeding, and comforting, may involve the parent, a partner, the child, and significant others (Olson, 2004); the activities inherent in this social interaction are reciprocal, interactive, and nested co-occupations (Dunlea, 1996; Esdaile & Olson, 2004). Consideration of co-occupations supports an integrated view of the client's engagement in context in relationship to significant others.

Occupational participation occurs individually or with others. It is important to acknowledge that clients can be independent in living regardless of the amount of assistance they receive while completing activities. Clients may be considered independent when they perform or direct the actions necessary to participate, regardless of the amount or kind of assistance required, if they are satisfied with their performance. In contrast with definitions of independence that imply a level of physical interaction with the environment or objects within the environment, occupational therapy practitioners consider clients to be independent whether they perform the component activities by themselves, perform the occupation in an adapted or modified environment, use various devices or alternative strategies, or oversee activity completion by others (AOTA, 2002a). For example, people with a spinal cord injury who direct a personal care assistant to assist them with their ADLs are demonstrating independence in this essential aspect of their lives.

Occupational therapy practitioners recognize that health is supported and maintained when clients are able to engage in home, school, workplace, and community life. Thus, practitioners are concerned not only with occupations but also with the variety of factors that empower and make possible clients' engagement and participation in positive health-promoting occupations (Wilcock & Townsend, 2014).

Client Factors

Client factors are specific capacities, characteristics, or beliefs that reside within the person and that influence performance in occupations (Table 2). Client factors are affected by the presence or absence of illness, disease, deprivation, disability, and life experiences. Although client factors are not to be confused with performance skills, client factors can affect performance skills. Thus, client factors may need to be present in whole or in part for a person to complete an action (skill) used in the execution of an occupation. In addition, client factors are affected by performance skills, performance patterns, contexts and environments, and performance and participation in activities and occupations. It is through this cyclical relationship that preparatory methods, activities, and occupations can be used to affect client factors and vice versa.

Values, beliefs, and spirituality influence a person's motivation to engage in occupations and give his or her life meaning. *Values* are principles, standards, or qualities considered worthwhile by the client who holds them. *Beliefs* are cognitive content held as true (Moyers & Dale, 2007). *Spirituality* is "the aspect of humanity that refers to the way individuals seek and express meaning and purpose and the way they experience their connectedness to the moment, to self, to others, to nature, and to the significant or sacred" (Puchalski et al., 2009, p. 887).

Body functions and *body structures* refer to the "physiological function of body systems (including psychological functions) and anatomical parts of the body such as organs, limbs, and their components," respectively (WHO, 2001, p. 10). Examples of body functions include sensory, musculoskeletal, mental (affective, cognitive, perceptual), cardiovascular, respiratory, and endocrine functions. Examples of body structures include the heart and blood vessels that support cardiovascular function (for additional examples, see Table 2). Body structures and body functions are interrelated, and occupational therapy practitioners must consider them when seeking to promote clients' ability to engage in desired occupations.

Moreover, occupational therapy practitioners understand that, despite their importance, the presence, absence, or limitation of specific body functions and body structures does not necessarily ensure a client's success or difficulty with daily life occupations. Occupational performance and various types of client factors may benefit from supports in the physical or social environment that enhance or allow participation. It is through the process of observing clients engaging in occupations and activities that occupational therapy practitioners are able to determine the transaction between client factors and performance and to then create adaptations and modifications and select activities that best promote enhanced participation.

Client factors can also be understood as pertaining to individuals at the group and population level. Although client factors may be described differently when applied to a group or population, the underlying tenets do not change substantively.

Performance Skills

Various approaches have been used to describe and categorize performance skills. The occupational therapy literature from research and practice offers multiple perspectives on the complexity and types of skills used during performance.

Performance skills are goal-directed actions that are observable as small units of engagement in daily life occupations. They are learned and developed over time and are situated in specific contexts and environments (Fisher & Griswold, 2014). Fisher and Griswold (2014) categorized performance skills as motor skills, process skills, and social interaction skills (Table 3). Various body structures, as well as personal and environmental contexts, converge and emerge as occupational performance skills. In addition, body functions, such as mental, sensory, neuromuscular, and movement-related functions, are identified as the capacities that reside within the person and also converge with structures and environmental contexts to emerge as performance skills. This description is consistent with WHO's (2001) *International Classification of Functioning, Disability and Health.*

Performance skills are the client's demonstrated abilities. For example, praxis capacities, such as imitating, sequencing, and constructing, affect a client's motor performance skills. Cognitive capacities, such as perception, affect a client's process performance skills and ability to organize actions in a timely and safe manner. Emotional regulation capacities can affect a client's ability to effectively respond to the demands of occupation with a range of emotions. It is important to remember that many body functions underlie each performance skill.

Performance skills are also closely linked and are used in combination with one another as a client engages in an occupation. A change in one performance skill can affect other performance skills. Occupational therapy practitioners observe and analyze performance skills to understand the transactions among client factors, context and environment, and activity or occupational demands, which support or hinder performance skills and occupational performance (Chisholm & Boyt Schell, 2014; Hagedorn, 2000).

In practice and in some literature, underlying body functions are labeled as *performance skills* and are seen in various combinations such as perceptual–motor skills and social–emotional skills. Although practitioners may focus on underlying capacities such as cognition, body structures, and emotional regulation, the *Framework* defines performance skills as those that are observable and that are key aspects of successful occupational participation. Table 3 provides definitions of the various skills in each category.

Resources informing occupational therapy practice related to performance skills include Fisher (2006); Polatajko, Mandich, and Martini (2000); and Fisher and Griswold (2014). Detailed information about the ways performance skills are used in occupational therapy practice may be found in the literature on specific theories and models such as the Model of Human Occupation (Kielhofner, 2008), the Cognitive Orientation to Daily Occupational Performance (Polatajko & Mandich, 2004), the Occupational Therapy Intervention Process Model (Fisher, 2009), sensory integration theory (Ayres, 1972, 2005), and motor learning and motor control theory (Shumway-Cook & Woollacott, 2007).

Performance Patterns

Performance patterns are the habits, routines, roles, and rituals used in the process of engaging in occupations or activities that can support or hinder occupational performance. *Habits* refers to specific, automatic behaviors; they may be useful, dominating, or impoverished (Boyt Schell, Gillen, & Scaffa, 2014b; Clark, 2000; Dunn, 2000). *Routines* are established sequences of occupations or activities that provide a structure for daily life; routines also can promote or damage health (Fiese, 2007; Koome, Hocking, & Sutton, 2012; Segal, 2004).

Roles are sets of behaviors expected by society and shaped by culture and context; they may be further conceptualized and defined by a client (person, group, or population). Roles can provide guidance in selecting occupations or can be used to identify activities connected with certain occupations in which a client engages.

When considering roles, occupational therapy practitioners are concerned with how clients construct their occupations to fulfill their perceived roles and identity and whether their roles reinforce their values and beliefs. Some roles lead to stereotyping and restricted engagement patterns. Jackson (1998a, 1998b) cautioned that describing people by their roles can be limiting and can promote segmented rather than enfolded occupations.

Rituals are symbolic actions with spiritual, cultural, or social meaning. Rituals contribute to a client's identity and reinforce the client's values and beliefs (Fiese, 2007; Segal, 2004).

Performance patterns develop over time and are influenced by all other aspects of the occupational therapy domain. Practitioners who consider clients' performance patterns are better able to understand the frequency and manner in which performance skills and occupations are integrated into clients' lives. Although clients may have the ability to engage in skilled performance, if they do not embed essential skills in a productive set of engagement patterns, their health, well-being, and participation may be negatively affected. For example, a client who has the skills and resources to engage in appropriate grooming, bathing, and meal preparation but does not embed them into a consistent routine may struggle with poor nutrition and social isolation. Table 4 provides examples of performance patterns for persons and groups or populations.

Context and Environment

Engagement and participation in occupation take place within the social and physical environment situated within context. In the literature, the terms *environment* and *context* often are used interchangeably. In the *Framework,* both terms are used to reflect the importance of considering the wide array of interrelated variables that influence performance. Understanding the environments and contexts in which occupations can and do occur provides practitioners with insights into their overarching, underlying, and embedded influences on engagement.

The *physical environment* refers to the natural (e.g., geographic terrain, plants) and built (e.g., buildings, furniture) surroundings in which daily life occupations occur. Physical environments can either support or present barriers to participation in meaningful occupations. Examples of barriers include doorway widths that do not allow for wheelchair passage or absence of healthy social opportunities for people abstaining from alcohol use. Conversely, environments can provide supports and resources for service delivery

March/April 2014, Volume 68(Supplement 1)

(e.g., community, health care facility, home). The *social environment* consists of the presence of, relationships with, and expectations of persons, groups, and populations with whom clients have contact (e.g., availability and expectations of significant individuals, such as spouse, friends, and caregivers).

The term *context* refers to elements within and surrounding a client that are often less tangible than physical and social environments but nonetheless exert a strong influence on performance. Contexts, as described in the *Framework,* are cultural, personal, temporal, and virtual.

The *cultural context* includes customs, beliefs, activity patterns, behavioral standards, and expectations accepted by the society of which a client is a member. The cultural context influences the client's identity and activity choices, and practitioners must be aware, for example, of norms related to eating or deference to medical professionals when working with someone from another culture and of socioeconomic status when providing a discharge plan for a young child and family. *Personal context* refers to demographic features of the individual, such as age, gender, socioeconomic status, and educational level, that are not part of a health condition (WHO, 2001). *Temporal context* includes stage of life, time of day or year, duration or rhythm of activity, and history.

Finally, *virtual context* refers to interactions that occur in simulated, real-time, or near-time situations absent of physical contact. The virtual context is becoming increasingly important for clients as well as occupational therapy practitioners and other health care providers. Clients may require access to and the ability to use technology such as cell or smartphones, computers or tablets, and videogame consoles to carry out their daily routines and occupations.

Contexts and environments affect a client's access to occupations and influence the quality of and satisfaction with performance. A client who has difficulty performing effectively in one environment or context may be successful when the environment or context is changed. The context within which the engagement in occupations occurs is specific for each client. Some contexts are external to clients (e.g., virtual), some are internal to clients (e.g., personal), and some have both external features and internalized beliefs and values (e.g., cultural).

Occupational therapy practitioners recognize that for clients to truly achieve an existence of full participation, meaning, and purpose, clients must not only function but also engage comfortably with their world, which consists of a unique combination of contexts and environments (Table 5).

Interwoven throughout all contexts and environments is the concept of *occupational justice,* defined as "a justice that recognizes occupational rights to inclusive participation in everyday occupations for all persons in society, regardless of age, ability, gender, social class, or other differences" (Nilsson & Townsend, 2010, p. 58). Occupational justice describes the concern that occupational therapy practitioners have with the ethical, moral, and civic aspects of clients' environments and contexts. As part of the occupational therapy domain, practitioners consider how these aspects can affect the implementation of occupational therapy and the target outcome of participation.

Several environments and contexts can present occupational justice issues. For example, an alternative school placement for children with psychiatric disabilities could provide academic support and counseling but limit opportunity for participation in sports, music programs, and organized social activities. A residential facility could offer safety and medical support but provide little opportunity for engagement in the role-related activities that were once a source of meaning for residents. Poor communities that lack accessibility and resources make participation especially difficult and dangerous for people with disabilities. Occupational therapy practitioners may recognize areas of occupational injustice and work to support policies, actions, and laws that allow people to engage in occupations that provide purpose and meaning in their lives.

By understanding and addressing the specific justice issues within a client's discharge environment, occupational therapy practitioners promote therapy outcomes that address empowerment and self-advocacy. Occupational therapy's focus on engagement in occupations and occupational justice complements WHO's (2001) perspective on health. In an effort to broaden the understanding of the effects of disease and disability on health, WHO recognized that health can be affected by the inability to carry out activities and participate in life situations caused both by environmental barriers and by problems that exist in body structures and body functions. The *Framework* identifies occupational justice as both an aspect of contexts and environments and an outcome of intervention.

Process

This section operationalizes the process undertaken by occupational therapy practitioners when providing services to clients. Exhibit 2 identifies the aspects of the process, and Figure 2 illustrates the dynamic interrelatedness among them. The *occupational therapy process* is

Evaluation
Occupational profile—The initial step in the evaluation process, which provides an understanding of the client's occupational history and experiences, patterns of daily living, interests, values, and needs. The client's reasons for seeking services, strengths and concerns in relation to performing occupations and daily life activities, areas of potential occupational disruption, supports and barriers, and priorities are also identified.
Analysis of occupational performance—The step in the evaluation process during which the client's assets and problems or potential problems are more specifically identified. Actual performance is often observed in context to identify supports for and barriers to the client's performance. Performance skills, performance patterns, context or environment, client factors, and activity demands are all considered, but only selected aspects may be specifically assessed. Targeted outcomes are identified.

Intervention
Intervention plan—The plan that will guide actions taken and that is developed in collaboration with the client. It is based on selected theories, frames of reference, and evidence. Outcomes to be targeted are confirmed.
Intervention implementation—Ongoing actions taken to influence and support improved client performance and participation. Interventions are directed at identified outcomes. The client's response is monitored and documented.
Intervention review—Review of the intervention plan and progress toward targeted outcomes.

Targeting of Outcomes
Outcomes—Determinants of success in reaching the desired end result of the occupational therapy process. Outcome assessment information is used to plan future actions with the client and to evaluate the service program (i.e., program evaluation).

Exhibit 2. Process of occupational therapy service delivery.
The process of service delivery is applied within the profession's domain to support the client's health and participation.

the client-centered delivery of occupational therapy services. The process includes evaluation and intervention to achieve targeted outcomes, occurs within the purview of the occupational therapy domain, and is facilitated by the distinct perspective of occupational therapy practitioners when engaging in clinical reasoning, analyzing activities and occupations, and collaborating with clients. This section is organized into four broad areas: (1) an overview of the process as it is applied within the profession's domain, (2) the evaluation process, (3) the intervention process, and (4) the process of targeting outcomes.

Overview of the Occupational Therapy Process

Many professions use a similar process of evaluating, intervening, and targeting intervention outcomes. However,

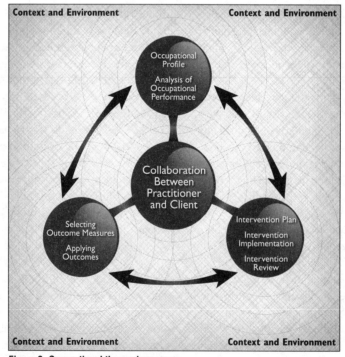

Figure 2. Occupational therapy's process.

only occupational therapy practitioners focus on the use of occupations to promote health, well-being, and participation in life. Occupational therapy practitioners use therapeutically selected occupations and activities as primary methods of intervention throughout the process (Table 6).

To help clients achieve desired outcomes, occupational therapy practitioners facilitate interactions among the client, his or her environments and contexts, and the occupations in which he or she engages. This perspective is based on the theories, knowledge, and skills generated and used by the profession and informed by available evidence (Clark et al., 2012; Davidson, Shahar, Lawless, Sells, & Tondora, 2006; Glass, de Leon, Marottoli, & Berkman, 1999; Jackson, Carlson, Mandel, Zemke, & Clark, 1998; Sandqvist, Akesson, & Eklund, 2005).

Analyzing occupational performance requires an understanding of the complex and dynamic interaction among client factors, performance skills, performance patterns, and contexts and environments, along with the activity demands of the occupation being performed. Occupational therapy practitioners attend to each aspect and gauge the influence of each on the others, individually and collectively. By understanding how these aspects influence each other, practitioners can better evaluate how each aspect contributes to clients' performance-related concerns and potentially contributes to interventions that support occupational performance.

For ease of explanation, the *Framework* describes the occupational therapy process as being linear. In reality, the process does not occur in a sequenced, step-by-step fashion. Rather, it is fluid and dynamic, allowing occupational therapy practitioners and clients to maintain their focus on the identified outcomes while continually reflecting on and changing the overall plan to accommodate new developments and insights along the way.

The broader definition of *client* included in this document is indicative of the profession's increasing involvement in providing services not only to a person but also to groups and populations. When working with a group or population, occupational therapy practitioners consider the collective occupational performance abilities of the members. Whether the client is a person, group, or population, information about the client's wants, needs, strengths, limitations, and occupational risks is gathered, synthesized, and framed from an occupational perspective.

Service Delivery Models

Occupational therapy practitioners provide services to clients directly, in settings such as hospitals, clinics, industry, schools, homes, and communities, and indi-

rectly on behalf of clients through consultation. Direct services include interventions completed when in direct contact with the individual or group of clients. These interventions are completed through various mechanisms such as meeting in person with a client, leading a group session, or interacting with clients and families through telehealth systems (AOTA, 2013c).

When providing services to clients indirectly on their behalf, practitioners provide consultation to entities such as teachers, multidisciplinary teams, and community planning agencies. Occupational therapy practitioners also provide consultation to community organizations such as park districts and civic organizations that may or may not include people with disabilities. In addition, practitioners consult with businesses regarding the work environment, ergonomic modifications, and compliance with the Americans With Disabilities Act of 1990 (Pub. L. 101–336).

Occupational therapy practitioners can indirectly affect the lives of clients through advocacy. Common examples of advocacy include talking to legislators about improving transportation for older adults or improving services for people with mental or physical disabilities to support their living and working in the community of their choice.

Regardless of the service delivery model, the individual client may not be the exclusive focus of the intervention. For example, the needs of an at-risk infant may be the initial impetus for intervention, but the concerns and priorities of the parents, extended family, and funding agencies are also considered. Occupational therapy practitioners understand and focus intervention to include the issues and concerns surrounding the complex dynamics among the client, caregiver, and family. Similarly, services addressing independent living skills for adults coping with serious and persistent mental illness may also address the needs and expectations of state and local services agencies and of potential employers.

Clinical Reasoning

Throughout the process, occupational therapy practitioners are continually engaged in clinical reasoning about a client's occupational performance. Clinical reasoning enables practitioners to

- Identify the multiple demands, required skills, and potential meanings of the activities and occupations and
- Gain a deeper understanding of the interrelationships between aspects of the domain that affect performance and that support client-centered interventions and outcomes.

Occupational therapy practitioners use theoretical principles and models, knowledge about the effects of conditions on participation, and available evidence of the effectiveness of intervention to guide their reasoning. Clinical reasoning ensures the accurate selection and application of evaluations, interventions, and client-centered outcome measures. Practitioners also apply their knowledge and skills to enhance clients' participation in occupations and promote their health and well-being regardless of the effects of disease, disability, and occupational disruption or deprivation.

Therapeutic Use of Self

An integral part of the occupational therapy process is *therapeutic use of self,* which allows occupational therapy practitioners to develop and manage their therapeutic relationship with clients by using narrative and clinical reasoning; empathy; and a client-centered, collaborative approach to service delivery (Taylor & Van Puymbroeck, 2013). *Empathy* is the emotional exchange between occupational therapy practitioners and clients that allows more open communication, ensuring that practitioners connect with clients at an emotional level to assist them with their current life situation.

Occupational therapy practitioners use narrative and clinical reasoning to help clients make sense of the information they are receiving in the intervention process, to discover meaning, and to build hope (Peloquin, 2003; Taylor & Van Puymbroeck, 2013). Clients have identified the therapeutic relationship as critical to the outcome of occupational therapy intervention (Cole & McLean, 2003).

Occupational therapy practitioners develop a collaborative relationship with clients to understand their experiences and desires for intervention. The collaborative approach used throughout the process honors the contributions of clients along with practitioners. Through the use of interpersonal communication skills, occupational therapy practitioners shift the power of the relationship to allow clients more control in decision making and problem solving, which is essential to effective intervention.

Clients bring to the occupational therapy process their knowledge about their life experiences and their hopes and dreams for the future. They identify and share their needs and priorities. Occupational therapy practitioners bring their knowledge about how engagement in occupation affects health, well-being, and participation; they use this information, coupled with theoretical perspectives and clinical reasoning, to critically observe, analyze, describe, and interpret human performance. Practitioners and clients, together with caregivers, family members, community members, and other

stakeholders (as appropriate), identify and prioritize the focus of the intervention plan.

Activity Analysis

Activity analysis is an important process occupational therapy practitioners use to understand the demands a specific activity places on a client:

> *Activity analysis* addresses the typical demands of an activity, the range of skills involved in its performance, and the various cultural meanings that might be ascribed to it. . . . Occupation-based activity analysis places the person in the foreground. It takes into account the particular person's interests, goals, abilities, and contexts, as well as the demands of the activity itself. These considerations shape the practitioner's efforts to help the . . . person reach his/her goals through carefully designed evaluation and intervention. (Crepeau, 2003, pp. 192–193)

Occupational therapy practitioners analyze the demands of an activity or occupation to understand the specific body structures, body functions, performance skills, and performance patterns that are required and to determine the generic demands the activity or occupation makes on the client.

Activity and occupational demands are the specific features of an activity and occupation that influence its meaning for the client and the type and amount of effort required to engage in it. Activity and occupational demands include the following (see Table 7 for definitions and examples):

- *The tools and resources needed to engage in the activity*—What specific objects are used in the activity? What are their properties, and what transportation, money, or other resources are needed to participate in the activity?
- *Where and with whom the activity takes place*—What are the physical space requirements of the activity, and what are the social interaction demands?
- *How the activity is accomplished*—What process is used in carrying out the activity, including the sequence and timing of the steps and necessary procedures and rules?
- *How the activity challenges the client's capacities*—What actions, performance skills, body functions, and body structures are the individual, group, or population required to use during the performance of the activity?
- *The meaning the client derives from the activity*—What potential symbolic, unconscious, and metaphorical meanings does the individual attach to the activity (e.g., driving a car equates with independence, preparing a holiday meal connects with family tradition, voting is a rite of passage to adulthood)?

Activity and occupational demands are specific to each activity. A change in one feature of an activity may change the extent of the demand in another feature. For example, an increase in the number or sequence of steps in an activity increases the demand on attention skills.

Evaluation Process

The evaluation process is focused on finding out what a client wants and needs to do; determining what a client can do and has done; and identifying supports and barriers to health, well-being, and participation. Evaluation occurs during the initial and all subsequent interactions with a client. The type and focus of the evaluation differ depending on the practice setting.

The evaluation consists of the occupational profile and an analysis of occupational performance. The occupational profile includes information about the client's needs, problems, and concerns about performance in occupations. The analysis of occupational performance focuses on collecting and interpreting information to more specifically identify supports and barriers related to occupational performance and identify targeted outcomes.

Although the *Framework* describes the components of the evaluation process separately and sequentially, the exact manner in which occupational therapists collect client information is influenced by client needs, practice settings, and therapists' frames of reference or practice models. Information related to the occupational profile is gathered throughout the occupational therapy process.

Occupational Profile

The *occupational profile* is a summary of a client's occupational history and experiences, patterns of daily living, interests, values, and needs. Developing the occupational profile provides the occupational therapy practitioner with an understanding of a client's perspective and background.

Using a client-centered approach, the practitioner gathers information to understand what is currently important and meaningful to the client (i.e., what he or she wants and needs to do) and to identify past experiences and interests that may assist in the understanding of current issues and problems. During the process of collecting this information, the client, with the assistance of the occupational therapy practitioner, identifies priorities and desired targeted outcomes that will lead to the client's engagement in occupations that support participation in life. Only clients can identify the occupations that give meaning to their lives and select the goals and priorities that are important to them. By valuing and respecting clients' input, practitioners help foster their involvement and can more efficiently guide interventions.

Occupational therapy practitioners collect information for the occupational profile at the beginning of contact with clients to establish client-centered outcomes. Over time, practitioners collect additional information, refine the profile, and ensure that the additional information is reflected in changes subsequently made to targeted outcomes. The process of completing and refining the occupational profile varies by setting and client. The information gathered in the profile may be completed in one session or over a longer period while working with a client. For clients who are unable to participate in this process, their profiles may be compiled through interaction with family members or other significant people in their lives.

Obtaining information for the occupational profile through both formal interview techniques and casual conversation is a way to establish a therapeutic relationship with clients and their support network. The information obtained through the occupational profile leads to an individualized approach in the evaluation, intervention planning, and intervention implementation stages. Information is collected in the following areas:

- Why is the client seeking service, and what are the client's current concerns relative to engaging in occupations and in daily life activities?
- In what occupations does the client feel successful, and what barriers are affecting his or her success?
- What aspects of his or her environments or contexts does the client see as supporting engagement in desired occupations, and what aspects are inhibiting engagement?
- What is the client's occupational history (i.e., life experiences)?
- What are the client's values and interests?
- What are the client's daily life roles?
- What are the client's patterns of engagement in occupations, and how have they changed over time?
- What are the client's priorities and desired targeted outcomes related to occupational performance, prevention, participation, role competence, health and wellness, quality of life, well-being, and occupational justice?

After collecting profile data, occupational therapists view the information and develop a working hypothesis regarding possible reasons for the identified problems and concerns. Reasons could include impairments in client factors, performance skills, and performance patterns or barriers within the context and environment. Therapists then work with clients to establish preliminary goals and outcome measures. In addition, therapists note strengths and supports within all areas because these can inform the intervention plan and affect future outcomes.

Analysis of Occupational Performance

Occupational performance is the accomplishment of the selected occupation resulting from the dynamic transaction among the client, the context and environment, and the activity or occupation. In the *analysis of occupational performance,* the client's assets and problems or potential problems are more specifically identified through assessment tools designed to observe, measure, and inquire about factors that support or hinder occupational performance. Targeted outcomes also are identified. The analysis of occupational performance involves one or more of the following activities:

- Synthesizing information from the occupational profile to focus on specific occupations and contexts that need to be addressed
- Observing a client's performance during activities relevant to desired occupations, noting effectiveness of performance skills and performance patterns
- Selecting and using specific assessments to measure performance skills and performance patterns, as appropriate
- Selecting and administering assessments, as needed, to identify and measure more specifically the contexts or environments, activity demands, and client factors that influence performance skills and performance patterns
- Selecting outcome measures
- Interpreting the assessment data to identify supports and hindrances to performance
- Developing and refining hypotheses about the client's occupational performance strengths and limitations
- Creating goals in collaboration with the client that address the desired outcomes
- Determining procedures to measure the outcomes of intervention
- Delineating a potential intervention approach or approaches based on best practices and available evidence.

Multiple methods often are used during the evaluation process to assess client, environment or context, occupation or activity, and occupational performance. Methods may include an interview with the client and significant others, observation of performance and context, record review, and direct assessment of specific aspects of performance. Formal and informal, structured and unstructured, and standardized criterion- or norm-referenced assessment tools can be used. Standardized assessments are preferred, when available, to provide objective data about various aspects of the domain influencing engagement and performance. The use of valid and reliable assessments for obtaining trustworthy information can also help support and justify the need for occupational therapy services (Doucet & Gutman, 2013; Gutman, Mortera, Hinojosa, & Kramer, 2007).

Implicit in any outcome assessment used by occupational therapy practitioners are clients' belief systems and underlying assumptions regarding their desired occupational performance. Occupational therapists select outcome assessments pertinent to clients' needs and goals, congruent with the practitioner's theoretical model of practice and based on knowledge of the psychometric properties of standardized measures or the rationale and protocols of nonstandardized yet structured measures and the available evidence. In addition, clients' perception of success in engaging in desired occupations is vital to any outcomes assessment (Bandura, 1986).

Intervention Process

The intervention process consists of the skilled services provided by occupational therapy practitioners in collaboration with clients to facilitate engagement in occupation related to health, well-being, and participation. Practitioners use the information about clients gathered during the evaluation and theoretical principles to direct occupation-centered interventions. Intervention is then provided to assist clients in reaching a state of physical, mental, and social well-being; identifying and realizing aspirations; satisfying needs; and changing or coping with the environment. Types of occupational therapy interventions are discussed in Table 6.

Intervention is intended to promote health, well-being, and participation. *Health promotion* is "the process of enabling people to increase control over, and to improve, their health" (WHO, 1986). Wilcock (2006) stated,

> Following an occupation-focused health promotion approach to well-being embraces a belief that the potential range of what people can do, be, and strive to become is the primary concern, and that health is a by-product. A varied and full occupational lifestyle will coincidentally maintain and improve health and well-being if it enables people to be creative and adventurous physically, mentally, and socially. (p. 315)

Interventions vary depending on the client—person, group, or population—and the context of service delivery (Moyers & Dale, 2007). The actual term used for clients or groups of clients receiving occupational therapy varies among practice settings and delivery models. For example, when working in a hospital, the person or group might be referred to as a *patient* or *patients,* and in a school, the clients might be *students.* When providing consultation to an organization, clients may be called *consumers* or *members.* The term *person* includes others who may help or be served indirectly, such as caregiver, teacher, parent, employer, or spouse.

Interventions provided to groups and populations are directed to all the members collectively rather than individualized to specific people within the group. Practitioners direct their interventions toward current or potential disabling conditions with the goal of enhancing the health, well-being, and participation of all group members collectively. The intervention focus often is on health promotion activities, self-management, educational services, and environmental modification. For instance, occupational therapy practitioners may provide education on falls prevention and the impact of fear of falling to a group of residents in an assisted living center or provide support to people with psychiatric disability as they learn to use the Internet to identify and coordinate community resources that meet their needs. Practitioners may work with a wide variety of populations experiencing difficulty in accessing and engaging in healthy occupations because of conditions such as poverty, homelessness, and discrimination.

The intervention process is divided into three steps: (1) intervention plan, (2) intervention implementation, and (3) intervention review. During the intervention process, information from the evaluation is integrated with theory, practice models, frames of reference, and evidence. This information guides occupational therapy practitioners' clinical reasoning in the development, implementation, and review of the intervention plan.

Intervention Plan

The *intervention plan,* which directs the actions of occupational therapy practitioners, describes selected occupational therapy approaches and types of interventions to be used in reaching clients' identified outcomes. The intervention plan is developed collaboratively with clients or their proxies and is directed by

- Client goals, values, beliefs, and occupational needs;
- Client health and well-being;
- Client performance skills and performance patterns;
- Collective influence of the context and environment, activity demands, and client factors on the client;

- Context of service delivery in which the intervention is provided; and
- Best available evidence.

The selection and design of the intervention plan and goals are directed toward addressing clients' current and potential situation related to engagement in occupations or activities. Intervention planning includes the following steps:

1. Developing the plan, which involves selecting
   - Objective and measurable occupation-focused goals and related time frames;
   - The occupational therapy intervention approach or approaches, such as create or promote, establish or restore, maintain, modify, and prevent (Table 8); and
   - Methods for service delivery, including who will provide the intervention, types of interventions, and service delivery models to be used.
2. Considering potential discharge needs and plans.
3. Making recommendations or referrals to other professionals as needed.

Intervention Implementation

Intervention implementation is the process of putting the intervention plan into action. Interventions may focus on a single aspect of the domain, such as a specific occupation, or on several aspects of the domain, such as context and environment, performance patterns, and performance skills.

Given that aspects of the domain are interrelated and influence one another in a continuous, dynamic process, occupational therapy practitioners expect that a client's ability to adapt, change, and develop in one area will affect other areas. Because of this dynamic interrelationship, evaluation and intervention planning continue throughout the implementation process.

Intervention implementation includes the following steps:

1. Determining and carrying out the occupational therapy intervention or interventions to be used (see Table 6), which may include the following:
   - Therapeutic use of occupations and activities
   - Preparatory methods (e.g., splinting, assistive technology, wheeled mobility) and preparatory tasks
   - Education and training
   - Advocacy (e.g., advocacy, self-advocacy)
   - Group interventions.
2. Monitoring a client's response to specific interventions on the basis of ongoing evaluation and reevaluation of his or her progress toward goals.

Intervention Review

Intervention review is the continuous process of reevaluating and reviewing the intervention plan, the effectiveness of its delivery, and progress toward outcomes. As during intervention planning, this process includes collaboration with the client on the basis of identified goals and progress toward the associated outcomes. Reevaluation and review may lead to change in the intervention plan.

The intervention review includes the following steps:

1. Reevaluating the plan and how it is implemented relative to achieving outcomes
2. Modifying the plan as needed
3. Determining the need for continuation or discontinuation of occupational therapy services and for referral to other services.

Targeting of Outcomes

Outcomes are the end result of the occupational therapy process; they describe what clients can achieve through occupational therapy intervention. The benefits of occupational therapy are multifaceted and may occur in all aspects of the domain of concern. Outcomes are directly related to the interventions provided and to the occupations, client factors, performance skills, performance patterns, and contexts and environments targeted. Outcomes may also be traced to the improved transactional relationship among the areas of the domain that result in clients' ability to engage in desired occupations secondary to improved abilities at the client factor and performance skill level (Table 9).

In addition, outcomes may relate to clients' subjective impressions regarding goal attainment, such as improved outlook, confidence, hope, playfulness, self-efficacy, sustainability of valued occupations, resilience, and perceived well-being. An example of a subjective outcome of intervention is parents' greater perceived efficacy about their parenting through a new understanding of their child's behavior after receiving occupational therapy services (Cohn, 2001; Cohn, Miller, & Tickle-Degnen, 2000; Graham, Rodger, & Ziviani, 2013).

Interventions can also be designed for caregivers of people with dementia to improve quality of life for both care recipient and caregiver. Caregivers who received intervention reported fewer declines in occupational performance, enhanced mastery and skill, improved sense of self-efficacy and well-being, and less need for help with care recipients (Gitlin & Corcoran, 2005; Gitlin, Corcoran, Winter, Boyce, & Hauck, 2001; Gitlin et al., 2003, 2008; Graff et al., 2007).

Outcomes for groups may include improved social interaction, increased self-awareness through peer support, a larger social network, or increased workplace productivity with fewer injuries. Outcomes for populations may include health promotion, occupational justice and self-advocacy, and access to services. The impact of outcomes and the way they are defined are specific to clients and to other stakeholders such as payers and regulators. Specific outcomes and documentation of those outcomes vary by practice setting and are influenced by the stakeholders in each setting.

The focus on outcomes is woven throughout the process of occupational therapy. Occupational therapists and clients collaborate during evaluation to identify initial client outcomes related to engagement in valued occupations or daily life activities. During intervention implementation and reevaluation, clients, occupational therapists, and, when appropriate, occupational therapy assistants may modify outcomes to accommodate changing needs, contexts, and performance abilities. As further analysis of occupational performance and the development of the intervention plan occur, therapists and clients may redefine the desired outcomes.

Implementation of the outcomes process includes the following steps:

1. Selecting types of outcomes and measures, including but not limited to occupational performance, prevention, health and wellness, quality of life, participation, role competence, well-being, and occupational justice (see Table 9). Outcome measures are
   - Selected early in the intervention process (see "Evaluation Process" section);
   - Valid, reliable, and appropriately sensitive to change in clients' occupational performance;
   - Consistent with targeted outcomes;
   - Congruent with clients' goals; and
   - Selected on the basis of their actual or purported ability to predict future outcomes.
2. Using outcomes to measure progress and adjust goals and interventions by
   - Comparing progress toward goal achievement to outcomes throughout the intervention process and
   - Assessing outcome use and results to make decisions about the future direction of intervention (e.g., continue intervention, modify intervention, discontinue intervention, provide follow-up, refer for other services).

Outcomes and the other aspects of the occupational therapy process are summarized in Exhibit 3.

Evaluation		Intervention			Targeting of Outcomes
Occupational Profile ⟷	**Analysis of Occupational Performance**	**Intervention Plan**	**Intervention Implementation**	**Intervention Review**	**Outcomes**

Identify the following:
• Why is the client seeking service, and what are the client's current concerns relative to engaging in activities and occupations?
• In what occupations does the client feel successful, and what barriers are affecting his or her success?
• What aspects of the contexts or environments does the client see as supporting and as inhibiting engagement in desired occupations?
• What is the client's occupational history?
• What are the client's values and interests?
• What are the client's daily life roles?
• What are the client's patterns of engagement in occupations, and how have they changed over time?
• What are the client's priorities and desired targeted outcomes related to occupational performance, prevention, participation, role competence, health and wellness, quality of life, well-being, and occupational justice?
	• Synthesize information from the occupational profile to focus on specific occupations and contexts.
	• Observe the client's performance during activities relevant to desired occupations.
	• Select and use specific assessments to identify and measure contexts or environments, activity and occupational demands, client factors, and performance skills and patterns.
	• Select outcome measures.
	• Interpret assessment data to identify supports for and hindrances to performance.
	• Develop and refine hypotheses about the client's occupational performance strengths and limitations.
	• Create goals in collaboration with the client that address desired outcomes.
	• Determine procedures to measure the outcomes of intervention.
	• Delineate a potential intervention based on best practices and available evidence.
		1. Develop the plan, which involves selecting
		  • Objective and measurable occupation-focused goals and related time frames;
		  • Occupational therapy intervention approach or approaches, such as create or promote, establish or restore, maintain, modify, or prevent; and
		  • Methods for service delivery, including who will provide the intervention, types of intervention, and service delivery models.
		2. Consider potential discharge needs and plans.
		3. Recommend or refer to other professionals as needed.
			1. Determine and carry out occupational therapy intervention or interventions, which may include the following:
			  • Therapeutic use of occupations and activities
			  • Preparatory methods and tasks
			  • Education and training
			  • Advocacy
			  • Group interventions
			2. Monitor the client's response through ongoing evaluation and reevaluation.
				1. Reevaluate the plan and implementation relative to achieving outcomes.
				2. Modify the plan as needed.
				3. Determine the need for continuation or discontinuation of occupational therapy services and for referral.
					1. Early in the intervention process, select outcomes and measures that are
					  • Valid, reliable, sensitive to change, and consistent with outcomes
					  • Congruent with client goals
					  • Based on their actual or purported ability to predict future outcomes
					2. Apply outcomes to measure progress and adjust goals and interventions.
					  • Compare progress toward goal achievement to outcomes throughout the intervention process.
					  • Assess outcome use and results to make decisions about the future direction of intervention.

←——————— Continue to renegotiate intervention plans and targeted outcomes. ———————→

←——— Ongoing interaction among evaluation, intervention, and outcomes occurs throughout the process. ———→

Exhibit 3. Operationalizing the occupational therapy process.

Conclusion

The *Framework* describes the central concepts that ground occupational therapy practice and builds a common understanding of the basic tenets and distinct contribution of the profession. The occupational therapy domain and process are linked inextricably in a transactional relationship, as illustrated in Figure 3. An understanding of this relationship supports and guides the complex decision making required in the daily practice of occupational therapy and enhances practitioners' ability to define the reasons for and direct interventions to clients (persons, groups, and populations), family members, team members, payers, and policymakers. The *Framework* highlights the distinct value of occupation and occupational therapy in contributing to client health, well-being, and participation in life.

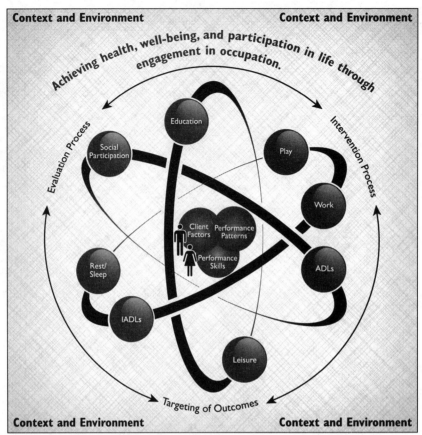

Figure 3. Occupational therapy domain and process.

TABLE 1. OCCUPATIONS

Occupations are various kinds of life activities in which individuals, groups, or populations engage, including activities of daily living, instrumental activities of daily living, rest and sleep, education, work, play, leisure, and social participation.

Category	Description
■ **ACTIVITIES OF DAILY LIVING (ADLs)**—Activities oriented toward taking care of one's own body (adapted from Rogers & Holm, 1994). ADLs also are referred to as *basic activities of daily living (BADLs)* and *personal activities of daily living (PADLs)*. These activities are "fundamental to living in a social world; they enable basic survival and well-being" (Christiansen & Hammecker, 2001, p. 156).	
Bathing, showering	Obtaining and using supplies; soaping, rinsing, and drying body parts; maintaining bathing position; and transferring to and from bathing positions
Toileting and toilet hygiene	Obtaining and using toileting supplies, managing clothing, maintaining toileting position, transferring to and from toileting position, cleaning body, and caring for menstrual and continence needs (including catheter, colostomy, and suppository management), as well as completing intentional control of bowel movements and urination and, if necessary, using equipment or agents for bladder control (Uniform Data System for Medical Rehabilitation, 1996, pp. III-20, III-24)
Dressing	Selecting clothing and accessories appropriate to time of day, weather, and occasion; obtaining clothing from storage area; dressing and undressing in a sequential fashion; fastening and adjusting clothing and shoes; and applying and removing personal devices, prosthetic devices, or splints
Swallowing/eating	Keeping and manipulating food or fluid in the mouth and swallowing it; *swallowing* is moving food from the mouth to the stomach
Feeding	Setting up, arranging, and bringing food [or fluid] from the plate or cup to the mouth; sometimes called *self-feeding*
Functional mobility	Moving from one position or place to another (during performance of everyday activities), such as in-bed mobility, wheelchair mobility, and transfers (e.g., wheelchair, bed, car, shower, tub, toilet, chair, floor). Includes functional ambulation and transportation of objects.
Personal device care	Using, cleaning, and maintaining personal care items, such as hearing aids, contact lenses, glasses, orthotics, prosthetics, adaptive equipment, glucometers, and contraceptive and sexual devices
Personal hygiene and grooming	Obtaining and using supplies; removing body hair (e.g., using razor, tweezers, lotion); applying and removing cosmetics; washing, drying, combing, styling, brushing, and trimming hair; caring for nails (hands and feet); caring for skin, ears, eyes, and nose; applying deodorant; cleaning mouth; brushing and flossing teeth; and removing, cleaning, and reinserting dental orthotics and prosthetics
Sexual activity	Engaging in activities that result in sexual satisfaction and/or meet relational or reproductive needs
■ **INSTRUMENTAL ACTIVITIES OF DAILY LIVING (IADLs)**—Activities to support daily life within the home and community that often require more complex interactions than those used in ADLs.	
Care of others (including selecting and supervising caregivers)	Arranging, supervising, or providing care for others
Care of pets	Arranging, supervising, or providing care for pets and service animals
Child rearing	Providing care and supervision to support the developmental needs of a child
Communication management	Sending, receiving, and interpreting information using a variety of systems and equipment, including writing tools, telephones (cell phones or smartphones), keyboards, audiovisual recorders, computers or tablets, communication boards, call lights, emergency systems, Braille writers, telecommunication devices for deaf people, augmentative communication systems, and personal digital assistants
Driving and community mobility	Planning and moving around in the community and using public or private transportation, such as driving, walking, bicycling, or accessing and riding in buses, taxi cabs, or other transportation systems
Financial management	Using fiscal resources, including alternate methods of financial transaction, and planning and using finances with long-term and short-term goals
Health management and maintenance	Developing, managing, and maintaining routines for health and wellness promotion, such as physical fitness, nutrition, decreased health risk behaviors, and medication routines
Home establishment and management	Obtaining and maintaining personal and household possessions and environment (e.g., home, yard, garden, appliances, vehicles), including maintaining and repairing personal possessions (e.g., clothing, household items) and knowing how to seek help or whom to contact

(Continued)

TABLE 1. OCCUPATIONS

(Continued)

Category	Description
Meal preparation and cleanup	Planning, preparing, and serving well-balanced, nutritious meals and cleaning up food and utensils after meals
Religious and spiritual activities and expression	Participating in *religion,* "an organized system of beliefs, practices, rituals, and symbols designed to facilitate closeness to the sacred or transcendent" (Moreira-Almeida & Koenig, 2006, p. 844), and engaging in activities that allow a sense of connectedness to something larger than oneself or that are especially meaningful, such as taking time out to play with a child, engaging in activities in nature, and helping others in need (Spencer, Davidson, & White, 1997)
Safety and emergency maintenance	Knowing and performing preventive procedures to maintain a safe environment; recognizing sudden, unexpected hazardous situations; and initiating emergency action to reduce the threat to health and safety; examples include ensuring safety when entering and exiting the home, identifying emergency contact numbers, and replacing items such as batteries in smoke alarms and light bulbs
Shopping	Preparing shopping lists (grocery and other); selecting, purchasing, and transporting items; selecting method of payment; and completing money transactions; included are Internet shopping and related use of electronic devices such as computers, cell phones, and tablets
▓ **REST AND SLEEP**—Activities related to obtaining restorative rest and sleep to support healthy, active engagement in other occupations.	
Rest	Engaging in quiet and effortless actions that interrupt physical and mental activity, resulting in a relaxed state (Nurit & Michal, 2003, p. 227); included are identifying the need to relax; reducing involvement in taxing physical, mental, or social activities; and engaging in relaxation or other endeavors that restore energy and calm and renew interest in engagement
Sleep preparation	(1) Engaging in routines that prepare the self for a comfortable rest, such as grooming and undressing, reading or listening to music to fall asleep, saying goodnight to others, and engaging in meditation or prayers; determining the time of day and length of time desired for sleeping and the time needed to wake; and establishing sleep patterns that support growth and health (patterns are often personally and culturally determined). (2) Preparing the physical environment for periods of unconsciousness, such as making the bed or space on which to sleep; ensuring warmth or coolness and protection; setting an alarm clock; securing the home, such as locking doors or closing windows or curtains; and turning off electronics or lights.
Sleep participation	Taking care of personal needs for sleep, such as ceasing activities to ensure onset of sleep, napping, and dreaming; sustaining a sleep state without disruption; and performing nighttime care of toileting needs and hydration; also includes negotiating the needs and requirements of and interacting with others within the social environment such as children or partners, including providing nighttime caregiving such as breastfeeding and monitoring the comfort and safety of others who are sleeping
▓ **EDUCATION**—Activities needed for learning and participating in the educational environment.	
Formal educational participation	Participating in academic (e.g., math, reading, degree coursework), nonacademic (e.g., recess, lunchroom, hallway), extracurricular (e.g., sports, band, cheerleading, dances), and vocational (prevocational and vocational) educational activities
Informal personal educational needs or interests exploration (beyond formal education)	Identifying topics and methods for obtaining topic-related information or skills
Informal personal education participation	Participating in informal classes, programs, and activities that provide instruction or training in identified areas of interest
▓ **WORK**—"Labor or exertion; to make, construct, manufacture, form, fashion, or shape objects; to organize, plan, or evaluate services or processes of living or governing; committed occupations that are performed with or without financial reward" (Christiansen & Townsend, 2010, p. 423).	
Employment interests and pursuits	Identifying and selecting work opportunities based on assets, limitations, likes, and dislikes relative to work (adapted from Mosey, 1996, p. 342)
Employment seeking and acquisition	Advocating for oneself; completing, submitting, and reviewing appropriate application materials; preparing for interviews; participating in interviews and following up afterward; discussing job benefits; and finalizing negotiations
Job performance	Performing the requirements of a job, including work skills and patterns; time management; relationships with coworkers, managers, and customers; leadership and supervision; creation, production, and distribution of products and services; initiation, sustainment, and completion of work; and compliance with work norms and procedures
Retirement preparation and adjustment	Determining aptitudes, developing interests and skills, selecting appropriate avocational pursuits, and adjusting lifestyle in the absence of the worker role

(Continued)

TABLE 1. OCCUPATIONS

(Continued)

Category	Description
Volunteer exploration	Determining community causes, organizations, or opportunities for unpaid work in relationship to personal skills, interests, location, and time available
Volunteer participation	Performing unpaid work activities for the benefit of selected causes, organizations, or facilities
▨ **PLAY**—"Any spontaneous or organized activity that provides enjoyment, entertainment, amusement, or diversion" (Parham & Fazio, 1997, p. 252).	
Play exploration	Identifying appropriate play activities, including exploration play, practice play, pretend play, games with rules, constructive play, and symbolic play (adapted from Bergen, 1988, pp. 64–65)
Play participation	Participating in play; maintaining a balance of play with other occupations; and obtaining, using, and maintaining toys, equipment, and supplies appropriately
▨ **LEISURE**—"Nonobligatory activity that is intrinsically motivated and engaged in during discretionary time, that is, time not committed to obligatory occupations such as work, self-care, or sleep" (Parham & Fazio, 1997, p. 250).	
Leisure exploration	Identifying interests, skills, opportunities, and appropriate leisure activities
Leisure participation	Planning and participating in appropriate leisure activities; maintaining a balance of leisure activities with other occupations; and obtaining, using, and maintaining equipment and supplies as appropriate
▨ **SOCIAL PARTICIPATION**—"The interweaving of occupations to support desired engagement in community and family activities as well as those involving peers and friends" (Gillen & Boyt Schell, 2014, p. 607); involvement in a subset of activities that involve social situations with others (Bedell, 2012) and that support social interdependence (Magasi & Hammel, 2004). Social participation can occur in person or through remote technologies such as telephone calls, computer interaction, and video conferencing.	
Community	Engaging in activities that result in successful interaction at the community level (e.g., neighborhood, organization, workplace, school, religious or spiritual group)
Family	Engaging in activities that result in "successful interaction in specific required and/or desired familial roles" (Mosey, 1996, p. 340)
Peer, friend	Engaging in activities at different levels of interaction and intimacy, including engaging in desired sexual activity

TABLE 2. CLIENT FACTORS

Client factors *include (1) values, beliefs, and spirituality; (2) body functions; and (3) body structures that reside within the client that influence the client's performance in occupations.*

▧ **VALUES, BELIEFS, AND SPIRITUALITY**—Clients' perceptions, motivations, and related meaning that influence or are influenced by engagement in occupations.

Category and Definition	Examples
Values—Acquired beliefs and commitments, derived from culture, about what is good, right, and important to do (Kielhofner, 2008)	*Person:* • Honesty with self and others • Commitment to family *Group:* • Obligation to provide a service • Fairness *Population:* • Freedom of speech • Equal opportunities for all • Tolerance toward others
Beliefs—Cognitive content held as true by or about the client	*Person:* • One is powerless to influence others. • Hard work pays off. *Group and population:* • Some personal rights are worth fighting for. • A new health care policy, as yet untried, will positively affect society.
Spirituality—"The aspect of humanity that refers to the way individuals seek and express meaning and purpose and the way they experience their connectedness to the moment, to self, to others, to nature, and to the significant or sacred" (Puchalski et al., 2009, p. 887)	*Person:* • Daily search for purpose and meaning in one's life • Guidance of actions by a sense of value beyond the personal acquisition of wealth or fame *Group and population:* • Common search for purpose and meaning in life • Guidance of actions by values agreed on by the collective

▧ **BODY FUNCTIONS**—"The physiological functions of body systems (including psychological functions)" (WHO, 2001, p. 10). This section of the table is organized according to the classifications of the *International Classification of Functioning, Disability and Health (ICF);* for fuller descriptions and definitions, refer to WHO (2001).

Category	Description (not an all-inclusive list)
Mental functions (affective, cognitive, perceptual)	
Specific mental functions	
Higher-level cognitive	Judgment, concept formation, metacognition, executive functions, praxis, cognitive flexibility, insight
Attention	Sustained shifting and divided attention, concentration, distractibility
Memory	Short-term, long-term, and working memory
Perception	Discrimination of sensations (e.g., auditory, tactile, visual, olfactory, gustatory, vestibular, proprioceptive)
Thought	Control and content of thought, awareness of reality vs. delusions, logical and coherent thought
Mental functions of sequencing complex movement	Mental functions that regulate the speed, response, quality, and time of motor production, such as restlessness, toe tapping, or hand wringing, in response to inner tension
Emotional	Regulation and range of emotions; appropriateness of emotions, including anger, love, tension, and anxiety; lability of emotions
Experience of self and time	Awareness of one's identity, body, and position in the reality of one's environment and of time
Global mental functions	
Consciousness	State of awareness and alertness, including the clarity and continuity of the wakeful state
Orientation	Orientation to person, place, time, self, and others
Temperament and personality	Extroversion, introversion, agreeableness, conscientiousness, emotional stability, openness to experience, self-control, self-expression, confidence, motivation, impulse control, appetite

(Continued)

TABLE 2. CLIENT FACTORS
(Continued)

Category	Description (not an all-inclusive list)
Energy and drive	Energy level, motivation, appetite, craving, impulse control
Sleep	Physiological process, quality of sleep
Sensory functions	
Visual functions	Quality of vision, visual acuity, visual stability, and visual field functions to promote visual awareness of environment at various distances for functioning
Hearing functions	Sound detection and discrimination; awareness of location and distance of sounds
Vestibular functions	Sensation related to position, balance, and secure movement against gravity
Taste functions	Association of taste qualities of bitterness, sweetness, sourness, and saltiness
Smell functions	Sensing odors and smells
Proprioceptive functions	Awareness of body position and space
Touch functions	Feeling of being touched by others or touching various textures, such as those of food; presence of numbness, paresthesia, hyperesthesia
Pain (e.g., diffuse, dull, sharp, phantom)	Unpleasant feeling indicating potential or actual damage to some body structure; sensations of generalized or localized pain (e.g., diffuse, dull, sharp, phantom)
Sensitivity to temperature and pressure	Thermal awareness (hot and cold), sense of force applied to skin
Neuromusculoskeletal and movement-related functions	
Functions of joints and bones	
Joint mobility	Joint range of motion
Joint stability	Maintenance of structural integrity of joints throughout the body; physiological stability of joints related to structural integrity
Muscle functions	
Muscle power	Strength
Muscle tone	Degree of muscle tension (e.g., flaccidity, spasticity, fluctuation)
Muscle endurance	Sustaining muscle contraction
Movement functions	
Motor reflexes	Involuntary contraction of muscles automatically induced by specific stimuli (e.g., stretch, asymmetrical tonic neck, symmetrical tonic neck)
Involuntary movement reactions	Postural reactions, body adjustment reactions, supporting reactions
Control of voluntary movement	Eye–hand and eye–foot coordination, bilateral integration, crossing of the midline, fine and gross motor control, and oculomotor function (e.g., saccades, pursuits, accommodation, binocularity)
Gait patterns	Gait and mobility considered in relation to how they affect ability to engage in occupations in daily life activities; for example, walking patterns and impairments, asymmetric gait, stiff gait
Cardiovascular, hematological, immunological, and respiratory system functions (*Note.* Occupational therapy practitioners have knowledge of these body functions and understand broadly the interaction that occurs among these functions to support health, well-being, and participation in life through engagement in occupation.)	
Cardiovascular system functions Hematological and immunological system functions	Maintenance of blood pressure functions (hypertension, hypotension, postural hypotension), heart rate and rhythm
Respiratory system functions	Rate, rhythm, and depth of respiration
Additional functions and sensations of the cardiovascular and respiratory systems	Physical endurance, aerobic capacity, stamina, fatigability
Voice and speech functions; digestive, metabolic, and endocrine system functions; genitourinary and reproductive functions (*Note.* Occupational therapy practitioners have knowledge of these body functions and understand broadly the interaction that occurs among these functions to support health, well-being, and participation in life through engagement in occupation.)	
Voice and speech functions	Fluency and rhythm, alternative vocalization functions

(Continued)

TABLE 2. CLIENT FACTORS

(Continued)

Category	Description (not an all-inclusive list)
Digestive, metabolic, and endocrine system functions	Digestive system functions, metabolic system and endocrine system functions
Genitourinary and reproductive functions	Urinary functions, genital and reproductive functions

Skin and related structure functions
(*Note.* Occupational therapy practitioners have knowledge of these body functions and understand broadly the interaction that occurs among these functions to support health, well-being, and participation in life through engagement in occupation.)

Skin functions Hair and nail functions	Protection (presence or absence of wounds, cuts, or abrasions), repair (wound healing)

■ **BODY STRUCTURES:** "Anatomical parts of the body, such as organs, limbs, and their components" that support body function (WHO, 2001, p. 10). The "Body Structures" section of the table is organized according to the *ICF* classifications; for fuller descriptions and definitions, refer to WHO (2001).

Category	Examples not delineated in the "Body Structure" section of this table
Structure of the nervous system **Eyes, ear, and related structures** **Structures involved in voice and speech** **Structures of the cardiovascular, immunological, and respiratory systems** **Structures related to the digestive, metabolic, and endocrine systems** **Structures related to the genitourinary and reproductive systems** **Structures related to movement** **Skin and related structures**	(*Note.* Occupational therapy practitioners have knowledge of body structures and understand broadly the interaction that occurs between these structures to support health, well-being, and participation in life through engagement in occupation.)

Note. The categorization of body function and body structure client factors outlined in Table 2 is based on the *ICF* proposed by WHO (2001). The classification was selected because it has received wide exposure and presents a language that is understood by external audiences. WHO = World Health Organization.

March/April 2014, Volume 68(Supplement 1)

TABLE 3. PERFORMANCE SKILLS

Performance skills *are observable elements of action that have an implicit functional purpose; skills are considered a classification of actions, encompassing multiple capacities (body functions and body structures) and, when combined, underlie the ability to participate in desired occupations and activities. This list is not all inclusive and may not include all possible skills addressed during occupational therapy interventions.*

Skill	Definition
■ **MOTOR SKILLS**—"Occupational performance skills observed as the person interacts with and moves task objects and self around the task environment" (e.g., activity of daily living [ADL] motor skills, school motor skills; Boyt Schell, Gillen, & Scaffa, 2014a, p. 1237).	
Aligns	Interacts with task objects without evidence of persistent propping or persistent leaning
Stabilizes	Moves through task environment and interacts with task objects without momentary propping or loss of balance
Positions	Positions self an effective distance from task objects and without evidence of awkward body positioning
Reaches	Effectively extends the arm and, when appropriate, bends the trunk to effectively grasp or place task objects that are out of reach
Bends	Flexes or rotates the trunk as appropriate to the task to grasp or place task objects out of reach or when sitting down
Grips	Effectively pinches or grasps task objects such that the objects do not slip (e.g., from the person's fingers, between teeth)
Manipulates	Uses dexterous finger movements, without evidence of fumbling, when manipulating task objects (e.g., manipulating buttons when buttoning)
Coordinates	Uses two or more body parts together to manipulate, hold, and/or stabilize task objects without evidence of fumbling task objects or slipping from one's grasp
Moves	Effectively pushes or pulls task objects along a supporting surface, pulls to open or pushes to close doors and drawers, or pushes on wheels to propel a wheelchair
Lifts	Effectively raises or lifts task objects without evidence of increased effort
Walks	During task performance, ambulates on level surfaces without shuffling the feet, becoming unstable, propping, or using assistive devices
Transports	Carries task objects from one place to another while walking or moving in a wheelchair
Calibrates	Uses movements of appropriate force, speed, or extent when interacting with task objects (e.g., not crushing objects, pushing a door with enough force that it closes)
Flows	Uses smooth and fluid arm and wrist movements when interacting with task objects
Endures	Persists and completes the task without showing obvious evidence of physical fatigue, pausing to rest, or stopping to catch one's breath
Paces	Maintains a consistent and effective rate or tempo of performance throughout the entire task
■ **PROCESS SKILLS**—"Occupational performance skills [e.g., ADL process skills, school process skills] observed as a person (1) selects, interacts with, and uses task tools and materials; (2) carries out individual actions and steps; and (3) modifies performance when problems are encountered" (Boyt Schell et al., 2014a, p. 1239).	
Paces	Maintains a consistent and effective rate or tempo of performance throughout the entire task
Attends	Does not look away from what he or she is doing, interrupting the ongoing task progression
Heeds	Carries out and completes the task originally agreed on or specified by another
Chooses	Selects necessary and appropriate type and number of tools and materials for the task, including the tools and materials that the person was directed to use or specified he or she would use
Uses	Applies tools and materials as they are intended (e.g., uses a pencil sharpener to sharpen a pencil but not to sharpen a crayon) and in a hygienic fashion
Handles	Supports or stabilizes tools and materials in an appropriate manner, protecting them from being damaged, slipping, moving, and falling
Inquires	(1) Seeks needed verbal or written information by asking questions or reading directions or labels and (2) does not ask for information when he or she was fully oriented to the task and environment and had immediate prior awareness of the answer
Initiates	Starts or begins the next action or step without hesitation
Continues	Performs single actions or steps without interruptions such that once an action or task is initiated, the person continues without pauses or delays until the action or step is completed
Sequences	Performs steps in an effective or logical order and with an absence of (1) randomness or lack of logic in the ordering and (2) inappropriate repetition of steps
Terminates	Brings to completion single actions or single steps without inappropriate persistence or premature cessation
Searches/locates	Looks for and locates tools and materials in a logical manner, both within and beyond the immediate environment
Gathers	Collects related tools and materials into the same work space and regathers tools or materials that have spilled, fallen, or been misplaced

(Continued)

TABLE 3. PERFORMANCE SKILLS

(Continued)

Skill	Definition
Organizes	Logically positions or spatially arranges tools and materials in an orderly fashion within a single work space and between multiple appropriate work spaces such that the work space is not too spread out or too crowded
Restores	Puts away tools and materials in appropriate places and ensures that the immediate work space is restored to its original condition
Navigates	Moves the arm, body, or wheelchair without bumping into obstacles when moving in the task environment or interacting with task objects
Notices/responds	Responds appropriately to (1) nonverbal task-related cues (e.g., heat, movement), (2) the spatial arrangement and alignment of task objects to one another, and (3) cupboard doors and drawers that have been left open during task performance
Adjusts	Effectively (1) goes to new work spaces; (2) moves tools and materials out of the current work space; and (3) adjusts knobs, dials, or water taps to overcome problems with ongoing task performance
Accommodates	Prevents ineffective task performance
Benefits	Prevents problems with task performance from recurring or persisting
■ **SOCIAL INTERACTION SKILLS**—"Occupational performance skills observed during the ongoing stream of a social exchange" (Boyt Schell et al., 2014a, p. 1241).	
Approaches/starts	Approaches or initiates interaction with the social partner in a manner that is socially appropriate
Concludes/disengages	Effectively terminates the conversation or social interaction, brings to closure the topic under discussion, and disengages or says good-bye
Produces speech	Produces spoken, signed, or augmentative (i.e., computer-generated) messages that are audible and clearly articulated
Gesticulates	Uses socially appropriate gestures to communicate or support a message
Speaks fluently	Speaks in a fluent and continuous manner, with an even pace (not too fast, not too slow) and without pauses or delays during the message being sent
Turns toward	Actively positions or turns the body and face toward the social partner or person who is speaking
Looks	Makes eye contact with the social partner
Places self	Positions self at an appropriate distance from the social partner during the social interaction
Touches	Responds to and uses touch or bodily contact with the social partner in a manner that is socially appropriate
Regulates	Does not demonstrate irrelevant, repetitive, or impulsive behaviors that are not part of social interaction
Questions	Requests relevant facts and information and asks questions that support the intended purpose of the social interaction
Replies	Keeps conversation going by replying appropriately to question and comments
Discloses	Reveals opinions, feelings, and private information about self or others in a manner that is socially appropriate
Expresses emotion	Displays affect and emotions in a way that is socially appropriate
Disagrees	Expresses differences of opinion in a socially appropriate manner
Thanks	Uses appropriate words and gestures to acknowledge receipt of services, gifts, or compliments
Transitions	Handles transitions in the conversation smoothly or changes the topic without disrupting the ongoing conversation
Times response	Replies to social messages without delay or hesitation and without interrupting the social partner
Times duration	Speaks for reasonable periods given the complexity of the message sent
Takes turns	Takes his or her turn and gives the social partner the freedom to take his or her turn
Matches language	Uses a tone of voice, dialect, and level of language that are socially appropriate and matched to the social partner's abilities and level of understanding
Clarifies	Responds to gestures or verbal messages signaling that the social partner does not comprehend or understand a message and ensures that the social partner is following the conversation
Acknowledges and encourages	Acknowledges receipt of messages, encourages the social partner to continue interaction, and encourages all social partners to participate in social interaction
Empathizes	Expresses a supportive attitude toward the social partner by agreeing with, empathizing with, or expressing understanding of the social partner's feelings and experiences
Heeds	Uses goal-directed social interactions focused on carrying out and completing the intended purpose of the social interaction
Accommodates	Prevents ineffective or socially inappropriate social interaction
Benefits	Prevents problems with ineffective or socially inappropriate social interaction from recurring or persisting

Source. From "Performance Skills: Implementing Performance Analyses to Evaluate Quality of Occupational Performance," by A. G. Fisher and L. A. Griswold, in *Willard and Spackman's Occupational Therapy* (12th ed., pp. 252–254), by B. A. B. Schell, G. Gillen, M. E. Scaffa, and E. S. Cohn (Eds.), 2014, Philadelphia: Wolters Kluwer/Lippincott Williams & Wilkins; http://lww.com. Copyright © 2014 by Wolters Kluwer/Lippincott Williams & Wilkins. Adapted with permission.

TABLE 4. PERFORMANCE PATTERNS

Performance patterns are the habits, routines, roles, and rituals used in the process of engaging in occupations or activities; these patterns can support or hinder occupational performance.

Category	Description	Examples
■ PERSON		
Habits	"Acquired tendencies to respond and perform in certain consistent ways in familiar environments or situations; specific, automatic behaviors performed repeatedly, relatively automatically, and with little variation" (Boyt Schell, Gillen, & Scaffa, 2014a, p. 1234). Habits can be useful, dominating, or impoverished and can either support or interfere with performance in occupations (Dunn, 2000).	• Automatically puts car keys in the same place • Spontaneously looks both ways before crossing the street • Always turns off the stove burner before removing a cooking pot • Activates the alarm system before leaving the home
Routines	Patterns of behavior that are observable, regular, and repetitive and that provide structure for daily life. They can be satisfying, promoting, or damaging. Routines require momentary time commitment and are embedded in cultural and ecological contexts (Fiese, 2007; Segal, 2004).	• Follows a morning sequence to complete toileting, bathing, hygiene, and dressing • Follows the sequence of steps involved in meal preparation • Follows a daily routine of dropping children off at school, going to work, picking children up from school, doing home-work, and making dinner
Rituals	Symbolic actions with spiritual, cultural, or social meaning contributing to the client's identity and reinforcing values and beliefs. Rituals have a strong affective component and consist of a collection of events (Fiese, 2007; Fiese et al., 2002; Segal, 2004).	• Uses an inherited antique hairbrush to brush hair 100 strokes nightly as her mother had done • Prepares holiday meals with favorite or traditional accoutre-ments using designated dishware • Kisses a sacred book before opening the pages to read • Attends a spiritual gathering on a particular day
Roles	Sets of behaviors expected by society and shaped by culture and context that may be further conceptualized and defined by the client.	• Mother of an adolescent with developmental disabilities • Student with a learning disability studying computer technology • Corporate executive returning to work after a stroke
■ GROUP OR POPULATION		
Routines	Patterns of behavior that are observable, regular, and repetitive and that provide structure for daily life. They can be satisfying, promoting, or damaging. Routines require momentary time commitment and are embedded in cultural and ecological contexts (Segal, 2004).	• Follows health practices, such as scheduled immunizations for children and yearly health screenings for adults • Follows business practices, such as provision of services for disadvantaged populations (e.g., loans to underrepresented groups) • Follows legislative procedures, such as those associated with the Individuals With Disabilities Education Improvement Act of 2004 (Pub. L. 108–446) or Medicare • Follows social customs for greeting
Rituals	Shared social actions with traditional, emotional, purposive, and technological meaning contributing to values and beliefs within the group or population.	• Holds cultural celebrations • Has parades or demonstrations • Shows national affiliations or allegiances • Follows religious, spiritual, and cultural practices, such as touching the mezuzah or using holy water when leaving and entering or praying while facing Mecca
Roles	Sets of behaviors by the group or population expected by society and shaped by culture and context that may be further con-ceptualized and defined by the group or population.	• Nonprofit civic group providing housing for people with mental illness • Humanitarian group distributing food and clothing donations to refugees • Student organization in a university educating elementary school children about preventing bullying

TABLE 5. CONTEXT AND ENVIRONMENT

Context *refers to a variety of interrelated conditions that are within and surrounding the client. Contexts include cultural, personal, temporal, and virtual. The term* environment *refers to the external physical and social conditions that surround the client and in which the client's daily life occupations occur.*

Category	Definition	Examples
■ CONTEXTS		
Cultural	Customs, beliefs, activity patterns, behavioral standards, and expectations accepted by the society of which a client is a member. The cultural context influences the client's identity and activity choices.	• *Person:* A person delivering Thanksgiving meals to home-bound individuals • *Group:* Employees marking the end of the work week with casual dress on Friday • *Population:* People engaging in an afternoon siesta or high tea
Personal	"Features of the individual that are not part of a health condition or health status" (WHO, 2001, p. 17). The personal context includes age, gender, socioeconomic status, and educational status and can also include group membership (e.g., volunteers, employees) and population membership (e.g., members of society).	• *Person:* A 25-year-old unemployed man with a high school diploma • *Group:* Volunteers working in a homeless shelter • *Population:* Older drivers learning about community mobility options
Temporal	The experience of time as shaped by engagement in occupations; the temporal aspects of occupation that "contribute to the patterns of daily occupations" include "rhythm . . . tempo . . . synchronization . . . duration . . . and sequence" (Larson & Zemke, 2003, p. 82; Zemke, 2004, p. 610). The temporal context includes stage of life, time of day or year, duration and rhythm of activity, and history.	• *Person:* A person retired from work for 10 years • *Group:* A community organization's annual fundraising campaign • *Population:* People celebrating Independence Day on July 4
Virtual	Environment in which communication occurs by means of airwaves or computers and in the absence of physical contact. The virtual context includes simulated, real-time, or near-time environments such as chat rooms, email, video conferencing, or radio transmissions; remote monitoring via wireless sensors; or computer-based data collection.	• *Person:* Friends who text message each other • *Group:* Members who participate in a video conference, telephone conference call, instant message, or interactive white board use • *Population:* Virtual community of gamers
■ ENVIRONMENTS		
Physical	Natural and built nonhuman surroundings and the objects in them. The natural environment includes geographic terrain, plants, and animals, as well as the sensory qualities of the surroundings. The built environment includes buildings, furniture, tools, and devices.	• *Person:* Individual's house or apartment • *Group:* Office building or factory • *Population:* Transportation system
Social	Presence of, relationships with, and expectations of persons, groups, or populations with whom clients have contact. The social environment includes availability and expectations of significant individuals, such as spouse, friends, and caregivers; relationships with individuals, groups, or populations; and relationships with systems (e.g., political, legal, economic, institutional) that influence norms, role expectations, and social routines.	• *Person:* Friends, colleagues • *Group:* Occupational therapy students conducting a class get-together • *Population:* People influenced by a city government

Note. WHO = World Health Organization.

March/April 2014, Volume 68(Supplement 1)

TABLE 6. TYPES OF OCCUPATIONAL THERAPY INTERVENTIONS

Occupational therapy interventions *include the use of occupations and activities, preparatory methods and tasks, education and training, advocacy, and group interventions to facilitate engagement in occupations to promote health and participation. The examples provided illustrate the types of interventions occupational therapy practitioners provide and are not intended to be all inclusive.*

Category	Description	Examples
▪ **OCCUPATIONS AND ACTIVITIES**—Occupations and activities selected as interventions for specific clients and designed to meet therapeutic goals and address the underlying needs of the mind, body, and spirit of the client. To use occupations and activities therapeutically, the practitioner considers activity demands and client factors in relation to the client's therapeutic goals, contexts, and environments.		
Occupations	Client-directed daily life activities that match and support or address identified participation goals.	The client • Completes morning dressing and hygiene using adaptive devices • Purchases groceries and prepares a meal • Visits a friend using public transportation independently • Applies for a job in the retail industry • Plays on a playground with children and adults • Participates in a community festival by setting up a booth to sell baked goods • Engages in a pattern of self-care and relaxation activities in preparation for sleep • Engages in a statewide advocacy program to improve services to people with mental illness
Activities	Actions designed and selected to support the development of performance skills and performance patterns to enhance occupational engagement. Activities often are components of occupations and always hold meaning, relevance, and perceived utility for clients at their level of interest and motivation.	The client • Selects clothing and manipulates clothing fasteners in advance of dressing • Practices safe ways to get into and out of the bathtub • Prepares a food list and practices using cooking appliances • Reviews how to use a map and transportation schedule • Writes answers on an application form • Climbs on and off playground and recreation equipment • Greets people and initiates conversation in a role-play situation • Develops a weekly schedule to manage time and organize daily and weekly responsibilities required to live independently • Uses adaptive switches to operate the home environmental control system • Completes a desired expressive activity (e.g., art, craft, dance) that is not otherwise classified • Plays a desired game either as a solo player or in competition with others
▪ **PREPARATORY METHODS AND TASKS**—Methods and tasks that prepare the client for occupational performance, used as *part of a treatment session* in preparation for or concurrently with occupations and activities or provided to a client as a home-based engagement to support daily occupational performance.		
Preparatory methods	Modalities, devices, and techniques to prepare the client for occupational performance. Often preparatory methods are interventions that are "done to" the client without the client's active participation.	The practitioner • Administers physical agent modalities to decrease pain, assist with wound healing or edema control, or prepare muscles for movement • Provides massage • Performs manual lymphatic drainage techniques • Performs wound care techniques, including dressing changes
Splints	Construction and use of devices to mobilize, immobilize, and support body structures to enhance participation in occupations.	The practitioner • Fabricates and issues a splint or orthotic to support a weakened hand and decrease pain • Fabricates and issues a wrist splint to facilitate movement and enhance participation in household activities
Assistive technology and environmental modifications	Identification and use of assistive technologies (high and low tech), application of universal design principles, and recommends changes to the environment or activity to support the client's ability to engage in occupations. This preparatory method includes assessment, selection, provision, and education and training in use of devices.	The practitioner • Provides a pencil grip and slant board • Provides electronic books with text-to-speech software • Recommends visual supports (e.g., a social story) to guide behavior • Recommends replacing steps with an appropriately graded ramp • Recommends universally designed curriculum materials
Wheeled mobility	Use of products and technologies that facilitate a client's ability to maneuver through space, including seating and positioning, and that improve mobility, enhance participation in desired daily occupations, and reduce risk for complications such as skin breakdown or limb contractures.	The practitioner • Recommends, in conjunction with the wheelchair team, a sip-and-puff switch to allow the client to maneuver the power wheelchair independently and interface with an environmental control unit in the home

(Continued)

849

TABLE 6. TYPES OF OCCUPATIONAL THERAPY INTERVENTIONS

(Continued)

Category	Description	Examples
Preparatory tasks	Actions selected and provided to the client to target specific client factors or performance skills. Tasks involve active participation of the client and sometimes comprise engagements that use various materials to simulate activities or components of occupations. Preparatory tasks themselves may not hold inherent meaning, relevance, or perceived utility as stand-alone entities.	The client • Refolds towels taken from a clean linen cart to address shoulder range of motion • Participates in fabricated sensory environment (e.g., through movement, tactile sensations, scents) to promote alertness • Uses visual imagery and rhythmic breathing to promote rest and relaxation • Performs a home-based conditioning regimen using free weights • Does hand-strengthening exercises using therapy putty, exercise bands, grippers, and clothespins • Participates in an assertiveness training program to prepare for self-advocacy

▨ EDUCATION AND TRAINING

Category	Description	Examples
Education	Imparting of knowledge and information about occupation, health, well-being, and participation that enables the client to acquire helpful behaviors, habits, and routines that may or may not require application at the time of the intervention session	The practitioner • Provides education regarding home and activity modifications to the spouse or family member of a person with dementia to support maximum independence • Educates town officials about the value of and strategies for making walking and biking paths accessible for all community members • Educates providers of care for people who have experienced trauma on the use of sensory strategies • Provides education to people with mental health issues and their families on the psychological and social factors that influence engagement in occupation
Training	Facilitation of the acquisition of concrete skills for meeting specific goals in a real-life, applied situation. In this case, *skills* refers to measurable components of function that enable mastery. Training is differentiated from education by its goal of enhanced performance as opposed to enhanced understanding, although these goals often go hand in hand (Collins & O'Brien, 2003).	The practitioner • Instructs the client in how to operate a universal control device to manage household appliances • Instructs family members in the use and maintenance of the father's power wheelchair • Instructs the client in the use of self range of motion as a preparatory technique to avoid joint contracture of wrist • Instructs the client in the use of a handheld electronic device and applications to recall and manage weekly activities and medications • Instructs the client in how to direct a personal care attendant in assisting with self-care activities • Trains parents and teachers to focus on a child's strengths to foster positive behaviors

▨ ADVOCACY—Efforts directed toward promoting occupational justice and empowering clients to seek and obtain resources to fully participate in daily life occupations. The outcomes of advocacy and self-advocacy support health, well-being, and occupational participation at the individual or systems level.

Category	Description	Examples
Advocacy	Advocacy efforts undertaken by the practitioner.	The practitioner • Collaborates with a person to procure reasonable accommodations at a work site • Serves on the policy board of an organization to procure supportive housing accommodations for people with disabilities • Serves on the board of a local park district to encourage inclusion of children with disabilities in mainstream district sports programs when possible • Collaborates with adults who have serious mental illness to raise public awareness of the impact of stigma • Collaborates with and educates staff at federal funding sources for persons with disabling conditions
Self-advocacy	Advocacy efforts undertaken by the client, which the practitioner can promote and support.	• A student with a learning disability requests and receives reasonable accommodations such as textbooks on tape. • A grassroots employee committee requests and procures ergonomically designed keyboards for their work computers. • People with disabilities advocate for the use of universal design principles with all new public construction. • Young adults contact their Internet service provider to request support for cyberbullying prevention.

(Continued)

March/April 2014, Volume 68(Supplement 1)

TABLE 6. TYPES OF OCCUPATIONAL THERAPY INTERVENTIONS

(Continued)

Category	Description	Examples
■ **GROUP INTERVENTIONS**—Use of distinct knowledge and leadership techniques to facilitate learning and skill acquisition across the life span through the dynamics of group and social interaction. Groups may also be used as a method of service delivery.		
Groups	Functional groups, activity groups, task groups, social groups, and other groups used on inpatient units, within the community, or in schools that allow clients to explore and develop skills for participation, including basic social interaction skills, tools for self-regulation, goal setting, and positive choice making.	• A group for older adults focuses on maintaining participation despite increasing disability, such as exploring alternative transportation if driving is no longer an option and participating in volunteer and social opportunities after retirement. • A community group addresses issues of self-efficacy and self-esteem as the basis for creating resiliency in preadolescent children at risk for being bullied. • A group in a mental health program addresses establishment of social connections in the community.

851

TABLE 7. ACTIVITY AND OCCUPATIONAL DEMANDS

Activity and occupational demands *are the components of activities and occupations that occupational therapy practitioners consider during the clinical reasoning process. Depending on the context and needs of the client, these demands can be deemed barriers to or supports for participation. Specific knowledge about the demands of activities and occupations assists practitioners in selecting activities for therapeutic purposes. Demands of the activity or occupation include the relevance and importance to the client, objects used and their properties, space demands, social demands, sequencing and timing, required actions and performance skills, and required underlying body functions and body structures.*

Type of Demand	Description	Examples
Relevance and importance to client	Alignment with the client's goals, values, beliefs, and needs and perceived utility	• Driving a car equates with independence. • Preparing a holiday meal connects with family tradition. • Voting is a rite of passage to adulthood.
Objects used and their properties	Tools, supplies, and equipment required in the process of carrying out the activity	• Tools (e.g., scissors, dishes, shoes, volleyball) • Supplies (e.g., paints, milk, lipstick) • Equipment (e.g., workbench, stove, basketball hoop) • Inherent properties (e.g., heavy, rough, sharp, colorful, loud, bitter tasting)
Space demands (related to the physical environment)	Physical environmental requirements of the activity (e.g., size, arrangement, surface, lighting, temperature, noise, humidity, ventilation)	• Large, open space outdoors for a baseball game • Bathroom door and stall width to accommodate wheelchair • Noise, lighting, and temperature controls for a library
Social demands (related to the social environment and virtual and cultural contexts)	Elements of the social environment and virtual and cultural contexts that may be required by the activity	• Rules of the game • Expectations of other participants in the activity (e.g., sharing supplies, using language appropriate for the meeting, appropriate virtual decorum)
Sequencing and timing	Process required to carry out the activity (e.g., specific steps, sequence of steps, timing requirements)	• *Steps to make tea:* Gather cup and tea bag, heat water, pour water into cup, let steep, add sugar. • *Sequence:* Heat water before placing tea bag in water. • *Timing:* Leave tea bag to steep for 2 minutes. • *Steps to conduct a meeting:* Establish goals for meeting, arrange time and location, prepare agenda, call meeting to order. • *Sequence:* Have people introduce themselves before beginning discussion of topic. • *Timing:* Allot sufficient time for discussion of topic and determination of action items.
Required actions and performance skills	Actions (performance skills—motor, process, and social interaction) required by the client that are an inherent part of the activity	• Feeling the heat of the stove • Gripping a handlebar • Choosing ceremonial clothes • Determining how to move limbs to control the car • Adjusting the tone of voice • Answering a question
Required body functions	"Physiological functions of body systems (including psychological functions)" (WHO, 2001, p. 10) required to support the actions used to perform the activity	• Mobility of joints • Level of consciousness • Cognitive level
Required body structures	"Anatomical parts of the body such as organs, limbs, and their components" that support body functions (WHO, 2001, p. 10) and are required to perform the activity	• Number of hands or feet • Olfactory or taste organs

TABLE 8. APPROACHES TO INTERVENTION

Approaches to intervention *are specific strategies selected to direct the process of evaluation and intervention planning, selection, and implementation on the basis of the client's desired outcomes, evaluation data, and evidence. Approaches inform the selection of practice models, frames of references, or treatment theories.*

Approach	Description	Examples
Create, promote (health promotion)	An intervention approach that does not assume a disability is present or that any aspect would interfere with performance. This approach is designed to provide enriched contextual and activity experiences that will enhance performance for all people in the natural contexts of life (adapted from Dunn, McClain, Brown, & Youngstrom, 1998, p. 534).	• Create a parenting class to help first-time parents engage their children in developmentally appropriate play • Provide a falls prevention class to a group of older adults at the local senior center to encourage safe mobility throughout the home
Establish, restore (remediation, restoration)	An intervention approach designed to change client variables to establish a skill or ability that has not yet developed or to restore a skill or ability that has been impaired (adapted from Dunn et al., 1998, p. 533).	• Restore a client's upper-extremity movement to enable transfer of dishes from the dishwasher into the upper kitchen cabinets • Develop a structured schedule, chunking tasks to decrease the risk of being overwhelmed when faced with the many responsibilities of daily life roles • Collaborate with a client to help establish morning routines needed to arrive at school or work on time
Maintain	An intervention approach designed to provide the supports that will allow clients to preserve the performance capabilities they have regained, that continue to meet their occupational needs, or both. The assumption is that without continued maintenance intervention, performance would decrease, occupational needs would not be met, or both, thereby affecting health, well-being, and quality of life.	• Provide ongoing intervention for a client with amyotrophic lateral sclerosis to address participation in desired occupations through provision of assistive technology • Maintain independent gardening for people with arthritis by recommending tools with modified grips, long-handled tools, seating alternatives, and raised gardens • Maintain safe and independent access for people with low vision by increasing hallway lighting in the home
Modify (compensation, adaptation)	An intervention approach directed at "finding ways to revise the current context or activity demands to support performance in the natural setting, [including] compensatory techniques . . . [such as] enhancing some features to provide cues or reducing other features to reduce distractibility" (Dunn et al., 1998, p. 533).	• Simplify task sequence to help a person with cognitive impairments complete a morning self-care routine • Consult with builders to design homes that will allow families to provide living space for aging parents (e.g., bedroom and full bath on the main floor of a multilevel dwelling) • Modify the clutter in a room to decrease a client's distractibility
Prevent (disability prevention)	An intervention approach designed to address the needs of clients with or without a disability who are at risk for occupational performance problems. This approach is designed to prevent the occurrence or evolution of barriers to performance in context. Interventions may be directed at client, context, or activity variables (adapted from Dunn et al., 1998, p. 534).	• Aid in the prevention of illicit chemical substance use by introducing self-initiated routine strategies that support drug-free behavior • Prevent social isolation of employees by promoting participation in after-work group activities • Consult with a hotel chain to provide an ergonomics educational program designed to prevent back injuries in housekeepers

TABLE 9. OUTCOMES

Outcomes *are the end result of the occupational therapy process; they describe what clients can achieve through occupational therapy intervention. The outcomes of occupational therapy can be described in two ways. Some outcomes are measurable and are used for intervention planning, monitoring, and discharge planning. These outcomes reflect the attainment of treatment goals that relate to engagement in occupation. Other outcomes are experienced by clients when they have realized the effects of engagement in occupation and are able to return to desired habits, routines, roles, and rituals. The examples listed specify how the broad outcome of health and participation in life may be operationalized and are not intended to be all inclusive.*

Category	Description	Examples
Occupational performance	Act of doing and accomplishing a selected action (performance skill), activity, or occupation (Fisher, 2009; Fisher & Griswold, 2014; Kielhofner, 2008) and results from the dynamic transaction among the client, the context, and the activity. Improving or enabling skills and patterns in occupational performance leads to engagement in occupations or activities (adapted in part from Law et al., 1996, p. 16).	See "Improvement" and "Enhancement," below.
Improvement	Outcomes targeted when a performance limitation is present. These outcomes reflect increased occupational performance for the person, group, or population.	• A child with autism playing interactively with a peer (person) • An older adult returning to a desired living situation in the home from a skilled nursing facility (person) • Decreased incidence of back strain in nursing personnel as a result of an in-service education program in body mechanics for carrying out job duties that require bending, lifting, and so forth (group) • Construction of accessible playground facilities for all children in local city parks (population)
Enhancement	Outcomes targeted when a performance limitation is not currently present. These outcomes reflect the development of performance skills and performance patterns that augment existing performance in life occupations.	• Increased confidence and competence of teenage mothers in parenting their children as a result of structured social groups and child development classes (person) • Increased membership in the local senior citizen center as a result of expanding social wellness and exercise programs (group) • Increased ability of school staff to address and manage school-age youth violence as a result of conflict resolution training to address bullying (group) • Increased opportunities for older adults to participate in community activities through ride-share programs (population)
Prevention	Education or health promotion efforts designed to identify, reduce, or prevent the onset and reduce the incidence of unhealthy conditions, risk factors, diseases, or injuries (AOTA, 2013b). Occupational therapy promotes a healthy lifestyle at the individual, group, community (societal), and governmental or policy level (adapted from AOTA, 2001).	• Appropriate seating and play area for a child with orthopedic impairments (person) • Implementation of a program of leisure and educational activities for a drop-in center for adults with severe mental illness (group) • Access to occupational therapy services in underserved areas regardless of cultural or ethnic background (population)
Health and wellness	Resources for everyday life, not the objective of living. For individuals, *health* is a state of physical, mental, and social well-being, as well as a positive concept emphasizing social and personal resources and physical capacities (WHO, 1986). Health for groups and populations includes these individual aspects but also includes social responsibility of members to the group or population as a whole. *Wellness* is "an active process through which individuals [or groups or populations] become aware of and make choices toward a more successful existence" (Hettler, 1984, p. 1117). Wellness is more than a lack of disease symptoms; it is a state of mental and physical balance and fitness (adapted from *Taber's Cyclopedic Medical Dictionary*, 1997, p. 2110).	• Participation by a person with a psychiatric disability in an empowerment and advocacy group to improve services in the community (person) • Implementation of a company-wide program for employees to identify problems and solutions regarding the balance among work, leisure, and family life (group) • Decreased incidence of childhood obesity (population)

(Continued)

TABLE 9. OUTCOMES

(Continued)

Category	Description	Examples
Quality of life	Dynamic appraisal of the client's life satisfaction (perceptions of progress toward goals), hope (real or perceived belief that one can move toward a goal through selected pathways), self-concept (the composite of beliefs and feelings about oneself), health and functioning (e.g., health status, self-care capabilities), and socioeconomic factors (e.g., vocation, education, income; adapted from Radomski, 1995).	• Full and active participation of a deaf child from a hearing family during a recreational activity (person) • Residents being able to prepare for outings and travel independently as a result of independent living skills training for care providers (group) • Formation of a lobby to support opportunities for social networking, advocacy activities, and sharing of scientific information for stroke survivors and their families (population)
Participation	Engagement in desired occupations in ways that are personally satisfying and congruent with expectations within the culture.	• A person recovering the ability to perform the essential duties of his or her job after a flexor tendon laceration (person) • A family enjoying a vacation while traveling cross-country in their adapted van (group) • All children within a state having access to school sports programs (population)
Role competence	Ability to effectively meet the demands of roles in which the client engages.	• An individual with cerebral palsy being able to take notes or type papers to meet the demands of the student role (person) • Implementation of job rotation at a factory that allows sharing of higher demand tasks to meet the demands of the worker role (group) • Improved accessibility of polling places to all people with disabilities to meet the demands of the citizen role (population)
Well-being	Contentment with one's health, self-esteem, sense of belonging, security, and opportunities for self-determination, meaning, roles, and helping others (Hammell, 2009). *Well-being* is "a general term encompassing the total universe of human life domains, including physical, mental, and social aspects" (WHO, 2006, p. 211).	• A person with amyotrophic lateral sclerosis being content with his ability to find meaning in fulfilling the role of father through compensatory strategies and environmental modifications (person) • Members of an outpatient depression and anxiety support group feeling secure in their sense of group belonging and ability to help other members (group) • Residents of a town celebrating the groundbreaking of a school during reconstruction after a natural disaster (population)
Occupational justice	Access to and participation in the full range of meaningful and enriching occupations afforded to others, including opportunities for social inclusion and the resources to participate in occupations to satisfy personal, health, and societal needs (adapted from Townsend & Wilcock, 2004).	• An individual with an intellectual disability serving on an advisory board to establish programs offered by a community recreation center (person) • Workers having enough break time to have lunch with their young children in their day care center (group) • Increased sense of empowerment and self-advocacy skills for people with persistent mental illness, enabling them to develop an antistigma campaign promoting engagement in the civic arena (group) and alternative adapted housing options for older adults to age in place (population)

References

Accreditation Council for Occupational Therapy Education. (2012). 2011 Accreditation Council for Occupational Therapy Education (ACOTE®) standards. *American Journal of Occupational Therapy, 66,* S6–S74. http://dx.doi.org/10.5014/ajot.2012.66S6

American Heritage dictionary of the English language (4th ed.). (2003). Retrieved from http://www.thefreedictionary.com/framework

American Occupational Therapy Association. (1979). *Occupational therapy product output reporting system and uniform terminology for reporting occupational therapy services.* (Available from American Occupational Therapy Association, 4720 Montgomery Lane, PO Box 31220, Bethesda, MD 20824-1220; pracdept@aota.org)

American Occupational Therapy Association. (1989). *Uniform terminology for occupational therapy* (2nd ed.). (Available from American Occupational Therapy Association, 4720 Montgomery Lane, PO Box 31220, Bethesda, MD 20824-1220; pracdept@aota.org)

American Occupational Therapy Association. (1994). Uniform terminology for occupational therapy (3rd ed.). *American Journal of Occupational Therapy, 48,* 1047–1054. http://dx.doi.org/10.5014/ajot.48.11.1047

American Occupational Therapy Association. (2001). Occupational therapy in the promotion of health and the prevention of disease and disability statement. *American Journal of Occupational Therapy, 55,* 656–660. http://dx.doi.org/10.5014/ajot.55.6.656

American Occupational Therapy Association. (2002a). Broadening the construct of independence [Position Paper]. *American Journal of Occupational Therapy, 56,* 660. http://dx.doi.org/10.5014/ajot.56.6.660

American Occupational Therapy Association. (2002b). Occupational therapy practice framework: Domain and process. *American Journal of Occupational Therapy, 56,* 609–639. http://dx.doi.org/10.5014/ajot.56.6.609

American Occupational Therapy Association. (2006). Policy 1.44: Categories of occupational therapy personnel. In *Policy manual* (2007 ed., pp. 33–34). Bethesda, MD: Author.

American Occupational Therapy Association. (2008). Occupational therapy practice framework: Domain and process (2nd ed.). *American Journal of Occupational Therapy, 62,* 625–683. http://dx.doi.org/10.5014/ajot.62.6.625

American Occupational Therapy Association. (2009). Guidelines for supervision, roles, and responsibilities during the delivery of occupational therapy services. *American Journal of Occupational Therapy, 63,* 797–803. http://dx.doi.org/10.5014/ajot.63.6.797

American Occupational Therapy Association. (2010). Standards of practice for occupational therapy. *American Journal of Occupational Therapy, 64*(Suppl.), S106–S111. http://dx.doi.org/10.5014/ajot.2010.64S106

American Occupational Therapy Association. (2011). *Definition of occupational therapy practice for the AOTA Model Practice Act.* Retrieved from http://www.aota.org/~/media/Corporate/Files/Advocacy/State/Resources/PracticeAct/Model%20Definition%20of%20OT%20Practice%20%20Adopted%2041411.ashx

American Occupational Therapy Association. (2013a). Guidelines for documentation of occupational therapy. *American Journal of Occupational Therapy, 67*(Suppl.), S32–S38. http://dx.doi.org/10.5014/ajot.2013.67S32

American Occupational Therapy Association. (2013b). Occupational therapy in the promotion of health and well-being. *American Journal of Occupational Therapy, 67*(Suppl.), S47–S59. http://dx.doi.org/10.5014/ajot.2013.67S47

American Occupational Therapy Association. (2013c). Telehealth. *American Journal of Occupational Therapy, 67*(Suppl.), S69–S90. http://dx.doi.org/10.5014/ajot.2013.67S69

Americans With Disabilities Act of 1990, Pub. L. 101–336, 42 U.S.C. § 12101.

Ayres, A. J. (1972). *Sensory integration and learning disorders.* Los Angeles: Western Psychological Services.

Ayres, A. J. (2005). *Sensory integration and the child.* Los Angeles: Western Psychological Services.

Bandura, A. (1986). *Social foundations of thought and action: A social cognitive theory.* Englewood Cliffs, NJ: Prentice Hall.

Bedell, G. M. (2012). Measurement of social participation. In V. Anderson & M. H. Beauchamp (Eds.), *Developmental social neuroscience and childhood brain insult: Theory and practice* (pp. 184–206). New York: Guilford Press.

Bergen, D. (Ed.). (1988). *Play as a medium for learning and development: A handbook of theory and practice.* Portsmouth, NH: Heinemann.

Boyt Schell, B. A., Gillen, G., & Scaffa, M. (2014a). Glossary. In B. A. Boyt Schell, G. Gillen, & M. Scaffa (Eds.), *Willard and Spackman's occupational therapy* (12th ed., pp. 1229–1243). Philadelphia: Lippincott Williams & Wilkins.

Boyt Schell, B. A., Gillen, G., & Scaffa, M. (Eds.). (2014b). *Willard and Spackman's occupational therapy* (12th ed.). Philadelphia: Lippincott Williams & Wilkins.

Chisholm, D., & Boyt Schell, B. A. (2014). Overview of the occupational therapy process and outcomes. In B. A. Boyt Schell, G. Gillen, & M. Scaffa (Eds.), *Willard and Spackman's occupational therapy* (12th ed., pp. 266–280). Philadelphia: Lippincott Williams & Wilkins.

Christiansen, C. H., & Baum, M. C. (Eds.). (1997). *Occupational therapy: Enabling function and well-being.* Thorofare, NJ: Slack.

Christiansen, C., Baum, M. C., & Bass-Haugen, J. (Eds.). (2005). *Occupational therapy: Performance, participation, and well-being.* Thorofare, NJ: Slack.

Christiansen, C. H., & Hammecker, C. L. (2001). Self care. In B. R. Bonder & M. B. Wagner (Eds.), *Functional performance in older adults* (pp. 155–175). Philadelphia: F. A. Davis.

Christiansen, C. H., & Townsend, E. A. (2010). *Introduction to occupation: The art and science of living* (2nd ed.). Cranbury, NJ: Pearson Education.

Clark, F. A. (2000). The concept of habit and routine: A preliminary theoretical synthesis. *OTJR: Occupation, Participation and Health, 20,* 123S–137S.

Clark, F., Jackson, J., Carlson, M., Chou, C. P., Cherry, B. J., Jordan-Marsh, M., . . . Azen, S. P. (2012). Effectiveness of a lifestyle intervention in promoting the well-being of independently living older people: Results of the Well Elderly 2 Randomised Controlled Trial. *Journal of Epidemiology and Community Health, 66,* 782–790. http://dx.doi.org/10.1136/jech.2009.099754

Cohn, E. S. (2001). Parent perspectives of occupational therapy using a sensory integration approach. *American Journal of Occupational Therapy, 55,* 285–294. http://dx.doi.org/10.5014/ajot.55.3.285

Cohn, E. S., Miller, L. J., & Tickle-Degnen, L. (2000). Parental hopes for therapy outcomes: Children with sensory modulation disorders. *American Journal of Occupational Therapy, 54,* 36–43. http://dx.doi.org/10.5014/ajot.54.1.36

Cole, B., & McLean, V. (2003). Therapeutic relationships redefined. *Occupational Therapy in Mental Health, 19,* 33–56. http://dx.doi.org/10.1300/J004v19n02_03

Collins, J., & O'Brien, N. P. (2003). *Greenwood dictionary of education.* Westport, CT: Greenwood Press.

Crepeau, E. (2003). Analyzing occupation and activity: A way of thinking about occupational performance. In E. Crepeau, E. Cohn, & B. A. Boyt Schell (Eds.), *Willard and Spackman's occupational therapy* (10th ed., pp. 189–198). Philadelphia: Lippincott Williams & Wilkins.

Davidson, L., Shahar, G., Lawless, M. S., Sells, D., & Tondora, J. (2006). Play, pleasure, and other positive life events: "Non-specific" factors in recovery from mental illness. *Psychiatry, 69,* 151–163.

Dickie, V., Cutchin, M., & Humphry, R. (2006). Occupation as transactional experience: A critique of individualism in occupational science. *Journal of Occupational Science, 13,* 83–93. http://dx.doi.org/10.1080/14427591.2006.9686573

Doucet, B. M., & Gutman, S. A. (2013). Quantifying function: The rest of the measurement story. *American Journal of Occupational Therapy, 67,* 7–9. http://dx.doi.org/10.5014/ajot.2013.007096

Dunlea, A. (1996). An opportunity for co-adaptation: The experience of mothers and their infants who are blind. In R. Zemke & F. Clark (Eds.), *Occupational science: The evolving discipline* (pp. 227–342). Philadelphia: F. A. Davis.

Dunn, W. (2000). Habit: What's the brain got to do with it? *OTJR: Occupation, Participation and Health, 20*(Suppl. 1), 6S–20S.

Dunn, W., McClain, L. H., Brown, C., & Youngstrom, M. J. (1998). The ecology of human performance. In M. E. Neistadt & E. B. Crepeau (Eds.), *Willard and Spackman's occupational therapy* (9th ed., pp. 525–535). Philadelphia: Lippincott Williams & Wilkins.

Dunton, W. R. (1934). The need for and value of research in occupational therapy. *Occupational Therapy and Rehabilitation, 13,* 325–328.

Esdaile, S. A., & Olson, J. A. (2004). *Mothering occupations: Challenge, agency, and participation.* Philadelphia: F. A. Davis.

Fiese, B. H. (2007). Routines and rituals: Opportunities for participation in family health. *OTJR: Occupation, Participation and Health, 27,* 41S–49S.

Fiese, B. H., Tomcho, T. J., Douglas, M., Josephs, K., Poltrock, S., & Baker, T. (2002). A review of 50 years of research on naturally occurring family routines and rituals: Cause for celebration. *Journal of Family Psychology, 16,* 381–390. http://dx.doi.org/10.1037/0893-3200.16.4.381

Fisher, A. (2006). Overview of performance skills and client factors. In H. Pendleton & W. Schultz-Krohn (Eds.), *Pedretti's occupational therapy: Practice skills for physical dysfunction* (pp. 372–402). St. Louis, MO: Mosby/Elsevier.

Fisher, A. G. (2009). *Occupational Therapy Intervention Process Model: A model for planning and implementing top-down, client-centered, and occupation-based interventions.* Fort Collins, CO: Three Star Press.

Fisher, A. G., & Griswold, L. A. (2014). Performance skills: Implementing performance analyses to evaluate quality of occupational performance. In B. A. Boyt Schell, G. Gillen, & M. Scaffa (Eds.), *Willard and Spackman's occupational therapy* (12th ed., pp. 249–264). Philadelphia: Lippincott Williams & Wilkins.

Gillen, G., & Boyt Schell, B. (2014). Introduction to evaluation, intervention, and outcomes for occupations. In B. A. Boyt Schell, G. Gillen, & M. Scaffa (Eds.), *Willard and Spackman's occupational therapy* (12th ed., pp. 606–609). Philadelphia: Lippincott Williams & Wilkins.

Gitlin, L. N., & Corcoran, M. A. (2005). *Occupational therapy and dementia care: The Home Environmental Skill-Building Program for individuals and families.* Bethesda, MD: AOTA Press.

Gitlin, L. N., Corcoran, M. A., Winter, L., Boyce, A., & Hauck, W. W. (2001). A randomized controlled trial of a home environmental intervention to enhance self-efficacy and reduce upset in family caregivers of persons with dementia. *Gerontologist, 41,* 15–30. http://dx.doi.org/10.1093/geront/41.1.4

Gitlin, L. N., Winter, L., Burke, J., Chernett, N., Dennis, M. P., & Hauck, W. W. (2008). Tailored activities to manage neuropsychiatric behaviors in persons with dementia and reduce caregiver burden: A randomized pilot study. *American Journal of Geriatric Psychiatry, 16,* 229–239.

Gitlin, L. N., Winter, L., Corcoran, M., Dennis, M. P., Schinfeld, S., & Hauck, W. W. (2003). Effects of the Home Environmental Skill-Building Program on the caregiver–care recipient dyad: 6-month outcomes from the Philadelphia REACH Initiative. *Gerontologist, 43,* 532–546. http://dx.doi.org/10.1093/geront/43.4.532

Glass, T. A., de Leon, C. M., Marottoli, R. A., & Berkman, L. F. (1999). Population based study of social and productive activities as predictors of survival among elderly Americans. *British Medical Journal, 319,* 478–483. http://dx.doi.org/10.1136/bmj.319.7208.478

Graff, M. J., Vernooij-Dassen, M. J., Thijssen, M., Dekker, J., Hoefnagels, W. H., & Olderikkert, M. G. (2007). Effects of community occupational therapy on quality of life, mood, and health status in dementia patients and their caregivers: A randomized controlled trial. *Journals of Gerontology, Series A: Biological Sciences and Medical Sciences, 62,* 1002–1009. http://dx.doi.org/10.1093/gerona/62.9.1002

Graham, F., Rodger, S., & Ziviani, J. (2013). Effectiveness of occupational performance coaching in improving children's and mothers' performance and mothers' self-competence. *American Journal of Occupational Therapy, 67,* 10–18. http://dx.doi.org/10.5014/ajot.2013.004648

Gutman, S. A., Mortera, M. H., Hinojosa, J., & Kramer, P. (2007). Revision of the *Occupational Therapy Practice Framework*. *American Journal of Occupational Therapy, 61,* 119–126. http://dx.doi.org/10.5014/ajot.61.1.119

Hagedorn, R. (2000). *Tools for practice in occupational therapy: A structured approach to core skills and processes.* Edinburgh: Churchill Livingstone.

Hakansson, C., Dahlin-Ivanoff, S., & Sonn, U. (2006). Achieving balance in everyday life. *Journal of Occupational Science, 13,* 74–82. http://dx.doi.org/10.1080/14427591.2006.9686572

Hammell, K. W. (2009). Self-care, productivity, and leisure, or dimensions of occupational experience? Rethinking occupational "categories." *Canadian Journal of Occupational Therapy, 76,* 107–114. http://dx.doi.org/10.1177/000841740907600208

Hettler, W. (1984). Wellness—The lifetime goal of a university experience. In J. D. Matarazzo, S. M. Weiss, J. A. Herd, N. E. Miller, & S. M. Weiss (Eds.), *Behavioral health: A handbook of health enhancement and disease prevention* (pp. 1117–1124). New York: Wiley.

Hildenbrand, W. C., & Lamb, A. J. (2013). Health Policy Perspectives—Occupational therapy in prevention and wellness: Retaining relevance in a new health care world. *American Journal of Occupational Therapy, 67,* 266–271. http://dx.doi.org/10.5014/ajot.2013.673001

Hinojosa, J., & Blount, M.-L. (2009). Occupation, purposeful activities, and occupational therapy. In J. Hinojosa & M.-L. Blount (Eds.), *The texture of life: Purposeful activities in context of occupation* (3rd ed., pp. 1–19). Bethesda, MD: AOTA Press.

Hinojosa, J., Kramer, P., Royeen, C. B., & Luebben, A. (2003). The core concepts of occupation. In P. Kramer, J. Hinojosa, & C. B. Royeen (Eds.), *Perspectives in human occupation: Participation in life* (pp. 1–17). Philadelphia: Lippincott Williams & Wilkins.

Hooper, B., & Wood, W. (2014). The philosophy of occupational therapy: A framework for practice. In B. A. Boyt Schell, G. Gillen, & M. Scaffa (Eds.), *Willard and Spackman's occupational therapy* (12th ed., pp. 35–46). Philadelphia: Lippincott Williams & Wilkins.

Individuals With Disabilities Education Improvement Act of 2004, Pub. L. 108–446, 20 U.S.C. § 1400 et seq.

Jackson, J. (1998a). Contemporary criticisms of role theory. *Journal of Occupational Science, 5,* 49–55. http://dx.doi.org/10.1080/14427591.1998.9686433

Jackson, J. (1998b). Is there a place for role theory in occupational science? *Journal of Occupational Science, 5,* 56–65. http://dx.doi.org/10.1080/14427591.1998.9686434

Jackson, J., Carlson, M., Mandel, D., Zemke, R., & Clark, F. (1998). Occupation in lifestyle redesign: The Well Elderly Study occupational therapy program. *American Journal of Occupational Therapy, 52,* 326–336. http://dx.doi.org/10.5014/ajot.52.5.326

James, A. B. (2008). Restoring the role of independent person. In M. V. Radomski & C. A. Trombly Latham (Eds.), *Occupational therapy for physical dysfunction* (pp. 774–816). Philadelphia: Lippincott Williams & Wilkins.

Kielhofner, G. (2008). *The model of human occupation: Theory and application* (4th ed.). Philadelphia: Lippincott Williams & Wilkins.

Koome, F., Hocking, C., & Sutton, D. (2012). Why routines matter: The nature and meaning of family routine in the context of adolescent mental illness. *Journal of Occupational Science, 19,* 312–325. http://dx.doi.org/10.1080/14427591.2012.718245

Larson, E., & Zemke, R. (2003). Shaping the temporal patterns of our lives: The social coordination of occupation. *Journal of Occupational Science, 10,* 80–89. http://dx.doi.org/10.1080/14427591.2003.9686514

Law, M., Baum, M. C., & Dunn, W. (2005). *Measuring occupational performance: Supporting best practice in occupational therapy* (2nd ed.). Thorofare, NJ: Slack.

Law, M., Cooper, B., Strong, S., Stewart, D., Rigby, P., & Letts, L. (1996). Person–Environment–Occupation Model: A transactive approach to occupational performance. *Canadian Journal of Occupational Therapy, 63,* 9–23. http://dx.doi.org/10.1177/000841749606300103

Law, M., Polatajko, H., Baptiste, W., & Townsend, E. (1997). Core concepts of occupational therapy. In E. Townsend (Ed.), *Enabling occupation: An occupational therapy perspective* (pp. 29–56). Ottawa, ON: Canadian Association of Occupational Therapists.

Magasi, S., & Hammel, J. (2004). Social support and social network mobilization in African American woman who have experienced strokes. *Disability Studies Quarterly, 24*(4). Retrieved from http://dsq-sds.org/article/view/878/1053

Meyer, A. (1922). The philosophy of occupational therapy. *Archives of Occupational Therapy, 1,* 1–10.

Moreira-Almeida, A., & Koenig, H. G. (2006). Retaining the meaning of the words *religiousness* and *spirituality:* A commentary on the WHOQOL SRPB group's "A Cross-Cultural Study of Spirituality, Religion, and Personal Beliefs as Components of Quality of Life" (62: 6, 2005, 1486–1497). *Social Science and Medicine, 63,* 843–845. http://dx.doi.org/10.1016/j.socscimed.2006.03.001

Mosey, A. C. (1996). *Applied scientific inquiry in the health professions: An epistemological orientation* (2nd ed.). Bethesda, MD: American Occupational Therapy Association.

Moyers, P. A.; American Occupational Therapy Association. (1999). The guide to occupational therapy practice. *American Journal of Occupational Therapy, 53,* 247–322. http://dx.doi.org/10.5014/ajot.53.3.247

Moyers, P. A., & Dale, L. M. (2007). *The guide to occupational therapy practice* (2nd ed.). Bethesda, MD: AOTA Press.

Nelson, D., & Jepson-Thomas, J. (2003). Occupational form, occupational performance, and a conceptual framework for therapeutic occupation. In P. Kramer, J. Hinojosa, & C. B. Royeen (Eds.), *Perspectives in human occupation: Participation in life* (pp. 87–155). Philadelphia: Lippincott Williams & Wilkins.

Nilsson, I., & Townsend, E. (2010). Occupational justice—Bridging theory and practice. *Scandinavian Journal of Occupational Therapy, 17,* 57–63. http://dx.doi.org/10.3109/11038120903287182

Nurit, W., & Michal, A. B. (2003). Rest: A qualitative exploration of the phenomenon. *Occupational Therapy International, 10,* 227–238. http://dx.doi.org/10.1002/oti.187

Olson, J. A. (2004). Mothering co-occupations in caring for infants and young children. In S. A. Esdaile & J. A. Olson

(Eds.), *Mothering occupations* (pp. 28–51). Philadelphia: F. A. Davis.

Parham, L. D., & Fazio, L. S. (Eds.). (1997). *Play in occupational therapy for children.* St. Louis, MO: Mosby.

Peloquin, S. M. (2003). The therapeutic relationship: Manifestations and challenges in occupational therapy. In E. B. Crepeau, E. S. Cohn, & B. A. Boyt Schell (Eds.), *Willard and Spackman's occupational therapy* (10th ed., pp. 157–170). Philadelphia: Lippincott Williams & Wilkins.

Pierce, D. (2001). Untangling occupation and activity. *American Journal of Occupational Therapy, 55,* 138–146. http://dx.doi.org/10.5014/ajot.55.2.138

Polatajko, H., & Mandich, A. (2004). *Enabling occupation in children: The Cognitive Orientation to Daily Occupational Performance (CO–OP) approach.* Ottawa, ON: CAOT Publications.

Polatajko, H. J., Mandich, A., & Martini, R. (2000). Dynamic performance analysis: A framework for understanding occupational performance. *American Journal of Occupational Therapy, 54,* 65–72. http://dx.doi.org/10.5014/ajot.54.1.65

Puchalski, C., Ferrell, B., Virani, R., Otis-Green, S., Baird, P., Bull, J., . . . Sulmasy, D. (2009). Improving the quality of spiritual care as a dimension of palliative care: The report of the Consensus Conference. *Journal of Palliative Medicine, 12,* 885–904. http://dx.doi.org/10.1089/jpm.2009.0142

Radomski, M. V. (1995). There is more to life than putting on your pants. *American Journal of Occupational Therapy, 49,* 487–490. http://dx.doi.org/10.5014/ajot.49.6.487

Rand, K. L., & Cheavens, J. S. (2009). Hope theory. In S. J. Lopez & C. R. Snyder (Eds.), *The Oxford handbook of positive psychology* (2nd ed., pp. 323–334). Oxford, England: Oxford University Press.

Reed, K. L. (2005). An annotated history of the concepts used in occupational therapy. In C. H. Christiansen, M. C. Baum, & J. Bass-Haugen (Eds.), *Occupational therapy: Performance, participation, and well-being* (3rd ed., pp. 567–626). Thorofare, NJ: Slack.

Rogers, J. C., & Holm, M. B. (1994). Assessment of self-care. In B. R. Bonder & M. B. Wagner (Eds.), *Functional performance in older adults* (pp. 181–202). Philadelphia: F. A. Davis.

Sandqvist, G., Akesson, A., & Eklund, M. (2005). Daily occupations and well-being in women with limited cutaneous systemic sclerosis. *American Journal of Occupational Therapy, 59,* 390–397. http://dx.doi.org/10.5014/ajot.59.4.390

Segal, R. (2004). Family routines and rituals: A context for occupational therapy interventions. *American Journal of Occupational Therapy, 58,* 499–508. http://dx.doi.org/10.5014/ajot.58.5.499

Shumway-Cook, A., & Woollacott, M. H. (2007). *Motor control: Translating research into clinical practice* (3rd ed.). Philadelphia: Lippincott Williams & Wilkins.

Slagle, E. C. (1924). A year's development of occupational therapy in New York State hospitals. *Modern Hospital, 22,* 98–104.

Spencer, J., Davidson, H., & White, V. (1997). Help clients develop hopes for the future. *American Journal of Occupational Therapy, 51,* 191–198. http://dx.doi.org/10.5014/ajot.51.3.191

Taber's cyclopedic medical dictionary. (1997). Philadelphia: F. A. Davis.

Taylor, R. R., & Van Puymbroeck, L. (2013). Therapeutic use of self: Applying the intentional relationship model in group therapy. In J. C. O'Brien & J. W. Solomon (Eds.), *Occupational analysis and group process* (pp. 36–52). St. Louis, MO: Elsevier.

Townsend, E., & Wilcock, A. A. (2004). Occupational justice and client-centred practice: A dialogue in progress. *Canadian Journal of Occupational Therapy, 71,* 75–87. http://dx.doi.org/10.1177/000841740407100203

Trombly, C. A. (1995). Occupation: Purposefulness and meaningfulness as therapeutic mechanisms (Eleanor Clarke Slagle Lecture). *American Journal of Occupational Therapy, 49,* 960–972. http://dx.doi.org/10.5014/ajot.49.10.960

Uniform Data System for Medical Rehabilitation. (1996). *Guide for the Uniform Data Set for Medical Rehabilitation (including the FIM instrument).* Buffalo, NY: Author.

Unruh, A. M. (2004). Reflections on: "So . . . what do you do?" Occupation and the construction of identity. *Canadian Journal of Occupational Therapy, 71,* 290–295. http://dx.doi.org/10.1177/000841740407100508

Wilcock, A. A. (2006). *An occupational perspective of health* (2nd ed.). Thorofare, NJ: Slack.

Wilcock, A. A., & Townsend, E. A. (2014). Occupational justice. In B. A. Boyt Schell, G. Gillen, & M. Scaffa (Eds.), *Willard and Spackman's occupational therapy* (12th ed., pp. 541–552). Philadelphia: Lippincott Williams & Wilkins.

World Federation of Occupational Therapists. (2012). *Definition of occupation.* Retrieved from http://www.wfot.org/aboutus/aboutoccupationaltherapy/definitionofoccupationaltherapy.aspx

World Health Organization. (1986, November 21). *The Ottawa Charter for Health Promotion (First International Conference on Health Promotion, Ottawa).* Retrieved from http://www.who.int/healthpromotion/conferences/previous/ottawa/en/print.html

World Health Organization. (2001). *International classification of functioning, disability and health.* Geneva: Author.

World Health Organization. (2006). *Constitution of the World Health Organization* (45th ed.). Retrieved from http://www.afro.who.int/index.php?option=com_docman&task=doc_download&gid=19&Itemid=2111WHO 2006

Zemke, R. (2004). Time, space, and the kaleidoscopes of occupation (Eleanor Clarke Slagle Lecture). *American Journal of Occupational Therapy, 58,* 608–620. http://dx.doi.org/10.5014/ajot.58.6.608

Zemke, R., & Clark, F. (1996). *Occupational science: An evolving discipline.* Philadelphia: F. A. Davis.

Authors

THE COMMISSION ON PRACTICE:

Deborah Ann Amini, EdD, OTR/L, CHT, FAOTA,
Chairperson, 2011–2014

Kathy Kannenberg, MA, OTR/L, CCM,
Chairperson-Elect, 2013–2014

Stefanie Bodison, OTD, OTR/L

Pei-Fen Chang, PhD, OTR/L

Donna Colaianni, PhD, OTR/L, CHT

Beth Goodrich, OTR, ATP, PhD

Lisa Mahaffey, MS, OTR/L, FAOTA

Mashelle Painter, MEd, COTA/L

Michael Urban, MS, OTR/L, CEAS, MBA, CWCE

Dottie Handley-More, MS, OTR/L,
SIS Liaison

Kiel Cooluris, MOT, OTR/L,
ASD Liaison

Andrea McElroy, MS, OTR/L,
Immediate-Past ASD Liaison

Deborah Lieberman, MHSA, OTR/L, FAOTA,
AOTA Headquarters Liaison

for

THE COMMISSION ON PRACTICE

Deborah Ann Amini, EdD, OTR/L, CHT, FAOTA,
Chairperson

Adopted by the Representative Assembly 2013DecCO11

Note. This document replaces the 2008 *Occupational Therapy Practice Framework: Domain and Process* (2nd ed.).

Acknowledgments

The Commission on Practice (COP) expresses sincere appreciation to all those who participated in the development of the *Occupational Therapy Practice Framework: Domain and Process.*

In addition to those named below, the COP wishes to thank everyone who has contributed to the dialogue, feedback and concepts presented in the document. Sincerest appreciation is extended to Madalene Palmer for all her support and to AOTA's policy and regulatory affairs staff. Further appreciation and thanks is extended to Mary Jane Youngstrom, MS, OTR, FAOTA; Susanne Smith Roley, OTD, OTR/L, FAOTA; Anne G. Fisher, PhD, OTR, FAOTA; and Deborah Pitts, PhD, OTR/L, BCMH, CPRP.

The COP wishes to acknowledge the authors of the second edition of this document: Susanne Smith Roley, MS, OTR/L, FAOTA, *Chairperson (2005–2008);* Janet V. DeLany, DEd, OTR/L, FAOTA; Cynthia J. Barrows, MS, OTR/L; Susan Brownrigg, OTR/L; DeLana Honaker, PhD, OTR/L, BCP; Deanna Iris Sava, MS, OTR/L; Vibeke Talley, OTR/L; Kristi Voelkerding, BS, COTA/L, ATP; Deborah Ann Amini, MEd, OTR/L, CHT, FAOTA, *SIS Liaison;* Emily Smith, MOT, *ASD Liaison;* Pamela Toto, MS, OTR/L, BCG, FAOTA, *Immediate-Past SIS Liaison;* Sarah King, MOT, OTR, *Immediate-Past ASD Liaison;* and Deborah Lieberman, MHSA, OTR/L, FAOTA, *AOTA Headquarters Liaison;* With contributions from M. Carolyn Baum, PhD, OTR/L, FAOTA; Ellen S. Cohn, ScD, OTR/L, FAOTA; Penelope A. Moyers Cleveland, EdD, OTR/L, BCMH, FAOTA; and Mary Jane Youngstrom, MS, OTR, FAOTA.

The COP also wishes to acknowledge the authors of the first edition of this document: Mary Jane Youngstrom, MS, OTR, FAOTA, *Chairperson (1998–2002);* Sara Jane Brayman, PhD, OTR, FAOTA, *Chairperson-Elect (2001–2002);* Paige Anthony, COTA; Mary Brinson, MS, OTR/L, FAOTA; Susan Brownrigg, OTR/L; Gloria Frolek Clark, MS, OTR/L, FAOTA; Susanne Smith Roley, MS, OTR; James Sellers, OTR/L; Nancy L. Van Slyke, EdD, OTR; Stacy M. Desmarais, MS, OTR/L, *ASD Liaison;* Jane Oldham, MOTS, *Immediate-Past ASCOTA Liaison;* Mary Vining Radomski, MA, OTR, FAOTA, *SIS Liaison;* and Sarah D. Hertfelder, MEd, MOT, OTR, FAOTA, *National Office Liaison.*

Appendix A. Glossary

A

Activities

Actions designed and selected to support the development of performance skills and performance patterns to enhance occupational engagement.

Activities of daily living (ADLs)

Activities oriented toward taking care of one's own body (adapted from Rogers & Holm, 1994). ADLs also are referred to as *basic activities of daily living (BADLs)* and *personal activities of daily living (PADLs)*. These activities are "fundamental to living in a social world; they enable basic survival and well-being" (Christiansen & Hammecker, 2001, p. 156; see Table 1).

Activity analysis

Analysis of "the typical demands of an activity, the range of skills involved in its performance, and the various cultural meanings that might be ascribed to it" (Crepeau, 2003, p. 192).

Activity demands

Aspects of an activity or occupation needed to carry it out, including relevance and importance to the client, objects used and their properties, space demands, social demands, sequencing and timing, required actions and performance skills, and required underlying body functions and body structures (see Table 7).

Adaptation

Occupational therapy practitioners enable participation by modifying a task, the method of accomplishing the task, and the environment to promote engagement in occupation (James, 2008).

Advocacy

Efforts directed toward promoting occupational justice and empowering clients to seek and obtain resources to fully participate in their daily life occupations. Efforts undertaken by the practitioner are considered advocacy, and those undertaken by the client are considered self-advocacy and can be promoted and supported by the practitioner (see Table 6).

Analysis of occupational performance

The step in the evaluation process in which the client's assets and problems or potential problems are more specifically identified through assessment tools designed to observe, measure, and inquire about factors that support or hinder occupational performance and in which targeted outcomes are identified (see Exhibit 2).

Assessments

"Specific tools or instruments that are used during the evaluation process" (American Occupational Therapy Association [AOTA], 2010, p. S107).

B

Body functions

"Physiological functions of body systems (including psychological functions)" (World Health Organization [WHO], 2001, p. 10; see Table 2).

Body structures

"Anatomical parts of the body, such as organs, limbs, and their components" that support body functions (WHO, 2001, p. 10; see Table 2).

C

Client

Person or persons (including those involved in the care of a client), group (collective of individuals, e.g., families, workers, students, or community members), or population (collective of groups or individuals living in a similar locale—e.g., city, state, or country—or sharing the same or like concerns).

Client-centered care (client-centered practice)

Approach to service that incorporates respect for and partnership with clients as active participants in the therapy process. This approach emphasizes clients' knowledge and experience, strengths, capacity for choice, and overall autonomy (Boyt Schell et al., 2014a, p. 1230).

Client factors

Specific capacities, characteristics, or beliefs that reside within the person and that influence performance in occupations. Client factors include values, beliefs, and spirituality; body functions; and body structures (see Table 2).

Clinical reasoning

"Process used by practitioners to plan, direct, perform, and reflect on client care" (Boyt Schell et al., 2014a, p. 1231). The term *professional reasoning* is sometimes used and is considered to be a broader term.

Collaborative approach

Orientation in which the occupational therapy practitioner and client work in the spirit of egalitarianism and mutual participation. Collaboration involves encouraging clients to describe their therapeutic concerns, identify their own goals, and contribute to decisions regarding therapeutic interventions (Boyt Schell et al., 2014a).

Context

Variety of interrelated conditions within and surrounding the client that influence performance, including cultural, personal, temporal, and virtual contexts (see Table 5).

Co-occupation

Occupation that implicitly involves two or more people (Boyt Schell et al., 2014a, p. 1232).

Cultural context

Customs, beliefs, activity patterns, behavioral standards, and expectations accepted by the society of which a client is a member. The cultural context influences the client's identity and activity choices (see Table 5).

D

Domain

Profession's purview and areas in which its members have an established body of knowledge and expertise.

E

Education

- *As an occupation:* Activities involved in learning and participating in the educational environment (see Table 1).

- *As an intervention:* Activities that impart knowledge and information about occupation, health, well-being, and participation, resulting in acquisition by the client of helpful behaviors, habits, and routines that may or may not require application at the time of the intervention session (see Table 6).

Engagement in occupation

Performance of occupations as the result of choice, motivation, and meaning within a supportive context and environment.

Environment

External physical and social conditions that surround the client and in which the client's daily life occupations occur (see Table 5).

Evaluation

"Process of obtaining and interpreting data necessary for intervention. This includes planning for and documenting the evaluation process and results" (AOTA, 2010, p. S107).

G

Goal

Measurable and meaningful, occupation-based, long-term or short-term aim directly related to the client's ability and need to engage in desired occupations (AOTA, 2013a, p. S35).

Group

Collective of individuals (e.g., family members, workers, students, community members).

Group intervention

Skilled knowledge and use of leadership techniques in various settings to facilitate learning and acquisition by clients across the life span of skills for participation, including basic social interaction skills, tools for self-regulation, goal setting, and positive choice making, through the dynamics of group and social interaction. Groups may be used as a method of service delivery (see Table 6).

H

Habilitation

Health care services designed to assist people in acquiring, improving, minimizing the deterioration of, compensating for an impairment of, or maintaining (partially or fully) skills, function, or performance for participation in occupation and daily life activities (AOTA policy staff, personal communication, December 17, 2013).

Habits

"Acquired tendencies to respond and perform in certain consistent ways in familiar environments or situations; specific, automatic behaviors performed repeatedly, relatively automatically, and with little variation" (Boyt Schell et al., 2014a, p. 1234). Habits can be useful, dominating, or impoverished and can either support or interfere with performance in areas of occupation (Dunn, 2000; see Table 4).

Health

"State of complete physical, mental, and social well-being, and not merely the absence of disease or infirmity" (WHO, 2006, p. 1).

Health promotion

"Process of enabling people to increase control over, and to improve, their health. To reach a state of complete physical, mental, and social well-being, an individual or group must be able to identify and realize aspirations, to satisfy needs, and to change or cope with the environment" (WHO, 1986).

Hope

"Perceived ability to produce pathways to achieve desired goals and to motivate oneself to use those pathways" (Rand & Cheavens, 2009, p. 323).

I

Independence

"Self-directed state of being characterized by an individual's ability to participate in necessary and preferred occupations in a satisfying manner irrespective of the amount or kind of external assistance desired or required" (AOTA, 2002a, p. 660).

Instrumental activities of daily living (IADLs)

Activities that support daily life within the home and community and that often require more complex interactions than those used in ADLs (see Table 1).

Interdependence

"Reliance that people have on one another as a natural consequence of group living" (Christiansen & Townsend, 2010, p. 419). "Interdependence engenders a spirit of social inclusion, mutual aid, and a moral commitment and responsibility to recognize and support difference" (Christiansen & Townsend, 2010, p. 187).

Interests

"What one finds enjoyable or satisfying to do" (Kielhofner, 2008, p. 42).

Intervention

"Process and skilled actions taken by occupational therapy practitioners in collaboration with the client to facilitate engagement in occupation related to health and participation. The intervention process includes the plan, implementation, and review" (AOTA, 2010, p. S107; see Table 6).

Intervention approaches

Specific strategies selected to direct the process of interventions on the basis of the client's desired outcomes, evaluation data, and evidence (see Table 8).

L

Leisure

"Nonobligatory activity that is intrinsically motivated and engaged in during discretionary time, that is, time not committed to obligatory occupations such as work, self-care, or sleep" (Parham & Fazio, 1997, p. 250; see Table 1).

M

Motor skills

"Occupational performance skills observed as the person interacts with and moves task objects and self around the task environment" (e.g., activity of daily living [ADL] motor skills, school motor skills; Boyt Schell et al., 2014a, p. 1237; see Table 3).

O

Occupation

Daily life activities in which people engage. Occupations occur in context and are influenced by the interplay among client factors, performance skills, and performance patterns. Occupations occur over time; have purpose, meaning, and perceived utility to the client; and can be observed by others (e.g., preparing a meal) or be known only to the person involved (e.g., learning through reading a textbook). Occupations can involve the execution of multiple activities for completion and can result in various outcomes. The *Framework* identifies a broad range of occupations categorized as activities of daily living, instrumental activities of daily living, rest and sleep, education, work, play, leisure, and social participation (see Table 1).

Occupational analysis

See *activity analysis.*

Occupational demands

See *activity demands.*

Occupational identity

"Composite sense of who one is and wishes to become as an occupational being generated from one's history of occupational participation" (Boyt Schell et al., 2014a, p. 1238).

Occupational justice

"A justice that recognizes occupational rights to inclusive participation in everyday occupations for all persons in society, regardless of age, ability, gender, social class, or other differences" (Nilsson & Townsend, 2010, p. 58). Access to and participation in the full range of meaningful and enriching occupations afforded to others, including opportunities for social inclusion and the resources to participate in occupations to satisfy personal, health, and societal needs (adapted from Townsend & Wilcock, 2004).

Occupational performance

Act of doing and accomplishing a selected action (performance skill), activity, or occupation (Fisher, 2009; Fisher & Griswold, 2014; Kielhofner, 2008) that results from the dynamic transaction among the client, the context, and the activity. Improving or enabling skills and patterns in occupational performance leads to engagement in occupations or activities (adapted in part from Law et al., 1996, p. 16).

Occupational profile

Summary of the client's occupational history and experiences, patterns of daily living, interests, values, and needs (see Exhibit 2).

Occupational therapy

Therapeutic use of everyday life activities (occupations) with individuals or groups for the purpose of enhancing or enabling participation in roles, habits, routines, and rituals in home, school, workplace, community, and other settings. Occupational therapy practitioners use their knowledge of the transactional relationship among the person, his or her engagement in valued occupations, and the context to design occupation-based intervention plans that facilitate change or growth in client factors (values, beliefs, and spirituality; body functions, body structures) and performance skills (motor, process, and social interaction) needed for successful participation. Occupational therapy practitioners are concerned with the end result of participation and thus enable engagement through adaptations and modifications to the environment or objects within the environment when needed. Occupational therapy services are provided for habilitation, rehabilitation, and promotion of health and wellness for clients with disability- and non–disability-related needs. These services include acquisition and preservation of occupational identity for those who have or are at risk for developing an illness, injury, disease, disorder, condition, impairment, disability, activity limitation, or participation restriction (adapted from AOTA, 2011).

Organization

Entity composed of individuals with a common purpose or enterprise, such as a business, industry, or agency.

Outcome

End result of the occupational therapy process; what clients can achieve through occupational therapy intervention (see Table 9).

P

Participation

"Involvement in a life situation" (WHO, 2001, p. 10).

Performance patterns

Habits, routines, roles, and rituals used in the process of engaging in occupations or activities; these patterns can support or hinder occupational performance (see Table 4).

Performance skills

Goal-directed actions that are observable as small units of engagement in daily life occupations. They are learned and developed over time and are situated in specific contexts and environments (Fisher & Griswold, 2014; see Table 3).

Person

Individual, including family member, caregiver, teacher, employee, or relevant other.

Personal context

"Features of the individual that are not part of a health condition or health status" (WHO, 2001, p. 17). The personal context includes age, gender, socioeconomic and educational status and may also include membership in a group (i.e., volunteers, employees) or population (i.e., members of a society; see Table 5).

Physical environment

Natural and built nonhuman surroundings and the objects in them. The natural environment includes geographic terrain, plants, and animals, as well as the sensory qualities of the natural surroundings. The built environment includes buildings, furniture, tools, and devices (see Table 5).

Play

"Any spontaneous or organized activity that provides enjoyment, entertainment, amusement, or diversion" (Parham & Fazio, 1997, p. 252; see Table 1).

Population

Collective of groups of individuals living in a similar locale (e.g., city, state, country) or sharing the same or like characteristics or concerns.

Preparatory methods and tasks

Methods and tasks that prepare the client for occupational performance, used either as part of a treatment session in preparation for or concurrently with occupations and activities or as a home-based engagement to support daily occupational performance. Often preparatory methods are interventions that are done to clients without their active participation and involve modalities, devices, or techniques.

Prevention

Education or health promotion efforts designed to identify, reduce, or prevent the onset and reduce the incidence of unhealthy conditions, risk factors, diseases, or injuries (AOTA, 2013b).

Process

Way in which occupational therapy practitioners operationalize their expertise to provide services to clients. The occupational therapy process includes evaluation, intervention, and targeted outcomes; occurs within the purview of the occupational therapy domain; and involves collaboration among the occupational therapist, occupational therapy assistant, and client.

Process skills

"Occupational performance skills [e.g., ADL process skills, school process skills] observed as a person (1) selects, interacts with, and uses task tools and materials; (2) carries out individual actions and steps; and (3) modifies performance when problems are encountered" (Boyt Schell et al., 2014a, p. 1239; see Table 3).

Q

Quality of life

Dynamic appraisal of life satisfaction (perception of progress toward identified goals), self-concept (beliefs and feelings about oneself), health and functioning (e.g., health status, self-care capabilities), and socioeconomic factors (e.g., vocation, education, income; adapted from Radomski, 1995).

R

Reevaluation

Reappraisal of the client's performance and goals to determine the type and amount of change that has taken place.

Rehabilitation

Rehabilitation services are provided to persons experiencing deficits in key areas of physical and other types of function or limitations in participation in daily life activities. Interventions are designed to enable the achievement and maintenance of optimal physical, sensory, intellectual, psychological, and social functional levels. Rehabilitation services provide tools and techniques needed to attain desired levels of independence and self-determination.

Rituals

Sets of symbolic actions with spiritual, cultural, or social meaning contributing to the client's identity and reinforcing values and beliefs. Rituals have a strong affective component (Fiese, 2007; Fiese et al., 2002; Segal, 2004; see Table 4).

Roles

Sets of behaviors expected by society and shaped by culture and context that may be further conceptualized and defined by the client (see Table 4).

Routines

Patterns of behavior that are observable, regular, and repetitive and that provide structure for daily life. They can be satisfying and promoting or damaging. Routines

require momentary time commitment and are embedded in cultural and ecological contexts (Fiese et al., 2002; Segal, 2004; see Table 4).

S

Self-Advocacy

Advocating for oneself, including making one's own decisions about life, learning how to obtain information to gain an understanding about issues of personal interest or importance, developing a network of support, knowing one's rights and responsibilities, reaching out to others when in need of assistance, and learning about self-determination.

Service delivery model

Set of methods for providing services to or on behalf of clients.

Social environment

Presence of, relationships with, and expectations of persons, groups, and populations with whom clients have contact (e.g., availability and expectations of significant individuals, such as spouse, friends, and caregivers; see Table 5).

Social interaction skills

"Occupational performance skills observed during the ongoing stream of a social exchange" (Boyt Schell et al., 2014a, p. 1241; see Table 3).

Social participation

"Interweaving of occupations to support desired engagement in community and family activities as well as those involving peers and friends" (Gillen & Boyt Schell, 2014, p. 607) or involvement in a subset of activities that involve social situations with others (Bedell, 2012) and that support social interdependence (Magasi & Hammel, 2004). Social participation can occur in person or through remote technologies such as telephone calls, computer interaction, and video conferencing (see Table 1).

Spirituality

"Aspect of humanity that refers to the way individuals seek and express meaning and purpose and the way they experience their connectedness to the moment, to self, to others, to nature, and to the significant or sacred" (Puchalski et al., 2009, p. 887; see Table 2).

T

Task

What individuals do or have done (e.g., drive, bake a cake, dress, make a bed; A. Fisher, personal communication, December 16, 2013).

Temporal context

Experience of time as shaped by engagement in occupations. The temporal aspects of occupations that "contribute to the patterns of daily occupations" include "rhythm . . . tempo . . . synchronization . . . duration . . . and sequence" (Larson & Zemke, 2003, p. 82; Zemke, 2004, p. 610). The temporal context includes stage of life, time of day, duration and rhythm of activity, and history (see Table 5).

Transaction

Process that involves two or more individuals or elements that reciprocally and continually influence and affect one another through the ongoing relationship (Dickie, Cutchin, & Humphry, 2006).

V

Values

Acquired beliefs and commitments, derived from culture, about what is good, right, and important to do (Kielhofner, 2008); principles, standards, or qualities considered worthwhile or desirable by the client who holds them (Moyers & Dale, 2007).

Virtual context

Environment in which communication occurs by means of airwaves or computers in the absence of physical contact. The virtual context includes simulated, real-time, or near-time environments such as chat rooms, email, video conferencing, and radio transmissions; remote monitoring via wireless sensors; and computer-based data collection (see Table 5).

W

Well-being

"General term encompassing the total universe of human life domains, including physical, mental, and social aspects" (WHO, 2006, p. 211).

Wellness

"Perception of and responsibility for psychological and physical well-being as these contribute to overall satisfaction with one's life situation" (Boyt Schell et al., 2014a, p. 1243).

Work

"Labor or exertion; to make, construct, manufacture, form, fashion, or shape objects; to organize, plan, or evaluate services or processes of living or governing; committed occupations that are performed with or without financial reward" (Christiansen & Townsend, 2010, p. 423).

Appendix B. Preparation and Qualifications of Occupational Therapists and Occupational Therapy Assistants

Who Are Occupational Therapists?

To practice as an occupational therapist, the individual trained in the United States

- Has graduated from an occupational therapy program accredited by the Accreditation Council for Occupational Therapy Education (ACOTE®) or predecessor organizations;
- Has successfully completed a period of supervised fieldwork experience required by the recognized educational institution where the applicant met the academic requirements of an educational program for occupational therapists that is accredited by ACOTE or predecessor organizations;
- Has passed a nationally recognized entry-level examination for occupational therapists; and
- Fulfills state requirements for licensure, certification, or registration.

Educational Programs for the Occupational Therapist

These include the following:

- Biological, physical, social, and behavioral sciences
- Basic tenets of occupational therapy
- Occupational therapy theoretical perspectives
- Screening, evaluation, and referral
- Formulation and implementation of an intervention plan
- Context of service delivery
- Management of occupational therapy services (master's level)
- Leadership and management (doctoral level)
- Scholarship
- Professional ethics, values, and responsibilities.

The fieldwork component of the program is designed to develop competent, entry-level, generalist occupational therapists by providing experience with a variety of clients across the lifespan and in a variety of settings. Fieldwork is integral to the program's curriculum design and includes an in-depth experience in delivering occupational therapy services to clients, focusing on the application of purposeful and meaningful occupation and/or research, administration, and management of occupational therapy services. The fieldwork experience is designed to promote clinical reasoning and reflective practice, to transmit the values and beliefs that enable ethical practice, and to develop professionalism and competence in career responsibilities. Doctoral-level students also must complete a doctoral experiential component designed to develop advanced skills beyond a generalist level.

Who Are Occupational Therapy Assistants?

To practice as an occupational therapy assistant, the individual trained in the United States

- Has graduated from an occupational therapy assistant program accredited by ACOTE or predecessor organizations;
- Has successfully completed a period of supervised fieldwork experience required by the recognized educational institution where the applicant met the academic requirements of an educational program for occupational therapy assistants that is accredited by ACOTE or predecessor organizations;
- Has passed a nationally recognized entry-level examination for occupational therapy assistants; and
- Fulfills state requirements for licensure, certification, or registration.

Educational Programs for the Occupational Therapy Assistant

These include the following:

- Biological, physical, social, and behavioral sciences
- Basic tenets of occupational therapy
- Screening and assessment
- Intervention and implementation
- Context of service delivery
- Assistance in management of occupational therapy services
- Scholarship
- Professional ethics, values, and responsibilities.

The fieldwork component of the program is designed to develop competent, entry-level, generalist occupational therapy assistants by providing experience with a variety of clients across the lifespan and in a variety of settings. Fieldwork is integral to the program's curriculum design and includes an in-depth experience in

---

Note. The majority of this information is taken from ACOTE (2012).

delivering occupational therapy services to clients, focusing on the application of purposeful and meaningful occupation. The fieldwork experience is designed to promote clinical reasoning appropriate to the occupational therapy assistant role, to transmit the values and beliefs that enable ethical practice, and to develop professionalism and competence in career responsibilities.

Regulation of Occupational Therapy Practice

All occupational therapists and occupational therapy assistants must practice under federal and state law. Currently, 50 states, the District of Columbia, Puerto Rico, and Guam have enacted laws regulating the practice of occupational therapy.

March/April 2014, Volume 68(Supplement 1)

Subject Index

Note: Page numbers in *italic* refer to exhibits, figures and tables.

A

accessibility, 479
accuracy, 783–784
activities of daily living (ADLs), narrowing of occupation to, 148–149
activity
    nature of, 589
    philosophical ideas, 84–85
activity analysis, 593–596
ADA (Americans with Disabilities Act) (1990), *449*
adaptation
    definition, 722
    and environment, 337–339
adversity
    flow in, 240–241
    overcoming, 407–417
    Parable of Two Frogs, 797
affiliation, 412
Age of Enlightenment, 16–17
aging-in-place, 445
alternative medicine, 621–623
Americans with Disabilities Act (ADA) (1990), *449*
Aristotle, 84
artful practice, 711
arts and crafts, 601–603, *604*
assessment, 542, 551–552
assumptions, occupational therapy, 191–196, 587, 739
asylums, 9–11
asynchronous technologies, 640
attention, 176–177
attitude, 177
authenticity, 690–691
autonomy/choice, 478
autotelic personalities, 240

B

balance
    attaining, 264–266
    balanced lifestyle, 211–212
    defining, 259
    epidemiological perspective, 263–264
    need-based approach, 282–283
    occupational perspective, 260–263, 264
    perspectives on, 259–260
    proposed model of, 279–289
    role in occupational health, 401–402
balanced lifestyle. *See* balance
Baldwin, B. T., model of practice, 120–121
Barton, George Edward, 24–25, 39–41
Bing, Robert K., *Occupational Therapy Revisited: A Paraphrastic Journey—Eleanor Clarke Slagle Lecture (1981)*, 17–33
biological need for occupation, 392–395, *393, 394*
built environments, 523

C

CAM (complementary and alternative medicine), 621–623
caring
    influences on, 462
    relationships, 469–475
case application, top-down approach to evaluation, 152–155
CCPE (Client-centred Process Evaluation), 576
Centennial Vision, 711
children
    comprehensive health care for, 750–752
    health promotion, 270–271
    and leisure, 270–272
    telehealth service delivery for, 644
choice, 478, 768–771
Christiansen, Charles H., *Defining Lives: Occupation as Identity: An Essay on Competence, Coherence, and the Creation of Meaning—Eleanor Clarke Slagle Lecture (1999)*, 425–436

circadian rhythm, 254. *See also* sleep
Circle of Friends, 331–332, *332. See also* inclusive communities
Clarke, C. K., 86
client-centered performance context, 136–138
client-centered practice
    overview, 477–478
    assumptions, 479–480
    barriers to, 575–576
    concepts, 478–479
    definitions, 479–480
    facilitating, 579–580
    family-centered care, 485–493, *488*
    framework for, 576–583, *577*
    illustration, *485*
    impact of practice realities on, 463
    implementation, 481
    implications for occupational therapy practice, 480–482
    and occupational justice, 353–362, *361, 362*
    practice settings, 580–581
    relationship-centered care model, *491*
Client-centred Process Evaluation (CCPE), 576
client-centered theory, 373–374
clinical reasoning
    narrative nature of, 565–573
    process of, 541–554
    study on, 555–562
    therapeutic emplotment, 570–573
coalition advocacy, 582–583
codes of ethics, 610–612
cognitive appraisal process, 408–409, 512. *See also* adversity
cognitive disabilities, Allen's model of, 122–123
coherence, and identity, 434
collaborative approach
    effectiveness of, 585–586
    methods for, 589–591
collaborative research, 705–706

communities. *See* inclusive communities
community, definition, 757
community development, 757–762
community organizing, 581–582
compensatory model, selecting, 141
competence, definition, 722
complementary and alternative medicine (CAM), 621–623
component-driven practice, 148–149
conditional reasoning, 560–562
conscious use of self, 461–465
contexts
    and health and participation, 447–456, *451–454*
    organizational, 767–768
    personal, 765–766
    professional, 766–767
contextual congruence, 479
continuous passive motion (CPM), 617–618
corporate asylums, 8
court cases related to occupational therapy practice, 448–450
CPM (continuous passive motion), 617–618
crafts, 601–603, *604*
critical occupational therapy, 367–374
critical reflexivity, 519–527
cross-cultural awareness, 214–215. *See also* cultural contexts of occupation
cryotherapy, 617–618
cultural contexts of occupation, 212–215, 297–302, 305–313
culture, and occupational therapy, 192–193

D

DC (direct current), 617–618
decision-making, ethical, 609–614
"Decorative Therapeutics" (poem), 46
deep thermal agents, 617–618
Defining Lives: Occupation as Identity: An Essay on Competence, Coherence, and the Creation of Meaning, Eleanor Clarke Slagle Lecture (1999), 425–436
direct current (DC), 617–618
disabilities
    and built environments, 523
    constructions of, 521–524
    and identity adaptations, 433–434
    and inclusion, 334–337
    perspectives on, 520–521
    and telehealth, 645
discordant assumptions, 76

disease perspective, 558
disruption, law of, 408–409. *See also* adversity
diversity, 479
Dix, Dorothea Lynde, 22
Dunton, William Rush, 25–26
Dunton's Principles of Occupational Therapy, 1
dynamic sizing skills, 312. *See also* cultural contexts of occupation

E

early hypothesis generation, 556
efficiency perspective, and health-care management, 733–734
eHealth, 643
Eleanor Clarke Slagle Lectures. *See also* Slagle, Eleanor Clarke
    Defining Lives: Occupation as Identity: An Essay on Competence, Coherence, and the Creation of Meaning (1999), 425–436
    Embracing Our Ethos, Reclaiming Our Heart (2005), 789–803
    A Fork in the Road: An Occupational Hazard? (2013), 807–816
    Occupation: Purposefulness and Meaningfulness as Therapeutic Mechanisms (1995), 159–170
    Occupational Therapy Can Be One of the Great Ideas of 20th-Century Medicine (1961), 93–101
    Occupational Therapy Revisited: A Paraphrastic Journey (1981), 17–33
    Our Mandate for the New Millennium: Evidence-Based Practice (2000), 661–672
    Professional Responsibility in Times of Change (1967), 749–755
    Resilience and Human Adaptability: Who Rises Above Adversity? (1990), 407–417
    Tools of Practice: Heritage or Baggage? (1986), 599–607
    Uniting Practice and Theory in an Occupational Framework (1998), 131–142
    Why the Profession of Occupational Therapy Will Flourish in the 21st Century (1996), 109–113
electrotherapeutic agents, 617–618
Embracing Our Ethos, Reclaiming Our Heart, Eleanor Clarke Slagle Lecture (2005), 789–803
emic approach, 499. *See also* ethnographic approach
enablement, 479

ends, occupation as, 150–151
engagement
    cultural contexts, 212–215, 297–302, 305–313
    personal contexts, 218–222
    role in occupational health, 400
    sociopolitical contexts, 215–218, 331–345
    temporal contexts, 209–212, 227–233
environment
    and adaptation, 337–339
    and health and participation, 447–456, *448–450, 451–454*
    role in theories of occupation, 370–372
epidemiological perspective on balance, 263–264
ESTR (high-voltage galvanic stimulation for tissue and wound repair), 617–618
ethical decision making, 609–614, 630
ethnographic approach
    case example, 500–502
    implications for occupational therapy practice, 502–503
    principles of, 498–500, *498, 500*
    and the use of self, 463
ethos, of occupational therapy, 789–803
eudaimonic well-being, 381–386
evidence-based practice
    client perspective, 682–683
    levels of evidence, 675–678
    mandate for, 661–672
    methods, 682
    process of, 681–686, *684*
    therapist perspective, 683–684
excellence perspective, and health-care management, 734–735

F

family-centered care, 485–493, *488*
Farrar, C. B., 86
Federal Nursing Home Reform Act (1987), *449*
FES (functional electrical stimulation), 617–618
Fine, Susan B., *Resilience and Human Adaptability: Who Rises Above Adversity?*—Eleanor Clarke Slagle Lecture (1990), 407–417
Fisher, Anne G., *Uniting Practice and Theory in an Occupational Framework*—Eleanor Clarke Slagle Lecture (1998), 131–142
flexibility, 479

flow
conceptualizations of, 175–177
literature review, 237–243
relevance to occupational
engagement, 177–178
research on, 178
and temporal contexts of
occupation, 209–212
two-dimensional model, *176*
*A Fork in the Road: An Occupational
Hazard?* Eleanor Clarke Slagle
Lecture (2013), 807–816
*Framework. See Occupational Therapy
Practice Framework*
frogs, parable of, 797
functional electrical stimulation
(FES), 617–618

G

generalizability, 512–513
Gillen, Glen, *A Fork in the Road: An
Occupational Hazard?* Eleanor
Clarke Slagle Lecture (2013),
807–816

H

habit training models of practice, 120
halfway houses, 21
Hall, Herbert J., 51–53
haptic technology, 643
hardy personality, 403–404
health, and occupation, 399–405
health and wellness, 645
health informatics, 643
health promotion, and leisure, 270–
271
health care
for children, 750–752
current demands, 586
environment, 474–475
health care management
efficiency perspective, 733–734
excellence perspective, 734–735
high-voltage galvanic stimulation for
tissue and wound repair (ESTR),
617–618
high-voltage pulsed current (HVPC),
617–618
Holm, Margo B., 661–672
hope, 412. *See also* adversity
hospital-based models of practice,
124–125
human beings
pragmatist views of, 70–71
structuralist views of, 72–73
human rights
and occupations, 372
Position Statement on, 441–442

and well-being, 368
humanistic models of practice, 121–
122
HVPC (high-voltage pulsed current),
617–618
hydrotherapy, 617–618

I

IDEA (Individuals with Disabilities
Education Improvement Act)
(2004), *448*
identity
and disabilities, 433–434
occupation as, 425–436
illness perspective, 558
impression management, 433
inclusion, occupational therapy's
commitment to, 443–444
inclusive communities, 215–218,
331–345, 349
independence, Position Paper on, 207
independent living movement, 124,
450
individualism, 195–196
individualizing treatment, 558
Individuals with Disabilities
Education Improvement Act
(IDEA) (2004), *448*
industry, and telehealth, 645–646
insanity, perception of, 8
intactness, 780–783
integration, definition, 722
integrative medicine, 622
intention, 176
intentional use of self, 461–465
interactive reasoning, 558–560, 562
*International Classification of Function-
ing, Disability and Health* (ICF),
183
interpersonal intelligence, 559
Intervention Process Model, 136–142
invalid occupation, 46
invalids. *See also* Tracy, Susan
Elizabeth, occupations for, 23–24
iontophoresis, 617–618

J

Johnson, Susan Cox, 53–54

K

Kawa model
box and arrow rendition, *318*
and cultural contexts of
occupation, 214–215
origins, 319–320, *320*
structure and components, 320–
325, *321, 323*

Kidner, Thomas Bessell, 54–56
kinetic behaviors, 299
knowledge
pragmatist views of, 71
pragmatist–structuralist
conversation, 75–76
structuralist views of, 73
Koori time, 232. *See also* time

L

legal issues, and ethical decision
making, 610–612
legislation and court cases related to
occupational therapy practice,
448–450
leisure
assumptions, 194–195
and health promotion, 270–271
importance of, 269
and occupational therapy practice,
270
levels of evidence, 675–678
lifestyle balance. *see* balance
livable communities, AOTA's Societal
Statement on, 445

M

macroflow, 241. *See also* flow
maldistributed labor, 347. *See also*
occupational deprivation
meaningfulness, as therapeutic
mechanisms, 159–170
means, occupation as, 151–152,
163–169
mechanical devices, 617–618
medical model, 465
Medicare, *449*
medium, 599–607, *600, 604*
mental health, 645
mental institutions, 8–11
methods, 599–607, *600, 604*
Meyer, Adolf
address in honor of Slagle, 105–107
biographical sketch of, 27–28
influence on OT, 85
mHealth, 643
microflow activities, 241. *See also* flow
Mill, John Stuart, 85
mindfulness
and flow, 176–177
relevance to occupational
engagement, 177–178
research on, 178–179
model, of the patient, 549–550
models of practice
cognitive disabilities, 122–123
future roles, 124–125
habit training, 120

humanistic, 121–122
motor control and motor learning, 123
multicontext approach
    to perceptual cognitive impairments, 123
physical dysfunction, 160–162
psychodynamic, 120–121
recommendations for, 125–127
restoration of movement, 120–121
sensory integrative, 122
modifier, definition, 643
monism, 201
moral treatment
    asylums, 9–11
    contexts for, 8–9
    decline of, 11–14, 23
    defined, 7–8
    and Pinel, 19–20
mortality, 404
motion study, and occupational therapy, 594–595
motor control and motor learning models of practice, 123

N

National Center for Complementary and Alternative Medicine (NCCAM), 621–623
National Society for the Promotion of Occupational Therapy (NSPOT), 56–58, 594–595
Nelson, David L., *Why the Profession of Occupational Therapy Will Flourish in the 21st Century*—Eleanor Clarke Slagle Lecture (1996), 109–113
neuro-muscular electrical stimulation (NMES), 617–618
No Child Left Behind Act (NCLB) (2001), *448*
nondisabled, notion of, 521–522
nondiscrimination, occupational therapy's commitment to, 443–444
non-human environment, 299
normalcy, 808–816

O

OAA (Older Americans Act) (1965), *449*
occupation
    conceptual framework for, 117–119
    cultural contexts, 212–215, 297–302, 305–313
    definitions, 116–117, 442
    as ends, 150–151, 162–163
    and flow, 237–243
    and health, 399–405

as identity, 425–436
as means, 151–152, 163–169
nesting of levels, *162*
personal contexts, 218–222
philosophical ideas, 84–85
within a practice context, 134–136
relationship with well-being, 369
and sleep, 250–252
sociopolitical contexts, 215–218, 331–345
temporal contexts, 209–212, 227–233
theory of the human need for, 391–397
as treatment, 85–86
Occupation: Purposefulness and Meaningfulness as Therapeutic Mechanisms, Eleanor Clarke Slagle Lecture (1995), 159–170
occupational alienation, 357–358
occupational analysis, 606–607
occupational deprivation, 217, 345–350, 358–359
occupational disruption, 346. *see also* occupational deprivation
occupational dysfunction, 346. *see also* occupational deprivation
occupational imbalance, 360
occupational justice
    and client-centered practice, 353–362, *361, 362*
    exploratory theory of, *357*
    foundations to explore, *354*
    and sociopolitical contexts of occupation, 215–218
occupational marginalization, 359–360
occupational nurses, use of term, 23
occupational performance, conceptualization of, *161*
occupational perspective on balance, 260–263, *264*
occupational rights
    and critical occupational therapy, 368
    relationship with well-being, 369–370
occupational therapists
    Clinical Reasoning Study, 555–562
    and positioning, 192–193
occupational therapy
    American perspective, 739–742
    assumptions, 191–196, 587, 739
    asylums, *2*
    Canadian perspective, 743–747
    and client-centered practice, 480–482
    commitment to nondiscrimination and inclusion, 443–444

and community development, 757–762
court cases related to, 448–450
and culture, 192–193
definitions, 28–29
ethnographic approach, 502–503
ethos of, 789–803
and eudaimonic well-being, 383–384
evolution of, 724–728
future of, 728–731, 739–742, 743–747
history of, 37–56
as identity building, 435
influences, 83–84
at its best, *718*
legitimate activities for, 135–136
lessons learned, 31–33
monistic approaches, 202–204
and motion study, 594–595
National Society for the Promotion of Occupational Therapy, 56–58
phases of, 27
philosophy of, 63–67, 103
pluralistic approaches, 205–206
pragmatist readings of, 71–72
principles of, 1–5, *1*, 28–29, 46
profession of, 201–206
public knowledge of, 588–589
and rehabilitation, 87–88
role in World War I, 46–50
second generation, 29–31
and spirituality, 422–423
structuralist readings of, 73–74
theory, 191–192
traditional thinking, 587–588
as a unique service, 93–101
Occupational Therapy Can Be One of the Great Ideas of 20th-Century Medicine, Eleanor Clarke Slagle Lecture (1961), 93–101
Occupational Therapy Intervention Process Model, 136–142
Occupational Therapy Practice Framework, relevance of theory to, 111
Occupational Therapy Revisited: A Paraphrastic Journey, Eleanor Clarke Slagle Lecture (1981), 17–33
occupational well-being
    overview, 184–186
    addressing, 187
    background, 181–182
    case examples, 187–188
    factors influencing, 186–187
occupation-based practice
    models of, 119–122
    theoretical and conceptual frameworks, 109–113

occupations
    assumptions, 193–196
    within the asylum context, 10–11
occupatiotemporality, 230–231. *See also* time
Older Americans Act (OAA) (1965), *449*
Olmstead v. L.C. and E. W. (1999), *450*
Omnibus Budget Reconciliation Act (1987), *449*
ordeals, 409. *See also* adversity
Our Mandate for the New Millennium: Evidence-Based Practice, Eleanor Clarke Slagle Lecture (2000), 661–672
overt behaviors, 299

P

PAMs (physical agent modalities), 617–618
Parable of Two Frogs, 797
participation
    cultural contexts, 212–215, 297–302, 305–313
    personal contexts, 218–222
    in research, 707–708
    sociopolitical contexts, 215–218, 331–345
    and telehealth, 645
    temporal contexts, 209–212, 227–233
partnership, 478–479
patient care, excellence in, 733–737
paying attention, 176–177
peak experiences, 241. *See also* flow
Peloquin, Suzanne M., *Embracing Our Ethos, Reclaiming Our Heart* Eleanor Clarke Slagle Lecture (2005), 789–803
perceived self-efficacy, 507–516
perceptual cognitive impairments, Toglia's multicontext approach, 123
personal community, 333. *See also* inclusive communities
personal contexts of occupation, 218–222
personal performance accomplishments, 511–512
personal reflection, 576–579
persuasion, 512
philosophy of occupational therapy, 63–67, 103
phonophoresis, 617–618
physical agent modalities (PAMs), 617–618
physical dysfunction, models of practice, 160–162
physiological state, 512

Pinel, Philippe, 19–20
Plato, 84
plausibility, 691
pluralism, 201
political action, 582–583
positioning, and occupational therapists, 192–193
posttraumatic stress disorder (PTSD), 645
practice, and theory, 131–142
pragmatism
    overview, 70–72
    pragmatist–structuralist conversation, 74–77
privacy officer, definition, 643
probabilities, of effectiveness, 676
procedural reasoning, 556–558, 562
productive aging, 644
productivity, 194–195
professional ethos, 789–803
professional identity, 201–206
Professional Responsibility in Times of Change, Eleanor Clarke Slagle Lecture (1967), 749–755
protocol, definition, 643
psychiatrists, emergence of, 23
psychodynamic models of practice, 120–121
psychological well-being, and perceived self-efficacy, 511
PTSD (posttraumatic stress disorder), 645
public health, models of practice, 124
purpose, identification of, 413
purposefulness, as therapeutic mechanisms, 159–170
putting it all together, 562

Q

qualitative research, evaluating, 689–697

R

reasoning, types of, 555–562
reciprocity of motives, 559
Reed, Kathlyn L., *Tools of Practice: Heritage or Baggage?* Eleanor Clarke Slagle Lecture (1986), 599–607
reflexivity, critical, 519–527
refugeeism, 347–348. *See also* occupational deprivation
rehabilitation
    models of, 88–89
    and occupational therapy, 87–88
    and telehealth, 645
Rehabilitation Act (1973), *448*
Reilly, Mary, *Occupational Therapy Can Be One of the Great Ideas of 20th-*

Century Medicine, Eleanor Clarke Slagle Lecture (1961), 93–101
reintegration, law of, 408–409. *See also* adversity
relationship-centered care model, 490–492, *491*
research
    evaluating, 689–697
    politics and practices of, 703–708
resilience, 410–412. *See also* adversity
Resilience and Human Adaptability: Who Rises Above Adversity? Eleanor Clarke Slagle Lecture (1990), 407–417
responsibility, 478–479
restoration of movement models of practice, 120–121
The Retreat for Persons Afflicted With Disorders of the Mind, 20–21
Rush, Benjamin, 21–22
Rusk, H., 87–88

S

sanding blocks, 603–605, *604*
satisfaction, role in occupational health, 400–401, *400*
scholarship, of practice, 649–656, *650, 651*
scientific-mindedness, 312. *See also* cultural contexts of occupation
self
    conscious use of, 461–465
    relationships with, 472–473
self-care, 194–195
self-efficacy, 507–516
selfhood, interpersonal nature of, 429–430
self-monitoring analysis and reporting technology (SMART), 640
self-reflection, 499. *See also* ethnographic approach
sensory integrative models of practice, 122
short-wave diathermy, 617–618
Slagle, Eleanor Clarke. *See also* Eleanor Clarke Slagle Lectures
    address in honor of, 105–107
    biographical sketch of, 26–27, 50–51
    model of practice, 120
sleep
    literature review, 247–253
    regulating the sleep–wake cycle, 254
    scientific study of, 253–254
    and temporal contexts of occupation, 211
social model of disability, 465

social positions, 192–193
social responsibility, 610–612
Social Security Amendments (1965), *449*
social support, 412
sociocultural need for occupation, 395–397, *397*
sociopolitical contexts of occupation, 215–218, 331–345
spirituality, 220, 421–423
stigma, 433
storytelling, and illness, 565–567
stress, 283. *See also* balance
structuralism
   overview, 72–74
   pragmatist–structuralist conversation, 74–77
Studies in Invalid Occupations (Tracy 1913), 41–43
superficial thermal agents, 617–618
synchronous technologies, 640

T

technology
   and future models of practice, 124
   impact of, 346–347
telehealth, 627–646, *642*, *647–648*
temporal adaptation, 231–232. *See also* time
temporal contexts of occupation, 209–212, 227–233
temporal dysfunction, 231. *See also* time
TENS (transcutaneous electrical nerve stimulation), 617–618
theory, and practice, 131–142
therapeutic arts, 84
therapeutic emplotment, 570–573
therapeutic goals, 685–686
therapeutic power, 777–784, *778*
therapeutic relationships, 473–474
therapeutic ultrasound, 617–618
therapists, Clinical Reasoning Study, 555–562

time. *See also* temporal contexts of occupation
   and the concept of occupatiotemporality, 230–231
   as a context for occupation, 230
   historical perspective on, 227–229
   Koori time, 232
   meaningful use of, 348
   occupation as a consumer of, 229–230
   temporal adaptation, 231–232
   temporal dysfunction, 231
   white time, 232
Tools of Practice: Heritage or Baggage? Eleanor Clarke Slagle Lecture (1986), 599–607
Tracy, Susan Elizabeth, 23–24, 41–43
transcendence, role in occupational health, 403
transcutaneous electrical nerve stimulation (TENS), 617–618
trauma, 409–410. *See also* adversity
treating the whole person, 562
Trombly, Catherine A., *Occupation: Purposefulness and Meaningfulness as Therapeutic Mechanisms—* Eleanor Clarke Slagle Lecture (1995), 159–170
Tuke, William, 20
two frogs, parable of, 797

U

unique service, occupational therapy as, 93–101
Uniting Practice and Theory in an Occupational Framework, Eleanor Clarke Slagle Lecture (1998), 131–142
use of self, 461–465

V

values, meaning of, 722–723
vasopneumatic devices, 617–618
vicarious experience, 512

videoconferencing, 640
virtual reality (VR), 641
Vocational Rehabilitation Act, 215
vocational training, 46
Voltaire, 84–85
VR (virtual reality), 641

W

well-being
   and critical occupational therapy, 368–370
   eudaimonic well-being, 381–386
wellness, 645
wellness models of practice, occupational therapy, 124
West, Wilma L., *Professional Responsibility in Times of Change*, Eleanor Clarke Slagle Lecture (1967), 749–755
WFOT (World Federation of Occupational Therapists), position on human rights, 441–442
white time, 232. *See also* time
whole person, treating, 562
Why the Profession of Occupational Therapy Will Flourish in the 21st Century, Eleanor Clarke Slagle Lecture (1996), 109–113
will to overcome, 412. *See also* adversity
women patients, 21
work, and telehealth, 645–646
work-related programs, 605–606
World Federation of Occupational Therapists (WFOT), position on human rights, 441–442
World War I, role of OT in, 46–50

Y

York Retreat, 20–21
youth, telehealth service delivery for, 644

Citation Index

A

Aalten, P., 814
Abbott, M., 604
Abdel-Hafez, N., 177
Abler, R. R., 160
Abreu, B., 668, 669, 671, 799
Abreu, B. A., 799
Abu-Lughod, L., 309
Achat, H., 284
Achermann, P., 253
Acierno, R., 645
Acker, J., 694
Ada, L., 812
Adam, B., 228, 233
Adamovich, S. V., 641
Adams, J., 630
Adams, J. E., 413, 414
Adams, N. E., 160, 284, 432, 507, 509, 514, 515
Adang, E., 454
Addams, J., 602
Adelson, H. L., 356
Adlai-Gail, W., 240
Adler, M., 84
Agnew NM, Pyke SW, 549
Agostino, P., 271
Agras, W. S., 586
Ahles, T. A., 645
Ahlschwede, K., 75, 536
Aitchison, C., 195
Albert, M., 284
Albert, S., 78
Albert, S. M., 497, 499
Albrecht, G., 382, 384
Alderman, N., 814
Aldridge, D., 422
Alessi, C. A., 780
Alford, C., 247
Algado, S. S., 192, 384, 385, 386, 757, 761
Allebrandt, K., 254
Allen, C. K., 814
Allen, E., 287
Allen, J., 694

Allen, J. K., 507, 514, 515
Allport, G. W., 552
Alsaker, S., 229
Altheide, D. L., 697
Altman, I., 781
Amar, J., 593
Ambrosi, E., 86, 87
Amoroso, B., 183, 184, 185, 187, 383, 761
Amundson, S. J. C., 123
Amy, C., 260
Anderson, A., 175
Anderson, E., 381, 382
Anderson, J., 462
Anderson, M. L., 792
Andi, R., 72
Andonian, L., 305
Anedda, A., 271
Anson, C. A., 196
Anthony, E. J., 408, 411
Antonovsky, A., 285, 286, 434
Applebaum, R. A., 435
Arai, S., 385
Arand, D. L., 254
Arendt, J. F., 254
Argyle, A., 402, 403
Argyris, C., 725
Aristotle, 84, 85
Arluke, A., 87, 134, 605
Armstrong, D., 693, 695
Armstrong, H., 356
Árnadóttir, G., 813, 814
Arnsten, S. M., 461
Asaba, E., 183, 185, 186, 383
Asarnow, R. F., 142
Ash, A., 485, 488
Asplund, K., 142
Astin, J., 176, 177
Astin, J. A., 623
Atchison, B. T., 815
Athenes, S., 165, 166
Atkinson, P., 690
Attree, E. A., 641
Aubin, G., 250
Austin, J. T., 676

Austin, N., 734
Aveni, A., 232
Aviles, A., 453
Avrech-Bar, M., 186, 247, 385
Avsec, A., 175
Ayele, H., 422
Ayrer, K., 185
Ayres, A. J., 75, 122, 132, 167, 649, 781
Aytch, L. S., 451
Azari, R., 485, 492

B

Baarends, E. M., 814
Bach, R., 744
Bachmann, K. D., 279
Backman, C., 285, 286, 346, 348, 434, 758
Backman, C. L., 645
Backman, L., 126
Bacon, N., 537
Badiani, C., 453
Baer, B., 802
Baer, R., 175
Baer, R. A., 179
Bagnall, J., 783
Bailey, D., 610, 612, 613
Bailey, D. B., 451
Bailey, G., 192
Bailey, S., 454
Baird, P., 422
Baker, N., 628, 646
Bakhtin, M. M., 309
Baksh, L., 229
Bakshi, R., 168
Baldwin, B. T., 86, 87, 594, 595
Balfour, J. L., 263
Baltes, P. B., 499
Bandura, A., 160, 284, 432, 507, 508, 509, 510, 511, 512, 513, 514, 515
Banko, K., 282
Banks, S., 757
Baptiste, S., 138, 242, 305, 348, 462, 477, 478, 479, 481, 483, 485, 489, 514, 516, 575, 758

Baptiste, W., 622
Barlow, I. G., 628, 645
Barnes, C., 358, 692, 694, 697
Barnes, K. J., 452
Barnes, P. M., 621
Barney, K. F., 213, 305
Barnitt, R., 693, 694, 697
Barrett, L., 69
Barrett-Bernstein, S., 814, 815
Barriatua, R. D., 482
Barris, R., 300, 513
Barrows, M., 159, 160
Barry, K., 694
Bartlett, J., 779
Barton, G. E., 38, 40, 41, 52, 54, 56,
    121, 211, 605, 793, 795
Bass, S. L., 272
Bassett, H., 421
Bass-Haugen, J., 109, 757, 758
Batavia, A. I., 433, 450
Bateson, M. C., 184, 425
Bauer, J., 384, 386
Baum, A., 284
Baum, C., 109, 124, 125, 136, 149,
    157, 160, 162, 229, 230, 237, 247,
    248, 250, 251, 252, 261, 273, 306,
    461, 475, 514, 575, 670, 758, 798,
    814
Baum, C. M., 814
Baum, S., 162, 163, 402
Bauman, A., 645
Bauman, Z., 193
Baumeister, R. F., 426, 428, 431, 432,
    434, 435
Baxendale, B., 479
Baxter, J., 287, 691, 692, 693, 696,
    697
Beagan, B., 757
Bean, J., 175
Bean, J. P., 260
Beck, A. J., 452
Beck, A. T., 85
Becker, D. M., 507, 514, 515
Becker, H., 510, 515
Beckett, L., 284
Beckung, E., 272, 273
Bedell, G., 681, 683
Bedell, G. M., 273
Beers, C. W., 45
Beilock, S. L., 814
Beisecker, A. E., 488, 492
Beisecker, T. D., 492
Beisser, A., 399, 400, 403, 741
Bejerholm, U., 229, 230
Belcham, C., 423
Belenky, M. F., 559
Belk, S. S., 511
Bell, L. V., 7, 8, 9, 12, 13, 14

Bell, R. A., 485, 492
Bellardinelli, R., 271
Belle Brown, J., 490
Bellin, B., 653
Bendixen, H., 229
Bendixen, R., 644, 645
Benedict, R. H. B., 142
Benloucif, S., 254
Benner, P., 499, 568, 569
Bennett, B., 644, 645
Bennett, J., 652
Bennett, R. L., 604
Bennett, S., 652, 814, 815
Bennett, T. L., 815
Berckman, L., 284
Beresford, S., 248
Berger, P., 559
Bergman, U., 142
Berkeley, G., 381
Berkey, C., 284
Berkman, L., 284
Bernard, J., 259
Bernard, P. M., 272
Bernard, S. L., 453, 458
Bernheimer, L. P., 451
Bernspång, B., 142, 401
Bernstein, N., 164
Bernstein, R. J., 559
Berry, J. W., 306
Bertaux, D., 693
Betteridge, D., 271
Betz, K., 645
Bhagwanjee, A., 196
Bhakta, P., 195
Bhambhani, Y., 168
Bhavnani, K.-K., 694, 697
Bibas, G., 814, 815
Bibeau, D., 582
Bickenbach, J., 213, 400, 405
Bielby, D. D., 260
Bielby, W. T., 260
Biffi, A., 271
Biley, F. C., 492
Billings, A., 408
Billingsley, F. F., 452
Bindon, J. R., 306
Bing, R. K., 7, 38, 215, 434, 790
Birch, D., 704
Birnbaum, R., 272, 273
Bissell, J., 534
Bittman, M., 347
Black, R. M., 305, 609
Blain, J., 477
Blair, D., 259
Blair, S., 534
Blair, S. E., 358
Blau, L., 809
Bleiberg, J., 254

Blesedell Crepeau, E., 248
Bliese, P., 285
Bliwise, D. L., 780
Bloch, M. W., 169
Block, P., 526
Blodgett, M. L., 604
Blok, H., 451
Bloom, B., 621
Bloomer, J. S., 586
Blute, R., 179
Boake, C., 813
Bockhoven, J. S., 23, 83
Boeshart, L. K., 809
Boian, R., 641
Boian, R. F., 641
Boissiere, L., 273
Boisvenu, M., 362
Bok, D., 382
Bolin, R., 411
Bond, J., 279, 454
Bonder, B., 311
Bonder, B. R., 307, 311, 312, 514
Bondoc, S., 537
Bonham, A., 229
Boniface, G., 382, 653
Bonilla, J. M., 645
Boninger, M. L., 628, 641
Bonnell, C., 696
Bonner, G., 178
Bonnet, M. H., 254
Booker, C., 807, 808, 809, 810
Booth, A., 669
Booth, M. L., 272
Bootzin, R., 179
Borbely, A. A.F., 253
Borell, L., 183, 185, 186, 280, 286,
    355, 356, 358, 383
Bores, A., 356
Borg, B., 109, 461
Borgetto, B., 653
Borkovec, T. D., 586
Borlund, K., 696
Borris, E., 602
Borson, S., 142
Borstad, A., 628, 645
Borthwick, B., 644, 645
Boshoff, K., 186
Bosma, H., 263
Boua, X. M., 347, 348
Bouchard, S., 645
Boud, D., 783
Bourdieu, P., 519
Bourke-Taylor, H., 213, 214
Bouwens, S. F., 814
Bouzit, M., 629
Bowen, R., 462, 575
Bowen, R. E., 138, 139
Bowman, M., 809

Bow-Thomas, C. C., 452
Boyd, K., 483
Boyd, R., 274, 537
Boyer, E., 783
Boyers, L., 487, 490
Boyt Schell, B. A., 248
Bracciano, A. G., 617
Brach, T., 176, 177
Brachtesende, A., 622
Bradford, D. L., 735
Bramwell, D. B., 716
Bränholm, I. B., 163
Branneck, R., 645
Brannen, J., 694, 697
Brannon, J. A., 628, 629, 632, 633
Braverman, H., 392
Brayman, S. J., 814
Brechin, A., 191, 692, 693, 697
Breines, E. B., 70, 125, 237, 766
Brennan, D., 628, 630
Brennan, M. C., 604
Brewer, B. R., 641
Brewer, B. W., 435
Brienza, D., 628
Brienza, D. M., 628, 629, 641, 645
Briffad, T., 645
Brigham, A., 7, 10
Brighton, C., 142
Brintnell, E. S., 765
Brintnell, S., 87, 88, 477
Britt, T., 285
Britton, B., 286
Brock, L., 585
Brodie, M., 650
Brontë, E., 343
Brooke, M., 666
Brookfield, J., 483
Brooks, R. H., 142
Broome, K., 229, 230
Broomfield, N. M. F., 253, 254
Brosnan, S., 537
Brouillard, 509
Brown, A. K., 665
Brown, C., 109, 136, 140, 209, 230,
    411, 413, 462, 479, 575, 662, 667
Brown, G., 282
Brown, G. D., 630
Brown, J., 628, 630, 757
Brown, K. W., 175, 176, 178
Brown, L., 185, 287
Brown, S., 382
Brown, S. M., 462
Browne, J., 519
Browne, S. E., 411
Broyard, A., 414
Bruce, A., 178
Bruce, C., 645
Bruce, H., 84

Bruce, M. A., 109, 461
Bruder, M., 451
Bruner, J., 162, 163, 167, 430, 559,
    565, 566
Brunner, E., 263
Brunnstrom, S., 131
Brunyate, R., 210, 215, 809, 812
Bryant, W., 422
Bryce, J., 175
Bryze, K., 815
Buchler, J., 560
Buck, M. M., 52, 53, 298, 794, 799
Bucknill, J. C., 22
Bull, J., 422
Bundy, A. C., 132, 779
Bunting, M., 195, 196
Burdea, G., 641
Burdea, G. C., 629, 641
Burgess, P. W., 814
Burgio, L. D., 666, 811
Burke, J., 711
Burke, J. P., 44, 74, 75, 83, 84, 89,
    148, 150, 209, 238, 247, 299, 452,
    565, 599, 740
Burket, A., 213
Burkhardt, A., 621, 622
Burnett, C. N., 163, 497
Burnett, S., 741
Burr, V., 520
Burright, R. G., 813
Bursell, J., 421, 423
Burton, D., 630
Burton, S., 693, 697
Bury, T., 662, 667, 668
Bush, M. A., 168
Butler, C., 810
Butler, S., 259
Butterfield, T., 628, 645
Buurke, J. H., 810
Buysse, D., 287
Buysse, V., 451
Bye, R. A., 667

C

Cabot, R., 734
Cacciatore, J., 139, 143
Cacioppo, J. T., 284
Cafferata, G. L., 497
Cain, C., 306, 308, 309, 310
Calfas, K., 271
Callahan, L. F., 142
Cameron, C., 524
Cameron, J., 282
Cameron, K., 272
Cameron, R. G., 160
Camilli, G., 663, 664
Campbell, A. V., 422
Campbell, D., 685

Campbell, D. T., 676
Campbell, J., 384
Campbell, M., 361, 628, 630
Campbell, P. H., 123
Camporese, R., 279
Cancian, F. M., 691
Canning, C. G., 812
Cannon, J., 252
Cantin, N., 183, 184, 185, 187, 383, 761
Cara, E., 248
Cardona, C. E., 757, 761
Cardwell, M. T., 765
Cardwell, T., 87, 88, 90
Carli, M., 238, 239, 240, 241, 242
Carlisle, S., 381, 383, 385
Carlon, R., 271
Carlova, J., 49, 51, 792, 794, 800
Carlson, E. T., 7, 8
Carlson, G., 192
Carlson, L., 176, 177
Carlson, M., 75, 175, 238, 239, 241,
    242, 251, 435, 776
Carlson, M. E., 126, 133, 151, 160,
    162, 251, 775
Carmer, D. R., 534
Carmody, J., 175, 179
Caron, J. S., 758
Caron, S., 359, 362
Caron Santha, J., 184
Caron-Parker, L. M., 478
Carpenter, C., 690, 691, 692, 694,
    695, 696, 697
Carpenter, S., 694, 695, 696
Carr, J. H., 126
Carr, T. H., 814
Carreon, D., 454
Carrier, J., 287
Carrigan, M., 230
Carroll, R. S., 792
Carrougher, G. J., 641
Carskadon, M. A., 247, 780
Carstensen, L. L., 287
Carswell, A., 138, 348, 481, 483, 579
Carswell-Opzoomer, A., 242, 478,
    514, 516
Carter, M., 260
Carter, W. B., 482
Cartwright, D. S., 586
Cartwright, R. D., 586
Casals, P., 473
Case, T., 273
Case-Smith, J., 667
Cason, J., 537, 627, 628, 629, 632,
    633, 640, 642, 644
Cassidy, A., 582
Cassidy, C. M., 622
Cassidy, J., 711
Cassidy, T., 269, 271

Cermak, S., 744
Cermak, S. A., 664, 667
Cerulo, K. A., 306
Cervaro, R. M., 361
Cervero, R., 532
Chacham, A., 142
Chamberlain, K., 285
Chambers, N., 286
Chan, W. K., 622
Chandler, C., 423
Chang, R. H., 260
Channon, S., 814
Chaplin, J. P., 606
Chapman, R. M., 249
Chapman, S., 269, 270
Chapparo, C. J., 185
Charles, C., 485
Charles, J. R., 811
Charmaz, K., 433
Charmé, S. L., 192
Chaytor, N., 814
Cherryholmes, C. H., 71, 73, 74
Chesney, M. A., 677
Chess, S., 411
Cheung, C. K., 621
Chiang, M., 192
Childs, P., 191
Chilingaryan, G., 272, 273
Chilton, H., 765
Chinnan, A., 811
Chiou, I. L., 163, 497
Chiu, T., 537
Chochinov, H., 422
Chokron, N., 273
Chow, S., 381
Christiana, D., 628, 630
Christiansen, C., 75, 109, 116, 125,
    136, 151, 160, 162, 184, 185, 186,
    195, 212, 213, 229, 230, 233, 247,
    248, 250, 251, 252, 254, 261, 279,
    280, 283, 284, 286, 287, 306, 358,
    422, 489, 513, 514, 599, 757, 758,
    759, 779
Christiansen, C. H., 251, 285, 286,
    346, 348, 434
Chronister, K., 645
Chu, K. Y., 526
Chubon, R. A., 193
Chumbler, N., 645
Chung, J., 381
Churchill, L. R., 789
Ciardi, J., 469
Cioffi, D., 509
Cipriani, J., 185
Clark, C., 497
Clark, F., 75, 150, 161, 162, 175, 184,
    193, 229, 230, 237, 238, 239, 241,
    242, 247, 250, 251, 346, 347, 395,
    435, 759, 775, 776

Clark, F. A., 72, 126, 133, 138, 151,
    160, 162, 232, 233, 251, 288, 339,
    489, 490, 603, 652, 711, 775, 776,
    781, 782
Clark, F. P., 134
Clark, G. F., 356
Clark, J., 358, 461, 575, 576
Clark, L., 576, 579
Clark, P. G., 628
Clarke, C. K., 86
Clayton, D. K., 704
Clayton, K. S., 193
Cleary, P. D., 78
Cleary-Guida, M. B., 623
Clements, E., 262, 263
Clemson, L., 305, 306, 309
Cleveland, M., 411
Clifford, J., 308, 311
Clinchy, B. M., 559
Clipp, E. C., 411
Close, J., 665
Clouston, T., 381
Coakle, E., 284
Coates, L. M. A., 814
Cockburn, L., 757, 759, 760, 761
Coelho, G. V., 413, 414
Coffey, M. S., 596
Cohen, A. R., 735
Cohen, D., 779
Cohen, F., 411
Cohen, L., 628
Cohler, B. J., 408, 411, 415
Cohn, E., 462
Cohn, E. S., 248, 447, 452, 558, 664
Colditz, G., 284
Cole, J. M., 164
Coleman, P., 422
Coles, R., 411, 413, 565, 735
Collins, C., 497
Collins, E., 692
Collins, E. L., 808, 809
Collins, J. C., 796, 798
Collins, K., 279
Collins, P. H., 192, 193, 693
Colman, W., 88
Colver, A., 272, 273
Colver, A. F., 271, 273, 274
Condillac, E. B., 18, 19
Connaughton, J. A., 664
Connor, A., 758
Connor, L. T., 814
Connors, C., 524
Connors, D., 411
Conroy, B., 628, 645
Conti, R., 383, 384
Cook, A., 621, 622
Cook, E. W., 811
Cook, J., 575, 697
Cook, J. A., 696

Cook, J. V., 133, 185, 359, 462, 485,
    490, 579, 695, 697
Cook, T. D., 676
Cookson, R., 356
Cooley, C. H., 429
Cooper, A., 650
Cooper, B., 141, 209, 338, 369, 370,
    761
Cooper, B. A., 454
Cooper, G., 48, 220, 222, 792
Cooper, J., 248
Cooper, L., 489
Cooper, M., 279
Cooper, R., 628
Cooper, R. A., 628, 641
Copeland, B., 361
Copley, F. B., 733
Corbin, J., 691
Corcoran, M., 454, 497, 498, 500
Corcoran, M. A., 497, 502
Corcos, D. M., 164
Coren, S., 779, 780, 781
Corr, S., 382
Corring, D. J., 462, 485, 490, 579,
    695, 697
Costello, A., 814
Coster, W., 73, 75, 663, 744, 775, 776,
    784
Cottrell, R. P., 215, 373, 835, 837
Coughlin, L. D., 556
Coulter, I. D., 622
Cousins, N., 411, 413, 473
Covalt, D. A., 809, 812
Cox, D., 645
Cox, D. L., 249, 254
Cox, J., 422
Coyte, M. E., 422
Crabree, J., 356
Crabtree, J., 611
Crabtree, J. L., 478
Craft, L., 284
Crago, J. E., 811
Craik, C., 229, 230, 250
Craik, J., 520
Crane, B. T., 793, 794
Crawford, D., 272, 734
Creek, J., 194, 248, 381, 383, 386
Crepeau, E. B., 447
Cress, E., 142
Crewe, N. M., 404
Crichton, A., 373
Crist, P. A. H., 514
Cross, G., 779
Crotty, M., 520
Crow, L., 520, 521
Crowe, T., 537
Crowe, T. K., 209
Crowne, D. P., 432
Csikszentmihalyi, I., 239, 240

Csikszentmihalyi, M., 84, 175, 176, 177, 178, 238, 239, 240, 241, 242, 261, 265, 287, 393, 401, 403, 739, 781, 803
Cubie, S. H., 596
Cullimore, A. R., 791
Cummings, R. G., 665
Cummins, R. A., 281
Curtin, L., 799
Curtin, M., 652
Cusick, A., 652, 653
Cusick, C. P., 453
Cuskelly, M., 274
Cwiek, M. A., 632
Cynkin, S., 151, 163, 164, 167, 213, 237, 596, 599, 600, 776, 784

D

Dahlin-Ivanoff, S., 281
Dain, N., 7, 8, 9, 10, 11, 13
Dale, A. E., 690
Dale, L. M., 220
Daloz, L., 337
Daly, K., 230
Damiano, D., 810
Dance, F., 331, 340
D'Andrade, R., 306
Daniels, N., 356
Darkins, A., 645
Darnell, J. L., 127
Darnell, R., 195
Darr, K., 609, 611
Darragh, A. R., 461, 462
Darrah, J., 810
Dashiell J F, 392
Daub, M., 508
Davidson, G., 332, 334
Davidson, H. A., 138
Davidson, M., 521, 523
Davies, B., 178, 519
Davies, G. K., 799
Davies, P., 228
Davis, C., 665
Davis, E. U., 605
Davis, J., 183, 184, 185, 186, 187, 383, 758, 761, 779
Davis, J. A., 274
Davis, L. A., 454
Davis, L. J., 521, 522
Davis, R. B., 623
Davis-Berman, J., 511
Davison, J., 454
Dawson, D. R., 814
Dawson, P., 454
Dawson, S. J., 628, 645
Day, D., 183
Day, K., 454
De Laat, D., 421, 422
de Saint-Exupéry, A., 796, 797, 803

Deal, A. G., 356, 490
Deal, T. E., 734, 735
Dean, A. H., 809
Debats, D. L., 428
deBrisay, A., 3
DeBusk, R. F., 512
Deci, E. L., 280, 282, 283, 284, 285, 287, 383, 384, 385
Deegan, P., 354, 356, 362
DeGrazia, J., 287
Deitz, J., 452
Dekker, J., 454
DeKuiper, W. P., 169
Delbridge, A., 259
Delle Fave, A., 238, 239, 240, 242
Delvecchio-Good, M. J., 567
Dement, W. C., 247, 780
Demos, E. V., 411
Denney-Wilson, E., 272
Dennis, M., 454
Dennis, M. P., 454
Denzin, N. K., 70
DePoy, E., 497
Derwent, G., 641
Desmarais, G., 273
Deutsch, A., 8, 9, 11, 12
Deutsch, J. E., 641
Deveney, R., 213
Devereaux, E., 462
Devers, K. J., 689
Devlieger, P., 382, 384
Devlin, R., 195
Dew, M., 287
Dewey, J., 70, 71, 76, 559
Dhanani, S., 644
D'Huyvetter, K., 622
Di Sante, E., 599
Diamond, B. J., 645
Diamond, P. M., 452
Diana-Rigby, G., 666
Dickie, V., 214, 758, 759, 779, 781
Dickinson, H. O., 272, 273
Dicocco, M., 452
Diener, E., 383, 432
Dierette, D., 652, 653
Dietz-Waschkowski, B., 179
Digby, A., 7, 12
Dige, M., 381
Dillard, M., 305
Diller, J., 610
Dimsdale, J. E., 411
Dipboye, R. L, Phillips, A. P., 286
Dishman, R., 284
do Rozario, L., 242
Dobbins, T., 272
Dobkin, P., 178
Doble, S., 112, 184, 381, 383, 386, 478, 758
Dodder, R. A., 260

Dokecki, P. R., 478
Dolan, P., 356, 382, 383, 385
Donald, A., 681, 686
Donnelly, C., 579
Donner, A., 490
Donovan, J. M., 209
Donovick, P. J., 813
Dorsch, S., 812
Dosse, F., 72, 73
Dott, N., 650, 716
Doucet, A., 695
Downs, M. L., 271
Dray, H., 567
Dray, W., 567
Dressler, W. W., 306
Dreyer, K. A., 628
Dreyer, N. C., 628
Dreyfus, H. L., 176, 559, 565
Dreyfus, S. E., 559, 565
Driver, M., 604
Dromerick, A. W., 814
Drost, J., 428
Drouin, M. S., 645
Drucker, P. F., 733, 734
Dubos, R., 724, 725, 726, 728, 730
Dubouloz, C.-J., 670, 671, 683
Dubus, A., 741
Dudgeon, K., 284
Dugan, T. F., 411, 413
Dugas, C., 165, 166
Duncan, E., 382
Duncan, E. A. S., 196
Duncan, M., 248, 356
Duncombe, L., 237, 238
Dunn, W., 109, 123, 136, 140, 209, 230, 362, 479, 612, 613, 649
Dunst, C., 451
Dunst, C. J., 356, 483, 490
Dunton, W. R. J., 1, 2, 4, 18, 24, 25, 40, 41, 43, 44, 45, 46
Duran, L., 141
Dyck, I., 305, 359, 362, 525

E

Eakman, A., 758
Eastabrook, S., 229
Edelman, G., 739
Edgar, D., 260
Edgerton, W. B., 587
Edmonson, E., 645
Edwards, C., 695
Edwards, D. F., 814
Edwards, R., 695
Eeg-Olofsson, A., 362
Efran, J. S., 585
Eftekhar, P., 758
Egan, M., 382, 421, 422, 670, 671, 683
Egendorf, A., 411

Eide, H., 490, 492
Einstein, A., 228
Eisenberg, D. M., 623
Eisenberg, L., 567
Ekirch, A. R., 252
Eklund, M., 185, 195, 229, 230, 247, 254, 280, 285, 286
Elbaum, B., 452
Elder, G. H. Jr., 411
Ellis, M., 665
Ellis, M. G., 667
Ellis, W. C., 21
Elrod, M., 644
Elstein, A., 556
Emanuel, E. J., 356, 485, 486, 487, 489, 492
Emanuel, L. L., 485, 486, 487, 489, 492
Emerson, R. W., 70, 71, 210
Emery, G., 85
Ende, J., 485, 488
Engel, G. L., 195
Engel, J. D., 689, 695
Engelhardt, H. T., 7, 83, 339, 586
Engelke, P., 359
Engel-Yager, B., 272
Engeser, S., 210
England, K., 694
Englehardt, T., 425, 436
English, C. B., 599
Engquist, D., 421, 422
Enticknap, A., 641
Epstein, R., 176, 179
Eriksen, E. L., 272
Erikson, E. H., 287, 428, 560
Eriksson, S., 142
Erklandsson, L. K., 232, 233
Erlandsson, L., 247, 254, 286
Erlandsson, L. K., 195, 280
Erlandsson, L-K., 185, 229, 280
Escandi, J. P., 724, 725, 726, 728, 730
Espie, C. A., 253, 254
Esseveld, J., 694
Estroff, S. E., 433
Ettner, S. L., 623
Eva, G., 196, 692
Evans, D, 284
Evans, G., 781
Evans, J., 480
Evans, K., 133, 237
Evans, R., 697
Everly, G. S. Jr., 409
Evert, M. M., 305
Ewart, C. K., 507, 508, 509, 512, 514, 515
Eyles, J., 691, 692, 693, 696, 697

F

Faderman, L., 347
Fagan, M., 641

Faig, S., 185
Falardeau, M., 361, 489, 490
Fanchiang, S. P. C., 782
Fang, M., 644
Fange, A., 453
Farb, N. A., 175
Farber, S., 649
Fardeau, M., 433
Faris, P. D., 142
Farnworth, L., 227, 229, 231, 232, 233, 250, 252, 537
Farrar, C. B., 86
Farrar, J. E., 422
Farrell, K. H., 666
Fasick, S. B., 453, 458
Fatima, Z., 175
Fauconnier, J., 272, 273
Favill, J., 602
Fawcett, L. C., 668
Fazio, L., 362, 779
Fearing, V., 358, 461, 575, 576, 579
Fearing, V. G., 768
Fedden, T., 382
Fee, M., 622
Feeney, L., 421
Feinstein, A. R., 556
Feletti, G., 783
Ferguson-Paré, M., 768
Fernandez, R., 645
Fernie, G. R., 433
Ferraro, G., 192
Ferrell, B., 422
Fetters, L., 142
Fidler, G., 1, 109, 121, 230, 535, 719, 792
Fidler, G. S., 84, 122, 209, 219, 237, 299, 431, 559, 779
Fidler, J. W., 84, 122, 209, 219, 237, 299, 431, 559
Fiebert, M., 282
Fiechtl, B., 644
Figueredo, A., 179
Fine, M., 526
Fine, S. B., 75, 220, 497, 498, 502, 588, 797
Finger, A., 195
Finkel, S. I., 254
Finlay, L., 248, 252
Finlayson, M., 765
Finn, G., 216, 795
Finset, A., 490, 492
Fiorentino, M. R., 73, 599, 649
Firouzan, P., 633
Fisher, A. C., 479
Fisher, A. G., 75, 110, 132, 133, 134, 138, 139, 140, 141, 252, 779, 792, 814, 815
Fisher, G., 711, 761
Fiske, D., 685

Fitzgerald, M. H., 305, 306, 309
Fitzgerald, S., 628
Fitzpatrick, M., 384
Fitzpatrick, R., 272
Flach, F., 408
Flachs, E. M., 272
Flaherty, J. F., 287
Fleharty, K., 121
Fleming, M., 69, 75, 152, 478, 502, 776, 783
Fleming, M. A., 502
Fleming, M. H., 168, 416, 500, 555, 558, 559
Fleming-Castaldy, R., 833, 835, 837
Fleming-Castaldy, R. P., 215, 649, 650, 652, 655
Fletcher, B. L., 550
Fliers, E., 781
Flores, O., 305
Flower, J., 768, 771
Flynn, M., 696
Fogler, H. S., 783
Foley, J. P., 743
Folger, T., 228
Folkman, S., 408, 411, 514
Follett, M. P., 734
Fonow, M. M., 696
Fontane, C., 121
Forbes, C., 814
Forbes, E. S., 604
Ford, L. H., 427
Forducey, P. G., 645
Forster, E. M., 566
Forster, L., 645
Forsyth, K., 649, 650, 651, 655, 656, 761
Forsyth, R. J., 271, 273, 274
Fortenberry, J. D., 497
Forwell, S., 305
Fossey, E., 227, 462
Foucault, M., 12, 707, 782
Fougeyrollas, P., 272, 273
Fourie, M., 758
Fox, M., 734
Frampton, G., 665
Franits, L. E., 526
Frank, A. W., 524
Frank, E., 287
Frank, G., 126, 133, 151, 160, 161, 162, 193, 237, 238, 242, 251, 425, 656, 695, 775, 781
Frank, J. D., 586
Frank, L., 359
Frankel, R. M., 692
Frankl, V. E., 285, 403, 413
Franks, D. D., 426, 432
Frantis, L., 653
Freedman, B., 176, 177
Freedman, S. B., 645

Freguja, C., 279
Freidland, J., 534
Freire, P., 520, 527
French, D., 269
French, S., 195
Fretz, B. R., 160
Freud, S., 403, 472
Frey, B. S., 421
Fricke, J., 229
Friedland, J., 5, 85, 237, 362
Friedman, I., 534
Friedson, E., 89, 90
Friesema, J., 711
Fritz, B., 175
Froehlich, J., 88
Fromm, E., 97, 349, 471
Frone, M., 279
Fuchs, H. A., 142
Fugl-Meyer, A. R., 142, 163
Fujita, F., 432
Fukkink, R., 451
Fulford, B., 422
Fuller, C. A., 780, 781
Furlong, B., 215

G

Gable, S. L., 280
Gabriel, L., 215
Gafni, A., 485
Gage, M., 432, 464, 507, 513, 514, 579
Gal, R., 413
Galanti, G., 307
Galheigo, S. M., 215, 525
Galinsky, E., 279
Gallagher, T. E., 644
Gallew, H., 230
Gallimore, R., 451
Galt, J. M., 9, 10, 11
Galvin, B., 667
Galvin, E., 487, 490
Gannon, S., 519
Gardner, H., 559, 560, 566
Garmezy, N., 411
Garry, H., 645
Gassaway, J., 810
Gebhardt, E., 451
Geertz, C., 306, 559, 778
Gell, A., 228
Gellner, E., 779
Genender, E., 411
George, S., 478, 480
Georgopoulos, A. P., 165
Gergen, K. J., 430
Gergen, M. M., 430
Gerhardt, K. A., 453
Germain, V., 645
Gheorghiu, S., 422
Giada, F., 271

Gibson, J. J., 287
Gideon, P., 665
Giese, T., 621, 622
Gifford, A. L., 677
Gilbert, P., 422
Gilbreth, F. B., 593, 594
Gilbreth, L. M., 593, 594, 595
Gilfoyle, E., 84, 116, 331, 337, 339, 461, 653, 718, 795
Gilfoyle, E. M., 813
Gill, A., 411, 412
Gill, C., 334, 335
Gillen, G., 649, 650, 652, 655, 717, 718
Gillette, N., 649
Gillette, N. P., 531, 555
Gilligan, C., 559
Gillilan, R. E., 507, 508, 509, 514, 515
Gilpin, A., 768, 769, 771
Girard, P., 629, 645
Giroux, H., 347
Gist, M., 512, 515
Gitlin, L., 454, 497
Gitlin, L. N., 454, 497, 498, 500, 502, 503
Gladwell, M., 766
Glanz, K., 582
Glaser, R., 284
Glass, R. M., 492
Glass, T., 284
Glegg, S. M. N., 650, 652
Glei, D., 284
Glendinning, C., 526
Gliner, J., 421, 422
Gliner, J. A., 693
Glucksman, E., 665
Godbey, G., 233, 279, 286
Godfrey, A., 381
Goertzel, M. G., 411
Goertzel, V., 411
Goffman, E., 433, 524
Goldberg, M., 284
Goldberger, N. R., 559
Goldman, N., 284
Goldstein, B., 692
Goldstein, M., 628
Goleman, D., 408
Golledge, J., 251, 758
Gonzales, V. M., 677
Good, B., 567, 690
Goode, W. J., 280
Goodman, N., 779
Gordijn, M., 254
Gordon, A. M., 811
Gorelick, S., 693
Gosling, A., 693, 695
Grabowecky, B. R., 369
Grady, A., 331, 337, 339

Grady, A. P., 75, 216, 339, 813
Graef, R., 241
Graff, M., 454
Graham, G., 670
Graham, R., 284
Grammenos, S., 356
Granieri, E., 666
Grant, S., 451
Graugaard, P., 490, 492
Gray, J. A. M., 662, 663, 665, 666, 667, 668, 669, 681, 686
Gray, J. M., 148, 151, 353, 662, 665, 670, 776, 784
Green, A., 249
Green, L., 282
Greenfield, P. M., 313
Greenfield, S., 482, 483
Greenhalgh, T., 683
Greenhaus, J., 279
Greenleaf, R. K., 770
Greeno, J., 559
Greenwald, A. G., 429
Greenwood, D. J., 708
Griffin, M. R., 665
Griffin, S., 361
Griffiths, P., 628, 645
Gritzer, G., 87, 134, 605
Grob, G. N., 7, 8, 10, 11, 12, 13
Groce, N., 334
Groff, D. G., 271
Groomes, T. E., 811
Gros, D. F., 645
Grossman, P., 179
Grossman, W., 582
Guadagnoli, E., 485, 490, 492
Guay, S., 645
Guba, E. G., 690, 691, 694
Gubrium, J. F., 497
Guihan, M., 692
Gullone, E., 281
Gums, J., 800
Gunn, M., 263
Gupta, J., 215
Gurney, G. W., 604
Gurung, R., 284
Gutierrez-Mayka, M., 497
Gutman, S., 1, 5, 109, 652, 653, 711
Guy, J. R., 353
Guyatt. G., 483
Guyton, A. C., 779
Guze, B., 287
Gwyer, J., 696

H

Haas, L. J., 83, 159, 595, 611
Haber, S., 733
Haberman, D. L., 70
Hachey, R., 250
Hack, L. M., 696

Hafsteinsdóttir, T., 652
Hagedorn, R., 139, 231, 250, 251
Hagen, A. S., 282
Hagerty, M., 282
Hahn, M., 814
Hahn, T., 644
Håkansson, C., 281
Halcon, L. L., 621
Hales, J. W., 630
Haley, W., 454
Hall, E. T., 781, 782
Hall, H., 54, 121, 533, 602, 603, 605,
    714, 795
Hall, H. J., 52, 53, 298, 794, 799
Hall, J. A., 482
Haltiwanger, E., 536
Hamburg, D. A., 413, 414
Hamby, D., 451
Hamilton Halcomb, J., 240
Hammal, D., 273
Hammell, K. W., 184, 186, 191, 192,
    193, 194, 270, 271, 362, 369, 381,
    382, 384, 385, 386, 519, 520, 525,
    526, 654, 689, 690, 691, 692, 693,
    694, 695, 696, 697, 759, 761
Hammer, G. S., 433
Hammersley, M., 691, 696
Hammond, A., 248
Hammond, K. H., 559
Han, S., 240, 241
Handwerker, W. P., 306
Handzo, G., 422
Hanh, T. N., 260
Hanlon, P. W., 381, 383, 385
Hanna, S., 271, 272, 273
Hansen, R. A., 610, 611, 790
Hansen P., 428
Hansson, L., 229, 230
Hantla, M. R., 645
Harada, N. D., 644
Hardin, J. M., 666
Harding, S., 691
Hardwig, J., 488
Hardy, L. L., 272
Hardy, T., 252
Harel, Z., 411
Hargraves, K., 628, 645
Harland, R., 72, 73
Harré, R., 431
Harris, A. E., 142
Harris, J., 765, 779
Harris, P. B., 497
Harrison, A., 641
Harrison, P. A., 271
Hartley, S. D., 696
Harvey, A., 286, 758
Harvey, S., 697
Haskell, W. L., 623
Haslam, G., 767

Hasselkus, B., 489, 782, 784
Hasselkus, B. R., 184, 250, 349, 358,
    489, 492, 497, 498, 499, 502, 676,
    689, 692, 693, 779, 790
Hassler, J. K., 798
Hauck, W., 454
Hauck, W. W., 454
Haugen, J. B., 123, 136, 149, 152, 164,
    810
Havighurst, R., 287
Hawking, S. W., 164, 228, 765
Hawkins, C., 248
Haworth, J., 175
Haybron, D., 178
Hayes, J., 359
Haymes, M., 282
Haynes, R. B., 653, 662, 663, 667,
    668, 669, 675, 676, 678, 681, 683,
    686
Hayward, R. S., 669
Hazboun, V. P., 121
Head, B., 757
Heah, T., 273
Healy, C., 779
Heap, I., 622
Heaphy, T., 667
Heater, S. L., 127
Heatherton, T. F., 432
Heaton, R. K., 814
Hebb, D.O., 743
Hebert, J., 179
Hebert, M., 362, 761
Hegel, M. T., 645
Heidegger, M., 176, 177, 178, 179
Heimerl, S., 644
Heitman, E., 356
Hektner, J., 177
Hektner, M., 177
Helen, S., 650
Helfrich, C., 453
Heller, J., 411, 413
Heller, K., 284
Helminski, K. E., 177
Hemingway, H., 263
Hemmingsson, H., 183, 356
Henderson, A., 744
Henderson, D. K., 209, 650
Henderson, G., 381, 383, 385
Henderson, J., 537
Henderson, J. N., 497
Henderson, M. L., 757
Hendrick, I., 100
Hendrickson, C., 307
Hendrix, I., 537
Henriksson, C., 362
Henry-Kohler, E., 382, 386
Hentz, V. R., 629
Heriot, C. S., 421
Herman, P. M., 622

Hermann, V., 537
Hermann, V. H., 645
Hermans, H. J. M., 306
Hersch, G. I., 596
Herz, N., 537
Herzing, D. L., 408
Herzog, M., 645
Hesse, P. W., 383
Heuser, A., 628
Hicks, J., 249
Hightower, M. D., 604
Hill, C. A., 426
Hill, G., 248
Hill, J. H., 309
Hill, R. F., 497
Hillman, A., 185
Hilton, I., 717
Hinojosa, J., 1, 5, 109, 461, 462, 535,
    653, 711, 716
Hobson, J. A., 779
Hobson, S. J. G., 579
Hoch, C., 287
Hochschild, A. R., 279
Hocking, C., 229, 349, 382, 840
Hodder, I., 781
Hodge, B. G., 628
Hodge, C., 70
Hoenig, H., 628, 645
Hoffmann, A. J., 704
Hoffman, C., 179
Hoffman, H. G., 641
Hoffmann, T., 628, 645, 814, 815
Hofherr, M., 645
Hofland, B., 611
Holahan, C. J., 511
Holahan, C. K., 511
Holland, D., 306, 308, 309, 310
Hollender, M. C., 485, 486, 487, 489
Hollis, L. I., 808
Holm, M. B., 628, 629, 645, 651, 652,
    653, 666, 668, 675, 676
Holman, H. R., 509, 514
Holmes, B., 733
Holmes, O. W., 70
Holohan, C. J., 781
Holsti, L., 650, 652
Holtzer, R., 813
Home, A., 263
Honan, E., 519
Hooks, B., 697
Hooper, B., 69
Hooper, R., 665
Hopkins, H. H., 51, 52, 809
Hopkins, H. L., 596
Hoppes, S., 454
Horak, F. B., 164, 810
Horger, M., 781
Hori, M., 644
Horn, K., 644

Horn, K. R., 645
Horn, S. D., 810
Horna, J., 195
Horowitz, B., 537, 609, 610, 611, 612
Horowitz, M. J., 410
Hoskinson, K., 287
Houck, P., 287
Houston, B. K., 408
Howard, B., 711
Howard, L. A., 165
Howe, M. C., 116, 242
Howell, D., 186, 247, 249
Howland, G. W., 87, 356
Hoxie, R. F., 733
Hoyland, M., 423
Hsu, C., 666
Hubbard, S., 525, 526, 527, 632, 790
Hudson, D., 213, 214
Hughes, A., 383, 386
Hughes, M. B., 666
Hughes, M. T., 452
Hui, P. M., 622
Huizinga, J., 779
Hull, H. H., 51
Hull, J. G., 645
Humbert, T. K., 213
Humphry, R., 462
Huntzinger, C., 452
Hurd, M. M., 666
Hurley, M., 272, 273
Hurley, P., 271
Hurst, H., 382
Hurt, S., 74
Huss, A. J., 75, 809
Huston, T., 287
Hutchinson, S. L., 522
Hutzler, Y., 142
Hvalsøe, B., 185

I

Idank, D., 666
Ignatieff, M., 356
Ikai, T., 666
Ilott, I., 649, 650, 652, 653, 656, 660
Imms, C., 269, 272, 273
Imperatore Blanche, E., 382, 386
Ingraham, C., 692
Inui, T. S., 482
Irani, K. D., 356
Irving, J., 178
Isaacs, W., 772
Isacsson, Å., 195, 285
Ivarsson, A.-B., 382
Iwama, M., 214, 215, 757
Iwama, M. K., 192, 194, 195, 196, 356, 385, 421
Iwarsson, S., 247, 254, 286, 453
Iwasaki, Y., 271
Izutsu, Satoru, 754

J

Jack, D., 641
Jackson, H., 815
Jackson, J., 75, 126, 133, 151, 160, 161, 162, 175, 193, 237, 238, 242, 251, 435, 775, 776
Jackson, S., 176, 178, 239, 241, 242, 665
Jackson, T., 760
Jacobs, K., 175, 177, 239, 241, 242, 628, 646
Jagust, W. J., 142
Jahoda, M., 402, 403
Jakobson, K., 229
James, N., 650
James, W., 70, 71, 429, 798
Jang, Y., 310, 311
Janoff-Bulman, R., 408, 416
Janovic, A., 382
Janssen, I., 254
Jantzen, A. C., 471, 599
Jaramazovic, E., 652
Jarjobski, D., 179
Jarman, J., 354
Jarus, T., 272
Jarvelin, M. R., 271
Jarvis, S., 273
Jarvis, S. N., 271, 273, 274
Jary, D., 691
Jary, J., 691
Jaworski, J., 770, 771
Jeannerod, M., 165, 166
Jebsen, R. H., 165
Jeffers, S., 769
Jefferson, P., 248
Jensen, B., 770
Jensen, G. M., 696
Jessel, A. S., 641
Jette, D. U., 810
Jewell, A., 422
Johansson, M., 231
Johnson, B., 713
Johnson, E., 287
Johnson, J., 38, 237, 238, 794
Johnson, J. A., 124, 599
Johnson, J. M., 697
Johnson, J. S., 85, 90, 186
Johnson, K., 582, 694, 696
Johnson, N.C., 185
Johnson, R., 489
Johnson, S., 769
Johnson, S. C., 53, 54
Johnston, D., 422, 423
Johnston, M. V., 645, 666
Jomsson, L., 454
Jones, B., 346
Jones, J. C., 783
Jones, K. B., 815

Jones, M. W., 487, 490
Jongbloed, L., 142, 373
Jonsson, H., 183, 210, 269, 280, 286
Jordan, R., 645
Jordan, W., 740, 742
Jorgensen, H. S., 142
José Durand, M., 361
Josephsson, S., 185, 186, 196, 280, 385
Juda, M., 254
Judge, J. O., 142

K

Kabat-Zinn, 176
Kabat-Zinn, J., 176, 179
Kagan, J., 399, 427
Kagawa-Singer, M., 196
Kahana, B., 411
Kahana, E., 411
Kahneman, D., 383
Kairy, D., 645
Kajihara, H. K., 665
Kallen E, 165
Kang, C., 382
Kanny, E., 683
Kantermann, T., 254
Kapci, E. G., 435
Kaplan, B. J., 142
Kaplan, R., 507, 509, 514, 515, 781
Kaplan, R. M., 478, 479, 667
Kaplan, S., 781
Kaplan, S. H., 482, 483
Karges, J., 810, 811
Karp, D. A., 435
Kasch, M., 124
Katbamna, S., 195
Katz, N., 641
Katz, N. R., 482
Kaufert, J., 581
Kaufman, P., 645
Kaufman, S. R., 497
Kawachi, I., 284, 356
Kaye, G., 582
Kaye, J. J., 142
Kayser, B., 271
Kazis, L., 485, 488
Keefe, E. B., 209
Keenan, B., 250
Kegan, R., 337, 338, 340, 559
Kelemen, M. D., 507, 508, 509, 514, 515
Kelemen, M. H., 507, 508, 509, 514, 515
Keller, A., 427
Keller, S., 779
Kelly, G., 192, 214, 383, 385
Kelly, J. R., 193, 195
Kelly, L., 693, 697
Kelly, S. J., 248

Kelso, G., 644
Kempen, H. J. G., 306
Kennedy, A. A., 734, 735
Kennedy, B. L., 148
Kennedy, B. P., 356
Kennedy, E., 270
Kennedy, K., 213
Kenny, R. A., 454
Keogh, B. K., 451
Keppel, F., 749
Kermode, F., 570
Kerr, N., 421, 422
Kersig, S., 179
Kertoy, S., 272, 273
Kestenbaum, V., 558
Ketkar, M., 461, 462
Keyes, C., 383
Keynes, J. M., 396
Khorsan, R., 622
Kidner, T. B., 55, 56, 120, 220, 531, 650, 791, 793, 837
Kiecolt-Glaser, J., 284
Kiecolt-Glaser, J. K., 284
Kielhofner, G., 1, 44, 69, 74, 83, 84, 89, 109, 119, 122, 125, 131, 132, 133, 135, 138, 140, 148, 150, 162, 163, 168, 184, 186, 187, 194, 209, 229, 231, 232, 237, 238, 247, 250, 251, 280, 299, 346, 348, 421, 461, 462, 489, 513, 519, 525, 526, 561, 570, 586, 599, 600, 649, 650, 651, 655, 656, 727, 728, 730, 744, 758, 761, 775, 790
Kihara, T., 644
Kim, A.-H., 452
Kim, J. B., 641
Kimiecik, I., 240, 242
Kinébanian, A., 185, 186, 196, 310, 385
King, G., 142, 271, 272, 273, 480, 482, 578, 580
King, J. C., 248
King, L. J., 44, 109
King, S., 271, 480, 482, 578, 580
Kinoshita, A., 644
Kinsella, E. A., 519, 578
Kipper, D., 241
Kirby, T. F., 814
Kircher, M. A., 169
Kiresuk, T., 579
Kirkbride, T. S., 7, 10, 11
Kirsch, G. E., 692, 694, 695, 696, 697
Kiuzik, J., 142
Kiyak, H. A., 142
Kizony, R., 641
Klapp, O., 402
Klatzky, R. L., 641
Kleiber, D. A., 522
Klein, S., 228

Kleiner, A., 578
Kleinman, A., 410, 415, 416, 497, 558, 565, 567
Kleinman, L., 644
Klinger, E., 285
Kloppenberg, J. T., 74, 78
Kluckhohn, F. R., 311
Klumb, P., 280
Knight, B. G., 497
Kobasa, S. C., 403, 404, 412, 434
Kobb, R., 644, 645
Koberg, D., 783
Koch, V., 667
Koerner, L., 526
Koestler, A., 559
Koh, C. L., 814, 815
Kohn, A., 799
Kokkonen, J., 271
Kollen, B. J., 810
Kondo, D., 430
Konner, M., 740
Konosky, K., 121
Konrad, R. T., 453, 458
Koomar, J. A., 452
Kornblau, B., 612
Korner-Bitensky, N., 270, 814, 815
Kornfield, J., 176, 177
Kornwolf, J. D., 602
Korotkov, D. L., 434
Kouzes, J., 734, 735
Kouzes, J. M., 735
Kramer, P., 1, 109, 461
Krause, J. S., 196, 404
Krause, M. S., 586
Kravitz, R. L., 485, 492
Kreeger, M. H., 217
Krefting, D. V., 305
Krefting, L., 310, 497, 498
Krefting, L. H., 305, 308, 313, 690, 693, 696
Kremer, E., 237, 238
Kremer, J., 284
Krieger, S. R., 461, 462
Kris, E., 431
Krishnagiri, S., 269, 270
Kroksmark, U., 229
Kronenberg, E., 355, 360
Kronenberg, F., 192, 215, 373, 384, 385, 386, 704, 758
Krupa, T., 229
Krupat, E., 485, 492
Kubota, M., 644
Kuehnle, T., 254
Kuhn, T. S., 565, 682
Kumas-Tan, Z., 757
Kunc, N., 333
Kunkel, S. R., 435
Kuper, A., 305, 306, 308, 309, 310, 311, 313

Kupfer, D., 287
Kupfer, D. J., 287
Kupperman, J. J., 193, 194
Kupych-Woloshyn, N., 249
Kurinczuk, J. J., 272
Kusznir, A., 579
Kutchins, H., 610
Kuzel, A. J., 689, 695
Kwakkel, G., 810
Kyler, P., 462, 463, 490, 491
Kyler-Hutchison. P., 611, 612, 613

L

Labonte, R., 356, 581, 757
Labovitz, O. R., 461
Lacaille, D., 645
Lach, L., 272
Lachicotte, W., 306, 308, 309, 310
Lai, L., 305
Laliberte, D., 238
Laliberte-Rudman, D., 185, 186
LaMore, K. L., 168
Lamport, N. K., 596
Lancaster, A. E., 645
Landers, D., 284
Landry, A., 362
Landry, G., 534
Landry, J., 757
Landry, J. E., 759
Lane, A. E., 271, 272
Lane, J. P., 124
Lang, E. M., 168
Langa, K., 382
Langbein, E., 692
Langer, E., 176, 179
Langer, E. J., 285, 431
Langer, N., 421
Langhammer, B., 652
Langille, L., 354, 704
Langley, J., 704
Langthaler, M., 558, 559
Laporte, D., 362
Larson, B. A., 757
Larson, C., 331, 340
Larson, E., 231, 232, 233, 247, 250, 251, 782
Larson, R., 238, 239
Lasley, E., 283
Lassiter, R. A., 606
Lateur, B., 666
Latham, N. K., 810
Lather, P., 694, 696
Lau, A. L. D., 281
Lauckner, H., 757, 762
Lauderdale, D., 628, 645
Laudin, H., 303
Laurent, D. D., 677
Lave, J., 739
LaVela, S., 692

Laverack, G., 757
Law, M., 1, 75, 138, 141, 142, 175, 196, 209, 242, 271, 272, 273, 274, 338, 348, 361, 369, 370, 422, 461, 462, 477, 478, 479, 480, 481, 483, 485, 489, 490, 491, 514, 516, 575, 576, 579, 581, 622, 670, 675, 676, 683, 692, 693, 694, 695, 696, 697, 711, 718, 761, 775, 782, 784
Lawlor, K., 273
Lawlor, M. C., 462, 485, 761
Laws, C., 519
Lawson, V., 696
Lawton, M. P., 288
Lazarus, R. S., 408, 411, 413, 514
Le Vesconte, H., 461
Lears, T. J. J., 602
Leavitt, R. L., 192
LeBlanc, S. E., 783
Lech-Boura, J., 621, 622
Leclair, L., 175, 196, 579, 692, 693, 694, 695, 696
Leclair, L. L., 714, 715
Ledbetter, N., 452
Lee, A., 628, 630
Lee, D. N., 165
Lee, E., 736
Lee, F., 737
Lee, S. W., 461, 462, 761
Lee, T. D., 812
Lefcourt, H. M., 414
LeFevre, J., 239, 242
Legro, M., 692
Lehoux, P., 645
Leitenberg, H., 586
Lennon, S., 810
Lepage, C., 272, 273
Lerner, M., 95, 97
Leseman, P., 451
Letts, L., 209, 338, 369, 370, 757, 760, 761
Letts, S., 141
Leufstadius, C., 185, 229
Leuret, J., 44
LeVesconte, H., 86
Levi, P., 409, 413, 414
Levin, M., 708
Levine, P., 645
Levine, R., 768
Levine, R. E., 83, 228, 229, 237, 305, 503, 601
Levine, S., 284
Levit, K., 123
Levy, C., 610, 644, 645
Levy, H., 780
Levy, L. L., 248
Levy-Storms, L., 284
Lewis, J. A., 641
Leys, R., 70, 71, 72

Li, Z., 645
Liang, B., 612
Licht, B., 121
Licht, S., 38, 40, 41, 42, 43, 44, 45, 46, 50, 51, 53, 54, 56, 73, 87, 534, 595, 649, 650, 790
Lichtenberg, P. A., 142
Lichtenberg, J., 229, 230
Lidz, C. W., 667
Lifton, R. J., 409, 411
Likroeber, A. l., 300
Lilja, M., 355
Lim, K. H., 195
Lin, K., 663
Lin, K. C., 166
Lin, S. H., 649, 655, 656, 660
Lin, Y., 284
Lincoln, Y. S., 70, 690, 691, 694
Lindeman, E., 652
Linder, L. H., 585
Lindsay, W. R., 622
Linton, S., 521, 527
Linville, P., 280
Lippincott, P., 482
Lippman, W., 70
Liptak, G. S., 272
Little, B. R., 285, 286, 287, 346, 348, 434
Liu, L., 628, 645
Ljubica, T., 345
Llorens, L., 534
Llorens, L. A., 109, 139, 159, 164, 299, 596
Lloyd, C., 421
Lloyd-Smith, W., 683
Lo, B., 610
Lobo, F., 347
Locke, C., 768
Locke, J., 18, 353
Locker, S., 161, 162
Loevenger, J., 431
Logan, P., 240, 241
Logan, R., 178
Logsdon, R., 78
Lohman, H., 215
Lollar, D. J., 491
Lomont, J. F., 585
Lonner, W. J., 306
Lopez, A., 179
Lopez, A. D., 279, 435
Lorenz, K., 391, 393
Lorig, K., 509, 514
Lorig, K. R., 677
Lougher, L., 248
Love, G., 284
Low, S. M., 781
Lowney, M. E. P., 160
Lozano, B. E., 645
Lu, F., 737

Luckman, T., 559
Ludwig, F. M., 168
Luera, M., 260
Lundberg, N. R., 271
Luria, A. R., 165
Lusignolo, T., 284
Lutfiyya, Z. M., 271
Luther, J., 602
Lutz, B. J., 645
Lutzky, S. M., 497
Lynch, H., 229
Lynch, R. D., 641
Lyons, B., 810
Lyons, K. D., 645
Lyons, M., 185, 186
Lysack, C., 581

M

Ma, H., 453, 513, 514
Maas, F., 664
Macan, T. H., 286
MacCleod, C., 177
MacDermid, S., 287
MacDermid, S. M., 260, 261, 262, 279, 280
Macdonald, R., 214, 215
MacFarlane, J., 249
Macfarlane, S., 704
MacKay, K. J., 271
MacKenzie, C. L., 165, 166
MacKinlay, E., 422
MacLaurey, R. E., 309
Macofsky-Urban, F., 497
MacRae, A., 248, 305
Mactavish, J. B., 271
Madge, B., 669
Madill, H., 87, 88, 168
Madill, H. M., 765
Magasi, S., 656
Magnus, E., 229
Maguire, M. C., 260
Maher, C. A., 271, 272
Mahon, M. J., 271
Mailloux, Z., 534
Mairs, N., 412
Majnemer, A., 212, 213, 271, 272, 273, 274
Majumdar, M., 179
Malouin, F., 270
Manchester, D., 815
Mandel, D., 75, 175, 435, 776
Mandich A., 273
Manguno, J., 534
Mankhetwit, S., 462
Manley, J. D., 507, 508, 509, 514, 515
Mann, H. S., 192
Mann, L., 649, 650, 651, 655, 656
Mann, W., 644
Mann, W. C., 124, 629, 644, 645

Mannell, R., 230
Mannheim, B., 308, 311, 313
Maples, N. J., 452
Mapp, R. H., 585
Maquet, A., 414
Marcelli, M., 272, 273
March, J., 734
Marchal, F., 433
Marchand, A., 645
Marcusson, J., 362
Marie, A., 623
Marino-Schorn, J. A., 279
Markow, T., 142
Marks, D., 520, 521, 523
Marks, S., 287
Marks, S. R., 260, 261, 262, 279, 280
Markus, H., 287, 431, 432
Marlowe, D., 432
Marmar, E. R., 410
Marmot, M., 263
Marmot, M. G., 263
Marolla, J., 426, 432
Marques, K., 666
Marr, D., 667
Marshall, C., 691, 693, 696
Marshall, H. M., 704
Marteau, T., 693, 695
Marteniuk, R. G., 165, 166
Martin, J. H., 779
Martin, L., 307, 311, 312
Martin, P., 253
Martin, R. A., 414
Marx, K., 392, 402
Masagatani, G., 556
Maslow, A., 175, 282, 283, 285, 394, 725, 779
Mason, M., 382
Massimini, A., 238, 239, 240, 241, 242
Massimini, F., 238, 239, 240, 242
Masten, A. S., 411
Masunaka-Noriega, M., 347
Matel, J. L. S., 683
Matheis-Kraft, C., 478, 480
Mathews, A., 177
Mathews, T., 604
Mathieu, J., 273
Mathiowetz, V., 123, 136, 149, 152, 164, 810
Mathiowetz, V. G., 165, 167
Matsuoka, Y., 641
Matsutsuyu, J. S., 156, 339
Mattingly, C., 69, 75, 152, 310, 312, 462, 464, 478, 497, 498, 502, 531, 532, 555, 558, 559, 561, 565, 776, 783
Mattingly, C. F., 462, 485
Mattingly C., 502
Matusaka, K., 212, 229, 233, 247, 279, 280

Matuska, K., 212, 213, 233, 283, 757
Matusow, L., 633
Mauthner, N., 695
May, H., 381, 382
Mayberg, H., 175
Mayberry, W., 508
Mayers, C., 422, 423
Mayers, C. A., 421, 423
Mayhan, Y. D., 668
Maynard, M., 691, 695, 696
Mays, N., 691
Mazer, B., 270
McManus, V., 272
McAdams, D., 384, 386
McAdams, D. P., 287, 430, 431
McArthur, C., 549
McAuley, D., 164
McAvoy, E., 381
McCall, M. A., 242, 478, 514, 516
McCluskey, A., 652, 653
McColl, M., 220, 221, 382, 384, 385, 386, 422, 477, 483, 489
McColl, M. A., 138, 348, 386, 481
McConachie, H., 271, 273, 274
McConnell, R. L., 88
McCormick, J. A., 142
McCuaig, M., 425
McCue, M., 645
McDonald, N. B., 645
McDowell, B. J., 666
McElroy, K., 582
McEwen, B., 283
McFarlane, H., 192, 214, 383, 385
McGarry, J., 534
McGlynn, F. D., 585
McGrath, M., 410
McGregor, I., 287
McGuigan, A., 109, 136, 140, 209, 479
McGuire, B., 273
McGuire, L., 284
McHale, K., 667
McHugh Pendleton, H., 230, 248
McKay, S., 356
McKean, M., 286
McKenna, K., 229, 230, 814, 815
McKeon, D., 175
McKieran, F., 422
McKinnon, A, L., 162, 362
McKnight, J. L., 356, 704
McLaughlin, C., 332, 334
McLaughlin-Gray, J., 758
McLean, H., 229
McLean, M., 451
McManus, V., 272, 273
McMurtrie, D., 209
McNary, H., 74, 587, 603
McNay, H., 222
McQuay, H., 662, 663, 665, 666, 667, 668

McSherry, A., 269, 270
McSherry, W., 422
McWhinney, I. R., 490
McWilliams, P., 332
Meacham, J. A., 427
Mead, G. H., 70, 429, 430
Mead, J., 662, 667, 668, 692, 696, 697
Meade, M., 284
Meador, K. G., 665
Mealiea, E. L., 585
Mee, J., 175
Mei-Ha Wong, M., 238, 239, 240
Meijer, O. G., 169
Meisel, A., 667
Melchoir, M., 284
Melrose, A. H., 3
Melzer, K., 271
Menashe, A., 802
Menchetti, B. M., 273
Mendes de Leon, C., 284
Menninger, W., 469, 471
Menon-Nair, A., 814, 815
Menzies, H., 228, 231, 233
Mercer, G., 694
Mercier, C., 250
Merians, A. S., 641
Merleau-Ponty, M., 176
Merquior, J. G., 72, 74
Merrell, R. C., 632
Merrill, S., 238
Merrow, M., 254
Merton, R. K., 94, 725
Mervau- Scheidel, D., 166
Metz, T., 356
Mew, M. M., 462
Meyer, A., 3, 27, 28, 45, 50, 71, 74, 85, 162, 163, 164, 227, 232, 237, 241, 247, 249, 260, 339, 356, 400, 401, 404, 436, 513, 603, 741, 791, 793, 808, 809, 810
Michelsen, S. I., 272, 273
Michie, A., 622
Middleton, B. F., 254
Mihaylov, S., 273
Milburn, K., 695
Mill, J. S., 85, 610
Miller, A., 411, 414
Miller, A. D., 48, 411
Miller, J. M., 630
Miller, L., 169, 273
Miller, L. J., 452, 462
Miller, N. E., 811
Miller, R., 109
Miller, S. B., 586
Miller, T. W., 630
Miller, V., 411
Mills, J., 462, 479, 485, 489, 575, 581
Mills, M., 422
Milton, B. R., 629, 644

Minear, R. H., 411
Minkler, M., 581
Minkowski, H., 228
Minuk, T., 666
Miracle, A. W., 307
Mirkopoulos, C., 305
Mirrey, L. M., 713
Misenheimer, A. M., 814
Misra, R., 286
Missiuna, C., 273
Mitcham, M. D., 669
Mitchell, D., 385
Mitchell, S., 760
Mitchell, T., 512, 515
Mitgang, L., 783
Mocellin, G., 191, 192, 193, 197
Mock, H. E., 49, 50, 795
Modell, S. J., 273
Moeini, S., 633
Mohler, M. J., 622
Moldoveanu, M., 176, 179
Molineux, M., 250, 349
Monette, P., 414
Monk, T., 287
Monk, T. H., 287
Monks, J., 433
Montgomery, D., 733
Montgomery, M. A., 740
Moodie, C., 41, 461, 793, 794
Mooney, P., 487, 490
Moorad, A., 628
Moorcroft, W. H., 780
Moore, A., 662, 663, 665, 666, 667, 668
Moore, J., 331, 337, 339
Moore, J. C., 75
Moore, R. C., 586
Moore, S. L., 428
Moore-Ede, M. C., 780, 781
Moorhead, K., 479
Moos, R., 408
Moos, R. H., 408
Morasso, P., 164
Morey, M., 645
Moriarty, A., 411
Morodan, J., 645
Morris, C., 272
Morris, D., 382
Morris, J., 520, 521, 522, 526
Morris, W., 599
Morrison, T., 814
Morse, H., 534, 535
Mortenson, P., 359, 362
Mortenson, W. B., 525
Mortera, M., 1, 109
Mosey, A., 799
Mosey, A. C., 109, 119, 135, 139, 141,
      142, 209, 229, 231, 232, 461, 534,
      559, 596, 711, 775, 790
Moskowitz, M. A., 485, 488

Moxley-Haegert, L., 482
Moyers, P. A., 220, 671, 790, 796
Mu, K., 230
Mueller, J., 452
Mueller- Rockstroh, B., 519
Mulder, R. M., 166
Mullavey-O'Byrne, C., 305, 306, 309
Müllersdorf, M., 382
Mulligan, S., 664
Mulligan, T., 422
Mullins, L., 734
Muncie, W., 71, 76
Munenori, 772
Muñoz, J. P., 213, 214
Murphy, G., 98
Murphy, J. S., 534
Murphy, L. B., 411
Murphy, R. F., 410, 415, 741, 742
Murphy, S. L., 649, 655, 656, 660
Murray, C. J. L., 279, 435
Murray, E., 744
Murray, E. A., 132, 779
Myers, C. M., 47

N

Nadeau, L., 273
Naditz, A., 629
Nagle, S., 185, 359
Nahemow, L. Yeh, T., 288
Nahin, R., 621
Nakamura, J., 240
Nakayama, H., 142
Namaste, K., 692
Nanna, M., 142
Narayan, G., 271
National Commission on Continued
      Competency in Occupational
      Therapy, 668
Nawas, M. M., 585
Naylor, G., 601, 602
Needham, G., 696, 697
Neill, G., 382
Neisser, U., 781
Neistadt, M., 138, 142
Neistadt, M. E., 164, 480, 575, 666
Nelson, C. E., 161
Nelson, D., 75, 110, 116, 126, 133,
      138, 160, 165, 237, 238, 488, 649,
      775, 810
Nelson, D. L., 121, 166, 168, 169, 736
Nelson, M., 628, 645
Nelson-Becker, H., 422
Neubeck, L., 645
Neville, A., 232
Newell, A., 556
Newell, K. M., 164
Newer, K., 121
Newman, J., 185, 186
Newton, I. G., 594

Nguyen, A., 285, 286, 346, 348, 434
Nicholls, V., 422
Nicholson, A. C., 263
Nicol, M. M., 664
Niedhammer, I., 284
Niemiec, C. P., 280
Nightlinger, K. M., 452
Nimigon, J., 272
Nishikawa, J., 669
Noble, M. O., 649, 650, 656
Nolan, C., 411, 413, 414
Nordell, K., 229
Noreau, L., 272, 273
Norris, M., 799
Northrup, F. M., 37
Nowicki, V., 809, 812
Noyes, J., 356
Nuechterlein, K. H., 142
Nurius, P. S., 431
Nuse-Clark, P, 299
Nutt, D., 250, 254
Nygård, L., 231, 358

O

Oakley, A., 696
Oakley, F, 694, 695, 696
Oakley, F., 513
Oates, J., 490
O'Brien, M., 183
O'Brien, P., 359, 362
O'Connor, P., 284
Odawara, E., 213
Odom, A. L., 451
Odom, S. L., 451
Ogilvie, D. M., 432
Ogourtsova, T., 814, 815
O'Hara, P., 249
Öhman, A, Nygård, L., 185
Ohta, R., 497
Okely, A. D., 272
Okoye, R. L., 596
Okvat, H. A., 623
Olds, T., 271, 272
O'Leary, A., 509, 514
Olesen, V., 696
Olinger, M. J., 478, 480
Olive, E., 644
Oliveau, D. C., 586
Oliver, M., 520, 696, 697
Oliver, S., 692, 696
Olowu, T., 526
Olsen, N. J., 142
Olsen, S., 644
Olsen, T. S., 142
Olson, E., 411
Oltjenbruns, K., 421, 422
Omstein, R., 392
O'Neill, E., 665
Opie, A., 696, 697

Opzoomer, A., 477
Orbeta, L., 254
O'Reilly, M., 570, 571, 572, 573
Oritz, R., 254
Orozovic, N., 185, 186
Ortiz, L. P. A., 421
Ory, M. G., 453, 458
Otis-Green, S., 422
Ottenbacher, K., 668, 669, 671, 799
Ottenbacher, K. J., 664, 676
Ouslander, J. G., 780
Owen, S. V., 452
Owens, A. C., 652
Oz, M. C., 623

P

Page, S. J., 645
Paget, M., 559
Paicheler, H., 433
Paisley, A., 73, 74
Pajouhandeh, P., 185, 186
Paley, J., 196
Pals, J., 384
Palsbo, S. E., 628
Papadimitriou, C., 656
Pape, T., 692
Parel, A. J., 260
Parham, D., 126, 133, 151, 160, 161,
    162, 193, 237, 238, 242, 251, 775
Parham, L. D., 452, 779
Park, H., 238
Park, J., 178
Park, R., 779
Park, S., 479
Parker, G., 195
Parker, I., 694, 695, 696
Parker, J. A., 621, 622
Parker, L. D., 734
Parkes, J., 272
Parkinson, K. N., 271, 273, 274
Parks, A. C., 382, 384
Parmanto, B., 628
Parr, J., 696
Parsons, S. E., 159
Partiman, T. S., 781
Partridge, C., 693, 694, 697
Pasquinelli-Estrada, S., 513
Passmore, A., 269
Patel, V. L., 556
Patterson, A., 331, 332, 486
Patterson, D. R., 641
Patterson, M., 757, 762
Patterson-Rudolph, C., 331
Pattison, H. A., 28
Pavot, W., 432
Payton, O. D., 161
Peachey-Hill, C., 695
Peacock, E. J., 285
Pearlman, R. A., 667

Peasgood, T., 382, 383, 385
Peck, E. C., 411
Pedlar, A., 385
Pedretti, L. W., 513
Peirce, C. S., 70, 71, 682, 683, 684
Pellegrino, E. D., 541
Pelletier, K. R., 408, 623
Peloquin, S. M., 3, 44, 83, 85, 229,
    260, 286, 422, 461, 478, 479, 490,
    533, 589, 656, 668, 669, 671, 711,
    716, 717, 791, 794, 797, 798, 799,
    800, 801, 802
Pender, N., 279
Pendleton, M. G., 814
Penn, H., 193
Pentland, M., 382, 384, 385, 386
Pentland, W., 286, 757, 762
Peoples, J., 192
Pepitone, A., 306
Perez, I., 667
Perkin, H., 801
Perlow, L. A., 279
Perraz, M., 280
Perrin, T., 381, 382
Perrow, C., 733
Perry, W., 559
Persson, D., 195, 210, 232, 233, 247,
    254, 285, 286
Persson, H., 269
Peters, C., 1, 2
Peters, D. J., 696
Peters, P., 259
Peters, R. S., 790
Peters, T., 734
Petersen, E. B., 519
Petersen, J., 802
Petrenchik, T., 271
Pew–Fetzer Task Force, 490, 491, 492
Pfeiffer, D., 694, 695, 696
Phelps, C., 382
Philip, I., 675, 676, 683
Phillip, A., 650
Phillips, R. S., 623
Piaget, J., 427
Picard, R., 273
Picard-Greffe, H., 765
Pichard, C., 271
Pierce, D., 126, 133, 151, 160, 161, 162,
    184, 186, 193, 194, 229, 230, 237,
    238, 242, 247, 249, 251, 280, 362,
    382, 395, 716, 758, 775, 776, 777,
    778, 779, 780, 781, 782, 783, 784
Pierce, W., 282
Piergrossi, J. C. Gibertoni, C., 769
Pilkington, K., 179
Pincus, T., 142
Pinel, P. H., 8, 10, 19, 20, 478, 479
Pippin, K., 433
Piškur, B., 185, 186, 196, 385

Pizzi, M., 123
Plummer, K., 692
Pogge, T. W., 356
Poizner, H., 641
Polatajko, H., 89, 133, 138, 175, 183,
    184, 185, 187, 191, 193, 194, 196,
    242, 270, 273, 348, 354, 370, 383,
    432, 464, 477, 478, 481, 483, 514,
    516, 622, 745, 747, 758
Polatajko, H. J., 142, 185, 274, 359,
    520, 761
Polgar, J. M., 759
Polkinghorne, D., 430, 776
Pollard, N., 192, 215, 373, 384, 385,
    386, 704, 758
Pollock, H., 649, 650, 651, 652
Pollock, N., 138, 142, 242, 273, 348,
    361, 386, 462, 477, 478, 481, 483,
    485, 490, 514, 516, 575, 697
Ponsolle-Mays, M., 801
Popay, J., 689, 695, 696
Pope, C., 691
Pope-Davis, D. B., 305
Pope-Davis, S. A., 305
Popescu, V. G., 629
Pörn, I., 399, 401
Porras, J., 796, 798
Porter, C., 683
Portney, L. G., 665
Posluszny, D., 284
Posner, B., 734, 735
Posner, B. Z., 735
Posner, M., 177
Post, M. L., 628
Poter, D. L., 482
Pothier, D., 195
Potocki, E. R., 409
Poulin, C., 272, 273, 274
Poulin, M., 382
Poulin, V., 814, 815
Poulsen, A. A., 274
Powe, N., 489
Powers, C., 537
Pramuka, M., 628, 629, 645
Pratt, C., 714
Press, V. R., 809
Presseller, S. R., 76
Pridham, K.R., 745
Priestley, N., 815
Priestly, M., 524
Prieto, L. R., 305
Prigerson, H., 287
Prigogine, I., 148
Prihoda, T. J., 452
Primeau, L., 242, 395
Primeau, L. A., 195, 229, 358, 775,
    778, 779
Prince-Paul, M., 422
Prior, S., 185, 186

Privette, G., 175
Puchalski, C., 422
Pugliese, K., 422
Puller, L. B., 741
Punch, M., 694
Purdie, L., 183, 184, 185, 187, 383, 761
Purdum, H. D., 159
Purtilo, R., 609, 610, 611, 612, 613
Putnam, H., 74, 565
Putnam, T., 176
Pynoos, J., 497

Q

Qamar, A., 632
Quera, V., 490, 492
Questad, K., 666
Quetsch, J. L., 630
Quigley, P., 645
Quintana, L. A., 149
Quiroga, V. A., 1, 3, 76, 115, 134, 213, 782

R

Raab, M., 451
Raaschau, H. O., 142
Radner, G., 407
Rafiq, A., 632
Rahe, R. H., 411
Rais, H., 5
Rand, D., 641
Rappaport, H., 586
Rappaport, J., 746
Rasch, N., 644
Rathunde, K., 240
Ravaud, J. F., 433
Ravaud, J-F., 193
Ravetz, C., 651
Rawls, J., 356
Ray, I., 9, 13
Ray, W. A., 665
Reagon, C., 382, 653
Rebeiro, K., 196, 353, 355, 369, 422, 489, 575, 580, 697
Rebeiro, K. L., 183, 694
Redfern, J., 645
Redmond, J. D., 369
Reed, B. R., 142
Reed, J. L., 282
Reed, K., 1, 2, 53, 54, 56, 57, 85, 87, 227, 228, 250, 252, 260, 261, 587, 588, 594, 790, 791
Reed, K. L., 73, 534, 649, 655
Reese, L. B., 512
Regan, L., 693, 697
Reich, R. B., 733, 734
Reid, D. T., 111, 175, 179, 180
Reilly, M., 5, 31, 72, 84, 90, 122, 151, 237, 243, 299, 355, 399, 402, 727,

728, 730, 740, 782, 792, 807, 808, 810
Reindal, S. M., 196
Reis, H. T., 280
Reitz, M., 714
Reker, G. T., 285, 435
Rennie, D., 662
Rensink, M., 652
Repetti, R., 284
Restall, G., 361, 532, 533, 575, 576, 578, 580, 757, 760
Reverby, S. M., 48
Reyes-Ortiz, C., 422
Reyna, S., 306
Reynolds, C., 287
Reynolds, E. J., 585
Reynolds, F., 185, 186
Rhodes, M., 610
Ribbens, J., 695
Ricafrente-Biazon, M., 526
Riccio, C. M., 168
Rice, J., 347
Rice, S. G., 271
Richarde, R. S., 507, 510, 514, 515
Richards, J., 356
Richardson, J., 179
Richardson, P., 628, 645
Richardson, W. S., 653, 662, 663, 667, 668, 669, 675, 676, 678, 681, 683, 686
Ricoeur, P., 570
Rider, R. A., 273
Riemersma-Van Der Lek, R. F., 254
Ries, A., 507, 509, 514, 515
Rifkin, J., 400
Rigby, P., 141, 209, 338, 369, 370, 761
Riger, S., 697
Ripat, J., 361, 532, 533, 576, 578, 580, 757, 760
Ripat, J. D., 369
Ripley, D., 354
Ritch, J., 452
Riveria, G., 835
Roback, A. A., 790
Roberts, C., 578
Robertson, D., 650
Robertson, J. A. F., 253, 254
Robertson, L., 664
Robinault, I. P., 809
Robinson, A., 740
Robinson, A. M., 151, 163, 164, 167, 237, 596
Robinson, H. A., 74
Robinson, I., 83, 86, 87, 88, 501, 739
Robinson, I. M., 765
Robinson, J. C., 649, 655, 656, 660
Robinson, J. P., 233, 279, 286
Robles, T., 284
Robson, C., 691, 692, 695

Rochberg-Halton, E., 781
Rochon, S., 361, 462, 485, 490, 575
Rodin, J., 285, 431
Rodin, J. C., 435
Rodrigue, M. M., 271
Roenneberg, T., 254
Rogers, A., 695, 696
Rogers, C. R., 477, 485, 486, 559
Rogers, J., 251
Rogers, J. C., 76, 142, 150, 163, 169, 204, 432, 510, 556, 570, 666, 790, 795
Rogers, S., 704
Rogers J. C., 570
Rögnvaldsson, T., 229, 280
Rood, M. S., 75, 110, 131, 649, 655, 809
Rorty, R., 74, 565
Rosa, S., 489, 782, 784
Rosaldo, R. I., 309, 313
Rose, A., 421
Rose, D., 645
Rose, F. D., 641
Rosen, G. M., 585, 586
Rosenau, P. M., 689
Rosenau, P. V., 356
Rosenbaum, P., 142, 271, 272, 273, 274, 480, 482, 578, 580
Rosenbaum, P. L., 272
Rosenberg, L., 183, 185, 186, 383
Rosenberg, W., 653, 663, 675, 676, 678, 681, 683, 686
Rosenberg, W. M., 662, 667, 668, 669, 681, 686
Rosenfeld, M. S., 124, 409
Rosensweig, P., 179
Rosner, T., 411
Rosser, B., 578
Rossman, G. B., 691, 693, 696
Roter, D., 489
Rothbart, M., 177
Rothman, D. J., 8, 9, 10, 11, 12
Rothman, J., 760, 761
Rowles, G. D., 311, 381
Roy, M. A., 270
Royeen, C., 356, 381, 781, 783
Rozich, A., 652, 653
Rubin, E., 534
Rubin, T., 779
Ruble, D., 427
Rudman, D. L., 133
Ruggles, O., 49, 51, 792, 794, 800
Rule, S., 644
Rumney, P., 644, 645
Rush, J., 85
Rusk, H., 83, 87, 88, 89
Russell, D., 142
Russell, M., 279
Russell, T., 628, 630, 645

Russo, A., 526
Ruwe, W. D., 645
Ryan, P., 645
Ryan, R. M., 175, 176, 178, 280, 282, 283, 284, 285, 287, 383, 384, 385
Ryan, S., 537
Ryff, C., 282, 283, 284, 285
Ryff, C. D., 195, 282, 383

S

Sabbadini, L. L., 279
Sabol, P., 453
Sachs, O., 461
Sackett, D. L., 653, 662, 663, 667, 668, 669, 675, 676, 678, 681, 683, 686
Sacks, O., 409, 410, 413, 416
Sadla, G., 178
Sadlo, G., 210, 231, 280, 286, 355
Sahagian-Whalen, S., 697
Sahlins, M., 311
Said, E. W., 191, 192, 196, 197, 697
Sakellariou, D., 215, 373, 704, 758
Sakzewski, L., 274
Saleh, M. N., 270
Salkeld, G., 665
Salmon, J., 272
Salmon, T. W., 57, 109
Sample, P. L., 461, 462
Sandelowski, M., 690, 691, 696
Sanderson, S., 53, 54, 56, 57, 85, 87, 227, 228, 250, 252, 260, 261, 587, 588, 594, 790, 791
Sands, D., 510, 515
Sandywell, B., 519
Sanford, J., 483, 628, 645
Sanford, J. A., 645
Sangl, J., 497
Sankar, A., 497
Santha, J., 112, 381, 383, 386
Sapir, E., 306
Sapolsky, R. M., 283
Saptono, A., 628, 629, 645
Sartre, J-P., 192
Sato, I., 239, 242
Savard, L., 628, 645
Saxe, G., 179
Sbordone, R. J., 815
Scaffa, M., 714
Scaletti, R., 757, 760
Scarry, E., 802
Schaaf, R. C., 452
Schaefer, J. A., 408
Schechtman, K., 142
Scheideman-Miller, C., 628, 645
Schein, R. M., 628, 629, 645
Schell, B., 532
Schell, B. A., 447

Schemm, R. L., 85, 213, 711
Scheper, M., 810
Schilling, D. L., 452
Schindehette, S., 744
Schinfeld, S., 454
Schkade, J., 109, 209, 775
Schleien, S. J., 271
Schmeler, M. R., 628, 629, 645
Schmidt, J., 177
Schmidt, R. A., 812
Schmidt, W. H., 735
Schmitter-Edgecombe, M., 814
Schmoll, B. J., 696
Schmuckler, M. A., 814
Schneider, D. M., 307
Schneider, J. A., 811
Schneiderman, L. J., 667
Schnelle, J. F., 780
Schoeneman, T. J., 429
Schoenfeld, H. B., 452
Schön, D., 242, 334, 339, 341, 559, 565, 578, 725, 783
Schopp, L. H., 630
Schrauger, J. S., 429
Schult, M.-L., 183, 185, 186, 383
Schultz, S., 109, 209, 775
Schultz, V., 356
Schultz-Krohn, W., 230, 248
Schulz, E., 421, 422
Schulz, R., 497
Schutz, A., 559
Schutz, M. E., 745
Schuurmans, M., 652
Schwartz, C. E., 196
Schwartz, G., 178, 179
Schwartz, K., 85, 339
Schwartz, K. B., 1, 86, 87
Schwartz, P. K., 487, 490
Schwartz, R., 453, 458
Schwartz, S. J., 383, 384
Schwartzberg, S., 610, 612, 613
Schwartzberg, S. L., 116, 242
Schwarz, N., 383
Schwimmer, P., 588
Scott, A. D., 596
Scott, A. H., 622
Scott, E., 185, 186, 579
Scott, P., 696
Scott. R., 609, 611, 612, 614
Scull, A., 8, 9
Seab, J. P., 142
Searls, D., 768
Sechrist, K., 279
Secker, J., 695
Seeman, T., 284, 285
Segal, R., 759, 781
Segal Z. V., 175
Segall, M. H., 306

Sekulic, A., 628, 645
Seleen, D., 280, 286
Self, H., 694, 695, 696
Seligman, M. E., 382, 384
Seligman, M. E. P., 421
Sellar, B., 186
Selye, H., 392, 408
Semans, S., 131
Semeniuk, B., 183
Sendor, M., 196
Senge, P. M., 578
Serbin, L. A., 482
Serrett, K. D., 70, 71, 72, 76, 260
Service, E. R., 311
Sewell, W. H., 311, 313
Seydel, E., 507, 510, 514, 515
Shaffer, H., 507
Shahani, C., 286
Shakespeare, T., 520, 694, 697
Shakir, M., 305
Shannon, P., 1, 711, 790
Shannon, R., 164
Shapcott, N., 628
Shapiro, C. M., 249
Shapiro, J., 334, 335
Shapiro, S., 176, 177, 178, 179
Sharrott, G. W., 167, 300
Shaw, B., 85
Shaw, C. N., 45, 213, 465, 713
Shaw, D., 652, 653
Shaw, D. K., 628
Shaw, J., 279, 652, 653
Shaw, R., 287
Shaw, S. M., 195
Sheehan, S., 411
Sheldon, K. M., 280
Sheldon, S., 780
Shelton, T., 333
Shengold, L., 411
Shenk, D., 662
Shepard, K. F., 696
Shepherd, R. B., 126
Sheridan, T. B., 641
Sherman, R., 579
Sherr Klein, B., 362
Sherry, K., 370, 371
Sherzer, J. A., 308
Shevell, M., 272, 273, 274
Shi, D. E., 602
Shiflet, S., 779
Shikako-Thomas, K., 272, 273
Shin, J., 757, 759, 760, 761
Shoor, S., 509, 514
Short, M. J., 814
Short-DeGraff, M., 138, 421, 422
Shreve, G. M., 645
Shulman, L., 556
Shunk, D., 507, 510, 514, 515

Sidell, M., 191, 692, 693, 697
Sidey, H., 32
Siebers, T., 521
Siegel, D., 176, 179
Siegel, Z., 176
Siegler, C. C., 558
Sietsema, J. M., 166
Sigerist, H. E., 392
Silberman, J., 179
Silcox, L., 248
Silverman, W. A., 662
Simeonsson, R. J., 491
Simmons, S. F., 780
Simo Algado, S., 355, 360
Simon, H., 556
Simon, R. I., 519
Simpson, J. A., 789, 798
Singer, B., 195, 282, 284
Skinner, D., 306, 307, 308, 309, 310, 451
Skully, D., 284
Skurla, E., 142
Slagle, E. C., 51, 74, 120, 127, 159, 162, 712, 741, 782, 792, 794
Slater, M., 510, 515
Slavin, M. D., 810
Sloan, C. V. M., 452
Sloan, S., 230
Sloman, J., 269
Smallfield, S., 810, 811
Smeltzer, S., 628
Smith, B. F., 260
Smith, B. J., 578
Smith, D., 382
Smith, D. A., 169, 736
Smith, D. E., 782
Smith, H. D., 596
Smith, J., 179, 499
Smith, N. M., 649, 650
Smith, N. R., 163
Smith, P., 51
Smith, R., 274
Smith, R. S., 411
Smith, S., 422
Smout, R. J., 810
Smyth, G., 461, 465, 575, 580
Smyth, K. A., 497
Snider, L., 270
Snoke, A. W., 733
Snyder, C., 347
Sobei, D., 392
Sokolov, J., 462, 534, 794
Sokoly, M. M., 478
Somerville, M., 770
Sommer, K. L., 431
Sommerville, J., 214
Sonn, U., 281
Spackman, C. S., 47, 809, 810, 812, 813

Spainhower, G., 532, 534
Spearritt, K., 260
Speck, P., 422
Spencer, J., 310, 497, 498
Spencer, J. C., 138, 502
Spiegel, A. H., 735
Spire, J., 780
Spitzer, S., 452
Sprafka, A., 556
Sprague, J., 359
Sprang, R., 630
Sproat, C. T., 462
Sridhar, D., 452
St. Clair, V. W., 361
Stacey, J., 696
Stacey, S., 142
Stachey, J., 431
Staisey, N., 477
Stalker, K., 524
Stanghelle, J. K., 652
Stanley, M., 229
Stansfeld, S. A., 263
Stanwyck, D. J., 196
Staples, A. R., 88
Stark, S., 453
Starr, P., 474, 733
Stattel, F. M., 37, 649, 650, 795
Stearns, S. C., 453, 458
Steckler, A., 582
Steel, K., 645
Steen, I. N., 454
Steen, T., 382, 384
Steger, M. B., 194
Stein, A., 692
Stein, C., 161, 162, 193, 237, 238, 242
Stein, F., 536
Stein, G., 240, 242
Stein, H. F., 497
Stein, J. G., 359, 361
Stein, R. B., 433
Steinbeck, T. M., 169
Steinmetz, H., 238
Steinwender, S., 175, 196, 579, 692, 693, 694, 695, 696
Stengers, I., 148
Stepanek, J., 333
Stepanski, E. J., 252
Stern, M., 361, 532, 575, 576, 578, 580, 757, 760
Stern, N., 411
Sternberg, E., 279
Sterritt, M., 433
Stevenson, L., 70
Stew, G., 178, 210, 231
Stewart, D., 183, 184, 185, 187, 209, 338, 369, 370, 383, 697, 761
Stewart, K. J., 507, 508, 509, 514, 515
Stewart, M., 490

Stewart, P., 229, 230, 250
Stewart, R., 196
Stewart, S., 141
Stiller, C., 789
Stockmeyer, S. A., 131
Stoffel, V. C., 514
Stomph, M., 310
Stone, B. M., 254
Stone, E., 696
Stone, R., 497
Storman, W., 195
Storr, A., 400, 403
Stratton, A., 382
Straub, C. C., 783
Strauss, A., 691
Strauss, S. E., 653, 675, 676, 678, 681, 683, 686
Strodtbeck, F. L., 311
Strong, J., 249, 254
Strong, L., 282
Strong, S., 209, 338, 369, 370, 761
Strong S., 141
Stuifbergen, A., 510, 515, 704
Stump, C., 454
Sturrock, J., 72
Stutzer, A., 421
Suckle, H. M., 809
Sud, S., 526
Sudsawad, P., 649
Sue, S., 312
Sullivan, W. M., 801
Sulmasy, D., 422
Sulzman, F. M., 780, 781
Summerfield, L. M., 649, 650, 651, 655, 656, 761
Sumner, W. G., 70
Sumsin, T., 485, 489, 490
Sumsion, T., 175, 461, 462, 465, 478, 575, 576, 580
Sunderland, T., 142
Suto, M., 191, 195
Sutton, B., 37
Sutton, D., 177
Svensson, V. W., 604
Sviden, G. A., 355
Swaab, D. F., 781
Swaim, L. T., 160
Swain, J., 195, 524
Swanberg, J., 279
Swank, R. T., 507, 514, 515
Swann, W. B., 426
Swanson, L., 483
Swarbrick, P., 714
Swedersky, J., 382
Swift, C., 665
Swigonski, M. E., 192
Syme, S. L., 263
Symons, F., 451

Szasz, T. S., 485, 486, 487, 489
Szeinberg, A., 142
Szmigin, I., 230
Szonyi, G., 665
Szuba, M., 287

T

Taal, E., 507, 510, 514, 515
Taanila, A., 271
Taffs, L., 666
Takahashi, R., 644
Tamiki, H., 412
Tamm, M., 490
Tang, P., 629
Tarule, J. M., 559
Tate, B., 361
Taub, E., 811
Taylor, C., 519, 527
Taylor, C. B., 509, 512
Taylor, D. P., 163
Taylor, E., 462, 534
Taylor, F. W., 593
Taylor, G., 191
Taylor, J., 765, 770, 771
Taylor, J. A., 665
Taylor, M. C., 683
Taylor, N., 165
Taylor, R., 382, 386, 461, 761
Taylor, R. R., 461, 462
Taylor, S., 284, 285
Taylor, S. E., 735
Taylor, W., 271
Teasdale, J., 176
Tedlock, D., 308, 311, 313
Teetzel, H., 667
Teitelman, J., 186
Telford, A., 272
Teri, L., 142
Tesser, A., 286
Thapa, P. B., 665
Thayer, A., 794
Thelen, E., 739
Theodoros, D., 628, 630
Thera, N., 176
Thibeault, R., 362, 757, 760, 761
Thibodeaux, C. S., 168
Thijssen, M., 454
Thom, T., 485, 492
Thomas, A., 411
Thomas, J., 192
Thomas, L., 469, 472
Thomas, M., 665
Thomasma, D. C., 541
Thompson, C. V., 809
Thompson, D., 454
Thompson, L., 628, 645
Thompson, M., 534
Thompson, M. G., 284
Thomson, A., 650

Thomson, N., 214, 215
Thorpe, D., 271
Tice, D. M., 434
Tickle-Degnen, L., 139, 462, 489, 663, 664, 676, 678, 681, 683, 744
Timko, C., 408, 416
Timperio, A., 272
Tindale, J., 358
Tindall, L., 628, 630
Ting, W., 623
Tinning, R., 69
Tkachuck, J., 628, 645
Toal, C., 697
Tobey, C., 632
Toch, H., 346
Toffler, A., 739, 740, 746, 765
Toglia, J. P., 123, 149
Tolentino, M., 812
Tolle, E., 176
Tomes, N., 7, 9, 10, 13, 14
Tomlin, G., 653
Tomlinson, J., 346
Torrance, E. P., 409
Torrance, M., 125
Toshima, M., 507, 509, 514, 515
Toth-Cohen, S., 421
Toulmin, S., 346
Townsend, E., 84, 89, 175, 183, 185, 186, 191, 193, 194, 196, 217, 229, 250, 254, 270, 287, 349, 353, 354, 355, 357, 360, 361, 370, 383, 477, 478, 490, 525, 622, 704, 757, 759, 760, 761, 840
Townsend, E. A., 520
Tracy, S. E., 41, 42, 43, 51, 121, 538, 711, 712, 715, 791, 793, 795
Trainer, P., 411
Tremaine, M., 641
Trentham, B., 757, 759, 760, 761
Tresolini, C. P., 490, 491, 492
Trieschmann, R. B., 165
Trillin, A. S., 411
Trivette, C., 451
Trivette, C. M., 356, 483, 490
Trochim, W., 670
Trombly, C., 744
Trombly, C. A., 75, 111, 133, 138, 139, 141, 148, 149, 150, 151, 152, 160, 163, 164, 166, 169, 453, 513, 514, 596, 649, 776, 781, 784
Tropman, J., 760, 761
Trotter, M., 165
Tsai, P. L., 164
Tse, S., 421
Tuckett, A. G., 789
Tuerk, P. W., 645
Tugwell, P., 663
Tuke, D. H., 22
Turner, A., 207, 382

Turner, H., 269, 270
Twigg, J., 359
Tyler, E. J., 704
Tylor, E. B., 306

U

Ubel, P., 382
Uchino, B. N., 284
Udell, L., 423
Uldall, P., 272
Unruh, A. M., 421, 422
Unsworth, C., 229, 230
Upham, E. G., 52, 134, 605, 795
Urban, G. A., 308
Urbanowski, R., 422
Urguhart, L., 645
Urquhart, K., 812
Urwick, L., 734

V

Vaillant, G. E., 411, 414
Valenti, S. A., 507, 508, 509, 514, 515
Vallerand, J., 670, 671, 683
van der Meer, A. L. H., 165
Van der Weel, F. R., 165
van Heugten, C. M., 814
van Menxel, D. A., 814
Van Someren, E. J. W., 254
Vancouver, J. B., 676
VanLeit, B. J., 209
Vargas, S., 663, 664
Vargo, J., 422
Varrier-Jones, P. J., 218
Vash, C. L., 403
Vaughn, S., 452
Vaux, C. L., 51
Velde, B., 230
Velde, B. P., 305, 312, 779
Velligan, D. I., 452
Velozo, C. A., 479
Venables, T., 629
Verbrugge, L. M., 280
Verburg, G., 644, 645
Verdonck, M., 537
Vergara, E., 123
Verhey, F. R., 814
Vernooij-Dassen, M., 454
Versnel, J., 421, 422, 757
Viau, S., 652, 653
Village, J., 645
Ville, I., 193, 433
Vincent, A., 628, 645
Vincent, C., 645
Virani, R., 422
Virey, 394
Visintin, M., 645
Vogel, K. A., 452
Vogel, S., 411, 413

von Eye, A., 231
von Zweck, C., 670, 671, 683
Vrkljan, B., 358
Vygotsky, L. S., 427

W

Wacker, W., 765, 770, 771
Wacquant, L., 519
Wade, B. D., 587
Wade, J. W., 783
Wagenaar, R. C., 169
Wagner, C., 602
Wagner, N., 629
Wakefield, B., 645
Wakeford, L., 629
Walach, H., 179
Walens, D., 453
Walker, C., 230
Walker, J. S., 286
Walker, K., 109
Walker, S., 279
Wallace, A. F. C., 306
Walley, M., 433
Walloch, C., 179, 215
Walter, C., 581
Walter, S., 142
Walters, K. S., 799
Walton, R. E., 734
Wan, M., 622
Wang, A., 507, 510, 514, 515
Wang, M., 452
Ward, L., 696
Ward, L. F., 70
Ward, P., 485, 490, 492
Ware, J. E., 482, 483
Warms, C. A., 704
Warwick, J., 487, 490
Washington, K., 452
Wassem, R., 507, 509, 514, 515
Wasserman, R. C., 482
Waterman, A. S., 383, 384
Waterman, M., 84
Waterman, R., 734
Waterman, R. H., 734
Watkins, M. P., 665
Watson, D., 761
Watson, D. E., 139
Watson, J., 695
Watson, R., 758
Watson, R. M., 385
Watts, J., 269, 270
Watts, J. H., 163, 186
Watzlaf, V., 633
Waygood, S., 382
Waylonis, G. W., 666
Weaver, F. M., 692
Weaver, G., 410
Webb, R., 121
Weekes, R., 249

Wehr T. A., 253, 254
Weick, K., 176
Weinberg, N., 433
Weinberger, D., 768
Weinblatt, N., 186, 247, 385
Weiner, E. S. C., 789, 798
Weiner E. Brown, A., 765
Weinman, J., 693, 695
Weinstein, M., 284
Weisner, T. S., 451
Weiss, P. L., 641
Weiss, P. T., 641
Welles, C., 57
Wells, A., 239, 242
Wells, A. J., 287
Wells, L., 359
Wells, S. A., 305, 609
Welsh, B., 273
Wendell, S., 520, 521, 522, 523, 524,
    526, 692
Wendland, T., 693
Wenston, S., 612
Werner, E. E., 411
Wernick, R., 242
Wescott, G., 744
West, M., 603
West, N. L., 75, 535
West, W., 72, 84, 88, 89, 126, 536,
    711, 790
Westbury, C., 665
Westhorp, P., 211, 213, 247
Weston, D., 534
Weston, W. W., 490
Wheatley-Smith, L., 810
Whelan, L., 629
Whelan, T., 485
Whitaker, C. M., 305
Whitcombe, S., 381
White, B. E., 166, 169
White, H., 570
White, M., 382, 383, 385
White, R. W., 84, 159, 160, 409, 413,
    415, 431, 432
White, S., 519, 527
White, V. K., 138
White G., 422
Whiteford, G., 229, 233, 287, 348,
    349, 356, 358, 361, 381, 519, 525,
    840
Whiteford, G. E., 192, 526
Whiteneck, G. G., 453
Wicker, F. W., 282
Wideman, J. E., 301
Wiegman, O., 507, 510, 514, 515
Wiehe, J. A., 282
Wiemer, R. B., 75, 535
Wierenga, S. A., 814
Wiesel, E., 412, 413
Wilcock, A., 194, 217, 353, 357, 760

Wilcock, A. A., 69, 72, 175, 183, 184,
    186, 192, 194, 218, 219, 227, 229,
    249, 253, 260, 261, 262, 264, 281,
    345, 346, 347, 348, 349, 353, 354,
    355, 356, 359, 368, 381, 383, 385,
    422, 526, 757, 758, 760, 761, 781,
    790, 791
Wild, J., 84
Wilding, C., 381
Wilkins, S., 361, 462, 485, 490, 575
Wilkins, W., 586
Wilkinson, R., 263
Willard, H. S., 809, 810, 813
Willeman, P., 312
Willi, V., 694, 695, 696
Williams, C. W., 585
Williams, G., 520, 689, 695, 696
Williams, J., 177
Williams, M., 176, 801
Williams, M. T., 271, 272
Williams, P., 191
Williams, R., 666
Williamson, G. M., 497
Wilson, A. L., 361
Wilson, B., 183
Wilson, B. N., 142
Wilson, I. B., 78
Wilson, M. C., 669
Wilson, S., 247, 249, 250, 253, 254,
    534, 761
Wilson, S. A., 761
Wilson, S. C., 50, 51, 210
Wilson, W., 111
Wilson L., 421, 422
Wimbush, E., 695
Winefield, H., 479
Winkle, M., 537
Winkler, D., 230
Winnicott, D., 337, 338
Winter, L., 454
Winters, J. M., 628
Wirz, S. L., 696
Wiseman, J. O., 274
Wish-Baratz, S., 87
Wittman, P., 305, 312
Wittman, P. P., 628
Wolery, M., 451
Wolfe, R. J., 126, 133, 151, 160, 162,
    251, 775
Wolff, T., 582
Wolfman, B. R., 260
Wolfs, C. A., 814
Wolsko, P. M., 623
Wong, P. T. P., 285
Wong, P. T. P., 238, 285, 434
Wood, R., 507, 509, 510, 513, 514,
    515
Wood, W., 148, 149, 247, 250, 251,
    349, 652, 711, 775, 784, 790, 798

Woods, S., 248
Woodside, H. H., 39
Wooten, J., 799
Woy, J. R., 585
Wressle, E., 362
Wright, B., 404
Wright, B. A., 550
Wright, D. E., 586
Wright, J., 178, 210, 231
Wright, M., 760
Wu, C., 663
Wu, C. Y., 166
Wyatt, J. K., 252
Wyman, J. F., 621

Y

Yager, A., 287
Yalmambirra, 232
Yalom, Y. D., 285
Yamagishi, M., 142
Yamshon, L. J., 809, 812
Yankelovitch, D., 332
Yasuda, Y. L., 248
Yerxa, E., 38, 72, 84, 88, 89, 122, 124,
    161, 162, 175, 219, 220, 237, 238,
    288, 333, 337, 339, 348, 355, 369,
    381, 461, 653, 655, 711, 713, 718,
    777, 790, 793, 801
Yerxa, E. J., 161, 162, 163, 193, 237,
    238, 242, 402, 741, 775
Yoder, M., 645
Yoder, R. M., 169, 736
York, L., 478, 480
Yoshida, K., 694, 695, 696
Yost, E., 593
Young, B., 347
Young, I. M., 356, 357
Young, J. A., 812
Young, N., 272, 273
Young, R. J. C., 191, 195
Youngstedt, S., 284
Youngstom, M., 230
Yu, B., 185, 186
Yung, P. M., 622

Z

Zabriskie, R. B., 271
Zaccaria, R., 164
Zanetti, V., 356
Zecha, D., 164
Zee, P. C., 254
Zemke, R., 75, 126, 133, 148, 150,
    151, 160, 162, 175, 184, 193, 229,
    230, 231, 232, 233, 251, 346, 435,
    759, 775, 776, 777, 781, 782, 784,
    795
Zemkè, R., 161, 162, 237, 238, 242
Zeppilli, P., 271
Zerubavel, E., 288, 782
Zika, S., 285
Zimmerman, D., 183, 184, 185, 187,
    383
Ziviani, J., 274
Ziviani, J. M., 274
Zorowitz, R. D., 666
Zuzanek, J., 229, 230